D1162157

Advances in Pain Research and Therapy
Volume 9

PROCEEDINGS OF THE FOURTH WORLD CONGRESS ON PAIN

Seattle

Advances in Pain Research and Therapy
Volume 9

Proceedings of the Fourth World Congress on Pain

Seattle

Editors

Howard L. Fields, M.D., Ph.D.

Member of Council of IASP
Professor
Department of Neurology
University of California
San Francisco, California

Ronald Dubner, D.D.S.

Member of Council of IASP
Chief, Neurobiology and
Anesthesiology Branch
National Institute of Dental Research
National Institutes of Health
Bethesda, Maryland

Fernando Cervero, M.D., Ph.D.

Department of Physiology
University of Bristol
Medical School
Bristol, England

Associate Editor
Louisa E. Jones, B.S.

Executive Officer
IASP
Seattle, Washington

Raven Press ■ New York

Raven Press, 1140 Avenue of the Americas, New York, New York 10036

Made in the United States of America

Library of Congress Cataloging in Publication Data

World Congress on Pain (4th: 1984: Seattle, Wash.)
Proceedings of the Fourth World Congress on Pain.

(Advances in pain research and therapy; v.9)
Meeting held Aug. 31–Sept. 5, 1984.
Includes bibliographies and index.
1. Pain—Congresses. 2. Analgesia—Congresses.
I. Fields, Howard L. II. Dubner, Ronald. III. Cervero, Fernando. IV. Title. V. Series. [DNLM: 1. Pain—congresses. W1 AD706 v.9 / WL 704 W927 1984p]
RB127.W67 1984 616′0472 83-14307
ISBN 0-88167-121-5

Preface

It is just over a decade since John Bonica convened the first major assembly in Issaquah, Washington of scientists and clinicians interested in pain. It was clear to those of us who attended the Issaquah conference, and the 1984 meeting in Seattle, that there have been dramatic advances. Although there had been major advances in the understanding of both pain mechanisms and pain treatment prior to that time, the field had no clear identity. There were psychologists, physiologists, anatomists, and a variety of other scientists and clinicians, but each reported to and interacted with their own group. Research and clinical care were equally fragmented and progress was slow. As this volume documents, the field of pain research is maturing rapidly. Pain researchers are now asking increasingly sophisticated questions and answering them more rigorously and in more detail.

This volume presents information on selected areas where progress has been particularly rapid in the past five years. One area of great progress is our understanding of the peripheral nociceptors. By correlating anatomical, physiological, behavioral, and psychophysical studies in animals and man, it is now possible to associate particular classes of peripheral nociceptors with certain aspects of pain sensation in man. Of particular interest are the reports of the nociceptor changes that occur with receptor or nerve damage or experimental inflammation. These latter studies open the way to understanding processes that occur with a time course of days or weeks and may be of great relevance to clinical conditions such as cancer, arthritis, and painful peripheral neuropathy. Steady progress also characterizes research on central nociceptive pathways with recent focus on the dorsal horn, thalamus, and somatosensory cortex.

Another area of dramatic progress presented herein is in our understanding of where and how opiates act on the brain to relieve pain. The pharmacokinetics of opiate analgesics and the neuroanatomy of cellular actions of opioid peptides are much better known than ten years ago. The use of intrathecal opiates represents an important clinical advance that arose directly from research into basic mechanisms and hopefully portends future improvements in clinical pain management.

This volume also contains information on the assessment of pain in man using both psychometric approaches, i.e., the visual analog scale and questionnaires, and physiologic measures such as the cerebral evoked potential.

Several chapters examine psychological factors contributing to the development of chronic pain, and several chapters evaluate pain management using behavioral, surgical, and nonnarcotic drug therapies.

The content of this volume accurately reflects both the increasing quality of pain research and the continued excitement of a field that is still growing. The seed planted by John Bonica in Issaquah has grown into a well-established tree that promises increasing productivity as it enters its second decade.

The Editors
June, 1985

Acknowledgments

The editors of this volume and the officers and members of the Council of the International Association for the Study of Pain wish to express their deepest appreciation to the many persons whose contributions were critical to the success of the Fourth World Congress on Pain and this book.

Professor B. Raymond Fink, chairman of the Local Arrangements Committee and his colleagues, John A. Bokan, Kenneth D. Craig, Louisa E. Jones, Karen Loeser, L. Brian Ready, Mark M. Schubert, and Margo Wyckoff, took care of the hundreds of details and completed the many tasks that assured the success of the congress. Special thanks are due to Mrs. Gwen Bell, secretary to Professor Fink, for her considerable efforts on behalf of the Local Arrangements Committee.

Ruth Olson and Dave Full and their associates at the Office of Conferences and Institutes of the University of Washington, working with the Local Arrangements Committee, ensured the smooth running of the scientific sessions and the many social events enjoyed by the participants.

We also thank our colleagues on the Scientific Program Committee, Mohammed L. Abdelmoumene, Allan I. Basbaum, Robert A. Boas, Jorgen Boivie, Stephen H. Butler, B. Raymond Fink, Mary Ellen Jeans, John C. Liebeskind, Joel E. Seres, Vittorio Ventafridda, and Toshikatsu Yokota, for helping us develop a most exciting, informative, and comprehensive program of speakers and a balanced selection of topics. Mr. Steve Guinn, administrative assistant to Professor Fields, deserves special thanks for his untiring work on behalf of the committee.

The editors express sincere thanks and appreciation to the members of the Editorial Panel for their excellent job of carefully reviewing the abstracts and selecting the short papers included in this volume and for their help in the final preparation of this book.

The work of the public relations consultants for the congress, Eugene and Estelle Kone, deserves special recognition. As a result of their efforts, the congress received extensive coverage by radio, television, newspapers, and magazines, not only in the United States but throughout the world.

On behalf of the Council and members of IASP, the editors also acknowledge and wish to express special appreciation for the financial support given the Fourth World Congress on Pain by the following:

Anonymous
Ives Laboratories, Inc.
Merck Sharp & Dohme
National Cancer Institute, USA
National Institute of Dental Research, USA
National Institute of Neurological and Communicative Disorders and Stroke, USA (NIH Grant: 1 R13 CA/NS/DE/DA/TW 38442-01)
Ortho Pharmaceutical Corporation
Wyeth International Limited
Ayerst Laboratories
Boehringer Ingelheim KG
The Boeing Company
Boots Pharmaceuticals Inc.
Burroughs Wellcome Company
CIBA-GEIGY Corporation
Eli Lilly and Company
Hoffman La Roche
ICI International
McNeil Pharmaceutical
Medtronic, Inc.
Merck'Sche Gesellschaft für Kunst und Wissenschaft
Pan American World Airways
A. H. Robbins Company
Sterling Drug Inc.
The Upjohn Company
United Airlines
Wellcome Research Laboratories
Abbott Laboratories
Breon Laboratories Inc.
Parke-Davis

Contents

Central Mechanisms of Nociception

Spinal Cord Dorsal Horn and Trigeminal Nucleus

Thalamocortical Mechanisms

Clinical Assessment

Painful Injury of Peripheral Nerve: Clinical Features and Neural Mechanisms

Central Nervous System Mechanisms of Analgesia

Cancer Pain

Special Section on Ethics

Pain Management

Opiate Analgesics

Nonopiate Drugs

Contributors

Introduction: Science, Pain, and Politics

Ainsley Iggo

From its inception, the International Association for the Study of Pain (IASP) has had several major objectives that are clearly expressed in its articles of association. These objectives include fostering research on pain mechanisms, promoting education and training in the field of pain, disseminating new information, and advising international and national agencies.

The World Congresses on Pain held every three years bear eloquent witness to the way in which biomedical sciences contribute substantially to the attempt by researchers "to help to improve the management of patients with acute and chronic pain." In this respect it must be appreciated that the problems science is asked to attack emerge from often inspired and always conscientious study and evaluation of the clinical condition of patients. The interaction is symbiotic, because science requires clear formulation of real problems arising in the practice of medicine, and medicine benefits from the results that flow from biomedical research.

The fruitful interaction of science and pain must be seen in the wider context of the real world, and thus politics, defined as the "art of the possible," assumes an important role. This need for active involvement of IASP in the wider scene of everyday politics is also clearly enshrined in our articles of association, where we acknowledge a responsibility to inform the public of the results and implications of current research and also to advise international and national bodies. At the political level, however, IASP has much more to do because it is not only directly concerned with alleviating one of humanity's major scourges but it is also closely involved with a serious ethical issue: the use of animals in biological research.

Biomedical science draws on many disciplines in science. To illustrate its role in the study of pain mechanisms and its multidisciplinary character, it is only necessary to read the reports presented to the Fourth World Congress and published in this volume.

It is useful to sharpen the distinction between the perception of pain and the subcortical or nonperceptual aspects that are components of the mechanisms of nociception. The term "nociception" is derived from the term "nociceptor," first used by Sir Charles Sherrington to define a sensory receptor that is sensitive to damaging or potentially tissue-damaging natural stimuli. Many physiological studies are indeed concerned with nociception, as even a cursory scrutiny of the contents of this volume will amply testify.

Politics and Pain

The wide range of pain studies reported in this volume involve not only multidisciplinary expertise but also international collaboration, often calling on the special skills and facilities in several laboratories in different countries and indirectly on the "Bank of International Science." This last aspect introduces the topic of politics, because not only does it require an acceptance at the governmental level of the need for such international collaboration but also it requires an acceptance of the need "to will the means as well as the ends"—in other words, to make adequate financial provision to allow the ends to be achieved. Two very important components of the needs are: (a) accessible stores of knowledge (these exist as libraries or as data banks in universities or research institutes, costly but vital) and (b) the provision of research facilities and funds to enable investigators to move among and utilize these data sources. University laboratories, usually through central government funding, are able to supply and equip laboratories with basic resources, together with the necessary library facilities. Such basic funding must be supplemented by the provision, from governmental sources (via research councils) and from private charitable sources, of additional funds needed for the special costs of specific research projects. Significant new international initiatives, such as the European Science Foundation's funding research visits through twinning grants, are making international collaboration possible. Even in a period of economic recession it is evident that governments, constrained though they may be by their particular economic and political ideals, nevertheless recognize the need for both fundamental and applied research in the field of pain.

World Congresses on Pain provide an opportunity for IASP to stress, in the face of continually escalating costs of research, the need for continued funding. The costs are rising steeply, for two principal reasons: inflation and technological sophistication. The latter is the more serious because valuable effort can be wasted in doing experiments with antiquated technology. IASP is also able at its congresses to show that past support has yielded rewards of immense value to society. This was demonstrably evident in the spectacular array of new work presented in 20 plenary lectures and more than 600 individual presentations as communications and posters by nearly 1,500 investigators. Advances in knowledge of pain mechanisms and analgesia come from rigorous application of science to these age-old problems. The new knowledge then finds its application in the clinic, in fulfillment of one of the major aims of IASP "to help to improve the management of patients with acute and chronic pain." Congresses, in addition to providing a forum for the presentation in set-pieces of new results, also afford a unique opportunity for discussion and interaction among investigators working in many disciplines from all parts of the world.

The message is clear and unambiguous: Not only do problems in pain and analgesia exist; they are being investigated vigorously and fruitfully. In many cases the investigators responsible for advances in this work were able to do their work and expose their ideas to critical scrutiny only because at the political level there was recognition of the need for this work to continue. The important conclusion is that science, pain, and politics have important linkages; the use of both science and politics will be necessary for realization of the goal of pain relief.

There are two other aspects of politics in relation to pain that merit particular consideration: ethics and education. Ethical considerations are important politically because the study of pain mechanisms requires application of potentially painful stimuli and the use of laboratory animals as well as human subjects. The sophistication of scientific methodology emphasizes one inescapable fact in relation to studies of pain: Further progress requires rigorously controlled experimentation. Compelling constraints on human experimentation, imposed by legislation and by moral considerations, force investigators to turn to the use of animals. In turn, this calls into question, as is increasingly evident in the media, the validity of human use (referred to pejoratively as exploitation) of animals for experimentation. An important function of the IASP is to present to the public and to politicians, clearly and unambiguously, the case for use of animals for investigation of pain, antinociception, and analgesia. The case can be argued at several levels: philosophical, sociological, and the severely practical.

At the philosophical or ethical level, we are at once faced with the difficulty that no agreed philosophical basis exists. Broadly stated, two kinds of approaches exist. The first one is based on *ex cathedra* statements of the kind enshrined in the biblical Ten Commandments couched in the form "Thou shalt not . . . ." The problem here is in establishing the primary authority for the directives. The second is based on the idea that one's conduct and actions should on balance be benevolent rather than malevolent. In this case, we must act according to our judgment of the consequences of our actions, rather than to a given set of inflexible injunctions. Adopting this latter approach, I find no real difficulty in advancing a rational case for achieving the greater good by the use of animals in laboratory-based experiments, while at the same time promoting the general idea of human and animal welfare. Indeed, both humans and animals can be expected to benefit from controlled animal experimentation. It is on such a view that a case can be presented to the general public and the politicians. At the more practical and mundane level, the case for animal experiments is overwhelmingly supported by endless examples that could be cited to illustrate the benefits to humans and animals alike, such as the development of new pharmaceutical agents.

My final example of the relation between pain and politics concerns education. IASP's articles of incorporation stress the need to promote education and training in the field of pain. This is an area of very considerable political importance because its implementation calls for an acceptance by the body politic of the need for education in the field of pain. The general membership of IASP realizes the need because the members are all actively engaged in one way or another in the investigation, teaching, or practice of pain relief in one form or another. The distribution of our membership on a global basis gives an indication of the current awareness and level of educational knowledge in the field. Taking the membership figures at their face value would lead to the conclusion that the clinical and scientific aspects of pain are best understood in the Western world (comprising Europe, North America, and Australasia) and in Japan. Even in these areas it is possible to be critical of the level of educational awareness, at least as judged by specific references to pain in teaching curricula in medical schools. Much more significant is the implication that pain, in the Western sense, is inadequately understood and treated in other regions. An important challenge to IASP can be identified here.

And, indeed, IASP, through its Education Committee, is seizing the opportunity and actively seeking ways to promote its educational objectives. Professor Sven Andersson and his Committee on Education are currently producing a handbook on chronic pain for devleoping countries. This project is well advanced and on completion should be of immense benefit because it seeks to express the basic ideas and practices in a clear and informative style. Another interesting aspect of their work has been to promote teaching activities in developing countries. This, too, is an enterprise that relies heavily on the willing cooperation of national governments as well as other national agencies in the countries concerned.

These last examples, then, once more add point to the general theme developed in this introduction: that the way forward is through active and willing cooperation of the sciences, on the one hand, and politics, broadly defined, on the other, in advancing closer to the goal of mastering one of the scourges of mankind: pain.

Advances in Pain Research and Therapy
Volume 9

Advances in Pain Research and Therapy, Vol. 9, edited by H. L. Fields et al. Raven Press, New York © 1985.

Unraveling the Story of Pain

Edward R. Perl

Department of Physiology, University of North Carolina, Chapel Hill, North Carolina 27514

Until a few years ago patients complaining of persistent pain for which no cause was obvious or for which the cause could not be eliminated had a bleak future. Typical therapy consisted of stupefying and addicting drugs and/or surgery. All too often therapeutic manipulations were ineffectual, resulting in iatrogenic additions to misery and a substantial bend to the psyche. Although miraculous solutions still are not available, the prospects are better for providing persons suffering from pain with an improved quality of life. To some extent the happier clinical outlook is due to a better understanding of pain mechanisms, but it is also the result of the foresight and proselytism of John Bonica and those who followed his lead. As a clinician he recognized that chronic pain is not a simple problem. He argued that regardless of etiology, persistence of pain complicates the relationship between the original cause and subsequent symptoms, and he championed the idea of bringing several therapeutic specialists into one clinic to design a coordinated plan for therapy. On the whole this approach has been a great improvement over traditional ones for treating such patients.

The lesson from the clinic concerning the complexities of pain needs to be applied to our research: Only when the kinds of thinking and the techniques of several disciplines are applied at the same time will we find new, important insights into the mechanisms, consequences, and treatment of pain. The virtues and advantages of a broad approach to a subject as complicated as pain are readily justified and have an apparent logic. Yet, as Lewis Carroll's Alice learned in her Wonderland, things are not always as they seem. Research does not become interdisciplinary simply by borrowing the tools and techniques of another discipline. In other words, while molecular biology or pharmacology can provide evidence on the presence or binding of a substance, the insights of anatomy and physiology must be used before such results can be properly interpreted. Similarly, prior to attaching an appropriate functional significance to discharges of a neuron, it is necessary to appreciate the teaching of psychology on the behavioral relationships and end points that apply. The wreckage of doctrinaire theories—old and recent—on the obstinate rocks of ignored evidence bears witness to the futility of any lesser approach.

PAIN MECHANISMS: WHAT HAVE WE LEARNED?

Along with the invitation to write this chapter, came the suggestion that I might write about the peripheral basis of pain and discuss how we have come to learn about nociceptors and their relationship to pain. Some years ago, I pointed out that the relevance of particular sense organs to a sensation cannot be understood in the absence of the larger perspective afforded by the functional organization of the related central neural apparatus and lessons from behavior (56). Therefore, my story shall touch on central as well as peripheral neural systems associated with pain.

Some have held that there are no new developments in our understanding of pain, or, alternately, that nothing old is meaningful to present thinking. Neither extreme fits even a casual view of history. What really has been learned about the afferent apparatus underlying pain in the three or so decades since John Bonica started expressing his concerns about pain management? Let us first consider from where we have come, and then end by speculating upon where we could or should go next in order to untangle the mysteries of this most common of medical complaints.

If 1950 is taken as a point of departure, in my view there have been four major developments in understanding the neural machinery underlying pain. Firstly, it has become clear that mammals have specialized peripheral sense organs for detecting the usual pain-causing stimuli or events. Secondly, in part, the information provided by these specialized sense organs is manipulated and transmitted rostrally by neurons forming a special subset of afferent systems projecting to the somatosensory cerebral cortex. Thirdly, the ascending projection of afferent information for all modalities of somatic sensation, including pain, are subject to modulation by activity descending from rostral levels. Fourthly, the mediation of activity between neurons and the modulation of neuronal excitability is part of a rich system of chemical signalling whose features and operation are just beginning to come to light.

Nociceptors: Sense Organs for Tissue Damage

Direct evidence for the essential part played by peripheral afferent fibers of smaller diameter in pain mechanisms began to accumulate about fifty years ago. The compound action potential and the relationship of its components to speed of conduction and fiber diameter was one of the tools. In the early 1930s Thomas Lewis and his associates (44) and Yngve Zotterman (85) tested the loss of function of a nerve's fibers on sensory capacity by partially blocking conduction using pressure and anoxemia or dilute local anesthetics. In that same era, Heinbecker, Bishop, and O'Leary (18) compared the progressive activation of subsets of a nerve's afferent fiber spectrum by graded electrical shocks to verbal descriptions of sensation (Fig. 1). From these and comparable studies in animals, by the mid 1930s it was widely accepted that unmyelinated and slowly-conducting myelinated afferent fibers of peripheral nerve were essential for transmission of activity initiating pain and related reactions. Such work indicated that discrimination of warmth and cold also depended upon the integrity of a similar, but not identical, part of the peripheral nerve fiber population. These conclusions were destined to be confirmed and extended years later by Landau and Bishop (41) and by Collins, Nulsen, and Randt (8) using similar techniques, and by Dyck, Lambert, and Nichols (12) using analysis of nerve defects in developmental or degenerative diseases. However, in the late 1930s a long period of uncertainty about this interpretation began.

In a sense, Adrian and Zotterman's (2) description of the first recordings from individual sensory nerve fibers nearly 60 years ago, by failing to note activation of a unique group of peripheral afferent fibers in response to pain-causing stimuli, contributed to the controversy over whether there were specialized afferent fibers for pain. However, several years later in a brief report that was never elaborated on, Adrian (1) described that acid dropped on a frog's skin (which elicited vigorous avoidance reactions) evoked action potentials of smaller amplitude than those initiated by an innocuous brushing contact. In other words, a noxious stimulus activated a different group of afferent fibers than an innocuous one.

In 1939, Zotterman (86) published a detailed paper on the discharges of individual cutaneous afferent fibers that included observations on slowly-conducting myelinated and unmyelinated fibers. He reported that intense stimulation of the skin did evoke activity in slowly-conducting fibers, but as Fig. 2 from his paper shows so did quite gentle stimulation. Thus a conundrum existed in the 1940s and 1950s. Based on work with compound

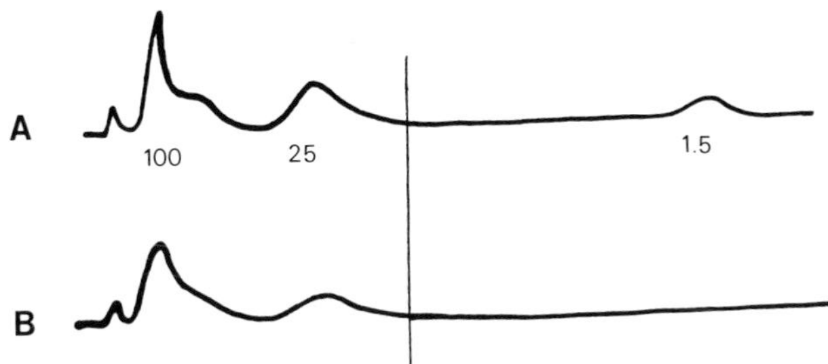

FIG. 1. Compound action potential of human cutaneous nerve. **A:** Activity evoked by a stimulus strong enough to excite all the fibers in the nerve. **B:** Activity evoked by a stimulus that caused painful sensations in human beings. (From Heinbecker et al., ref. 18, with permission.)

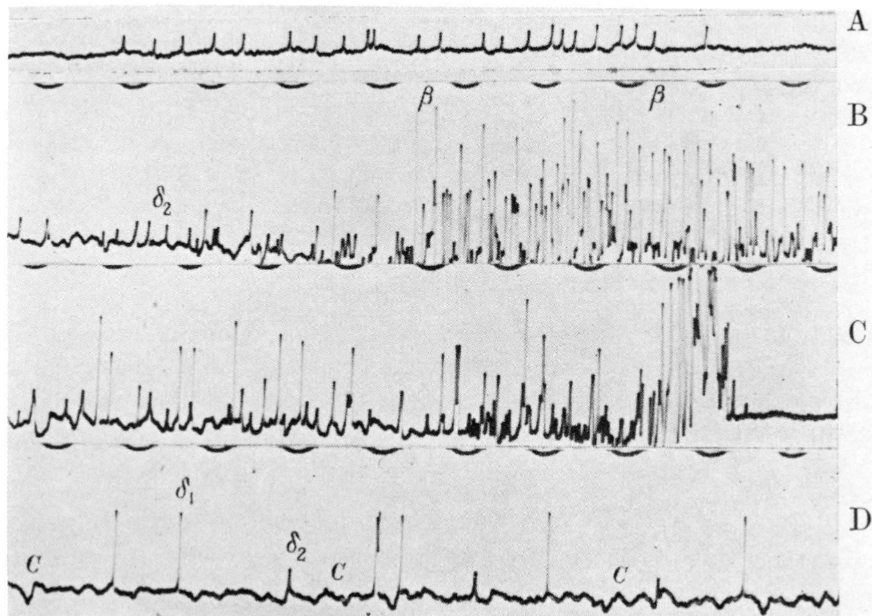

FIG. 2. Recordings from fine filaments dissected from cutaneous nerves of cat (to be read from the right). **A:** Response of δ2 fibers to a very light contact with cotton-wool. **B:** The end of a firm stroke with a smooth probe. **C:** A needle prick. **D:** 4 sec after needle pressure (52 g) on the skin began. Time: 1/50 sec. (From Zotterman, ref. 86, with permission.)

action potentials, slowly-conducting fibers were deemed essential for pain and temperature sensations and related reactions, yet single fiber discharges recorded from cutaneous nerves in experimental animals gave uncertain evidence for correlating the activity of a specific class of receptors with slowly conducting fibers and the usual pain-causing stimuli. This controversy was heightened by the experiments of Douglas and Ritchie (11) in which they used an ingenious collision technique for determining the component of the compound action potential that was associated with fibers activated by particular forms of natural stimulation. Douglas and Ritchie concluded that the majority of the unmyelinated (C) afferent fibers in cat cutaneous nerve were excited by gentle mechanical stimulation of the skin. Those who argued against specificity of function for afferent fibers leading to pain took courage from these apparently conflicting data and strongly maintained that pain, at least, was not associated with a specific set of sense organs in the periphery (50,68). These arguments persisted into the 1960s even though observations to the contrary had begun to appear. For example, Fig. 3, taken from the 1959 paper of Iggo (27), one of the early single unit recordings from a C-afferent fiber, shows discharges evoked in a fiber by heat; this unit's threshold to skin warming was quite elevated compared to

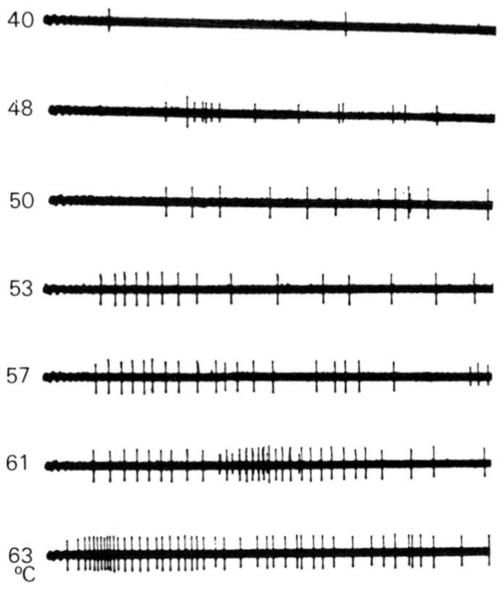

FIG. 3. Responses of a C-fiber primary afferent unit (large impulses) when a brass rod (10-mm diameter) was held in contact with the skin. Rod temperatures were as indicated. The small impulses in the *upper two tracings* are from a mechanoreceptive unit in response to mechanical contact. The C-fiber receptor did not respond to a thermally neutral mechanical stimulus. Time-seconds at the 40° trace at the top. (From Iggo, ref. 27, with permission.)

those of the usually observed thermoreceptors of the region. The next year, Iggo (28) reported that the thresholds to mechanical stimulation for individual cutaneous C fiber receptors ranged from very low to quite high, an observation interpreted to suggest a continuum. Even though descriptions of a few other primary afferent units excited only by stimuli so strong as to make them candidates for "pain" receptors appeared, on the whole developments to this time provided grist for the mill of those who were unconvinced of specificity of sense organ function for pain. Thus, in the early 1960s there were two reasons for skepticism about specificity of sense organs for pain. In the 40 years after the pioneering observations of Adrian and Zotterman, thousands of recordings had been made of the activity of single primary afferent fibers from skin, muscle, and other tissue, but the number of reports on primary afferent fibers from sense organs with elevated thresholds or with signalling characteristics suggestive of a selective responsiveness to pain-causing stimuli was truly quite small. The characteristics described for those few high-threshold, or otherwise unusual peripheral afferent units, were not consistent and thus differed from those which had been established for other specialized sense organs.

This was when Burgess and I decided to restudy the functional makeup of the population of thin primary afferent fibers. Our method differed in two ways from that used in previous work. An unbiased survey of receptive characteristics was essential; in the selection of units to be studied it seemed crucial to avoid the often seductive lure of ease of identification of a receptive field or the most effective stimulus. The sole criterion for selection of afferent fibers was speed of conduction. Fibers in the slowly-conducting myelinated range were examined first because we had perfected a procedure for stably recording the discharges of such elements in complete isolation from other activity by the use of fine capillary microelectrodes inserted into the nerve. The second feature was an operational definition of what might be considered a pain fiber. The basis was a logic set down generations earlier by Sherrington (67). He had pointed out that although pain might be caused by a diversity of circumstances, it was common experience that it was usually associated with injury to tissue. He defined stimuli or events capable of causing tissue damage as noxious, and a sense organ that would detect and uniquely signal tissue damage as a "nociceptor." This definition has now become widely employed. It is important to bear in mind that noxious stimuli are not absolutes; what is noxious for one tissue (e.g., the lips or skin in protected areas) may not be for another (e.g., the sole of a foot). To reliably decide what is noxious and what is not, adequate tests for responses to stimuli appropriate to the tissue and to natural history are essential. After all, sensory systems evolved in a world presenting certain environmental situations and general behavioral patterns. An appropriate test stimulus (e.g., displacement, moving contact, temperature change, etc.) must be employed to decide upon afferent characteristics. A survey based upon these approaches led to the discovery of the kind of cutaneous sense organ with responses of the type illustrated in Fig. 4; the unit did not respond to substantial pressure against the skin with a blunt rounded object (Fig. 4A) but discharged repeatedly to pinch with a serrated forceps (Fig. 4B). The latter

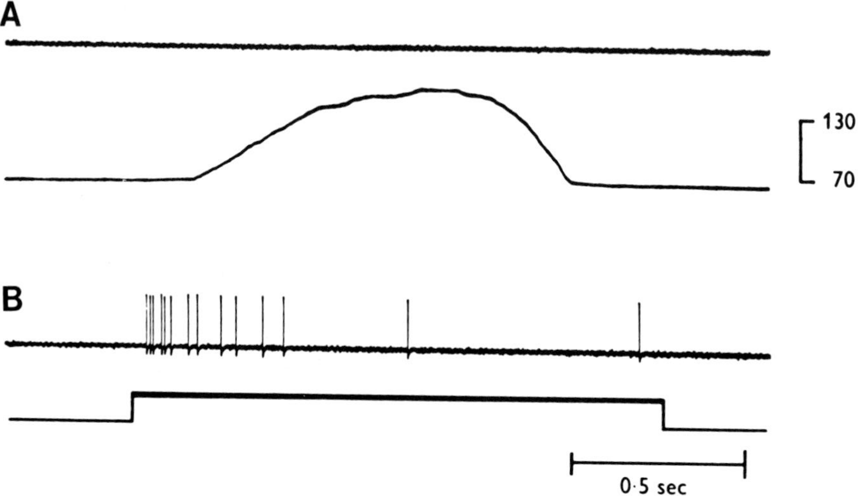

FIG. 4. Response of cutaneous mechanical nociceptor to mechanical stimuli. Afferent fiber conduction velocity: 25 m/sec. **A:** A fold of skin was squeezed between smooth plates at force shown on *lower trace* (calibration on right in g). **B:** Same fold of skin firmly squeezed by serrated forceps for duration of upward deflection on *lower trace*. (From Burgess and Perl, ref. 6, with permission.)

stimulus was clearly noxious; it produced punctures in the skin. A small but consistent fraction of slowly conducting myelinated fibers in cat cutaneous nerves were of this type, exhibiting intensity thresholds for mechanical stimuli many times greater than those of the more common mechanically excitable sensory units. They were unresponsive, at least initially, to thermal stimulation. Another feature that distinguished these units from other sensory units with afferent fibers of similar conduction velocity was the nature of their cutaneous receptive fields which consisted of a number (5 to 25) of quite small, spot-like areas separated by much larger areas from which equivalent stimuli were ineffectual in eliciting a response. Graded, intense mechanical stimulation of each spot evoked responses proportionately graded by the number and frequency of discharges (Fig. 5). Thus these afferent units were capable of signalling not only the presence but also the intensity of noxious stimuli. Although the thresholds for evoking a first impulse from such elements vary substantially, they are always considerably higher than those of other mechanoreceptors in the same skin areas. In cat and experimental primate the conduction velocities of their afferent fibers cover a considerable part of the lower end of the myelinated spectrum (5 to 40+ m/sec). It turns out that such high-threshold mechanoreceptors (HTM) of the skin are a feature of all mammalian species so far studied, including human beings (6,14,35,55).

The small size of the individual punctate areas of the peripheral receptive fields provided an opportunity to learn something of the morphology of the HTM cutaneous terminals. Kruger, Sedivec, and I (37) did a study in which very small slivers of metal were placed into the skin to bracket the punctate excitable regions determined by electrophysiological recording from HTM afferent fibers. The marked skin areas were then analyzed at the light microscopic and electron microscopic levels. A consistent pattern was found in the delineated regions. A thinly myelinated fiber lost its myelin covering in

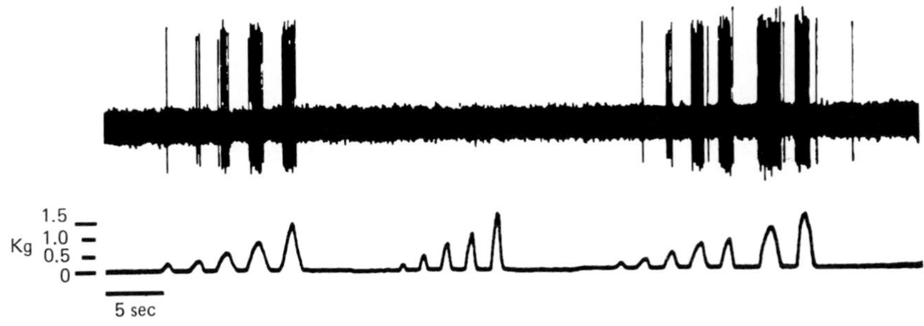

FIG. 5. Responses of a myelinated fiber nociceptor to graded mechanical stimulation. **Lower trace** shows forces used to press a 1-mm probe: *left,* one spot of receptive field: *middle,* an unresponsive zone; *right,* another spot 5 mm from the first. (From Kruger et al., ref. 37, with permission.)

the dermis, then branched, covered by a Schwann cell process with a basal lamina. The complex contacted the epidermis and the basal lamina of the Schwann-nerve fiber complex and that of the epidermis fused. The nerve process still largely covered by Schwann cell processes terminated between keratinocytes of the epidermis (37). One could theorize that the envelopment of the terminal branch by the Schwann cell and its ending between sturdy cells of the epidermis, insulated the terminal from stresses produced by mechanical stimuli. This insulation may provide the high-threshold characteristic to sensory units of this class.

It has also been possible to learn something about the morphology of the central terminals of this particular type of mechanical nociceptor. Light and I (47) stained the primary afferent fibers from functionally identified myelinated HTM units with horseradish peroxidase (HRP) iontophoresed from a microelectrode used to record the fiber's electrical signals. HRP is moved by axoplasmic transport throughout central ramifications of the fiber. After histochemical reaction HRP produces a light and electron dense mark, permitting the fiber's distribution to be traced. A two-dimensional rendering of the three-dimensional distribution in the spinal cord of a marked HTM fiber from the monkey is shown in Fig. 6. The central distributions of these mechanical nociceptors proved to be remarkably stereotyped, with many terminals in lamina I of the dorsal horn and extensions into the outer part of lamina II, branches in lamina V, and often a branch crossing the midline that distributes terminals near the central canal and to the contralateral lamina V. This pattern is totally different from that of the low-threshold mechanoreceptors with either large or small diameter myelinated fibers.

The picture of the central termination of the myelinated fiber HTM has been expanded a step further with observations on the synaptic contacts made by these sensory units. Réthelyi joined us (65) in analyzing the ultrastructure of central synaptic contacts of the myelinated HTM units labelled intracellularly with HRP. We found that their synaptic contacts appeared only at enlargements which typically had a notably scalloped appearance in lamina I, as in the example of Fig. 7 and were filled with clear, round vesicles. The question of vesicles in central terminals will be addressed again later.

Thus far we have only touched on recent studies of single fibers of the thinly myelinated population. Similar surveys of unmyelinated (C) afferent fiber receptive characteristics helped resolve some of the apparent inconsistencies and uncertainties in the older literature. We analyzed the cutaneous C-fiber population in cat using two methods. One method was the classic technique of splitting peripheral nerve into fine filaments to permit the recording of action potentials identifiable as originating from single fibers (5,38). The other method consisted of recording with microelectrodes from the cell bodies in dorsal root ganglia (4). Both techniques indicated that between 40 and 50% of cat cutaneous C-afferent fibers in hairy skin areas

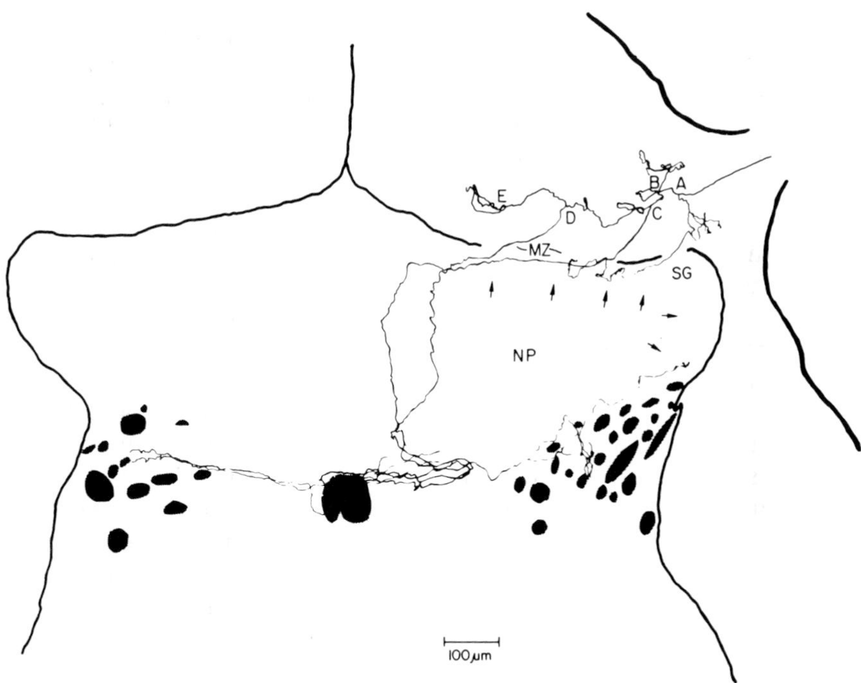

FIG. 6. Camera lucida drawing of a stained central fiber from a cutaneous high threshold mechanoreceptor in monkey spinal cord. Conduction velocity: 28 m/sec. A–D are branch points, A,C, and D terminal collaterals. At B a branch of the main fiber turned caudally and at E the main branch coursed rostrally in the dorsal columns. *Arrow heads* indicate the boundary between substantia gelatinosa (SG) and nucleus proprius (NP). Laterally placed *dark areas* represent longitudinally oriented myelinated fibers at the base of the nucleus proprius. (From Light and Perl, ref. 47, with permission.)

are associated with nociceptors whose characteristics differ importantly from those of the myelinated mechanical nociceptors. In addition, these surveys in cat and similar ones in monkey confirmed earlier conclusions that the unmyelinated afferent fibers are related not only to nociceptors or highly selective thermal receptors but also to low-threshold mechanoreceptors; the latter were present in relatively large numbers in carnivore, although this may be a feature of mammals with a fur-covered skin. Thus, both the unmyelinated and the thinly myelinated afferent fibers are mixed populations, consisting of low-threshold mechanoreceptors, thermoreceptors, and nociceptors.

The observations just mentioned, as well as subsequent work, emphasize that tissue such as skin, muscle, and ligaments contains more than one type of nociceptive sense organ. This is most clearly established for the skin. In addition to the myelinated fiber mechanical nociceptor found in the skin of many mammalian species, there is an equally ubiquitous nociceptor with an

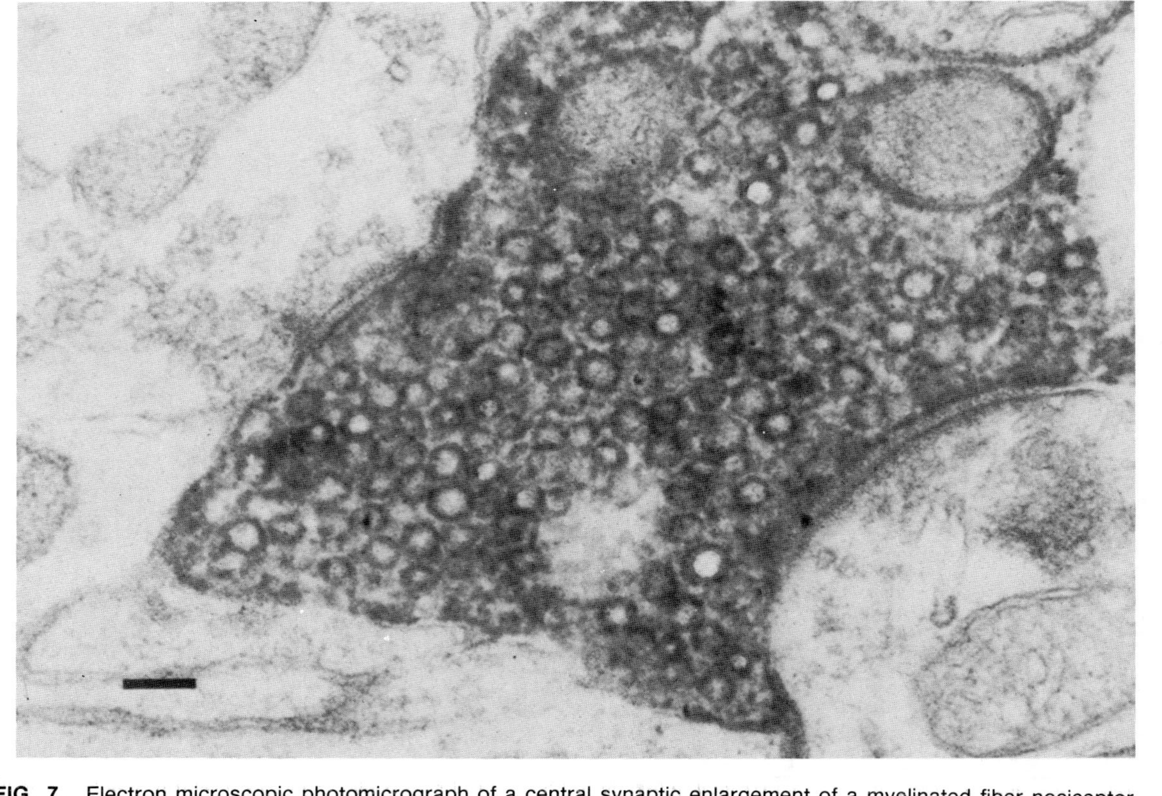

FIG. 7. Electron microscopic photomicrograph of a central synaptic enlargement of a myelinated fiber nociceptor. Horseradish peroxidase was iontophoresed intracellularly into a dorsal root fiber after functional characterization based upon electrophysiological recording. Bar: 200 nm. (From Réthelyi et al., *unpublished observations.*)

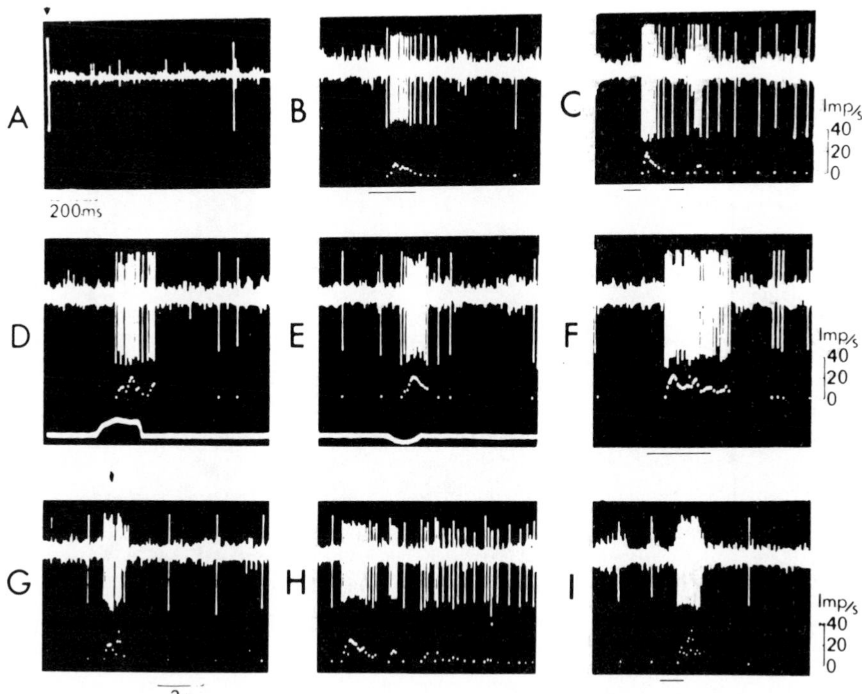

FIG. 8. Discharges recorded by a percutaneously inserted microelectrode from human C-fiber polymodal nociceptor. Duration of stimuli indicated beneath the records by bars or deflections in a strain gauge signal. **A:** Response evoked by a single electric shock in the cutaneous receptive field on the big toe. **B:** Sustained pressure with a stiff von Frey hair, 2 g, which was perceived as 'itch.'' **C:** Repeated firm strokings with a small wooden stick, reported as ''slight aching, followed by nonpainful after-sensations.'' **D:** Pressure (15 g) with a blunt probe to a 1-mm area of skin, indicated by the upward deflection of the strain gauge signal and described as ''pressure.'' **E:** Pressure (5 g) to a 0.1-mm area of skin with a sharp probe, indicated as a downward deflection of the strain gauge signal. Reported as ''slight pain.'' **F:** Needle penetration through skin, perceived as ''pricking and delayed pain.'' **G:** Burst following application of itch powder, reported as ''burning itch.'' **H:** Activity appearing after the skin was touched with a nettle leaf. Subject reported ''pain followed by itch.'' **I:** Large, intense burst of impulses initiated by touching skin with a glowing match. Reported by subject as ''pricking followed by burning pain.'' (From Torebjörk, ref. 72, with permission.)

unmyelinated afferent fiber. This common C-fiber nociceptor responds not only to strong mechanical stimulation, but also to noxious heat and to irritant chemical agents. The broad receptiveness for noxious stimuli led us (5) to coin the etymologically unfortunate but expressive name, polymodal nociceptor. Although polymodal nociceptors are excited by several kinds of noxious stimuli that buffet the skin, this responsiveness is not global since cooling, even to low temperatures, is normally not an effective stimulus. C-fiber polymodal nociceptors occur not only in cat, where they were first seen, but also in monkey, rat, rabbit, and humans. We know of their presence in

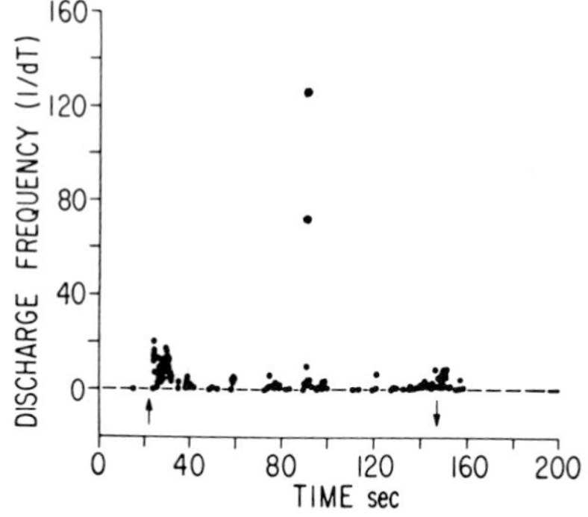

FIG. 9. Response of a polymodal nociceptor to dilute acid on unbroken skin (from cat). Conduction velocity: 0.8 m/sec. (From Bessou and Perl, ref. 5, with permission.)

humans as the result of observations with percutaneous neural recording. Figure 8, from Torebjörk (72), illustrates the effectiveness of various stimuli in exciting them. I stress the responsiveness of polymodal nociceptors to chemical agents; in our laboratory, Szolcsányi (70) found that pain-producing chemicals such as capsaicin and bradykinin excite polymodal nociceptors at concentrations at least an order of magnitude less than that which will cause activity in any other kind of sense organ found in the same afferent nerves. Figure 9 illustrates the low frequency, persisting discharge evoked from a polymodal nociceptor by acid placed upon the intact skin. Not only are the receptive properties of C-fiber polymodal nociceptors different from those of the mechanical nociceptors, but so are their receptive fields; C-fiber polymodal nociceptors typically have a receptive field consisting of a single small area ranging in size from somewhat less than 1 mm^2 to 3–5 mm^2. Multiple, separated, receptive fields of the type seen with the

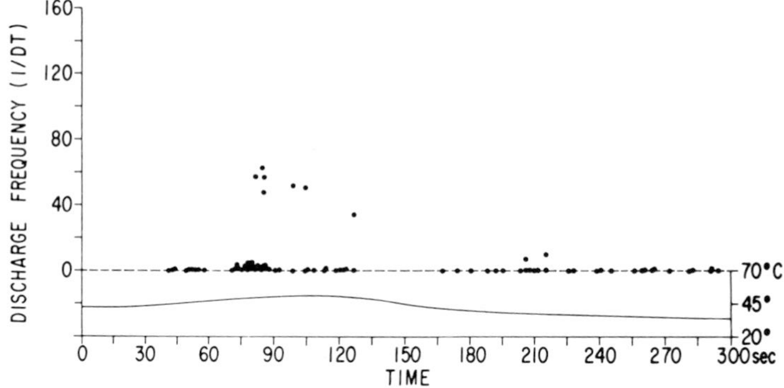

FIG. 10. Development of background discharge by a C-fiber polymodal nociceptor from cat hairy skin. Each recorded discharge is plotted as a *dot.* Below the *dashed line,* a *continuous line* graphs the temperature of a small (3-mm^2) contact thermode centered on the receptive field. The first heating of the receptive field is shown; no background discharge was recorded in the previous 5 min. The first discharges appeared at temperatures of 42–43°C; the peak temperature was approximately 52°C. (From Perl, ref. 57, with permission.)

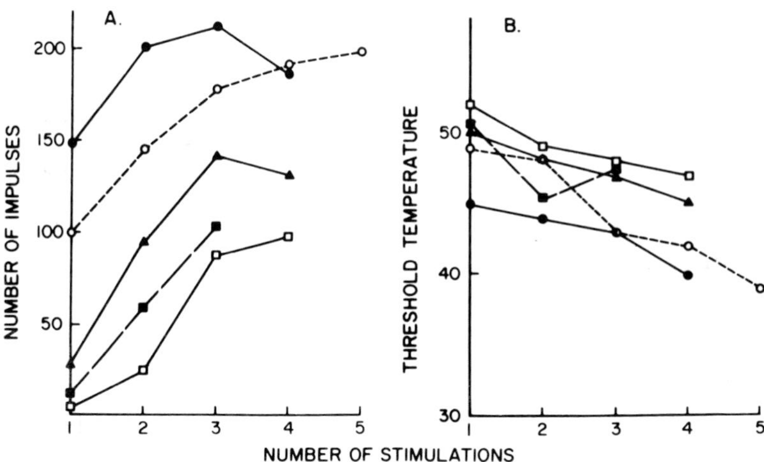

FIG. 11. Changes in number of discharges and threshold by C-fiber polymodal nociceptors upon repeated stimulation with noxious heat. The receptive field was repeatedly heated every 200 sec with a small contact probe. The maximal temperature was approximately 53°C. Each symbol refers to a different unit, and a given symbol identifies the same unit in **A** and **B. A:** Total impulses recorded during each of the sequential heating cycles are plotted as a function of the stimulation cycle. Noxious heat was used for the first time with cycle 1. **B:** Threshold temperature for an evoked discharge. (From Kumazawa and Perl, ref. 38, with permission.)

myelinated high-threshold mechanoreceptors are not found, and only a small proportion of C-fiber polymodal nociceptors have receptive fields consisting of more than one small area.

The responsiveness of C-polymodal nociceptors of hairy skin changes upon repeated noxious stimulation of the skin. In striking contrast to most somatic sense organs, a large proportion of polymodal nociceptors "sensitize" after one or two exposures to moderately intense noxious stimuli. This sensitization is reflected in part by the development of ongoing discharge, activity continuing after cessation of the stimulus. Figure 10 illustrates an example of the appearance of ongoing discharge after the first instance of contact heating of the skin to noxious levels. Sensitization is also manifested by enhanced responsiveness as depicted by the graphs in Fig. 11 for five primate polymodal nociceptors; note that both the number of discharges and the threshold can shift significantly upon repeated stimulation. The process producing sensitization can spread some distance (several mm or more) from the actual point of cutaneous noxious stimulation, as units with a receptive field located near to, but not coextensive with, a damaged skin area often exhibit evidence of sensitization. Fitzgerald and Lynn (14) showed that a similar sensitization also occurs with the myelinated HTM and that these initially selectively mechanoreceptive units develop a responsiveness to heat upon prolonged exposure to skin-damaging high temperatures. One cannot help but think of correlations between nociceptor sensitization and the hyperalgesia described by Lewis (43; see also "primary" hyperalgesia in ref. 17) and of the clinical significance of such changes. Parenthetically, sensitization may also help explain vagaries in the interpretation of experimental results when peripheral tissue is subjected to noxious stimulation.

Finally, direct evidence on the relationship between nociceptors and pain has emerged from experiments in conscious human subjects in which single afferent fibers were stimulated electrically through percutaneously inserted microelectrodes. Excitation of the afferent fibers of nociceptors, but not those of low-threshold mechanoreceptors, evoked reports of pain-like sensations (35,73). Other interesting observations have been made upon nociceptors of skin and subcutaneous tissue in the past decade or so but space in this chapter is too limited to discuss them. To summarize this brief overview of the primary afferent apparatus associated with pain, several points need to be emphasized. High-threshold sense organs, i.e., nociceptors, are a part of the normal innervation of most tissues, and many tissues have more than one type. The different nociceptors of a given tissue have different functional and chemical responsivenesses, including probable differences in their pharmacological reactivities. Nociceptors have a tendency to sensitize as a consequence of persisting or repeated noxious events. Sensitization is manifested by "spontaneous" activity and an increase of responsiveness (decrease in threshold and/or increased discharge) for given intensities of stimulation.

Selectively Nocireceptive Central Neurons

Sense organs specialized for stimuli that ordinarily cause pain, or if you will, warn of circumstances deleterious to tissue, do not necessarily imply an equally selective central organization. Thus, confirmation of central arrangements that preserve a substantial degree of the selectivity observed in the periphery was of great importance, and convincing evidence in this regard has really only been found in the past 25 years. Many have given Christensen and me (7) credit for discovering neurons selectively excited by nociceptors and noxious stimulation at the spinal level. Actually, Kolmodin and Skoglund (34) preceded us by a decade in making observations of this type; although their selectively nocireceptive neurons were located deep in the dorsal horn and those we described were in the marginal zone, the principle was the same. The point is that at least part of the central nervous organization is arranged so that the sense organs excited by noxious stimuli convey their activity to central cells in such a way that the selectivity of effective excitatory stimulation seen in the periphery is retained in some central pathways. To be sure, in the transmission of information from primary afferent to central neurons some features change. Receptive fields become more complex and interactions between stimuli applied to various regions are added. Our initial studies of spinal projections in cat (7) noted

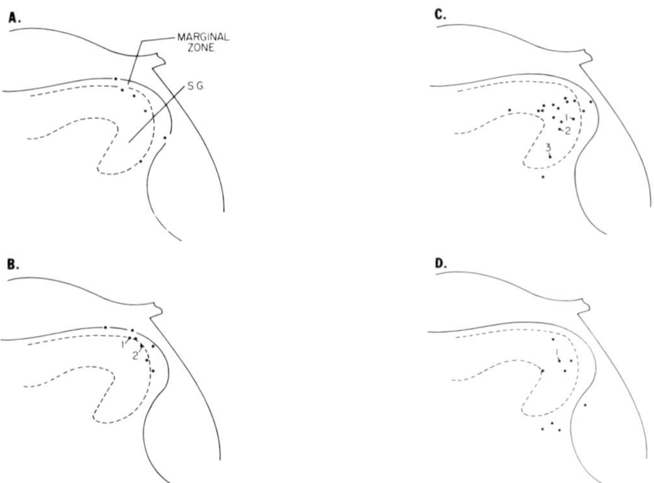

FIG. 12. Recording loci in monkey superficial dorsal horn categorized by the kind of effective excitatory stimulation. Each *dot* represents the recording locus determined by histological recovery of dye after iontophoresis from the recording micropipette. **A:** Units dominated by excitation from slowly-conducting myelinated afferent fibers originating in high-threshold mechanoreceptors (mechanical nociceptors). **B:** Units dominated by excitation from slowly-conducting myelinated afferent fibers originating in low-threshold thermoreceptors. **C:** Units dominated by excitation from cutaneous polymodal nociceptors; all evinced strong excitation by C fibers and most responded to volleys in the slower myelinated fibers. **D:** Units dominated by excitation from low-threshold mechanoreceptors; all evinced strong excitation by C fibers, and all but one responded to volleys in the range of Aδ myelinated fibers. (From Kumazawa and Perl, ref. 39, with permission.)

two categories of selectively nocireceptive neurons in the superficial dorsal horn: one receiving a dominant input from the myelinated high-threshold mechanoreceptors of the skin, and the other excited by both A and C fibers and responsive to noxious heat, mechanical, and chemical stimulation. The nocireceptive neurons of the superficial layers were positioned very near or adjacent to others that had equally selective thermoreceptive characteristics. When this analysis was extended to monkey, with its thicker substantia gelatinosa and more clearly defined marginal zone, a separation became apparent between the typical locations of recording sites for neurons dominated by myelinated nociceptors and those for neurons receiving potent C-fiber excitation. The former tended to be in lamina I and the latter in lamina II (39). The substantia gelatinosa also was found to contain neurons with innocuous mechanoreceptive characteristics (Fig. 12).

Willis and his colleagues (15,74,75,79–82) have done much to establish the cells of origin of the spinothalamic tract. They have shown that spinal neurons projecting to the thalamus, particularly contralaterally, include selectively nocireceptive neurons, some of which are located in the superficial portion of the dorsal horn. Recently it has become evident that the

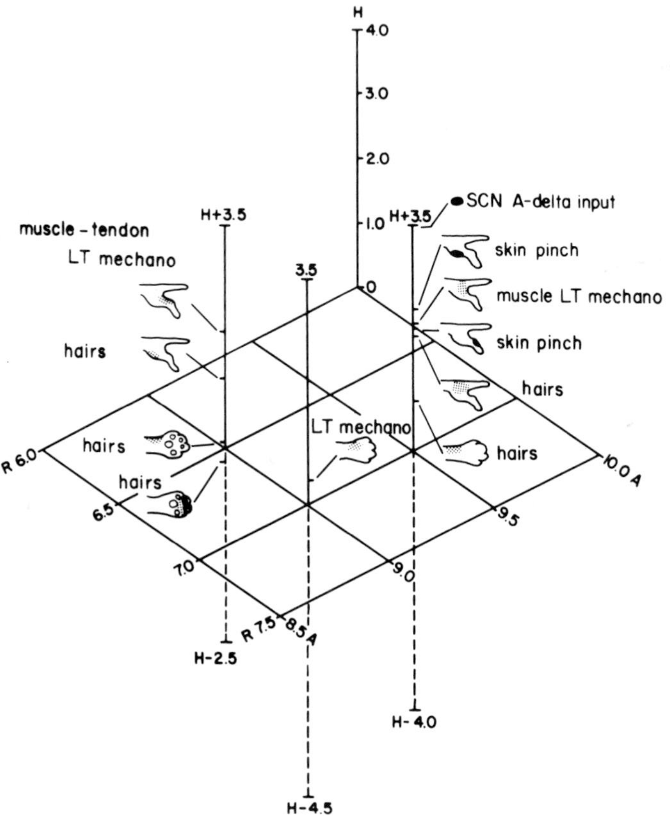

FIG. 13. Diagram showing observations made during three penetrations through the cat VPL hindlimb region. Numbers refer to Horsley-Clarke (HC) stereotaxic coordinates (mm). The grid indicates the HC horizontal plane. *A:* anterior; *R:* right (lateral axis); *H:* vertical. The approximate location and size of the receptive fields of units encountered in the vertical penetrations appear on the outline drawings. *Solid black* designates high threshold units, and *shading* indicates the units that responded to gentle mechanical stimulation. (From Honda et al., ref. 25, with permission.)

selectively nocireceptive projection of information also includes specific neurons of the ventral posterior lateral thalamus. Actually, at about the time that Kolmodin and Skoglund made their observations on selective spinal nocireceptive cells, Whitlock and I (60) noted the presence of a few selectively nocireceptive neurons in the thalamus of cats and monkeys with lesions of dorsally located spinal tracts. This early work on specific thalamic neurons could be legitimately criticized since it was done on a reduced preparation from which it was difficult to extrapolate to arrangements in an organism with undamaged pathways. However, it now has been shown that a selectively nocireceptive organization is a feature of the lateral thalamus of intact animals (25,33). Selectively nocireceptive neurons, as illustrated by

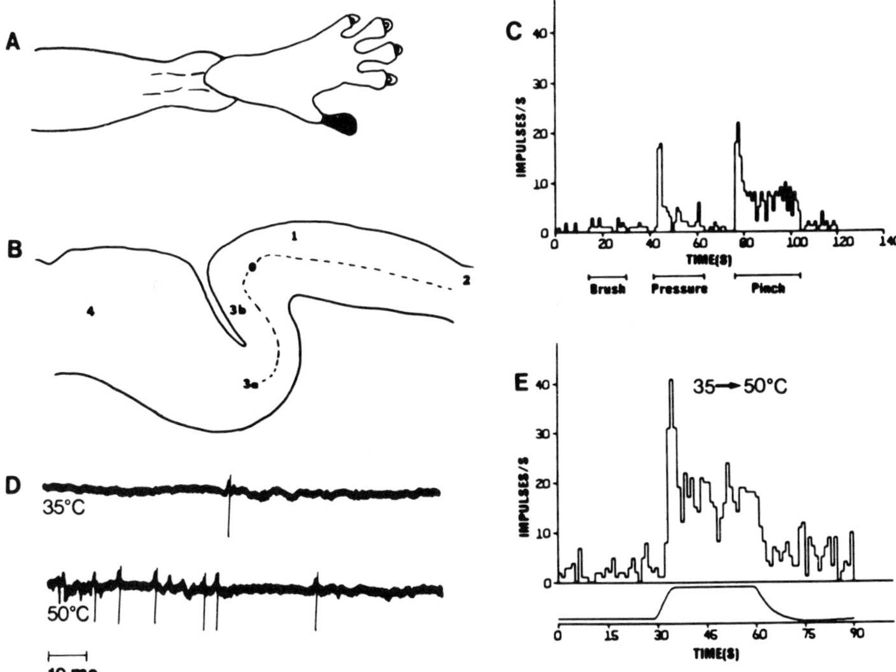

FIG. 14. Responses of a high-threshold S1 cortical neuron to mechanical and thermal stimuli. **A:** Receptive field (glabrous skin of the hallux). **B:** The recording site was in layer 4. **C:** Histogram showing the responses to a graded series of mechanical stimuli. **D:** Action potentials before *(upper trace)* and during *(lower trace)* a heat pulse rating temperature from 35–50°C. **E:** Histogram of response to a noxious heat pulse (stimulus timing indicated above abscissa). Bin width was 1 sec for all peristimulus time histograms. (From Kenshalo and Isensee, ref. 32, with permission.)

Fig. 13, appear in a rim outside the mechanoreceptive core of the ventral-posterior lateral (VPL) nucleus.

Given the importance of the VPL as a source of projections to the somatosensory cortex it is not surprising that selectively nocireceptive neurons are part of the organization of this cortical region. An example is shown in Fig. 14 for a cortical area 3b cell in the monkey, from work by Kenshalo and Isensee (32); comparable results have been reported for the rat by Lamour et al. (40). Thus, there is a projection system from primary afferent neurons to the cortex that provides two nocireceptive-specific kinds of information: a) The presence of a particular subset of neurons selectively excited by noxious stimuli insures that the information contained by their activity will be at least partially separated from other messages and provides an unambiguous signal about the presence of a noxious event. b) The circumscribed and relatively small receptive fields of neurons in this system indicate with cer-

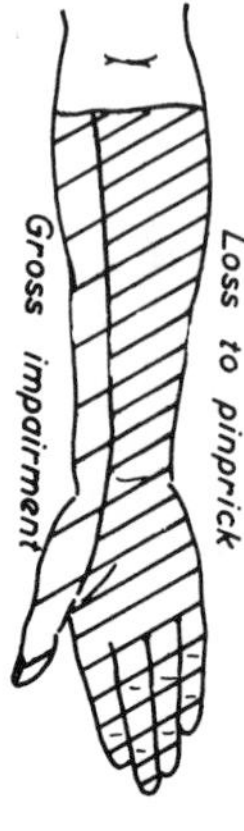

FIG. 15. Areas of impaired sensibility to pinprick in a subject who had suffered a localized parietal cortex injury 34 years previously. (From Marshall, ref. 48, with permission.)

tainty the part of the body stimulated; the population of such neurons, each representing a body region, provides a central map of the represented parts.

How do these data fit with what we know about the normal individual's capacity to recognize and localize pain-causing stimuli? I submit that if we had read the literature well these recent observations on the forebrain representation of nociception and its probable relationship to pain could have been anticipated. In 1951 Marshall (48), a British neurologist, published a remarkable study in which he tracked down a number of ex-soldiers who, during the two World Wars had suffered limited injury of the cerebral cortex and who, at the time of triage, had a loss of capacity to recognize painful stimuli. He excluded cases with persisting loss of consciousness or evidence of appreciable subcortical damage. Figure 15 shows the defect in sensibility in one of these patients 36 years after a penetrating skull wound caused a parietal cortical lesion. After many years the individual continued to have a severe defect in the ability to recognize pain-causing stimuli applied to skin or deep tissue. Marshall provides details on a number of similar cases. In my view, selective nocireceptive projections have much to do with both the recognition and localization of tissue-damaging stimuli as pain sensation.

Nonselective or Multireceptive Neurons and Pain

To this point, I have stressed the presence of a selective detection and central signalling system for noxious events. However, the repeated documentation of neurons with quite different characteristics, but whose overall functional features imply a nocireceptive function, is another of the important findings of the past several decades. Kolmodin and Skoglund (34) and Hunt and Kuno (26) independently reported spinal interneurons evincing excitatory inputs from a mixture of afferent sources. This kind of arrangement was neglected until attention was called to such elements by the

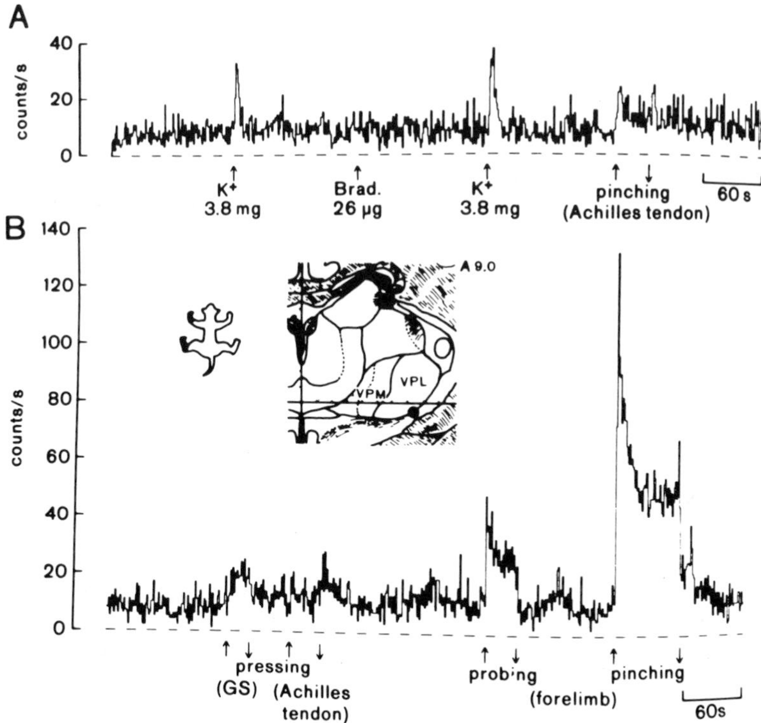

FIG. 16. Multireceptive type of VPL thalamic neuron. The neuron responded to intra-arterial injection of K^+, but was only weakly excited by mechanical stimulation (pinching, pressing) of tendon and muscle (**A**). Cutaneous receptive fields were present on both the forelimb and the hindlimb. Stimulation of the former region was more effective in evoking responses than stimulation of the latter. The recording site was at the ventral border of VPL (inset in **B**). (From Kniffki and Mizumura, ref. 33, with permission.)

reports of Mendell and Wall (53), Mendell (52), and Price and Wagman (63). Neurons receiving excitation from both myelinated and unmyelinated primary afferent fibers and showing a marked augmentation of activity upon addition of input of the latter to that of the former were labelled by Mendell (52) as "wide-dynamic range." That designation also stemmed from the enhanced responsiveness of such neurons to noxious stimuli as compared to innocuous mechanical stimulation. As Price and Dubner (62) pointed out, many multireceptive neurons respond vigorously to noxious heat, a type of stimulus that in cat excites few receptors other than C-fiber nociceptors. Multireceptive neurons are found not only at the spinal level, but also at every synaptic station in somatosensory pathways (Fig. 16). Some have argued that these broadly receptive neurons are the means by which painful stimuli are discerned (49,62); however, these neuronal responses can only differentiate innocuous (mechanical or other) stimuli from noxious events by frequency of discharge and total number of impulses. These measures are constantly modulated by other intercurrent activity from primary afferent neurons, local interneurons, and descending input from rostral centers. Thus, depending upon other influences, a particular level of activity could represent the presence of either innocuous or noxious events. This flexibility makes multireceptive neurons unlikely candidates for making reliable, qualitative distinctions. Furthermore, the extensive and often fragmented receptive fields described for multireceptive neurons are hard to reconcile with the recognized capacity of mammals to localize irritating and pain-causing stimulations (9,10,25,58,59).

Several functions have been proposed for multireceptive neurons other than the perception and cognition of pain. Wall (76) has suggested that they modulate descending control systems operating upon pain mechanisms. To me, such neurons are part of an arrangement with a more global significance. This opinion derives from the observation that multireceptive or cross-modality (e.g., neurons receiving excitation from somatic and auditory inputs) elements are not unique to the spinothalamic projection or any system essential for pain; they exist in all ascending sensory systems and have their parallels in the neural organization associated with the special senses. I propose that multireceptive neurons in ascending sensory systems are part of the mechanism that adjusts (enhances) sensitivity of the neural apparatus associated with a sensation and concomitantly the focus of attention (59). An enhanced capacity to recognize and discriminate stimuli when attention is directed at their presence and locus is common experience. Therefore, the idea is that such broadly responsive neurons help set the underlying excitability of their parallel, more selective brethren, and, in this fashion, may be part of mechanisms augmenting peripheral capacity for detection. To borrow an engineering concept, these multireceptive neurons act to modify the ratio between signal and noise. In this arrangement the function of multireceptive neurons would be other than simple recognition and modulation. Nonetheless, the parallel projection implied by the presence of such neurons and those selective for a particular submodality of sensation in ascending systems may be very important in the pathophysiology of sensation.

Descending Control

Any book of neuroanatomy should be a convincing testimony to the intricacy and detail of the structural organization of the central nervous system. Such detail is reproduced in each individual typical of the species and is remarkably similar between species. However, from a functional standpoint, the nervous system of mammals is not a rigid structure; in fact, its most striking characteristic may be its plasticity—the ability to modify output or reactions as a result of experience and circumstances. Some thirty years ago Hagbarth and Kerr (16) demonstrated that afferent activity ascending from the spinal cord in the classical systems and projecting to the cerebellum or to the cerebral cortex could be suppressed by stimulation of brain stem structures, the cerebral somatosensory regions, and parts of the cerebellum. This observation was an important step in understanding how central structures could modulate ascending somatosensory messages, again an organizational feature that is replicated in the apparati associated with the special senses. Melzack and Wall (51) focused attention on such descending modulation in sensory arrangements for pain, work which was extended by observations made by Reynolds (66), Liebeskind (45,46), Fields (13), Basbaum et al. (3), Willis and his colleagues (77,78), and many others. Other chapters in this volume deal in depth with this issue. Let me reiterate, however, that descending modification of ascending sensory signals occurs not only with activity related to pain; it operates as well for tactile messages and probably for most modalities of sensation. Thus, ideas about its functional significance must be put into the perspective that higher center control of afferent projection is a general feature of sensory organization in the mammal.

Chemical Mediators and the Nocireceptive Systems

The hunt for chemical mediators of neural activity is an old one, but 35 years ago, only a few transmitters had been reasonably identified and then only for the peripheral nervous system. Now, it seems that almost every week brings us a new candidate for a neurotransmitter in the central nervous system. This topic will be the subject of detailed consideration in other presentations; however, some general comments seem appropriate. The explosion in the number of putative chemical mediators for synapses has occurred largely because of new technologies allowing the identification of a molecular structure by agents that bind to it, carrying either a radioactive or otherwise recognizable substance as a marker. Binding by radioactive analogs helped to characterize the opiate receptors, which, in turn, then led to the discovery of the endogenous ligands for such receptors ("receptor" here means a biologically active complex in or on the cell surface membranes adapted to mate with a particular compound). By now all of us have read and will read more about enkephalins and endorphins and the many ideas that are currently afloat about how they might act. Opiate binding sites do exist upon primary afferent neurons, but their functional significance in this location is as yet unclear.

Understanding the potential involvement of peptides in synaptic transmission represents one of the major developments in the past 30 years. Of equal importance has been the recognition that many of the peptides of possible importance for synaptic activity in the peripheral central nervous system also serve a mediator function in endocrine regulation. Otsuka and his colleagues (54) called attention to a peptide in dorsal roots that depolarized central neurons. The peptide subsequently was shown to be similar or identical to substance P (71). Interestingly, Lembeck (42) nearly twenty years earlier had suggested that substance P might be a mediator for primary afferent fibers.

Immunohistochemical studies of the type pioneered by Hökfelt and his colleagues (21–24) indicate that peptides like substance P and somatostatin are concentrated in the superficial part of the dorsal horn of the spinal cord. These two peptides can be localized by immunocytochemistry to largely separate populations of dorsal root ganglion cells. Substance P was linked to the C-fiber population in part because the dorsal root ganglion neurons reacting with antibodies against substance P were small and C fibers were presumed to terminate in the superficial dorsal horn. When it was found that iontophoretically applied substance P selectively excited spinal interneurons that were also excited by activity in polymodal nociceptors, it was then hypothesized that substance P was contained in the C fibers associated with cutaneous polymodal nociceptors. This hypothesis seemed to be supported by experiments that used a clever technique for sampling cerebral spinal fluid developed by Yaksh. Yaksh et al. (83,84) showed that when peripheral nerves were stimulated repetitively at C-fiber intensities, substance P was released into the cerebral spinal fluid, a release which was inhibited by opiates. About the time that the latter observations were reported, there was excitement about the effects of capsaicin, the pungent chemical in red pepper, because it suppressed the activity or development of neurons containing substance P (29,31). Substance P content in the spinal dorsal horn could be reduced by treating young rats with capsaicin; such animals showed decreased reaction to noxious thermal stimulation. Despite the circumstantial nature of this evidence, many, including the authors of textbooks, embraced the idea that substance P is *the* synaptic transmitter for the afferent fibers causing pain.

This conclusion about the role of substance P in peripheral signalling is now recognized to have been premature. Immunohistochemical studies do show that some small-diameter dorsal root ganglion cells react as if they contained substance P. Studies at the electron microscopic level also show that in synaptic enlargements in the substantia gelatinosa substance P reactivity appears most closely associated with the dense core vesicles and not with the clear round vesicles visible at the same terminals (61). Thus, it seems likely that the substance P found in terminals in the substantia gelatinosa and perhaps in other places coexists with another synaptic chemical mediator stored in clear, round, small vesicles. Remember that the identified central terminals of the mechanical nociceptors with myelinated afferent fibers (HTM) contain few or no dense core vesicles.

Still another problem has been the nature of effects produced by substance P iontophoresis upon neurons of the dorsal horn (19,20,64). The excitatory action of substance P differs substantially from that of other iontophoretically applied, putative synaptic agents. Substance P action begins after a relatively long latency and has a prolonged duration of action when compared to other presumed chemical mediators or the actual recorded synaptic potentials from neurons excited by C-afferent fibers.

There are other difficulties with the concept that substance P is the principal chemical mediator for nociceptors. Substance P and another peptide, cholecystokinin-8, have been shown by Hökfelt's laboratory to coexist in certain nerve terminals (24). Moreover, Jancsó et al. (30) demonstrated that capsaicin administration, while clearly decreasing the number of dorsal root ganglion neurons that contain substance P, also suppressed immunoreactivity for cholecystokinin, somatostatin, and vasoactive intestinal peptide (VIP). Immunoreactivity to antibodies generated against cholecystokinin, VIP, and somatostatin all appear concentrated in the superficial part of the dorsal horn. Although neonatal capsaicin treatment clearly modifies substance P content in spinal cord and dorsal root ganglion neurons and suppresses pain reactivity in rats, the changes in other peptide substances must also be taken into account. In summary, at this time, substance P is only one of several putative synaptic mediators for peripheral nociceptors. Moreover, it seems likely that some nociceptors probably do not utilize substance P as a mediator. One of the more interesting ideas that has evolved out of this story is the possibility that substance P and perhaps certain other chemical constituents of nerve terminals may act as modulators of synaptic action rather than actual mediators of impulse traffic between neurons (36).

SPECULATIONS AND SUGGESTIONS FOR THE FUTURE

What better efforts can be made in the future to help the patient who is suffering from pain? I believe improvements can come at two levels. The first is at the scientific level where we have really only begun to sort out the neural basis of pain. Its unraveling requires an understanding of the basic principles through which a neural system encodes information and the mysteries of interneuronal communication. The challenge at this level is to gain insight into the neural bases of perception, discrimination, and emotion such as suffering. Fundamental pieces of knowledge about brain function are still missing. The second level of needed progress must occur at the juncture with the clinic. The gap in time between basic discoveries and eventual practical application is more often long than not.

Much is still to be learned about sense organs. For instance, what is the structure of C-polymodal nociceptors or nociceptors in subcutaneous tissues? Why do they have high thresholds to ordinary stimuli? I believe that a significant clinical contribution will be made by determining the mechanisms of enhanced responsiveness, i.e., sensitization, which is a feature of nociceptors. All indications are that sensitization is the product of interaction between chemical agents and nerve terminals in the peripheral tissue. If the chemical agents underlying this enhanced responsiveness can be identified, there will be better opportunities for developing more effective and more selective agents to suppress the pain associated with damaging changes in peripheral tissue. The pain of acute injury is one problem, and the pain of chronic damage and associated inflammation may be another. Chronic inflammation and acute inflammation are both marked by hyperalgesia, and drugs to combat hyperalgesia now are shots in the dark—largely developed or used empirically. Much of our drug armamentarium for treating causes of pain in the periphery is aimed at suppressing prostaglandin formation. Are prostaglandins the only chemical factors to be considered?

Another obvious research opportunity exists at the central terminations of the primary afferent neurons: the synaptic contacts of these neurons in the central nervous system and the brain stem. What are the synaptic mediators for nociceptors? Are there dual mediators for certain primary afferent fibers? Most of our effective drug manipulation of central nervous system function is the result of effects produced at synapses. Targeting drugs to suppress pain of peripheral origin will become more effective only if we fully understand the agents and processes at the central synapses. We are close to learning the nature of central synaptic mediation for primary afferent fibers, and when that happens the door for a new and effective pharmacology will surely open.

I can think of no better place for examining the central organization related to pain than the superficial dorsal horn. The neuropil of the substantia gelatinosa and the marginal zone to some extent intertwine, and the wiring diagram that exists in this region is clearly related to the sensory function of the region. We have several, sometimes conflicting, hypotheses but no direct experiments to test the effect of activity of one neuron of the region upon that of another. Such tests must be done to explain how afferent information enters and is modulated and processed in or by this area, with its rich supply of peptides and opioid receptors. If we learn what goes on in the superficial dorsal horn, I predict we will know much more about phenomena such as secondary hyperalgesia and some of the puzzling aberrations of pain that follow nerve root avulsion or spinal injury.

What is the function of multireceptive neurons with nocireceptive features? The several reasonable explanations are untested. Are such multireceptive neurons the cause of aberrant pain in lesions of peripheral nerve or dorsal root? Are changes in their function a possible explanation for the pain that is produced by normally innocuous stimulation as occurs in tic douloureux and some other painful syndromes? This is not an easy proposition to attack, yet the problem is there and begging for an answer.

Now that we recognize that there is a selective projection of nocireceptive information to the cerebral cortex and that discrete lesions to the cerebral cortex can produce persisting analgesia, are there opportunities for us in the clinic? From the days of Spiller and Martin (69) we have intervened in the central nervous system of human beings to take away awful pain. If, as the last resort, we must make lesions in the central nervous system to make life more bearable for a person with persisting pain, are there better places than those currently used? In other words, now that there is a better understanding of the functional organization of the nocireceptive system, are there untested opportunities for relieving intractable pain by more selective neural lesions?

ACKNOWLEDGMENTS

I am grateful to Ms. Marianna Chambless for her editorial and bibliographic assistance and to Mr. David Maloof for his help in preparing the typescript. Thanks are also due to Dr. Elizabeth Bullitt for her helpful suggestions on the manuscript. The manuscript preparation was supported by grant NS-10321 from the National Institute of Neurological and Communicative Disorders and Stroke of the U.S. Public Health Service.

REFERENCES

1. Adrian, E. D. (1930): Impulses in sympathetic fibres and in slow afferent fibres (Abstract). *J. Physiol. (Lond.),* 70:xx–xxi.
2. Adrian, E. D., and Zotterman, Y. (1926): The impulses produced by sensory nerve endings. Part 3. Impulses set up by touch and pressure. *J. Physiol. (Lond.),* 61:465–483.
3. Basbaum, A. I., Clanton, C. H., and Fields, H. L. (1978): Three bulbospinal pathways from the rostral medulla of the cat: an autoradiographic study of pain modulating systems. *J. Comp. Neurol.,* 178:209–224.
4. Bessou, P., Burgess, P. R., Perl, E. R., and Taylor, C. B. (1971): Dynamic properties of mechanoreceptors with unmyelinated (C) fibers. *J Neurophysiol.,* 34:116–131.
5. Bessou, P., and Perl, E. R. (1969): Response of cutaneous sensory units with unmyelinated fibers to noxious stimuli. *J. Neurophysiol,* 32:1025–1043.
6. Burgess, P. R., and Perl, E. R. (1967): Myelinated afferent fibres responding specifically to noxious stimulation of the skin. *J. Physiol. (Lond.),* 190:541–562.
7. Christensen, B. N., and Perl, E. R. (1970): Spinal neurons specifically excited by noxious or thermal stimuli: marginal zone of the dorsal horn. *J. Neurophysiol.,* 33:293–307.
8. Collins, W. F., Jr., Nulsen, F. E., and Randt, C. T. (1960): Relation of peripheral nerve fiber size and sensation in man. *Arch. Neurol. (Chicago),* 3:381–385.
9. Craig, A. D., and Kniffki, K.-D. (1985): The multiple representation of nociception in the spinothalamic projection of lamina I cells in the cat. In: *Development, Organization and Processing in Somatosensory Pathways,* edited by M. Rowe and W. Willis, pp. 347–353, Alan Liss, New York.
10. Craig, A. D., and Kniffki, K.-D. (1985): Spinothalamic lumbosacral lamina I cells responding to skin and muscle stimulation in the cat. *J. Physiol. (Lond.). (in press).*
11. Douglas, W. W., and Ritchie, J. M. (1957): A technique for recording functional activity in specific groups of medullated and non-medullated fibres in whole nerve trunks. *J. Physiol. (Lond.),* 138:19–30.
12. Dyck, P. J., Lambert, E. H., and Nichols, P. C. (1971): Quantitative measurement of sensation related to compound action potential and number and sizes of myelinated and unmyelinated fibers of sural nerve in health, Friedreich's ataxia, hereditary sensory neuropathy, and tabes dorsalis. *Electroencephalogr. Clin. Neurophysiol.,* 9:83–118.

13. Fields, H. L., Basbaum, A. I., Clanton, C. H., and Anderson, S. D. (1977): Nucelus raphe magnus inhibition of spinal cord dorsal horn neurons. *Brain Res.,* 126:441–453.
14. Fitzgerald, M., and Lynn, B. (1977): The sensitization of high threshold mechanoreceptors with myelinated axons by repeated heating. *J. Physiol. (Lond.),* 365:549–563.
15. Foreman, R. D., Applebaum, A. E., Beall, J. E., Trevino, D. L., and Willis, W. D. (1975): Responses of primate spinothalamic tract neurons to electrical stimulation of hindlimb peripheral nerves. *J. Neurophysiol.,* 38:132–145.
16. Hagbarth, K.-E., and Kerr, D. I. B. (1954): Central influences on spinal afferent conduction. *J. Neurophysiol.,* 17:295–307.
17. Hardy, J. D., Wolff, H. G., and Goodell, H. (1952): *Pain Sensations and Reactions.* Williams and Wilkins, Baltimore.
18. Heinbecker, P., Bishop, G. H., and O'Leary, J. (1933): Pain and touch fibers in peripheral nerves. *Arch. Neurol. Psychiatry,* 29:771–789.
19. Henry, J. L. (1976): Effects of substance P on functionally identified units in cat spinal cord. *Brain Res.,* 114:439–451.
20. Henry, J. L., Krnjević, K., and Morris, M. E. (1975): Substance P and spinal neurones. *Can. J. Physiol. Pharmacol.,* 53:423–432.
21. Hökfelt, T., Elde, R., Johansson, O., Luft, R., Nilsson, G., and Arimura, A. (1976): Immunohistochemical evidence for separate populations of somatostatin-containing and substance P-containing primary afferent neurons in the rat. *Neuroscience,* 1:131–136.
22. Hökfelt, T., Kellerth, J. O., Nilsson, G., and Pernow, B. (1975): Substance P: localization in the central nervous system and in some primary sensory neurons. *Science,* 190:889–890.
23. Hökfelt, T., Ljungdahl, A., Terenius, L., Elde, R., and Nilsson, G. (1977): Immunohistochemical analysis of peptide pathways possibly related to pain and analgesia: enkephalin and substance P. *Proc. Natl. Acad. Sci. USA,* 74:3081–3085.
24. Hökfelt, T., Vincent, S., Dalsgaard, C.-J., Skirboll, L., Johansson, O., Schultzberg, M., Lundberg, J. M., Rosell, S., Pernow, B., and Jancsó, G. (1982): Distribution of substance P in brain and periphery and its possible role as a co-transmitter. In: *Substance P in the Nervous System,* edited by R. Porter and M. O'Connor, pp. 84–106. Pitman, London.
25. Honda, C.N., Mense, S., and Perl, E. R. (1983): Neurons in ventrobasal region of cat thalamus selectively responsive to noxious mechanical stimulation. *J. Neurophysiol.,* 49:662–673.
26. Hunt, C. C., and Kuno, M. (1959): Background discharge and evoked responses of spinal interneurones. *J. Physiol. (Lond.),* 147:364–384.
27. Iggo, A. (1959): Cutaneous heat and cold receptors with slowly conducting (C) afferent fibres. *Q. J. Exp. Physiol.,* 44:362–370.
28. Iggo, A. (1960): Cutaneous mechanoreceptors with afferent C fibres. *J. Physiol. (Lond.),* 152:337–353.
29. Jancsó, N. (1960): Role of the nerve terminals in the mechanism of inflammatory reactions. *Bull. Millard Fillmore Hosp.,* 7:53–77.
30. Jancsó, G., Hökfelt, T., Lundberg, J. M., Király, E., Halász, N., Nilsson, G., Terenius, L., Rehfeld, J., Steinbusch, H., Verhofstad, A., Elde, R., Said, S., and Brown, M. (1981): Immunohistochemical studies on the effect of capsaicin on spinal and medullary peptide and monoamine neurons using antisera to substance P, gastrin/CCK, somatostatin, VIP, enkephalin, neurotensin and 5-hydroxytryptamine. *J. Neurocytol.,* 10:963–980.
31. Jancsó, G., Király, E., and Jancsó-Gábor, A. (1977): Pharmacologically induced selective degeneration of chemosensitive primary sensory neurones. *Nature (London)* 270:741–743.
32. Kenshalo, D. R., Jr., and Isensee, O. (1983): Effects of noxious stimuli on primate SI cortical neurons. In: *Advances in Pain Research and Therapy, Vol. 5,* edited by J. J. Bonica, U. Lindblom, and A. Iggo, pp. 139–145. Raven Press, New York.
33. Kniffki, K.-D., and Mizumura, K. (1983): Responses of neurons in VPL and VPL-VL region of the cat to algesic stimulation of muscle and tendon. *J. Neurophysiol.,* 49:649–661.
34. Kolmodin, G. M., and Skoglund, C. R. (1960): Analysis of spinal interneurons activated by tactile and nociceptive stimulation. *Acta Physiol. Scand.,* 50:337–355.
35. Konietzny, F., Perl, E. R., Trevino, D., Light, A., and Hensel, H. (1981): Sensory experiences in man evoked by intraneural electrical stimulation of intact cutaneous afferent fibers. *Exp. Brain Res.,* 42:219–222.

36. Krivoy, W. A., Couch, J. R., Henry, J. L., and Stewart, J. M. (1979): Synaptic modulation by substance P. *Fed. Proc.,* 38:2344–2347.
37. Kruger, L., Perl, E. R., and Sedivec, M. J. (1981): Fine structure of myelinated mechanical nociceptor endings in cat hairy skin. *J. Comp. Neurol.,* 198:137–154.
38. Kumazawa, T., and Perl, E. R. (1977): Primate cutaneous sensory units with unmyelinated (C) afferent fibers. *J. Neurophysiol.,* 40:1325–1338.
39. Kumazawa, T., and Perl, E. R. (1978): Excitation of marginal and substantia gelatinosa neurons in the primate spinal cord: indications of their place in dorsal horn functional organization. *J. Comp. Neurol.,* 177:417–434.
40. Lamour, Y., Willer, J. C., and Guilbaud, G. (1983): Rat somatosensory (SmI) cortex: I. Characteristics of neuronal responses to noxious stimulation and comparison with responses to non-noxious stimulation. *Exp. Brain Res.,* 49:46–54.
41. Landau, W., and Bishop, G. H. (1953): Pain from dermal, periosteal, and fascial endings and from inflammation. *Arch. Neurol. Psychiatry,* 69:490–504.
42. Lembeck, F. (1953): Zur Frage der zentralen Übertragung afferenter Impulse. III. Das Vorkommen und die Bedeutung der Substanz P in den dorsalen Wurzeln des Rückenmarks. *Arch. Exp. Pathol. Pharmakol.,* 219:197–213.
43. Lewis, T. (1942): *Pain.* Macmillan, New York.
44. Lewis, T., Pickering, G. W., and Rothschild, P. (1931): Centripetal paralysis arising out of arrested bloodflow to the limb, including notes on a form of tingling. *Heart,* 16:1–32.
45. Liebeskind, J. C., Guilbaud, G., Besson, J.-M., and Oliveras, J.-L. (1973): Analgesia from electrical stimulation of the periaqueductal gray matter in the cat: behavioral observations and inhibitory effects on spinal cord interneurons. *Brain Res.,* 50:441–446.
46. Liebeskind, J. C., Mayer, D. J., and Akil, H. (1974): Central mechanisms of pain inhibition: studies of analgesia from focal brain stimulation. *Adv. Neurol.,* 4:261–268.
47. Light, A. R., and Perl, E. R. (1979): Spinal termination of functionally identified primary afferent neurons with slowly conducting myelinated fibers. *J. Comp. Neurol.,* 186:133–150.
48. Marshall, J. (1951): Sensory disturbances in cortical wounds with special reference to pain. *J. Neurol. Neurosurg. Psychiatry,* 14:187–204.
49. Mayer, D. J., Price, D. D., and Becker, D. P. (1975): Neurophysiological characterization of the anterolateral spinal cord neurons contributing to pain perception in man. *Pain,* 1:51–58.
50. Melzack, R., and Wall, P. D. (1962): On the nature of cutaneous sensory mechanisms. *Brain,* 85:331–356.
51. Melzack, R., and Wall, P. D. (1965): Pain mechanisms: a new theory. *Science,* 150:971–979.
52. Mendell, L. M. (1966): Physiological properties of unmyelinated fiber projection to the spinal cord. *Exp. Neurol.,* 16:316–332.
53. Mendell, L. M., and Wall, P. D. (1965): Responses of single dorsal cord cells to peripheral cutaneous unmyelinated fibres. *Nature (London),* 206:97–99.
54. Otsuka, M., Konishi, S., and Takahashi, T. (1972): The presence of a motoneuron-depolarizing peptide in bovine dorsal roots of spinal nerves. *Proc. Jpn. Acad.,* 48:342–346.
55. Perl, E. R. (1968): Myelinated afferent fibres innervating the primate skin and their response to noxious stimuli. *J. Physiol. (Lond.),* 197:593–615.
56. Perl, E. R. (1971): Is pain a specific sensation? *J. Psychiatr. Res.,* 8:273–287.
57. Perl, E. R. (1976): Sensitization of nociceptors and its relation to sensation. In: *Advances in Pain Research and Therapy, Vol. 1,* edited by J. J. Bonica and D. Albe-Fessard, pp. 17–28. Raven Press, New York.
58. Perl, E. R. (1984): Pain and nociception. In: *Handbook of Physiology. The Nervous System,* edited by I. Darian-Smith, pp. 915–975. The American Physiological Society, Bethesda, MD.
59. Perl, E. R. (1984): Why are selectively responsive and multireceptive neurons both present in somatosensory pathways? In: *Somatosensory Mechanisms,* edited by C. von Euler, O. Franzén, U. Lindblom, and D. Ottoson, pp. 141–161. The Macmillan Press, London.

60. Perl, E. R., and Whitlock, D. G. (1961): Somatic stimuli exciting spinothalamic projections to thalamic neurons in cat and monkey. *Exp. Neurol.,* 3:256–296.
61. Pickel, V. M., Reis, D. J., and Leeman, S. E. (1977): Ultrastructural localization of substance P in neurons of rat spinal cord. *Brain Res.,* 122:534–540.
62. Price, D. D., and Dubner, R. (1977): Neurons that subserve the sensory-discriminative aspects of pain. *Pain,* 3:307–338.
63. Price, D. D., and Wagman, I. H. (1970): Physiological roles of A and C fiber inputs to the spinal dorsal horn of *Macaca mulatta. Exp. Neurol.,* 29:383–399.
64. Randić, M., and Miletić, V. (1977): Effect of substance P in cat dorsal horn neurones activated by noxious stimuli. *Brain Res.,* 128:164–169.
65. Réthelyi, M., Light, A. R., and Perl, E. R. (1982): Synaptic complexes formed by functionally defined primary afferent units with fine myelinated fibers. *J. Comp. Neurol.,* 207:381–393.
66. Reynolds, D. V. (1969): Surgery in the rat during electrical analgesia induced by focal brain stimulation. *Science,* 164:444–445.
67. Sherrington, C. S. (1906): *The Integrative Action of the Nervous System.* Scribner, New York.
68. Sinclair, D. C. (1955): Cutaneous sensation and the doctrine of specific energy. *Brain,* 78:584–614.
69. Spiller, W. G., and Martin, E. (1912): The treatment of persistent pain of organic origin in the lower part of the body by division of the anterolateral column of the spinal cord. *J. Am. M. A.,* 58:1489–1490.
70. Szolcsányi, J. (1980): Effect of pain-producing chemical agents on the activity of slowly conducting afferent fibres. *Acta Physiol. Acad. Sci. Hung.,* 56:86.
71. Takahashi, T., and Otsuka, M. (1975): Regional distribution of substance P in the spinal cord and nerve roots of the cat and the effect of dorsal root section. *Brain Res.,* 87:1–11.
72. Torebjörk, H. E. (1974): Afferent C units responding to mechanical, thermal and chemical stimuli in human non-glabrous skin. *Acta Physiol. Scand.,* 92:374–390.
73. Torebjörk, E., and Ochoa, J. (1983): Selective stimulation of sensory units in man. In: *Advances in Pain Research and Therapy, Vol. 5,* edited by J. J. Bonica, U. Lindblom, and A. Iggo, pp. 99–104. Raven Press, New York.
74. Trevino, D. L., Coulter, J. D., Maunz, R. A., and Willis, W. D. (1974): Location and functional properties of spinothalamic cells in the monkey. *Advan. Neurol.,* 4:167–170.
75. Trevino, D. L., Coulter, J. D., and Willis, W. D. (1973): Location of cells of origin of spinothalamic tract in lumbar enlargement of the monkey. *J. Neurophysiol.,* 36:750–761.
76. Wall, P. D. (1980): The substantia gelatinosa. A gate control mechanism set across a sensory pathway. *Trends Neurosci.,* 3:221–224.
77. Willis, W. D. (1982): *Control of Nociceptive Transmission in the Spinal Cord. Progress in Sensory Physiology 3,* edited by H. Autrum, D. Ottoson, E. R. Perl, and R. F. Schmidt. Springer-Verlag, Berlin.
78. Willis, W. D, Haber, L. H., and Martin, R. F. (1977): Inhibition of spinothalamic tract cells and interneurons by brain stem stimulation in the monkey. *J. Neurophysiol.,* 40:968–981.
79. Willis, W. D., Kenshalo, D. R., Jr., and Leonard, R. B. (1979): The cells of origin of the primate spinothalamic tract. *J. Comp. Neurol.,* 188:543–573.
80. Willis, W. D., Leonard, R. B., and Kenshalo, D. R. (1978): Spinothalamic tract neurons in the substantia gelatinosa. *Science,* 202:986–988.
81. Willis, W. D., Maunz, R. A., Foreman, R. D., and Coulter, J. D. (1975): Static and dynamic responses of spinothalamic tract neurons to mechanical stimuli. *J. Neurophysiol.,* 38:587–600.
82. Willis, W. D., Trevino, D. L., Coulter, J. D., and Maunz, R. A. (1974): Responses of primate spinothalamic tract neurons to natural stimulation of hindlimb. *J. Neurophysiol.,* 37:358–372.
83. Yaksh, T. L., Farb, D. H., Leeman, S. E., and Jessell, T. M. (1979): Intrathecal capsaicin depletes substance P in the rat spinal cord and produces prolonged thermal analgesia. *Science,* 206:481–483.

84. Yaksh, T. L., Jessell, T. M., Gamse, R., Mudge, A. W., and Leeman, S. E. (1980): Intrathecal morphine inhibits substance P release from mammalian spinal cord, *in vivo. Nature London,* 286:155–157.
85. Zotterman, Y. (1933): Studies in the peripheral nervous mechanism of pain. *Acta Med. Scand.,* 80:185–242.
86. Zotterman, Y. (1939): Touch, pain and tickling: an electrophysiological investigation on cutaneous sensory nerves. *J. Physiol. (Lond.),* 95:1–28.

Advances in Pain Research and Therapy, Vol. 9, edited by H. L. Fields et al. Raven Press, New York © 1985.

Fast and Slow Excitatory Transmitters at Primary Afferent Synapses in the Dorsal Horn of the Spinal Cord

Thomas M. Jessell and Craig E. Jahr

Department of Neurobiology, Harvard Medical School, Boston, Massachusetts 02115

ORGANIZATION OF THE SUPERFICIAL DORSAL HORN

The mechanisms that underlie the processing of cutaneous sensory information in the dorsal horn of the spinal cord remain poorly understood despite substantial clarification, over the last decade, of the anatomical organization of afferent fiber input. Much of this anatomical information is due to the development of techniques for mapping the terminal arbors of single, functionally characterized sensory fibers after intraaxonal injection of horseradish peroxidase (HRP) (4,24). These studies have revealed that the central terminals of functionally distinct classes of cutaneous afferent fibers are segregated in a precise laminar pattern. Low-threshold myelinated afferents that innervate hair follicles and both slowly and rapidly adapting mechanoreceptors terminate relatively deep within the dorsal horn, predominantly in laminae III and IV (4). Although these classes of low-threshold myelinated afferents all terminate within laminae III and IV, each can be distinguished by the mediolateral extent of its terminal arborization and by the spacing of collateral branches that give rise to the terminal fields (4). In contrast, myelinated afferents that respond to high-threshold mechanical stimuli project to lamina I and also have collaterals that terminate in lamina V (17,27).

The vast majority of unmyelinated afferents, of which between 50 and 70% correspond to polymodal nociceptors (19), terminate within laminae I and II (27). Lamina II can be subdivided according to morphological and ultrastructural features of the neuropil (25,29). Polymodal nociceptors appear to project to the outer region of lamina II, whereas C fibers innervating low-threshold mechanoreceptors are thought to project to inner lamina II (18).

The responses of superficial dorsal horn neurons to sensory stimuli

(11,30,32) reflect the peripheral receptive properties of afferent fibers that project to specific dorsal horn laminae. High proportions of neurons in lamina I and outer lamina II are activated by noxious peripheral stimuli (2,18). Some superficial dorsal horn neurons respond selectively to noxious stimuli, whereas others have been reported to be activated by both innocuous and noxious stimuli, suggesting a convergence of afferent fiber input (2,26). Convergence of afferent input is more marked within deeper regions of the dorsal horn, in particular onto lamina V neurons that contribute axons to the spinothalamic tract (16).

These anatomical and physiological observations have emphasized the crucial role of the primary afferent synapse in the transfer of specific cutaneous sensory stimuli from the periphery to the central nervous system (CNS). However, the identity of the chemical mediators at afferent synapses and characterization of their postsynaptic actions have not been resolved. There are still fewer clues about the molecular events that result in the formation of appropriate synaptic connections between primary sensory neurons and their spinal cord targets (8).

NEUROTRANSMITTERS AT PRIMARY AFFERENT SYNAPSES IN THE DORSAL HORN

The processing and integration of sensory information conveyed by the functionally diverse classes of primary afferent fibers that terminate within the dorsal horn have raised several questions about the nature of chemical transmitters at afferent synapses. It is possible that many or all functionally distinct classes of afferent fibers release different chemical transmitters. The specificity of information transfer at afferent synapses would thus be dependent on both the synaptic circuitry in the dorsal horn and the chemical specificity at the afferent synapse. Alternatively, all primary afferent fibers might release the same synaptic transmitter, independent of the sensory modality carried by each fiber type. In that event, the specificity of sensory coding would depend to a much greater extent on the neuronal circuitry formed by each class of afferent fiber. Some sensory fibers could also release more than one chemical transmitter at afferent synapses in the dorsal horn. Recent physiological, morphological, and biochemical studies have begun to resolve some of these possibilities.

Morphological and Physiological Analysis

Ultrastructural studies of the superficial dorsal horn in rodents, cats, and primates have revealed that all primary afferent terminals contain small, clear synaptic vesicles (25,29). In some cases ultrastructural analysis of single identified HRP-filled afferents has also been possible, demonstrating that both low- and high-threshold myelinated afferents appear to possess, exclusively, small clear vesicles in their synaptic terminals (1,26,28). However, many afferent terminals in the superficial dorsal horn also contain a second class of larger vesicles with dense cores (25,29). In other regions of the CNS, the presence of dense-core vesicles has been associated with storage of transmitters that are chemically distinct from those contained within small clear vesicles. Ultrastructural evidence therefore suggests that some primary afferents that project to the superficial dorsal horn can store and release more than one class of transmitter.

Complementary physiological studies have provided evidence that synaptic transmitters released from sensory afferents may produce qualitatively different responses in a single postsynaptic dorsal horn neuron. Intracellular recording from neurons in the superficial dorsal horn in a slice preparation of rat spinal cord has demonstrated that a single stimulus applied to the dorsal root elicits a fast excitatory postsynaptic potential (EPSP) that can be detected in most dorsal horn neurons (31). Increasing the frequency of dorsal root stimulation, however, evokes a second type of synaptic potential that is slow in onset and prolonged in duration (31). Although the sensory origin and chemical identity of the transmitter mediating the slow synaptic response have not been established conclusively, one explanation of these results is that there is release of both fast and slow excitatory transmitters by primary sensory neurons.

A more detailed description of the characteristics of monosynaptic transmission at identified afferent synapses has been provided by analysis of excitatory postsynaptic currents recorded from cat spinal motoneurons with Ia afferent input (9). Studies of synaptic connections between dorsal root ganglion (DRG) neurons and unidentified spinal neurons in dissociated cell culture have also provided evidence on the postsynaptic actions of sensory transmitters (20). However, the complexities of neural circuitry in the dorsal horn *in vivo* and even in slice preparations has prevented a similar analysis of transmission at cutaneous afferent synapses.

Identification of Fast Excitatory Transmitters at Sensory Synapses

In order to determine the chemical identity of primary sensory transmitters with rapid postsynaptic actions, we have developed methods to examine the monosynaptic excitatory connections formed by DRG neurons grown in co-culture with dorsal horn neurons (14). Examination of the chemosensitivity of cultured dorsal horn neurons has thus far identified only two classes of compounds, excitatory amino acids and nucleotides, that have excitatory actions consistent with their roles as fast excitatory sensory transmitters (7,13,14).

Application of ATP (1–10 μM) produces a rapid and marked depolarization (5–35 mV) of approximately 25% of dorsal horn neurons examined (13). The response to ATP is frequently accompanied by one or more action potentials superimposed at the peak of the depolarization. Other dorsal horn neurons are unaffected by ATP at concentrations up to 100 μM. Although the majority of dorsal horn neurons receive spontaneous synaptic input, the ATP response does not depend on intact synaptic transmission. Superfusion of cultures with $CdCl_2$ (200 μM) completely abolishes all spontaneous synaptic activity but does not decrease the response to ATP.

The depolarization of dorsal horn neurons is elicited only by ATP and closely related nucleotide analogs. Adenosine, AMP, GTP, and UTP produce no effect on dorsal horn neurons, whereas ADP and CTP are less than one-tenth as active as ATP. Adenosine tetraphosphate and the slowly hydrolyzable ATP analogs AMP-PNP and β-γ-methylene ATP also depolarize dorsal horn neurons, indicating that the ATP-induced excitation of dorsal horn neurons is unlikely to require hydrolysis of the triphosphate chain. The relative potencies of nucleosides and nucleotides also make it unlikely that the actions of ATP are mediated by adenosine receptors (5). In support of this, superfusion of dorsal horn neurons with 8-phenyltheophylline at a concentration sufficient to block adenosine receptors did not decrease the depolarization produced by ATP (13).

It has been suggested that Ca^{2+} chelation is responsible for the excitatory action of ATP on cuneate neurons *in vivo.* However, we found that the disodium, magnesium, calcium, and Tris salts of adenosine triphosphate (ATP) were equally effective in depolarizing dorsal horn neurons. Furthermore, the chelators EDTA (10^{-5} M) and inorganic pyrophosphate (10^{-4} M) were without effect on dorsal horn neurons that were sensitive to ATP (7).

The depolarization of dorsal horn neurons by ATP is accompanied by an increase in membrane conductance that persists when the membrane potential is voltage-clamped to the resting potential. The increase in conductance therefore reflects the action of ATP itself and does not result from voltage-dependent membrane rectification. Hyperpolarization of dorsal horn neurons by intracellular injection of current greatly increases the depolarization elicited by ATP even in neurons that exhibit inward rectification. This indicates that the reversal potential of the ATP response is positive to the resting potential (7). Additional studies using patch-clamp recording techniques have suggested that the depolarization of dorsal horn neurons by ATP is likely to be due to an increase in Na^+ and K^+ conductance (C. E. Jahr, *unpublished observations*).

Several important criteria remain to be fulfilled before a sensory transmitter role for ATP in the spinal cord can be established. Whereas biochemical studies have demonstrated a selective release of ATP from the dorsal horn of the spinal cord (34), the neuronal elements in the dorsal horn that release ATP remain to be identified. There is also an urgent need for specific receptor antagonists in order to provide a more critical assessment of the role of ATP in sensory transmission. Recent studies by Fyffe and Perl (10), however, have provided additional support for the concept that ATP may be released as a sensory transmitter. They found that a subset of cat dorsal horn neurons with A- and C-fiber-sensitive mechanoreceptor input were selectively excited by ATP.

ATP cannot be the only fast excitatory transmitter released from primary sensory neurons, because many dorsal horn neurons that receive sensory input are insensitive to ATP (13,14). Several lines of evidence have suggested that the fast excitation of some spinal cord neurons evoked by afferent fiber stimulation is mediated by glutamate or by compounds with similar postsynaptic actions. Application of glutamate depolarizes the majority of spinal neurons with a reversal potential similar to that of the afferent-evoked synaptic potential (9,21). However, the excitation by glutamate of virtually all spinal neurons and the difficulty of examining monosynaptic interactions in the intact spinal cord has made it difficult to establish the role of excitatory amino acids as sensory transmitters.

To provide information on the role of glutamate and other excitatory amino acids as primary afferent transmitters, we have studied the actions of amino acid agonists and antagonists at monosynaptic sensory synapses formed in culture (14). Application of L-glutamate produces a potent excitation of all cultured dorsal horn neurons that receive monosynaptic DRG-evoked synaptic potentials. Moreover, both the monosynaptic EPSP elicited by sensory neuron stimulation and the depolarization evoked by L-glutamate are abolished by the amino acid antagonist kynurenate (14), suggesting that amino acids are likely to be sensory transmitters released at a substantial fraction of primary afferent synapses. Because of the accessibility to primary afferent synapses formed in culture, it has also been possible to block, selectively, the *N*-methyl-D-aspartate (NMDA) class of excitatory amino acid receptor by addition of high levels of Mg^{2+} (22). Under these conditions, L-aspartate has little or no action on glutamate-sensitive dorsal horn neurons that receive a sensory-neuron-evoked EPSP (14). It is likely, therefore, that L-glutamate, or a closely related compound, but not L-aspartate, is the fast transmitter at sensory synapses examined in these experiments. A similar pharmacological analysis at identified Ia afferent synapses in the intact neonatal spinal cord has suggested that L-glutamate may also be the transmitter at Ia synapses (14a).

Slow Excitatory Transmitters at Sensory Synapses

In addition to transmitters that mediate fast synaptic potentials at afferent synapses, there is increasing evidence that several of the neuropeptides identified within subsets of cutaneous sensory neurons (15) may act as slow synaptic transmitters in the dorsal horn. Approximately one-third of small-diameter sensory neurons have thus far been shown to contain neuropeptides. Substance P (and probably the structurally related tachykinin, substance K) is present within 10 to 20% of DRG neurons, somatostatin is present within a separate population of 5 to 10% of cells, and vasoactive intestinal polypeptide (VIP) can be found in a few scattered neurons within sensory ganglia. A peptide related to but not identical with cholecystokinin (CCK) is also present within a subpopulation of sensory ganglion cells (12). Recent studies have shown that many of the CCK-like immunoreactive cells also contain substance P (12). Consistent with this overlap, the central-terminal fields of substance P and CCK containing sensory neurons are strikingly similar and are confined predominantly to lamina I and to outer lamina II (12). Somatostatin neurons of sensory origin project more ventrally and terminate almost exclusively in the central region of lamina II, whereas VIP immunoreactive terminals are located predominantly within lamina I. Some sensory neurons that project to lamina II of the dorsal horn may also contain an angiotensin-like peptide (12).

Of the peptides localized in sensory ganglia, the role of substance P has been studied in greatest detail. Substance P immunoreactivity is associated with large, dense-core vesicles in the central terminals of sensory neurons in laminae I and II of the dorsal horn (3,6) that also contain small clear vesicles, suggesting that tachykinin peptides may be present in afferent terminals that release fast sensory transmitters.

The release of substance P from sensory terminals in the dorsal horn has been demonstrated *in vitro* (15,23) and *in vivo* (33). Experiments in which the release of substance P into the spinal subarachnoid space has been measured after intrathecal superfusion of the cat spinal cord have shown that substance P release is evoked selectively by recruitment of peripheral sensory fibers that have conduction velocities in the $A\delta$- and C-fiber range (33).

It has been difficult to correlate the postsynaptic actions of substance P with the responses of dorsal horn neurons to noxious peripheral stimuli. *In vivo,* iontophoretic application of substance P produces a slow and prolonged activation of dorsal horn neurons that is in many cases slower in onset than the response of the same neuron to peripheral noxious stimuli (15). Intracellular recording from dorsal horn neurons in spinal cord slices has demonstrated a slow synaptically mediated depolarization following high-frequency dorsal root stimulation (31). A similar depolarization can be produced by application of substance P to dorsal horn neurons. Moreover, synthetic peptide analogs of substance P block the slow depolarization of dorsal horn neurons evoked by both dorsal root stimulation and substance P application (31). Thus, substance P and perhaps many of the other peptides found within primary sensory neurons may be released as slow synaptic transmitters in the dorsal horn. The release of peptides from specific classes of afferent fibers may play an important physiological role in regulating the excitability of subsets of dorsal horn neurons that receive synaptic input mediated by fast sensory transmitters such as L-glutamate or ATP.

The functional roles of other peptides in primary sensory neurons are also uncertain. Somatostatin has been reported to inhibit nociceptive dorsal horn neurons, whereas CCK and VIP have excitatory actions (15,31).

CONCLUSIONS

The studies outlined here suggest that there are likely to be two major classes of synaptic transmitters released by primary sensory neurons in the mammalian spinal cord. Many, and probably all, primary sensory neurons appear to release synaptic transmitters with fast excitatory postsynaptic actions on spinal neurons. Although the identity of fast sensory transmitters is still not established, L-glutamate, or a closely related compound, is likely to be a sensory transmitter at synapses formed between DRG and dorsal horn neurons maintained in culture and also at Ia afferent synapses. Pharmacological studies in culture and *in vivo* have provided evidence that is consistent with the concept that ATP may be a fast transmitter at some cutaneous afferent synapses, possibly those mediating low-threshold mechanical stimuli conveyed by C fibers. In addition to the fast excitatory sensory transmitters, several peptides have been shown to exist in subsets of primary sensory neurons that project to the superficial dorsal horn. Substance P and related tachykinins are likely to be slow excitatory transmitters released following activation of high-threshold afferent fibers. The physiological functions of substance P and other peptides in the processing of sensory information are still uncertain. However, it seems likely that the release of peptides may modify the responses of certain classes of dorsal horn neurons to other rapidly acting sensory transmitters. Future studies on the interactions between different sensory transmitter candidates should provide information on some of the mechanisms underlying the integration of sensory information that takes place at primary afferent synapses in the dorsal horn.

ACKNOWLEDGMENTS

The work from the authors' laboratory described in this chapter was supported by grants from the National Institutes of Health, the McKnight Foundation, The Muscular Dystrophy Association, and the Rita Allen Foundation.

REFERENCES

1. Bannatyne, B. A., Maxwell, D. J., Fyffe, R. E. W., and Brown, A. G. (1984): Fine structure of primary afferent axon terminals of slowly adapting cutaneous receptors in the cat. *Q.J. Exp. Physiol.,* 69:547–557.
2. Bennett, G. J., Abdelmonmene, M., Hayashi, H., and Dubner, R. (1980): Physiology and morphology of substantia gelatinosa neurones intracellularly stained with horseradish perioxidase. *J. Comp. Neurol.,* 194:809–827.

3. Bresnahan, J. C., Ho, R. H., and Beattie, M. S. (1984): A comparison of the ultrastructure of substance P and enkephalin-immunoreactive elements in the nucleus of the dorsal lateral funiculus and laminae I and II of the rat spinal cord. *J. Comp. Neurol.,* 229:497–511.
4. Brown, A. G. (1982): The dorsal horn of the spinal cord. *Q.J. Exp. Physiol.,* 67:193–212.
5. Burnstock, G. (1978): Purninergic receptors. *J. Theor. Biol.,* 62:491–499.
6. DiFiglia, M., Aronin, N., and Leeman, S. (1982): Light microscopic and ultrastructural localization of immunoreactive substance P in the dorsal horn of the monkey spinal cord. *Neuroscience,* 7:1127–1139.
7. Dodd, J., Jahr, C. E., Hamilton, P., Heath, M., Matthew, W. D., and Jessell, T. M. (1983): Cytochemical and physiological properties of sensory and dorsal horn neurons that transmit cutaneous sensation. *Cold Spring Harbor Symp. Quant. Biol.,* 48:685–695.
8. Dodd, J., Solter, D., and Jessell, T. M. (1984): Monoclonal antibodies against carbohydrate differentiation antigens identify subsets of primary sensory neurons. *Nature,* 311:469–472.
9. Finkel, A. S., and Redman, S. J. (1983): The synaptic current evoked in cat spinal motoneurons by impulses in single group Ia axons. *J. Physiol. (Lond.),* 342:615–632.
10. Fyffe, R. E. W., and Perl, E. R. (1984): Is ATP a central synaptic mediator for certain primary afferent fibres from mammalian stain? *Proc. Natl. Acad. Sci. U.S.A.,* 81:6890–6893.
11. Hentall, I. (1977): A novel class of unit in the substantia gelatinosa of the spinal cat. *Exp. Neurol.,* 57:792–806.
12. Hökfelt, T., Skirboll, L., Lundberg, J. M., Dalsgaard, C. J., Johansson, D., Pernow, B., and Jancso, G. (1983): Neuropeptides and pain pathways. *Adv. Pain Res. Ther.,* 5:227–246.
13. Jahr, C. E., and Jessell, T. M. (1983): ATP excites a subpopulation of rat dorsal horn neurons. *Nature,* 304:730–733.
14. Jahr, C. E., and Jessell, T. M. (1985): Synaptic transmission between cultured dorsal root ganglion and dorsal horn neurons: antagonism of glutamate excitation and monosynaptic EPSP's by kynurenate. *J. Neurosci. (in press)*
14a. Jahr, C. E., and Yoshioka, K. (1985): 1a Afferent excitation of motoneurons in the newborn rat spinal cord is selectively antagonized by Kynurenate. *J. Physiol.* (*in press*)
15. Jessell, T. M. (1983): Nociception. In: *Brain Peptides,* edited by D. Krieger, M. Brownstein, and J. B. Martin, pp. 315–332. Wiley, New York.
16. Kenshalo, D. R., Leonard, R. B., Chung, J. M., and Willis, W. D. (1979): Responses of primate spinothalamic tract neurons to graded and repeated noxious heat stimuli. *J. Neurophysiol.,* 42:1370–1389.
17. Light, A. R., and Perl, E. R. (1979): Spinal termination of functionally identified primary afferent fibres with slowly conducting myelinated fibres. *J. Comp. Neurol.,* 186:133–150.
18. Light, A. R., Trevino, D. L., and Perl, E. R. (1979): Morphological features of functionally defined neurons in the marginal zone and substantia gelatinosa of the spinal dorsal horn. *J. Comp. Neurol.,* 186:151–172.
19. Lynn, B., and Carpenter, S. E. (1982): Primary afferent units from the hairy skin of the rat hind limb. *Brain Res.,* 238:29–43.
20. MacDonald, R. C., Pun, R. Y. K., Neale, E. A., and Nelson, P. G. (1983): Synaptic interactions between mammalian central neurons in cell culture. I. Reversal potential for excitatory post-synaptic potentials. *J. Neurophysiol.,* 49:1428–1441.
21. Mayer, M. L., and Westbrook, G. L. (1984): Mixed agonist action of excitatory amino acids on mouse spinal cord neurons under voltage clamp. *J. Physiol. (Lond.),* 354:29–53.
22. Mayer, M. L., Westbrook, G. L., and Guthrie, P. B. (1984): Voltage dependent block by Mg^{++} of NMDA responses in spinal cord neurons. *Nature,* 309:261–263.
23. Otsuka, M., Konishi, S., Yanagisawa, M., Tsunoo, A. and Akagi, H. (1982): Role of substance P as a sensory transmitter in spinal cord and sympathetic ganglia. *Ciba Found. Symp.,* 91:13–34.
24. Perl, E. R. (1983): Characterization of nociceptors and their activation of neurons in the superficial dorsal horn: First steps for the sensation of pain. *Adv. Pain Res. Ther.,* 6:23–51.
25. Ralston, J. H., III (1979): Distribution of dorsal root axons in laminae I, II and III of the macaque spinal cord. *J. Comp. Neurol.,* 184:643–684.
26. Ralston, J. H., Light, A. R., Ralston, D. D., and Perl, E. R. (1984): Morphology and synaptic relationships of physiologically identified low-threshold dorsal root axons stained with intra-axonal horseradish peroxidase in the cat and monkey, *J. Neurophysiol.,* 51:777–792.

27. Rethelyi, M. (1977): Preterminal and terminal axon arborizations in the substantia gelatinosa of cat's spinal cord. *J. Comp. Neurol.* 172:511–528.
28. Rethelyi, M., Light, A. R., and Perl., E. R. (1982): Synaptic complexes formed by functionally defined primary afferent units with fine myelinated fibers. *J. Comp. Neurol.,* 207:381–393.
29. Ribiero DaSilva, A., and Coimbra, A. (1982): Two types of synaptic glomeruli and their distribution in laminae I–III of the rat spinal cord. *J. Comp. Neurol.,* 209:176–189.
30. Steedman, W. M., Iggo, A., Molony, V., Korogod, S., and Zachary, S. (1983): Statistical analysis of ongoing activity of neurons in the substantia gelatinosa and in lamina III of cat spinal cord. *Q.J. Exp. Physiol.,* 68:733–746.
31. Urban, and Randic, M. (1984): Slow excitatory transmission in rat dorsal horn: Possibly mediation by peptides. *Brain Res.,* 290:336–341.
32. Wall, P. D., Merrill, E. G., and Yaksh, T. L. (1979): Responses of single units in laminae II and III of cat spinal cord. *Brain Res.,* 160:245–260.
33. Yaksh, T. L., Jessell, T. M., Gamse, R., Mudge, A. W., and Leeman, S. E. (1980): Intrathecal morphine inhibits substance P release from mammalian spinal cord in vivo. *Nature,* 286:155–157.
34. Yoshioka, K., and Jessell, T. M. (1984): ATP release from the dorsal horn of rat spinal cord. *Soc. Neurosci. Abst.,* 10:993.

Advances in Pain Research and Therapy, Vol. 9, edited by H. L. Fields et al. Raven Press, New York © 1985.

Role of Sensory Neuronal Peptides in Nociception

J. D. Leah, A. A. Cameron, and P. J. Snow

Anatomy Department, Queensland University, St. Lucia, Australia 4067

Since the localization by immunohistochemical techniques of the neuroactive peptides substance P (SP), somatostatin (SS), cholecystokinin (CCK), and vasoactive intestinal polypeptide (VIP) in small primary sensory neurons there has been considerable speculation that these compounds may be involved in the transmission of noxious information to the spinal cord (7,8,12). If these peptides are indeed involved in such primary afferent transmission, either by acting as transmitter compounds or by modulating the actions of a coexistent transmitter, then there arises the interesting possibility that they may relate specifically to the modality or submodality of the afferent neuron.

The evidence for the involvement of these peptides in primary afferent transmission and in nociception includes their localization in approximately 25% of the small-diameter sensory neurons, their release from spinal cord following electrical stimulation of C fibers, the inhibition of this release by opioid compounds, and their ability to alter the activity of dorsal horn neurons that respond to noxious input (12). Additionally, SP antagonists appear to reduce the depolarization of dorsal horn neurons that is produced by both SP and by stimulation of C fibers and to elevate behaviorally assessed nociceptive thresholds (11,13). However, such evidence that the peptides are contained in, and released by, the nociceptive primary afferents is largely indirect. Some of the foregoing effects could, for instance, arise from the peptides concerned being released from dorsal horn interneurons rather than from the primary afferent fibers.

To determine whether or not the sensory neurons containing these peptides are in fact the nociceptive afferents, we made intracellular recordings from single cutaneous C and Aδ fibers (1,3), determined their modality, and injected them with Lucifer yellow. We then used PAP immunochemistry to examine the peptide content of these neurons. Our results show that there is no clear correlation between the neuropeptide content of sensory fibers and the modality they subserve. This raises the important question of the general role of these neuroactive peptides within the nervous system.

METHODS

Experiments were performed on 40 adult cats. Twenty-four hours prior to recording, the L7, S1, and S2 ganglia were treated with 20% colchicine (in Hartmann's solution) for 1 hr to cause accumulation of the peptides in the cell bodies. The animals were then reanesthetized with α-chloralose (70 mg/kg i.v.) and prepared for recording as detailed elsewhere (10). Cells in the ganglia were impaled with microelectrodes containing Lucifer yellow CH (5% to 0.5-M LiCl, 80–200 megohm), and the receptive modality of those having peripheral axons conducting in the C or A range was carefully determined using procedures outlined by previous workers (1,3). The cells were then injected with dye, and the ganglia were excised and fixed by immersion in 4% paraformaldehyde in 0.1-M phosphate buffer, followed by overnight immersion in 5% sucrose in phosphate-buffered saline (pH 7.4). The ganglia were then embedded in wax; 5-μm serial sections were cut, and the sections through the injected cell were located and photographed. Each section through the cell was then immunostained by the PAP technique using antiserum to one of the peptides (Immunonuclear, Amersham, or Bioproducts) SP, SS, CCK, and VIP.

RESULTS

On examining the cutaneous receptive characteristics of more than 120 C and Aα neurons, we found that the modalities could be classified into one of the following previously described (1,3) types: (a) polymodal receptors that responded to both noxious mechanical (NM) and noxious thermal (NT) stimuli (sometimes in addition to chemical irritants); (b) receptors that responded to NM stimuli; (c) receptors that responded to innocuous mechanical (IM) stimuli; (d) receptors that were responsive to both IM stimuli and skin cooling. The Aδ fibers responded to down hairs or to NM stimuli.

When the peptide contents of 26 of these cells were examined it was clear that there was no correlation between the peptide content and the modality subserved (Table 1). Indeed, few of these cells contained peptides; notably, in only 2 of the 12 cells that responded to noxious stimuli could we detect immunostaining for SP. To ensure that the injection of cells with Lucifer yellow did not in some manner initiate lysis of these peptides, we also injected 10 neurons for which we could not locate a cutaneous receptive field but which we considered to be C-fiber somata on the basis of their perinuclear diameter and the shape and duration of their action potentials. All these cells were found to contain immunoreactivity to at least one peptide, and 8 of the 10 showed immunoreactivity to SP.

TABLE I. *Peptide contents of identified cutaneous C-fiber and Aδ-fiber somata and unidentified C-fiber somata*

Fiber	Peptide content			
	SP	SS	CCK	VIP
C fibers: noxious mechanical and noxious thermal	−	−	+	0
	+	+	+	0
	−	−	−	−
	−	−	−	−
	−	−	−	0
C fibers: innocuous mechanical and skin cooling	−	−	−	−
	−	−	+	+
	+	−	+	−
	−	−	−	−
	−	−	−	−
	+	−	−	−
	−	−	+	−
	+	+	−	−
	−	−	0	−
C fibers: noxious mechanical	+	+	−	0
	−	−	−	−
	−	−	+	−
	−	−	−	−
	−	−	−	0
	−	−	−	−
	−	−	−	−
C fibers: without cutaneous receptive fields	−	0	+	+
	+	−	+	+
	+	+	+	−
	+	−	−	−
	+	−	−	−
	+	+	−	−
	+	−	+	−
	+	−	+	−
	+	−	−	+
	−	−	+	−
Aδ fibers: down hairs	−	−	0	+
	0	−	−	+
	−	−	−	−
Aδ fibers: noxious mechanical	−	0	−	−
	−	−	0	0

The modalities of C and Aδ fibers, the somata of which were injected intracellularly with Lucifer yellow CH and shown to contain immunoreactivity to SP, SS, CCK, and VIP. The symbols under the peptides indicate instances in which there was definite immunoreactivity (+), instances in which there was no immunoreactivity even though other uninjected cells in the same section showed clear positive immunoreactivity (−), and instances in which the presence or absence of immunoreactivity could not be confirmed because the cell was not present in the section, or other cells in the section did not show sufficiently strong immunoreactivity, or because the section was damaged during processing (0).

DISCUSSION

Our results, showing that SP is not present in the majority of sensory neurons that respond to noxious cutaneous stimulation, do not support the hypothesis that SP is involved in the transmission of cutaneous noxious information to spinal neurons. Thus, other roles for SP in primary sensory neurons need to be considered. It has been suggested (6,14) that SP may have trophic effects on the circuitry of dorsal horn neurons, but such an effect remains to be clearly established. The finding of SP in many sensory neurons with noncutaneous fields is suggestive of a role in autonomic function. Certainly primary afferent fibers containing SP as well as those containing VIP project not only to the dorsal horn but also to the intermediolateral nucleus in the spinal cord (8). There is evidence that in the central nervous system, neurons containing CCK and VIP act to coordinate local blood flow and neuronal activity (9). A similar role may therefore be postulated for these peptides in sensory neurons by suggesting that they increase blood flow in the locality of the central terminals of the afferent and as a consequence in the locality of the spinal cells that those terminals influence. Thus, perhaps a certain class of primary afferent fibers (those containing these substances) might be regarded as controlling local blood flow in addition to effecting the transmission of sensory information as do other sensory neurons.

Another striking finding from the present experiments was that even those fine-caliber primary cutaneous afferents that subserve identical modalities contain widely varying and sometimes complex combinations of neuropeptides (Table 1). In relation to this, it is possible that the levels of these neuropeptides in sensory neurons may be determined by some extrinsic factor such as the past history of electrical activity in a neuron. Certainly the number of autonomic neurons containing detectable levels of SP and SS can be increased by depolarization (2). Thus, sensory neurons having peripheral nociceptors may indeed synthesize SP and SS, but possibly the levels of these substances reach concentrations detectable by immunohistochemical techniques only after these neurons are subjected to a high level of electrical activity. Such a mechanism could endow the fine-caliber primary afferents with the capacity to exert a variable influence on spinal neurons.

A final point that needs some consideration arises from the findings of Edwards (5) that differential release of a peptide or a coexistent classic neurotransmitter from autonomic neurons can be achieved by different patterns of electrical stimulation. By such a mechanism, the release of one substance from an afferent fiber that contains a host of neuroactive agents may be coded for by a specific discharge pattern that itself arises from a specific form or intensity of natural stimulation. In the present study we did not detect marked differences in the temporal patterning of action potentials in the responses of those sensory neurons that were sensitive to identical modalities. Nevertheless, these neurons often contained markedly different combinations of neuropeptides. Although it may be that a highly quantitative study of the impulse patterns in the responses would have produced a correlation with neuropeptide content, we consider this an unlikely possibility. Consequently, we believe that the question of the general role (if any) of the neuropeptides in synaptic transmission must be approached by studying the pharmacology of transmission between single physiologically and neurochemically identifiable afferent neurons and those neurons on which they make synapses.

ACKNOWLEDGMENTS

We wish to thank Ms. Wendy Kelly and Mr. Ron Hume for their skilled assistance and Dr. Michael Landry for his technical assistance in preparing the manuscript. This work was supported by grants from the NH & MRC, the Utah Foundation, and the Queensland Brain Research Fund, and by a Commonwealth Postgraduate Scholarship to A. A. Cameron.

REFERENCES

1. Bessou, P., and Perl, E. R. (1969): Responses of cutaneous sensory units with unmyelinated fibres to noxious stimuli. *J. Neurophysiol.,* 32:1025–1043.
2. Black, I. B., Kessler, J. A., Alder, J. E., and Bohn, M. C. (1982): Regulation of substance P expression and metabolism in vivo and in vitro. In: *Substance P in the Nervous System,* CIBA Foundation Symposium 91, edited by R. Porter and M. O'Connor, pp. 107–118. Pittman, London.
3. Burgess, P. R., and Perl, E. R. (1973): Cutaneous mechanoreceptors and nociceptors. In: *Handbook of Sensory Physiology—II. Somatosensory System,* edited by A. Iggo, pp. 29–78. Springer, Heidelberg.
4. Cameron, A., Leah, J., and Snow, P. (1984): Electrophysiology, morphology, and modality of feline DRG cells. *Proc. Aust. Physiol. Pharmacol. Soc.,* 15:90P.
5. Edwards, A. V. (1982): Adrenal catecholamine output in response to stimulation of the splanchnic nerve in bursts in the conscious calf. *J. Physiol. (Lond.),* 327:409–419.
6. Fitzgerald, M. (1983): Capsaicin and sensory neurones—a review. *Pain,* 25:109–130.
7. Hökfelt, T., Johansson, O., Ljungdahl, A., Lundberg, J. M., and Schultzberg, N. (1980): Peptidergic neurones. *Nature (Lond.),* 287:515–521.
8. Hökfelt, T., Skirboll, L., Lundberg, J. M., Dalsgaard, C.-J., Johansson, O., Pernow, B., and Jansco, A. (1983): Neuropeptides and pain pathways. In: *Advances in Pain Research and Therapy,* Vol. 5, edited by J. J. Bonica, U. Lindblom, and A. Iggo, pp. 227–246. Raven Press, New York.
9. McCulloch, J. (1983): Peptides and the microregulation of blood flow in the brain. *Nature,* 304:210.
10. Meyers, D. E. R., and Snow, P. J. (1981): The responses to somatic stimuli of deep spinothalamic tract cells in the lumbar spinal cord of the cat. *J. Physiol. (Lond.),* 329:355–371.
11. Rodriguez, R. E., Salt, T. E., Cahusac, P. M. B., and Hill, R. G. (1983): The behavioural effects of intrathecally administered [D-Pro2 D-Trp7,9]-substance P, an analogue with presumed antagonist actions, in the rat. *Neuropharmacology,* 22:173–176.
12. Salt, T. E., and Hill, R. G. (1983): Neurotransmitter candidates of somatosensory primary afferent fibres. *Neuroscience,* 10:1083–1103.

13. Stoppini, L., Baertschi, A. J., Mathison, R., and Barja, F. (1983): Neural actions of several substance P antagonists in the rat spinal cord. *Neurosci. Lett.,* 37:279–283.
14. Wall, P. D., and Fitzgerald, M. (1982): If substance P fails to fulfill the criteria as a neurotransmitter in somatosensory afferents, what might be its function? In: *Substance P in the Nervous System,* CIBA Foundation Symposium 91, edited by R. Porter and M. O'Connor, pp. 249–261. Pittman, London.

Advances in Pain Research and Therapy, Vol. 9, edited by H. L. Fields et al. Raven Press, New York © 1985.

Assessment of the Antinociceptive Activity of Three Substance P Antagonists

Jeffry L. Vaught and Linda J. Post

Department of Biological Research, McNeil Pharmaceutical, Spring House, Pennsylvania 19477

The undecapeptide, substance P, is localized in high concentrations in the dorsal horn of the spinal cord in thin afferent fibers associated with the transmission of noxious information (1,5). Substance P, administered intrathecally (i.t.), has been reported on several occasions to produce a transient hyperalgesia and to induce behavioral responses suggested to be characteristic of noxious stimulation (3,4). These pieces of evidence all support the suggestion that substance P has an excitatory role in neural transmission involving spinal nociceptive pathways (5).

The substance P analogs [D-Pro^{2},D-Trp^{7,9}]-substance P (DPDT), [D-Pro^{2},D-Phe^{7},D-Trp^{9}]-substance P (DPDPDT), and [D-Pro^{4},D-Trp^{7,9,10}]-substance P octapeptide (DPDT-8) have been suggested to be specific antagonists of substance P (2,9). If substance P is involved in the transmission of noxious information, then blockade of its neural transmission should result in antinociception. Thus, one would expect DPDT, DPDPDT, and DPDT-8 to be analgesic agents. To date, only a few studies have examined this hypothesis (6,7).

We now report that despite adequate blockade of central tachykinin receptors (as evidenced by inhibition of substance-P-induced behaviors), only DPDT displays antinociceptive activity. Thus, mere blockade of central tachykinin receptors does not invariably result in antinociception.

METHODS

In all experiments, male Swiss CD-1 mice (18–24 g) were used.

Dr. L. J. Post's present address is BOC Health Care Group, 100 Mt. Avenue, Murray Hill, New Jersey 07974.

Inhibition of Substance-P-Induced Scratching

Substance P (Peninsula) was injected at a dose of 10 ng i.t. (max. volume 5μl) to mice as described by Hylden and Wilcox (4). Following the injection, the mice were transferred to a clear Plexiglas chamber and observed (5 min) for the presence or absence of the characteristic substance-P-induced reciprocal hindlimb scratching response. Animals were scored as either positive (scratching behavior evident) or negative (no scratching behavior). Ten animals were used per group, and the percentage of animals scratching (of the total) was recorded. Bombesin-induced (5 ng, Peninsula) scratching was similarly evaluated. It should be noted that the vehicle (0.01-N acetic acid) produced no abnormal behavior. The SD_{50} values (the dose of agonist that caused 50% of the animals to scratch) for substance P and bombesin were 5.8 (3.9–9.6) and 2.4 (1.3–3.7) ng per mouse, respectively.

DPDT, DPDPDT, and DPDT-8 (all from Peninsula) were injected i.t. either simultaneously with substance P or bombesin or at various times prior to substance P (peptides dissolved in 0.01-N acetic acid). The percentage of animals scratching in the presence of antagonist was then compared with the percentage in a control group (Fisher's exact probability test).

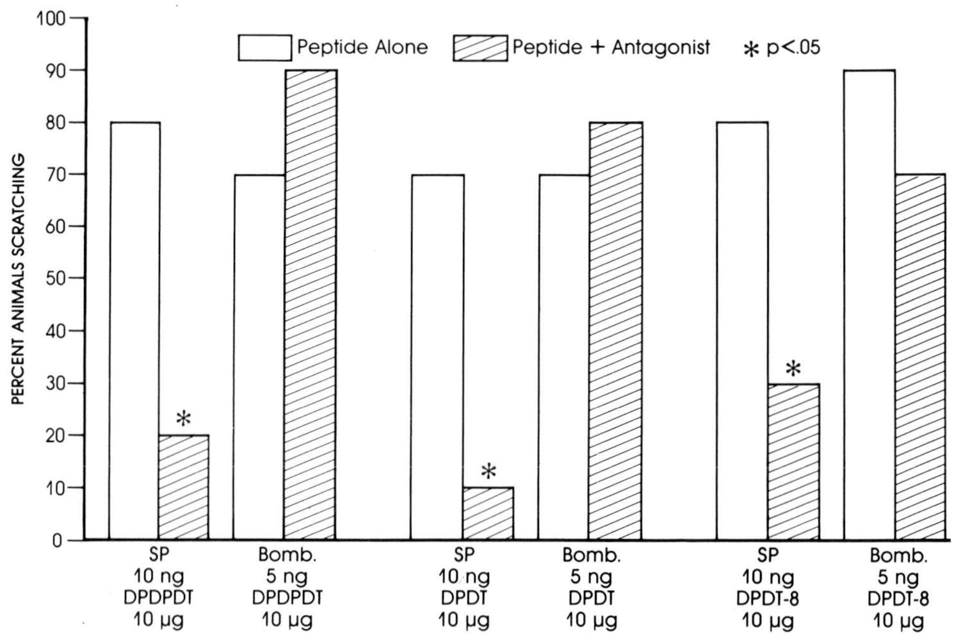

FIG. 1. Effects of substance P (SP) antagonists on SP-induced scratching. Substance P or bombesin (Bomb.) was administered by the i.t. route alone or simultaneously with antagonist. The two treatment groups were then compared by Fisher's exact probability test ($^*p < 0.05$).

Assessment of Antinociceptive Activity

The mouse tail-flick and hot-plate (48°C) assays were used to assess the antinociceptive activity of the three substance P antagonists (6,7). Drugs were injected i.t., and at 2, 5, 15, and 30 min later, the reaction times were redetermined. In each instance the criterion for an analgesic response was a drug-induced increase in reaction time greater than three standard deviations from the predrug control reaction time for all the animals in the group. Ten animals were used per dose, and a minimum of three doses was used to construct dose–response curves. A probit analysis was used to generate values for ED_{50} and 95% confidence limits.

A tail-pinch assay was also used to assess analgesic activity. An artery clamp (precalibrated to deliver 400 g pressure) was placed on the base of the tail. If an animal failed to bite at the clip within 30 sec, it was considered analgesic (vehicle-treated animals responded within 10 sec). ED_{50} and 95% confidence limits were determined as described for the tail-flick and hot-plate assays.

To eliminate analgesic bias, groups of mice given vehicle alone were included in each antinociceptive evaluation. In general, reaction times of vehicle-treated animals varied <10% from their preinjection control times.

RESULTS

Effects of DPDT, DPDPDT, and DPDT-8 on Substance-P- and Bombesin-Induced Scratching

DPDT, DPDPDT, and DPDT-8 all blocked the scratching and biting produced by substance P (but not that produced by bombesin) (Fig. 1). None of these analogs displayed any agonist-like activity following i.t. injection.

Of particular interest are the durations of action for the three antagonists. DPDT and DPDT-8 significantly blocked the behavioral syndrome elicited by substance P for more than 60 min, whereas DPDPDT had a considerably shorter duration of action (<30 min) (Fig. 2).

Analgesic Assessment of DPDT, DPDPDT, and DPDT-8

In all three analgesic tests, DPDT was found to produce a consistent antinociceptive effect (Fig. 3). In all instances it was approximately 50 times less potent than morphine. DPDT-8 was without activity in these nociceptive assays. DPDPDT, for the most part, was similarly inactive. On occasion, modest (30–40%) analgesic activity could be detected at the highest doses (10–20 μg). These effects were inconsistent and were not dose related.

DPDT-induced analgesia was quite easy to detect, usually resulting in a twofold or threefold increase in reaction times as compared with control

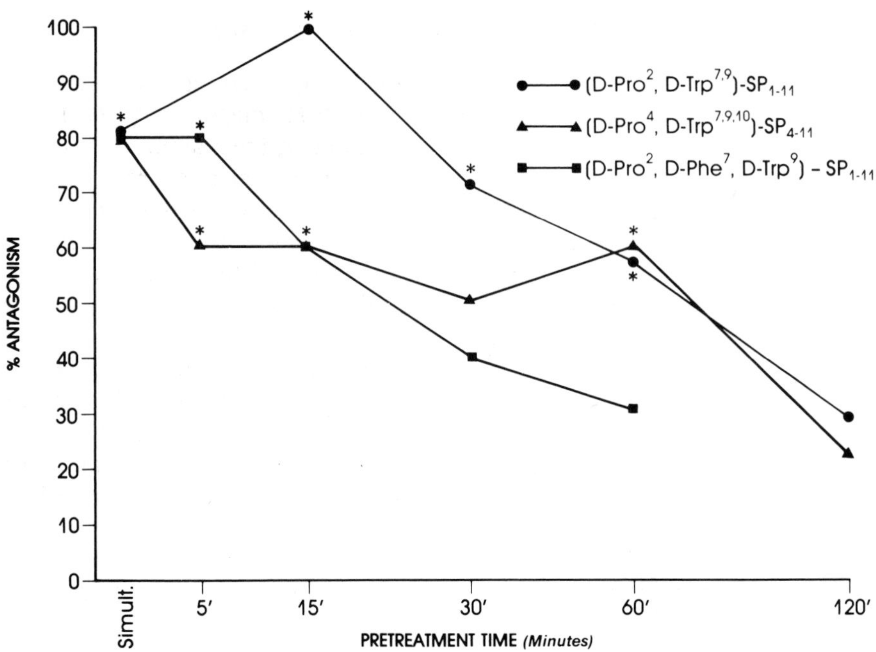

FIG. 2. Substance P antagonist (10 μg) administered i.t. simultaneously or 5, 15, 30, 60, or 120 min prior to i.t. substance P (10 ng). *Significantly different from the control group at that time ($p < 0.05$, Fisher's exact probability test).

reaction times. However, in comparison to the prolonged antagonism by DPDT of substance-P-induced behaviors, its antinociceptive activity peaked at 2 to 5 min and was absent 30 min after drug administration (Fig. 4). Naloxone (2 mg/kg i.p., 15 min prior), at a dose that completely blocked i.t. morphine-induced antinociception, had no effect on DPDT-induced antinociception (data not shown).

		DPDT	DPDPDT	DPDT-8	MORPHINE
Tail Flick	IT	6.53 μg (4.39 – 9.79) 2′***	NDR*	>20 μg	0.15 μg (.04 – .58) 5′
Hot Plate	IT	4.85 (2.62 – 7.88) 5′	NDR*	>20 μg	NT**
Haffner	IT	5.4 (3.2 – 10.8) 5′	>10 μg	NT**	0.14 (0.07 – 0.22) 5′

FIG. 3. Comparisons of analgesic responses induced by substance P antagonists and morphine: ED_{50} (95% confidence limits). *Not dose-related; **not tested; ***time of peak effect.

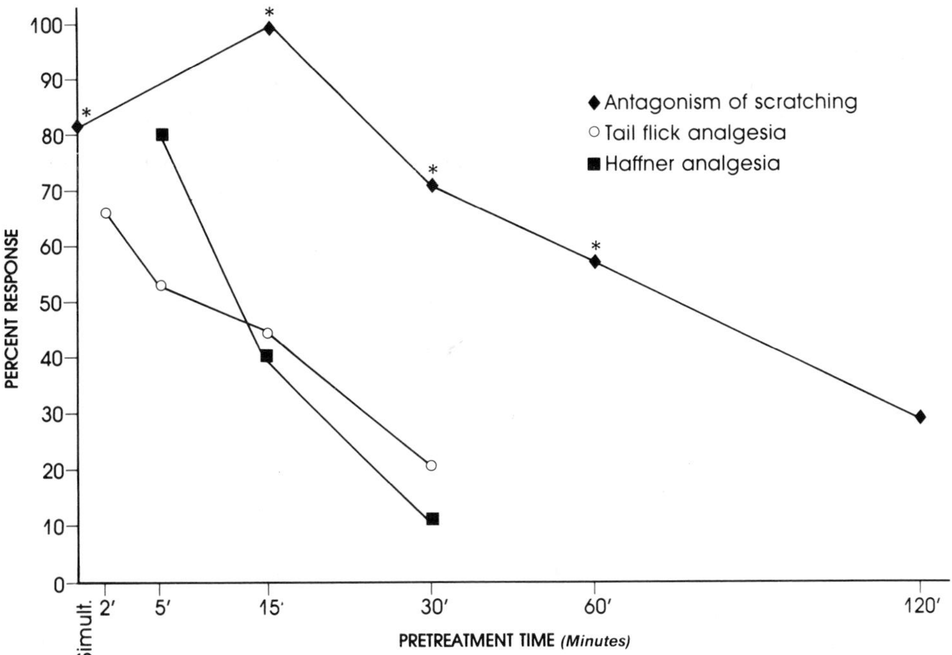

FIG. 4. DPDT (10 μg) administered i.t., simultaneously or 5, 15, 30, 60, or 120 min prior to i.t. substance P (10 ng); percentage response = percentage antagonism of scratching. *Significantly different from control group at that time ($p < 0.05$; Fisher's exact probability test). DPDT (10 μg) effects on nociception at various times post drug (percentage response = percentage analgesia).

DISCUSSION

DPDT, DPDPDT, and DPDT-8 all produced selective blockage of the scratching and biting behaviors produced by substance P. Interestingly, despite their marked potency differences *in vitro* (2,9), *in vivo* they appeared to be equipotent in the ability to block substance-P-induced scratching. Previously reported differences between the central and peripheral actions of substance P, fragments of substance P, and substance P antagonists, coupled with these observations, lend further support to the concept of differences between peripheral and central tachykinin receptors (8). The dose of antagonist required to block these substance-P-mediated behaviors is 1,000 times the dose of substance P necessary to produce them, indicating very poor antagonist efficacy.

Despite the apparent central antagonist qualities of the three agents, only DPDT displayed antinociceptive activity. The lack of activity by the other antagonists does not appear to be due to a short half-life, because all had durations of action 30 min or greater. It is of particular interest that DPDT displayed antinociceptive activity for <15 min, despite the continued presence of antagonist (as evidenced by its ability to block scratching). This is the first report of the antinociceptive evaluation of DPDT-8, and our data for DPDT and DPDPDT provide an extension of previous reports (6,7).

In summary, all three substance P antagonists were devoid of agonist-like activity when injected i.t. in mice (i.e., they produced no scratching behavior) and selectively blocked substance-P-induced scratching (i.e., no block of bombesin-induced scratching). All three substance P antagonists produced prolonged antagonism of scratching, indicating resistance to degradation. However, only DPDT displayed antinociceptive activity. Thus, mere blockade of a central tachykinin receptor by a substance P antagonist (as evidenced by inhibition of scratching) does not invariably result in antinociceptive activity.

ACKNOWLEDGMENT

The authors wish to express their appreciation to Mrs. Cathy Braun for her careful preparation of this manuscript.

REFERENCES

1. Barber, R. P., Vaughn, J. E., Siemmon, J. R., Salvaterra, P. M., Roberts, E., and Leeman, S. E. (1979): The origin, distribution and synaptic relationships of substance P in the rat spinal cord. *J. Comp. Neurol.,* 84:331–351.
2. Bjorkroth, U., Rosell, S., Xu, J. C., and Folkers, K. (1982): Pharmacological characterization of four related substance P antagonists. *Acta Physiol. Scand.,* 116:167–173.
3. Hayes, A. G., and Tyers, M. B. (1979): Effects of intrathecal and intracerebroventricular injections of substance P on nociception in the rat and mouse. *Br. J. Pharmacol.,* 66:488–493.
4. Hylden, J. L. K., and Wilcox, G. L. (1981): Intrathecal substance P elicits caudally-directed biting and scratching behavior in mice. *Brain Res.,* 217:2169–2178.
5. Leeman, S. E., and Mroz, E. A. (1980): Minireview: Substance P. *Life Sci.,* 15:2033–2044.
6. Lembeck, F., Folkers, K., and Donnerer, J. (1981): Analgesic effect of antagonists of substance P. *Biochem. Biophys. Res. Commun.,* 103:1318–1321.
7. Piercey, M. F., Schroeder, L. A., Folkers K., Xu, J. C., and Horig, J. (1981): Sensory and motor functions of spinal cord substance P. *Science,* 214:1361–1363.
8. Post, L. J., and Vaught, J. L. (1983): Substance P antagonists: Analgesia and inhibition of SP-induced scratching. *Pharmacologist,* 25:183.
9. Regoli, D., Escher, E., Drapeau, G., D'Orleans-Juste, P., and Mizrahi, J. (1984): Receptors for substance P. III. Classification by competitive antagonists. *Eur. J. Pharmacol.,* 97:179–189.

Advances in Pain Research and Therapy, Vol. 9, edited by H. L. Fields et al. Raven Press, New York © 1985.

Peripheral Neural Mechanisms of Cutaneous Hyperalgesia

*†Richard A. Meyer, †James N. Campbell, and **Srinivasa N. Raja

**Applied Physics Laboratory, †Departments of Neurosurgery, and **Anesthesiology and Critical Care Medicine, The Johns Hopkins University, Baltimore, Maryland 21205*

Cutaneous hyperalgesia is the perceptual companion of cutaneous injury, inflammation, certain nerve injuries, and certain neuropathies. It is characterized by one or more of the following symptoms: (a) a decrease in the threshold for eliciting pain; (b) enhanced pain produced by suprathreshold stimuli; (c) spontaneous pain. Two of the forerunners of modern research in pain, Lewis (34) and Hardy (25), dedicated much effort to understanding the basis of hyperalgesia. Research in recent years has served to extend and to some extent modify the conclusions of these authors. In this chapter, this recent work will be reviewed, with particular emphasis on peripheral neural mechanisms.

Experimental investigations of the neural mechanism of hyperalgesia have focused on changes in sensation and neural response following injury to the skin. Various types of skin injury lead to hyperalgesia, including freezing, cutting, and crushing the skin, as well as the commonly experienced ultraviolet irradiation of the skin (i.e., sunburn). In this review we shall focus on the most frequently studied injury: the burn resulting from exposure to intense heat.

Two distinct types of cutaneous hyperalgesia have been identified and will be discussed separately. They are characterized by different changes in sensation and are thought to be coded by different neural mechanisms. *Primary hyperalgesia* refers to changes that occur within the site of injury, whereas *secondary hyperalgesia* refers to changes that occur outside the site of injury.

PAIN AND NORMAL SKIN

Before considering the mechanisms of hyperalgesia, it will be useful to review peripheral neural mechanisms of pain sensation in the normal state. Studies in humans, monkeys, and other species have shown that there exist specialized classes of myelinated (A fiber) and unmyelinated (C fiber) afferents in the peripheral nerves, termed nociceptors, that encode the occurrence, intensity, duration, and location of noxious and near-noxious stimuli (1,3–5,7,9–11,13,16–21,23,27–31,37,39–42,44,50,51,53–57). This in itself provides a convincing basis for assuming that nociceptor activity signals pain sensation. It is apparent, however, that there are different types of nociceptors and that the contributions of each need to be considered separately.

Nociceptors have been classified by three criteria: (a) conduction velocity (i.e., A fiber versus C fiber); (b) modalities to which nociceptors respond; and (c) differences in the characteristics of the responses to stimuli. Although nociceptors responding only to noxious heat or mechanical stimuli have been described, the majority appear to respond to both modalities (21). In this review, A-fiber nociceptors sensitive to intense mechanical and heat stimuli are called *AMHs,* and C-fiber nociceptors sensitive to both stimuli are called *CMHs.* Many, if not most, of these nociceptors respond to noxious chemical irritants and thus may be considered to be polymodal (5). A separate subdivision also responds to intense cooling (29). In most quantitative studies, heat stimuli have been used, so that comparatively little is known about responses to other stimuli. Finally, nociceptors may be classified in terms of the characteristics of their responses to stimuli. For example, CMHs have been shown to display either a quickly adapting or a slowly adapting response to step heat stimuli (39). Whether this distinction correlates with responses to other modes of stimulation (e.g., mechanical stimuli) remains to be determined. As will be described in detail below, AMHs also can be subclassified by their responses to heat.

A large amount of evidence indicates that nociceptors code for pain from heat stimuli. For the uninjured glabrous skin of the hand, only two receptor types respond to heat up to 49°C: CMHs and "warm" fibers. The heat threshold for AMHs on glabrous skin is typically above 49°C (11). A correlation of responses to heat by CMHs and warm fibers with responses of humans given similar stimuli indicates that the CMHs, not the warm fibers, code for the pain (28). The threshold of the CMHs and the pain threshold in humans are similar (about 43°C), and responses to suprathreshold heat stimuli increase in each case monotonically with stimulus intensity. In contrast, warm fibers are exquisitely sensitive to gentle warming of the skin (14), and the response of warm fibers to stimuli greater than 43°C does not increase monotonically (28). Warm fibers are well suited to code exclusively for the sensation of warmth (14,15,26).

The technique of magnitude estimation in psychophysical studies allows direct comparisons with neurophysiological studies. Because the responses in each case can be analyzed in terms of a ratio scale, normalized stimulus–response functions can be constructed for comparison. This was done for a sample of CMHs and human subjects; they were each given a randomized series of 10 stimuli for 3 sec at 41°C to 49°C. The first stimulus in each stimulus sequence was 45°C, the response to which served as the denominator for normalizing subsequent responses. As shown in Fig. 1, there is a remarkable correspondence between the two stimulus–response functions.

Additional evidence to support the role of CMHs in coding for pain in uninjured skin includes the following observations: (a) Selective A-fiber ischemic blocks or C-fiber (local anesthetic) blocks indicate that C-fiber function is sufficient for thermal pain perception near the pain threshold (41,47,52). (b) Stimulus interaction effects observed in psychophysical experiments are also observed in recordings from CMHs (28). (c) The latency to pain sensation on glabrous skin following step temperature

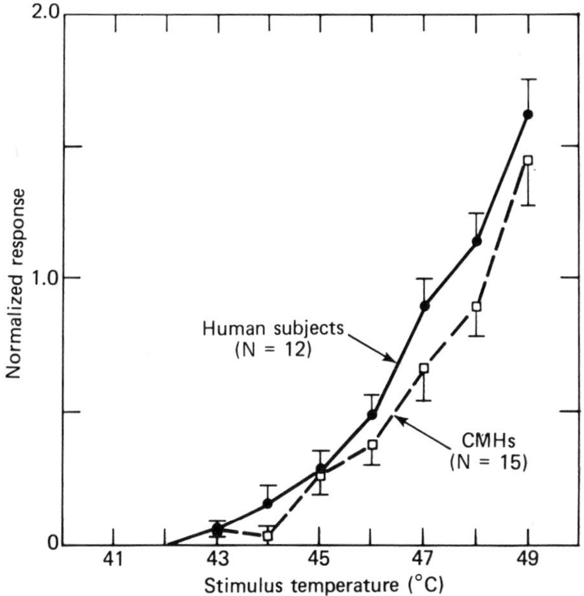

FIG. 1. Normalized responses of human subjects and CMHs exposed to identical heat stimuli on glabrous skin. The close match between the curves supports a role of CMHs in pain sensation. The skin was not previously stimulated with heat. A laser thermal stimulator was used to apply noncontact constant-temperature stimuli (43). The first stimulus of the heat sequence was always 45°C. The remaining nine stimuli ranged from 41°C to 49°C in 1°C increments and were presented in random order. The stimuli were 3 sec in duration and were presented every 30 sec. A base temperature of 38°C was applied 1 min before the first stimulus and between stimuli. Human judgments of pain were measured with the magnitude-estimation technique (48): Subjects assigned an arbitrary number (the modulus) to the magnitude of pain evoked by the first 45°C stimulus of the first run and judged the painfulness of all subsequent stimuli relative to this modulus. Standard techniques (9) were used to record from single fibers of the median and ulnar nerves of monkeys anesthetized with pentobarbital. The response to a given stimulus was normalized by dividing by the modulus for each human subject or by the average response to the first 45°C stimulus of the first run for the CMHs. The response to the first 45°C stimulus of each run is not included in this figure or in Figs. 3 and 6, which also use this stimulus paradigm. (From Meyer and Campbell, ref. 40, with permission.)

changes is long enough that C fibers could be responsible (8). (d) Intraneural electrical stimulation of presumed single identified CMHs in humans elicits pain (56). (e) The heat threshold for activating CMHs recorded for awake humans is usually just below the pain threshold (23,57). (f) A linear relationship exists between responses of CMHs recorded in awake humans and ratings of pain over the temperature range 39°C to 51°C (55).

AMHs also contribute to heat pain. There appear to be two distinct classes of AMHs (Table 1) that we call type I and type II (10,18). Type I AMHs have a high threshold to heat stimuli—generally greater than 49°C. They are found on both glabrous and hairy skin. Some investigators call these receptors high-threshold mechanoreceptors (HTMs) in deference to their high threshold to heat (16). Type II AMHs have not been reported in the glabrous skin of the hand. On hairy skin, type II AMHs are found less frequently than type I AMHs and have a sensitivity to heat (18) that is similar to that for CMHs (threshold near 43°C). Several examples of the responses of type I and type II AMHs to a 53°C 30-sec stimulus are shown in Fig. 2. The type I AMHs have a long receptor utilization time (time between stimulus onset and initiation of action-potential activity), and the response lasts throughout the 30-sec stimulus. In contrast, type II AMHs have a short receptor utilization time and display a quickly adapting response.

One of the roles of type I AMHs is apparent from comparison of human ratings for a sustained high-intensity heat stimulus with responses of type I AMHs and CMHs (41). As shown in Fig. 3, a 53°C 30-sec stimulus applied to the glabrous skin of the hand evoked a sustained high level of pain. The CMHs responded vigorously only in the initial few seconds of this stimulus, whereas the type I AMHs responded vigorously beginning several seconds into the stimulus. It is likely, therefore, that type I AMHs play an important role in signaling the sustained pain during such a stimulus.

Stepped increments of skin temperature up to 51°C, when applied to the hairy (i.e., nonglabrous) portion of the hand and forearm, evoke a double

TABLE 1. *Comparison of type I and type II AMHs*

Characteristic	Type I AMH	Type II AMH
Skin type	Glabrous and hairy	Hairy only
Receptor utilization time (to heat)	Long (>500 msec)	Short (<200 msec)
Heat-response characteristic	Slowly adapting[a]	Quickly adapting[c]
Median heat threshold	>49°C[a]	43°C[b]
Median mechanical threshold	1.3 g[b]	0.4 g [b]
Median conduction velocity	31.1 m/sec[a]	15.2 m/sec[b]

[a]From Campbell et al. (11).
[b]From Dubner et al. (18).
[c]From Campbell and Meyer (10).

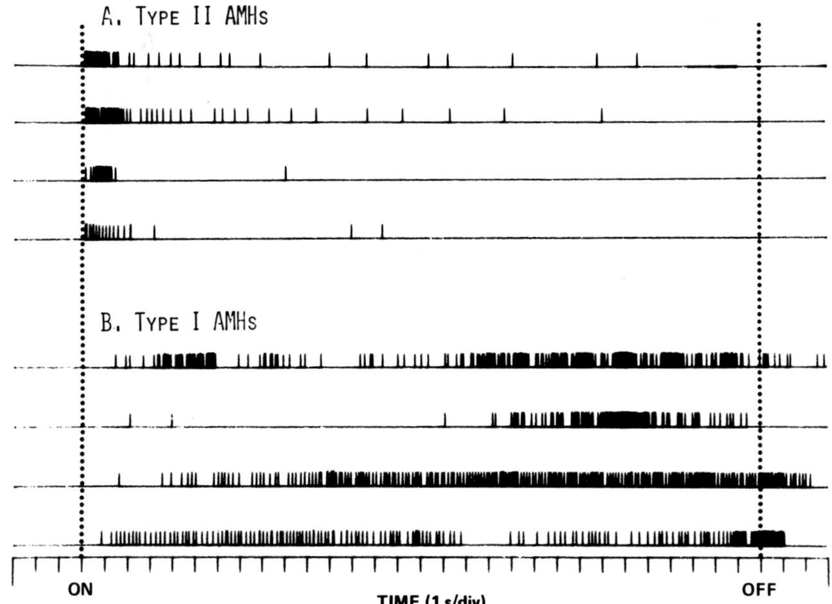

FIG. 2. Responses to a 53°C 30-sec stimulus of four type I and type II AMHs. **A:** Type II AMHs have a short receptor utilization time and show a quickly adapting response to a stepped temperature stimulus. **B:** Type I AMHs have a long receptor utilization time and respond throughout the stimulus. Each horizontal line corresponds to a different fiber, and each vertical tick corresponds to an action potential.

pain sensation (35). Latency measurements of the first pain sensation in human subjects indicate that the responsible afferents must have conduction velocities greater than 6 m/sec and thus must be A fibers (8). The low heat threshold, short utilization time, and burst response to heat of type II AMHs (Fig. 2) make them ideal candidates for subserving first pain sensation (10,18). Notably, the first-pain/second-pain sequence in humans has not been observed when stimuli up to 51°C are presented to the glabrous skin of the hand, which is in keeping with the failure to find type II AMHs in the glabrous skin of the monkey hand.

Whereas the pain threshold of humans and the response threshold of CMHs to heat stimuli are similar, this is not the case for mechanical stimuli. The mechanical threshold for the nociceptors (28) is 6.0 ± 0.6 bars for CMHs (mean ± SEM) and 3.5 ± 0.3 bars for type I AMHs (11), but the mechanical threshold for pain on glabrous skin (45) is 12.0 ± 1.1 bars (1 bar = 10^6 dynes/cm^2). In single-nerve recordings obtained from awake humans, mechanically evoked C-fiber discharges even up to 10 spikes/sec were not accompanied by pain sensation, but a much lower discharge (less than 2 spikes/sec) evoked by heat did result in strong pain (57). One possibility is that the punctate mechanical stimulus evokes a discharge in fewer

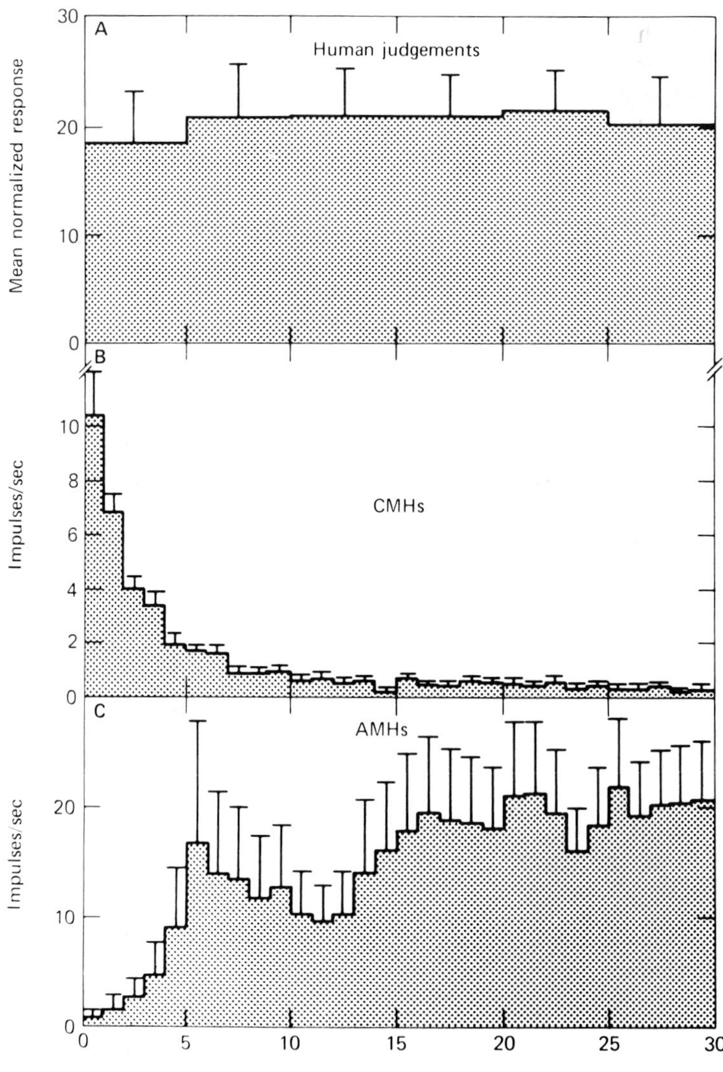

FIG. 3. Pain ratings of human subjects during a 53°C 30-sec heat stimulus to the glabrous hand are compared with responses of CMHs and type I AMHs. **A:** Pain was intense throughout the stimulus ($N = 8$). **B:** The brisk response of the CMHs at the beginning of the stimulus changed to a low rate of discharge after 5 sec ($N = 15$). **C:** The responses of the AMHs increased during the first 5 sec and remained high throughout the stimulus ($N = 14$). (From Meyer and Campbell, ref. 41, with permission. Copyright 1981 by the AAAS.)

nociceptors than does the broader heat stimulus. As with warmth, spatial summation could be an important coding mechanism for pain intensity (22). Another possible explanation for this discrepancy is that mechanical stimulation also activates low-threshold mechanoreceptors that have an inhibitory influence in the central nervous system on the nociceptive input. This hypothesis is supported by the observation that pain induced by intraneural electrical stimulation at C-fiber strength can be substantially reduced by vibration of the skin within the area of projected pain (6). As will be discussed later, a decrease in this inhibitory influence following an injury might account for secondary hyperalgesia.

CHARACTERISTICS OF PRIMARY HYPERALGESIA

To characterize quantitatively the hyperalgesia that arises at the site of an injury, the responses of human volunteers to mechanical and heat stimuli were determined before and after a burn to the glabrous skin of the hand (41,45). The burn consisted of a 53°C 30-sec stimulus over a 7.5-mm-diameter spot, which resulted in a blister after several hours in approximately 50% of subjects. This burn led to prominent primary hyperalgesia within minutes. The base temperature (38°C) evoked pain, indicating that the pain threshold decreased markedly. In addition, the response to suprathreshold stimuli increased dramatically (Fig. 4A). For example, the 41°C stimulus was not painful before the burn, but the painfulness of this stimulus after the burn was at least as great as that of the 49°C stimulus before the burn. The threshold for mechanically induced pain, as tested by von Frey probes, decreased from 12.6 ± 1.9 bars before the burn to 5.4 ± 0.5 bars after the burn (45). Thus, primary hyperalgesia following a burn to the glabrous skin is characterized by augmented pain from both mechanical and heat stimuli.

As indicated in Fig. 5A, the characteristics of primary hyperalgesia following a burn to the hairy skin are not the same as for the glabrous skin. Whereas a marked decrease in pain threshold is still observed, the response to suprathreshold heat stimuli (e.g., 49°C) after a 50°C 100-sec injury to hairy skin is not greatly different from the response before the burn (30). Similar characteristics of primary hyperalgesia following a 53°C 30-sec heat injury to hairy skin have also been observed (R. A. Meyer and J. N. Campbell, *unpublished observations*).

PERIPHERAL NEURAL MECHANISMS OF PRIMARY HYPERALGESIA

To determine whether CMHs or type I AMHs account for the primary hyperalgesia following a burn to the glabrous skin, the responses to heat stimuli of CMHs and AMHs innervating glabrous skin were determined before and after a burn using the same protocol as described in Fig. 4A for

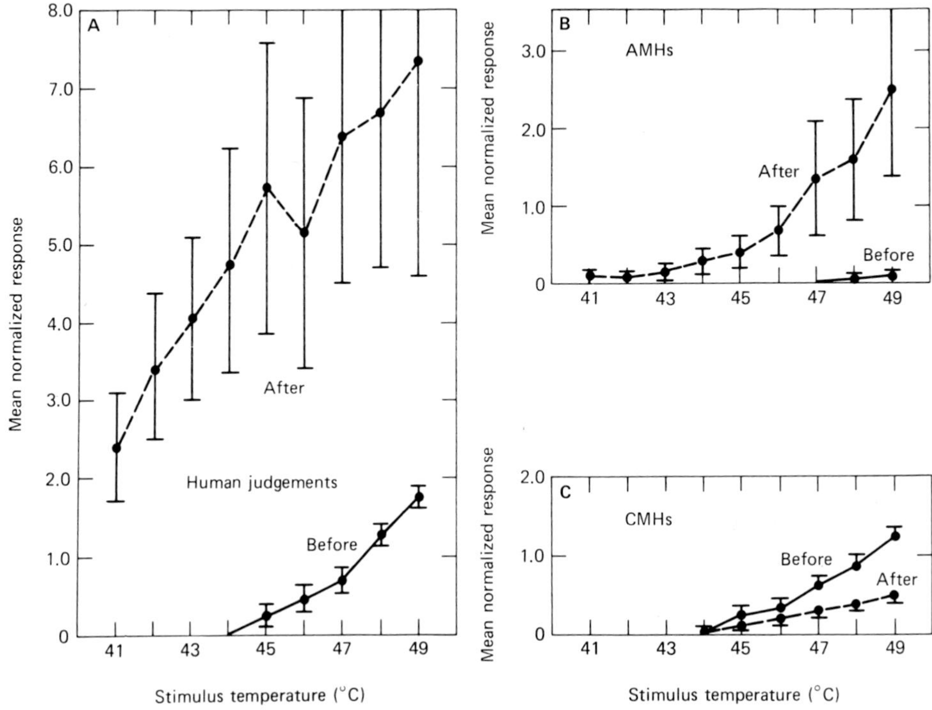

FIG. 4. Normalized responses to heat sequence (described in Fig. 1) 5 min before and 10 min after a 53°C 30-sec burn to the glabrous skin of the hand. The burn resulted in increases in the magnitude of pain (hyperalgesia) in human subjects that were matched by enhanced responses (sensitization) in the type I AMHs. In contrast, the burn resulted in decreased sensitivity in the CMHs. **A:** Human judgments (N = 8). **B:** A-fiber nociceptive afferents (type I AMHs) in monkeys (N = 14). Because the AMHs did not respond to the 45°C stimulus before the burn, the data were normalized by dividing by the response to the first 45°C stimulus after the burn. **C:** C-fiber nociceptive afferents (CMHs) in monkeys (N = 15). Standard-error bars are shown. (From Meyer and Campbell, ref. 41, with permission. Copyright 1981 by the AAAS.)

the psychophysical studies (41). As shown in Fig. 4B, the threshold for type I AMH response to heat was greatly decreased after the burn, and the response to suprathreshold stimuli was increased. Similar sensitization of AMHs by heat has been reported by others (11,18,20). In contrast, the CMHs showed an increased heat threshold and a decreased response to suprathreshold stimuli following the burn (Fig. 4C). Similar hyperalgesia in human subjects and lack of sensitization of CMHs in monkeys were observed by LaMotte et al. (30) following at 50°C 100-sec burn to glabrous skin.

As an alternate means to determine if A fibers or C fibers are responsible for the hyperalgesia to heat stimuli following a glabrous skin burn, a pressure cuff inflated to a level above systolic pressure was placed on the upper

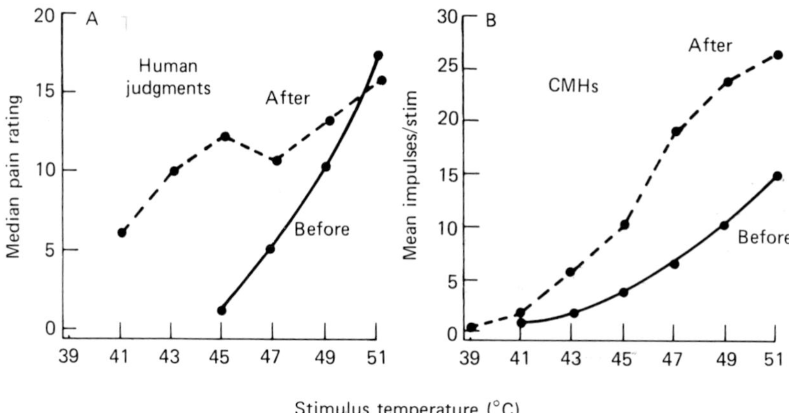

FIG. 5. Responses to heat stimuli immediately before and 10 min after a 50°C 100-sec burn to the hairy skin of the forearm. The burn resulted in a decrease in the pain threshold and an increase in the painfulness to mild heat stimuli (e.g., 43°C), but a decrease in painfulness to intense heat stimuli (e.g., 51°C). In contrast, the burn resulted in enhanced responses of the CMHs at all temperatures. The heat test consisted of an ascending sequence of seven stimuli ranging from 39°C to 51°C in 2°C increments. The stimuli were 5 sec in duration and were presented every 30 sec. **A:** Median maximum pain rating for 13 human subjects. **B:** Mean total number of impulses per stimulus in 12 CMHs recorded from anesthetized monkey. (Adapted from LaMotte et al., ref. 30.)

arm after the burn to obtain an A-fiber block (41). Motor function and sensitivity to light touching and coolness were gone 40 min after inflation of the cuff, indicating that the action-potential activity in A fibers was at least partially blocked. Hyperalgesia to heat stimuli at the injury site was markedly decreased, although the pain evoked by the heat stimuli applied to uninjured skin 5 cm from the burn was not reduced, indicating intact C-fiber function. These results support the hypothesis that A fibers play an important role in signaling the hyperalgesia to heat that follows a burn to the glabrous skin.

It might be expected that sensitization of nociceptors to heat stimuli following injury of their receptive fields must be accompanied by sensitization to mechanical stimuli. However, the threshold for response to mechanical stimuli of CMHs and AMHs appears not to be altered reliably by a heat injury (11,20,50,51). Although injury can lead to sensitization to mechanical stimuli of a proportion of CMHs (5,37), others become desensitized, and the net change for the whole population is small (37). The effects of injury on the responses to suprathreshold mechanical stimuli have not been tested quantitatively.

These results indicate that AMHs, not CMHs, account for the dramatic hyperalgesia to heat stimuli following a burn to the glabrous skin. However, it may well be that the hyperalgesia to mechanical stimuli is not mediated by sensitization of nociceptors.

The failure to find sensitization of CMHs after heat injury to the glabrous skin caused confusion concerning the role of CMHs in view of previous observations that CMHs may, in certain instances, sensitize to heat (4,5,12,19,27,30,31,37,44,50,51,54,55). This confusion seems to have been resolved by the finding that sensitization of CMHs in monkeys varies with skin type (9). The CMHs that innervate hairy skin sensitize readily, whereas those that innervate the glabrous skin of the hand will not sensitize regardless of the heat stimuli used. The fact that CMHs that innervate hairy skin sensitize lends support to the possibility that CMHs might play a role in primary hyperalgesia in hairy skin. The responses of CMHs on hairy skin before and after a burn are shown in Fig. 5B (30). The CMHs become sensitized following the burn and show a decreased threshold and an increased response to suprathreshold stimuli. The decreased threshold in the CMHs correlates with the decreased pain threshold in human subjects (31). However, the increased responses at the higher temperatures (e.g., 49°C) did not correlate with the unchanged painfulness in humans at these temperatures (Fig. 5A). This apparent discrepancy between the sensitization of monkey CMHs on hairy skin and the hyperalgesia in humans may be due to species differences. For example, only 1 of 8 CMHs on hairy skin recorded from awake humans became notably sensitized after a 50°C 100-sec injury (55). Another possibility is that the anesthetic state of the monkey alters the sensitization properties of the CMHs. For example, halothane, a general anesthetic, increases the response to heat of CMHs and AMHs in a dose-dependent manner (12). It should be noted that type I AMHs (11) and type II AMHs (18; R. A. Meyer and J. N. Campbell, *unpublished observations*) on hairy skin also become sensitized by intense heat stimuli. The role of type II AMHs in hyperalgesia on hairy skin has not been studied. It appears that the relative roles of CMHs and type I AMHs may be dictated by the intensity of the injury (31).

CHARACTERISTICS OF SECONDARY HYPERALGESIA

Whereas there is general agreement regarding the characteristics of primary hyperalgesia described earlier, disagreement exists concerning the characteristics of secondary hyperalgesia (24,25,32–34). Hyperalgesia to heat stimuli was not found by Lewis, whereas Hardy observed increased pain from suprathreshold heat stimuli without a change in pain threshold. With regard to mechanical stimuli, Lewis reported a lower threshold and increased pain from suprathreshold stimuli, whereas Hardy reported only increased pain from suprathreshold mechanical stimuli, without a decrease in threshold. Some of these differences can be attributed to different experimental designs, artifacts of the experimental technique, and semantics (e.g., definition of threshold).

In the psychophysical studies described in Fig. 4, light brushing of the skin caused burning pain when applied to an area next to a burn, indicating an obvious decrease in the pain threshold. However, pain in response to heat stimuli to the same area was not enhanced. Postulating that the injury was perhaps insufficient to bring out hyperalgesia to heat in the secondary area, the paradigm illustrated in Fig. 6A was adopted (45). Burns consisting of 53°C for 30 sec were applied to two locations (spots A and D), leaving enough room between the stimuli to do psychophysical testing on uninjured skin (spot B). Within minutes the skin became tender to touch (mechanical hyperalgesia). When a nylon monofilament probe was dragged across the skin, there was a clear point of demarcation between normal skin and hyperalgesic skin. Light brushing of the skin never evoked pain prior to injury, but consistently did so after injury in both the primary and secondary hyperalgesia areas. Pain thresholds, measured at sites A, B, and C using von Frey hairs, decreased after the burn (Fig. 6B). Notably, the decreases were similar within and outside the area of injury; i.e., the mechanical hyperalgesia was uniform in the primary and secondary hyperalgesia areas. The zone of mechanical hyperalgesia and the maximum area of flare evident to visual inspection are shown in Fig. 6A for a typical subject. In all subjects, the area of mechanical hyperalgesia (20.1 ± 3.6 cm^2) was larger than the area of flare (8.3 ± 0.8 cm^2).

The responses to heat stimuli at sites A, B, and C were also tested (Fig. 6C–E). Marked hyperalgesia to heat (thermal hyperalgesia) was observed at site A, the injury site, where ratings of pain increased more than fourfold (Fig. 6C). Between the two burns, the painfulness of the heat stimuli actually decreased by 50% (Fig. 6D). At site C, the ratings of pain from heat were comparable to those before injury (Fig. 6E). Thus, at both sites B and C, thermal hyperalgesia did not occur, despite the observation that there was concurrent mechanical hyperalgesia. Of note, site B was *hypalgesic* to heat, while being hyperalgesic to mechanical stimuli.

The conclusion seems inescapable that the characteristics of secondary hyperalgesia and primary hyperalgesia differ. In the primary region there is hyperalgesia to both mechanical and heat stimuli, whereas in the secondary region there is hyperalgesia to only mechanical stimuli. Because the mechanical hyperalgesias observed in the primary and secondary regions are similar (Fig. 6B), we speculate that the neural mechanism is the same. Therefore, it might be more appropriate in the future to discuss hyperalgesia in terms of the modality (heat versus mechanical) rather than in terms of the site (primary versus secondary).

NEUROPHYSIOLOGICAL BASIS FOR SECONDARY HYPERALGESIA

Lewis (34) proposed that secondary hyperalgesia was due to spread of sensitization to adjoining pain receptors by way of the nocifensor system. The

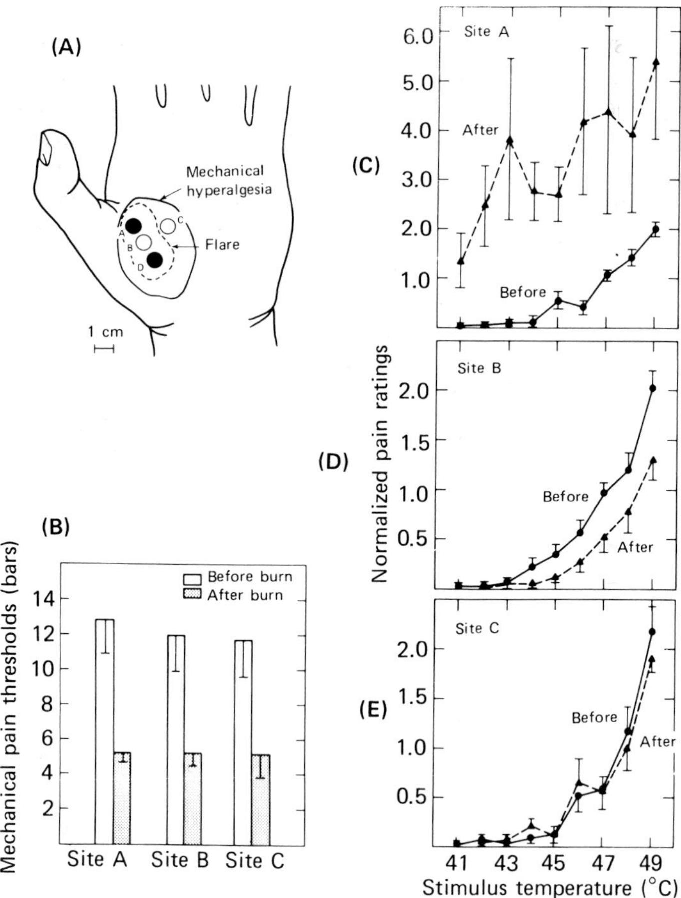

FIG. 6. Measurements of mechanical and heat sensitivities in the areas of primary and secondary hyperalgesia following burns to the glabrous skin of the hand. Hyperalgesia to mechanical stimuli was observed in both areas. Hyperalgesia to heat stimuli was observed only in the primary area. **A:** Mechanical thresholds for pain and ratings of pain to heat stimuli were recorded at sites A, B, and C before and after burns at sites A and D. The burns consisted of a 53°C 30-sec stimulus at both sites. The areas of flare and mechanical hyperalgesia following the burns in one subject are also shown. In all subjects, the area of mechanical hyperalgesia was larger than the area of flare. Mechanical hyperalgesia was present even after the flare disappeared. **B:** Mean mechanical thresholds for pain before and after burns are shown for 7 subjects. The mechanical threshold for pain was significantly decreased following the burn. The mechanical hyperalgesias were of similar magnitude at each of the three test spots (A, B, C). Error bars correspond to SEM. **C–E:** Mean normalized ratings of painfulness of heat stimuli (same as described in Fig. 1) before and after burns are shown. **C:** At site A, all the characteristics of thermal hyperalgesia (i.e., decrease in pain threshold, increased pain to suprathreshold stimuli, and spontaneous pain) were observed after the burns ($N = 8$). **D:** At site B, pain ratings decreased after the burns. Thus, thermal hyperalgesia was observed ($N = 9$). **E:** At site C, pain ratings before and after the burns were not significantly different ($N = 8$). (From Raja et al., ref. 45, with permission.)

nocifensor system was viewed to be independent of sensory afferents and autonomic nerve fibers. Activation of nociceptors triggered a response reflexively (the axon reflex) in the nocifensor system that branched into adjoining tissue. Activation of these nocifensor branches led to release from their terminals of substances that in turn sensitized and activated the nociceptors that innervated the adjoining area, thus leading to secondary hyperalgesia. A key observation in the formulation of Lewis was that electrical stimulation of a nerve trunk led to hyperalgesia to mechanical stimuli in the distribution of that nerve, even if the proximal end of the nerve was blocked with a local anesthetic during the stimulation period (34). In contrast, Hardy reported that antidromic nerve stimulation led to *hypalgesia* in the distribution of the nerve and hyperalgesia only to the skin that was directly stimulated and presumably injured (24,25). Hardy postulated that changes accounting for secondary hyperalgesia occurred in the dorsal horn of the spinal cord.

Fitzgerald (19) reported that antidromic nerve stimulation of a population of 10 CMHs on hairy skin of rabbits resulted in heat thresholds that were significantly lower than those of CMHs in a control population. She did not report the effects of antidromic stimulation on mechanical sensitivity of nociceptors. In preliminary experiments we measured the responses to heat stimuli of CMHs and AMHs on the hairy skin of monkeys before and after electrical nerve stimulation (R. A. Meyer and J. N. Campbell, *unpublished observations*). The test heat stimuli (1-sec duration, ranging from 39°C to 49°C) were chosen such that they did not in themselves result in sensitization (9). The electrical stimulus was of low frequency (2–10 Hz for 5 min) and of sufficient intensity to excite C fibers (i.e., sufficient to cause gooseflesh in the distribution of the nerve). There was no decrease in threshold and no increase in response to suprathreshold heat stimuli when the stimulating electrode was proximal to the recording electrode. A transient *increase* in threshold and *decrease* in suprathreshold response (i.e., suppression) occurred when the stimulating electrode was distal to the recording electrode. Other than the differences among species and our within-fiber control, we cannot account for the discrepancy between these results and those of Fitzgerald (19). In future experiments we plan to determine if antidromic electrical stimulation alters the responses of CMHs and AMHs to mechanical stimuli, because psychophysical studies suggest that hyperalgesia to mechanical, but not heat, stimuli occurs (34).

To determine if an injury to half of the receptive field of a nociceptor might lead to spread of sensitization to the other half, Thalhammer and LaMotte (50,51) applied a 56°C 7-sec burn to half the receptive fields of AMHs and CMHs located on hairy skin (Fig. 7). Sensitization to heat was observed only in the receptive-field half that was burned, not in the other half. No significant changes in mechanical threshold were observed in either half, though a slight enlargement of the receptive field within the area of

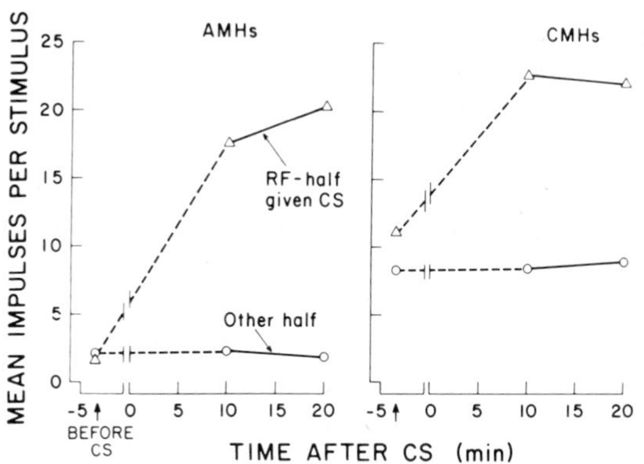

FIG. 7. Mean responses of 7 type I AMHs and 4 CMHs innervating hairy skin to a 51°C 5-sec stimulus before and after a conditioning stimulus (CS), which was a 56°C 7-sec stimulus applied to half of the receptive field. Sensitization was observed only for the receptive-field half directly exposed to the conditioning stimulus *(triangles)*, not for the other half *(circles)*. No significant change in mechanical sensitivity was observed. (From Thalhammer and LaMotte, ref. 51, with permission.)

injury was sometimes observed (50). Similar results were obtained with a more substantial injury: a 53°C 30-sec burn (J. N. Campbell and R. A. Meyer, *unpublished observations*). In preliminary experiments we found that the responses to heat of CMHs before and after a scalpel cut surrounding three sides of its receptive field (no cut on proximal side) did not differ. Scalpel cuts on the volar forearm of human subjects resulted in hyperalgesia to heat stimuli within but not adjacent to the area of injury (J. N. Campbell, R. A. Meyer, and S. N. Raja, *unpublished observations*). In contrast, Fitzgerald (19) reported that the population of CMHs that had a cut beside their receptive field before heat testing had lower heat thresholds than the control population. Fitzgerald did not report the effects of the cut on mechanical sensitivity.

Hyperalgesia to mechanical stimuli occurring within or adjacent to an injury does not appear to be mediated by changes in response of nociceptive afferents. It is of interest to note that the mechanical pain threshold in the region of secondary hyperalgesia (5.2 ± 0.5 bars) (Fig. 6B) is similar to the threshold for activating nociceptors before injury: 6.0 ± 0.6 bars for CMHs (28) and 3.5 ± 0.3 bars for type II AMHs (11). Thus, sensitization of nociceptors to mechanical stimuli is not necessary to explain mechanical hyperalgesia. Instead, a decrease in central inhibition of the mechanically induced nociceptive input could account for the secondary hyperalgesia. Indeed, Woolf (59) has reported evidence for increased excitability of spinal cord neurons to C-fiber input following a severe injury (75°C for 60 sec) to the rat foot. Another possible central mechanism that could account for the mechanical hyperalgesia is that signals in low-threshold mechanoreceptors may, after injury, excite central nociceptive neurons.

Secondary hyperalgesia and the flare response or reddening that surrounds an area of injury have been linked since Lewis's original description of these responses (32–34). The flare is part of the axon reflex and has been thought to result from antidromic invasion of axon branches following nociceptor activation. Although free nerve endings have been observed in the dermis and around capillaries, no axonal connection between these endings has been described. Recent neurophysiological evidence that coupling of action-potential activity occurs between unmyelinated fibers in the skin may provide a basis for the flare response (42). It has been suggested that the substances that induce the flare also sensitize nociceptors, thus leading to hyperalgesia. However, there is evidence against this hypothesis. Most important, certain agents such as histamine dihydrochloride, when injected intradermally, elicit flare, with little or no pain or hyperalgesia (2). Also, as noted earlier, the area of the flare following a burn is significantly less than that in mechanical hyperalgesia. Additionally, the flare may last only several minutes, whereas secondary hyperalgesia may last beyond several hours.

CUTANEOUS HYPERALGESIA FOLLOWING PERIPHERAL NERVE INJURY

Peripheral nerve injury may lead to disabling chronic pain and hyperalgesia (49). In general, mechanical hyperalgesia is easy to demonstrate in affected patients, whereas thermal hyperalgesia is less prominent. In some patients, movement even of hair follicles elicits pain. Responses to heat stimuli in these patients are variable (36). In some cases there seems to be exaggerated pain from suprathreshold heat stimuli, but there is no clear-cut decrease in the pain threshold. Perhaps the hyperalgesia in these patients is more like that of secondary hyperalgesia.

To determine whether A fibers or C fibers signal hyperalgesia in patients with nerve injuries in the upper extremities, we applied a tourniquet inflated above systolic pressure to the affected arm (46) to achieve an orderly loss of sensory function beginning with those functions subserved by the largest fibers. In 12 patients, hyperalgesia to mechanical stimuli began to disappear 7 to 15 min after application of the cuff and completely disappeared after 15 to 22 min. At that time, sensitivity to touch was altered, indicating loss of Aβ-fiber function, though sensitivity to warmth and cold was preserved.

These results suggest a prominent role of large fibers in signaling hyperalgesia in cases of nerve injury. Results from reaction-time experiments in chronic neuralgia patients by Lindblom and Verrillo (36) and differential-pressure-block experiments in reflex sympathetic dystrophy patients by Wallin et al. (58) also support this hypothesis. Whether the hyperalgesia results from activity in low-threshold mechanoreceptive afferents or from AMHs (mean conduction velocity 31 m/sec) (11) remains to be determined.

SUMMARY

Hyperalgesia, and hence its neural mechanism, should be considered in terms of several variables: (a) Changes within the site of injury are different from those surrounding the area of injury; i.e., primary and secondary hyperalgesias differ. (b) Hyperalgesia to mechanical stimuli may exist independent of hyperalgesia to heat stimuli. (c) The magnitude of hyperalgesia is influenced by skin type (i.e., hairy versus glabrous).

The marked primary hyperalgesia to heat following a burn to the glabrous skin is signaled by sensitization of A-fiber nociceptors. Glabrous-skin C-fiber nociceptors do not sensitize, regardless of the intensity of the heat injury. In contrast, the hyperalgesia to heat following a minor burn to the hairy skin appears to be signaled by sensitization of C-fiber nociceptors. More substantial injuries to hairy skin lead to sensitization of both A- and C-fiber nociceptors. Hyperalgesia to heat is not observed in the area surrounding an injury.

The exquisite hyperalgesia to mechanical stimuli observed at and surrounding an area of injury does not appear to be coded by sensitization of nociceptors to mechanical stimuli. It may be that this form of hyperalgesia is derived from changes within the central nervous system.

Studies in patients suffering from mechanical hyperalgesia secondary to peripheral nerve injury indicate that this hyperalgesia is signaled by A fibers. Whether this hyperalgesia is coded by activity in sensitized nociceptors or by low-threshold mechanoreceptors or by a disinhibition of nociceptive input remains to be determined.

ACKNOWLEDGMENTS

The efforts of numerous individuals contributed to this work. In particular, we wish to express appreciation for the technical assistance of Adil Khan, Trudy Lund, and Ronald Burke. This work was supported by USPHS grants NS-14447, NS-00519, and GM-33451 from the National Institutes of Health.

REFERENCES

1. Adriaensen, H., Gybels, J., Handwerker, H. O., and Van Hees, J. (1983): Response properties of thin myelinated (A-δ) fibers in human skin nerves. *J. Neurophysiol.,* 49:111–122.
2. Becerra-Cabal, L., LaMotte, R. H., Ngeow, J., and Putterman, G. J. (1983): Pain and hyperalgesia by intra-epidermal injection. *Soc. Neurosci. Abstr.,* 9:1063.
3. Beck, P. W., Handwerker, H. O., and Zimmerman, M. (1974): Nervous outflow from the cat's foot during noxious radiant heat stimulation. *Brain Res.,* 67:373–386.

4. Beitel, R. E., and Dubner, R. (1976): Response of unmyelinated (C) polymodal nociceptors to thermal stimuli applied to monkey's face. *J. Neurophysiol.,* 39:1160–1175.
5. Bessou, P., and Perl, E. R. (1969): Response of cutaneous sensory units with unmyelinated fibers to noxious stimuli. *J. Neurophysiol.,* 32:1025–1042.
6. Bini, G., Crucci, G., Hagbarth, K., Schady, W., and Torebjork, E. (1984): Analgesia effect of vibration and cooling on pain induced by intraneural electrical stimulation. *Pain,* 18:239–248.
7. Burgess, P. R., and Perl, E. R. (1967): Myelinated afferent fibers responding specifically to noxious stimulation of the skin. *J. Physiol. (Lond.),* 190:541–562.
8. Campbell, J. N., and LaMotte, R. H. (1983): Latency to detection of first pain. *Brain Res.,* 226:203–208.
9. Campbell, J. N., and Meyer, R. A. (1983): Sensitization of unmyelinated nociceptive afferents in monkeys varies with skin type. *J. Neurophysiol.,* 49:98–110.
10. Campbell, J. N., and Meyer, R. A. (1985): Primary afferents and hyperalgesia. In: *Functional Organization of Spinal Afferent Processing,* edited by T. L. Yaksh, Humana Press, Clifton, N.J. *(in press).*
11. Campbell, J. N., Meyer, R. A., and LaMotte, R. H. (1979): Sensitization of myelinated nociceptive afferents that innervate monkey hand. *J. Neurophysiol.,* 42:1669–1679.
12. Campbell, J. N., Raja, S. N., and Meyer, R. A. (1984): Halothane sensitizes cutaneous nociceptors in monkey. *J. Neurophysiol.,* 52:762–770.
13. Croze, S., Duclaux, R., and Kenshalo, D. (1976): The thermal sensitivity of the polymodal nociceptors in the monkey. *J. Neurophysiol.,* 263:539–562.
14. Darian-Smith, I., Johnson, K. O., LaMotte, C., Shigenaga, Y., Kenins, P., and Champness, P. (1979): Warm fibers innervating palmar and digital skin of the monkey: responses to thermal stimuli. *J. Neurophysiol.,* 42:1297–1315.
15. Darian-Smith, I., Johnson, K. O., LaMotte, C., Kenins, P., Shigenaga, Y., and Ming, V. C. (1979): Coding of incremental changes in skin temperature by single warm fibers in the monkey. *J. Neurophysiol.,* 42:1316–1331.
16. Dubner, R., and Bennett, G. J. (1983): Spinal and trigeminal mechanisms of nociception. *Annu. Rev. Neurosci.,* 6:381–418.
17. Dubner, R., and Hu, J. W. (1977): Myelinated (A-delta) nociceptive afferents innervating the monkey's face. *J. Dent. Res.,* 56:A16.
18. Dubner, R., Price, D. D., Beitel, R. E., and Hu, J. W. (1977): Peripheral neural correlates of behavior in monkey and human related to sensory-discriminative aspects of pain. In: *Pain in the Trigeminal Region,* edited by D. J. Anderson and B. Mathews, pp. 57–66. Elsevier, Amsterdam.
19. Fitzgerald, M. (1979): The spread of sensitization of polymodal nociceptors in the rabbit from nearby injuries and by antidromic nerve stimulation. *J. Physiol. (Lond.),* 297:207–216.
20. Fitzgerald, M., and Lynn, B. (1977): The sensitization of high threshold mechanoreceptors with myelinated axons by repeated heating. *J. Physiol. (Lond.),* 365:549–563.
21. Georgopoulos, A. P. (1976): Functional properties of primary afferent units probably related to pain mechanisms in primate glabrous skin. *J. Neurophysiol.,* 39:71–83.
22. Greene, L. C., and Hardy, J. D. (1958): Spatial summation of pain. *J. Appl. Physiol.,* 17:693–696.
23. Gybels, J., Handwerker, H. O., and Van Hees, J. (1979): A comparison between the discharges of human nociceptive nerve fibers and the subject's ratings of his sensations. *J. Physiol. (Lond.),* 292:193–206.
24. Hardy, J. D., Wolff, H. G., and Goodell, H. (1950): Experimental evidence on the nature of cutaneous hyperalgesia. *J. Clin. Invest.,* 29:115–140.
25. Hardy, J. D., Wolff, H. G., and Goodell, H. (1952): *Pain Sensation and Reactions,* Williams & Wilkins, Baltimore.
26. Johnson, K. O., Darian-Smith, I., LaMotte, C., Johnson, B., and Oldfield, S. (1979): Coding of incremental changes in skin temperature by a population of warm fibers in the monkey: Correlation with intensity discrimination in man. *J. Neurophysiol.,* 42:1322–1353.
27. Kumazawa, T., and Perl, E. R. (1977): Primate cutaneous sensory units with unmyelinated (C) afferent fibers. *J. Neurophysiol.,* 40:1325–1338.
28. LaMotte, R. H., and Campbell, J. N. (1978): Comparison of responses of warm and noci-

ceptive C-fiber afferents in monkey with human judgments of thermal pain. *J. Neurophysiol.,* 41:509–528.
29. LaMotte, R. H., and Thalhammer, J. G. (1982): Response properties of high-threshold cutaneous cold receptors in the primate. *Brain Res.,* 244:279–287.
30. LaMotte, R. H., Thalhammer, J. G., and Robinson, C. J. (1983): Peripheral neural correlates of magnitude of cutaneous pain and hyperalgesia: A comparison of neural events in monkey with sensory judgments in human. *J. Neurophysiol.,* 50:1–26.
31. LaMotte, R. H., Thalhammer, J. G., Torebjork, H. E., and Robinson, C. J. (1982): Peripheral neural mechanisms of cutaneous hyperalgesia following mild injury by heat. *J. Neurosci.,* 2:765–781.
32. Lewis, T. (1933): Clinical observations and experiments relating to burning pain in extremities and to so-called "erythromelageia" in particular. *Clin. Sci.,* 1:175–211.
33. Lewis, T. (1935): Experiments relating to cutaneous hyperalgesia and its spread through somatic nerves. *Clin. Sci.,* 2:373–423.
34. Lewis, T. (1942): *Pain.* Macmillan, New York.
35. Lewis, T., and Pochin, E. E. (1937): The double pain response of the human skin to a single stimulus. *Clin. Sci.,* 3:67–76.
36. Lindblom, V., and Verrillo, R. T. (1979): Sensory functions in chronic neuralgia. *J. Neurol. Neurosurg. Psychiat,* 42:422–435.
37. Lynn, B. (1979): The heat sensitization of polymodal nociceptors in the rabbit and its independence of the local blood flow. *J. Physiol. (Lond.),* 287:493–507.
38. McMahon, S. B., and Wall, P. D. (1984): Receptive fields of rat lamina 1 projection cells move to incorporate a nearby region of injury. *Pain,* 19:235–247.
39. Meyer, R. A., and Campbell, J. N. (1981): Evidence for two distinct classes of unmyelinated nociceptive afferents in monkey. *Brain Res.,* 224:149–152.
40. Meyer, R. A., and Campbell, J. N. (1981): Peripheral neural coding of pain sensation. *John Hopkins APL Technical Digest,* 2:167–171.
41. Meyer, R. A., and Campbell, J. N. (1981): Myelinated nociceptive afferents account for the hyperalgesia that follows a burn applied to the hand. *Science,* 213:1527–1529.
42. Meyer, R. A., Raja, S. N., and Campbell, J. N. (1984): Coupling of action potential activity between unmyelinated fibers in the peripheral nerve of monkey. *Science,* 227:184–187.
43. Meyer, R. A., Walker, R. E., and Mountcastle, V. B. (1976): A laser stimulator for the study of cutaneous thermal pain sensation. *IEEE Trans. Biomed. Eng.,* 23:54–60.
44. Perl, E. R., Kumazawa, T., Lynn B., and Kennins, P. (1976): Sensitization of high threshold receptors with unmyelinated (C) afferent fibers. In: *Progress in Brain Research,* Vol. 43, edited by A. Iggo and O. B. Ieyinsky, pp. 263–276. Elsevier, Amsterdam.
45. Raja, S. N., Campbell, J. N., and Meyer, R. A. (1984): Evidence for different mechanisms of primary and secondary hyperalgesia following heat injury to the glabrous skin. *Brain,* 107:1179–1188.
46. Raja, S. N., Campbell, J. N., Meyer, R. A., and Mackinnon, S. N. (1984): Hyperalgesia following nerve injury is signalled by myelinated fibers. *Pain,* [Suppl. 2:]S8.
47. Sinclair, D. C., and Hinshaw, J. R. (1950): A comparison of the sensory dissociation produced by procaine and by limb compression. *Brain,* 73:480–498.
48. Stevens, S. S., and Galanter, E. H. (1957): Ratio scales and category scales for a dozen perceptual continua. *J. Exp. Psych.,* 54:377–411.
49. Sunderland, S. (1978): *Nerves and Nerve Injuries.* Churchill Livingstone, New York.
50. Thalhammer, J. G., and LaMotte, R. H. (1982): Spatial properties of nociceptor sensitization following heat injury of the skin. *Brain Res.,* 231:257–265.
51. Thalhammer, J. G., and LaMotte, R. H. (1983): Heat sensitization of one-half of a cutaneous nociceptor's receptive field does not alter the sensitivity of the other half. In: *Advances in Pain Research and Therapy,* Vol. 5, edited by J. J. Bonica et al., pp. 71–75. Raven Press, New York.
52. Torebjork, H. E., and Hallin, R. G. (1973): Perceptual changes accompanying controlled preferential blocking of A and C fiber responses in intact human skin. *Exp. Brain Res.,* 16:321–332.
53. Torebjork, H. E., and Hallin, R. G. (1974): Responses in human A and C fibers to repeated electrical intradermal stimulation. *J. Neurol. Neurosurg. Psychiatry,* 37:653–664.
54. Torebjork, H. E., and Hallin, R. G. (1977): Sensitization of polymodal nociceptors with C fibers in man. *Proc. Int. Union Physiol. Sci.,* 13:758.

55. Torebjork, H. E., LaMotte, R. H., and Robinson, C. J. (1984): Peripheral neural correlates of magnitude of cutaneous pain and hyperalgesia: Simultaneous recordings in humans of sensory judgments of pain and evoked responses in nociceptors with C-fibers. *J. Neurophysiol.,* 51:325–339.
56. Torebjork, H. E., and Ochoa, J. (1980): Specific sensations evoked by activity in single identified sensory units in man. *Acta Physiol. Scand.,* 110:445–447.
57. Van Hees, J., and Gybels, J. (1981): C nociceptor activity in human nerve during painful and non painful skin stimulation. *J. Neurol. Neurosurg. Psychiatry,* 44:600–607.
58. Wallin, G., Torebjork, E., and Hallin, R. (1976): Preliminary observations on the pathophysiology of hyperalgesia in the causalgic pain syndrome. In: *Sensory Functions of the Skin in Primates,* edited by Y. Zotterman, pp. 489–499. Pergamon Press, Oxford.
59. Woolf, C. J. (1983): Evidence for a central component of post-injury pain hypersensitivity. *Nature,* 306:686–688.

Advances in Pain Research and Therapy, Vol. 9, edited by H. L. Fields et al. Raven Press, New York © 1985.

Neurophysiological Correlates of Posttraumatic Acute Pain

R. W. Beuerman, A. J. Rózsa, and D. L. Tanelian

Lions Eye Research Laboratories, LSU Eye Center, Louisiana State University School of Medicine, New Orleans, Louisiana 70112

Lesions of peripheral nerves are usually accompanied by sensations of pain. Even wounds of a superficial nature involving the distal terminal branches of a nerve can lead to paresthesia, extending through the acute phase of wounding and into the healing process. In 1930, Adrian (1) demonstrated that peripheral nerve damage is accompanied by prolonged spontaneous neural discharges in sensory fibers. Clearly, it could be suggested that this abnormal activity may be the basis of traumatic pain. However, Wall et al. (13) found only an initial-injury discharge in a mixed peripheral nerve, after which the fibers were silent. Recent advances in microneurography in awake humans have been used to compare patterns of neural activity conjointly with the perception elicited by a stimulus. Studies by Ochoa and Torebjork (9) suggested that a change in the perception of a stimulus is coincident with altered temporal patterns of action potentials in a population of axons. In skin, the complexities of this tissue make it difficult to isolate experimentally that region of the axon producing abnormal discharges (9). Although a number of animal models are available for studying modulation of neuronal excitability, they may not be relevant to human situations. Particularly, when the origin of pain sensation is at issue, the animal model should have relevance to human pain states. Moreover, evidence should be available that the animal perceives an abnormal sensation (11).

Our studies have focused on the change in the functional status of sensory nerves of the cornea at various times following a standard wound. Corneal injuries are commonly seen clinically, and they involve sensory fibers to the same extent as does the standard wound. Abrasion of the cellular epithelial layer of the cornea leads to distressing, unpleasant sensations that can be relieved by repeated applications of topical anesthetics (2). Such corneal

Dr. Tanelian's present address is Department of Anesthesiology, Stanford Medical Center, Stanford, California 94305.

defects are often painful until they are healed, which usually requires several days (7). Previous work from our laboratory has documented the anatomical changes in neural organization produced by a standard corneal wound using both light and electron microscopy (6,10). This system also allows correlations to be made between the functional characteristics of ciliary nerve axons during the growth of collateral sprouts within the corneal epithelium.

MATERIALS AND METHODS

These experiments were carried out with albino rabbits (2–3 kg). Following urethane anesthesia (1.5 g/kg i.p.), tracheotomy was performed, and the animals respired spontaneously. Body temperature was maintained by a heating pad with circulating water. The details of the procedure for obtaining the long ciliary nerve for action-potential recording have been described. (12). Briefly, the animal was positioned in a specially designed head holder, and the globe was secured by the conjunctiva to a stainless-steel ring. The vascular supply to the eye was not compromised. A chamber (1.5 ml) covered the cornea for superfusion of test solutions, and also limited exposure to the cornea. Action-potential responses were recorded via a platinum-iridium wire using conventional equipment. It should be noted that only the long ciliary nerve, a sensory nerve, was used for recording in all experiments.

Responsiveness of corneal afferents was tested by chemical, mechanical, and thermal stimuli in unwounded, normal animals and at various times after a corneal injury. The wound was made with a 4-mm-diameter corneal trephine and resulted in removal of a circular slab of tissue about 200 μm thick (10). The injury included approximately 11% of the area of the corneal surface. Topical corneal anesthesia was used prior to wounding when the animal had not been previously anesthetized systemically. The response properties of the corneal sensory receptors were explored at times after wounding that coincided with particular anatomical events uncovered in a previous study (10). These postwound intervals included the following: 5 min, 1 to 2 hr, 5 hr, 24 hr, 3 days, and 7 days. Mechanical stimulation was carried out with a set of calibrated filaments (40–570 dynes of force). Thermal stimulation (10°C, 23°C, 40°C) was accomplished with isotonic sodium chloride solutions. Chemical stimulation consisted of sodium chloride and sucrose solutions at several osmolarities, but isothermal to the cornea (31°C–32°C).

Action potentials were converted into uniform pulses and used to create frequency histograms. As found by other investigators, action-potential records following injury are temporally unpredictable and somewhat difficult to quantify (8). Therefore, an active circuit was constructed to initially rectify and then to perform a running-time average (t.c. 1.0 sec), which after amplification was displayed on a chart recorder. Data in this format can be directly measured and have been used extensively in sensory neurophysiology (3,4,8).

RESULTS

An advantage of using the cornea in these experiments is that the extent of neural damage and the subsequent neural reactions can be described by correlated anatomical and neurophysiological studies. The sensory axons supplying the rabbit cornea are predominantly unmyelinated (>70%), and there is an absence of myelinated axons greater than the Aδ range (5). Sensory nerve terminals are restricted to the outer epithelial layer and are represented only as morphologically unspecialized or free nerve endings; in addition, preterminal axons underlie the wound area (10). Therefore, at the margin of the wound, severed axons were directly exposed to the environment. However, surrounding the wound there was a border of initially normal-appearing epithelium and sensory terminals. Immediately following the wound, mechanical or electrical stimulation within the wound bed was not able to generate an action-potential response in the long ciliary nerve; however, these remained effective at the wound margin and surrounding the wound (6). Twenty-four hours after wounding, clumps of degenerating terminals were found in the epithelium around the wound. More striking was the appearance of radially oriented, collateral sprouts growing toward the wound margin (Fig. 1). Sprout length and density increased over the next several days. The wound became reepithelialized in about 3 days, and collateral sprouts grew into this covering, providing innervation for the anesthetic wound. Between 5 and 7 days after wounding, collateral sprouts began to degenerate, and sprout formation occurred at the severed preterminal axons.

In the normal cornea, spontaneous neural activity was unremarkable. Recording was interrupted for 3 to 5 min during the wounding procedure; however, after that time an immediate increase in spontaneous activity was observed in only 2 of 12 preparations. A single 10-sec thermal (warm) or osmotic stimulus was sufficient to initiate spontaneous firing. At times this could also be brought about by light mechanical stimulation of the wound margin with a smooth glass probe, which may mimic the action of the eyelids. After spontaneous firing began, it usually continued for several hours, but without maintaining an obvious pattern. During that time, short bursts as well as prolonged activity with a relatively constant frequency interval were observed. Maximal frequencies of a single-unit burst did not exceed 90 Hz and more commonly were between 40 and 60 Hz. Twenty-four hours following the wound, spontaneous activity had greatly decreased in comparison with that seen in the acute phase. Although preparations at later postoperative times (days 2–7) also exhibited some spontaneous activity, it was probably of a different origin.

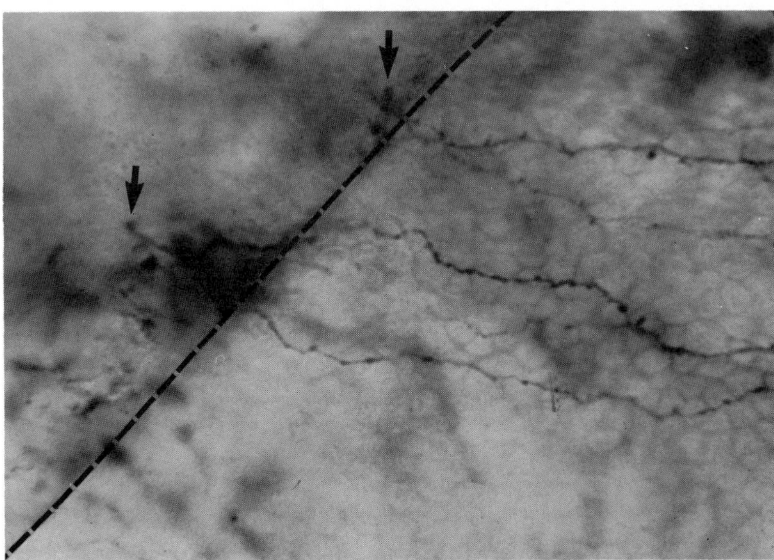

FIG. 1. Flat mount of corneal epithelium following gold chloride impregnation of nerves. This photomicrograph depicts the wound margin *(dashed line)* 48 hr after wounding. The growth-cone-tipped *(arrows)* collateral sprouts course in radial fashion from adjacent unwounded areas. ×650.

Abnormal sensory responses to thermal, chemical, and mechanical stimulations developed rapidly in the immediate postoperative period. There was an indication in several preparations that the initial stimulation following wounding could be less excitatory than normal. However, a subsequent stimulus application always showed that responsiveness was increased in intensity or persistence.

Application of warm (40°C) isotonic saline evoked a barrage of neural activity that continued beyond the duration of the stimulus (Fig. 2). It was not unusual for the residual excitation to be prolonged for 30 to 40 sec, slowly approaching a new level of spontaneous background activity over several minutes. A single cool stimulus (23°C) was sufficient to rapidly lower the frequency of the residual activity. A 10-sec exposure to 10°C isotonic saline quieted the spontaneous activity for several minutes. This excitatory warm activity was uniquely associated with the wound. Within 24 hr, excitation by warm stimulation was less frequent and less intense than immediately after wounding (Fig. 2). The effects of wounding on the responses to hyperosmotic, isothermal sodium chloride solutions were examined in the first 30 min after the injury. Two aspects of the response, amplitude and persistence, were both increased, as seen in Fig. 3. Hyperosmotic solutions of sucrose were tested but appeared to evoke little change in the response profile when compared with prewound values. In the normal cornea, the

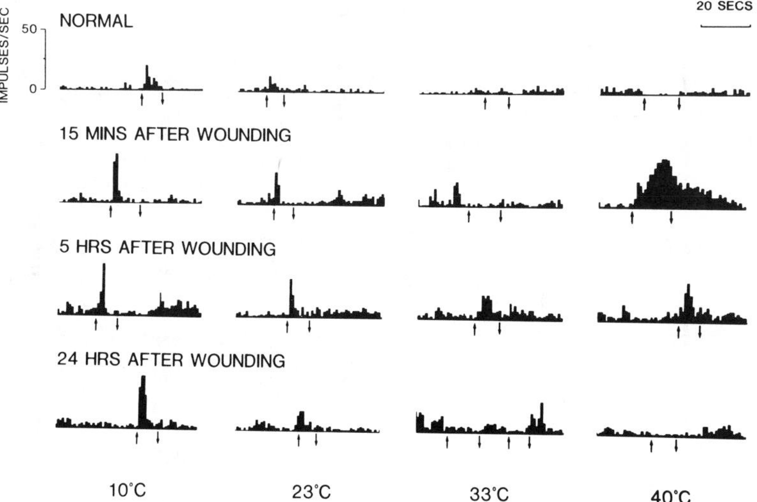

FIG. 2. Neural responses to thermal stimulation following a corneal wound. In the normal cornea, stimuli below the adapting temperature (33°C) were differentially excitatory; however, at 40°C these units were quieted. Following wounding and up to 24 hr, there were slight but consistently greater responses to stimulation at 10°C and 23°C. More striking was the vigorous discharge to 40°C isotonic saline that continued beyond the 10-sec stimulation period. However, this situation rapidly changed and at 24 hr was similar to the normal response. The base-line activity was sometimes irregular at several hours after wounding. This is reflected in the frequency histograms at the 33°C stimulation.

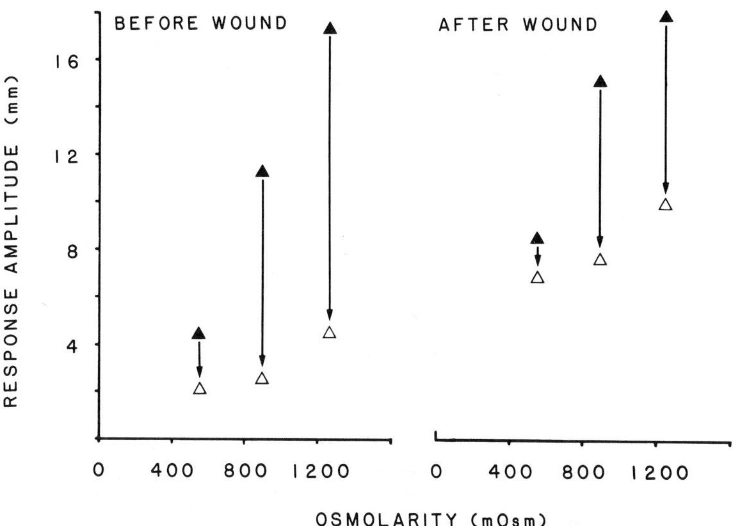

FIG. 3. Wounding affected both the amplitude *(closed triangles)* of the response to a 10-sec stimulus of a hyperosmotic sodium chloride solution and the residual excitation 10 sec after terminating the stimulus *(open triangles).* Each data point represents the mean of five stimulus applications in a series of five preparations.

response to punctate mechanical stimulation was stereotyped. The onset of the stimulus was accompanied by a brief burst that was rapidly adapting. As shown in Fig. 4, at greater forces an "off" response accompanied the release of a maintained stimulus. Following wounding, mechanical stimulation around the wound margin elicited a slowly adapting response that in some cases continued after cessation of the stimulus (Fig. 4). It was consistently noticed that the wound margin was exquisitely sensitive to even small stimuli (20 dynes), whereas in the center of the normal rabbit cornea the threshold was approximately 40 dynes. Unlike the response to thermal stimulation, the response to mechanical stimulation did not return to normal by 7 days after wounding.

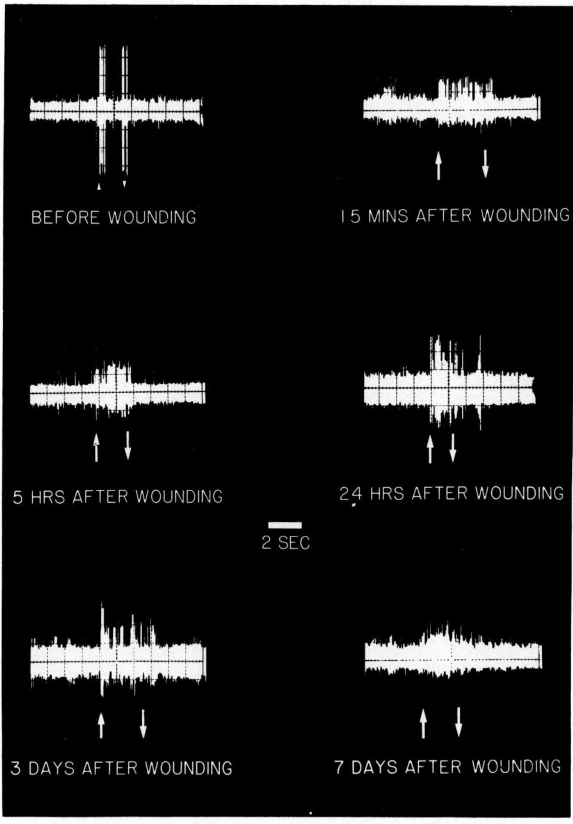

FIG. 4. Mechanical stimulation of the normal cornea elicited a rapidly adapting response and an "off" response when a stimulus of larger magnitude was maintained. Wounding led to a slowly adapting response that had not recovered 7 days after wounding.

DISCUSSION

In this study, the period immediately following an injury was defined by a change in the biophysical specificity and response characteristics of the sensory axons. Abnormal spontaneous activity subsequent to sensory stimulation continued at a vigorous and unpredictable level for several hours. The types of discharges observed in this study were similar to those described by others (1,9). However, it was clear that the ectopic activity was not a continuation of the injury discharge due to the wounding procedure. In agreement with the results of Wall et al. (13), immediately after the wound and prior to stimulation there was no abnormal excitation, and the fibers were quiet. The origin of this activity was at the preterminal or terminal endings of the axons, because a drop of a topical anesthetic on the cornea rapidly diminished all neural activity. This is somewhat different from the conclusion reached by Ochoa and Torebjork (9).

Because paresthesias also occur in conjunction with sensory stimulation, the response characteristics to several modes of stimulation were examined to determine how these were affected by wounding. In the normal rabbit, corneal axons that are responsive to particular forms of stimulation have been described (12). The loss of specificity to a warm stimulus and the appearance of cold inhibition parallel clinical experience, where a cold pack decreases pain from a corneal abrasion. The differences in traumatic and ischemic pain are underscored by the findings of Culp et al. (8) that warming decreases abnormal sensations. It may be suggested that hyperosmotic stimuli may lead to heightened and prolonged excitation by opening sealed axons around the wound margin. However, the effect is ionic in nature, because hyperosmotic sucrose solutions are minimally excitatory.

Initiation of the action potential probably occurs at the preterminal axon that underlies the corneal epithelium. Previous physiological studies indicated that this segment of the axon could be spatially extensive. However, within this layer, anatomical studies have found only unmyelinated axons, usually surrounded by Schwann processes (6). Discontinuities in the diameters of these preterminal axons have not been noted. Finally, the influence of substances produced by the inflammatory processes initiated by wounding must be considered in future experiments.

ACKNOWLEDGMENTS

This work was supported in part by USPHS grants EY-04074, EY-07073, and EY-02377 from the National Eye Institute and by the Louisiana Lions Eye Foundation.

REFERENCES

1. Adrian, E. D. (1930): The effects of injury on mammalian nerve fibers. *Proc. R. Soc. Lond. [Biol.]*, 106:596–618.
2. Behrendt, T. (1956): Experimental study of corneal lesions produced by topical anesthesia. *Am. J. Ophthalmol.*, 41:99–105.
3. Beidler, L. M. (1956): Properties of chemoreceptors of tongue of rat. *J. Neurophysiol.*, 16:595–607.
4. Beuerman, R. W. (1975): Slow potentials of the turtle olfactory bulb in response to odor stimulation of the nose. *Brain Res.*, 97:61–78.
5. Beuerman, R. W., Klyce, S. D., Kooner, S., Tanelian, D., and Rózsa, A. (1983): Dimensional analysis of rabbit ciliary nerve. *Invest. Ophthalmol. Vis. Sci.* [*Suppl.*], 24:261.
6. Beuerman, R. W., and Rózsa, A. J. (1984): Collateral sprouts are replaced by regenerating neurites in the wounded corneal epithelium. *Neurosci. Lett.*, 44:99–104.
7. Cavanagh, H. D., Philaja, D., Thoft, R. A., and Dohlman, C. H. (1976): The pathogenesis and treatment of persistent epithelial defects. *Trans. Am. Acad. Ophthalmol. Otolaryngol.*, 81:754–769.
8. Culp, W. J., Ochoa, J., and Torebjork, E. (1984): Ectopic impulse generation in myelinated sensory nerve fibers in man. In: *Abnormal Nerves and Muscles as Impulse Generators*, edited by W. J. Culp and J. Ochoa, Oxford University Press, New York.
9. Ochoa, J. L., and Torebjork, H. E. (1980): Paraesthesiae from ectopic impulse generation in human sensory nerve. *Brain*, 103:835–853.
10. Rózsa, A. J., Guss, R. B., and Beuerman, R. W. (1983): Neural remodeling following experimental surgery of the rabbit cornea. *Invest. Ophthalmol. Vis. Sci.*, 24:1033–1051.
11. Scadding, J. W. (1982): Ectopic impulse generation in experimental neuromas: Behavioral, physiological and anatomical correlates. In: *Abnormal Nerves and Muscles as Impulse Generators*, edited by W. J. Culp and J. Ochoa, pp. 533–552. Oxford University Press, New York.
12. Tanelian, D. L., and Beuerman, R. W. (1984): Responses of rabbit corneal nociceptors to mechanical and thermal stimulation. *Exp. Neurol.*, 84:165–178.
13. Wall, P. D., Waxman, S., and Basbaum, A. I. (1974): Ongoing activity in peripheral nerve: Injury discharge. *Exp. Neurol.*, 45:576–589.

Advances in Pain Research and Therapy, Vol. 9, edited by H. L. Fields et al. Raven Press, New York © 1985.

Sensory Changes in Joint-Capsule Receptors of Arthritic Rats: Effect of Aspirin

*G. Guilbaud, **A. Iggo, and †R. Tegnér

**Unité de Recherches de Neurophysiologie Pharmacologique de l'INSERM (U161), 75014 Paris, France; ** Department of Veterinary Physiology, Royal (Dick) School of Veterinary Studies, University of Edinburgh, Edinburgh EH9 1QH, Scotland; and †Department of Neurology, Karolinska Institutet, S-104 01 Stockholm, Sweden*

Rats with adjuvant-induced arthritis have been widely used for the evaluation of the antiinflammatory and analgesic properties of various compounds (10,27), and they now appear to provide a useful model for the study of "clinical" pain by comparison with experimental pain. This interest in their use has been underlined by several behavioral (6) and pharmacological (4,5,19,20,28) studies, and in particular it has been emphasized that these rats are very sensitive to morphine and naloxone.

In systematic electrophysiological experiments it was found that the responses of somatosensory neurons recorded in areas known to be involved in nociception are dramatically altered: in spinal dorsal horn (25), in thalamic nuclei (9,21), and in the somatomotor cortex (23). In these central nervous structures there is a decrease of neurons exclusively driven by intense cutaneous stimuli, as well as a striking increase in the sensitivity of the neurons to moderate mechanical stimulation of the inflamed joints and the adjacent cutaneous areas. It is a complex issue whether the various changes are exclusively due to the peripheral modifications of the sensory receptors or whether additional central processes also contribute. In an attempt to evaluate the peripheral mechanisms, we investigated in arthritic rats the responsiveness of the afferent fibers contained in an articular ramus innervating an inflamed ankle joint and compared the data with those obtained in a parallel investigation in normal rats. Moreover, to investigate further the functional implications of the joint-capsule fibers in a pathological situation, we tested the effects on their responses brought about by aspirin (ASA), an analgesic drug especially active in articular pain.

MATERIALS AND METHODS

Animals were injected with Freund's adjuvant into the tail and were selected as arthritic at the Centre d'Elevage of Charles Rivers, France. The rats used for this electrophysiological study weighed between 170 and 240 g at the time of the experiment, which was between 3 and 4 weeks after the injection of Freund's complete adjuvant. Indeed, the arthritic lesions were usually maximum at this time and tended to diminish by approximately 28 days. The arthritis, which has been described in detail in several studies (27), consisted of an acute or subacute polyarthritis affecting the ankles, wrists, and minor joints of the limbs. The inflamed paws disclosed swollen edematous hyperemic tissue. The ankle joint was selected for investigation because it is severely affected (circumference of the ankle: 21 mm in normals, versus 40–45 in arthritic rats).

Animals were anesthetized with sodium pentobarbitone (intraperitoneally). A branch of the medial plantar nerve, which we called the primary articulocutaneous ramus (PACR), supplying the ankle capsule was dissected. Afferent activity in the ankle-joint-capsule nerve fibers was recorded extracellularly after dissection of the PACR, as described elsewhere (14). The properties of the afferent units were assessed by the use of a variety of natural stimuli, including different intensities of pressure with probes ranging from fine von Frey hairs to stiff metal rods, as well as squeezing the tissues with metal dissecting forceps, both smooth-tipped and serrated. Quantitative mechanical stimuli were delivered using an electromechanical indentation generator with feedback control of position (Somedic AB, Stockholm).

For the conduction-velocity measurements, identification of the active axons was aided by the use of the collision technique (17), as modified by Brown and Iggo (2) for use in combination with an electromechanical transducer. Conduction velocity was calculated from the time required for conduction (from the stimulating electrode on the peripheral nerve to the recording electrodes) and the conduction distance, measured *in situ.* In addition, because of the short distances involved, the nerve was stimulated at the level of the receptor through a metal probe attached to the mechanical transducer that also acted as the stimulating cathode.

We tested the effects of aspirin (15–50 mg/kg i.v., aspirin equivalent) on responses to mechanical stimuli of nine fibers after a period of stable recording.

RESULTS

Electrophysiological Characteristics of Capsule Afferent Units

Thirty-three units were examined in 14 rats. Thirty units adapted slowly to sustained mechanical indentation (Fig. 1), and the other three responded

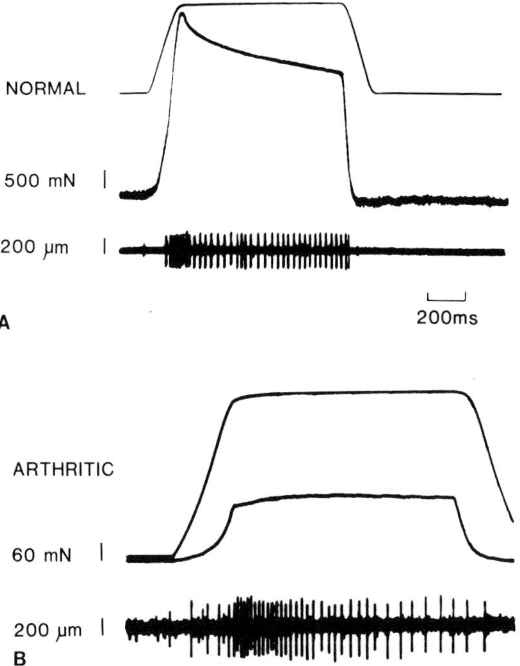

FIG. 1. Responses of joint-capsule receptors to controlled indentation of the capsule in normal and arthritic rats. In each record from above downward are displayed the indentation and the force applied in the capsule and the afferent discharge in the PACR.

only during the dynamic phase of indentation; i.e., they were rapidly adapting. These proportions were similar to those in normal rats.

Background Discharge

A low-frequency background discharge was present in 7 of the 30 slowly adapting (SA) receptors that had a high mechanical sensitivity. The mean threshold for these 7 units with background activity was 2.5 ± 1.1 mN. For the other 23 units the mean threshold was 6.9 ± 1.5 mN. However, the difference in sensitivity of the two groups was not statistically significant ($p > 0.05$).

Responses to Mechanical Stimulation

Natural stimuli, such as pressure on the joint, lateral compression of the joint, or small degrees of flexion or extension, were tested in 14 units in 7 rats. All yielded positive results, in striking contrast to the normal animals, in which movement of the joint was ineffective. Figure 2 illustrates the discharge in a joint-capsule receptor (threshold 1.7 mN) to mild lateral

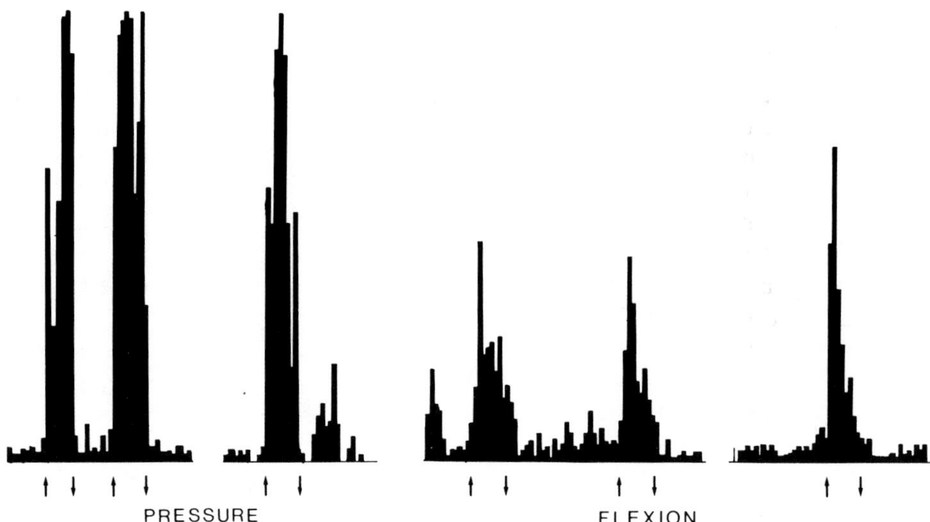

FIG. 2. Peristimulus histograms of the discharge of joint-capsule receptors in arthritic rat to mild compression and to slight flexion of the ankle joint (number of spikes counted in 1-sec period).

compression of the inflamed ankle and indicates the high rate of firing. The same receptor also responded to a slight flexion of the ankle, a further illustration of the enhanced sensitivity of joint receptors in arthritic animals.

The mechanical thresholds, measured with von Frey hairs, ranged from 0.4 to 46 mN. The range of thresholds is compared in Fig. 3 with that for joint-capsule receptors in normal animals, and the lower threshold for the arthritic animals is clearly evident. The capsular tissue of the ankle joint in arthritic animals was grossly enlarged and thickened in comparison with normal animals, and this influenced both receptive-field sizes and mechanical thresholds, as tested by stimuli applied to the exterior of the capsule. Dissection of the outer layers of the thickened capsule, under binocular microscopic control, while recording from the nerve, led to progressive

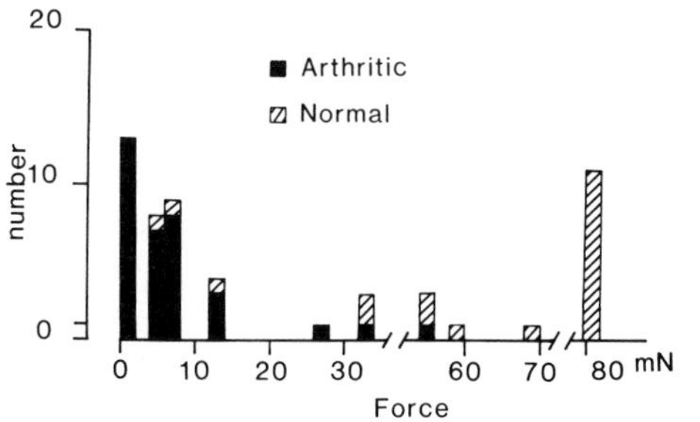

FIG. 3. Threshold values, measured with von Frey hairs, for mechanical stimulations of joint-capsule receptors in normal and arthritic rats.

reductions in both the threshold and receptive-field size as tissue was removed. For example, a receptor with a threshold of 7.5 mN became approximately 10 times more sensitive after exposure of the receptor by dissection, the threshold falling to 0.7 mN. For this standpoint, the range of thresholds cited earlier and illustrated in Fig. 3 is an overestimate of the actual local thresholds within the tissues.

When monitored mechanical stimuli were applied, there was an initial dynamic phase during the ramp indentation, followed by a continued slowly adapting discharge at a lower frequency during the maintained indentation (Fig. 1B). The stimulus–response relationship was best described by a power function, as in normal rats.

When the quantitatively controlled mechanical stimulus was repeated rapidly, the response to successive stimuli, tested in 10 units, fell very rapidly, almost to extinction, and the recovery was slower than in normal animals.

Conduction Velocities

Conduction velocities were measured in 17 units. The capsule receptors all had slowly conducting afferent fibers, the maximum velocity being 12 m/sec. The majority were slower than 6 m/sec, values that are at the lower end of the normal range. All the measurements were made for conduction from the stimulating cathode on the receptive field of a unit to the recording electrode on the PACR, and therefore these values are as shown in normal animals (14), underestimates of the conduction velocities in the main nerve trunk. In particular, the units with measured conduction velocities between 2.5 and 5 m/sec were probably all small myelinated axons at, and proximal to, the recording electrode, with conduction velocities in the main nerve of at least 6 m/sec. In the absence of further evidence it is not unreasonable to assume, on the basis of measurements made in the normal animals, that many of the units had axons that were myelinated in the tibial nerve but were unmyelinated in the articular branch of the PACR.

Action of Aspirin

With 5 min of injection of aspirin equivalent at 50 mg/kg, the discharge to a standard stimulus became less, and it continued to decline during the next 20 to 30 min to the point of extinction (Fig. 4). Thereafter, the response recovered gradually, although the fragility of the experimental preparation usually prevented satisfactory recording for longer than 50 to 70 min. The effect was dose-dependent, and 15 mg/kg was without a convincing effect (13).

The rate of decline of the response after the injection was linear when plotted on semilogarithmic coordinates. A similar result was obtained with

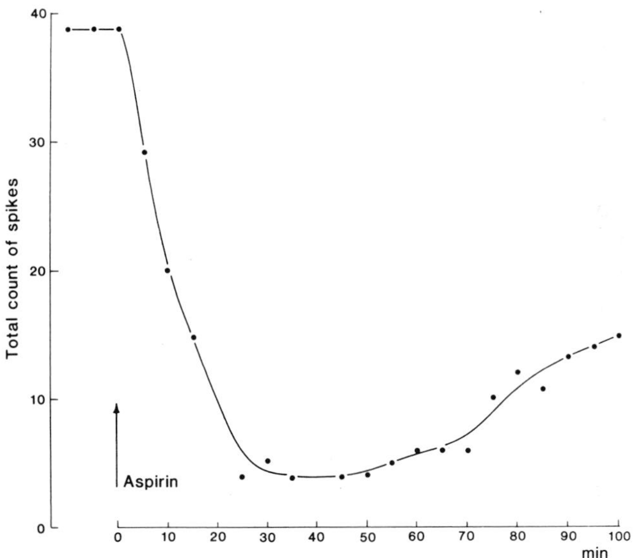

FIG. 4. Effects of 50 mg/kg aspirin equivalent (i.v.) on a stable response of a joint-capsule receptor induced by a monitored mechanical stimulation.

local application of aspirin, even when the circulation to the capsule was arrested. Threshold responses of the fibers were measured before and at the height of aspirin action; they were at least three times higher after drug administration.

DISCUSSION AND CONCLUSION

Probably the most striking feature of the joint-capsule receptors in the arthritic animals was their low threshold for mechanical stimulation, both those with small myelinated axons and those with nonmyelinated axons. The lowest thresholds, down to 0.4 mN, begin to approach the sensitivity of C mechanoreceptors in the skin (18). At these low thresholds the joint receptors also began to have a background discharge, in contrast to those in normal animals, and also a response to small movements of the joint. The joints were certainly much stiffer than in normal animals, so that passive movement required application of greater force than was normally needed, and this may have led to larger forces developing during movement of the arthritic joint. Nevertheless, the heightened sensitivity of the receptors would certainly be expected to play a part in the greater afferent discharge of the diseased-joint afferent units to flexion or extension of the joint. There is a parallel with the results of Coggeshall et al. (3), who reported that during acute inflammation of the knee joint in cats, the receptors of their categories

3 and 4 with fine afferent fibers developed a heightened mechanical sensitivity, a background discharge, and a previously absent sensitivity to joint movement. However, from our histological investigation as detailed elsewhere (14), there was no evidence for change in the number of axons in the PACR nerve and therefore no change in the nerve supply to the joint capsule.

Because aspirin is known to block cyclooxygenase irreversibly, and therefore the synthesis of prostaglandins (7,29), its action in depressing the enhanced sensitivity of arthritic-joint-capsule receptors indicates that prostaglandins, not leukotrienes produced locally in the inflamed tissues (11,16), probably are responsible for the hypersensitivity. Because prostaglandin E_2 (PGE_2) is relatively stable in the tissues, the time constants of decay and of hypersensitivity obtained experimentally further suggest that a thromboxane or prostaglandin with a short life, such as prostacyclin (7), may be the causative agent. This agent probably enhanced the responsiveness of the receptors to algogenic substances, such as bradykinin, that are also present in the inflammatory exudate (16). Indeed, bradykinin excited small afferent fibers of both cutaneous (1,8) and muscular (22,26) origin, and responses elicited by this substance were enhanced during continuous intravenous infusion of PGE_2 (15). The enhanced responses to bradykinin were prevented by ASA (15,26).

These results, if they cannot explain all the changes in responses observed for central neurons, can account for the great number of thalamic and cortical neurons that are easily driven by joint stimulation such as gentle pressure or movement (especially from the ankle) (9,21,23). It is also of interest to mention the relatively high fatigability of these central responses, because an interval of several minutes between peripheral stimuli or a shift in the stimulus locus is necessary to record stable and reproducible responses from the neurons (9,25).

Finally, the general similarities of the time course and extent of the aspirin effect in the capsule receptors and thalamic responses in arthritic rats (12) suggest that the depressive action observed at the thalamic level can be attributed in great part to the peripheral action of aspirin (7,29). Other changes in the properties of other sensory receptors (not studied in these experiments) that could also contribute are a matter for further experimental analysis.

REFERENCES

1. Beck, P. W., and Handwerker, H. O. (1974): Bradykinin and serotonin effects in various types of cutaneous fibres. *Pfluegers Arch.*, 347:209–222.
2. Brown, A. G., and Iggo, A (1967): A quantitative study of cutaneous receptors and afferent fibres in the cat and rabbit. *J. Physiol. (Lond.),* 193:707–733.
3. Coggeshall, R. E., Hong, K. A. P., Langford, L. A., Schaible, H. G., and Schmidt, R. F. (1983): Discharge characteristics of fine medial articular afferents at rest, during passive movements of inflamed knee joints. *Brain Res.,* 272:185–188.

4. Colpaert, F. C., De Whitte, P., Maroli, A. N., Awouters, F., Niemegeers, C. J. E., and Janssen, P. A. J. (1980): Self-administration of the analgesic suprofen in arthritic rats: Evidence of mycobacterium butyricum-induced arthritis as an experimental model of chronic pain. *Life Sci.* 27:921–928.
5. Colpaert, F. C., Meert, T., De Whitte, P., and Schmitt, P. (1982): Further evidence validating of adjuvant arthritis as an experimental model of chronic pain in the rat. *Life Sci.*, 31:67–75.
6. De Castro Costa, M., De Sutter, P., Gybels, J., and Van Hees, J. (1981): Adjuvant-induced arthritis in rats: A possible animal model of chronic pain. *Pain,* 10:173–185.
7. Ferreira, S. H. (1979): Site of analgesic action of aspirin-like drugs and opioids. In: *Mechanisms of Pain and Analgesic Compounds,* edited by R. F. Beers, Jr., and E. G. Bassett, pp. 309–321, Raven Press, New York.
8. Fjällbrant, N., and Iggo, A. (1961): The effect of histamine, 5-hydroxytryptamine and acetylcholine on cutaneous afferent fibres. *J. Physiol. (Lond.),* 156:578–590.
9. Gautron, M., and Guilbaud, G. (1982): Somatic responses of ventrobasal thalamic neurones in polyarthritic rats. *Brain Res.,* 237:459–471.
10. Gouret, C., Mocquet, G., and Raynaud, G. (1976): Use of Freund's adjuvant arthritis test in antiinflammatory drug screening in the rat: Value of animal selection and preparation at the breeding center. *Lab. Anim. Sci.,* 26:281–287.
11. Granström, E. (1983): Biochemistry of the prostaglandins, thromboxanes and leukotriens. In: *Advances in Pain Research and Therapy,* Vol. 5, edited by J. J. Bonica et al., pp. 605–615. Raven Press, New York.
12. Guilbaud, G., Benoist, J. M., Gautron, M., and Kayser, V. (1982): Aspirin clearly depressed responses of ventrobasal thalamus neurons to joint stimuli in arthritic rats. *Pain,* 13:153–163.
13. Guilbaud, G., and Iggo, A. (1985): The effects of aspirin on the mechanical sensitivity of joint-capsule sensory receptors in arthritic rats. *J. Physiol. (Lond.),* 357:29.
14. Guilbaud, G., Iggo, A., and Tegnér, R. (1985). Sensory receptors in ankle joint capsules in normal and arthritic rats. *Exp. Brain Res.,* 58:29–40.
15. Handwerker, H. O. (1976): Influences of algogenic substances and prostaglandins on the discharges of unmyelinated cutaneous nerve fibers identified as nociceptors. In: *Advances in Pain Research and Therapy,* Vol. 1, edited by J. J. Bonica and D. Albe-Fessard, pp. 41–46. Raven Press, New York.
16. Higgs, G. A., and Moncada, S. (1983): Interactions of arachidonate products with other pain mediators. In: *Advances in Pain Research and Therapy,* Vol. 5, edited by J. J. Bonica et al., pp. 617–626. Raven Press, New York.
17. Iggo, A. (1958): The electrophysiological identification of single nerve fibres; with particular reference to the slowest conducting vagal afferent fibres in the cat. *J Physiol. (Lond.),* 142:110–116.
18. Iggo, A. (1960): Cutaneous mechanoreceptors with afferent C fibers. *J. Physiol. (Lond.),* 152:337–353.
19. Kayser, V., and Guilbaud, G. (1981): Dose-dependent analgesic and hyperalgesic effects of systemic naloxone in arthritic rats. *Brain Res.,* 226:344–348.
20. Kayser, V., and Guilbaud, G. (1983): Effects of morphine, but not those of the enkephalinase inhibitor, Thiorphan, are enhanced in arthritic rats. *Brain Res.,* 267:131–138.
21. Kayser, V., and Guilbaud, G. (1984): Further evidence for changes in the responsiveness of somatosensory neurons in arthritic rats: A study of the posterior intralaminar region of the thalamus. *Brain Res.,* 323:144–147.
22. Kumazawa, T., and Mizumura, K. (1976): The polymodal C-fiber receptor in the muscle of the dog. *Brain Res.,* 101:589–593.
23. Lamour, Y., Guilbaud, G., and Willer, J. C. (1983): Altered properties and laminar distribution of neuronal responses to peripheral stimulation in the SmI cortex of the arthritic rat. *Brain. Res.,* 273:183–187.
24. Lim, R. K. S. (1966): Salicylate analgesia. In: *The Salicylates: A Critical Bibliography Review,* edited by M. J. H. Smith and P. K. Smith, pp. 155–202. Wiley, New York.
25. Menétrey, D., and Besson, J. M. (1982): Electrophysiological characteristics of dorsal horn cells in rats with cutaneous inflammation resulting from chronic athritis. *Pain,* 13:343–364.

26. Mense, S. (1977): Nervous outflow from skeletal muscle following chemical noxious stimulation. *J. Physiol. (Lond.),* 267:75–88.
27. Pearson, C. M., and Wood, F. D. (1959): Studies of arthritis and other lesions induced in rats by injection of mycobacterial adjuvant. I. General clinical and pathological characteristics and some modifying factors. *Arthritis Rheum.,* 2:440–459.
28. Pircio, W. A., Fedele, C. T., and Bierwagen, M. E. (1975): A new method for the evaluation of analgesic activity using adjuvant-induced arthritis in the rat. *Eur. J. Pharmacol.,* 31:207–215.
29. Vane, J. R. (1971): Inhibition of prostaglandin synthesis as a mechanism of action for aspirin-like drugs. *Nature* [*New Biol.*], 231:232–235.

Advances in Pain Research and Therapy, Vol. 9, edited by H. L. Fields et al. Raven Press, New York © 1985.

Effects of Prostaglandins E_1 and E_2 on the Mechanosensitivity of Group III Afferents from Normal and Inflamed Cat Knee Joints

B. Heppelmann, H.-G. Schaible, and R. F. Schmidt

Physiologisches Institut der Universität, D-8700 Würzburg, Federal Republic of Germany

The afferent innervation of the cat's knee joint is characterized by its high proportion of fine afferent fibers both in the group III (conduction velocity 2.5–20 m/sec) and in the group IV (conduction velocity <2.5 m/sec) fiber range (12,13). Recent studies of the receptive properties of fine afferent fibers in the medial articular nerve revealed that those fibers that were excited by local mechanical stimulation from small, often spot-like single or multiple receptive fields on the medial and anteromedial aspects of the joint could be classified into four categories according to their response behaviors to passive innocuous and noxious joint movements: (1) units that were excited by innocuous movements of the knee joint; (2) units that were only weakly excited by innocuous movements, whereas noxious movements led to pronounced discharges; (3) units that did not respond to any innocuous joint movements, but fired clearly and consistently to noxious ones; and (4) units that could not be excited by any joint movement. It was concluded from these data that articular mechanoreceptive units with fine afferent fibers are activated not only by noxious events but also by everyday innocuous local stimuli and by movements in the physiological working range of the joint (18–21).

An acute experimental arthritis of the cat's knee joint induces two major changes in many, although not all, fine afferent fibers of medial articular nerve. There is an appearance of resting activity (or marked enhancement of ongoing resting discharge) and an increased sensitivity to movement in the normal working range of the joint (2). Both effects may be seen in a given unit, or only one of the effects may appear. The increased sensitivity to movement manifests itself as either reduction in threshold or enhancement of movement-induced responses or both. All these changes were observed both in group IV units, which normally have a high percentage of fibers in categories 3 and 4, and in group III units, in which approximately 50% of the units belong to categories 1 and 2.

The changes in receptive properties that occur in fine articular afferents in the course of inflammation are thought to be due to the sensitizing actions of chemical mediators on their receptive terminals. Several such presumed mediators can be found in high concentrations in inflamed tissue, as reviewed elsewhere (15). Among them, the prostaglandins (PGs) have long been held responsible for sensitization of nociceptive units, for the following reasons: PGs occur regularly in inflamed tissue (4,8,11,15); they have sensitizing and algesic effects in humans (1,4,8,15); they induce signs of hyperalgesia in animals (4,8,9,15); in single-unit studies they have been shown to increase the responses of fine afferent fibers to bradykinin (14,17), to heat stimuli (5), and to mechanical stimuli (16).

This report deals with the actions of PGs E_1 and E_2 (PGE_1 and PGE_2) on the resting and evoked activities of medial articular group III units from normal and inflamed knee joints of cats. It will be shown that in most units from normal joints these PGs induced changes in receptive properties that were similar in character to those induced by inflammation (but much weaker in extent), and in units from inflamed joints, small to very small doses of PGs led to marked additional sensitization. These latter effects became particularly obvious when the arthritis-induced activity had been subdued by application of indomethacin or acetylsalicylic acid (6,7).

METHODS

The experiments were performed on cats of both sexes weighing 2.1 to 4.3 kg. The animals were anesthetized by intramuscular injection of ketamine hydrochloride (Ketanest) at 15 mg/kg, followed by intravenous injection of α-chloralose (10 mg/kg). Additional doses of chloralose (10 mg/kg i.v.) were given as required to maintain a deep level of anesthesia throughout the experiments. All animals were immobilized with pancuronium bromide (Pancuronium, Organon), 0.6 mg/hr i.v., and artificially ventilated. Blood pressure, end-expiratory CO_2, and body temperature were monitored and kept at physiological levels.

The right knee joint was used in all experiments. The dissection of the leg, the positioning of the animal on the mounting table, the performance of passive limb movements, and the mode of close intra-arterial (i.a.) application of test substances via a fine cannula in the saphenous artery have recently been described in detail (10,18–20). PGE_1 and PGE_2 were dissolved in Tyrode solution at room temperature. Each injection was done in the following way: The arterial catheter was filled with 0.3 ml of PG solution. The solution was injected with 1 ml Tyrode solution. The injection was completed in about 10 sec. Injection of another 1 ml of Tyrode solution cleaned the tube system of remaining traces of PG.

Prior to any application of PG and repeatedly in the course of the experiment a bolus injection of 1 ml Tyrode solution containing 1% Evans blue was given via the cannula in order to ascertain that the injection fluid reached the joint tissue innervated by the medial articular nerve (MAN). To test the accessibility of isolated single units via the blood vessels, injections of 0.3 ml of a twice-isotonic solution of KC1 (again with 1 ml Tyrode) were performed. Such an injection typically evokes a rapid burst of impulses at short latency in fine MAN units. In a few cases in which this short latency discharge was absent or in which i.a. injections of PGE_1 or PGE_2 did not have any obvious effects, further PG injections directly into the joint cavity were performed.

Single units of the MAN with conduction velocities from 2.5 to 20 m/sec were used. With the knee joint in mid-position, the receptive-field properties of each unit were determined by its responses to probing with a hand-held glass rod and a set of von Frey hairs (18). Thereafter, the responses to passive limb movements were recorded in order to classify the unit as belonging to one of the four distinct categories mentioned earlier. Further details of the mechanical testing procedure are available (19,20).

Acute experimental arthritis was induced by injecting into the joint cavity 0.5 ml of a 4% solution of kaolin, followed 1 hr later by 0.3 ml of a 2% solution of carrageenan. In an awake, freely moving cat, such an injection causes guarding of the leg and avoidance of movement or weight bearing on the joint starting after 2 to 4 hr and lasting at least 12 hr. Sometimes the body temperature rises. In an anesthetized animal, edema is significant. Histological examination reveals all signs of acute arthritis with marked cellular infiltration (2).

RESULTS

Normal Joints

Excitatory action of PGE_2. The effect of PGE_2 on the resting activity of group III units was tested in 12 single fibers in which no previous PG injection had been given (first injections of the day in 12 different cats). In 7 of the 12 units, application of PGE_2 led either to a prolonged evoked response in previously silent units or to a prolonged increase in resting activity for at least 3 min and up to 10 min or more (Figs. 1A and 2B). In 5 of the 7 fibers with this type of reaction, the effective dose of PGE_2 was 3 μg or less. In 3 of the 12 fibers, the PG-evoked response consisted of a few discharges or a brief increase in resting frequency. In the last 2 fibers, no evoked responses were seen, even after injection of 30 μg.

Regarding their response behavior to joint movements, the 10 fibers that showed PG-evoked responses were from all four categories, 5 of them being in the lowest threshold category, i.e., category 1. On the other hand, the 2

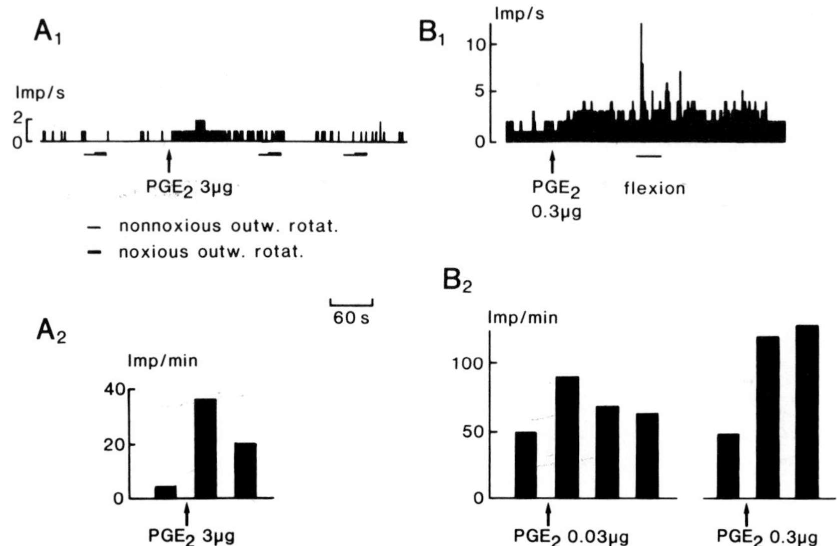

FIG. 1. Excitatory effects of PGE_2 on group III units from normal **(A)** and inflamed **(B)** joints. **A_1:** Peristimulus time histogram with an address advance rate of 1 sec showing activating action of PGE_2 on a group III unit (conduction velocity 2.8 m/sec). **A_2:** Numbers of impulses 1 min before and in the first 2 min after injection of PGE_2. **B_1:** Effect of 0.3 μg PGE_2 on the ongoing discharges of a group III unit (conduction velocity 8.4 m/sec) from an inflamed joint; 2.5 hr earlier the resting activity had been significantly reduced by treatment with ASA. **B_2:** Numbers of impulses per minute before and after injection of 0.03 μg PGE_2 and 0.3 μg PGE_2 (shown in B_1).

units that were not excited by PGE_2 were from two different categories, namely 1 and 2.

An excitatory effect could be combined with a sensitizing effect *(vide infra),* but (as in the unit shown in Fig. 1A) PG could activate afferent fibers without inducing changes in the reaction to the test movements.

Corresponding results were obtained in fibers that were isolated later in the experiments, i.e., in which PG injections had been given earlier. Similar observations were made when using PGE_1 injections (Fig. 2A). In summary, these PGs have definite excitatory actions on most group III units of all four categories, inducing on injection discharges in silent units and accelerating ongoing resting discharges for considerable periods of time.

The excitatory effects of PGs were pronounced in inflamed joints *(vide infra)* (Figs. 1B and 5B).

Sensitizing actions of PGE_1 and PGE_2. A common form of sensitization observed in articular group III units on close i.a. bolus injection of PGs is illustrated in Fig. 2. The unit, which had two receptive fields on the anteromedial aspects of the joint (Fig. 2D), responded to innocuous flexions of the joint, i.e., it belonged to category 1 (see the initial part of Fig. 2A). Appli-

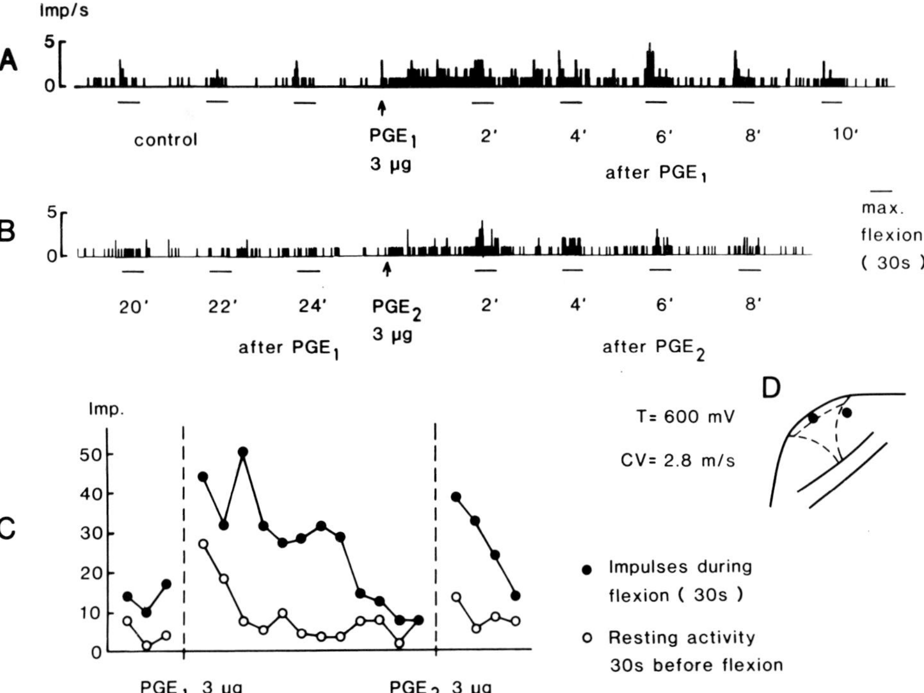

FIG. 2. Excitatory and sensitizing effects of PGE_1 and PGE_2 on a group III unit (conduction velocity 2.8 m/sec) of category 1. **A:** Peristimulus time histogram with an address advance rate of 1 sec illustrating the resting activity and the responses to maximum flexion before and after injection *(arrow)* of 3 μg PGE_1. **B:** Effects of a further injection, this time 3 μg PGE_2, 26 min after the first. **C:** Diagram showing total numbers of impulses 30 sec before and during each of the flexion movements shown in A and B. **D:** View of the medial aspect of the right knee joint giving the locations of the receptive fields of this unit. The electrical threshold of its afferent fiber was 600 mV.

cation of 3 μg PGE_1 increased the background resting discharge (excitatory action of PGs) and, in addition, enhanced the movement-induced responses to a level much higher than the control difference between the resting and movement-evoked discharges (Figs. 2A and 2C). A second injection of PGE_2 26 min later again had a direct excitatory effect as well as a sensitizing effect (Fig. 2B and right-hand part of Fig. 2C).

The sensitizing effects of PGs may also occur without an obvious excitatory component. This is illustrated in Fig. 3 for a group III unit of category 3 (excited only by noxious movements) that displayed no resting discharges. The unit had its receptive field in the patellar region (Fig. 3D) and responded with only a few impulses to noxious outward rotations (Fig. 3A). Injections of 3 μg and 30 μg PGE_2 regularly led to enhancement of the responses to such outward rotations without any direct excitatory action of

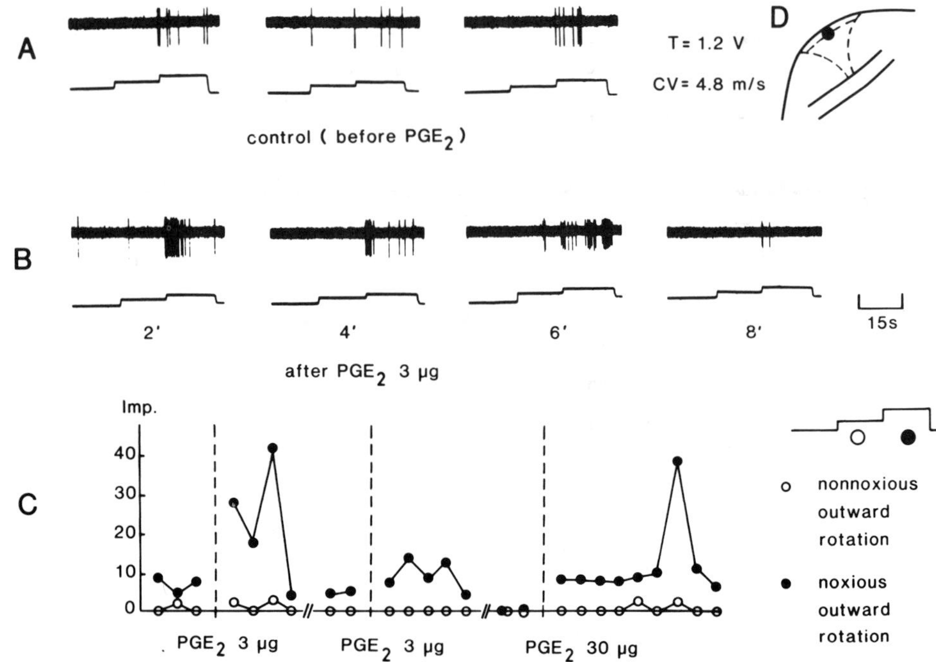

FIG. 3. Sensitizing effects of PGE_2 on a group III unit (conduction velocity 4.8 m/sec) of category 3 (activated only by noxious joint movements). **A:** Three specimen records showing responses to outward rotations and noxious outward rotations in mid-position of the joint. **B:** Responses to the same movements at the indicated times after close i.a. injection of 3 μg PGE_2. **C:** Diagram showing total numbers of impulses during innocuous *(open circles)* and noxious *(closed circles)* outward rotations before and after injections of 3 and 30 μg PGE_2. The unit had no resting activity at any time. **D:** Location of the receptive field. The electrical threshold of the afferent fiber was 1.2 V.

PGE_2 or the appearance of reproducible responses to innocuous movements (Fig. 3B–C). After further injections of PGE_2, a few impulses could be evoked by non-noxious movements.

The other form of sensitization was a change in the response behavior of a fiber. This is exemplified in Fig. 4, which shows a unit in which half extensions only occasionally evoked one or a few impulses under control conditions (Fig. 4A). After injection of PGE_1, marked responses to the same movement occurred for many minutes (Fig. 4B–C). Subsequent injection of PGE_2 had a similar but weaker effect (Fig. 4C).

Other types of sensitization included cases in which (a) injections of PGs plus bradykinin were necessary to observe sensitization and (b) i.a. injection of PGs remained ineffective, but injection of PGs into the joint cavity led to increased responses to movements.

Finally, it should also be pointed out that marked sensitization often required several injections of PGs, frequently at rather high doses (6–30

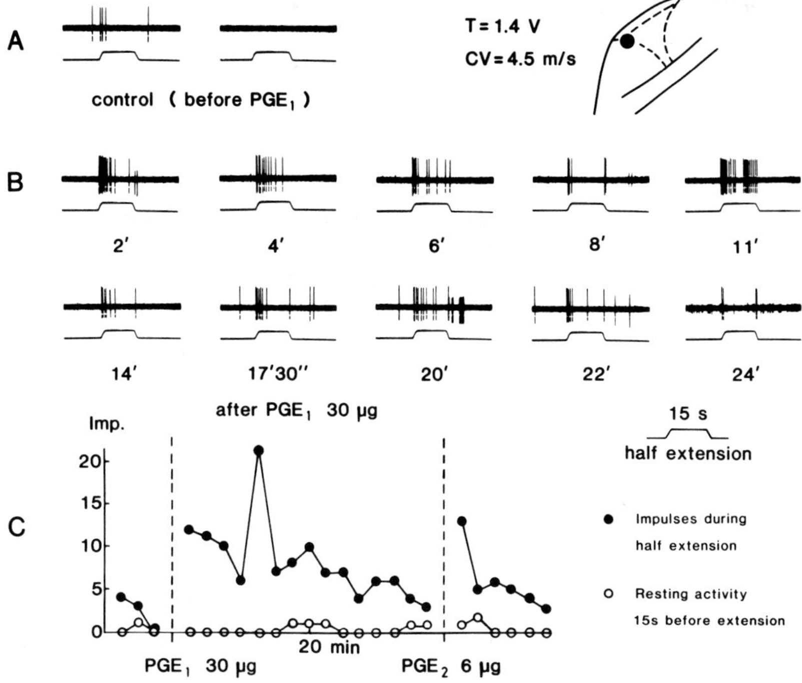

FIG. 4. Effects of PGE_1 and PGE_2 on a unit in which half extensions only occasionally evoked a few impulses under control conditions. **A:** Control movements. **B:** Same movements after injection of PGE_1, 30 μg. **C:** Recordings of A and B and effects of subsequent injection of PGE_2 (not illustrated) as quantified.

μg). No distinct differences could be seen between the effects of PGE_1 (a PG much in use in experimental studies of hyperalgesia, but probably not present in inflamed tissue) and PGE_2 (present at high concentrations in inflamed tissue).

Inflamed Joints

Although the effects of PGs on articular group III units are similar to those induced by experimental arthritis *(vide supra),* the magnitude was much weaker in the former than in the latter situation. Possibly, inflamed tissue provides a more favorable environment for action than normal tissue. To test this notion, experiments were carried out on single units from inflamed joints that when isolated displayed vigorous resting and evoked activity and that thereafter had been treated with indomethacin or acetylsalicylic acid (ASA) in order to decrease their activity (6,7). The specific point investigated was whether in an inflamed environment application of additonal PG had more powerful actions on group III units than in a normal environment.

The results of such an experiment are shown in Fig. 5. In this inflamed joint, indomethacin had been given 4 hr earlier. The depressive effect of the drug was observed in another group III fiber (conduction velocity = 4.6 m/sec) that had, in a control period of 70 min, stable ongoing discharges (80–90 impulses per minute). After intravenous application of indomethacin, the resting activity was reduced to 30 to 40 impulses per minute within 30 min, which was a typical time course in such experiments (6). After this pretreatment the unit shown in Fig. 5 had little resting or evoked activity (Fig. 5A). A small dose of PGE_2 (0.3 μg) induced an increase in ongoing discharges and powerful responses to movements (Fig. 5B–C) that lasted at least 1 hr.

Altogether, seven group III units from seven different inflamed joints were tested with PGE_2 in this way. In 4 cats, indomethacin and later PGE_2

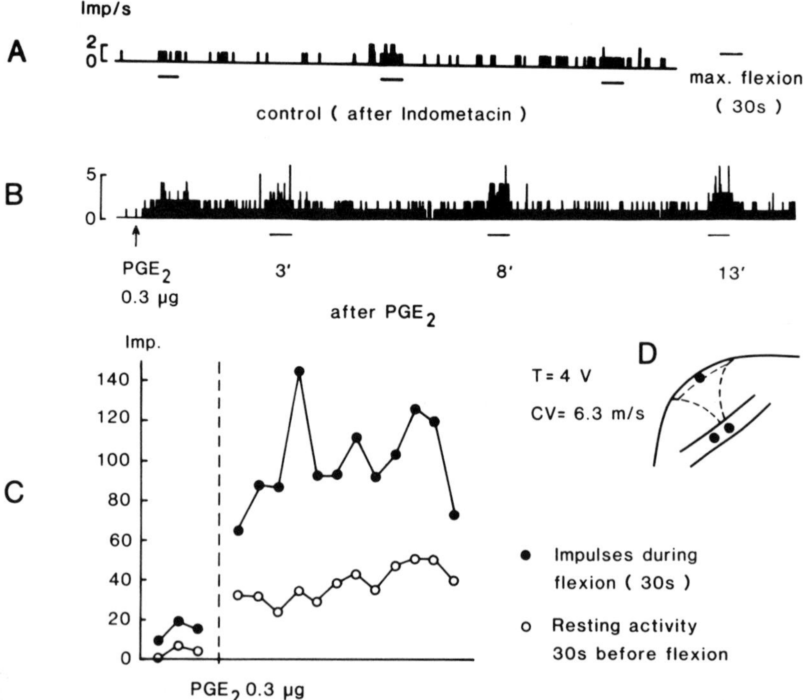

FIG. 5. Effects of 0.3 μg PGE_2 on a group III unit (conduction velocity 6.3 m/sec) from an inflamed joint. Histograms (A, B), diagram (C), and receptive fields (D) recorded and plotted as in Fig. 2. **A:** Resting and evoked activities after treatment with indomethacin applied systematically 4 hr before. **B:** Same, but after injection of 0.3 μg PGE_2 *(arrow)*. **C:** Total number of impulses 30 sec before *(open circles)* and during *(closed circles)* flexion.

were tested in one unit (Fig. 1B shows the effect of PGE_2 on such a unit); in 3 cats, different units had to be taken. The results were rather uniform. In two units, only 0.03 μg PGE_2 was necessary to obtain effects similar to those just described (Fig. 1B), and the highest dose necessary in two units to induce activation and sensitization similar to those seen before pretreatment with indomethacin or ASA was a single dose of 3 μg. Thus, the overall effects of PGs were much more obvious under these experimental conditions than under normal conditions.

DISCUSSION

These results show that PGs have a twofold action on articular group III units: a direct excitatory action (activation of silent units, acceleration of ongoing discharge) and a sensitizing action (lowering of threshold, more forceful responses to movements). Both effects usually occur in a given unit, but it was also observed in this study that sometimes only one or the other could be induced in a unit, even after repeated injections of high doses of PGs. Thus, the sensitization effects do not seem to be a consequence of the excitatory effects and vice versa. We should like to assume, therefore, that they reflect independent processes in the terminal receptive regions of these units.

PGs have long been suspected of modifying the receptive properties of nociceptive fine afferent units in the course of inflammation (4,8,9,15,22). But, as shown here, low-threshold group III afferent units (categories 1 and 2) are just as susceptible to PGs as those with higher thresholds (categories 3 and 4) that presumably have nociceptive functions (19–21). Actually, this observation is well in line with the finding that all categories of articular group III units can be excited by close i.a. injection of bradykinin (10). Similar findings have been obtained for fine afferents in other tissues, as reviewed elsewhere (10). Furthermore, an acute inflammatory process in the knee joint seems to influence not only fibers of categories 3 and 4 (which presumably have nociceptive functions according to their response behavior to mechanical testing in the normal joint) but also fibers of categories 1 and 2 (2; B. Heppelmann et al., *unpublished observations*). Therefore, "nonspecific" activation of receptors with different response properties to mechanical stimulation may be the typical situation in the case of an acute inflammation.

Similar to our results, it was found that PGE_1 induced sensitization of Aδ moderate-pressure mechanoreceptors supplying the skin of the rat hindlimb (16).

The lack of PG sensitivity of some units (which again is not related to their mechanosensitivity) is further evidence that the chemosensitivity of group III afferent units is not simply related to their response behavior to passive movements. Thus, in every aspect tested so far, group III articular afferents are anything but a homogeneous population of high-threshold units with fine free ("naked") terminals in the joint tissue. It may be that this variety in receptive properties is just as much a function of the terminal membrane properties as of the properties of the extraneural tissue in which the nerve endings are embedded (3,12).

In inflamed tissue, single injections of very small amounts of PGs induced much more powerful and long-lasting activation and sensitization of group III units than under normal conditions. This became particularly obvious when highly active units were pretreated with indomethacin or ASA (Fig. 5). Obviously, the changes induced in the unit's terminal environment by the inflammation, which presumably include increased levels of PGs (4,8,15,22), provide much more favorable conditions for the PG actions than those prevailing under normal circumstances. It will be fascinating to find out which of the substances present in inflamed tissue other than PGs themselves contribute to this increase in PG susceptibility.

We have not yet made more than a few observations on the effects of PGs on the mechanosensitivity of articular group IV (C-fiber) units. It appears that the excitatory actions of PGs on these units are similar to those reported here for group III units, but that the sensitizing effects are less pronounced, both in normal joints and in inflamed joints. These preliminary findings further support our contention that the activating and sensitizing effects of PGs have to be regarded as independent processes.

REFERENCES

1. Chahl, L. A. (1979): Pain induced by inflammatory mediators. In: *Mechanisms of Pain and Analgesic Compounds,* edited by R. F. Beers, Jr., and E. G. Bassett, pp. 273–284. Raven Press, New York.
2. Coggeshall, R. E., Hong, K. A. P., Langford, L. A., Schaible, H.-G., and Schmidt, R. F. (1983): Discharge characteristics of fine medial articular afferents at rest and during passive movements of inflamed knee joints. *Brain Res.,* 272:185–188.
3. Düring, M. von, Andres, K. H., and Schmidt, R. F. (1984): Ultrastructure of fine afferent fibre terminations in muscle and tendon of the cat. In: *Sensory Receptor Mechanisms (Mechanoreceptors, Thermoreceptors and Nociceptors),* edited by W. Hamann and A. Iggo. World Scientific, Singapore.
4. Ferreira, S. H. (1983): Prostaglandins: Peripheral and central analgesia. In: *Advances in Pain Research and Therapy,* Vol. 5, edited by J. J. Bonica, U. Lindblom, and A. Iggo, pp. 627–634. Raven Press, New York.
5. Handwerker, H. O. (1976): Influences of algogenic substances and prostaglandins on the discharges of unmyelinated cutaneous nerve fibers identified as nociceptors. In: *Advances in Pain Research and Therapy,* Vol. 1, edited by J. J. Bonica and D. G. Albe-Fessard, pp. 41–51. Raven Press, New York.
6. Heppelmann, B., Heuss, C., Schaible, H.-G., and Schmidt, R. F. (1984): ASA and indometacin reduce sensitivity to movements of fine articular afferent units of inflamed joints. *Pfleugers Arch.,* 402:R37.
7. Heppelmann, B., Schaible, H. -G., and Schmidt, R. F. (1984): Indometacin reduces resting activity of fine afferent units of inflamed knee joints. *Pfluegers Arch.,* 400:R16.
8. Higgs, G. A., and Moncada, S. (1983): Interactions of arachidonate products with other pain mediators. In: *Advances in Pain Research and Therapy,* Vol. 5, edited by J. J. Bonica, U. Lindblom, and A. Iggo, pp. 617–626. Raven Press, New York.

9. Juan, H. 91978): Prostaglandins as modulators of pain. *Gen. Pharmacol.,* 9:403–409.
10. Kanaka, R., Schaible, H. -G., and Schmidt, R. F. (1985): Activation of fine articular afferent units by bradykinin. *Brain Res.,* 327:81–90.
11. Kuehl, F. A., Jr., and Egan, R. W. (1980): Prostaglandins, arachidonic acid, and inflammation. *Science,* 210:978–984.
12. Langford, L. A., Schaible, H.-G., and Schmidt, R. F. (1984): Stucture and function of fine joint afferents; observations and speculations. In: *Sensory Receptor Mechanisms (Mechanoreceptors, Thermoreceptors and Nociceptors),* edited by W. Hamann and A. Iggo, pp. 241–252. World Scientific, Singapore.
13. Langford, L. A., and Schmidt, R. F. (1983): Afferent and efferent axons in the medial and posterior articular nerves of the cat. *Anat. Rec.,* 206:71–78.
14. Mense, S. (1981): Sensitization of group IV muscle receptors to bradykinin by 5-hydroxytryptamine and prostaglandin E_2. *Brain Res.,* 225:95–105.
15. Moncada, S., Ferreira, S. H., and Vane, J. R. (1979): Pain and inflammatory mediators. In: *Handbook of Experimental Pharmacology,* Vol. 50, *Part I, Inflammation,* edited by J. R. Vane and S. H. Ferreira, pp. 588–616. Springer, Berlin.
16. Pateromichelakis, S., and Rood, J. P. (1982): Prostaglandin E_1-induced sensitization of Aδ moderate pressure mechanoreceptors. *Brain Res.,* 232:89–96.
17. Schaible, H.-G. (1983): Bradykinin sensitivity of polymodal fine afferent joint units. Sensitization by prostaglandin E_1. *Naunyn Schmiedebergs Arch. Pharmacol.* [*Suppl.*], 322:R98.
18. Schaible, H.-G., and Schmidt, R. F. (1983): Activation of groups III and IV sensory units in medial articular nerve by local mechanical stimulation of knee joint. *J. Neurophysiol.,* 49:35–44.
19. Schaible, H.-G., and Schmidt, R. F. (1983): Responses of fine medial articular nerve afferents to passive movements of knee joint. *J. Neurophysiol.,* 49:1118–1126.
20. Schaible, H.-G., and Schmidt, R. F. (1984): Mechanosensibility of joint receptors with fine afferent fibers. In *Sensory-Motor Integration in the Nervous System,* edited by O. Creutzfeldt, R. F. Schmidt, and W. D. Willis. *Exp. Brain Res.* (Suppl. 9), 9:284–297.
21. Schaible, H.-G., and Schmidt, R. F. (1985): Coding of pain information from joints. In: *Development, Organization and Processing in Somatosensory Pathways,* edited by M. J. Rowe and W. D. Willis, pp. 309–316. Alan R. Liss, New York.
22. Vane, J. R. (1983): Pain of inflammation. In: *Advances in Pain Research and Therapy,* Vol. 5, edited by J. J. Bonica., U. Lindblom, and A. Iggo, pp. 597–603. Raven Press, New York.

Advances in Pain Research and Therapy, Vol. 9, edited by H. L. Fields et al. Raven Press, New York © 1985.

Nociceptive Role of Ventral Root Afferents

Jin Mo Chung, Kyu Ho Lee, and Richard E. Coggeshall

Marine Biomedical Institute, and Departments of Anatomy, and Physiology and Biophysics, The University of Texas Medical Branch, Galveston, Texas 77550-2772

It was previously thought that all somatic sensory axons entered the spinal cord via dorsal roots (7,12), but recent studies have shown a significant number of these fibers in ventral roots (3,5). Physiological recordings indicate that the majority of these axons, at least in lumbosacral segments of the cat, transmit nociceptive information (2,6). Activation of these fibers results in pressor or algesic responses (11,14), and it has been suggested that they may be an explanation for the failure of dorsal rhizotomy to relieve pain (4). Nevertheless, the functional importance of these fibers is not yet well understood. The study reported here shows that stimulation of these fibers increases the activity of neurons in the dorsal horn, which is a first step toward analyzing the central processing of information carried by these fibers.

METHODS

Fourteen adult cats (2.0–4.5 kg) of either sex were anesthetized with intraveneous injection of α-chloralose (70 mg/kg). After anesthesia was deep, a tracheotomy was done, gallamine triethiodide (4 mg/kg/hr) was administered, and artificial ventilation was begun. The level of end-tidal CO_2 was maintained between 3.5 and 4.5%, and body temperature was kept near 37.5°C. Laminectomy was performed to expose the L7 and S1 segments of spinal cord and corresponding roots. Ventral roots L7 and S1 were cut near the spinal cord, and each distal stump was placed on a pair of stimulating electrodes. An extra ground electrode was placed on the ventral root distal to the stimulating electrodes to prevent spread of electrical current to the spinal cord. Unit activity from dorsal horn neurons was recorded with a carbon-filament-filled glass microelectrode (1), and the amplified signal was fed into a window discriminator whose output was used to compile histograms by a computer. A diagram of the spinal cord, roots, and electrodes is shown in Fig. 1. Once a dorsal horn cell was found to be activated by

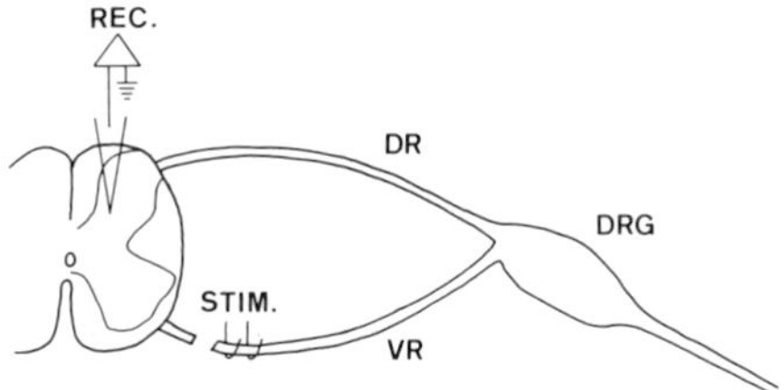

FIG. 1. Diagram showing arrangement of recording and stimulating electrodes. Activities of dorsal horn cells are recorded (REC.) while stimulating (STIM.) the distal end of the cut ventral root (VR). DR, dorsal root; DRG, dorsal root ganglion.

ventral root stimulation, the receptive field of the cell was mapped and characterized. In some experiments, responses of cells were studied after stimulation of a peripheral nerve that innervated the receptive field. Responses of the cell to noxious thermal stimulation were also studied by applying a heat pulse to the skin with a contact stimulator in the receptive field (Thermal Devices, LTS3).

At the end of the recording session, some cells were marked by passing a DC current (20–30 μA for 10 sec) through the recording electrode. A segment of the spinal cord that contained the mark was taken out at the end of the experiment and immersed in 10% formaldehyde. The tissue was then cut serially and the mark identified.

RESULTS

Results for 46 dorsal horn cells activated by ventral root stimulation were recorded in this study. An example of such a cell is shown in Fig. 2. This particular cell was located in the neck of the dorsal horn of the spinal cord at the junction between L7 and S1 (Fig. 2A). It had a large receptive field covering the skin over the entire hindlimb, with a more sensitive area around the foot (Fig. 2B). When mechanical stimuli of graded strength were applied to the receptive field, the cell did not respond to innocuous stimuli, but it responded very well to noxious mechanical stimuli (Fig. 2C). This cell was excited when the distal stump of the cut S1 ventral root was stimulated as shown in Fig. 2D. A much larger excitation was elicited by applying a train of pulses of the same strength. All recorded cells required this kind of temporal summation for maximum activation by ventral root stimulation. The threshold for activation of ventral root fibers that excite the dorsal horn cell was very high (3–5 V, 0.5–1 msec), so that it was approximately 300 to 500 times the threshold for activation of motor fibers in the ventral root.

The cutaneous receptive fields of our cells varied from a small spot to an entire hindlimb. Some cells could also be activated by pressure on deep tissue such as muscle. All of these cells responded strongly to noxious mechanical stimuli such as pinch and squeeze in the receptive field. Thirty-four cells had receptive-field properties that could be characterized. Nineteen of the 34 responded exclusively to noxious mechanical stimuli (high-threshold

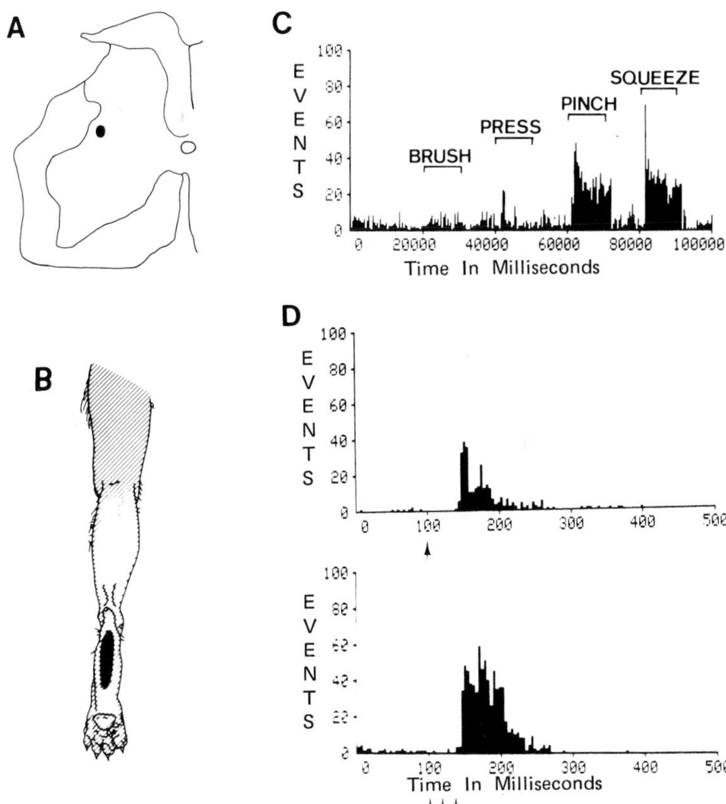

FIG. 2. Example of a dorsal horn cell that was activated by ventral root stimulation. **A:** Location of recorded cell is shown. **B:** The cutaneous receptive field of this cell is depicted by the shaded area. The more sensitive area is indicated by a black spot. **C:** Responses of the dorsal horn cell to graded mechanical stimuli applied to the skin in the receptive field. A single-pass peristimulus time histogram was made by a computer (bin width 400 msec) while brushing the skin repeatedly with a camel-hair brush (BRUSH), applying a large arterial clip (PRESS), applying a small arterial clip (PINCH), and squeezing a fold of skin with serrated forceps (SQUEEZE). The pinch and squeeze stimuli were painful when tried on a human subject. **D:** Responses of the dorsal horn cell to ventral root stimulation. Peristimulus time histograms were compiled (bin width 4 msec) from 20 consecutive stimulations of the distal stump of the S1 ventral root with a 10-V 1-msec single pulse *(top)* or a train of pulses *(bottom);* arrows indicate times at which stimulus pulses were applied.

cells), 1 responded exclusively to stimulation of deep tissue, and 14 responded to innocuous stimuli, such as brushing the skin with a camel-hair brush, as well as the noxious stimuli. For the last 14 cells, the responses to noxious stimuli were greater than those to innocuous stimuli (wide-dynamic-range cells). None of the cells responded to innocuous stimuli exclusively.

A total of 10 recorded cell bodies were located anatomically. These were distributed in the marginal layer and throughout the dorsal horn, but most were found in lamina V.

It was found that these neurons could also be activated by stimulation of unmyelinated fibers in the sciatic nerve, as shown in Fig. 3A. The evidence that this is a C-fiber response rather than a delayed polysynaptic activation from A fibers is that reducing the stimulus strength to the point where C fibers were not activated resulted in disappearance of the activity labeled C response in Fig. 3A. Some cells were also activated by noxious thermal stimuli applied to the skin in the receptive field, as shown in Fig. 3B. These results indicate that the dorsal horn cells that could be activated by ventral root stimulation receive nociceptive input from the periphery.

Because it requires a high intensity of stimulation of the ventral root to activate dorsal horn cells, prevention of current spread to the spinal cord is important. Thus, an extra ground electrode was placed on the ventral root between the stimulating electrodes and the spinal cord. In addition, in some cases the ventral root was crushed distal to the stimulating electrodes. As shown in Fig. 4, a dorsal horn cell could no longer be excited after crushing the ventral root distal to the stimulating electrodes (Fig. 4B), but the excitation reappeared when the root was stimulated distal to the crushed area

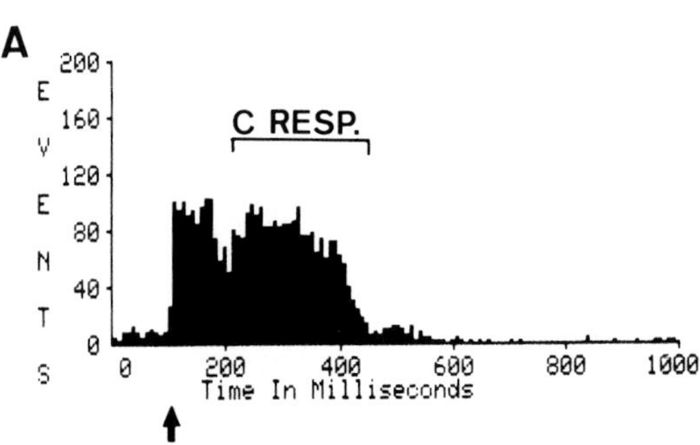

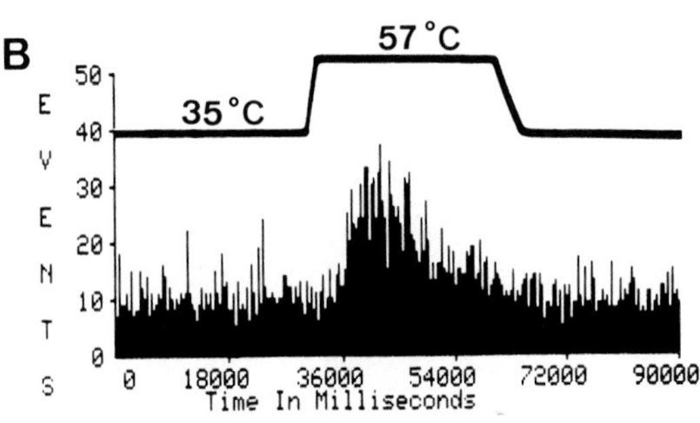

FIG. 3. A: Responses of a dorsal horn cell that was activated by ventral root and peripheral nerve stimulation. Once a dorsal horn cell was activated by ventral root stimulation, the sciatic nerve was stimulated (at the time indicated by an arrow) with a train of three pulses (20 V, 1 msec, 50 Hz internal frequency). The peristimulus time histogram was formed from 20 consecutive stimuli (bin width 8 msec). Note the marked C response to high-intensity peripheral nerve stimulation (indicated by a bracket). If a lower-intensity stimulus was used, the long latency response (C RESP.) was not seen. Distance from stimulating electrode to recording electrode was 130 mm. **B:** A single-pass peristimulus time histogram (bin width 360 msec) of a dorsal horn cell during application of a heat pulse to the skin of the receptive field. After adaptation to 35°C, a heat pulse of 57°C was delivered with a contact thermostimulator. The temperature tracing is shown above the histogram. Note the increased firing of the cell at the higher temperature.

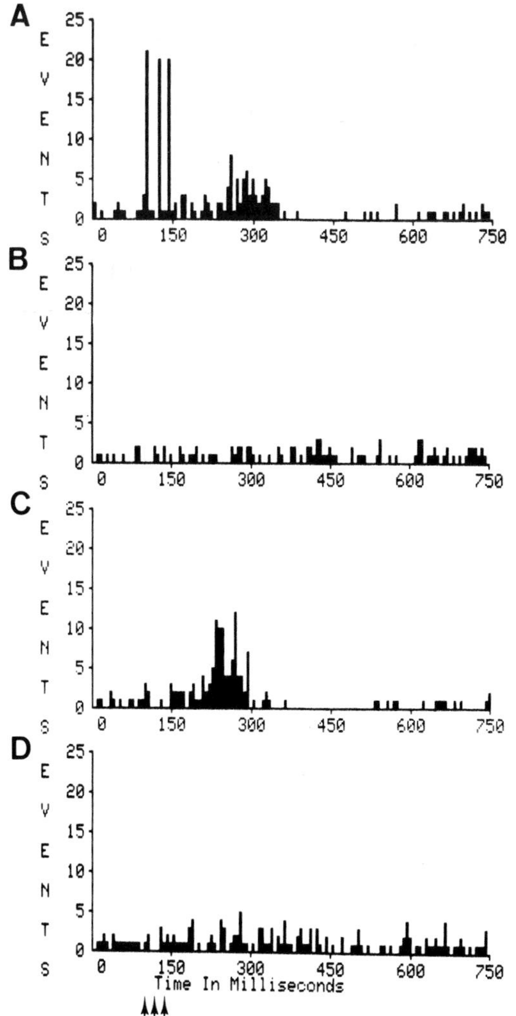

FIG. 4. Responses of a dorsal horn cell to stimulation of the distal stump of the cut ventral root of the conduction block. Peristimulus time histograms were made (bin width 6 msec) of responses to 20 consecutive stimuli to the L7 ventral root **(A).** The stimuli consisted of a train of three pulses (each 15 V for 0.5 msec) separated by 20-msec intervals *(arrows).* Note that the response was abolished after the ventral root was pinched just distal to the stimulation site **(B).** The response reappeared by stimulating the ventral root distal to the pinch **(C).** The response was again abolished when the L7 dorsal root was sectioned **(D).** Shock artifacts triggered the window discriminator in A.

(Fig. 4C). The response could then be abolished by cutting the dorsal root of the same segment (Fig. 4D). These crushing and stimulation experiments were repeated in seven other cells with the same results. This indicates that the excitation of the dorsal horn cell produced by ventral root stimulation is not due to electrical current spread to the spinal cord but rather to activation of fibers in the ventral root. This further indicates that the excitation is carried by fibers that enter the spinal cord in the dorsal root. Therefore, the conduction distance is the distance from the ventral root where stimulation was done to the dorsal root ganglion plus the distance from the dorsal root ganglion to the dorsal horn cell where the recording was made. The conduction velocity of the response was calculated on the basis of this distance and the latency between stimulus and the beginning of the apparent response in 44 cells. The conduction velocities ranged between 0.25 and 1.78 m/sec, with a mean of 0.91 ± 0.47 (SD) m/sec. Fibers that conduct at less than 2.5 m/sec are regarded as unmyelinated (10).

DISCUSSION

As long ago as 1822, Magendie (12) noted that manipulation of the ventral root caused an animal to behave as if it was experiencing pain. It was further shown that section of the dorsal roots eliminated these behavioral responses. Frykholm et al. (9) extended this work to conscious humans by showing that stimulation of the ventral root led to a deep dull ache and that this effect was abolished when the dorsal root was anesthetized locally. This phenomenon is known as recurrent sensibility, and the usual explanation is that some sensory fibers loop into the ventral root before they enter the spinal cord.

The present study demonstrates that stimulation of the ventral root increases the activity of neurons in the mammalian dorsal horn. These effects are due to activation of axons in the root, as indicated by the crush experiments, and the axons are presumed to be unmyelinated, as indicated by their conduction velocity. The stimulated axons enter the spinal cord through the dorsal root, as indicated by the absence of an effect after the dorsal root is cut. These results thus provide evidence at the single-cell level that bears on the mechanism of recurrent sensibility. Our data are most easily interpreted as indicating that unmyelinated sensory processes travel for some distance in the ventral root but ultimately enter the spinal cord through the dorsal root.

In our opinion, the most likely arrangements are (a) that axons from the periphery travel into the ventral root and then loop back to enter the spinal cord through the dorsal root (13) or (b) that fibers from the meninges and connective tissue at the base of the cord travel back to the dorsal root ganglion via the ventral root, and the central processes of these cells enter the spinal cord through the dorsal root (8). Probably both of these fiber arrangements exist, and further work will be necessary to determine the percentage of each.

Not all sensory fibers in the ventral root ultimately enter the spinal cord through the dorsal root. Retrograde transport of the neuronal marker horseradish peroxidase indicates that some axons from dorsal root ganglion cells enter the spinal cord through the ventral root. These are the axons that violate the separation of function of the spinal roots, and they may be responsible for the failure of dorsal rhizotomy to relieve segmental pain. The proportion of these axons, as compared with those that ultimately enter the spinal cord through the dorsal root, is not known. Thus, it can be seen that the sensory axons in the ventral root, as in the dorsal root, are a diverse population, and it will be important to obtain quantitative data on the functional types and different morphologic arrangements of the sensory axons in the ventral roots.

In summary, we provide evidence at the single-cell level to show that some of the unmyelinated afferents in the ventral roots provide the explanation of recurrent sensibility. Whether or not other sensory fibers in the ventral root are responsible for failure of dorsal rhizotomy to relieve segmental pain can only be determined by further research.

ACKNOWLEDGMENTS

This work was supported by NIH grants NS-10161, NS-17039, NS-18830, and NS-21266 and by grants from the Moody Foundation and the American Heart Association, Texas Affiliate.

REFERENCES

1. Anderson, C. W., and Cushman, M. R. (1981): A simple and rapid method for making carbon fiber microelectrodes. *J. Neurosci. Meth.,* 4:435–436.
2. Clifton, G. L., Coggeshall, R. E., Vance, W. H., and Willis, W. D. (1976): Receptive fields of unmyelinated ventral root afferent fibres in the cat. *J. Physiol. (Lond.),* 256:573–600.
3. Coggeshall, R. E. (1980): Law of separation of function of the spinal roots. *Physiol. Rev.,* 60:716–755.
4. Coggeshall, R. E., Applebaum, M. L., Fazen, M., Stubbs, T. B., III, and Sykes, M. T. (1975): Unmyelinated axons in human ventral roots, a possible explanation for the failure of dorsal rhizotomy to relieve pain. *Brain,* 98:157–166.
5. Coggeshall, R. E., Coulter, J. D., and Willis, W. D. (1974): Unmyelinated axons in the ventral roots of the cat lumbosacral enlargment. *J. Comp. Neurol.,* 153:39–58.
6. Coggeshall, R. E., and Ito, H. (1977): Sensory fibres in ventral roots L7 and S1 in the cat. *J. Physiol. (Lond.),* 267:215–235.
7. Cranefield, P. F. (1974): *The Way In and The Way Out.* Futura, Mount Kisco, N.Y.
8. Dalsgaard, C. -J., Risling, M., and Cuello, C. (1982): Immunohistochemical localization of substance P in the lumbosacral spinal pia mater and ventral roots of the cat. *Brain Res.,* 246:168–171.
9. Frykholm, R., Hyde, J., Norlen, G., and Skoglund, C. R. (1953): On pain sensations produced by stimulation of ventral roots in man. *Acta Physiol. Scand.* [*Suppl.*], 106:455–459.
10. Gasser, H. S. (1950): Unmedullated fibers originating in dorsal root ganglia. *J. Gen. Physiol.,* 33:651–690.
11. Longhurst, J. C., Mitchell, J. H., and Moore, M. B. (1980): The spinal cord ventral root: An afferent pathway of the hind-limb pressor reflex in cats. *J. Physiol. (Lond.),* 301:467–476.
12. Magendie, F. (1822): Experiences sur les functions des racines des nerfs qui naissent de la moelle epiniere. *J. Physiol. Exp. Pathol.,* 2:366–372.
13. Risling, M., and Hildebrand, C. (1982): Occurrence of unmyelinated axon profiles at distal, middle and proximal levels in the ventral root L7 of cats and kittens. *J. Neurol. Sci.,* 56:219–231.
14. Voorhoeve, P. E., and Nauta, J. (1983): Do nociceptive ventral root afferents exert central somatic effects? In: *Advances in Pain Research and Therapy,* Vol. 5, edited by J. J. Bonica, U. Lindbloom, and A. Iggo, pp. 105–110. Raven Press, New York.

Advances in Pain Research and Therapy, Vol. 9, edited by H. L. Fields et al. Raven Press, New York © 1985.

Specialization in Nociceptive Pathways: Sensory Discrimination, Sensory Modulation, and Neural Connectivity

Ronald Dubner

Neurobiology and Anesthesiology Branch, National Institute of Dental Research, National Institutes of Health, Bethesda, Maryland 20205

Recent technical advances and multidisciplinary approaches have increased our knowledge of the encoding of pain messages in the brain and how these messages can be modified by intrinsic neural control systems. For example, behavioral models such as the tail-flick test, the hot-plate test, or the shock titration method have been used to infer pain in animals and have been combined with brain electrical stimulation or microinjection of opiates to examine pain-suppressing sites in the central nervous system (50,77). The study of opiate receptors and their endogenous ligands has involved biochemical, neuropharmacological, and behavioral approaches (46). Correlative electrophysiological, anatomical, and immunocytochemical techniques have been employed to unravel neural circuitry in the brainstem (5).

Our studies[1] have focused on the roles of the medullary and spinal dorsal horns in nociception. We have combined behavioral and electrophysiological methods in awake animals to study transmission of pain messages in the dorsal horn and its modulation. In addition, we are interested in the cellular mechanisms responsible for the encoding of noxious information into perceived sensations and appropriate behavior. We have used correlative neuroanatomical and electrophysiological techniques to investigate this underlying neural substrate of nociception. This chapter discusses our research strategies and findings at these two levels of analysis in the dorsal horn.

[1]My many collaborators on these studies are cited in the appropriate references. They all made important contributions to the success of these projects.

STRATEGIES FOR ASSESSING SENSORY DISCRIMINATIVE CAPACITIES OF NOCICEPTIVE PATHWAYS

It is important to examine behavioral correlates of pain in animals to determine the capacity of the nervous system to extract features of noxious stimuli from the environment. Such sensory discriminative features include the quality of the stimulus as well as its spatial, temporal, and intensive aspects. It is empirically obvious that humans have the capacity to detect and discriminate different aspects of other somatic sensations such as touch. We easily report the location and intensity of a tactile stimulus and its movement across the surface of the skin. These stimulus features are encoded and transmitted by specialized neural pathways in the spinal cord, thalamus, and cerebral cortex. On the other hand, pain is produced by intense mechanical, thermal, or chemical stimuli that generally result in nonpain sensations at lower stimulus magnitudes. It is difficult to determine whether the sensory discriminative aspects of the sensation are related to the preceding innocuous stimulation or to the noxious stimulus itself. It has been proposed that neural pathways involved in signaling pain merely provide information about the threat of noxious stimulation, with minimal capacities for providing information about fine discriminative aspects of the stimulus; see Melzack (51) for a review. This interpretation has led to the idea that pain sensations are the result of excessive stimulation of all types of peripheral receptors and are not transmitted by specialized nociceptive pathways.

The capacity of the nervous system to transmit features of noxious stimuli and the roles of specialized neural pathways in this sensory coding process can be established when neural studies are combined with behavioral data related to the sensory discriminative aspects of pain. One strategy is to determine whether or not animals can make fine discriminations in the pain sensitivity range. Such evidence would strongly suggest that specialized peripheraland central neural pathways are essential for transmitting this information. A related strategy is to examine the response range of neurons activated by noxious stimuli and to determine which class or classes of neurons can provide the minimal amount of information necessary to account for a particular behavior related to pain. For example, if an animal can be trained to discriminate different intensities of noxious heat stimuli, and only one class of neuron exhibits similar or greater thermal sensitivity, then these neurons most likely are essential for that discriminative behavior.

The choice of an appropriate behavioral task to assess sensory discriminative capacities in the pain sensitivity range is crucial. Human verbal reports of pain often are accompanied by reflexive and more complex behaviors to avoid or to escape noxious stimulation. Animals exhibit the same motor behaviors in response to noxious stimulation, and from them we can infer that an animal is experiencing pain. An ideal behavioral model should have the following characteristics (17,18,20,70,71): (a) It should distinguish between responses to innocuous and noxious stimuli. Simple escape and titration tasks often allow an animal to escape innocuous stimuli in anticipation of increasing intensities of stimuli in the noxious range. Tasks in which animals are required to detect or discriminate noxious stimuli avoid this problem (16,18,41). (b) The animals' behavioral responses should vary in magnitude with changes in stimulus intensity in the noxious range and permit an evaluation of responses over a range of stimuli acceptable to the animal, i.e., the range from threshold to tolerance. (c) The modification of behavioral responses by nonsensory factors such as attention, motivation, and motor performance should be distinguishable from the behavioral effects of changes in stimulus parameters. (d) Multiple threshold and suprathreshold behavioral measures should be used to infer pain. Consistent responses across different measures increase the reliabililty of inferences about pain. (e) The model should be susceptible to behavioral and pharmacological manipulations that alter the sensory discriminative capacities of the animal. For example, the effects of attention on discriminability (15) or opiate drugs on sensory performance (53) should be measurable.

Of equal importance is the selection of an appropriate noxious stimulus (Table 1). It should be a natural, quantifiable stimulus that has a rapid onset and termination. Pain threshold and tolerance levels should be comparable across species so that inferences can be made from one animal model to another. If one is interested in correlating behavior with nervous system activity, the stimulus should excite a restricted group of primary afferent fibers and activate only receptors preferentially sensitive in the noxious range. Otherwise, it may be difficult to establish that the neuron is coding features of a noxious stimulus independent of its response to innocuous

TABLE 1. *Selection of an appropriate noxious stimulus*

Requirements	Thermal	Electrical	Mechanical
Natural quantified stimulus that can be varied between threshold and tolerance	++	−	+
Rapid onset and termination	+	++	++
Threshold and tolerance levels comparable across species	++	−	+
Stimulation activates a restricted group of nociceptors	++	−	−
Stimulation activates only nociceptors in the pain sensitivity range	++	−	−
Stimulus quality is constant across pain sensitivity range in humans	++	−	++
Stimulation does not produce tissue damage	+/−	++	+/−

++, Fully satisfactory; +, minimally satisfactory; −unsatisfactory.

stimuli. This is a major disadvantage of intense electrical and mechanical stimuli that activate Aβ low-threshold mechanoreceptive afferents in addition to nociceptive afferents. Finally, it is important that the noxious stimulus does not produce irreversible tissue damage over the pain sensitivity range. Noxious thermal stimuli (temperatures of 45°C or greater) appear to meet these requirements best (Table 1), although they tend to produce tissue damage with repeated stimulation near tolerance levels. We selected the intensity feature of noxious heat stimuli as the independent variable in our studies (22,25). Although some investigators favor electrical stimulation (70,71), it does not adequately satisfy the preceding criteria (Table 1). In addition, electrical stimulation produces synchronous activation of all primary afferent neurons, thereby distorting the temporal pattern of discharge produced by natural stimuli. Such distortions may mask important modulating events related to nociception.

SPECIALIZED NOCICEPTIVE PATHWAYS ESSENTIAL FOR PAIN DISCRIMINATION

Evidence that there are specialized neural pathways exclusively involved in the coding of stimulus features in the noxious range has come from recent findings that specific nociceptors in skin, muscle, and viscera provide information about the intensity and location of noxious stimuli, as reviewed elsewhere (19). Only two classes of peripheral nociceptors respond to noxious heat. Those in one class, the unmyelinated polymodal nociceptors, respond to intense thermal, mechanical, and chemical stimuli and have remarkably similar characteristics in many different species (12,19,54). Those in the other class, called heat nociceptors or mechanothermal nociceptors, have myelinated axons that conduct in the Aδ range. They have been found only in monkeys (19) and humans (1). Both Aδ heat nociceptors (AHNs) and C polymodal nociceptors (CPNs) respond differentially to temperatures in the 45°C to 49°C range (Fig. 1). However, from such findings alone, one cannot conclude that there are exclusive, specialized nociceptive pathways in the brain or that the central nervous system utilizes specific information about stimulus quality and intensity coded by nociceptors. The alternative interpretations, that pain sensations are coded by the combined activities of *all* afferent fibers activated by the stimulus or that nociceptive pathways merely provide information about the presence of noxious stimuli, cannot be ruled out.

We have developed a number of behavioral models to examine whether or not the central nervous system utilizes information about stimulus quality and intensity coded by peripheral nociceptors. In an early study we trained monkeys to discriminate and escape noxious thermal stimuli applied to the face (17,18). In that task, the monkey pressed a panel button to initiate a trial, and at the same time the temperature at the skin-thermode

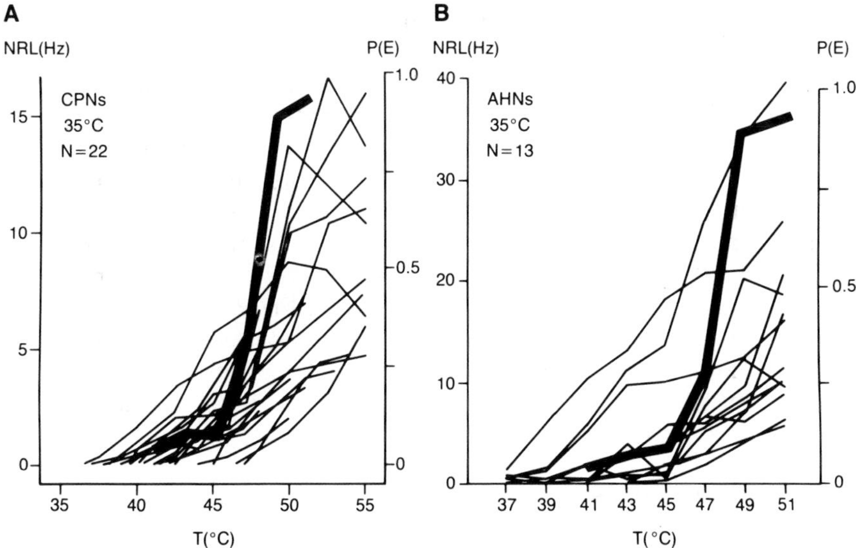

FIG. 1. Range of thermal sensitivity of 22 C polymodal nociceptors (CPNs) and 13 Aδ heat nociceptors (AHNs) compared with the temperature range over which 2 monkeys escaped noxious thermal stimuli. NRL(Hz) refers to the magnitude of the neuronal response expressed as the mean frequency of impulses in 3 sec (**A**) and 5 sec (**B**) plotted against final temperatures from 35°C adapting temperatures. The heavy line shows the escape probability, P(E). Neuronal data in A adapted from Beitel and Dubner (7), those in B from Dubner et al. (22). The escape probabilities are from Beitel and Dubner (7), and each data point is based on approximately 70 trials.

junction changed from 35°C to final temperatures varying from 37°C to 51°C. To receive a grape juice reward, the monkey continued to press the panel button until the temperature returned to the 35°C base line. If the temperature shift was aversive to the animal, it released the button and escaped the stimulus, but received no reward. Figure 1 shows that the temperature range over which 2 monkeys escaped noxious thermal stimuli (>45°C) corresponded closely to the range of maximum sensitivity of AHNs and CPNs studied in separate experiments. Escape probabilities ranged from approximately 10% at 45°C to 90% at 49°C and 51°C. A further examination of the escape latency distribution revealed that twice as many escapes occurred within 3.0 sec of stimulus onset during 51°C trials as during 49°C trials. Comparing this latency distribution to the latency of discharge of AHNs and CPNs revealed that these fast escapes were dependent on the discharge of AHNs (22). Within 2.5 sec of stimulus onset, only the cumulative discharge of AHNs on 51°C trials was significantly different from the discharge on 49°C trials. This difference occurred early enough to account for the higher proportion of fast escapes at 51°C than at 49°C. We conclude from these findings that AHNs are the only nociceptors that can provide the minimal information necessary for the monkeys' fast escapes. They provide unique and specific information about noxious thermal input that is essential in the performance of this learned behavior.

This behavioral escape task, however, does not provide information about the monkeys' ability to make fine thermal discriminations within the noxious heat range. Evidence for such discriminative capacity would clearly establish that nociceptive pathways code stimulus intensity and that such capabilities are dependent on the activity of specific nociceptors.

We addressed this question by having humans and one monkey perform two-choice discriminations between simultaneous thermal stimuli applied to both sides of the face (16,20). All subjects were presented stimulus pairs in the innocuous and noxious ranges and reported which stimulus was hotter. The humans received three standard stimuli, 39°C, 43°C, and 47°C, and the monkey received two standard stimuli, 39°C and 47°C. Each standard stimulus was paired with lesser-magnitude stimuli presented on the other side of the face. Human subjects and the monkey produced more accurate discriminations at 47°C than at 39°C, for every temperature difference greater than zero. The monkey's performance was virtually indistinguishable from that of the humans at 47°C. The mean difference threshold for humans of 0.31°C at 47°C was significantly different from the mean difference threshold for humans of 0.52°C at 39°C. The 47°C difference threshold of the monkey was 0.27°C, a value comparable to that for the human subjects.

These findings demonstrate that human subjects and monkeys can discriminate small differences between noxious thermal stimuli applied to the face and that the discriminative capabilities of the two species are quite similar within the noxious range. The results also suggest that the discriminative capacities of the two species are greater in the noxious thermal range than in the innocuous thermal range. Other studies have reported detection thresholds on human palmar skin of 0.1°C at 47°C (58) and on human digital pads of 0.3°C at 40°C (37), comparable to our results. It appears that thermal sensitivity in the noxious range is not peculiar to facial cutaneous zones, but rather is a general characteristic of thermal nociceptive pathways in primates.

The comparable discriminative abilities of humans and monkeys in the noxious thermal range suggest that heat sensitivity is coded by similar nociceptive afferents in both species. AHNs and CPNs innervating monkey facial skin are the only two afferent populations capable of providing this information (7,22). Warm fibers that exhibit maximum responses to warming of the skin are not sensitive to changes in stimulus intensity in this range and cannot provide such discriminative information (22,47).

The foregoing findings provide definitive evidence that activity in specific peripheral nociceptive pathways is essential for noxious heat discrimination. Specialized nociceptive pathways must also exist in the central nervous system and code heat intensity. Two general classes of neurons in the medullary and spinal dorsal horns receive input from peripheral nociceptors, as reviewed elsewhere (19,54,76). Those in one class, referred to as nociceptive-specific (NS) neurons, respond only to intense mechanical stimuli or mechanical, thermal, and other forms of noxious stimuli and receives input exclusively from different types of nociceptors. Those in the second class, called wide-dynamic-range (WDR) neurons, are activated by hair movement and weak mechanical stimuli, but respond maximally to intense and potentially tissue-damaging mechanical stimulation. Many WDR neurons respond to noxious heat. WDR neurons receive input from myelinated, low-threshold mechanoreceptors as well as from nociceptors. Some WDR and NS neurons send their axons directly to the thalamus, suggesting that they play a role in the perceived intensity of noxious stimuli.

What are the properties of these neurons in awake animals trained to detect and discriminate noxious stimuli? Do they code sensory discriminative information during behavioral tasks? We addressed these questions by examining the response properties of NS and WDR neurons while rhesus monkeys performed a modification of the discrimination task described earlier (14,45,49). In this task, each monkey had only one thermode on its face and was required to detect small temperature changes in the noxious heat range. The monkey pressed the panel button at the beginning of a trial. The thermode temperature then increased from 38°C to temperatures in the noxious heat range, remained at that level for a variable time period of 3 to 9 sec, and then increased an additional small step that was usually less than 1°C. The monkey was rewarded for releasing the button within 2 sec of this second temperature increase, and the temperature returned to the 38°C base line. Figure 2A shows that monkeys detected threshold second temperature shifts (T2) of approximately 0.1°C and 0.2°C from 46°C and 45°C temperatures (T1), respectively. Detection latencies were inversely related to the magnitude of suprathreshold T2 shifts and were dependent on the T1 level (Fig. 2B). Human subjects have similar detection thresholds and latencies in this task (14,15,58). These findings further substantiate that monkeys and humans can make fine discriminations in the pain sensitivity range. They also indicate that detection latencies provide a measure of the perceived intensity of small suprathreshold temperature shifts of 0.1°C to 1.0°C in the noxious heat range.

We recorded activities from projection and nonprojection WDR and NS neurons in the medullary dorsal horn while monkeys performed this detection task. There was a monotonic relationship between the magnitude of neuronal discharge and T2 intensity for almost all the neurons that were sensitive to temperature changes in the noxious heat range. Because both neuronal discharge and detection latencies were monotonically related to T2 levels, we directly compared them, as shown in Fig. 3. Note that the detection latency is inversely related to the magnitude of discharge from both the

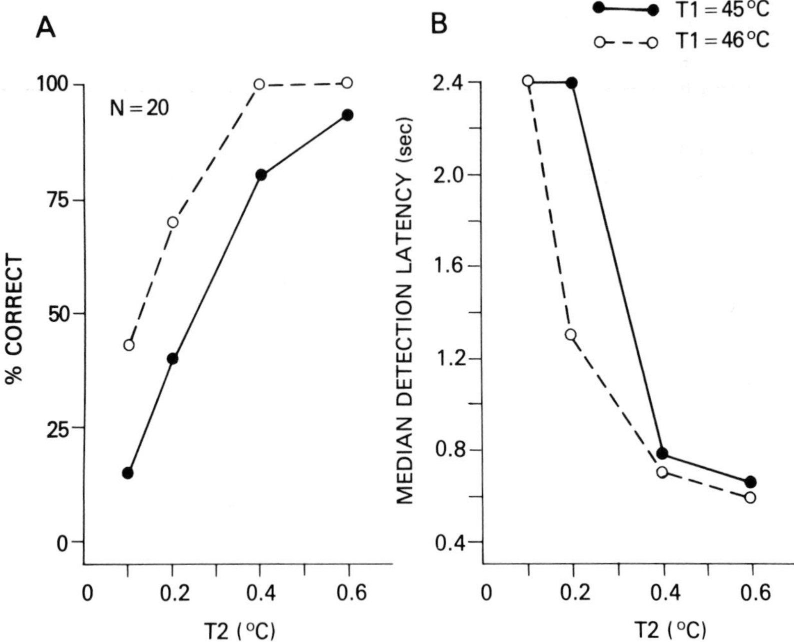

FIG. 2. Detection thresholds (**A**) and latencies (**B**) for 1 monkey from first temperature shifts (T1) of 45°C and 46°C. The detection threshold was approximately 0.13°C from 46°C and 0.25°C from 45°C. Note that detection latencies were inversely related to suprathreshold second temperature shifts (T2) and were dependent on T1 levels. Each point in A and B is based on 20 trials. Data from Kenshalo et al. (45).

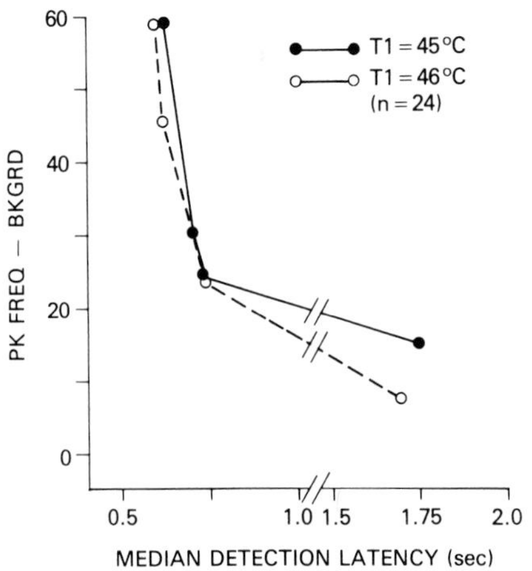

FIG. 3. Relationship between magnitude of neuronal discharge and median detection latencies from 45°C and 46°C first temperature shifts (T1). From 45°C, the T2 values were 0.4, 0.6, 0.8, and 1.5°C, and from 46°C, the T2 values were 0.2, 0.4, 0.6, and 0.8°C. Note that except for the near-threshold T2 values of 0.4 (45°C) and 0.2 (46°C), the relationship between peak discharge frequency (minus background) and detection latency was independent of T2 and T1 levels. Each point is the mean of 24 trials of neuronal data (four trials each from six WDR neurons). Median detection latencies were calculated from the same 24 trials. Data from Maixner et al. (49).

45°C and 46°C first temperature shifts. Furthermore, the magnitude of neuronal discharge predicts the behavioral detection latency, because the relationship is the same irrespective of the T1 or T2 levels. Intensities of T1 (45°C or 46°C) and T2 (0.2°C–0.8°C) that produced similar peak neuronal discharge frequencies also had similar detection latencies. These findings indicate that both WDR and NS neurons can provide the minimal information necessary for detection of small temperature changes in the noxious heat range and that these specialized central nociceptive pathways are essential for such fine discriminations.

We have some evidence that WDR neurons are better predictors of performance in the task than NS neurons. By comparing the magnitude of discharge on correctly detected trials with that on undetected trials of 0.2°C from a T1 of 46°C, we found that almost all WDR neurons showed greater activity on correctly detected trials. NS neurons did not show this difference. The findings suggest that WDR neurons are better predictors of the monkeys' ability to detect near-threshold changes from 45°C to 46°C temperatures. WDR neurons appear to code stimulus intensity in this range more precisely than NS neurons.

We conclude from these correlative behavioral and neural studies that nociceptive neurons in the medullary dorsal horn code stimulus intensity in the noxious heat range and that noxious heat discrimination is dependent on activation of this central nociceptive pathway projecting to the thalamus. The findings support the concept that pain is signaled by specialized central pathways that are exquisitely sensitive to stimulus features. They code stimulus intensity as precisely as non-nociceptive pathways involved in tactile and thermal discrimination. The idea that neural pathways signaling pain merely provide information about the threat of tissue-damaging stimulation can now be discarded.

BEHAVIORAL AND PHARMACOLOGICAL MANIPULATIONS THAT ALTER DISCRIMINATION IN THE NOXIOUS RANGE

One cannot conclude from the foregoing findings that activation of specialized nociceptive pathways always produces pain. There is evidence that these pathways are subject to considerable modulation. Behavioral factors are known to modify pain experience. For example, how humans respond to pain depends on the situation in which the pain occurs, previous pain experience, cultural background, and the belief that an analgesic treatment will be effective (24,51). Recent studies provide evidence that pain signals can be modified at the first central synapse in the spinal cord or the brainstem. The information transmitted by dorsal horn output pathways is not immutable and is subject to descending control from more rostral brainstem sites (4,19,75). Electrical stimulation or administration of opiate drugs activates these descending pathways and produces a profound behavioral analgesia. Naloxone, a specific opiate antagonist, reverses these effects. A number of reviews have provided evidence in support of these opioid-mediated systems (50,67,77). Other findings indicate that neuropeptides such as the enkephalins and the endorphins represent the endogenous opioid compounds that act at some of these sites (46). Activation of these pathways by stressful procedures (19) can also produce analgesia. In addition, nonopioid-related descending pathways have been identified and involve the release of neurotransmitters such as norepinephrine and serotonin in the medullary and spinal dorsal horns (19).

Effects of Behavioral Contingencies

What role do these descending control systems play in the processing of sensory information under more natural behavioral conditions? In our correlative behavioral and neural studies we examined whether or not behavioral variables such as attention and stimulus relevance modulate the thermal responses of medullary dorsal horn projection and nonprojection neurons (13,15,38). In these studies the term *attention* refers to a selective phenomenon that influences an animal's response to competing environmental stimuli. The effect of selective attention on behavioral responses to competing thermal and visual stimuli was assessed in monkeys. In one study (14,15) the monkeys were trained in the thermal detection task described earlier. Second temperature shifts (T2) that the monkeys could detect approximately 75% of the time were chosen. The monkeys also were trained to perform a visual detection task in which they were rewarded for releasing the response button within 2 sec of onset of a cue light. Visual and thermal trials were presented randomly, and the monkeys could not anticipate the relevant cue in a trial. To aid in the detection, on some thermal trials a signal was presented throughout the trial indicating that the reinforced cue was a temperature shift (T2). Similarly, on some visual trials a different signal was presented throughout the trial indicating that the reinforced cue was to be the cue light;. The signal lights allowed the monkeys to attend to the relevant cue on that trial, and we examined whether or not such information improved their performance of the task. Figure 4A shows that both monkeys tested in this attentional task responded with shorter mean latencies on signaled thermal trials than on unsignaled thermal trials. The mean percentage of undetected trials ("no responses") across sessions was smaller on signaled trials than on unsignaled trials (Fig. 4B). Thus, attentional manipulations influenced both the detectability of intensity changes in the noxious heat range and the latency of correct detections. Similar results were obtained when humans performed a selective attention task involving spatially separate thermal stimuli applied to both sides of the face (14). Although we do not know if these attentional effects on noxious heat detection are reflected in changes in activity of trigeminothalamic neurons,

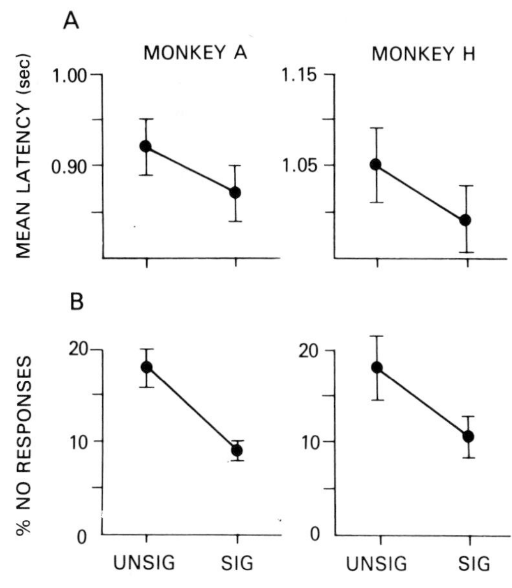

FIG. 4. Mean detection latency (**A**) and mean percentage "no response" (**B**) for 2 monkeys during unsignaled and signaled thermal conditions in the attentional task. Performances were averaged across 13 sessions of 160 trials each. *Vertical lines* show SEM. Differences between signaled and unsignaled conditions were statistically significant in all cases. (Adapted from Bushnell et al., ref. 14.)

the neural substrate of selective attention probably involves modulatory systems active in specialized trigeminal nociceptive pathways.

In an earlier study, we showed that behavioral contingencies, such as stimulus relevance, modulate the activity of medullary dorsal horn neurons (13,38). The responses to noxious heat during a task in which monkeys discriminated innocuous from noxious stimuli were compared with responses to similiar stimuli presented between trials and not related to the animal's behavior in the task. When the monkey was using the stimulus as a discriminative cue during the task, the magnitude of the neuronal discharge was greater and the neuronal response latency was shorter than when the stimulus was unrelated to the monkey's behavior. Because the monkeys attended to relevant noxious heat stimuli that led to reinforcement, attentional differences may be a major factor in the enhancement of the response of medullary dorsal horn neurons during these behavioral tasks. Such behavioral modulation may be related to descending pathways originating from more rostral brain sites.

Pharmacological Manipulations

Morphine and endogenous opioid substances activate descending pain modulatory pathways and act directly on dorsal horn nociceptive neurons (4,50,77). It is commonly assumed that morphine-like drugs produce clinical analgesia by altering the unpleasantness or aversiveness of pain sensations. Because dorsal horn neurons are part of specialized nociceptive pathways, these opiate drugs should also alter sensory discriminative aspects of pain. Fentanyl and morphine recently have been shown to reduce the intensity of pain sensations in humans (35,36). However, those studies did not elucidate the sites of action of opiates on discriminative ability in the noxious range. To further elucidate the actions of opiates, we microinjected morphine into the monkey medullary dorsal horn and examined its effects on the detection of noxious heat (53). Monkeys were trained in the thermal detection task described previously, and varying doses of morphine (1–15 μg in 0.2 μl) were injected. Figure 5 shows the effects of morphine on a monkey's ability to detect suprathreshold (approximately 90% correct detec-

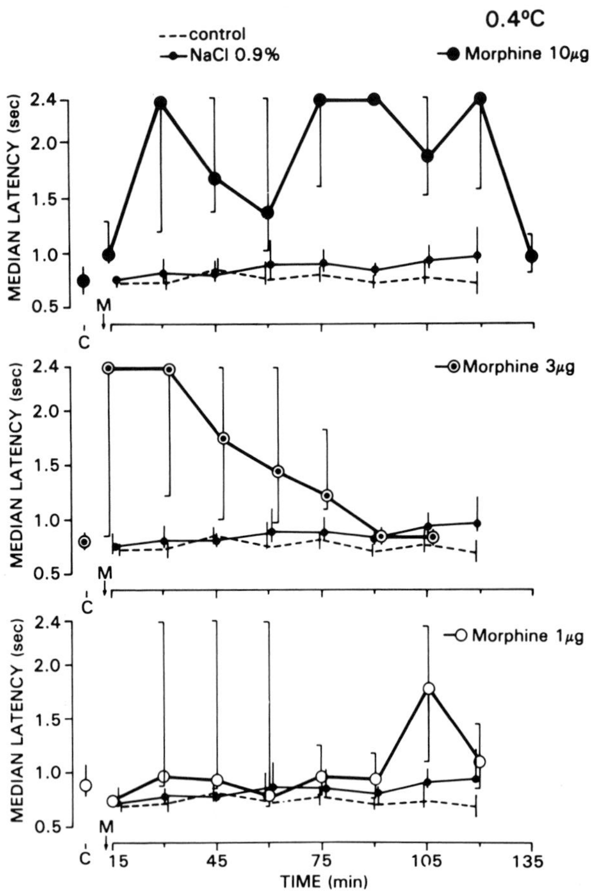

FIG. 5. Effects of morphine microinjection (1, 3, and 10 μg in 0.2 μl) into the medullary dorsal horn on a monkey's ability to detect 0.4°C second temperature shifts from a 46°C base line (first temperature shift). Abscissa shows the time after morphine microinjection. C = control point in each session. Data from control and saline sessions also are shown. Each point is the median of eight trials. A cutoff value of 2.4 sec was used on undetected trials. *Vertical lines* show semiinterquartile range. Data from Oliveras et al. (53).

tions) second temperature shifts (T2) of 0.4°C from a 46°C base line. There was a dose-dependent effect on detectability. Median detection latencies increased dramatically within 15 min of drug administration at the higher doses of 3 and 10 μg. The 1-μg dose produced an early increase in response variability, with larger increases in median latencies occurring within 1.5 to 2 hr. The effects of morphine microinjection persisted for up to 2 hr and could be reversed by systemic administration of the opiate receptor antagonist naloxone (0.5 mg/kg s.c.). These behavioral changes were not related to nonspecific attentional or motoric effects of morphine, because the monkeys were able to simultaneously perform an innocuous cooling detection task of similar difficulty with no change in detection latencies. The results confirm previous findings in humans suggesting that opiate drugs have a pharmacologically specific effect on sensory discriminative capacities in the noxious range (36). They also show that the site of action of these effects is at an early stage of sensory processing in the medullary dorsal horn. The findings provide additional support for a specialized role for dorsal horn neurons in coding stimulus intensity information in the noxious range.

Dorsal horn neurons involved in signaling noxious heat intensities receive input from AHNs or CPNs, or both. The increase in behavioral latencies produced by morphine in the thermal detection task suggests that neurons receiving input from AHNs are affected. If morphine's effects were exclusively on thermal nociceptive neurons receiving input only from the more slowly conducting CPNs, it is not likely that detection latencies would be changed. Evidence in support of this conclusion comes from studies of opiate effects on Aδ and C nociceptors using models of first and second pain in humans (56,71). Brief noxious heat or electrical stimuli to the hand or foot produce an initial sharp or "pricking" pain sensation that is followed approximately 1 sec later by a "burning" or "throbbing" sensation. These first and second pain sensations are attributable to activity in Aδ and C fibers, respectively. We have used brief noxious heat pulses (peak temperature 51.5°C) to evoke these sensations. Application of successive heat pulses at intervals of 3 sec or less produces a decrease in the intensity of first pain and an increase in the intensity of second pain. The suppression of first pain results in a progressive increase in reaction times after six to eight heat pulses that plateaus at latency values consistent with the report of second pain (56). Morphine, given to chronic pain patients in doses that reduced the intensity of their clinical pain, increased the latency of first and second pain in this model (R. H. Gracely et al., *unpublished observations*). There were more robust effects on CPN-evoked second pain than on AHN-evoked first pain. Nonspecific effects of morphine on attention, motivation, or motor behavior were ruled out by having patients provide reaction times to repetitive auditory stimuli. Morphine had no effect on the detection of auditory stimuli. Our findings are different from those of Vierck et al. (71), who reported that morphine suppressed only second pain sensations evoked by electrical stimuli. These differences may be related to the highly synchronous activation of primary afferent neurons produced by electrical stimulation, thereby masking any morphine effects on Aδ activity. Nevertheless, both studies support the notion that morphine influences noxious thermal discrimination.

ACTIVATION OF SPECIALIZED NOCICEPTIVE PATHWAYS BY STIMULI UNRELATED TO PAIN DISCRIMINATION

The presence of behaviorally and pharmacologically specific modulation of dorsal horn neuronal activity provides strong evidence that the output of these specialized nociceptive pathways is not immutable. Other findings suggest that these nociceptive pathways can be activated by behaviorally relevant stimuli that are unrelated to noxious thermal discrimination. Some medullary dorsal horn nociceptive neurons activated by noxious thermal stimuli exhibit additional responses during behavior that are independent of stimulus parameters or stimulus modality (13,21,26). These task-related responses sometimes occur at trial initiation and sometimes after the signal to release the response button, irrespective of whether the cue is an innocuous thermal or visual stimulus. Similar stimuli that do not have any behavioral relevance outside of the task do not produce these responses. Task-related responses are associated with sensory cues that are components of the sequence of behavioral events leading to reception of the reward. These responses occur in mechanoreceptive as well as in nociceptive neurons and are not necessarily related to the discrimination of noxious stimuli.

Figure 6 shows the excitatory and inhibitory task-related responses of two WDR neurons while a monkey performed a thermal discrimination task. When characterized outside of the behavioral task, these neurons were classified as WDR neurons, based on their responses to mechanical stimuli. In addition, neither cell had a thermal response to any temperature tested. Figure 6A illustrates the responses of a neuron that had an excitatory response during the trials and a response burst after the signal to release the key for reward. The neuron whose responses are shown in Fig. 6B exhibited an increase in activity associated with the light cue indicating that a trial could begin. As the monkey initiated the trial, neuronal activity was reduced and was completely suppressed throughout the trial. There was a return of activity just preceding release of the panel button for reward. Figure 6 also shows that there was little correlation between lip EMG activity and neuronal activity during the trials. Consequently, it is unlikely that these task-related responses were an artifact caused by mechanical stimulation of the face. Thermal nociceptive WDR and NS neurons also exhibited task-related responses to innocuous thermal and visual cues. These findings indicate that specialized nociceptive pathways are subject to modulation unrelated to noxious stimulation. Their activation, therefore, does not always produce pain. The same nociceptive neuron that exhibits sensory discriminative

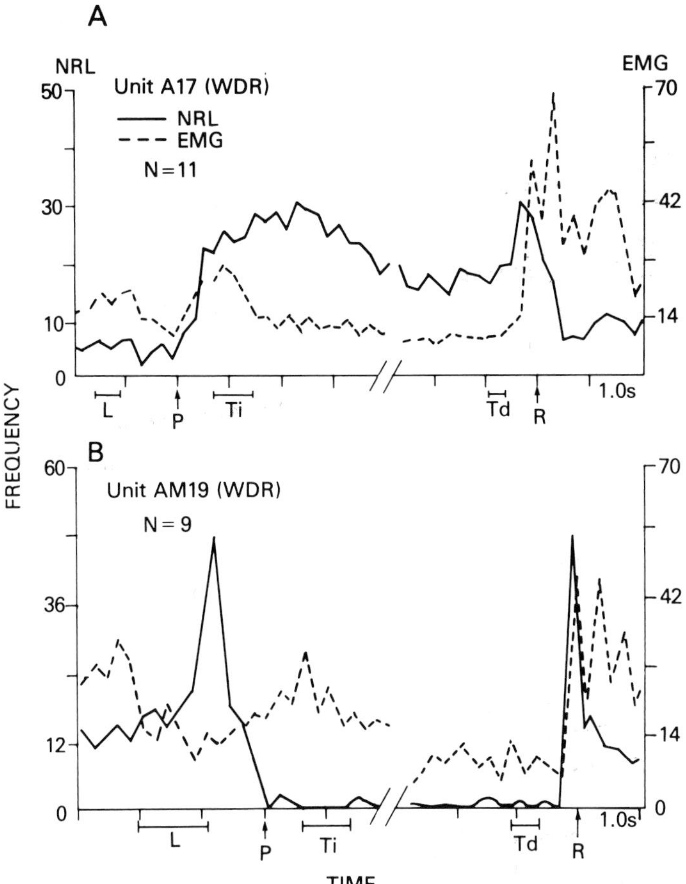

FIG. 6. Peristimulus histograms showing excitatory and inhibitory task-related responses of two WDR neurons while a monkey performed a thermal discrimination task. *Solid lines* (NRL) show neuronal activity, and *dashed lines* (EMG) show orbicularis oris activity. Each line represents the average of 11 trials in A and 9 trials in B. All temperatures were below the thermal threshold of the neurons. Histograms are synchronized around button press (P) and button release (R). Brackets under the abscissa mark the range of time of occurrence on individual trials of button light onset (L), temperature increase (Ti), and temperature decrease (Td). (**A** adapted from Bushnell et al., ref. 13, and **B** from Duncan et al., ref. 26.)

properties in response to noxious stimuli may also exhibit task-related responses independent of stimulus parameters.

NEURAL CIRCUITRY MEDIATING SENSORY DISCRIMINATION AND SENSORY MODULATION IN SPECIALIZED NOCICEPTIVE PATHWAYS

The performance of behavioral tasks such as those previously described approximates the demands placed on an animal in a natural environment in which extraction of significant stimulus features is necessary for survival. How is the behavioral context in which a stimulus is received recognized by the nervous system? What underlying cellular mechanisms and principles of neural connectivity account for the amplification of novel or behaviorally relevant signals?

Recent findings suggest that the broad repertoire of responses available to dorsal horn neurons involves the multiplicity of neurotransmitters or chemical messengers active at this site. The list of amino acids, amines, and peptides localized to the dorsal horn has grown rapidly in the last few years. The functional diversity of individual transmitters has led to a reevaluation of how chemical messengers act in the nervous system. Some neurochemicals such as gamma-aminobutyric acid (GABA) and glutamate act as conventional inhibitory and excitatory neurotransmitters in the dorsal horn, respectively. They produce changes in ionic conductances, with resulting membrane hyperpolarization or depolarization. On the other hand, many neuropeptides do not produce changes in membrane ionic permeability or membrane polarization but act only to enhance or reduce the effectiveness of another conventional chemical mediator. Their activity is often voltage-sensitive and dependent on membrane events produced by other transmitters. Some transmitters produce different effects even at the same locus. For example, enkephalin in the dorsal horn may alter specific ionic conductance like a conventional neurotransmitter or exert a modulatory role without any direct effect on membrane polarization or ionic permeability (78,79). The multiplicity of actions by different chemical messengers has led to new principles of neural connectivity in the dorsal horn and elsewhere. The same neurons may receive input from many neurotransmitters, and each neurotransmitter may have multiple actions. With these new principles in mind, we have explored the roles of different neurotransmitters in dorsal horn circuitry.

Similar to other relay pathways in the nervous system, the medullary and spinal dorsal horns consist of four major functional components: (a) the central terminals of primary afferent neurons that relay signals from distant sites; (b) the output neurons that transmit information to distant sites; (c) local circuit neurons that control transmission in a restricted region; and (d) the axon terminals of extrinsic neurons that arise from restricted sites but have multiple targets. We already have identified the trigeminothalamic tract and its counterpart at spinal levels as a major output system in specialized nociceptive pathways. Let us focus on the neuronal connectivity of dorsal horn lamina I where the cells of origin of the trigeminothalamic and spinothalamic tracts are highly concentrated (19,76). Primary nociceptive afferents terminate here and in the outer part of the substantia gelatinosa, lamina IIa. Lamina II consists almost entirely of local circuit neurons that can directly or indirectly modulate the output of the spinothalamic neurons in lamina I. The axon terminals of extrinsic neurons localized to the super-

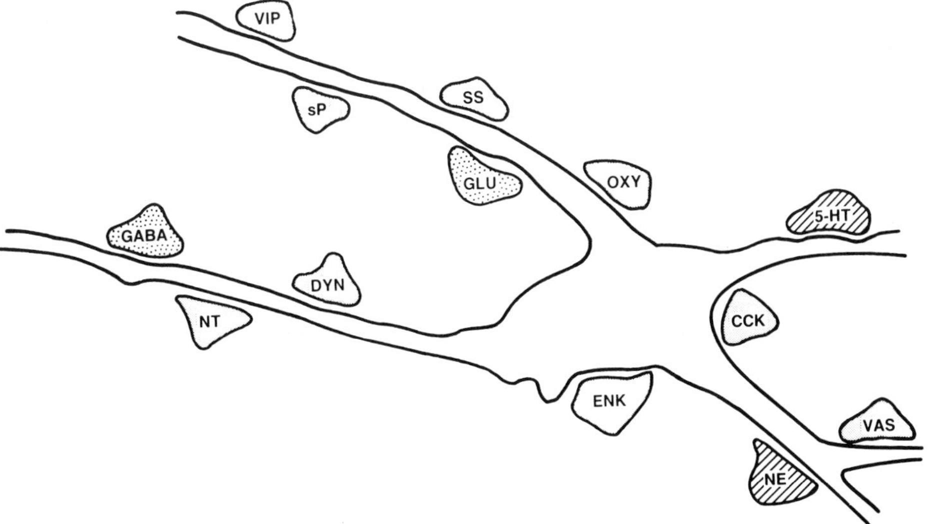

FIG. 7. Soma and proximal dendrites of a lamina I thalamic projection neuron showing candidate neurotransmitters that may directly modulate the output of such neurons: VIP, vasoactive intestinal polypeptide; sP, substance P; SS, somatostatin; GLU, glutamate; OXY, oxytocin; 5-HT, serotonin; CCK, cholecystokinin; GABA, gamma-aminobutyric acid; NT, neurotensin; DYN, dynorphin; ENK, enkephalin; NE, norepinephrine; VAS, vasopressin. The shadings indicate groups of amino acids *(large dots),* monamines *(stripes),* and peptides *(small dots).*

ficial dorsal horn arise from multiple brainstem sources. Figure 7 is a diagram showing most of the candidate neurotransmitters found in lamina I that could directly modulate the output of spinothalamic neurons. By utilizing immunocytochemistry in combination with the intracellular horseradish peroxidase (HRP) and retrograde HRP techniques, it is possible to examine the direct interaction of various neurochemically defined axon terminals with projection neurons and local circuit neurons in laminae I and II (23,60).

Afferents to Identified Laminae I and II Neurons

Evidence is accumulating that the peptide substance P is a neurotransmitter in small-diameter nociceptive afferents, as reviewed elsewhere (19). Substance P has been identified in small neurons in trigeminal and spinal ganglia and may be a neurotransmitter in some C polymodal nociceptors. The peptide is concentrated superficially in laminae I and IIa and in the neck of the dorsal horn (lamina V). Dorsal root transection markedly decreases substance P levels, indicating that most dorsal horn substance P originates from primary afferent axons. Substance P immunoreactive contacts have been found on lamina I thalamic projection neurons (57), lamina I nonprojection neurons (39), and lamina II stalked cells (R. Dubner, *unpublished observations*). It cannot be assumed, however, that these contacts originate only from primary afferent axons, because substance P is found in some laminae I and II neurons (28,43,48) and in descending axons arising from brainstem neurons (29,42). Following spinal cord transection there is a slight decrease in substance P levels in the superficial dorsal horn, indicating that descending substance P axons terminate there. Although it is known that substance P in primary axons acts as an excitatory transmitter, it is not known whether descending substance P axons have excitatory or inhibitory actions.

Essentially all of the serotonin (5-HT) found in the dorsal horn originates from descending brainstem neurons, because chronic spinal cord transection results in complete depletion of 5-HT below the lesion (62). We examined sites of interaction between descending 5-HT axons and lamina I neurons in two separate experiments. By combining 5-HT immunocytochemistry with the intracellular HRP method, we were able to correlate physiological properties with cell morphology and 5-HT input (40,52). The intracellular HRP method produces a Golgi-like staining of the neurons' dendritic arbor and permits an analysis of the distribution of 5-HT contacts on the soma and dendrites. HRP-filled lamina I neurons that were characterized physiologically ($N = 13$) were either nociceptive-specific or WDR neurons. The effect of nucleus raphe magnus stimulation was examined in 12 of these neurons, and all were inhibited. All lamina I neurons exhibited many 5-HT immunoreactive contacts (average of 74 contacts per cell, $N = 12$). The limits of light microscopy do not allow us to conclude unequivocally that these contacts are sites of synaptic interaction. However, electron microscopic studies using the same immunocytochemical techniques (64) indicated that 5-HT immunoreactive varicosities are in close apposition to dendritic profiles without intervening glia. Serial sections of these varicosities invariably revealed synaptic contacts with the apposing dendrite. Therefore, we conclude that the contacts observed with the light microscope most likely represent sites of synaptic interaction.

Although it was not directly determined in the previously cited study that the lamina I neurons had axons that projected to the thalamus, direct evidence for 5-HT contacts on thalamic projection neurons was obtained in a second double-label experiment in which the retrograde HRP method was combined with 5-HT immunocytochemistry (60,61). Retrogradely filled lamina I thalamic projection neurons of the monkey medullary and spinal dorsal horns exhibited variable numbers of 5-HT immunoreactive contacts on their somata and proximal dendrites. These contacts were shown to be sites of synaptic interaction at the ultrastructural level. These observations are in agreement with iontophoretic studies that suggest a postsynaptic inhibitory action of 5-HT on spinothalamic tract neurons (73). The findings suggest the presence of a long inhibitory pathway, without intervening inhibitory local circuit neurons, from the brainstem to dorsal horn output systems.

There also are numerous 5-HT immunoreactive contacts on some local circuit neurons in dorsal horn lamina II, the substantia gelatinosa layer. The most common local circuit neurons in lamina II are called stalked cells and islet cells. They have been found in the medullary and spinal dorsal horns of cat and monkey (8,32,55). The unmyelinated axon of the stalked cell arborizes profusely in lamina I, presumably synapsing on lamina I thalamic projection neurons. All stalked cells identified with the intracellular HRP method have been either NS or WDR nociceptive neurons (8,52). Gobel (32) has proposed that stalked cells function as excitatory local circuit neurons. Although there are data consistent with this hypothesis (8,55), the possibility that the stalked cell/lamina I synaptic linkage is inhibitory cannot be excluded.

Islet cells, the other major type of lamina II local circuit neurons, have their cell bodies located in laminae IIa or IIb. Islet cell axons are unmyelinated and arborize profusely within or near their dendritic trees. Islet cells are presumed to be inhibitory local circuit neurons (32). Islet cells in lamina IIa are nociceptive neurons (either WDR or NS), whereas lamina IIb islet cells respond exclusively to low-threshold mechanoreceptive input (8,52).

We used the intracellular HRP method in combination with 5-HT immunocytochemistry to study the 5-HT contact distribution on lamina II neurons (23,52). All stalked cells exhibited numerous 5-HT immunoreactive contacts (average of 63 contacts per cell, $N = 7$). The effect of nucleus raphe magnus stimulation on four of these neurons was examined, and all were inhibited. In contrast, nucleus raphe magnus stimulation had no effect on laminae IIa or IIb islet cells ($N = 5$). In addition, all tissue sections containing islet cells that were immunocytochemically stained with 5-HT antiserum ($N = 7$) had very few 5-HT immunoreactive contacts. It appears that direct descending 5-HT postsynaptic inhibition modifies the output of lamina II local circuit neurons as well as lamina I projection neurons. However, lamina II local circuit neurons are differentially affected; stalked cells, which can directly modulate the output of lamina I projection neurons, are heavily innervated, as are the lamina I projection neurons themselves. In contrast, islet cells whose axons are confined to lamina II have few 5-HT contacts.

Other studies have revealed the existence of a second neurochemically distinct monamine descending pathway terminating in the dorsal horn (5,19). Descending norepinephrine (NE) systems originate in the pons and mediate inhibition and possibly excitation in the dorsal horn. Axon terminals of pontine NE-containing cell groups have been localized in laminae I and II (72). However, it is not known if descending NE systems act directly on trigeminothalamic and spinothalamic neurons or if their effects are mediated via dorsal horn local circuit neurons.

Neurochemical Diversity of Identified Local Circuit Neurons

Since opioid mechanisms appear to be critical in modulating the sensory discriminative capacities of dorsal horn nociceptive pathways, it is important to determine the precise circuitry of endogenous opioids at this site. Which morphological types of neurons receive enkephalin or dynorphin input? What interactions are there between descending pathways and opioid-containing neurons?

By combining enkephalin (ENK) immunocytochemistry with the retrograde HRP method, it has been shown that ENK immunoreactive endings make direct synaptic contact with the soma and proximal dendrites of approximately one-third of lamina I thalamic projection neurons (59,63). The most densely innervated lamina I neurons often are the large Waldeyer cells. ENK immunoreactive contacts on thalamic projection neurons have been shown at the ultrastructural level to be sites of synaptic interaction (59,63). These findings suggest that opioid peptides act, at least in part, via postsynaptic mechanisms. Iontophoretic studies provide additional evidence that ENK inhibits the activity of thalamic projection neurons at postsynaptic sites (74).

Although some ENK appears to be localized to descending axons (11), studies of ENK in the dorsal horn following spinal transection reveal a negligible decrease in ENK immunoreactivity (43,62,65), suggesting that most of the ENK in the dorsal horn originates from intrinsic neurons. In cats treated with colchicine to enhance cell body staining, many ENK-containing neurons are found in laminae I and II (10,30,44).

ENK-containing lamina I neurons appear to be distinct from thalamic projection neurons. Using a fluorescent retrograde tracer in combination with ENK immunocytochemistry, Basbaum and colleagues (3) found no double labeling of lamina I thalamic projection neurons. In general, the thalamic projection neurons formed a thin band superficial to the ENK-containing, nonprojection, lamina I neurons. We suspect that nociceptive lamina I neurons with local axon collaterals are reasonable candidates for the ENK-containing lamina I neurons (9). Their axon terminals arborize in lamina I and probably synapse on the dendrites of lamina I thalamic projection neurons.

Some lamina IIa stalked cells and some lamina IIb islet cells are ENK-containing neurons (10,30,43,44). Because the axons of stalked cells arborize in lamina I among the dendrites of lamina I projection neurons, ENK-containing stalked cells are a second potential source of ENK input on thalamic projection neurons. Lamina IIb islet cell axons and dendrites are confined to lamina IIb and cannot directly influence output systems in lamina I. However, islet cell dendrites contain synaptic vesicles and probably synapse on the dendrites of stalked cells (33,34). Thus, islet cells may indirectly modulate the activity of lamina I neurons via the stalked cell/lamina I linkage.

Other evidence suggests that subpopulations of laminae I and II local circuit neurons are neurochemically diverse. In addition to ENK-containing lamina I neurons, other lamina I neurons contain GABA (2,6,43). It is likely that these GABA-containing neurons are in synaptic contact with thalamic projection neurons and mediate inhibitory interactions. The distribution of dynorphin, another opioid peptide, is concentrated in lamina I (5). The number of dynorphin-containing lamina I neurons far exceeds the number of ENK-containing neurons in the same region. The analgesia produced by intrathecal dynorphin likely is mediated via inhibition of superficial dorsal horn neurons (5).

In addition to ENK-containing stalked cells, other stalked cells may contain GABA (2,43) and inhibit the activity of thalamic projection neurons via their lamina I axonal arbors. The neurochemical diversity of islet cells is even more complex. Besides ENK-containing islet cells in lamina II, GABA (2,33,34) and neurotensin (66) have been suggested as neurotransmitters in islet cells. The list of peptides in otherwise unidentified lamina II neurons includes substance P (28,43), cholecystokinin (28), somatostatin (43), and neuropeptide Y (avian pancreatic polypeptide) (43).

Figure 8 is a schema of proposed dorsal horn circuitry based on identified connections between lamina I projection neurons and neurochemically defined axon terminals. Substance P is probably an excitatory neurotransmitter in some nociceptive afferents. Substance P axons synapse on thalamic projection neurons and laminae I and IIa local circuit neurons. Substance-P-containing descending axons (action unknown) also may synapse

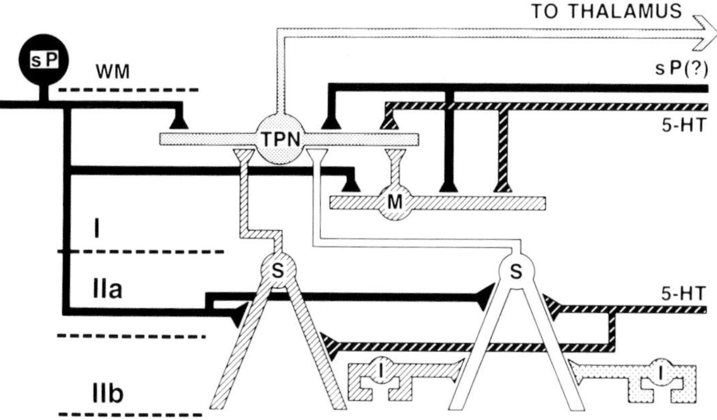

FIG. 8. Proposed dorsal horn circuitry in laminae I and II. Lamina borders and white matter (WM) are represented at the left. Primary afferent axons schematically enter at the left, and descending extrinsic axons enter at the right. TPN, thalamic projection neuron; M, lamina I local circuit neuron; S, stalked cell; I, islet cell; sP, substance P; 5-HT, serotonin. *Striped cells* are enkephalin-containing local circuit neurons; *cross-hatched cell* is a GABA-containing local circuit neuron. (See text for details.)

on thalamic projection neurons. It is established that ENK terminals synapse on lamina I thalamic projection neurons. This postsynaptic inhibitory input likely is provided directly by ENK-containing local circuit neurons in lamina I and ENK-containing stalked cells in lamina II. ENK-containing and GABA-containing lamina IIb islet cells form dendrodendritic synapses on other stalked cells (transmitter unknown) and thus indirectly influence the output of the thalamic projection neurons. Descending 5-HT axons can exert their effects directly on thalamic projection neurons without intervening local circuit neurons. The presence of 5-HT contacts on stalked cells supports recent findings of an ENK spinal link in descending 5-HT circuitry (31) and suggests that this pathway also influences lamina I output systems.

How does this proposed neural connectivity play a role in the neural transmission and recognition of behaviorally relevant sensory signals in the noxious range? Because the circuitry is obviously incompletely known, we can only begin to suggest mechanisms by which sensory information in nociceptive pathways is transmitted, enhanced, or suppressed. The four functional components of the superficial dorsal horn appear to utilize different chemical mediators. The input-output system relaying information between distant sites involves highly secure synaptic transmission. The conventional type of excitatory transmitter in this pathway is not known. Substance P is a slowly acting neurotransmitter in primary afferent neurons that may augment noxious signals by enhancing the effectiveness of the conventional transmitter. Local circuit neurons containing GABA and ENK may have inhibitory effects that sharpen the features of the stimulus through inhibitory surround and "signal-to-noise ratio" mechanisms. The multitargeted effects of descending 5-HT-containing and NE-containing neurons in the dorsal horn suggest that they provide a global enhancement or suppression of activity that enables nociceptive pathways to respond more effectively to incoming sensory information. Such mechanisms probably form the neural basis of behavioral constructs that we have termed attention, stimulus relevance, and task-relatedness. 5-HT pathways appear to increase motorneuron excitability and enhance organized motor behaviors associated with various stages of arousal (68,69). In preparation for such behaviors there probably is simultaneous suppression of extraneous incoming sensory signals in the dorsal horn, thereby enhancing the effectiveness of relevant signals. Ascending NE pathways have been shown to amplify novel and behaviorally relevant signals in the cerebral cortex and cerebellum (27). Descending NE pathways may have similar effects in the dorsal horn.

It is clear that the neurochemical diversity and the synaptic circuitry of the dorsal horn are sufficiently complex to account for the plasticity of the pain message that is sent to rostral brain centers. Although this plasticity is often thought of in terms of analgesia, it seems certain that a more fundamental aspect of central nervous system processing is being revealed.

ACKNOWLEDGMENTS

I am extremely grateful to all my colleagues who contributed to the research findings presented, to Drs. Bennett, Kenshalo, Maixner, and Ruda, who reviewed previous drafts, and to Edith Welty for preparation of the manuscript.

REFERENCES

1. Adriaensen, H., Gybels, J., Handwerker, H. O., and Van Hees, J. (1983): Response properties of thin myelinated (A-delta) fibers in human skin nerves. *J. Neurophysiol.,* 49:111–122.
2. Barber, R. P., Vaughn, J. E., and Roberts, E. (1982): The cytoarchitecture of gabaergic neurons in rat spinal cord. *Brain Res.,* 238:305–328.
3. Basbaum, A. I. (1982): Anatomical substrates for the descending control of nociception. In: *Brain Stem Control of Spinal Mechanisms,* edited by B. Sjöland and A. Björklund, pp. 119–133. Elsevier, Amsterdam.
4. Basbaum, A. I., and Fields, H. L. (1978): Endogenous pain control mechanisms: Review and hypothesis. *Ann. Neurol.,* 4:451–462.
5. Basbaum, A. I., and Fields, H. L. (1984): Endogenous pain control systems: Brain stem spinal pathways and endorphin circuitry. *Annu. Rev. Neurosci.,* 7:309–338.
6. Basbaum, A. I., Glazer, E. J., and Oertel, W. (1981): A light and EM analyses of immunoreactive glutamic acid decarboxylase (GAD) in the spinal and trigeminal dorsal horn of the cat. *Soc. Neurosci. Abstr.,* 7:528.
7. Beitel, R. E., and Dubner, R. (1976): Response of unmyelinated (C) polymodal nociceptors to thermal stimuli applied to monkey's face. *J. Neurophysiol.,* 39:1160–1175.
8. Bennett, G. J., Abdelmoumene, M., Hayashi, H., and Dubner, R. (1980): Physiology and morphology of substantia gelatinosa neurons intracellularly stained with horseradish peroxidase. *J. Comp. Neurol.,* 194:809–827.
9. Bennett, G. J., Abdelmoumene, M., Hayashi, H., Hoffert, M. J., and Dubner, R. (1981): Spinal cord layer I neurons with axon collaterals that generate local arbors. *Brain Res.,* 209:421–426.
10. Bennett, G. J., Ruda, M. A., Gobel, S., and Dubner, R. (1982): Enkephalin immunoreactive stalked cells and lamina IIb islet cells in cat substantia gelatinosa. *Brain Res.,* 240:162–166.
11. Bowker, R. M., Steinbusch, H. W. M., and Coulter, J. D. (1981): Serotonergic and peptidergic projections to the spinal cord demonstrated by a combined retrograde HRP histochemical and immunocytochemical staining method. *Brain Res.,* 211:412–417.
12. Burgess, P. R., and Perl, E. R. (1973): Cutaneous mechanoreceptors and nociceptors. In: *Handbook of Sensory Physiology, Somatosensory System,* Vol. 2, edited by A. Iggo, pp. 29–78. Springer, Heidelberg.
13. Bushnell, M. C., Duncan, G. H., Dubner, R., and He, L. F. (1984): Activity of trigeminothalamic neurons in medullary dorsal horn of awake monkeys trained in a thermal discrimination task. *J. Neurophysiol.,* 52:170–187.
14. Bushnell, M. C., Duncan, G. H., Dubner, R., Jones, R. L., and Maixner, W. (1985): Attentional influences on noxious and innocuous cutaneous heat detection in humans and monkeys. *J. Neurosci.* 5:1103–1110.
15. Bushnell, M. C., Jones, R. L., Duncan, G. H., and Dubner, R. (1983): Effects of attention on detection of noxious and innocuous thermal stimuli. *Soc. Neurosci. Abstr.,* 9:473.
16. Bushnell, M. C., Taylor, M. B., Duncan, G. H., and Dubner, R. (1983): Discrimination of innocuous and noxious thermal stimuli applied to the face in human and monkey. *Somatosensory Res.,* 1:119–129.
17. Dubner, R., and Beitel, R. E. (1976): Peripheral neural correlates of escape behavior in rhesus monkey to noxious heat applied to the face. In: *Advances in Pain Research and*

Therapy, Vol. 1, edited by J. J. Bonica and D. Albe-Fessard, pp. 155–160. Raven Press, New York.

18. Dubner, R., Beitel, R. E., and Brown, F. J. (1976): A behavioral animal model for the study of pain mechanisms in primates. In: *Pain: New Perspectives in Therapy and Research,* edited by M. Weisenberg and B. Tursky, pp. 155–170. Plenum Press, New York.
19. Dubner, R., and Bennett, G. J. (1983): Spinal and trigeminal mechanisms of nociception. *Annu. Rev. Neurosci.,* 6:381–418.
20. Dubner, R., Bushnell, M. C., and Duncan, G. H. (1983): Behavioral and neural correlates of nociception. In: *Current Topics in Pain Research and Therapy,* edited by T. Yokota and R. Dubner, pp. 45–55. Excerpta Medica, Amsterdam.
21. Dubner, R., Hoffman, D. S., and Hayes, R. L. (1981): Neuronal activity in medullary dorsal horn of awake monkeys trained in a thermal discrimination task. III. Task-related responses and their functional role. *J. Neurophysiol.,* 46:444–464.
22. Dubner, R., Price, D. D., Beitel, R. E., and Hu, J. W. (1977): Peripheral neural correlates of behavior in monkey and human related to sensory-discriminative aspects of pain. In: *Pain in the Trigeminal Region,* edited by D. J. Anderson and B. Matthews, pp. 57–66. Elsevier, Amsterdam.
23. Dubner, R., Ruda, M. A., Miletic, V., Hoffert, M. J., Bennett, G. J., Nishikawa, N., and Coffield, J. (1984): Neural circuitry mediating nociception in the medullary and spinal dorsal horns. In: *Advances in Pain Research and Therapy,* vol. 6, edited by L. Kruger and J. C. Liebeskind, pp. 151–166. Raven Press, New York.
24. Dubner, R., Sessle, B. J., and Storey, A. T. (1978): *The Neural Basis of Oral and Facial Function.* Plenum Press, New York.
25. Dubner, R., Sumino, R., and Starkman, S. (1974): Responses of facial cutaneous thermosensitive and mechanosensitive afferent fibers in the monkey to noxious heat stimulation. In: *Advances in Neurology,* Vol. 4, edited by J. J. Bonica, pp. 61–71. Raven Press, New York.
26. Duncan, G. H., Bushnell, M. C., Bates, R., and Dubner, R. (1983): Inhibitory task-related responses of monkey medullary dorsal horn neurons. *Soc. Neurosci. Abstr.,* 9:2.
27. Foote, S. L., Bloom, F. E., and Aston-Jones, G. (1983): The nucleus locus coeruleus: new evidence of anatomical and physiological specificity. *Physiol. Rev.,* 63:844–914.
28. Gibson, S. J., Polak, J. M., Bloom, S. R., and Wall, P. D. (1981): The distribution of nine peptides in rat spinal cord with special emphasis on the substantia gelatinosa and on the area around the central canal (lamina X). *J. Comp. Neurol.,* 201:65–79.
29. Gilbert, R. F. T., Emson, P. C., Hunt, S. P., Bennett, G. W., Marsden, C. A., Sandberg, B. E. B., Steinbusch, H. W. M., and Verhofstad, A. A. J. (1982): The effects of monoamine neurotoxins on peptides in the rat spinal cord. *Neuroscience,* 7:69–87.
30. Glazer, E. J., and Basbaum, A. I. (1981): Immunohistochemical localization of leucine-enkephalin in the spinal cord of the cat: Enkephalin-containing marginal neurons and pain modulation. *J. Comp. Neurol.,* 196:377–389.
31. Glazer, E. J., and Basbaum, A. I. (1984): Axons which take up [^{3}H]serotonin are presynaptic to enkephalin immunoreactive neurons in cat dorsal horn. *Brain Res.,* 298:386–391.
32. Gobel, S. (1978): Golgi studies of the neurons in layer II of the dorsal horn of the medulla (trigeminal nucleus caudalis). *J. Comp. Neurol.,* 180:395–414.
33. Gobel, S., Bennett, G. J., Allen, B., Humphrey, E., Seltzer, Z., Abdelmoumene, M., Hayashi, H., and Hoffert, M. J. (1982): Synaptic connectivity of substantia gelatinosa neurons with reference to potential termination sites of descending axons. In: *Brain Stem Control of Spinal Mechanisms,* edited by B. Sjöland and A. Björklund, pp. 135–158. Elsevier, Amsterdam.
34. Gobel, S., Falls, W. M., Bennett, G. J., Abdelmoumene, M., Hayashi, H., and Humphrey, E. (1980): An EM analysis of the synaptic connections of horseradish peroxidase-filled stalked cells and islet cells in the substantia gelatinosa of adult cat spinal cord. *J. Comp. Neurol.,* 194:781–807.
35. Gracely, R. H., and Dubner, R. (1981): Pain assessment in humans—a reply to Hall. *Pain,* 11:109–120.
36. Gracely, R. H., Dubner, R., and McGrath, P. A. (1979): Narcotic analgesia: fentanyl reduces the intensity but not the unpleasantness of painful tooth pulp sensations. *Science,* 203:1261–1263.

37. Handwerker. H. O., Keck, F. S., and Neermann, G. (1982): Detection of temperature increases in the operating range of warm receptors and of nociceptors. *Pain,* 14:11–20.
38. Hayes, R. L., Dubner, R., and Hoffman, D. S. (1981): Neuronal activity in medullary dorsal horn of awake monkeys trained in a thermal discrimination task. II. Behavioral modulation of responses to thermal and mechanical stimuli. *J. Neurophysiol.,* 46:428–443.
39. Hoffert, M. J., Miletic, V., Ruda, M. A., and Dubner, R. (1982): A comparison of substance P and serotonin axonal contacts on identified neurons in cat spinal dorsal horn. *Soc. Neurosci. Abstr.,* 8:805.
40. Hoffert, M. J., Miletic, V., Ruda, M. A., and Dubner, R. (1983): Immunocytochemical identification of serotonin axonal contacts on characterized neurons in laminae I and II of the cat dorsal horn. *Brain Res.,* 267:361–364.
41. Hoffman, D. S., Dubner, R., Hayes, R. L., and Medlin, T. P. (1981): Neuronal activity in medullary dorsal horn of awake monkeys trained in a thermal discrimination task. I. Responses to innocuous and noxious thermal stimuli. *J. Neurophysiol.,* 46:409–427.
42. Hökfelt, T., Ljungdahl, A., Steinbusch, H., Verhofstad, A. N., Nilsson, G., Brodin, E., Pernow, B., and Goldstein, M. (1978): Immunohistochemical evidence of substance P-like immunoreactivity in some 5-hydroxytryptamine containing neurons in the rat central nervous system. *Neuroscience,* 3:517–538.
43. Hunt, S. P., Kelly, J. S., Emson, P. C., Kimmel, J. R., Miller, R. J., and Wu, J.-Y. (1981): An immunohistochemical study of neuronal populations containing neuropeptides or gamma-aminobutyrate within the superficial layers of the rat dorsal horn. *Neuroscience,* 6:1883–1898.
44. Hunt, S. P., Nagy, J. I., and Ninkovic, M. (1982): Peptides and the organization of the dorsal horn. In: *Brain Stem Control of Spinal Mechanisms,* edited by B. Sjöland and A. Björklund, pp. 159–178. Elsevier, Amsterdam.
45. Kenshalo, D. R., Jr., Maixner, W., Oliveras, J. L., Bushnell, M. C., and Dubner, R. (1984): The activity of wide-dynamic-range neurons and not nociceptive specific neurons predicts the detection of small increments in noxious thermal stimuli in the primate. *Soc. Neurosci. Abstr.,* 10:798.
46. Kosterlitz, H. W. (1983): Opioid peptides and pain—an update. In: *Advances in Pain Research and Therapy,* Vol. 5, edited by J. J. Bonica, U. Lindblom, and A. Iggo, pp. 199–208. Raven Press, New York.
47. LaMotte, R. H., and Campbell, J. N. (1978): Comparison of responses of warm and nociceptive C-fiber afferents in monkey with human judgments of thermal pain. *J. Neurophysiol.,* 41:509–528.
48. Ljungdahl, A., Hökfelt, T., and Nilsson, G. (1978): Distribution of substance P immunoreactivity in the central nervous system of the rat. I. Cell bodies and nerve terminals. *Neuroscience,* 3:861–943.
49. Maixner, W., Kenshalo, D. R., Jr., Bushnell, M. C., Oliveras, J. L., and Dubner, R. (1984): Correlation of primate medullary dorsal horn neuronal responses with thermal detection in the noxious range. *Soc. Neurosci. Abstr.,* 10:797.
50. Mayer, D. J., and Price, D. D. (1976): Central nervous system mechanisms of analgesia. *Pain,* 2:379–404.
51. Melzack, R. (1973): *The Puzzle of Pain.* Basic Books, New York.
52. Miletic, V., Hoffert, M. J., Ruda, M. A., Dubner, R., and Shigenaga, Y. (1984): Serotonergic axonal contacts on identified cat spinal dorsal horn neurons and their correlation with nucleus raphe magnus stimulation. *J. Comp. Neurol.,* 228:129–141.
53. Oliveras, J. L., Maixner, W., Bushnell, M. C., Bates, R., and Dubner, R. (1984): Microinjection of morphine into the medullary dorsal horn attenuates noxious thermal discrimination in the behaving monkey. *Pain* [*Suppl.*], 2:S380.
54. Price, D. D., and Dubner, R. (1977): Neurons that subserve the sensory-discriminative aspects of pain. *Pain,* 3:307–338.
55. Price, D. D., Hayashi, H., Dubner, R., and Ruda, M. A. (1979): Functional relationships between neurons of marginal and substantia gelatinosa layers of primate dorsal horn. *J. Neurophysiol.,* 42:1590–1608.
56. Price, D. D., Hu, J. W., Dubner, R., and Gracely, R. H. (1977): Peripheral suppression of first pain and central summation of second pain evoked by noxious heat pulses. *Pain,* 3:57–68.

57. Priestley, J. V., and Cuello, A. C. (1983): Substance P immunoreactive terminals in the spinal trigeminal nucleus synapse with lamina I neurons projecting to the thalamus. In: *Substance P,* edited by P. Skraborek and D. Powell, pp. 251–252. Book Press, Dublin.
58. Robinson, C. J., Torbjörk, H. E., and LaMotte, R. H. (1983): Psychophysical detection and pain ratings of incremental thermal stimuli: A comparison with nociceptor responses in humans. *Brain Res.,* 274:87–106.
59. Ruda, M. A. (1982): Opiates and pain pathways: Demonstration of enkephalin synapses on dorsal horn projection neurons. *Science,* 215:1523–1525.
60. Ruda, M. A. (1985): The pattern and place of nociceptive modulation in the dorsal horn: A discussion of the anatomically characterized neural circuitry of enkephalin, serotonin and substance P. In: *Functional Organization of Spinal Afferent Processing,* edited by T. L. Yaksh, Plenum Press, New York.
61. Ruda, M. A., and Coffield, J. (1983): Light and ultrastructural immunocytochemical localization of serotonin synapses on primate spinothalamic tract neurons. *Soc. Neurosci. Abstr.,* 9:1.
62. Ruda, M. A., Coffield, J., Bennett, G. J., and Dubner, R. (1983): Role of serotonin (5-HT) and enkephalin (ENK) in trigeminal and spinal pain pathways. *J. Dent. Res.,* 62:691.
63. Ruda, M. A., Coffield, J., and Dubner, R. (1984): Demonstration of postsynaptic opioid modulation of thalamic projection neurons by the combined techniques of retrograde horseradish peroxidase and enkephalin immunocytochemistry. *J. Neurosci.,* 4:2117–2132.
64. Ruda, M. A., Coffield, J., and Steinbusch, H. W. M. (1982): Immunocytochemical analysis of serotonergic axons in laminae I and II of the lumbar spinal cord of the cat. *J. Neurosci.,* 2:1660–1671.
65. Seybold, V., and Elde, R. (1980): Immunohistochemical studies of peptidergic neurons in the dorsal horn of the spinal cord. *J. Histochem. Cytochem.,* 28:367–370.
66. Seybold, V. S., and Elde, R. P. (1982): Neurotensin immunoreactivity in the superficial laminae of the dorsal horn of the rat: I. Light microscopic studies of cell bodies and proximal dendrites. *J. Comp. Neurol.,* 205:89–100.
67. Sherman, J. E., and Liebeskind, J. C. (1980): An endorphinergic, centrifugal substrate of pain modulation: Recent findings, current concepts, and complexities. In: *Pain,* edited by J. J. Bonica, pp. 191–204. Raven Press, New York.
68. Trulson, M. E., and Jacobs, B. J. (1979): Raphe unit activity in freely moving cats: Correlation with level of behavioral arousal. *Brain Res.,* 163:135–150.
69. Vandermaelen, C. P., and Aghajanian, G. K. (1982): Serotonin-induced depolarization of rat facial motoneurons in vivo: Comparison with amino acid transmitters. *Brain Res.,* 239:139–152.
70. Vierck, C. J., Jr., and Cooper, B. Y. (1984): Guidelines for assessing pain reactions and pain modulation in laboratory animal subjects. In: *Advances in Pain Research and Therapy,* Vol. 6, edited by L. Kruger and J. C. Liebeskind, pp. 305–322. Raven Press, New York.
71. Vierck, C. J., Jr., Cooper, B. Y., Franzen, O., Ritz, L. A., and Greenspan, J. D. (1983): Behavioral analysis of CNS pathways and transmitter systems involved in conduction and inhibition of pain sensations and reactions in primates. In: *Progress in Psychobiology and Physiological Psychology,* Vol. 10, edited by J. Sprague and A. Epstein, pp. 113–165. Academic Press, New York.
72. Westlund, K. N., Bowker, R. M., Ziegler, M. G., and Coulter, J. D. (1984): Origins and terminations of descending noradrenergic projections to the spinal cord of monkey. *Brain Res.,* 292:1–16.
73. Willcockson, W. S., Chung, J. M., Hori, Y., Lee, K. H., and Willis, W. D. (1984): Effects of iontophoretically released amino acids and amines on primate spinothalamic tract cells. *J. Neurosci.,* 4:732–740.
74. Willcockson, W. S., Chung, J. M., Hori, Y., Lee, K. H., and Willis, W. D. (1984): Effects of iontophoretically released peptides on primate spinothalamic tract cells. *J. Neurosci.,* 4:741–750.
75. Willis, W. D. (1982): Control of nociceptive transmission in the spinal cord. In: *Progress in Sensory Physiology,* edited by D. Ottoson, pp. 1–159. Springer-Verlag, Heidelberg.
76. Willis, W. D., and Coggeshall, R. E. (1978): *Sensory Mechanisms of the Spinal Cord.* Plenum Press, New York.

77. Yaksh, T. L., and Rudy, T. A. (1978): Narcotic analgetics: CNS sites and mechanisms of action as revealed by intracerebral injection techniques. *Pain,* 4:299–359.
78. Yoshimura, M., and North, R. A. (1983): Substantia gelatinosa neurones hyperpolarized *in vitro* by enkephalin. *Nature,* 305:529–530.
79. Zieglgänsberger, W., and Tulloch, I. F. (1979): The effects of methionine- and leucine-enkephalin on spinal neurones of the cat. *Brain Res.,* 167:53–64.

Advances in Pain Research and Therapy, Vol. 9, edited by H. L. Fields et al. Raven Press, New York © 1985.

Synaptic Contacts on Physiologically Defined Neurons of the Superficial Dorsal Horn

*M. Réthelyi, **A. R. Light, and **E. R. Perl

**Second Department of Anatomy, Semmelweis University Medical School, Budapest, Hungary; and **Department of Physiology, University of North Carolina, Chapel Hill, North Carolina 27514*

Somatosensory primary afferent neurons constitute a functionally heterogeneous population differentiable on the bases of afferent fiber conduction velocity, the physiological stimuli that effectively excite them, and the nature of the receptive field in peripheral tissue. Intracellular marking of individual primary afferent fibers with horseradish peroxidase (HRP) has revealed such functionally distinguished classes of sensory units to have distinctive patterns of central terminations and synaptic articulations (1,5,7,9,11). In our studies of the superficial dorsal horn of the spinal cord (laminae I and II), nociceptors with fine, myelinated fibers were shown to terminate in lamina I and outer lamina II (IIo), and low-threshold cutaneous mechanoreceptors with similarly fine myelinated dorsal root fibers (D hair) were shown to have sparse terminations in inner lamina II (IIi) and extensive distributions in lamina III (5,11).

The same intracellular marking approach can be used to compare the physiological and morphological features of neurons whose cell bodies lie within the superficial dorsal horn (6). A number of neurons of this region receive excitation from a subset of primary afferent neurons with thin fibers. Christensen and Perl (3) found some lamina I neurons to be excited by cutaneous nociceptors and others to be selectively responsive to innocuous thermal stimulation. Neurons of the outer layers of the dorsal horn exhibiting a particular selective excitation were found to have major dendritic arborizations within certain laminae; for example, cells principally excited by cutaneous mechanical nociceptors with myelinated fibers had large dendritic arborizations in lamina I, whereas neurons dominated by excitation from low-threshold mechanoreceptors had a major dendritic distribution in lamina IIi and lamina III (6).

After histochemical reaction with diaminobenzidine, the reaction product of HRP is electron-dense, and the intracellularly marked neurons can be identified with the electron microscope. With this technique, detailed ultrastructural analyses were made for 18 physiologically characterized neurons of the superficial spinal dorsal horn. The principal aim of the study was to analyze relationships between functional characteristics of a neuron and the structural features of synaptic connections on dendrites and perikarya. This preliminary report summarizes the findings.

CLASSIFICATION OF NEURONS

Most of the 18 neurons in the study had perikarya in Rexed's laminae I and II, i.e., the superficial dorsal horn (2); however, 2 neurons had perikarya in lamina III contiguous to its junction with lamina II, and the perikaryon of 1 neuron was in the white matter just superficial to lamina I. Nine neurons were effectively excited only by noxious stimulation of the skin and were categorized as selectively nociceptive. Seven neurons responded vigorously to innocuous mechanical stimulation of the skin, and no greater activity could be evoked by noxious stimuli; these were categorized as selectively (low-threshold) mechanoreceptive. The remaining 2 neurons exhibited excitatory convergence from low-threshold mechanoreceptors and from nociceptors and were considered to be of the class defined as multireceptive (2). Both classes of selectively responsive neurons had small to medium-size perikarya, and their dendritic arborizations were generally elongated rostrocaudally. Eight of these, including examples from both the nociceptive and mechanoreceptive classes, fit Ramón y Cajal's description of limitrophe cells (10). Cells in lamina I that were of Cajal's central type were selectively nociceptive, and those of the same form in lamina II (also known as SG neurons) were selectively mechanoreceptive. Both of the multireceptive units were large Waldeyer neurons characteristic of lamina I and the adjacent white matter.

SYNAPTIC CONTACTS

Axosomatic, axodendritic, and dendrodendritic synapses were found in this sample of cells; however, not all of these arrangements appeared on a particular neuron or in each of the functional categories. Moreover, the synaptic arrangements varied within a functionally defined category.

Axosomatic Synapses

Most of the functionally selective neurons, that is, small and medium-size neurons, did not have axosomatic synapses. Two selectively nociceptive neurons located at the junction between laminae I and II were exceptions; they received synaptic contacts on perikarya or on short-necked perikaryal spines from scattered, small, axonic terminals containing pleomorphic syn-

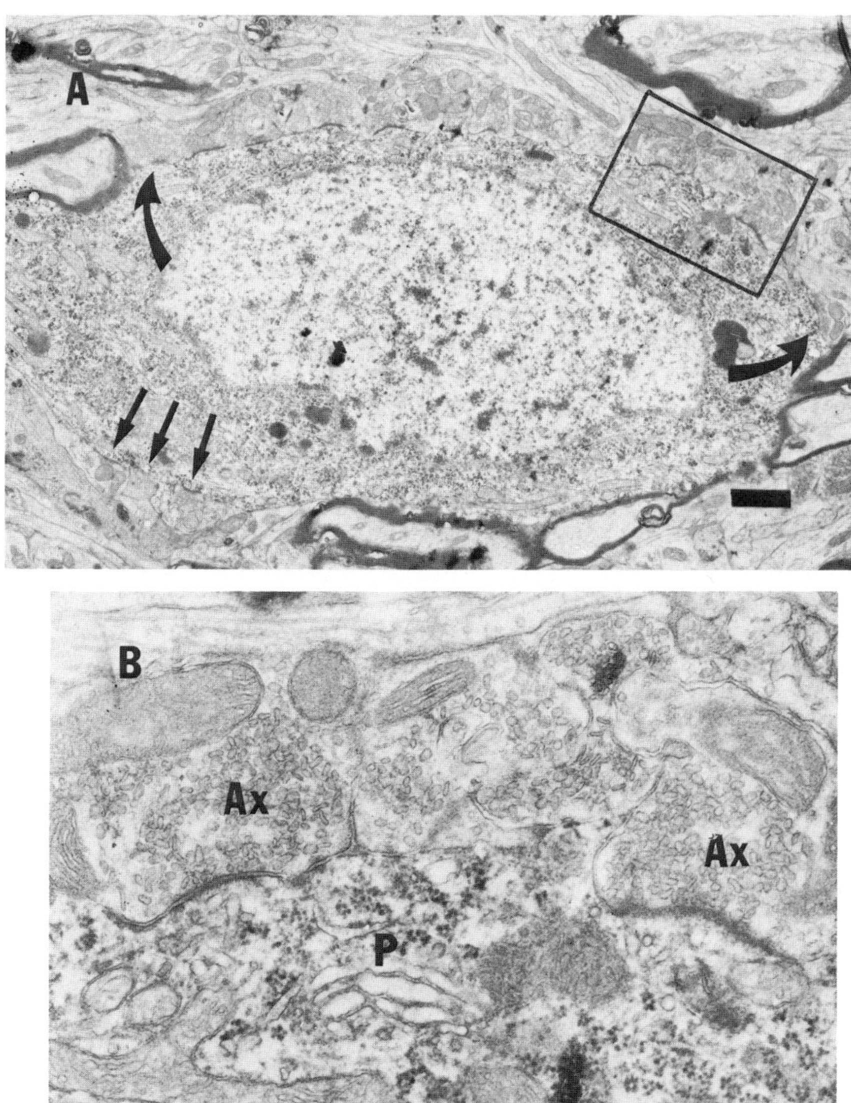

FIG. 1. A: Low-power electron micrograph showing an uninterrupted row of axosomatic synapses *(between curved arrows)* and some scattered synapses *(arrows)* on the surface of an HRP-stained mechanoreceptive-specific neuron. The perikaryon was located at the border between laminae II and III. **B:** Higher-power magnification of rectangular area in A. Axon terminals (Ax) contain flattened synaptic vesicles and form symmetrical synapses with the perikaryon (P). Scale: 1 μm.

aptic vesicles. Another exception was a selectively mechanoreceptive neuron of small size located in lamina II that was densely covered by uniform axonic terminals containing flattened vesicles (Fig. 1). In addition, both of the large, multireceptive neurons had axosomatic synapses; one had many direct contacts to the soma itself, and the other had axonic synapses on an elaborate system of unusually long protrusions from its perikarya. These observations of axosomatic contacts contrast with earlier descriptions suggesting a paucity of such synapses on perikarya in the superficial dorsal horn (8).

Axodendritic Synapses

The dendritic trees of the labeled neurons were generally confined to laminae I and II. In these laminae, primary afferent fibers commonly terminate in glomerular synaptic arrangements in which a central axon makes synaptic connections with a number of peripheral profiles representing both dendrites and small enlargements of other axons (12). Therefore, because it was presumed that the stained neurons in our sample were second-order, particular care was taken to look for glomerular synaptic arrangements involving dendrites of a labeled cell. The dendrites of three selectively nociceptive and five selectively mechanoreceptive neurons did participate in glomerular synapses. As illustrated in Figs. 2 and 3, the labeled dendritic spines of these

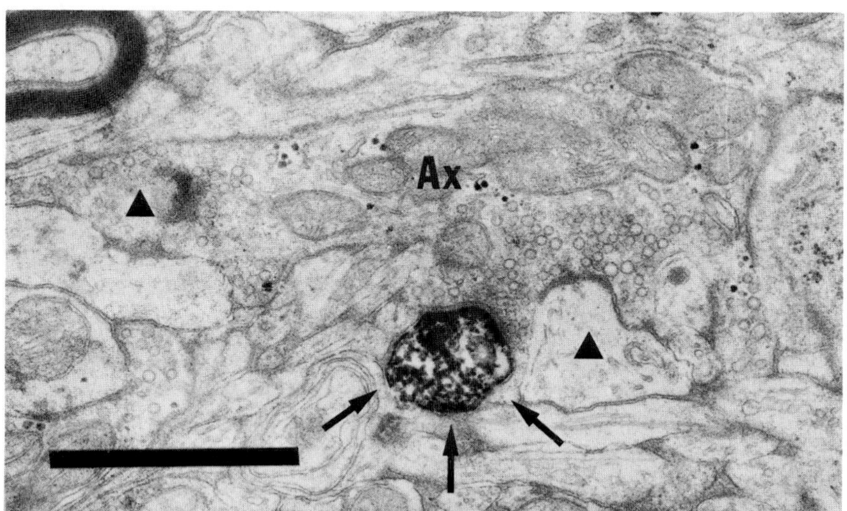

FIG. 2. Synaptic glomerulus in lamina I composed of a large axon ending (Ax) and three dendritic spine heads, one of which is labeled by HRP *(arrows)* and belongs to the dendritic arbor of a nociceptive-specific neuron. Unlabeled spine heads are marked by triangles. Scale: 1 μm.

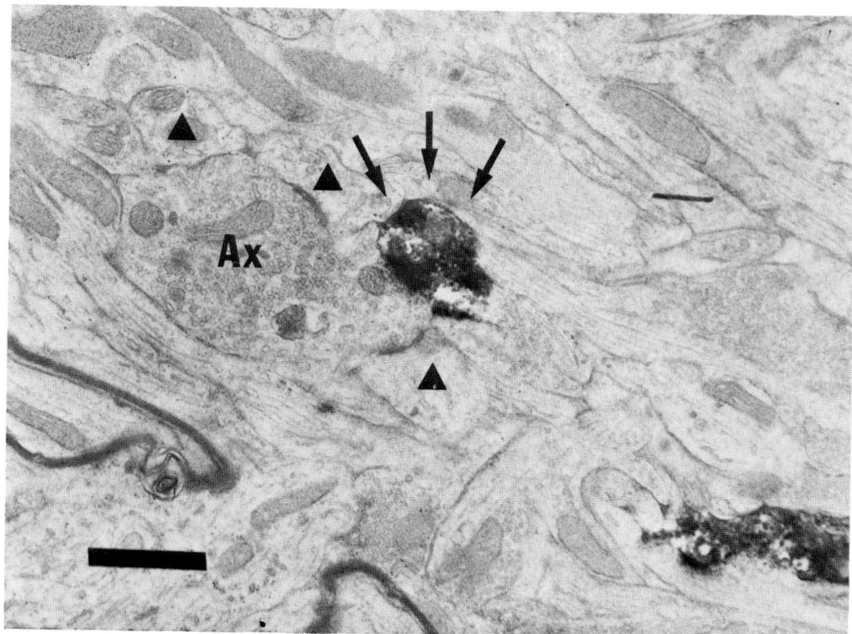

FIG. 3. Synaptic arrangement similar to that of Fig. 2, but in lamina II. A large axon ending (Ax) is in the center of the glomerulus, surrounded by an HRP-labeled spine head of a mechanoreceptive-specific neuron *(arrows)* and unlabeled profiles *(triangles)*. Scale: 1 μm.

eight neurons were common among the small, postsynaptic profiles in glomeruli. Dendritic shafts were also involved in such complex synaptic arrangements. Along their courses, the dendrites of a given cell repeatedly participated in similarly appearing glomerular synapses.

Exhaustive search of multiple runs of serial sections failed to uncover glomerular synaptic connections in the other eight selectively responsive neurons or the two multireceptive neurons. In these neurons without glomerular contacts, dendrites and dendritic protrusions were covered with axon terminals containing circular or ovoid synaptic vesicles that formed simple synaptic connections (Fig. 4). Many of the presynaptic axonic enlargements forming such simple contacts contained dense-core vesicles.

There were differences in the ways simple axodendritic contacts were distributed on the various cells. In some, presynaptic terminals were scattered along the dendritic surface, whereas in others they were closely packed, essentially covering the dendritic surface (Fig. 5). In one selectively nociceptive neuron, the main dendritic shafts were surrounded by many fine unmyelinated fibers that lay parallel to the dendrite and that periodically exhibited varicose enlargements that formed simple synapses on the labeled

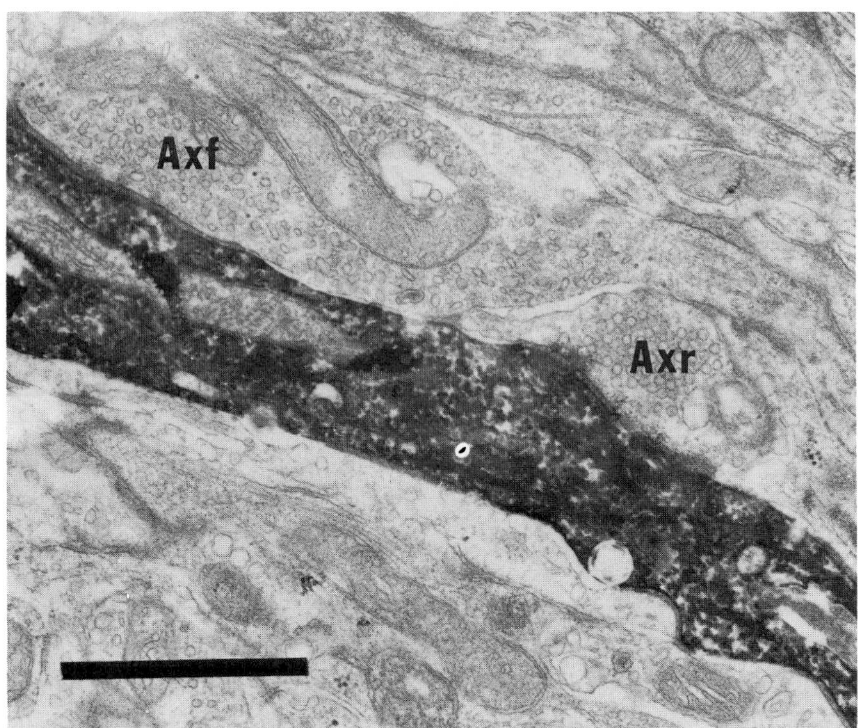

FIG. 4. Simple axodendritic synapses along the HRP-labeled dendritic shaft of a mechanoreceptive-specific neuron in lamina II. One of the axon endings contains round (Axr) and the other flattened (Axf) synaptic vesicles. Scale: 1 μm.

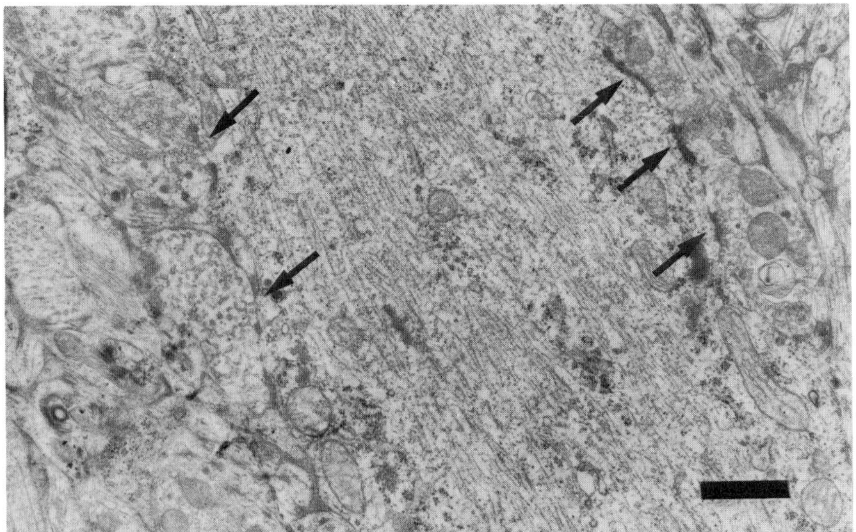

FIG. 5. Rows of synapsing axon endings *(arrows)* along the surface of an HRP-stained dendritic shaft in lamina I (multireceptive neuron). Scale: 1 μm.

shaft, or on either the head or the narrow neck of a protrusion from the shaft (Fig. 6).

Dendrodendritic Synapses

Dendritic-like profiles were seen to synapse on the dendrites of three selectively nocireceptive neurons. The presynaptic dendritic profiles contained only a small cluster of synaptic vesicles, largely pleomorphic, and synaptic contact was presumed on the basis of the membrane thickening between the two dendritic profiles (Fig. 7).

CONCLUSIONS

The observations on these 18 neurons do not support the idea that distinctive structural features can be associated with a particular type of excit-

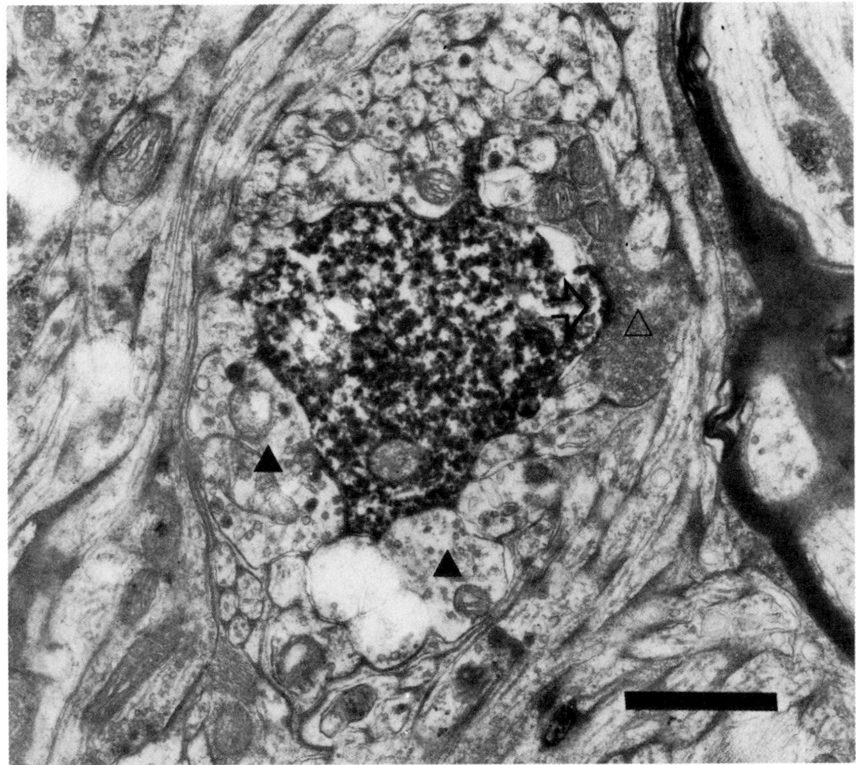

FIG. 6. HRP-stained dendritic shaft of a nociceptive-specific neuron in lamina II surrounded by a bundle of fine unmyelinated axons. Some of the axons show *en passant* enlargements *(triangles)* that synapse with the dendrite *(arrow).* Scale: 1 μm.

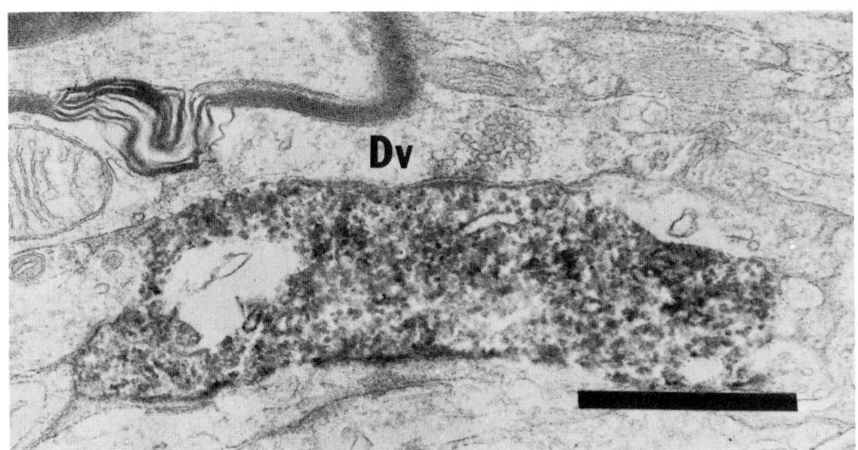

FIG. 7. Presumed dendrodendritic synaptic contact in lamina I between a vesicle-containing unlabeled dendrite (Dv) and the dendritic shaft of an HRP-labeled nociceptive-specific neuron. Scale: 1 μm.

atory projection to neurons of the superficial dorsal horn. The absence of unique correlations between structural and functional features in this region contrasts, therefore, with the arrangements found in the central distributions of primary afferent fibers. Functionally defined types of primary sensory units are seen to terminate in particular areas of the spinal cord, to manifest distinct patterns of arborization, and, in some instances, to have unique synaptic enlargements (11).

Although neurons with particular excitatory inputs may vary in form, in arrangement of dendritic tree, and in synaptic articulation, the present observations support the earlier conclusions by Light et al. (6) that the location of the major dendritic arborization reflects the dominant type of primary afferent excitation. Input from sources other than peripheral afferent fibers may explain the variety of axon terminals found to synapse on neurons with dendritic trees confined to particular territories in the superficial dorsal horn. The present observations do argue for selective connections between axon arborizations and dendritic trees, because individual neurons were not found to receive synapses from all kinds of axonic terminals existent within the confines of their dendritic arborization. Dendrites of a particular neuron apparently maintain a "microdomain" (4) by repeatedly receiving synapses from a limited number of types of axon profiles. Thus, the specificity of excitatory projections found in functional studies on the superficial dorsal horn may have a basis in a morphological selectivity of connections from primary afferent fibers similar to that established by Lichtman et al. (4) for motoneurons of the bullfrog.

In fact, the glomerular synaptic arrangements noted for the central terminations of certain kinds of primary afferent units in the superficial dorsal horn (11) were curiously missing on neurons that evidenced peripheral excitation from the sensory receptors in question. Therefore, it is possible that some stained neurons in the present sample were not second-order at all, but rather were a higher-order link in a modality-selective chain in which each element maintains a functional similarity. Finally, one could speculate that variability in structure and ultrastructure of neurons with a common functional feature results from their association with substantially different functions, i.e., ascending transmission, regional reflexes, or local integration.

ACKNOWLEDGMENTS

This research was supported by grant NS-10231, and some of the facilities were provided by grant NS-14899 from the National Institute for Neurological and Communicative Disorders and Stroke of the United States Public Health Service. The work was done under the auspices of a cooperative research agreement cosponsored by the Ministry of Health, Budapest, Hungary, and the National Institutes of Health, Bethesda, Maryland. We thank Marianna Chambless for her editorial assistance with the manuscript.

REFERENCES

1. Bannatyne, B. A., Maxwell, D. J., Fyffe, R. E. W., and Brown, A. G. (1984): Fine structure of primary afferent axon terminals of slowly adapting cutaneous receptors in the cat. *Q. J. Exp. Physiol.,* 69:547–557.
2. Brown, A. G., and Réthelyi, M. (editors) (1981): *Spinal Cord Sensation. Sensory Processing in the Dorsal Horn.* Scottish Academic Press, Edinburgh.
3. Christensen, B. N., and Perl, E. R. (1970): Spinal neurons specifically excited by noxious or thermal stimuli: Marginal zone of the dorsal horn. *J. Neurophysiol.,* 33:293–307.
4. Lichtman, J. W., Jhaveri, S., and Frank, E. (1984): Anatomical basis of specific connections between sensory axons and motor neurons in the brachial spinal cord of the bullfrog. *J. Neurosci.,* 4:1754–1763.
5. Light, A. R., and Perl, E. R. (1979): Spinal termination of functionally identified primary afferent neurons with slowly conducting myelinated fibers. *J. Comp. Neurol.,* 186:133–150.
6. Light, A. R., Trevino, D. L., and Perl, E. R. (1979): Morphological features of functionally defined neurons in the marginal zone and substantia gelatinosa of the spinal dorsal horn. *J. Comp. Neurol.,* 186:151–171.
7. Maxwell, D. J., Bannatyne, B. A., Fyffe, R. E. W., and Brown, A. G. (1982): Ultrastructure of hair follicle afferent fibre terminations in the spinal cord of the cat. *J. Neurocytol.,* 11:571–582.
8. Ralston, H. J., III (1968): The fine structure of neurons in the dorsal horn of the cat spinal cord. *J. Comp. Neurol.,* 132:275–302.
9. Ralston, H. J., III, Light, A. R., Perl, E. R., and Ralston, D. D. (1984): Morphology and synaptic relationships of physiologically identified low threshold dorsal root axons stained with intra-axonal horseradish peroxidase in the cat and monkey. *J. Neurophysiol.,* 51:777–792.
10. Ramón y Cajal, S. (1909): *Histologie du système nerveux de l'homme et des vertébrés.* Maloine, Paris.
11. Réthelyi, M., Light, A. R., and Perl, E. R. (1982): Synaptic complexes formed by functionally defined primary afferent units with fine myelinated fibers. *J. Comp. Neurol.,* 207:381–393.
12. Willis, W. D., and Coggeshall, R. E. (1978): *Sensory Mechanisms of the Spinal Cord.* Plenum Press, New York.

Advances in Pain Research and Therapy, Vol. 9, edited by H. L. Fields et al. Raven Press, New York © 1985.

Functional Analysis of the Cytochemistry of the Spinal Dorsal Horn

Allan I. Basbaum

Departments of Anatomy and Physiology, University of California San Francisco, San Francisco, California 94143

It is unusual that basic science observations have significant clinical implications soon after they are made. In most cases, potential clinical applications cannot even be envisioned. A notable exception concerns the rapid development and refinement of pain-control therapies that are based on anatomical, biochemical, and pharmacological analyses of the spinal dorsal horn. Some treatments have limited clinical application, e.g., intracerebral implantation of electrodes for relief of chronic intractable pain. In contrast, there has been rapid and widespread application of laboratory observations in the area of epidural and intrathecal administration of analgesics. In this review I shall focus on the cytochemical organization of the spinal dòrsal horn. The topic has been reviewed many times; nevertheless, there is considerable new information that bears directly on the transmission and control of nociceptive messages. This includes the organization of spinal cord dynorphin systems and the contribution of the gamma-aminobutyric acid (GABA) B receptor to antinociceptive controls exerted at the spinal cord level. To simplify the analysis of spinal circuitry, I shall try to relate the different cytochemical elements in the dorsal horn to output neurons. In most cases this is a nociceptive transmission neuron at the origin of a spinothalamic or spinoreticular tract axon.

The two major groups of nociceptive projection neurons of the dorsal horn are located in lamina I (the marginal zone) and, more ventrally, in lamina V. Most studies of dorsal horn cytochemistry, however, have focused on the superficial dorsal horn, lamina I and the underlying substantia gelatinosa (SG), which contain much greater concentrations of almost every peptide so far uncovered. This includes peptides associated with pain control, e.g., enkephalin, as well as transmission, e.g., substance P. Because it is certain that neurons of lamina V contribute to the transmission of the pain message, it is important to establish the functional significance of these cytochemical differences. One hypothesis is that lamina V cells, via interactions with their apically directed dendrites, receive inputs within and are controlled by peptidergic neurons of the SG. This may hold for some cells (47); however, the majority of spinothalamic tract neurons in lamina V do not have dendrites that penetrate the SG. A cascade of control sent ventrally from the SG to the lamina V neurons is, of course, possible, but this begs the question. Ralston and Ralston (131) have suggested that lamina V does not receive a direct C afferent input. This could account for much of the cytochemical distinction between the superficial and deep dorsal horn; i.e., the differences may reflect the differential central projections of Aδ and C primary afferent fibers.

Three major systems feed into and can control the output of the projection neuron: the primary afferents, the local interneurons of the dorsal horn, and supraspinal systems. It is confusing and almost impossible to be all-inclusive in an analysis of dorsal horn cytochemistry. Thus, this discussion will focus on those cytochemically characterized neuronal elements that have been implicated either in transmission or in control of pain. Very simple circuits that may influence the projection neurons will be illustrated. These are without doubt oversimplified; however, they offer some insight into the types of interactions that take place in the dorsal horn and, perhaps more important, provide pharmacologically characterized "synapses" on which to focus future studies aimed at development of more specific methods of pain control.

CYTOCHEMISTRY OF THE PRIMARY AFFERENT INPUT

Based on a variety of anatomical and physiological studies, we now have a reasonably detailed description of the organization of the afferent projections to the spinal dorsal horn. Of particular importance to nociception is the segregation of the inputs from small- and large-diameter fibers. Small myelinated (Aδ) and unmyelinated (C) fibers terminate superficially, in the marginal zone and in the SG. Large-diameter fibers terminate ventral to the SG. It has been suggested that although both Aδ and C fibers terminate in lamina I, there may be a relatively selective projection of C afferents to lamina II (115,130). There is also evidence for a subdivision of the C fiber input to the outer and inner parts of the SG (SGo and SGi, respectively). The outer part of the SG contains cells that respond either specifically to noxious peripheral stimulation or to both noxious and non-noxious peripheral stimulation (like the neurons of the overlying marginal layer) and probably receive a high-threshold C mechanoreceptor and C polymodal nociceptor input (21,29,102). In contrast, the inner part of the SG contains neurons more like those of the underlying nucleus proprius; i.e., they respond predominantly to non-noxious inputs. It is proposed that lamina IIi receives input from low-threshold C mechanoreceptors.

Several possibilities exist for the transmitter of the small-diameter afferent fibers. Small-diameter dorsal root ganglion (DRG) cells contain numerous, often nonoverlapping peptides, including substance P (SP), vasoactive intestinal polypeptide (VIP), cholecystokinin (CCK), somatostatin, bombesin, and gastrin (52,77). More recently, a calcitonin-gene-related peptide (CGRP) has been located in many of the smaller-diameter DRG cells. (For a review of DRG cytochemistry, see Chapter 2 in this volume.) I shall concentrate on the contribution of SP, because it provides the best example of a putative nociceptive transmitter.

Consistent with it being located in and possibly transmitting the nociceptive message, SP is found in approximately 20% of small-diameter DRG cells (77) and in high concentrations in terminals of lamina I and the outer part of the SG. Smaller quantities are found in lamina V. Capsaicin treatment, which destroys small-diameter afferent fibers, significantly decreases the quantities of SP in the dorsal horn (53,67,92). Most important, SP is located in the so-called C or central terminal of the glomerular arrangement that characterizes the superficial dorsal horn (7,40). The central terminal of the glomerulus is presumed to be derived from C and/or Aδ primary afferent fibers (62). It provides a presynaptic input to a variety of dorsal horn cell bodies and dendrites and most important is postsynaptic to many vesicle-filled axonal and dendritic profiles. Using labeled SP ligands, recent studies have documented SP binding sites autoradiographically (107,118,129). Not surprisingly, the density of binding sites parallels the distribution of immunoreactive SP.

Consistent with it being a primary afferent neurotransmitter, SP is released into the spinal CSF by high-intensity peripheral nerve stimulation (164) and excites spinal nociceptors, including spinothalamic tract neurons, when iontophoresed into the cord (71,156,157). Because peripheral nerve sectioning significantly reduces the level of SP in the dorsal horn (without loss of the peripheral-nerve electrically evoked response in dorsal horn neurons), it has been argued that SP could not be a critical primary afferent nociceptive transmitter (154). What remains after peripheral nerve section, however, probably reflects the postsynaptic effect generated by neurotransmitters that coexist with SP, possibly an amino acid transmitter. SP, in contrast, mediates a slow depolarization of dorsal horn neurons that is not routinely recorded in extracellular studies (114,153).

On the other hand, although the anatomical and electrophysiological studies are consistent with an SP contribution to the transmission of primary afferent nociceptive messages, there is controversy concerning the behavioral effects produced by injection of SP directly into the cord. For example, in rats, some authors have reported a hyperalgesic action of intrathecal administration of SP (67,111), which, interestingly, can antagonize the analgesic action of morphine, baclofen, or norepinephrine (142). Similar hyperalgesia was obtained in mice (145). Doi and Jurna (44), however, reported an antinociceptive effect of intrathecal SP and later found a concomitant depression of C-fiber-evoked spinal reflexes and decreased activity in ascending axons. The analgesic effect of SP, although naloxone-reversible, apparently did not involve an SP-activated endorphin intermediary (45). In contrast, Yashpal and Henry (166) demonstrated that intrathecal SP produces a short-lived hyperalgesia that is followed by a naloxone-reversible analgesia. They concluded that this resulted from feed-forward inhibition generated by SP activation of dorsal horn enkephalin interneurons. Tang et al. (151), in fact, reported that intrathecal injection of SP evokes the release of immunoreactive products of the proenkephalin precursor, specifically, methionine-enkephalin and methionine-enkephalin-arg-phe. The latter pharmacological studies are consistent with studies indicating that nociceptive stimuli can evoke release of enkephalins at the level of the spinal cord (30,31,163).

Figure 1 provides a simple circuit on which I shall try to build a working model of the dorsal horn cytochemical map. It should be pointed out that a direct primary afferent SP input to projection neurons has not been demonstrated. Thus, a possible relay via an excitatory interneuron in the SG has been included. In addition to activating the nociceptive projection neurons,

→

FIG. 1. Cytochemical circuitry in the dorsal horn. Excitatory and inhibitory connections are represented by open circles and filled circles, respectively. **A:** The three major inputs to dorsal horn nociceptive neurons, some of which are at the origin of spinothalamic tract (STT) axons. Excitatory afferent inputs (a) are illustrated as originating from an SP-containing primary afferent fiber. Descending inputs are typified by bulbospinal serotonin (5-HT) and norepinephrine (NE) axons that postsynaptically inhibit the STT neuron (b). Local interneurons also converge onto the projection neurons. The cross-hatched neuron represents an enkephalinergic (ENK) interneuron that postsynaptically inhibits the STT neuron (c). The SP excitatory and ENK inhibitory controls may be exerted through other excitatory interneurons of the dorsal horn (d). Finally, the broken line illustrates a possible enkephalinergic presynaptic control of the primary afferent fiber (e). **B:** An example of interactions that may occur between bulbospinal axons and interneurons of the dorsal horn. Two inhibitory interneurons are illustrated. The ENK *(cross-hatched)* and GABA *(dotted)* neurons postsynaptically inhibit the projection neuron (f, g, respectively). GABAergic neurons also presynaptically control the primary afferent input (h). This figure suggests that descending inhibitory control (from 5-HT or NE axons) may be exerted either by direct postsynaptic inhibition of the projection neuron (b) or by excitation of the inhibitory interneurons (i, j). The bulbospinal inhibition and excitation may derive from different populations of descending axons. **C:** A possible circuit whereby descending control is exerted by bulbospinal axons that are exclusively inhibitory. It is hypothesized that some GABAergic interneurons that presynaptically (k) or postsynaptically (l) inhibit the STT neurons are under tonic inhibitory control from ENK interneurons (m). Activation of the bulbospinal inhibitory axons would turn off the ENK control and release the GABAergic inhibition of the projection neurons. **D:** The complexity introduced by the presence of dynorphin (DYN)-containing neurons *(narrow cross-hatching)*. Some primary afferents are DYN immunoreactive. Their effect on the projection neurons is unknown (o). Conceivably, DYN exerts an effect opposite to that of a coexisting transmitter within the same primary afferent. Similarly, the action of the DYN-positive neurons in the dorsal horn is unclear. Direct effects on the projection neuron (p) are likely. It is also possible that DYN released either from primary afferents (q) or from spinal neurons (r) is the source of an opioid peptide control of primary afferent fibers. Finally, the figure illustrates that interactions between spinal ENK and DYN neurons need to be assessed (s), as does the possibility that some spinal DYN neurons have axons that ascend (t).

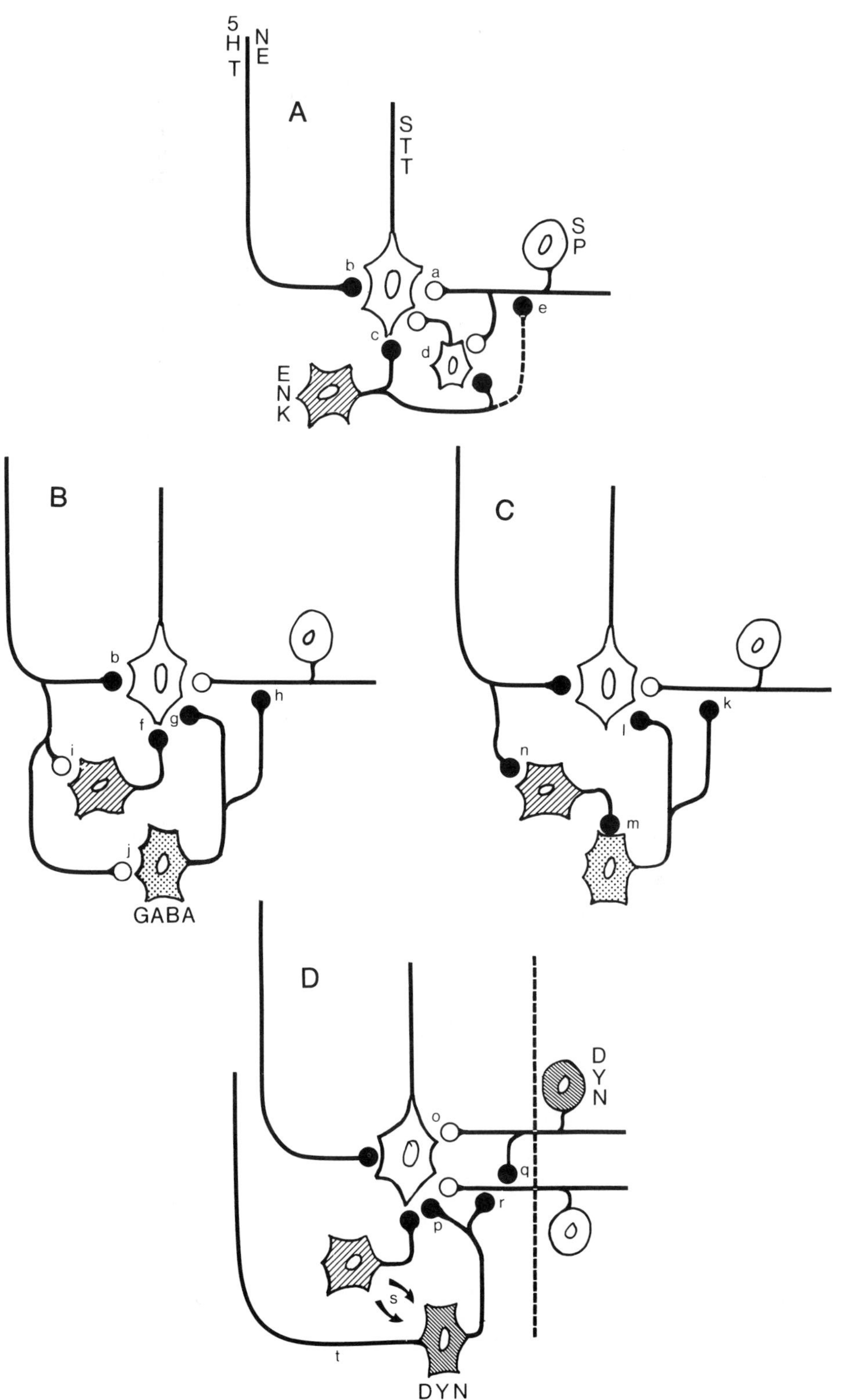
5
H
T
N
E
A
S
T
T
S
P
b
a
e
c
d
E
N
K
B
b
f
g
h
i
j
GABA
C
k
l
n
m
D
D
Y
N
o
q
r
p
s
t
DYN

SP-containing primary afferents probably feed onto a spinal enkephalin network. The nature of the enkephalin output and the contributions of other endorphins will be discussed later.

The projection neuron almost certainly receives a convergent excitatory input from other primary afferent peptide-containing neurons. It is of interest, however, that Seybold et al. (145) did not find that intrathecal injection of VIP, another peptide located in primary afferents, evoked "pain behavior" similar to that of SP. VIP is associated with small-diameter primary afferent fiber systems and is released into the spinal CSF by high-intensity peripheral nerve stimulation (162), but it does not exert equivalent algogenic effects. It may be significant in this regard that VIP has a much more restricted rostrocaudal spinal distribution and appears to be associated with afferents from pelvic viscera rather than from somatic structures (2,13,39,82). Furthermore, electrophysiological studies revealed a totally nonselective, albeit potent, excitation of nociceptive and non-nociceptive neurons by iontophoresis of VIP (90). Thus, although there are numerous peptides localized in small-diameter primary afferent systems, some may not be involved in the transmission of nociceptive information.

CYTOCHEMISTRY OF INTRINSIC NEURONS OF THE DORSAL HORN

Cytoarchitectural and Golgi studies have identified a relatively limited morphology of superficial dorsal horn neurons. With some exceptions, most neurons in this region fit into a few anatomical classes. Large and small fusiform and pyramidal cells predominate in the marginal layer; many of these are projection neurons (60). In general, the dendrites of marginal neurons arborize within lamina I; however, some medially located neurons in the primate arborize ventrally (19). In the SG, two cell types prodominate (61). The stalked cell has its cell body located at the lamina I/II border; its dendrites arborize ventrally through the SG and sometimes into lamina III. The axon of the stalked cell characteristically arborizes in lamina I. Both the inner and outer layers of the SG also contain small, fusiform neurons: the islet cells. Dendrites and axons of the islet cells arborize rostrocaudally, within the layer in which the cell body is found. Unfortunately, it has been difficult, if not impossible, to correlate the physiology of these neurons with their morphology (102,160). Furthermore, the same morphological cell type may contain one of a variety of putative neurotransmitter substances. Thus, any or all of these cytochemically different but morphologically similar neurons may contribute to the transmission and/or control of nociceptive messages. Perhaps what is significant is that differences in the terminal distributions of these compounds can be recognized (85). The task at hand is to characterize the functional significance of these cytochemically distinct neuronal classes.

Endorphins

Not surprisingly, most attention has focused on the endorphins. Initial studies indicated that there is dense opiate receptor binding in the superficial dorsal horn (4,99). These reports were followed by immunohistochemical studies of the spinal distribution of the enkephalins (56,79) and, most important, by pharmacological studies in animals and humans that demonstrated that epidural or intrathecal administration of narcotics generates a profound analgesia, as reviewed elsewhere (161).

A brief review of the distribution of the enkephalins in the dorsal horn is sufficient to introduce a discussion of the functional consequences of their organization. The enkephalins are synthesized on a single precursor molecule, proenkephalin A, which produces six copies of methionine-enkephalin (two of which are extended) and one of leucine-enkephalin, as reviewed by Höllt (81). Although some enkephalin immunoreactive bulbospinal axons project to the spinal cord (80), the vast majority of spinal enkephalin derives from intrinsic neurons of the dorsal horn.

Enkephalin terminals are concentrated in laminae I and II. Several studies have indicated that the inner part of the SG contains the highest density of enkephalin terminals (22,56). There is also relatively dense immunoreactive enkephalin terminal staining in lamina V, in lamina VII, and just lateral to the central canal. Enkephalin cell bodies are concentrated in similar places; however, there is also considerable perikaryal staining in lamina III, i.e., in a region where there are few enkephalin terminals *(vide infra).*

Two major modes of action of the spinal dorsal horn enkephalin neurons have been proposed. Early studies of the distribution of the opiate binding sites demonstrated high concentrations associated with primary afferents (50,73,99). Other studies reported a loss of opiate receptor binding in rats treated neonatally with capsaicin (54). Because capsaicin relatively selectively destroys small-diameter primary afferent axons, these data provided indirect evidence that the opiate binding site is located on unmyelinated, C, and possibly Aδ afferents. Furthermore, because capsaicin also renders rats analgesic (53,66,67,116), it is likely that afferent nociceptors, some of which contain SP, are opiate-receptor-laden. More important, these studies directed attention to a possible opioid peptide presynaptic control of primary afferent nociceptors.

First, Jessel and Iversen (91) demonstrated that opiates and opioid peptides block the potassium-evoked release of SP from slices of trigeminal nucleus caudalis (TNC), i.e., from the medullary dorsal horn. Later, Yaksh et al. (164) reported similar data in an *in vivo* preparation in which SP release was evoked by high-intensity electrical stimulation of peripheral Aδ and C nerve fibers. Finally, Mudge et al. (113) reported that enkephalins block the calcium spike of cultured DRG cells and concomitantly block the cells' release of SP. Taken together, these studies suggested that the release of the putative neurotransmitter SP from small-diameter, possibly nociceptive, afferents can be presynaptically controlled by opiate interactions with opiate receptors located on the primary afferents.

The major criticism of the presynaptic hypothesis reflects the failure of anatomical studies to demonstrate the predicted synaptic relationship. In general, one associates axoaxonic synapses with presynaptic control; however, unequivocal examples in which enkephalin terminals are presynaptic to primary afferent fibers (or, for that matter, to any other fiber) have never been found (3,33,57,84,97,98,148). The majority of enkephalin synapses are either axosomatic or axodendritic. The latter arrangement is consistent with a postsynaptic enkephalin control of spinal neurons. There is a small population of enkephalin terminals that are postsynaptic to vesicle-containing profiles. This, however, only suggests that enkephalin terminals themselves are presynaptically controlled.

A postsynaptic hypothesis finds additional support in other anatomical and physiological studies. First, some spinothalamic tract neurons of laminae I and V (some of which are likely to be nociceptive) are directly contacted by (i.e., are postsynaptic to) enkephalin terminals (134). Some of these neurons probably receive a convergent enkephalin and SP input (96). Furthermore, electrophysiological studies have established that enkephalin hyperpolarizes dorsal horn neurons via an increased potassium conductance (155,167,168). Figure 1 illustrates some circuits through which enkephalin neurons may control the output neuron. Both direct and indirect postsynaptic inhibitory controls are illustrated.

What remains of the presynaptic hypothesis? Three possibilities must be considered. It is conceivable that the opiate binding does not have the predicted biological function, i.e., that the binding site on the primary afferent is not a receptor. This would eliminate the presynaptic hypothesis completely. Alternatively, based on studies of peripheral peptidergic synapses (89), we have suggested that CNS peptide transmitters may not necessarily act at receptors in the immediate vicinity of the release site. The traditional model of the synapse, viz., the acetylcholine terminal at the neuromuscular junction, with its apposing presynaptic and postsynaptic elements, may be inappropriate for peptidergic synapses. A more diffuse, nonsynaptic release mechanism may operate. Evidence to this effect has, in fact, very recently been provided in studies of the ultrastructural distribution of the opiate binding site in the striatum (63). It was found that only 7% of the binding sites are located over synaptic densities. The vast majority, any of which may be a target of synaptically released enkephalin, were located on plasma membrane structures away from the density.

The third hypothesis is that other opioid peptides located in the dorsal horn provide the presynaptic input to the opiate receptor. With the discovery of the dynorphin family of opioid peptides and the report of profound analgesic effects of intrathecal administration of dynorphin

(15,17,65,123,127,128), we became interested in the possible relationship of spinal dynorphin systems to antinociceptive mechanisms in the spinal cord. We therefore initiated a detailed analysis of the distribution of immunoreactive dynorphin in the spinal cord of the cat (34,35). Fortunately, we have antisera that distinguish immunoreactive enkephalin and dynorphin, so that comparison of the distributions of the two opioid peptides was possible, without the immunocytochemical problem of antibody cross-reactivity.

Our studies were concentrated in the TNC and in the sacral spinal cord. We chose these areas because they are readily treated with colchicine, a drug necessary if one wishes to demonstrate the cellular as well as terminal distribution of most peptides in the nervous system. As will be described later, we found several striking differences in the anatomical distributions of immunoreactive enkephalin and dynorphin. Most important, the dynorphin staining pattern was consistent with it having a particularly significant contribution to nociceptive mechanisms.

In contrast to the dense enkephalin terminal distribution in laminae I and II, there is extremely limited dynorphin terminal staining. Moreover, it is restricted to lamina I and to the region of lamina V. Only a few scattered fibers were located in the outer part of the SG. In neither the TNC nor the spinal dorsal horn was there terminal staining in the inner part of the SG, where, as described earlier, enkephalin terminals are most heavily concentrated.

Colchicine treatment revealed that the dynorphin cells are also highly restricted to the marginal zone, lamina I, and to the region of lamina V (Fig. 2A). In fact, over 80% of the labeled dynorphin cells are located in those two sites. The remainder are scattered in the outer part of the SG and in laminae VI and VII. Not only is the dynorphin distribution more restricted, but the absolute number of dynorphin cells exceeds the enkephalin population in the marginal zone. In functional terms, the dynorphin cells are concentrated almost exclusively in areas in which neurons with nociceptive inputs predominate. Note that approximately 19% of enkephalin cells are found in lamina III, an area that, with some exceptions (26), contains neurons driven by non-noxious inputs. Dynorphin neurons are almost absent in lamina III.

Surprisingly, our initial analysis of the sacral cord suggested a much denser terminal staining pattern than observed in the TNC. Rather than deriving from local interneurons, however, we hypothesized that most of the dynorphin terminals in the sacral cord originate in primary afferent fibers. This proposal was based on the remarkable similarity of the dynorphin staining in the sacral cord to that revealed with antisera directed against VIP (15,17,82), a peptide that clearly originates in primary afferents, and to the spinal cord terminal arborization of pelvic visceral afferents demonstrated by the transganglionic transport of horseradish peroxidase (112).

Figure 2B illustrates the typical dynorphin staining pattern that one finds

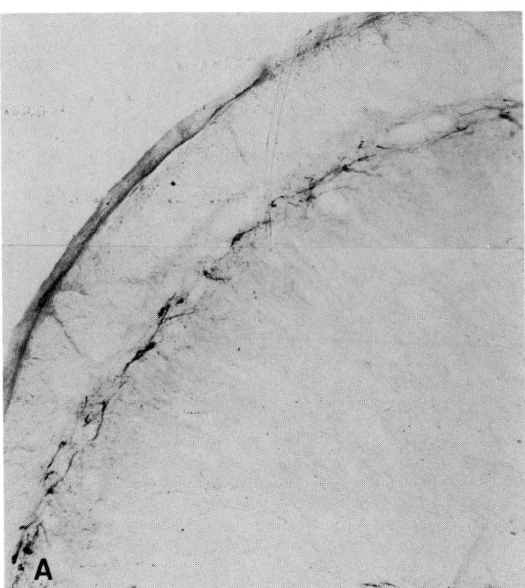

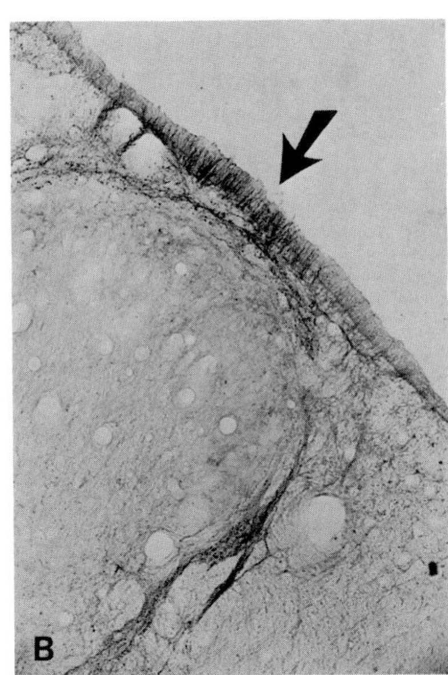

FIG. 2. Dynorphin immunoreactivity in the trigeminal nucleus caudalis (**A**) and sacral spinal dorsal horn (**B**). Large numbers of DYN perikarya are found in the marginal zone of the medullary dorsal horn (A); few labeled terminals are present. In the sacral dorsal horn, the dynorphin immunoreactive axons are concentrated in the tract of Lissauer *(arrow)* and along the dorsal and lateral borders of the marginal zone. The latter pattern of staining is similar to that found with antisera directed against vasoactive intestinal polypeptide. It is also characteristic of the central termination of pelvic visceral afferent fibers labeled by transganglionic transport of horseradish peroxidase.

in the sacral cord in normal cats. There is dense fiber staining in the tract of Lissauer; some of these fibers extend into an attached dorsal rootlet. Two major fiber branches appear to arise from the Lissauer tract. The largest arborizes in the part of the marginal zone that bends along the lateral border of the gray matter. From this branch, axons are given off medially, in the region of lamina V, across the base of the dorsal horn and around the central canal. A few fibers can be traced to the opposite side of the cord. The second branch is much smaller and distributes along the dorsal surface of the zone.

To more directly evaluate whether or not this staining pattern in fact derives from primary afferent fibers, we first tried various colchicine treatments of the sacral DRG to demonstrate cell body labeling. Despite evidence for staining of some cultured DRG cells with dynorphin antisera (150), we were not successful. Our subsequent studies, however, provided strong evidence that there is a significant primary afferent dynorphin projection. First we performed radioimmunoassay for dynorphin and demonstrated measurable levels in all DRG tested (18). This confirmed a previous analysis in rats and guinea pigs (23). Consistent with the histochemical analysis, the level of immunoreactivity was considerably higher in the sacral ganglia. We next evaluated the effects of dorsal rhizotomy on the staining patterns of various peptides in the dorsal horn in cats. Not surprisingly, unilateral deafferentation (L5-S3) produced a large ipsilateral drop in the staining of SP terminals. Enkephalin staining was unchanged. In contrast, the terminal dynorphin staining was also dramatically decreased. These data indicate that much of the terminal dynorphin in the sacral dorsal horn is, in fact, of primary afferent origin. Moreover, it suggests that it derives from the pelvic viscera. A visceral origin would, of course, explain why there was not a similar afferent projection to the TNC. A visceral dynorphin afferent input to the medulla would terminate in the nucleus of the solitary tract.

Given that there is an extrinsic source of dorsal horn dynorphin terminals, it follows that the concentration of dynorphin terminals in the spinal and medullary dorsal horn that derives from intrinsic neurons must be quite limited. This suggests that the axonal arborization of spinal dynorphin neurons is not in the immediate vicinity of the cell body, i.e., that some of the spinal dynorphin neurons project. When we first reported enkephalin neurons in the marginal zone (56), we raised the possibility that some may be projection neurons. We have, however, failed to double-label spinothalamic tract neurons with enkephalin antisera (A. I. Basbaum and M. Peschanksi, *unpublished observations*). On the other hand, we have not examined for propriospinal projections or for projections to the brainstem. Pickel et al. (122), in fact, have recently reported that some enkephalin neurons of the cord have axons that ascend in the lateral white matter. Because dynorphin terminals are so sparse, and because the distribution of dynorphin cells precisely overlaps with those at the origin of the spinothalamic and spinoreticular axons, it is clear that a study of possible dynorphin projections is necessary.

The possibility that dynorphin neurons of the dorsal horn provide a presynaptic opioid peptide input to the primary afferent cannot, however, be overlooked. Dynorphin is considered to be the endogenous ligand for the kappa opiate receptor (32). Although some authors report that mu and delta receptor subtypes predominate in the spinal cord (106), others find that kappa receptors account for more than 50% of the opiate binding in the dorsal horn (37). Moreover, autoradiographic studies of kappa binding reveal dense concentrations in the marginal zone and the SG (146), i.e., in that region that receives the densest small-diameter primary afferent fiber termination. It is also of interest that MacDonald and Werz (105) found that some DRG cells grown in culture are specifically inhibited by kappa ligands. Other DRG cells displayed mixed mu/delta sensitivity.

Perhaps most significant, the dynorphin effect has a different ionic basis from that of the enkephalins. The enkephalins produce a hyperpolarization that is mediated by an increased potassium conductance. This action has recently been reported in some SG neurons (167). Enkephalins also block the depolarizing action of iontophoretic application of glutamate (168), an effect consistent with a postsynaptic enkephalin action. Dynorphin, in contrast, reduces calcium conductance, resulting in reduced entry of calcium into the cell (105). This action would reduce primary afferent transmitter release and could underlie a presynaptic inhibitory control. As described earlier, Mudge et al. (113) originally demonstrated an enkephalin-mediated decrease in the calcium spike of DRG cells and concluded that that was its mode of presynaptic inhibitory control. Those studies were performed before dynorphin ligands or the kappa receptor had been discovered. Thus, it is possible that the doses used were large enough to have mimicked a kappa-receptor-mediated (i.e., dynorphin) action on primary afferents. Obviously electron microscopic studies will have to be performed to assess whether or not any dynorphin terminals are presynaptic to primary afferents. Interestingly, given the presence of dynorphin in some primary afferent fibers (in addition to second-order spinal neurons), such a synaptic arrangement would provide an anatomical basis for a presynaptic "autoreceptor." That is, the release of dynorphin from some primary afferent fibers could regulate its own transmitter release, or that from neighboring primary afferents. This is comparable to the presynaptic regulatory mechanisms that operate at catecholamine synapses. Figure 1 illustrates the complexity that is introduced by the possible interactions of both enkephalin and dynorphin opioid peptides.

Neurotensin

The evidence linking other dorsal horn peptidergic neurons to nociception is much less convincing. Recent interest, however, has been directed at neurotensin, a 13-amino-acid peptide (88,165) that has an analgesic effect after intrathecal injection. Like enkephalin, neurotensin terminals appear to derive exclusively from neurons located within the CNS. Neurotensin cell bodies, however, in contrast to those of the opioid peptides, are concentrated in laminae II and III of the dorsal horn (43,85,144). Consistent with the presence of dense neurotensin binding in the superficial dorsal horn (119), neurotensin terminals extend through laminae I, II, and III. Like enkephalin, neurotensin terminals predominantly form axosomatic or axodendritic synapses with dorsal horn neurons; however, some neurotensin immunoreactive terminals are also located presynaptic to an as-yet-unidentified vesicle-containing profile (43). Taken together with the report that intrathecal neurotensin produces analgesia to peripheral noxious stimuli, but does not block the algogenic effects of intrathecal SP (86), these anatomical data suggest that the neurotensin action is in part presynaptic. On the other hand, dorsal rhizotomy does not change the density of neurotensin binding in the dorsal horn (119). Furthermore, electrophysiological studies reveal a dose-dependent excitation of spinal neurons by neurotensin iontophoresis (109,147). Thus, it is unlikely that the analgesic effect of neurotensin is directly mediated by a presynaptic control of primary afferents. Rather, neurotensin may activate other intrinsic neurons of the dorsal horn that in turn presynaptically control the release of, for example, SP from primary afferent fibers.

Gamma-aminobutyric Acid

Although the majority of studies have focused on peptide and amine circuitry in the transmission and control of nociceptive messages, recent data have reintroduced the possible contribution of GABAergic systems. It has been known for many years that a presynaptic control of certain classes of primary afferent fibers is mediated by spinal GABAergic neurons. Those studies, however, focused on the presynaptic control of the large-diameter Ia afferents from muscle (36,42,120). Thus, the relevance of this control to analgesia production was justifiably questioned.

Biochemical and anatomical studies reveal very high concentrations of GABA in the superficial dorsal horn (110,121), specifically where there is dense input from small-diameter primary afferent fibers. Immunocytochemical studies with antibodies directed against the biosynthetic enzyme for GABA, specifically glutamic acid decarboxylase (GAD), suggest that the small-diameter primary afferent fibers that terminate in the SG are presynaptically controlled by spinal GABAergic neurons. The presynaptic anatomical relationship long sought for enkephalin is, in fact, common with GABA (6,14).

Despite the strong anatomical evidence for GABAergic control of nociceptive transmission, electrophysiological studies have only recently focused on the GABAergic presynaptic control of cutaneous afferents (59). Pharmacological evidence that would link GABA to spinal antinociceptive mechanisms is also limited. To my knowledge, GABA does not produce significant analgesia by intrathecal injection, and there is also little evidence that the GABA antagonist bicuculline reverses the analgesia produced by other compounds. In fact, the analgesic action of Baclofen, a molecule structurally related to GABA, is also not reversed by bicuculline (159). Its relevance to GABAergic systems was thus questioned. It appeared that spinal GABAergic neurons were neither directly nor indirectly involved in the pain-control circuits that operate at the level of the cord.

It has recently been established, however, that there are at least two different GABA receptors (24). The GABA A receptor is bicuculline-sensitive; the B type is not. Most important, Baclofen, while not an endogenous ligand, is the prototypic ligand for the GABA B receptor. (This is analogous to morphine or naloxone as prototypic ligands of the mu opiate receptor.)

Electrophysiological studies demonstrated that the bicuculline-insensitive GABA B receptor mediates a decreased Ca^{2+} conductance, which presumably could underlie a presynaptic inhibitory control (41). This contrasts with the GABA A receptor, which is a bicuculline- and picrotoxin-sensitive receptor that is coupled to Cl-conductance.

Studies of the distribution of GABA A and B binding sites in the spinal cord are particularly revealing. GABA A binding is found in all regions of the cord, but is most concentrated in the ventral horn. This would be expected if this receptor mediated the presynaptic control of inputs to motoneurons. In contrast, GABA B binding is most concentrated in the superficial dorsal horn, laminae I and II. Furthermore, there is a significant decrease in GABA B binding in rats treated neonatally with capsaicin (125). These data indicate that the GABA B receptor is probably located on small-diameter nociceptive primary afferents. In fact, Aδ and C primary afferent fibers probably have both types of GABA receptors on them (41).

Of particular interest are studies by Henry (69,70) that demonstrated an important bicuculline-insensitive effect of Baclofen on spinal nociceptive neurons. This consisted of a late, prolonged inhibitory effect on spontaneous and noxious-stimulus-evoked activity. Glutamate-evoked activity, notably, was not blocked by Baclofen, suggesting that the presumed GABA B receptor inhibitory action was presynaptic. In contrast to the putative enkephalin-SP presynaptic interactions described earlier (91), however, no blockade of K^+-evoked release of SP from spinal cord slices was found with Baclofen superfusion (140).

In light of the anatomical association of the GABA B receptor with nociceptive transmission systems, studies of the analgesic effects of spinal Baclofen clearly need to be reevaluated. Failure to reverse the analgesia with bicuculline may reflect activity at the GABA B receptor. It remains to be established that Baclofen analgesia involves mimickry of GABAergic circuitry. This is suggested, however, from studies that demonstrated a bicuculline-insensitive analgesic effect of GABA transaminase, a GABA degradative enzyme (141). This indicates that increased GABA levels in the cord could generate analgesia via interactions with the B-type receptor.

Baclofen, of course, has long been used clinically for the relief of spasticity. Although it is occasionally used for the treatment of paroxysmal pains (e.g., trigeminal neuralgia), it is not generally considered an effective analgesic. It is possible, however, that different doses are required to exert antispastic (presumably GABA A) and analgesic (GABA B) effects. Obviously the development of specific GABA B receptor agonists and antagonists will greatly facilitate the analysis of the GABA B receptor contribution to spinal antinociceptive mechanisms. Figure 1 illustrates possible GABAergic interactions that may operate in the dorsal horn to control the output of the projection neurons. Both presynaptic and postsynaptic controls are indicated.

CYTOCHEMISTRY OF DESCENDING CONTROL SYSTEMS

The third major source of the cytochemical complexity within the dorsal horn is the brainstem. There is now considerable evidence for the existence of powerful brainstem controls that are exerted on the nociceptive neurons of the dorsal horn. The best-analyzed descending control system originates in the midbrain periaqueductal gray (PAG) and, via interconnections in the rostral ventral medulla, inhibits the discharge of spinal neurons. This system has various endorphin and aminergic links and has been considered to underlie, at least in part, the analgesic actions of electrical brain stimulation and of systemic and intracerebral injections of narcotics (11,12).

What is of interest to this review is the cytochemistry of the descending connections and the circuitry through which they exert their analgesic effects within the dorsal horn. Although much emphasis has been placed on the contribution of the biogenic amines, specifically serotonin and norepinephrine, as reviewed elsewhere (15,17), there is now considerable evidence for the existence of multiple, pharmacologically distinct bulbospinal systems that probably all contribute to nociceptive transmission at the level of the spinal cord. For example, a variety of supraspinal peptide-containing systems project to the spinal cord (25). Among these are CCK-, thyrotropin-releasing hormone (TRH)-, enkephalin-, and SP-containing neurons of the medulla and oxytocin neurons from the hypothalamus. Of particular interest is that in many of the bulbospinal systems, more than one putative neurotransmitter is found (78), often coexisting with serotonin or norepinephrine. Unfortunately, little is known about the functional significance of these multiple-transmitter-containing systems.

The neurons of the medullary raphe and adjacent reticular formation project to the spinal cord via a pathway in the dorsolateral funiculus and terminate in laminae I, II, and V of the dorsal horn (9,18). There is an additional light projection to lamina VII and to the area surrounding the central canal. Part of this pathway is presumed to include a serotonergic projection from the nucleus raphe magnus (NRM). This descending pathway is thought to underlie the inhibition of dorsal horn nociceptors that results from raphe/reticular and/or PAG electrical stimulation (49,55,158). The 5-HT neurons of the NRM are also presumed to provide the serotonergic link in the controls exerted from more rostral sites in the diencephalon and forebrain (28).

The serotonin link in analgesia is not without its problems. Most significantly, although some studies indicate that depletion of 5-HT in the cord interrupts bulbospinal inhibition (133) and induces a hyperalgesia (126), other studies find that such treatments are only temporary or are without effect (83,126). Furthermore, Johannessen et al. (93) report that such treatments do not influence stimulation-produced or narcotic analgesia. The controversy is not yet resolved; however, a recent study of Fasmer et al. (48) is worth noting. They reported that after 80% depletion of 5-HT in the cord with 5,6-DHT, there was an initial decrease in the tail-flick latency (i.e., hyperalgesia) that returned to normal 6 days later. The recovery was apparently mediated by the surviving 5-HT axons, because metergoline, a 5-HT receptor blocker, again lowered the latencies. Clearly, in evaluating the contribution of aminergic systems to antinociception, one has to take into account the remarkable capacity of these systems to sprout after injury.

Despite the controversy as to the serotonin contribution to morphine- and stimulation-produced analgesia, it is certain that the distribution of 5-HT terminals is a component of the raphe-spinal termination (18,135). It has recently been claimed, however, that 5-HT axons do not course to the cord via the dorsolateral funiculus (DLF) (94), and thus the antagonistic effects of DLF lesions on opiate- and stimulation-produced analgesia (16) could not be due to interruption of 5-HT axons. Numerous other studies, however, have provided unequivocal evidence that there are 5-HT axons in the DLF (38), and we have recently demonstrated that after a DLF lesion there is a marked buildup of 5-HT immunoreactivity rostrally in the DLF. It is thus highly likely that the 5-HT terminals in the superficial dorsal horn derive from DLF projecting axons.

The majority of spinal 5-HT terminals form axosomatic and axodendritic synapses with neurons of the dorsal horn (97,98,101,108,136). In the primate, however, there is also evidence for a possible presynaptic 5-HT control of primary afferents (97,98). Thus, we again are faced with the question of presynaptic and/or postsynaptic control. The evidence for postsynaptic 5-HT-mediated inhibition is much firmer. Some projection neurons of the dorsal horn receive a direct 5-HT input (76), and 5-HT iontophoresis blocks glutamate-evoked excitation of spinothalamic tract neurons (156,157). Furthermore, because intrathecal 5-HT not only produces analgesia to external noxious stimuli (143) but also blocks the pain behavior evoked by intrathecal injection of SP, it was concluded that the 5-HT must, at minimum, have a postsynaptic inhibitory action (87). Carstens et al. (27), however, demonstrated that 5-HT iontophoresis in the region of primary afferent terminals evokes a dose-dependent increase in the threshold for antidromically activating afferent fibers. Similar results were described in an *in vitro* system (72). This would not be consistent with the primary afferent depolarization produced from stimulating the medulla, but it could underlie a presynaptic inhibitory control (via shunting of current during terminal hyperpolarization).

A second major question concerning serotonergic inhibitory control is whether or not it is exerted exclusively through inhibitory 5-HT synapses. Most studies indicate that 5-HT iontophoresis inhibits laminae I and V dorsal horn neurons (95,156,157); however, some deeper (lamina VI) neurons were excited (95). In contrast, Todd and Millar (152) found that the majority of SG neurons are excited by 5-HT iontophoresis, and Light (100) has reported both inhibitory and excitatory effects on SG interneurons. Obviously, a raphe-spinal inhibition of spinal nociceptors could be generated by a direct inhibition by 5-HT terminals, or through 5-HT excitation of some dorsal horn inhibitory interneurons. Despite the predominance of inhibitory effects from raphe stimulation, excitatory effects have been reported when 5-HT levels have been reduced with the synthesis inhibitor pCPA (133), or when dorsal horn neuron activity has been drastically altered, e.g., by deafferentation (74). Furthermore, Dubuisson and Wall (46) found strong excitatory effects of DLF stimulation on the firing of neurons of the SG, indicating that mixed excitatory and inhibitory effects are probably exerted from the medulla.

With a view to dissecting out the mechanisms of 5-HT control, Hoffert et al. (76) combined the intracellular recording and marking of superficial dorsal horn neurons with 5-HT immunocytochemistry and demonstrated that 5-HT axons are presynaptic both to marginal cells (presumably projection neurons) and to stalked cells, i.e., interneurons of the dorsal horn. In contrast, the islet cells of the SG had a much weaker 5-HT input. This innervation correlated with a predominant raphe inhibition of marginal and stalked cells but not of islet cells. The 5-HT inputs were predominantly on dendritic shafts; SP inputs, in contrast, were mainly on dendritic spines. These differences could underlie a selective nociceptive versus non-nociceptive control of wide-dynamic-range neurons, without invoking presynaptic mechanisms. These authors interpret their data as evidence for either a direct 5-HT postsynaptic inhibition of dorsal horn projection nociceptors or a 5-HT inhibition of excitatory, stalked cell interneurons. In other words, they presume that there is an exclusive 5-HT inhibitory input to the superficial dorsal horn.

Although that laboratory had previously proposed that the stalked cell is an excitatory interneuron that conveys inputs to overlying marginal projection neurons (124), it is now clear that the stalked cells are a heterogeneous population. Many contain either enkephalin or dynorphin. Because enkephalin neurons are probably uniformly inhibitory (117), it is possible that a raphe-spinal control is generated via activation of spinal enkephalin neurons through excitatory 5-HT descending axons. We have recently demonstrated that some 5-HT axons synapse on enkephalin neurons of the superficial dorsal horn (58). Moreover, Zorman et al. (169) reported that intrathecal naloxone can antagonize the analgesic action of low-intensity electrical stimulation of the midline raphe. Not surprisingly, intrathecal administration of the 5-HT antagonist methysergide had a similar effect (5).

Paralleling the descending 5-HT control is that exerted by norepinephrine (NE), as reviewed elsewhere (15,17). There is less information about the catecholamine circuitry in the cord, perhaps because the development of 5-HT antisera made the study of serotonergic circuitry simpler. NE terminals, nevertheless, are also found in high concentrations in association with spinal nociceptive neurons, and NE exerts very powerful inhibitory effects on those neurons (20,68,75,156,157). Through an alpha receptor, NE agonists generate a very profound analgesia on intrathecal injection (132). Intrathecal NE also blocks both the response to peripheral noxious stimuli and that produced by intrathecal SP, implying that postsynaptic mechanisms operate (88). In many ways, therefore, descending 5-HT and NE systems are organized in a comparable fashion. In fact, a component of the analgesic effects exerted by the 5-HT-containing raphe magnus involves bulbospinal NE systems (5,64).

Figure 1 illustrates some of the interactions through which bulbospinal controls (represented in this case by a 5-HT axon) may exert inhibitory effects on spinal nociceptive projection neurons. The simplest action would be a postsynaptic inhibition of the spinal projection neurons (which, we hypothesize, receive the direct primary afferent, possibly SP input). The postsynaptic controls could be direct, or through inhibition of excitatory interneurons. Although it is possible, we have not indicated that there is evidence for presynaptic 5-HT and NE controls. Again, these may be direct or indirect.

The presence of 5-HT-enkephalin synapses suggests that the descending controls may also be mediated via a 5-HT excitation of dorsal horn inhibitory interneurons. Similarly, the evidence for direct raphe-magnus-GABA interactions suggests that some 5-HT bulbospinal axons may be excitatory on GABAergic interneurons (104). On the other hand, if 5-HT and enkephalin axons are exclusively inhibitory, then one must postulate cascades of inhibitory neurons, so that the 5-HT-enkephalin interaction would result in inhibition of the projection neuron. We have provided one example, i.e., enkephalin inhibition of GABA interneurons. Such an arrangement would explain why Cesselin et al. (30) found no effect of 5-HT on enkephalin release in an *in vitro* slice preparation of rat spinal cord. Enkephalin-GABA interactions have, in fact, been found in several CNS systems, including the spinal dorsal horn (103).

Given such cascading inhibitory circuitry, one might predict excitatory effects of enkephalin iontophoresis. In fact, there are examples of enkephalin excitation (or naloxone inhibition) in the superficial dorsal horn (51,139). The latter group reported predominant excitatory effects of morphine or met-enkephalin iontophoresis on SG neurons. In contrast, neurons of the nucleus proprius were uniformly inhibited. Because opiates are presumed to exclusively exert inhibitory effects, it is possible that the excitatory enkephalin effects in the SG are indirectly mediated through inhibition of a GABAergic control, e.g., by blocking GABA-evoked IPSPs in spinal neurons (8). Comparable examples exist in the hippocampus and olfactory bulbs (117). The depression of primary afferent depolarization (PAD) by enkephalins (149) is conceivably a result of inhibition of a tonic GABAergic-mediated PAD. This schema may seem overly complicated; however, the lesson we have learned from cytochemical analyses of the dorsal horn is that its organization is not simple.

CONCLUSIONS

A brief review of descending controls emphasizes that no one system predominates. There are multiple, bulbospinal control systems that operate in parallel. They are pharmacologically distinct, and although seemingly redundant, they probably exert subtly different controls that adjust the level of firing in the spinal projection neurons. The controls interplay with the afferent input and the pharmacologically diverse segmental controls.

Although discussion sections often invoke the concept of "neuromodulatory" mechanisms, the majority of studies focus on all-or-nothing inhibitory events. That may be appropriate for analgesia-producing electrical brain stimulation, but it is unlikely that the brainstem controls operate that crudely in the awake animal. Conceivably, the peptidergic component of bulbospinal inhibitory systems provides the fine tuning of the descending control. As described earlier, peptide neurotransmitters exert actions on a time scale much longer than that of the amines or amino acid transmitters. In some cases this is manifested as late-occurring excitatory or inhibitory postsynaptic potentials. Some peptides also have a biochemical regulatory role. For example, Agnati et al. (1) reported that SP reduces the affinity and increases the number of 5-HT binding sites in spinal cord slices. Such changes could have prolonged and profound effects on bulbospinal controls exerted from the raphe. The behavioral consequences of strong electrical brain stimulation, e.g., of the raphe magnus, may only reflect the output of a limited number of transmitter classes that, in effect, function independent of the peptidergic actions. The latter may indeed operate in a different time frame. We do not yet have behavioral models to assess long-term peptide transmitter effects on the controls exerted by the more traditional neurotransmitter substances.

We have broken much new ground in the analysis of dorsal horn circuitry. Much remains to be done. It is perhaps most significant that the studies of spinal cord organization have not only led to the use of spinally directed narcotics and opioid peptides, but for the first time it is possible to precisely define the neural mechanisms underlying a powerful analgesic therapy. This is particularly important because it will permit refinements based not on trial and error but on identified cytochemical subtleties in the synaptic circuitry of the spinal cord.

ACKNOWLEDGMENTS

I am very grateful to Ms. Martine Hoch for typing this manuscript. Support was provided by USPHS grants NS-14627 and NS-16033.

REFERENCES

1. Agnati, L. F., Fuxe, K., Benfenati, F., Zini, I., and Hökfelt, T. (1983): On the functional role of coexistence of 5-HT and substance P in bulbospinal 5-HT neurons. Substance P reduces affinity and increases density of ^{3}H-5-HT binding sites. *Acta Physiol. Scand.*, 117:299–302.
2. Anand, P., Gibson, S. J., McGregor, G. P., Blank, M. A., Ghatei, M. A., Bacarese-Hamilton, A. J., Polak, J. M., and Bloom, S. R. (1983): A VIP-containing system concentrated in the lumbosacral region of human spinal cord. *Nature,* 305:143–145.
3. Aronin, N., Difiglia, M., Liotta, A. S., and Martin, J. B. (1981): Ultrastructural localization and biochemical features of immunoreactive leu-enkephalin in monkey dorsal horn. *J. Neurosci.,* 1:561–577.
4. Atweh, S. F., and Kuhar, M. (1977): Autoradiographic localization of opiate receptors in rat brain. I. Spinal cord and lower medulla. *Brain Res.,* 124:53–67.
5. Barbaro, N. M., Hammond, D. L., and Fields, H. L. (1983): Antagonism of microstimulation-produced analgesia by intrathecal injection of methysergide and yohimbine. *Neurosci. Abstr.,* 9:791.
6. Barber, R. P., Vaughn, J. E., Saito, K., McLaughlin, B. J., and Roberts, E. (1978): Gabaergic terminals are presynaptic to primary afferent terminals in the substantia gelatinosa of the rat spinal cord. *Brain Res.,* 141:35–55.
7. Barber, R. P., Vaughn, J. E., Slemmon, R. J., Salvaterra, P. M., Roberts, E., and Leeman, S. E. (1979): The origin, distribution and synaptic relationships of substance P axons in rat spinal cord. *J. Comp. Neurol.,* 184:331–352.
8. Barker, J. L., Smith, J. G., and Neale, J. H. (1978): Multiple membrane actions of enkephalin revealed using cultured spinal neurons. *Brain Res.,* 154:153–158.
9. Basbaum, A. I., Clanton, C. H., and Fields, H. L. (1978): Three bulbospinal pathways from the rostral medulla of the cat: An autoradiographic study of pain modulating systems. *J. Comp. Neurol.,* 178:209–224.
10. Basbaum, A. I., Cruz, L., and Weber, E. (1985): Immunoreactive dynorphin in sacral primary afferent fibers of the cat. *(Submitted for publication.)*
11. Basbaum, A. I., and Fields, H. L. (1978): Endogenous pain control mechanisms: Review and hypothesis. *Ann. Neurol.,* 4:451–462.
12. Basbaum, A. I., and Fields, H. L. (1984): Endogenous pain control systems: Brainstem spinal pathways and endorphin circuitry. *Annu. Rev. Neurosci.,* 7:309–338.
13. Basbaum, A. I., and Glazer, E. J. (1983): Immunoreactive vasoactive intestinal polypeptide is concentrated in sacral spinal cord: A possible marker for pelvic visceral afferent fibers. *Somatosensory Res.* 1:69–82.
14. Basbaum, A. I., Glazer, E. J., and Oertel, W. (1981): A light and EM analysis of immunoreactive glutamic acid decarboxylase (GAD) in the spinal and trigeminal dorsal horn of the cat. *Neurosci. Abstr.,* 7:528.
15. Basbaum, A. I., Jacknow, D., Mulcahy, J., and Levine, J. (1983): Studies on the contribution of different endogenous opioid peptides to the control of pain. In: *Current Topics in Pain Research and Therapy,* edited by T. Yokota and R. Dubner, pp. 118–120. Elsevier, Amsterdam.
16. Basbaum, A. I., Marley, N., O'Keefe, J., and Clanton, C. H. (1977): Reversal of opiate and stimulus produced analgesia by subtotal spinal cord lesions. *Pain,* 3:43–56.
17. Basbaum, A. I., Moss, M. S., and Glazer, E. J. (1983): Opiate and stimulation-produced analgesia: The contribution of the monoamines. *Adv. Pain Res. Ther.,* 5:323–339.
18. Basbaum, A. I., Ralston, D. D., and Ralston, H. J. (1985): Bulbospinal projections in the primate: A light and electron microscopic autoradiographic study of a pain modulating system. *(Submitted for publication.)*
19. Beal, J. A. (1979): The ventral dendritic arbor of marginal (lamina I) neurons in the adult primate spinal cord. *Neurosci. Lett.,* 14:201–206.
20. Belcher, G., Ryall, R. W., and Schaffner, R. (1978): The differential effects of 5-hydroxytryptamine, noradrenaline and raphe interneurons in the cat. *Brain Res.,* 151:307–323.
21. Bennett, G. J., Abdelmoumene, M., Hayashi, H., and Dubner, R. (1980): Physiology and morphology of substantia gelatinosa neurons intracellulary stained with horseradish peroxidase. *J. Comp. Neurol.,* 194:809–827.

22. Bennett, G. J., Ruda, M. A., Gobel, S., and Dubner, R. (1982): Enkephalin immunoreactive stalked cells and lamina IIb islet cells in cat substantia gelatinosa. *Brain Res.,* 240:162–166.
23. Botticelli, L. H., Cox, B. M., and Goldstein, A. (1981): Immunoreactive dynorphin in mammalian spinal cord and dorsal root ganglia. *Proc. Natl. Acad. Sci., U.S.A.,* 78:7783–7786.
24. Bowery, N. G. (1982): Baclofen: 10 years on. *Trends Pharm. Sci.,* 3:400–403.
25. Bowker, R. M., Steinbusch, H. W. M., and Coulter, J. D. (1981): Serotonergic and peptidergic projections to the spinal cord demonstrated by a combined retrograde HRP histochemical and immunocytochemical staining method. *Brain Res.,* 211:412–417.
26. Brown, A. G. (1982): The dorsal horn of the spinal cord. *Q. J. Exp. Physiol.,* 67:193–212.
27. Carstens, E., Klumpp, D., Randic, M., and Zimmermann, M. (1981): Effect of iontophoretically applied 5-hydroxytryptamine on the excitability of single primary afferent C- and A-fibers in the cat spinal cord. *Brain Res.,* 220:151–158.
28. Carstens, E., MacKinnon, J. D., and Guinan, M. J. (1983): Serotonin involvement in descending inhibition of spinal nociceptive transmission produced by stimulation of medial diencephalon and basal forebrain. *J. Neurosci.,* 3:2112–2120.
29. Cervero, F., and Iggo, A. (1980): The substantia gelatinosa of the spinal cord. A critical review. *Brain,* 103:717–772.
30. Cesselin, F., Bourgoin, S., Artaud, F., and Hamon, M. (1984): Basic and regulatory mechanisms of *in vitro* release of met-enkephalin from the dorsal zone of the rat spinal cord. *J. Neurochem.,* 43:763–774.
31. Cesselin, F., Le Bars, D., Bourgoin, S., Artaud, F., Gozlan, H., Clot, A. M., Besson, J. M., and Hamon, M. (1985): Spontaneous and evoked release of met-enkephalin-like material from the rat spinal cord *in vivo. Brain Res., (in press).*
32. Chavkin, D., James, I. F., and Goldstein, A. (1982): Dynorphin is a specific endogenous ligand of the κ opioid receptor. *Science,* 215:413–415.
33. Conrath-Verrier, M., Dietl, M., Arluison, M., Cesselin, F., Bourgoin, S., and Hamon, M. (1983): Localization of met-enkephalin within pain-related nuclei of brain stem and spinal cord in the cat. *Brain Res. Bull.,* 11:587–604.
34. Cruz, L., and Basbaum, A. I. (1985): Multiple opioid peptides and the modulation of pain. I. Immunohistochemical analysis of dynorphin and enkephalin in the trigeminal nucleus caudalis. *J. Comp. Neurol., (in press)*
35. Cruz, L., and Basbaum, A. I. (1985): Multiple opioid peptides and the modulation of pain. II. Immunohistochemical analysis of dynorphin and enkephalin in the spinal cord of the cat. *J. Comp. Neurol., (in press).*
36. Curtis, D. R., Lodge, D., and Brand, S. J. (1977): GABA and spinal afferent terminal excitibility in the cat. *Brain Res.,* 130:360–363.
37. Czlonkowski, A., Costa, T., Przewlocki, R., Pasi, A., and Herz, A. (1983): Opiate receptor binding sites in human spinal cord. *Brain Res.,* 267:392–396.
38. Dahlstrom, A., and Fuxe, K. (1964): Evidence for the existence of monoamine neurons in the central nervous system. II. Experimental demonstration of monoamines in the cell bodies of brain stem neurons. *Acta Physiol. Scand.* [*Suppl. 232*], 62:1–55.
39. de Groat, W. C., Kawatani, M., Hisamitsu, T., Lowe, I., Morgan, C., Roppolo, J., Booth, A. M., Nadelhaft, I., Kuo, D., and Thor, K. (1983): The role of neuropeptides in the sacral autonomic reflex pathways of the cat. *J. Autonom. Nerv. Syst.,* 7:339–350.
40. de Lanerolle, N. C., and LaMotte, C. C. (1983): Ultrastructure of chemically defined neuron systems in the dorsal horn of the monkey. I. Substance P immunoreactivity. *Brain Res.,* 274:31–49.
41. Désarmenien, M., Feltz, P., Occhipinti, G., Santangelo, F., and Schlichter, R. (1984): Coexistence of $GABA_a$ and $GABA_b$ receptors on A and C primary afferents. *Br. J. Pharmacol.,* 81:327–333.
42. Deschênes, M., Feltz, P., and Lamour, Y. (1976): A model for an estimate *in vivo* of the ionic basis of presynaptic inhibition: An intracellular analysis of the GABA-induced depolarization in rat dorsal root ganglia. *Brain Res.,* 118:486–493.
43. Difiglia, M., Aronin, N., and Leeman, S. E. (1984): Ultrastructural localization of immunoreactive neurotensin in the monkey superficial dorsal horn. *J. Comp. Neurol.,* 225:1–12.

44. Doi, T., and Jurna, I. (1981): Intrathecal substance P depresses the tail-flick response—antagonism by naloxone. *Naunyn Schmiedebergs Arch. Pharmacol.*, 317:135–139.
45. Doi, T., and Jurna, L. (1982): Intrathecal substance P depresses spinal motor and sensory responses to stimulation of nociceptive afferents—antagonism by naloxone. *Naunyn Schmiedebergs Arch. Pharmacol.*, 319:154–160.
46. Dubuisson, D., and Wall, P. D. (1980): Descending influences on receptive fields and activity of single units recorded in laminae 1, 2 and 3 of cat spinal cord. *Brain Res.*, 199:283–298.
47. Duggan, A. W., Hall, J. G., and Headly, P. M. (1976): Morphine, enkephalin and the substantia gelatinosa. *Nature,* 264:456–458.
48. Fasmer, O. B., Berge, O. G., Walther, B., and Hole, K. (1983): Changes in nociception after intrathecal administration of 5,6-dihydroxytryptamine in mice. *Neuropharmacology,* 22:1197–1201.
49. Fields, H. L., Basbaum, A. I., Clanton, C. H., and Anderson, S. D. (1977): Nucleus raphe magnus inhibition of spinal cord dorsal horn neurons. *Brain Res.,* 126:441–453.
50. Fields, H. L., Emson, P. C., Leigh, B. K., Gilbert, R. F. T., and Iversen, L. L. (1980): Multiple opiate receptor sites on primary afferent fibres. *Nature,* 284:351–353.
51. Fitzgerald, M., and Woolf, C. (1980): The stereospecific effect of naloxone on rat dorsal horn neurones: Inhibition in superficial laminae and excitation in deeper laminae. *Pain,* 9:293–306.
52. Fuxe, K., Agnati, L. F., McDonald, T., Locatelli, V., Hökfelt, T., Dalsgaard, C. J., Battistini, N., Yanaihara, N., Mutt, V., and Cuello, A. C. (1983): Immunohistochemical indications of gastrin releasing peptide—bombesin-like immunoreactivity in the nervous system of the rat. Codistribution with substance P-like immunoreactive nerve terminal systems and coexistence with substance P-like immunoreactivity in dorsal root ganglion cell bodies. *Neurosci. Lett.*, 37:17–22.
53. Gamse, R. (1982): Capsaicin and nociception in the rat and mouse. Possible role of substance P. *Naunyn Schmiedergs Arch. Pharmacol.*, 320:205–216.
54. Gamse, R., Holzer, P., and Lembeck, F. (1979): Indirect evidence for presynaptic location of opiate receptors on chemosensitive primary sensory neurons. *Naunyn Schmiedebergs Arch. Pharmacol.*, 308:281–285.
55. Gebhart, G. F., Sandkühler, J., Thalhammer, J. G., and Zimmermann, M. (1983): Inhibition of spinal nociceptive information by stimulation in midbrain of the cat is blocked by lidocaine microinjected in nucleus raphe magnus and medullary reticular formation. *J. Neurophysiol.*, 50:1446–1459.
56. Glazer, E. J., and Basbaum, A. I. (1981): Immunohistochemical localization of leucine-enkephalin in the spinal cord of the cat: Enkephalin-containing marginal neurons and pain modulation. *J. Comp. Neurol.*, 196:377–389.
57. Glazer, E. J., and Basbaum, A. I. (1983): Opioid neurons and pain modulation: An ultrastructural analysis of enkephalin in cat superficial dorsal horn. *Neuroscience,* 10:357–376.
58. Glazer, E. J., and Basbaum, A. I. (1984): Axons which take up ^{3}H-serotonin are presynaptic to enkephalin immunoreactive neurons in cat dorsal horn. *Brain Res.*, 298:386–391.
59. Gmelin, G., and Zimmermann, M. (1983): Effects of γ-aminobutyrate and bicuculline on primary afferent depolarization of cutaneous fibres in the cat spinal cord. *Neuroscience,* 10:869–874.
60. Gobel, S. (1978): Golgi studies of the neurons in layer I of the dorsal horn of the medulla (trigeminal nucleus caudalis). *J. Comp. Neurol.,* 180:378–394.
61. Gobel, S. (1978): Golgi studies of the neurons in layer II of the dorsal horn of the medulla (trigeminal nucleus caudalis). *J. Comp. Neurol.,* 180:395–414.
62. Gobel, S. (1979): Neural circuitry in the substantia gelatinosa of Rolando: Anatomical insights. *Adv. Pain Res. Ther.,* 3:175–195.
63. Hamel, E., and Beaudet, A. (1984): Electron microscopic localization of opioid receptors in rat neostriatum. *Nature,* 312:155–157.
64. Hammond, D. L., Levy, R. A., and Proudfit, H. K. (1980): Hypoalgesia induced by microinjection of a norepinephrine antagonist in the raphe magnus: Reversal by intrathecal administration of a serotonin antagonist. *Brain Res.,* 201:475–489.
65. Han, J. S., and Xie, C. W. (1982): Dynorphin: Potent analgesic effect in spinal cord of the rat. *Life Sci.,* 31:1781–1784.

66. Hayes, A. G., Skingle, M., and Tyers, M. B. (1981): Effects of single doses of capsaicin on nociceptive thresholds in the rodent. *Neuropharmocology,* 20:505–511.
67. Hayes, A. G., and Tyers, M. B. (1980): Effects of capsaicin on nociceptive heat, pressure and chemical thresholds and on substance P levels in the rat. *Brain Res.,* 189:561–564.
68. Headley, P. M., Duggan, A. W., and Griersmith, B. T. (1978): Selective reduction by noradrenaline and 5-hydroxytryptamine of nociceptive responses of cat dorsal horn neurones. *Brain Res.,* 145:185–189.
69. Henry, J. L. (1982): Effects of intravenously administered enantiomers of baclofen on functionally identified units in lumbar dorsal horn of the spinal cat. *Neuropharmacology,* 21:1073–1083.
70. Henry, J. L. (1982): Pharmacological studies on the prolonged depressant effects of baclofen on lumbar dorsal horn units in the cat. *Neuropharmacology,* 21:1085–1093.
71. Henry, J. L. (1976): Effects of substance P on functionally identified units in cat spinal cord. *Brain Res.,* 114:439–451.
72. Hentall, I. D., and Fields, H. L. (1983): Actions of opiates, substance P and serotonin on the excitability of primary afferent terminals and observations on interneuronal activity in the neonatal rat's dorsal horn *in vitro. Neuroscience,* 9:521–528.
73. Hiller, J. M., Simon, E. J., Crain, S. M., and Peterson, E. R. (1978): Opiate receptors in culture of fetal mouse dorsal root ganglia (DRG) and spinal cord: Predominance in DRG neurites. *Brain Res.,* 145:396–400.
74. Hodge, C. J., Jr., Apkarian, A. V., Owen, M. P., and Hanson, B. S. (1983): Changes in the effects of stimulation of locus coeruleus and nucleus raphe magnus following dorsal rhizotomy. *Brain Res.,* 288:325–329.
75. Hodge, C. J., Jr., Woods, C. C. I., and Delatizky, J. (1980): Noradrenalin, serotonin, and the dorsal horn. *J. Neurosurg.,* 52:674–685.
76. Hoffert, M. J., Miletic, V., Ruda, M. A., and Dubner, R. (1983): Immunocytochemical identification of serotonin axonal contacts on characterized neurons in laminae I and II of the cat dorsal horn. *Brain Res.,* 267:361–364.
77. Hökfelt, T., Johansson, O., Ljungdahl, A., Lundberg, J. M., and Schultzberg, M. (1980): Peptidergic neurones. *Nature,* 284:515–521.
78. Hökfelt, T., Ljungdahl, A., Steinbusch, H., Verhofstad, A. N., Nilsson, G., Brodin, E., Pernow, B., and Goldstein, M. (1978): Immunohistochemical evidence of substance P like immunoreactivity in some 5-hydroxytryptamine containing neurons in the rat central nervous system. *Neuroscience,* 3:517–538.
79. Hökfelt, T., Ljungdahl, A., Terenius, L., Elde, R., and Nilsson, G. (1977): Immunohistochemical analysis of peptide pathways possibly related to pain and analgesia: Enkephalin and Substance P. *Proc. Natl. Acad. Sci. U.S.A.,* 74:3081–3085.
80. Hökfelt, T., Terenius, T., Kuypers, H. G. J. M., and Dann, O. (1979): Evidence for enkephalin immunoreactive neurons in the medulla oblongata projecting to the spinal cord. *Neurosci. Lett.,* 14:55–60.
81. Höllt, V. (1983): Multiple endogenous opioid peptides. *Trends Neurosci.,* 16:24–26.
82. Honda, C. N., Rethelyi, M., and Petrusz, P. (1983): Preferential immunohistochemical localization of vasoactive intestinal polypeptide (VIP) in the sacral spinal cord of the cat: Light and electron microscopic observations. *J. Neurosci.,* 3:2183–2196.
83. Howe, J. R., and Yaksh, T. L. (1982): Changes in sensitivity to intrathecal norepinephrine and serotonin after 6-hydroxydopamine (6-OHDA), 5,6-dihydroxytryptamine (5,6-DHT) or repeated monoamine administration. *J. Pharmacol. Exp. Ther.,* 220:311–321.
84. Hunt, S. P., Kelly, J. S., and Emson, P. C. (1980): The electron microscopic localization of methionine-enkephalin within the superficial layers (I and II) of the spinal cord. *Neuroscience,* 5:1871–1890.
85. Hunt, S. P., Kelly, J. S., Emson, P. C., Kimmel, J. R., Miller, R. J., and Wu, J. Y. (1981): An immunohistochemical study of neuronal populations containing neuropeptides or γ-aminobutyrate within the superficial layers of the rat dorsal horn. *Neuroscience,* 6:1883–1898.
86. Hylden, J. L. K., and Wilcox, G. L. (1983): Antinociceptive action of intrathecal neurotensin in mice. *Peptides,* 4:517–520.
87. Hylden, J. L. K., and Wilcox, G. L. (1983): Intrathecal serotonin in mice: Analgesia and inhibition of a spinal action of substance P. *Life Sci.,* 33:789–795.

88. Hylden, J. L. K., and Wilcox, G. L. (1983): Pharmacological characterization of substance P-induced nociception in mice: Modulation by opioid and noradrenergic agonists at the spinal level. *J. Pharmacol. Exp. Ther.,* 226:398–404.
89. Jan, L. Y., and Jan, Y. N. (1982): Peptidergic transmission in sympathetic ganglion of the frog. *J. Physiol. (Lond.),* 324:219–246.
90. Jeftinija, S., Murase, K., Nedeljokov, V., and Randic, M. (1982): Vasoactive intestinal polypeptide excites mammalian dorsal horn neurons both *in vivo* and *in vitro. Brain Res.,* 243:158–164.
91. Jessel, T. M., and Iversen, L. L. (1977): Opiate analgesics inhibit substance P release from rat trigeminal nucleus. *Nature,* 268:549–551.
92. Jessel, T. M., Iversen, L. L., and Cuello, A. C. (1978): Capsaicin-induced depletion of substance P from primary sensory neurons. *Brain Res.,* 152:183–188.
93. Johannessen, J. N., Watkins, L. R., Carlton, S. M., and Mayer, D. J. (1982): Failure of spinal cord serotonin depletion to alter analgesia elicited from the periaqueductal gray. *Brain Res.,* 237:373–386.
94. Johannessen, J. N., Watkins, L. R., and Mayer, D. J. (1984): Non-serotonergic origins of the dorsolateral funiculus in the rat ventral medulla. *J. Neurosci.,* 4:757–766.
95. Jordan, L. M., Kenshalo, D. R., Jr., Martin, R. F., Haber, L. H., and Willis, W. D. (1979): Two populations of spinothalamic tract neurons with opposite responses to 5-hydroxytryptamine. *Brain Res.,* 164:342–346.
96. LaMotte, C. C., and de Lanerolle, N. C. (1981): Human spinal neurons: Innervation by both substance P and enkephalin. *Neuroscience,* 6:713–723.
97. LaMotte, C. C., and de Lanerolle, N. C. (1983): Ultrastructure of chemically defined neuron systems in the dorsal horn of the monkey. II. Methionine-enkephalin immunoreactivity. *Brain Res.,* 274:51–63.
98. LaMotte, C. C., and de Lanerolle, N. C. (1983): Ultrastructure of chemically defined neuron systems in the dorsal horn of the monkey. III. Serotonin immunoreactivity. *Brain Res.,* 274:65–77.
99. LaMotte, C., Pert, C. B., and Snyder, S. H. (1976): Opiate receptor binding in primate spinal cord. Distribution and changes after dorsal root section. *Brain Res.,* 112:407–412.
100. Light, A. R. (1983): Postsynaptic effects in spinal lamina I and II neurons produced by stimulating midline medulla and pons. *Neurosci. Abstr.,* 9:2.
101. Light, A. R., Kavookjian, A. M., and Petrusz, P. (1983): The ultrastructure and synaptic connections of serotonin-immunoreactive terminals in spinal laminae I and II. *Somatosensory Res.,* 1:33–50.
102. Light, A. R., Trevino, D. L., and Perl, E. R. (1979): Morphological features of functionally identified neurons in the marginal zone and substantia gelatinosa of the spinal dorsal horn. *J. Comp. Neurol.,* 186:151–171.
103. Lovick, T. A. (1983): Enkephalin blocks primary afferent depolarization of Aδ tooth pulp afferents evoked by stimulation in nucleus raphe magnus in the decerebrate cat. *Neurosci. Lett.,* 37:273–278.
104. Lovick, T. A., and Wolstencroft, J. H. (1980): Inhibition from nucleus raphe magnus of tooth pulp responses in medial reticular neurones of the cat can be antagonized by bicuculline. *Neurosci. Lett.,* 19:325–330.
105. MacDonald, R. L., and Werz, M. A. (1983): Dynorphin decreases calcium conductance of mouse cultured dorsal root ganglion neurons. *Neurosci. Abstr.,* 9:1129.
106. Mack, K. J., Killian, A., and Weyhenmeyer, J. A. (1984): Comparison of mu, delta and kappa opiate binding sites in rat brain and spinal cord. *Life Sci.,* 34:281–285.
107. Mantyh, P. M., Hunt, S. P., and Maggio, J. E. (1984): Substance P receptors: Localization by light microscopic autoradiography in rat brain using [^{3}H]SP as the radioligand. *Brain Res.,* 307:147–165.
108. Maxwell, D. J., Leranth, C. S., and Verhofstad, A. A. J. (1983): Fine structure of serotonin-containing axons in the marginal zone of the rat spinal cord. *Brain Res.,* 266:253–260.
109. Miletic, V., and Randic, M. (1979): Neurotensin excites cat spinal neurones located in laminae I–III. *Brain Res.,* 169:600–604.
110. Miyata, Y., and Otsuka, M. (1975): Quantitative histochemistry of γ-aminobutyric acid in cat spinal cord with special reference to presynaptic inhibition. *J. Neurochem.,* 24:239–244.

111. Moochhala, S. M., and Sawynok, J. (1984): Hyperalgesia produced by intrathecal substance P and related peptides: Desensitization and cross desensitization. *Br. J. Pharmacol.,* 82:381–388.
112. Morgan, C., Nadelhaft, I., and de Groat, W. C. (1981): The distribution of visceral primary afferents from the pelvic nerve to Lissauer's tract and the spinal gray matter and its relationship to the sacral parasympathetic nucleus. *J. Comp. Neurol.,* 201:415–440.
113. Mudge, A. W., Leeman, S. E., and Fischbach, G. D. (1979): Enkephalin inhibits release of substance P from sensory neurons in culture and decreases action potential duration. *Proc. Natl. Acad. Sci. U.S.A.,* 76:526–530.
114. Murase, K., and Randic, M. (1984): Actions of substance P on rat spinal dorsal horn neurones. *J. Physiol. (Lond.),* 346:203–217.
115. Nagy, J. I., and Hunt, S. P. (1983): The termination of primary afferents within the rat dorsal horn: Evidence for rearrangement following capsaicin treatment. *J. Comp. Neurol.,* 218:145–158.
116. Nagy, J. I., and Van Der Kooy, D. (1983): Effects of neonatal capsaicin treatment on nociceptive thresholds in the rat. *J. Neurosci.,* 3:1145–1150.
117. Nicoll, R. A., Alger, B. E., and Nicoll, R. A. (1980): Enkephalin blocks inhibitory pathways in the vertebrate CNS. *Nature,* 287:22–25.
118. Ninkovic, M., Beaujouan, J. C., Torrens, Y., Saffroy, M., Hall, M. D. and Glowinski, J. (1985): Differential localization of tachykinin receptors in rat spinal cord. *Eur. J. Pharmacol.,* 106:463–464.
119. Ninkovic, M., Hunt, S. P., and Kelly, J. S. (1981): Effect of dorsal rhizotomy on the autoradiographic distribution of opiate and neurotensin receptors and neurotensin-like immunoreactivity within the rat spinal cord. *Brain Res.,* 230:111–119.
120. Osorio, I., Hackman, J. C., and Davidoff, R. A. (1979): GABA or potassium: Which mediates primary afferent depolarization? *Brain Res.,* 161:183–186.
121. Patrick, J. T., McBride, W. J., and Felten, D. L. (1983): Distribution of glycine, GABA, aspartate and glutamate in the rat spinal cord. *Brain Res.,* 10:415–418.
122. Pickel, V. M., Miller, R., Chan, J., and Sumal, K. K. (1983): Substance P and enkephalin in transected axons of medulla and spinal cord. *Regul. Peptides,* 6:121–135.
123. Piercey, M. F., Lahti, R. A., Schroeder, L. A., Einspahr, E. J., and Barsuhn, C. (1982): U50488H, pure kappa receptor agonist with spinal analgesic loci in the mouse. *Life Sci.,* 31:1197–1200.
124. Price, D. D., Hayashi, H., Dubner, R., and Ruda, M. A. (1979): Functional relationships between neurons of the marginal and substantia gelatinosa layers of the primate dorsal horn. *J. Neurophysiol.,* 42:1590–1608.
125. Price, G. W., Wilkin, G. P., Turnbull, M. J., and Bowery, N. G. (1984): Are baclofen-sensitive $GABA_b$ receptors present on primary afferent terminals of the spinal cord? *Nature,* 307:71–74.
126. Proudfit, H. K., and Yaksh, T. L. (1980): Alterations in nociceptive threshold and morphine-induced analgesia following selective depletion of spinal cord monoamines. *Neurosci. Abstr.,* 6:433.
127. Przewlocki, R., Shearman, G. T., and Herz, A. (1983): Mixed opioid/nonopioid effects of dynorphin and dynorphin-related peptides after their intrathecal injection in rats. *Neuropeptides,* 3:233–240.
128. Przewlocki, R., Stala, L., Greczek, M., Shearman, G. T., Przewlocka, B., and Herz, A. (1983): Analgesic effects of μ-, and κ-opiate agonists and, in particular, dynorphin at the spinal level. *Life Sci.,* 33:649–652.
129. Quirion, R., Shults, C. W., Moody, T. W., Pert, C. B., Chase, T. N., and O'Donohue, T. L. (1983): Autoradiographic distribution of substance P receptors in rat central nervous system. *Nature,* 303:714–717.
130. Ralston, H. J., III, and Ralston, D. D. (1979): The distribution of dorsal root axons in laminae I, II and III of the macaque spinal cord: A quantitative electron microscope study. *J. Comp. Neurol.,* 184:643–684.
131. Ralston, H. J., III, and Ralston, D. D. (1982): The distribution of dorsal root axons to laminae IV, V, and VI of the macaque spinal cord: A quantitative electron microscopic study. *J. Comp. Neurol.,* 212:435–448.
132. Reddy, S. V. R., Maderdrut, J. L., and Yaksh, T. L. (1980): Spinal cord pharmacology of

adrenergic agonist-mediated antinociception. *J. Pharmacol. Exp. Ther.,* 213:525–533.
133. Rivot, J. P., Chaouch, A., and Besson, J. M. (1980): Nucleus raphe magnus modulation of response of rat dorsal horn neurons to unmyelinated fiber inputs: Partial involvement of serotonergic pathways. *J. Neurophysiol.,* 44:1039–1057.
134. Ruda, M. A. (1982): Opiates and pain pathways: Demonstration of enkephalin synapses on dorsal horn projection neurons. *Science,* 215:1523–1524.
135. Ruda, M. A., Allen, B., and Gobel, S. (1981): Ultrastructural analysis of medial brain stem afferents to the superficial dorsal horn. *Brain Res.,* 205:175–180.
136. Ruda, M. A., Coffield, J., and Steinbusch, H. W. M. (1982): Immunocytochemical analysis of serotonergic axons in laminae I and II of the lumbar spinal cord of the cat. *J. Neurosci.,* 2:1660–1671.
137. Ruda, M. A., and Gobel, S. (1980): Ultrastructural characterization of axonal endings in the substantia gelatinosa which take up [^{3}H]serotonin. *Brain Res.,* 184:57–83.
138. Sastry, B. R. (1979): γ-aminobutyric acid and primary afferent depolarization in feline spinal cord. *Can. J. Physiol. Pharmacol.,* 57:1157–1167.
139. Sastry, B. R., and Goh, J. W. (1983): Actions of morphine and met-enkephalin-amide on nociceptor driven neurones in substantia gelatinosa and deeper dorsal horn. *Neuropharmacology,* 22:119–122.
140. Sawynok, J., Kato, N., Havlicek, V., and LaBella, F. S. (1982): Lack of effect of baclofen on substance P and somatostatin release from the spinal cord in vitro. *Naunyn Schmiedergs Arch. Pharmacol.,* 319:78–81.
141. Sawynok, J., and LaBella, F. S. (1982): On the involvement of GABA in the analgesia produced by baclofen, muscimol and morphine. *Neuropharmacology,* 21:397–403.
142. Sawynok, J., Moochhala, S. M., and Pillay, D. J. (1984): Substance P, injected intrathecally, antagonizes the spinal antinociceptive effect of morphine, baclofen and noradrenaline. *Neuropharmacology,* 23:741–747.
143. Schmauss, C., Hammond, D. L., Ochi, J. W., and Yaksh, T. L. (1983): Pharmacological antagonism of the antinociceptive efforts of serotonin in the rat spinal cord. *Eur. J. Pharmacol.,* 90:349–357.
144. Seybold, V. S., and Elde, R. P. (1982): Neurotensin immunoreactivity in the superficial laminae of the dorsal horn of the rat: I. Light microscopic studies of cell bodies and proximal dendrites. *J. Comp. Neurol.,* 205:89–100.
145. Seybold, V. S., Hylden, J. L. K., and Wilcox, G. L. (1982): Intrathecal substance P and somatostatin in rats: Behaviors indicative of sensation. *Peptides,* 2:49–54.
146. Slater, P., and Patel, S. (1983): Autoradiographic localization of opiate κ receptors in the rat spinal cord. *Eur. J. Pharmacol.,* 92:159–160.
147. Stanzione, P., and Zieglgänsberger, W. (1983): Action of neurotensin on spinal cord neurons in the rat. *Brain Res.,* 268:111–118.
148. Sumal, K. K., Pickel, V. M., Miller, R. J., and Reis, D. J. (1982): Enkephalin-containing neurons in substantia gelatinosa of spinal trigeminal complex: Ultrastructural and synaptic interaction with primary sensory afferents. *Brain Res.,* 248:223–236.
149. Suzue, T., and Jessell, T. (1960): Opiate analgesics and endorphins inhibit rat dorsal root potential in vitro. *Neurosci. Lett.,* 16:161–166.
150. Sweetnam, P. M., Neale, J. H., Barker, J. L., and Goldstein, A. (1982): Localization of immunoreactive dynorphin in neurons cultured from spinal cord and dorsal root ganglia. *Proc. Natl. Acad. Sci. U.S.A.,* 79:6742–6746.
151. Tang, J., Chou, J., Yang, H. Y. T., and Costa, E. (1983): Substance P stimulates the release of met^5-enkephalin-arg^6-phe^7 and met^5-enkephalin from rat spinal cord. *Neuropharmacology,* 22:1147–1150.
152. Todd, A. J., and Millar, J. (1983): Receptive fields and responses to ionophoretically applied noradrenaline and 5-hydroxytryptamine of units recorded in laminae I–III of cat dorsal horn. *Brain Res.,* 288:159–167.
153. Urban, L., and Randic, M. (1984): Slow excitatory transmission in rat dorsal horn: Possible mediation by peptides. *Brain Res.,* 290:336–341.
154. Wall, P. D., Fitzgerald, M., and Gibson, S. J. (1981): The response of rat spinal cord cells to unmyelinated afferents after peripheral nerve section and after changes in substance P levels. *Neuroscience,* 5:2205–2215.

155. Werz, M. A., and MacDonald, R. L. (1983): Opioid peptides selective for mu- and delta-opiate receptors reduce calcium-dependent action potential duration by increasing potassium conductance. *Neurosci. Lett.,* 42:173–178.
156. Willcockson, W. S., Chung, J. M., Hori, Y., Lee, K. H., and Willis, W. D. (1984): Effects of iontophoretically released amino acids and amines on primate spinothalamic tract cells. *J. Neurosci.,* 4:732–740.
157. Willcockson, W. S., Chung, J. M., Hori, Y., Lee, K. H., and Willis, W. D. (1984): Effects of iontophoretically released peptides on primate spinothalamic tract cells. *J. Neurosci.,* 4:741–750.
158. Willis, W. D., Haber, L. H., and Martin, R. F. (1977): Inhibition of spinothalamic tract cells and interneurons by brain stem stimulation in the monkey. *J. Neurophysiol.,* 40:968–981.
159. Wilson, P. R., and Yaksh, T. L. (1978): Baclofen is antinociceptive in the spinal intrathecal space of animals. *Eur. J. Pharmacol.,* 51:323–330.
160. Woolf, C. J., and Fitzgerald, M. (1983): The properties of neurones recorded in the superficial dorsal horn of the rat spinal cord. *J. Comp. Neurol.,* 221:313–328.
161. Yaksh, T. L. (1981): Spinal opiate analgesia. Characteristics and principles of action. *Pain,* 11:293–346.
162. Yaksh, T. L., Abay, E. O., II, and Go, V. L. W. (1982): Studies on the location and release of cholecystokinin and vasoactive intestinal peptide in rat and cat spinal cord. *Brain Res.,* 242:279–290.
163. Yaksh, T. L., and Elde, R. P. (1981): Factors governing release of methionine enkephalin-like immunoreactivity from mesencephalon and spinal cord of the cat *in vivo. J. Neurophysiol.,* 46:1056–1075.
164. Yaksh, T. L., Jessell, T. M., Gamse, R., Mudge, A. W., and Leeman, S. E. (1980): Intrathecal morphine inhibits substance P release from mammalian spinal cord *in vivo. Nature,* 286:155–157.
165. Yaksh, T. L., Schmauss, C., Micevych, P. E., Obay, E. O., and G., V. L. W. (1982): Pharmacological studies on the application, disposition and release of neurotensin in the spinal cord. *Ann. N.Y. Acad. Sci.,* 400:228–242.
166. Yashpal, K., and Henry, J. L. (1983): Endorphins mediate overshoot of substance P-induced facilitation of a spinal nociceptive reflex. *Can. J. Physiol. Pharmacol.,* 61:303–307.
167. Yoshimura, M., and North, R. A. (1983): Substantia gelatinosa neurons hyperpolarized *in vitro* by enkephalin. *Nature,* 305:529–530.
168. Zieglgansberger, W., and Tulloch, I. F. (1979): The effects of methionine- and leucine-enkephalin on spinal neurones of the cat. *Brain Res.,* 167:53–64.
169. Zorman, G., Belcher, G., Adams, J. E., and Fields, H. L. (1982): Lumbar intrathecal naloxone blocks analgesia produced by microstimulation of the ventromedial medulla in the rat. *Brain Res.,* 236:77–84.

Advances in Pain Research and Therapy, Vol. 9, edited by H. L. Fields et al. Raven Press, New York © 1985.

Anginal-Like Pain: Spinal Mechanisms Underlying this Symptom in Gallbladder Disease

Robert D. Foreman and W. Steve Ammons

Department of Physiology and Biophysics, University of Oklahoma Health Sciences Center, Oklahoma City, Oklahoma 73190

Gallbladder disease is often associated with pain of the abdomen or back (18), but pain also may be referred to the chest and closely mimic angina pectoris (8,12,14) even though patients have no heart disease. Another population of patients has preexisting cardiac disease in addition to gallbladder disease (8,11). In these patients removal of the gallbladder often alleviates anginal-like pain. Several studies show that pain originating from visceral organs and referred to somatic structures, including the chest, results from convergence of visceral and somatic afferent fibers onto spinothalamic tract (STT) cells (5,7,9,13). Coronary artery occlusion or intracardiac injection of bradykinin activates T_1–T_5 spinothalamic tract neurons that also respond to somatic manipulation of the chest or left forearm (3, 4). Thus, angina pectoris probably results in excitation of STT cells whose somatic fields are located on the chest and arm. Based on these results, anginal-like pain of abdominal origin may result from abdominal sympathetic afferent excitation of STT neurons whose somatic fields also are located in the chest region. It is not known if abdominal visceral afferent fibers influence the T_1–T_5 STT neurons. Therefore, the primary goals of this study are to determine (a) if electrical stimulation of the left greater splanchnic nerve activates STT neurons and (b) if distention of the gallbladder alters the cell activity.

METHODS

Experiments were conducted on monkeys *(Macaca fascicularis)* tranquilized with ketamine (10–20 mg/kg) and anesthetized with α-chloralose (60–80 mg/kg). α-Chloralose (0.06–0.15 mg/kg/hr) and pancuronium bromide (0.15 μg/kg/hr) were infused constantly to maintain the plane of anesthesia and muscle paralysis, respectively. Catheters were placed in the femoral vein for fluid and drug injections and in the femoral artery for monitoring blood pressure. Artificial ventilation was used to maintain expiratory CO_2 between 3.5 and 4.5%.

After a left thoracotomy was performed, a bipolar platinum electrode was placed on the caudal ansa subclavia and on the sympathetic chain between the T_2 and T_3 rami communicantes to stimulate cardiopulmonary (CP) sympathetic afferent fibers. Another bipolar platinum electrode was placed on the left greater splanchnic (SPL) nerve as it emerged superior to the diaphragm (1).

A catheter was placed in the left atrium to inject bradykinin (4). After a midline abdominal incision, the cystic duct was ligated near its intersection with the common hepatic duct (2). A double-barrel polyethylene cannula was placed in the fundus of the gallbladder to monitor gallbladder pressure and to inject saline. Responses to gallbladder distention were examined during saline injections at one of the following pressures: 10, 20, 40, 60, 80, and 100 mm Hg.

After monkeys were placed in a stereotaxic frame, a laminectomy was performed to expose the T_1–T_5 spinal segments and a craniotomy was performed to allow placement of a concentric bipolar electrode in the right ventral posterior lateral nucleus (VPL) of the thalamus to activate antidromically spinothalamic tract cells in the upper thoracic cord. The left side of spinal gray matter was searched with a carbon filament glass microelectrode while stimulating VPL (10 Hz, 2 mA, 100 μsec duration). Standard criteria were used to demonstrate that all cells were antidromically activated.

After each cell was completely studied, DC current (50 μA, 20 sec) was passed through the electrode to mark the recording location. Thalamic sites were determined from lesions (20 μA, 20 sec) made at the end of the experiment. The brain and spinal segments were fixed in a 10% formalin solution; the tissue was frozen and cut in 60 μm sections. Sections containing the lesions were projected and drawn. All thalamic sites were in the VPL. Laminar locations were based on the descriptions for the laminae of the cat (16).

RESULTS

Recordings were made from 85 T_1–T_5 STT neurons. All the neurons responded to somatic manipulation of the triceps of the left forearm and the left chest and to electrical stimulation of the CP sympathetic afferent fibers. Every cell tested for SPL input received viscerosomatic inputs. Electrical stimulation of the SPL nerve excited 63 (74%) of the 85 neurons. Table 1 provides information about the number of SPL-responsive cells according to the type of somatic input they received. Cells were classified according to the type of somatic stimuli required to activate them. Wide dynamic range (WDR) cells were excited slightly during hair movement, but increased their discharge rate more during a pressure stimulus or noxious pinch. High-

TABLE 1. *STT cell responses to CP and SPL sympathetic stimulation*

			CP sympathetic response		SPL response	
Cell types	SPL inputs	No SPL input	Early only	Early plus late	Early only	Early plus late
WDR	29	6	22	13	15	14
HT	21	10	13	18	6	15[a]
HT_i	13	5	15	3	10[a]	3
LT	0	1	1	0	0	0
Total	63	22	51	34	31	32

HT, high-threshold cells; HT_i, high-threshold inhibitory cells; WDR, wide dynamic range cells; LT, low-threshold cell; SPL, left greater splanchnic nerve; CP, cardiopulmonary.

[a] $p < 0.05$ compared to corresponding early (HT) or early and late (HT_i) response.

threshold (HT) cells were excited only during noxious pinch. HT inhibitory cells (HT_i) required a noxious pinch to activate them, but hair movement inhibited the spontaneous activity. Low-threshold cells discharged maximally during hair movement or light touch. More WDR cells appeared to receive SPL input than the other three classes, but the distribution was not significantly different. Cells with SPL input were found in laminae I, IV, V, and VII (Fig. 1). A higher percentage of SPL-responsive cells tended to be found in the deeper laminae but the trend was insignificant because too few cells were found in laminae I and VII.

Comparison of Cell Responses to SPL and CP Sympathetic Stimulation

All 63 SPL-responsive cells exhibited early responses to both CP and SPL stimulation. In contrast to the cells responding to the early response, 51% of the cells exhibited late responses to SPL input and 40% had late responses

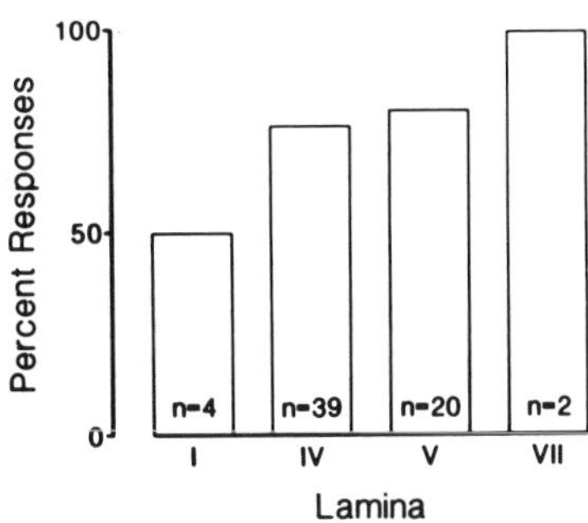

FIG. 1. Laminar locations of cells responding to SPL stimulation.

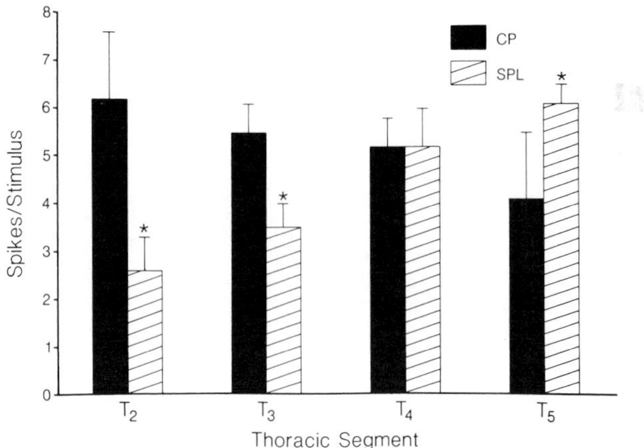

FIG. 2. STT cell responses to electrical stimulation of the CP and SPL nerves segregated according to segments. The maximum number of spikes per stimulus in the early peak was determined for each cell in the T_2–T_5 segments.*, $p < 0.05$.

to CP sympathetic input. Table 1 lists the number of cells with early and late responses classified according to the category of somatic input. HT cells were more likely to have early and late responses than the other categories, whereas HT_i cells were more likely to have only early responses.

The relationship of the maximum early burst discharge to CP and SPL stimulation changed according to the segment where the STT cells were found. Figure 2 shows that in T_2, STT cell responses to CP sympathetic stimulation were much greater than responses to SPL stimulation ($p < 0.01$). At more caudal segments the CP-evoked responses diminished and the SPL-evoked responses increased until they were nearly equal at segment T_4. In T_5, SPL responses were greater than the CP responses ($p < 0.05$). There was no apparent relationship between segmental location and magnitude of late responses to sympathetic afferent nerve stimulation.

Responses to Gallbladder Distention

Forty-four STT neurons were tested for their responses to gallbladder distention. Gallbladder distention increased the discharge rate of 16 (36%) cells, but none were inhibited. Figure 3 illustrates the response of a WDR neuron to a gallbladder distention of 100 mm Hg. The threshold for this cell was 50 mm Hg. This response was separated into an early phasic component and a later tonic component. Changes in cell activity that occurred during a change in gallbladder pressure, but adapted or were not maintained during the distention period, were considered phasic responses. A response was considered tonic if cell activity remained at an increased level for the duration of the distention (Fig. 4). The discharge rate of cells during the phasic

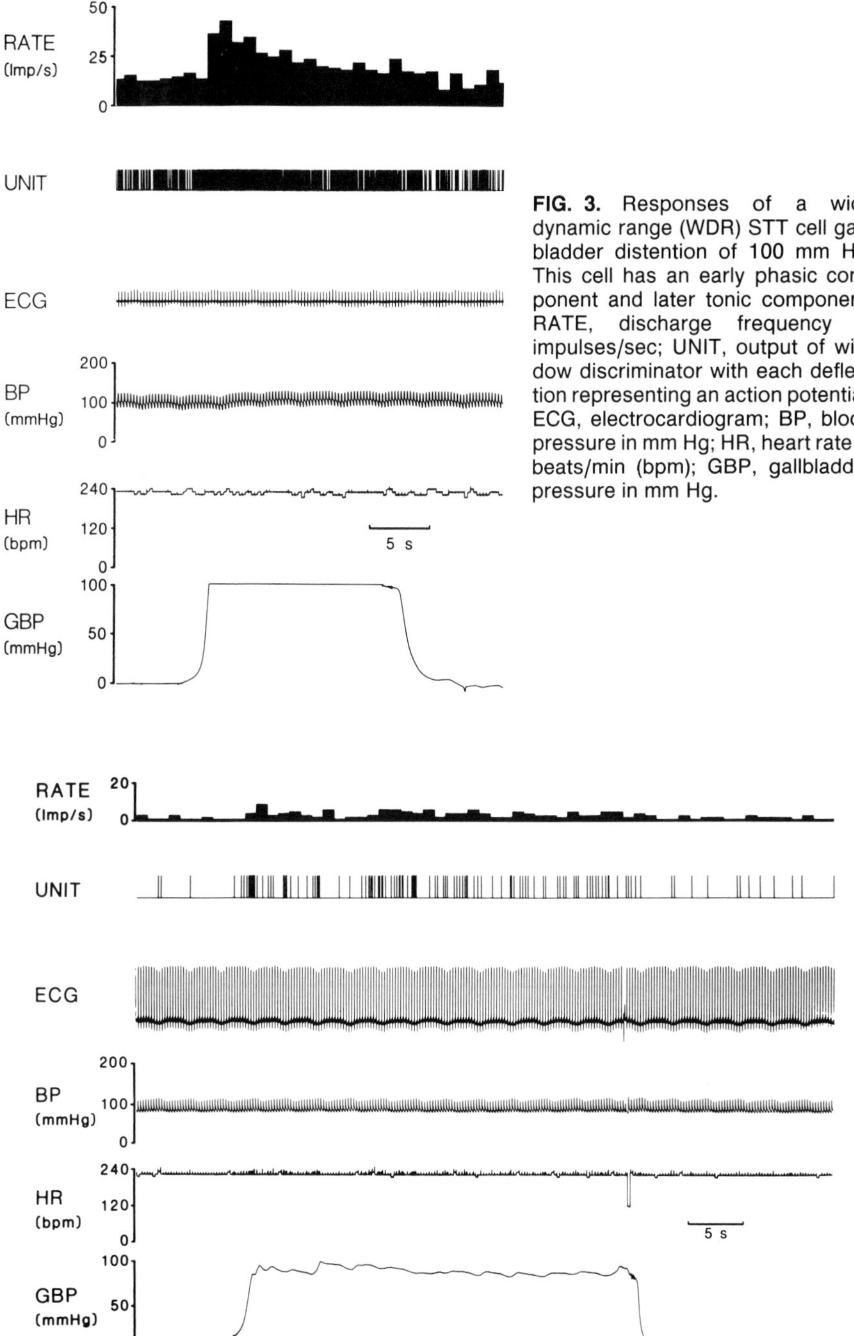

FIG. 3. Responses of a wide dynamic range (WDR) STT cell gallbladder distention of 100 mm Hg. This cell has an early phasic component and later tonic component. RATE, discharge frequency in impulses/sec; UNIT, output of window discriminator with each deflection representing an action potential; ECG, electrocardiogram; BP, blood pressure in mm Hg; HR, heart rate in beats/min (bpm); GBP, gallbladder pressure in mm Hg.

FIG. 4. Responses of a high threshold (HT) STT cell to gallbladder distention of 80 mm Hg. The abbreviations are the same as Fig. 3.

response was greater than for cells with the tonic response at distention pressures of 60, 80, and 100 mm Hg ($p < 0.05$).

Responses to Bradykinin

Bradykinin (2 μg/kg) was injected into the heart to determine its effect on the activity of 10 gallbladder-responsive and 21 nonresponsive cells to gallbladder distention. In this study the discharge rate of 20 (65%) cells increased after bradykinin injections. Of the 20 cells, 9 were responsive and 11 were nonresponsive to the gallbladder distention. Thus, 9 of 10 cells with response and 11 of 21 cells without response to gallbladder distention responded to bradykinin. The proportion of gallbladder-responsive cells was significantly greater than for the gallbladder-nonresponsive cells. Peak discharge rates obtained from gallbladder-responsive cells during bradykinin injections were significantly greater ($p < 0.05$) than for the nonresponsive cells (Fig. 5).

DISCUSSION

Splanchnic stimulation excites a large population of STT cells in the T_1 to T_5 segments of the spinal cord, in addition to STT cells of the lower thoracic spinal cord (7,9). T_1–T_5 cells also responded to manipulation of somatic structures, usually in the region of the left forelimb and left chest. All cells recorded in this study received input from the Aδ or Aδ and C sympathetic afferent fibers originating from the cardiopulmonary region.

The early response characteristics of STT cells to SPL and CP sympathetic afferent input were compared as a function of their inputs to cells in different segments. The maximum number of spikes per stimulus of the early peak

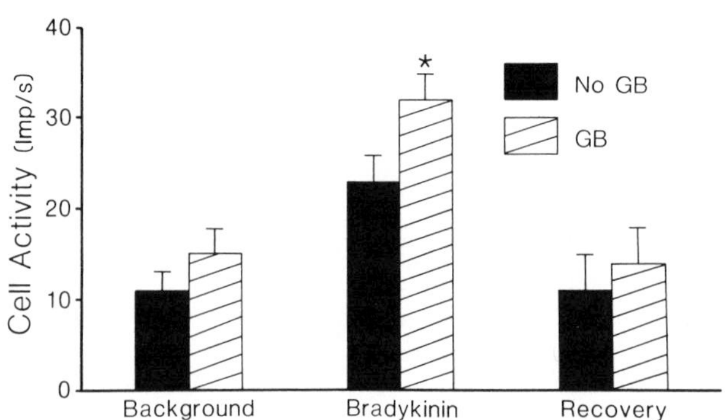

FIG. 5. Changes in activity of gallbladder-responsive and nonresponsive STT cells after injecting bradykinin into the left atrium. Bradykinin values represent the peak activity during the response.*, $p < 0.05$ compared to cells without gallbladder input.

decreased for CP afferent input and increased for SPL afferent input at more caudal segments; probably this trend continues as cells are examined in segments more caudal than T_5. This distribution of the response characteristics along the spinal cord may represent a mechanism the brain uses to localize the source of visceral pain. For example, acute gallbladder inflammation may increase cell activity in several segments of the spinal cord, but the majority of the input may be localized to the lower spinal cord. Since the cell activity of the lower spinal segments is greater than the activity of the upper segments, the brain may localize the source of the stimulus by comparing levels of activity according to the segments being most activated. There is a possibility that some patients with gallbladder disease may generate unusual patterns of input to the spinal cord so that the greatest activity may occur in the upper thoracic spinal cord.

This study is particularly relevant for providing an explanation of referred pain associated with gallbladder disease, because it provides further support for Ruch's (17) convergence-projection theory for referred pain. These results substantiate our hypothesis that anginal-like pain associated with gallbladder disease is the result of the convergence of gallbladder information with information from the somatic structures and the cardiopulmonary afferent fibers onto STT cells of the upper thoracic spinal cord.

Chest pain associated with gallbladder disease has many characteristics similar to that of angina pectoris (8,10,12,15). These similarities may exist because there is a population of T_1 to T_5 STT neurons that are particularly responsive to noxious stimulation of both the gallbladder and the heart, as demonstrated by intracardiac bradykinin injections. Since the marked increase in pressure associated with acute inflammatory gallbladder disease probably excites cells that also respond during myocardial ischemia, the anginal-like sensations of pain would be similar. These studies do not eliminate the possibility that this type of chest pain may result from reflexes altering cardiac performance, thereby leading to ischemia. It is still unclear why some patients experience anginal-like pain, whereas a majority of the patients experience pain in the somatic structures overlying the vicinity of the gallbladder, or the gallbladder responsive neurons of the lower thoracic spinal neurons are responsive to noxious stimulation of the abdominal wall (6).

SUMMARY AND CONCLUSIONS

The responses of 85 primate STT neurons were tested for electrical stimulation of the SPL nerve and distention of the gallbladder and chemical injections of bradykinin to the heart. We concluded that STT cells received both cardiac and gallbladder inputs, in addition to somatic inputs. These results supported our hypothesis that anginal-like pain associated with gallbladder disease resulted from the convergence of gallbladder information with information from the somatic structures and the cardiopulmonary afferent fibers onto STT T_1–T_5 cells.

ACKNOWLEDGMENTS

The authors thank Diana Holston for her expert technical assistance, Mary Martindale for technical support, Tammi Williams for preparing the figures, and Lula Rhoton for typing the manuscript. This research was supported by National Institutes of Health grant HL 22732 and HL 27260. W. S. Ammons is the recipient of National Institutes of Health postdoctoral fellowship NS 07114, and R. D. Foreman is the recipient of National Institutes of Health research career development award HL 00557.

REFERENCES

1. Ammons, W. S., Blair, R. W., and Foreman, R. D. (1984): Greater splanchnic excitation of primate T_1–T_5 spinothalamic neurons. *J. Neurophysiol.,* 51:592–603.
2. Ammons, W. S., Blair, R. W., and Foreman, R. D. (1984): Responses of primate T_1–T_5 spinothalamic neurons to gallbladder distention. *Am. J. Physiol.,* 247:R995–R1002.
3. Blair, R. W., Ammons, W. S., and Foreman, R. D. (1984): Responses of thoracic spinothalamic and spinoreticular cells to coronary artery occlusion. *J. Neurophysiol.,* 51:636–648.
4. Blair, R. W., Weber, R. N., and Foreman, R. D. (1982): Responses of thoracic spinothalamic neurons to intracardiac injections of bradykinin in the monkey. *Circ. Res.,* 51:83–94.
5. Blair, R. W., Weber, R. N., and Foreman, R. D. (1981): Characteristics of primate spinothalamic tract neurons receiving viscerosomatic convergent inputs in T_1–T_5 segments. *J. Neurophysiol.,* 46:797–811.
6. Cervero, F. (1983): Somatic and visceral inputs to the thoracic spinal cord of the cat: Effects of noxious stimulation of the biliary system. *J. Physiol. (Lond.),* 337:51–67.
7. Foreman, R. D., Hancock, M. B., and Willis, W. D. (1981): Responses of spinothalamic tract cells in the thoracic spinal cord of the monkey to cutaneous and visceral inputs. *Pain,* 11:149–162.
8. Hampton, A. G., Beckwith, J. R., and Wood, J. E. (1959): The relationship between heart disease and gallbladder disease. *Ann. Int. Med.,* 50:1135–1148.
9. Hancock, M. B., Foreman, R. D., and Willis W. D. (1975): Convergence of visceral and cutaneous input onto spinothalamic tract cells in the thoracic spinal cord of the cat. *Exp. Neurol.,* 47:240–248.
10. McArthur, S. W., and Wakefield (1945): Observations on the human electrocardiogram during experimental distention of the gallbladder. *J. Lab. Clin. Med.,* 30:349–351.
11. McLemore, G. A., and Levine, S. A. (1955): The possible therapeutic value of cholecystectomy in Adams-Stokes disease. *Am. J. Med. Sci.,* 229:386–391.
12. Miller, H. R. (1942): The interrelationship of disease of the coronary arteries and gallbladder. *Am. Heart J.,* 24:579–587.
13. Milne, R. J., Foreman, R. D., Giesler, G. J., Jr., and Willis, W. D. (1981): Convergence of cutaneous and pelvic visceral nociceptive inputs onto primate spinothalamic neurons. *Pain,* 11:163–183.
14. Ravdin, I. S., Fitzhugh, T., Wolferth, C. C., Barbier, E. A., and Ravdin, R. G. (1955): Relation of gallstone disease to angina pectoris. *Arch. Surg.,* 70:333–342.
15. Ravdin, I. S., Royster, H. P., and Sanders, G. B. (1942): Reflexes originating in the common duct giving rise to pain simulating angina pectoris. *Ann. Surg.,* 115:1055–1062.
16. Rexed, B. (1954): A cytoarchitechtonic organization of the spinal cord in the cat. *J. Comp. Neurol.,* 100:297–351.
17. Ruch, T. C. (1961): Pathophysiology of pain. In: *Neurophysiology,* edited by T. C. Ruch, H. D. Patton, J. W. Woodbury, and A. L. Towe, pp. 350–368. Saunders, Philadelphia.
18. Sherlock, S. (1981): *Diseases of the Liver and Biliary System.* Blackwell, Oxford.

Advances in Pain Research and Therapy, Vol. 9, edited by H. L. Fields et al. Raven Press, New York © 1985.

Nocireceptive Neurons in the Superficial Dorsal Horn of Cat Spinal Cord with an Inhibitory Input from Cutaneous Mechanoreceptors

Wilma M. Steedman and V. Molony

Department of Veterinary Physiology, University of Edinburgh, Edinburgh, Scotland EH9 1QH

There is a considerable body of evidence for segregation within the dorsal horn of the spinal cord, both of the afferent input arriving from specific sensory receptors in the skin and projecting to the spinal cord along identifiable axon groups, and of the patterns of response of the dorsal horn neurons themselves. In particular, it is well established that the superficial dorsal horn, made up of Rexed's laminae I and II, is a principal region of termination of fine myelinated (Aδ) afferent axons arising from cutaneous nociceptors (11,17) and of unmyelinated (C) axons (10,14,16). Electrophysiological recording has shown a population of cells first described by Christensen and Perl (5) that can be excited from the skin by noxious stimulation only. Some identified nociceptive neurons have been stained and characterized morphologically. These include large Waldeyer marginal neurons in lamina I (12,13,18) and neurons with small perikarya situated close to the lamina I/II border (1,12,13,18,21,22). Nociceptive neurons in the superficial dorsal horn are therefore heterogeneous morphologically; anatomical studies indicate that this diversity extends to the pattern of axonal projection. Some give rise to long ascending axons projecting to various supraspinal destinations including the thalamus (2,6), but the majority are interneurons projecting only a short distance within the dorsal horn.

Inhibition of nociceptive neurons in the superficial dorsal horn by afferent input in myelinated axons of cutaneous origin has been described by several laboratories (3,4,12,19,20); the opportunities thus exist for interaction between innocuous and noxious afferent inputs and modulation of the output of the neurons. A detailed knowledge of the nature of their responses to afferent stimulation is, therefore, an important requirement in reaching an understanding of their function. We have made prolonged, stable intracellular recordings from a small number of nocireceptive neurons in the superficial dorsal horn to analyze the responses, excitatory and inhibitory, to inputs from the skin and to electrical stimulation of peripheral nerves, and to obtain information on their morphology and axonal projection.

METHODS

Experiments were performed on adult cats anesthetized with chloralose and paralyzed with gallamine, and intracellular recordings made in the L6 and L7 segments of the spinal cord using fine glass microelectrodes containing horseradish peroxidase (HRP) which was ionophoresed into the neurons. Methods have been described in detail elsewhere (13). Thresholds and conduction times for different afferent fiber groups were established by stimulating the intact peroneal and tibial nerves at the ankle and recording the compound action potential from the dorsal root and the activity of afferent axons in the dorsal columns. Peripheral conduction velocities and central delays for individual inputs were calculated by comparing the responses of the dorsal horn neurons to stimulation of peripheral nerve and dorsal root. A range of innocuous mechanical stimuli was applied to the skin, and firm squeezing was the noxious mechanical stimulus. Receptive fields were identified but not mapped in detail.

RESULTS

The responses of ten neurons to afferent stimulation were examined in some detail. They were all located (by ionophoresis of HRP) around the lamina I/II border. Figure 1 shows one well-stained neuron reconstructed from several sections. It had a small cell body (maximum diameter 20 μm) located 95 μm below the border of the superficial dorsal horn. Its dendritic tree arose from three principal dendrites and was fan-shaped, extending 650 μm rostrocaudally, 280 μm dorsoventrally, and 200 μm mediolaterally. It resembled the "limitrophe" cells of Ramón y Cajal (15) or the "stalked" cells of Gobel (8,9). Its axon travelled 150 μm laterally before branching in lamina I outwith the limits of the dendritic tree, and, *en passant,* and terminal swellings were observed on the branches. Four other neurons with similarly shaped dendritic trees have been reconstructed. In one there was evidence of a parent axon travelling dorsolaterally into Lissauer's tract while the axons of the other three arborized locally, and swellings were observed on branches within laminae I and II. One well-stained neuron had a cylindrical dendritic tree oriented parallel to the lamina I/II border; two principal dendrites arose from the rostral and caudal poles of the soma and its axon remained within lamina II and terminated outwith the dendritic tree. It was a typical "islet" cell as described by Gobel (8,9).

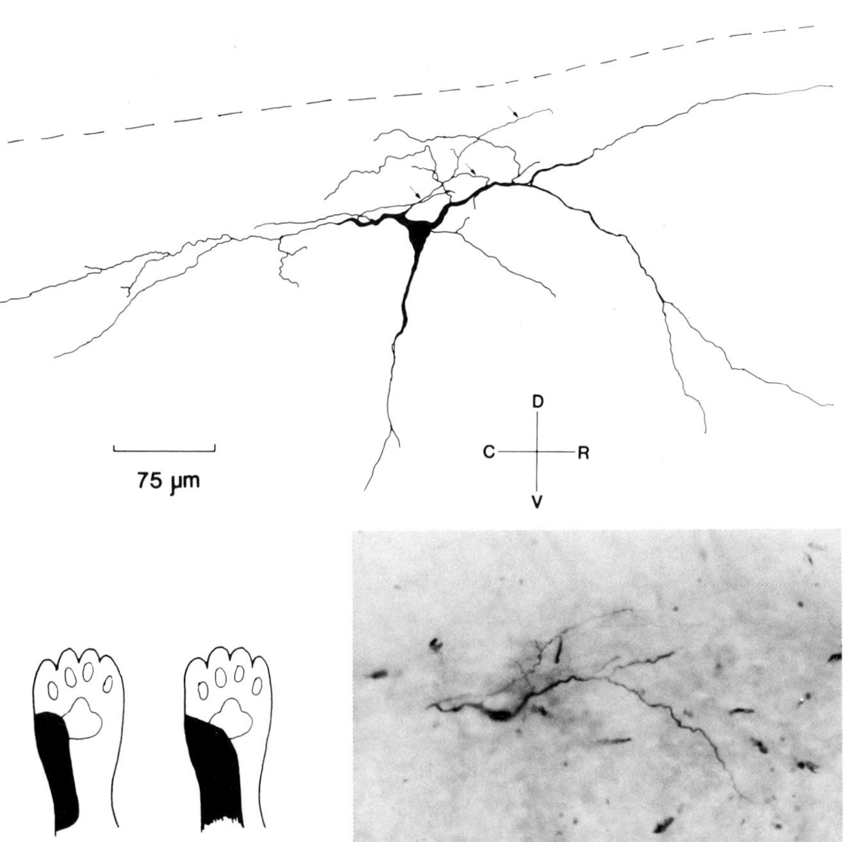

FIG. 1. Nocireceptive neuron in the superficial dorsal horn with receptive fields on the skin as shown. **Lower:** Photomicrograph. **Upper:** Reconstruction from five 50 μm serial parasagittal sections. The *broken line* represents the border between the dorsal columns and dorsal horn. The axon *(arrowed)* traveled 150 μm laterally before branching out with the dendritic tree.

Responses to Stimulation of the Skin

Excitatory receptive fields responding only to noxious stimulation were generally small, on the toes. One neuron, located laterally in the dorsal horn, had a relatively large excitatory field on the foot and leg (Fig. 1). Eight neurons had more extensive inhibitory receptive fields responding to innocuous mechanical stimuli, which frequently overlapped the excitatory fields. The excitatory stimulus caused depolarization of the membrane, maintained for the duration of the stimulus. Increased firing was abrupt in onset and lasted only for the duration of the stimulus. Action potentials arose singly from excitatory postsynaptic potentials (EPSPs); bursts of spikes arising from prolonged EPSPs were never recorded. The inhibitory stimulus evoked a less well-defined hyperpolarization and decreased firing. These responses have been previously described for other neurons in this region (19).

Responses to Electrical Stimulation of Peripheral Nerves

Electrical stimulation revealed considerable convergence of excitatory inputs along different fiber groups and different nerves, and strong low threshold inhibitory inputs along either or both peripheral nerves. Excitatory responses were short-lived, and occurred consistently in response to repeated stimulation. Central delay measurements for six neurons gave evidence of a monosynaptic Aδ input. Where a C-fiber input was present it evoked a regularly occurring constant-latency response as previously recorded extracellularly by Fitzgerald and Wall (7) who suggested that this was evidence for a monosynaptic input. Figure 2 shows the responses of a neuron to single pulse electrical stimulation of the peroneal nerve, showing a pronounced inhibition of background activity and a regular C-fiber evoked single spike response at 300 msec latency (for a conduction distance of 240 mm) with a maximum variation of ± 1 msec at threshold voltage. At 1.5 times "C" threshold four regularly occurring spikes were evoked.

All neurons received an inhibitory input, activated by electrical stimulation at the threshold for exciting Aβ fibers. This evoked hyperpolarization which increased in amplitude and duration with increasing stimulus strength (Fig. 3A). Both Aδ and C excitatory responses arose from a hyperpolarized membrane (Fig. 3B).

DISCUSSION

The neurons described form part of a group of small nocireceptive neurons in the superficial dorsal horn with locally projecting axons, small numbers of which have been reported from various laboratories (1,12,18).

The electrophysiological evidence for monosynaptic Aδ- and C-fiber inputs is in agreement with the known distribution of primary afferent terminations within the dorsal horn. Inhibition, whether in response to natural stimulation of the skin or electrical stimulation of the peripheral nerves, was associated with hyperpolarization and was, therefore, at least in part postsynaptic. These intracellular recordings show that the response of a neuron to noxious stimulation of the skin is influenced by concurrent innocuous mechanical stimulation; this is evidence that the onward transmission of noxious information from the superficial dorsal horn depends on the bal-

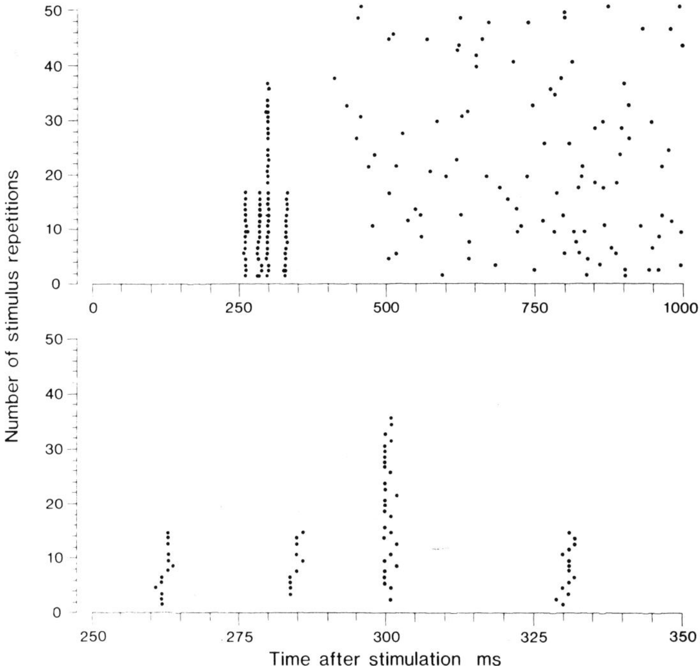

FIG. 2. Raster displays of spikes recorded from a nociceptive neuron in the superficial dorsal horn. The peroneal nerve was stimulated repeatedly (once every 4 sec) with single 1.2 msec pulses at voltages below threshold, at threshold, and at 1.5 times threshold for a single C-fiber evoked spike. **Upper:** Spikes recorded for 1 sec after the application of each stimulus. There was a prolonged inhibition, and a late C-fiber evoked excitatory response. **Lower:** The late excitatory response shown on a different time scale. Stimulation at threshold for C fibers evoked a single, constant-latency regularly occurring spike at 300 msec, and stimulation at 1.5 times C threshold evoked four regularly occurring spikes. Spikes were collected in 1 msec bins.

ance of these different primary afferent inputs. The presence of swellings, presumed to be boutons, on fine branches of axons within lamina I suggests that this processed nociceptive output may be transmitted to projecting neurons (e.g., spinothalamic tract) in lamina I. Swellings were also observed within lamina II, and as the majority of neurons in this area have locally projecting axons the output of these nociceptive neurons may be expected to affect reflex activity at the spinal level.

ACKNOWLEDGMENTS

This work was supported by a grant from the Wellcome Trust. We acknowledge gratefully the assistance of Mrs. A. Leask, Miss H. Hunter, Mr.

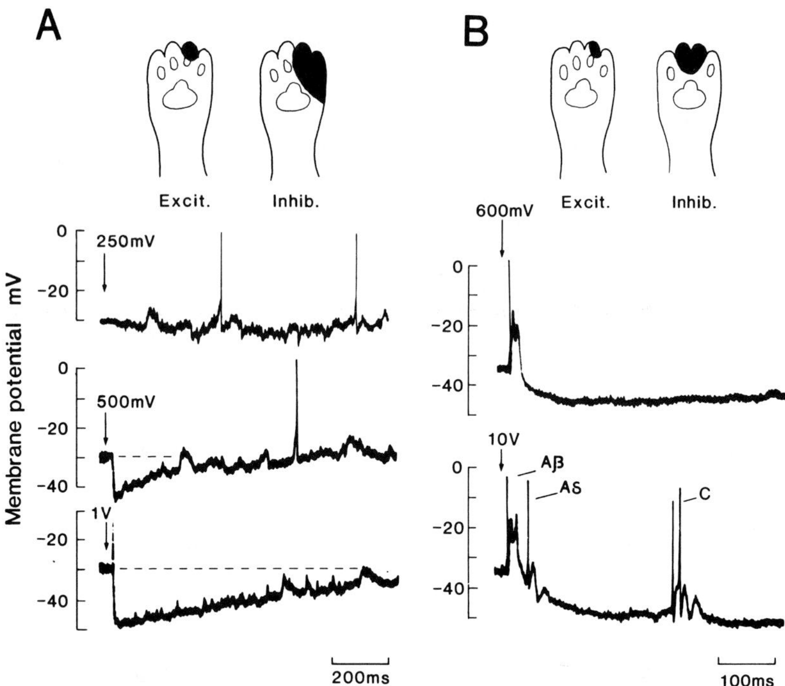

FIG. 3. Intracellular recordings of the responses of two nocireceptive superficial dorsal horn neurons to repeated single pulse stimulation of the nerve at the intensities shown. Cutaneous excitatory and inhibitory receptive fields are shown. **A:** The hyperpolarization evoked at low threshold increased in both amplitude and duration as stimulus strength was increased. **B:** The Aδ- and C-fiber evoked excitatory responses arose from a hyperpolarized membrane.

M. L. Graham, Mr. J. G. Greenhorn, and Mr. C. M. Warwick. Animals were held in the Wellcome Animal Research Unit of the Faculty of Veterinary Medicine.

REFERENCES

1. Bennett, G. J., Abdelmoumene, M., Hayashi, H., and Dubner, R. (1980): Physiology and morphology of substantia gelatinosa neurons intracellularly stained with horseradish perodixase. *J. Comp. Neurol.,* 194:809–827.
2. Carstens, E., and Trevino, D. L. (1978): Laminar origins of spinothalamic projections in the cat as determined by the retrograde transport of horseradish peroxidase. *J. Comp. Neurol.,* 182:151–166.
3. Cervero, F., Iggo, A., and Molony, V. (1979): An electrophysiological study of neurones in the substantia gelatinosa Rolandi of the cat's spinal cord. *Q. J. Exp. Physiol.,* 64:297–314.
4. Cervero, F., Iggo, A., and Ogawa, H. (1976): Nociceptor-driven dorsal horn neurones in the lumbar spinal cord of the cat. *Pain,* 2:5–24.
5. Christensen, B. N., and Perl, E. R. (1970): Spinal neurons specifically excited by noxious or thermal stimuli: marginal zone of the dorsal horn. *J. Neurophysiol.,* 33:293–307.

6. Craig, A. D., Jr., and Burton, H. (1981): Spinal and medullary lamina I projection to nucleus submedius in medial thalamus: a possible pain center. *J. Neurophysiol.,* 45:443–466.
7. Fitzgerald, M., and Wall, P. D. (1980): The laminar organization of dorsal horn cells responding to peripheral C fibre stimulation. *Exp. Brain Res.,* 41:36–44.
8. Gobel, S. (1975): Golgi studies of the substantia gelatinosa neurons in the spinal trigeminal nucleus. *J. Comp. Neurol.,* 162:397–415.
9. Gobel, S. (1978): Golgi studies of the neurons in layer II of the dorsal horn of the medulla trigeminal nucleus caudalis. *J. Comp. Neurol.,* 180:395–414.
10. Gobel, S., Falls, W. M., and Humphrey, E. (1981): Morphology and synaptic connections of ultrafine primary axons in lamina I of the spinal dorsal horn: candidates for the terminal axon arbors of primary neurons with unmyelinated (C) axons. *J. Neurosci.,* 1:1163–1179.
11. Light, A. R., and Perl, E. R. (1979): Spinal termination of functionally identified primary afferent neurons with slowly conducting myelinated fibers. *J. Comp. Neurol.,* 186:133–150.
12. Light, A. R., Trevino, D. L., and Perl, E. R. (1979): Morphological features of functionally defined neurons in the marginal zone and substantia gelatinosa of the spinal dorsal horn. *J. Comp. Neurol.,* 186:151–172.
13. Molony, V., Steedman, W. M., Cervero, F., and Iggo, A. (1981): Intracellular marking of identified neurones in the superficial dorsal horn of the cat spinal cord. *Q. J. Exp. Physiol.,* 66:211–223.
14. Perl, E. R. (1984): Characterization of nociceptors and their activation of neurons in the superficial dorsal horn: first steps for the sensation of pain. In: *Advances in Pain Research and Therapy, Vol. 6,* edited by L. Kruger and J. C. Liebeskind, pp. 23–51. Raven Press, New York.
15. Ramón y Cajal, S. (1909): *Histologie du Système nerveux de l'Homme et des Vertébrés, Vol. 1.* Maloine, Paris.
16. Réthelyi, M. (1977): Preterminal and terminal axon arborizations in the substantia gelatinosa of cat's spinal cord. *J. Comp. Neurol.,* 172:511–528.
17. Réthelyi, M., Light, A. R., and Perl, E. R. (1982): Synaptic complexes formed by functionally defined primary afferent units with fine myelinated fibers. *J. Comp. Neurol.,* 207:381–393.
18. Réthelyi, M., Light, A. R., and Perl, E. R. (1983): Synapses made by nociceptive laminae I and II neurons. In: *Advances in Pain Research and Therapy, Vol. 5,* edited by J. J. Bonica, U. Lindblom, and A. Iggo. Raven Press, New York.
19. Steedman, W. M., Iggo, A., Molony, V., Korogod, S., and Zachary, S. (1983): Statistical analysis of ongoing activity of neurones in the substantia gelatinosa and in lamina III of cat spinal cord. *Q. J. Exp. Physiol.,* 68:733–746.
20. Steedman, W. M., and Molony, V. (1983): Functional characteristics of substantia gelatinosa neurons in unanesthetized decerebrate cats. In: *Advances in Pain Research and Therapy, Vol. 5,* edited by J. Bonica, U. Lindblom, and A. Iggo, pp. 119–124. Raven Press, New York.
21. Steedman, W. M., and Molony, V. (1985): Small nociceptive neurones in the superficial dorsal horn of the cat. *Philos. Trans. R. Soc. Lond. (Biol),* B308:415.
22. Woolf, C. J., and Fitzgerald, M. (1983): The properties of neurones recorded in the superficial dorsal horn of the rat spinal cord. *J. Comp. Neurol.,* 221:313–328.

Advances in Pain Research and Therapy, Vol. 9, edited by H. L. Fields et al. Raven Press, New York © 1985.

Functional Plasticity of the Flexor Withdrawal Reflex in the Rat Following Peripheral Tissue Injury

Clifford J. Woolf

Department of Anatomy, University College London, London WC1E 6BT, United Kingdom

The relationship between noxious stimuli and the responses they generate, measured either as motor responses or as sensation, is exceedingly complex. Except where stimuli of an intensity insufficient to produce tissue injury are used, no simple power function can be found to describe this relationship. One reason for the complexity of the input/output coupling is that it is unlikely that the somatosensory system is organized as a series of labeled-line channels, which once activated simply relay the input to appropriate output centers. Instead, at each stage in the nociceptive system, there are a multitude of inhibitory controls modifying the sensory transfer. In the dorsal horn of the spinal cord, for example, both segmental and descending inhibitory systems control the access of different sensory inputs into the central nervous system. The presence of these inhibitory controls means that the response to a given stimulus does not depend only on the nature, intensity, and location of the stimulus, but also on all the factors which, directly or indirectly, either increase or decrease the activity of the inhibitory circuits. In other words, we must look to the central nervous system as well as to peripheral receptors to explain the consequences of noxious inputs.

Inhibitory mechanisms may not be, however, the only factor that can result in the same stimulus producing different responses at different times. The present series of experiments have set out to examine whether certain types of input can increase the excitability of the central nervous system for periods which outlast the duration of the stimulus. The rationale of this study is not just to find yet another element which contributes to the variability of noxious stimulus-response coupling but to try to identify whether the sensory disturbances that accompany acute or chronic peripheral tissue injury, such as hyperalgesia or allodynia, have a central component.

Sensation cannot be measured directly in animals, only changes in behavior can be observed. It is useful, therefore, when performing experiments in laboratory animals to study sensory input from the point of view of the motor response it elicits. We have used the flexor withdrawal reflex to study noxious stimulus-response relations in the spinal cord of the rat. The flexor reflex in a limb manifests as a self-limiting, explosive burst of activity in the motoneurons innervating the flexor muscles of the limb following adequate noxious stimuli. In man there is a good correlation between the elicitation of the flexor reflex and the perception of pain (6).

BEHAVIORAL EXPERIMENTS

The hindlimb flexor withdrawal reflex has been examined both in intact and in chronic decerebrate rats. The reason for using the decerebrated animals is simply that it permits the study of the consequences of peripheral injuries that cannot ethically be performed in the intact animal. The animals are decerebrated under barbiturate anesthesia by aspiration of all the cranial contents rostral to the mesencephalon. With careful nursing, body temperature control, and regular orogastric tube feeding the animals can survive for many weeks (8). The animals display an extensive behavioral repertoire including righting reflexes, grooming, locomotion, etc. Noxious stimuli at intensities insufficient to cause tissue injury evoke a brisk withdrawal reflex, orientation of the body to the site of the stimulus, and vocalization.

The flexor reflex has been examined by measuring the mechanical threshold necessary to elicit it (using von Frey hairs), the response time following immersion of the hindpaw in water at 49°C and finally by a qualitative assessment; the flexor sensitivity score (8). This is a range of scores from 0 for an unresponse foot to 5 where a sustained flexion is elicited by fine touch or brushing. In the absence of tissue injury the flexor reflex is remarkably stable in the decerebrate animals, although the mechanical thresholds are slightly less than that found in intact animals. An acute thermal injury (radiant heat) produces a short latency (minutes) fall in the mechanical threshold and a decrease in the thermal response time of the reflex (7) that returns to normal within 24 hr. Contact thermal injuries to the lateral edge of the foot or the subcutaneous injection of turpentine produce a mechanical hypersensitivity of the reflex which in the former case lasts for as long as 4 weeks and in the latter for 2 weeks (8). Figure 1 shows the changes in the reflex occurring following turpentine injection. A feature of the postinjury reflex hypersensitivity is that the reflex, instead of lasting for 1 or 2 sec following a standard pinch, can last up to 3 min as a sustained flexion. These changes in the reflex, a decrease in threshold and in increase in responsiveness, indicate that the chronic decerebrate animal is a useful preparation for studying changes that may be analogous to the postinjury sensory disturbances that occur in man.

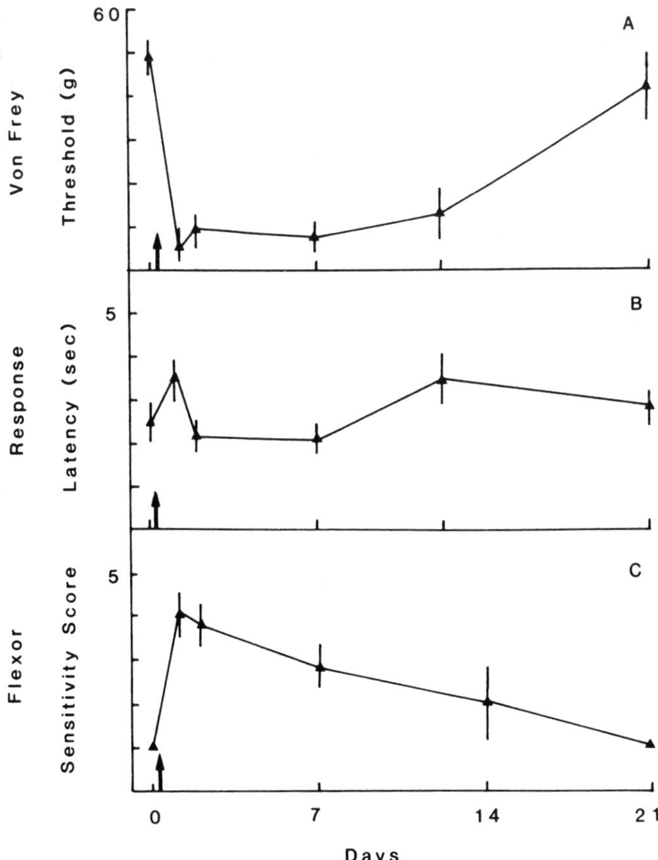

FIG. 1. Alterations in the hindlimb flexor reflex of chronic decerebrate rats following the injection of turpentine (0.1 ml) into the hindpaw at the time indicated by the *arrow.* **A** illustrates the change in the mechanical threshold of the reflex measured with von Frey hairs. **B** shows that there was no significant alteration in the response time following immersion in water at 49°C, while **C** indicates the qualitative increase in reflex sensitivity lasting for 14 days. (From ref. 8, with permission.)

ELECTROPHYSIOLOGICAL EXPERIMENTS

The response properties of single α-motoneurons innervating the posterior head of biceps femoris or semitendinosus have been studied by isolating single units in small filaments dissected from these muscle nerves in decerebrate and spinalized rats (initial anesthetic, Althesin). In this preparation the phasic flexor motoneurons have an absent spontaneous activity, very distinctive delayed and prolonged C-fiber evoked responses and stable cutaneous receptive fields responding to polymodal noxious stimuli (9).

The production of an acute thermal injury (radiant heat, 75°C for 60 sec) to the hindpaw ipsilateral to a hamstring motoneuron results in a decrease in the mechanical threshold of the existing cutaneous receptive field of the motoneuron, an increase in spontaneous activity, an expansion of the size of the cutaneous receptive field, and an increase in the amplitude and duration of the response evoked by a standard pinch (7).

This postinjury hypersensitivity of the flexor reflex results, at least in part, from changes in the excitability of the spinal cord, which are triggered but not sustained by the peripheral injury. The production of a sensory block at the site of the injury, with local anesthetic, does not result in the return of the reflex to its preinjury levels either in terms of the expanded receptive fields or in terms of the responses evoked by stimulation of the sural nerve (7) (Fig. 2). The afferent barrage generated by the thermal injury has altered the spinal cord such that the response to a standard input after the injury is much greater than that prior to the injury. The spinal cord has in effect a "memory" of the injury input. These central changes do not mean that the peripheral injury has not altered the properties of primary afferents in its vicinity producing sensitization (2). We have, in fact, found that a thermal injury identical to that used for the above experiments does alter C nociceptor responses, but that the changes are insufficient to account for the reflex hypersensitivity (3).

We have also investigated which types of primary afferent input can produce these prolonged alterations in the excitability of the spinal cord (5). A brief conditioning stimulus to the sural nerve (1 Hz, 20 sec) at C-fiber strength produces an increase in the excitability of the flexion reflex that lasts up to 10 min (Fig. 3). An identical conditioning stimulus applied to the nerve innervating the gastrocnemius-soleus produces an excitability increase lasting 40 min. These changes are only produced by conditioning stimuli at C-fiber strength and are suppressed by prior pretreatment of the sciatic nerve with capsaicin, a C-fiber neurotoxin. These results show that brief inputs from unmyelinated afferents innervating skin and muscle can generate prolonged changes in the excitability of the spinal cord and that this may underly the changes found with the acute thermal injury. We are currently investigating precisely where in the spinal cord these changes occur and why muscle afferents are more effective than cutaneous ones. It is interesting to speculate whether peptides such as substance P or cholecystokinin may be involved, since they can produce prolonged excitations (4). Apart from electrical conditioning stimuli and acute thermal injuries, we have also found that the application of mustard oil, a C-fiber irritant, to the skin and the production of tetany in muscles result in similar prolonged excitability increases.

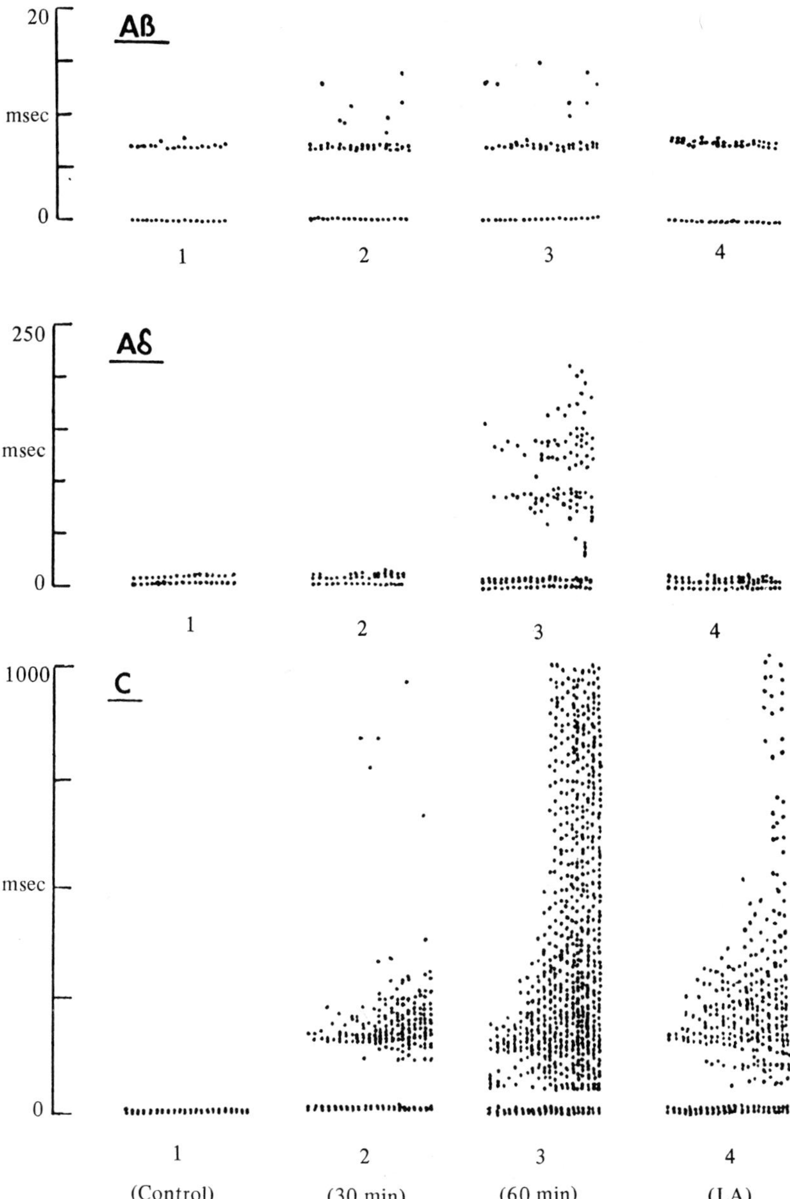

FIG. 2. Raster dot displays of a single biceps femoris motoneuron activated by stimulation of the sural nerve before an ipsilateral thermal injury (control), 30 and 60 min postinjury and 10 min after the injured foot had been completely anesthetized with xylocaine. Each *dot* is an action potential. The *vertical scale* is the latency of response, whereas the *horizontal scale* is real time with each stimulus repeat every 2 sec. The sural nerve was stimulated at strengths that only activated Aβ afferents, Aβ and Aδ afferents, and Aβ, Aδ, and C afferents. Note the different time scales. The injury resulted in an increase in the sural evoked response but sensory block of the site of the injury (LA) did not return the response to preinjury levels. (From ref. 7, with permission.)

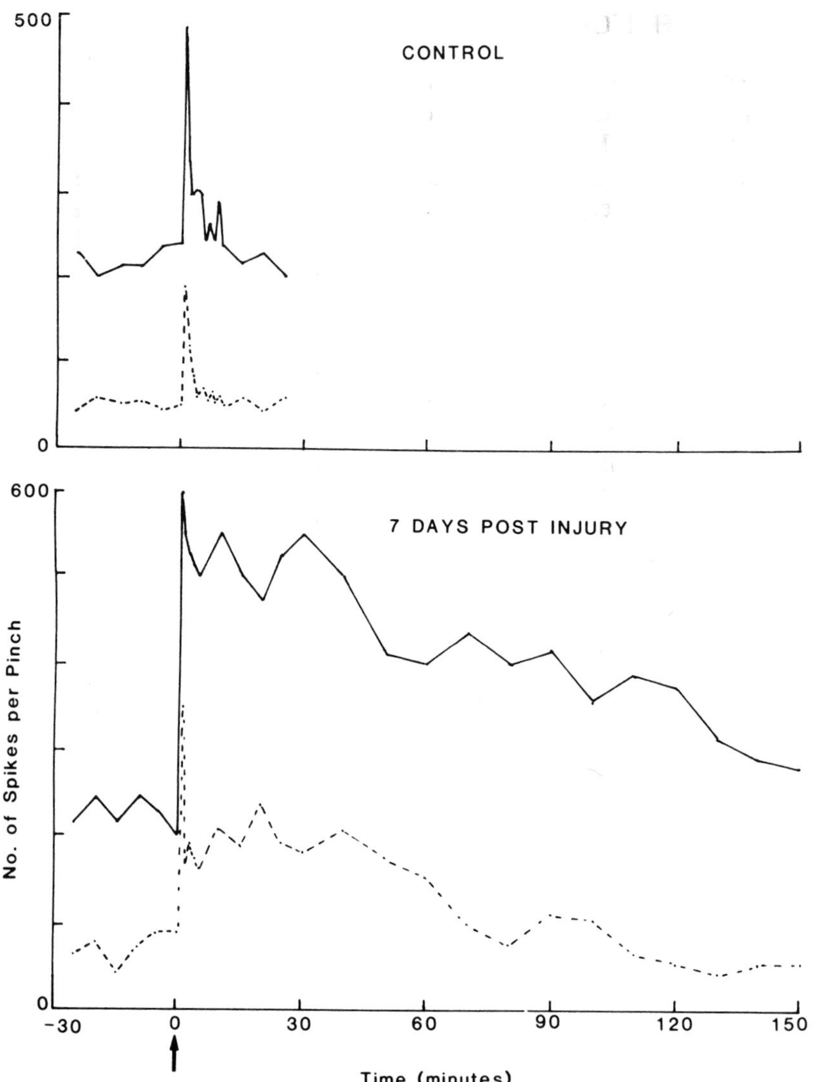

FIG. 3. Changes in the excitability of the flexor reflex measured by counting the total number of spikes evoked in a flexor motoneuron by a standard 3-sec suprathreshold pinch to the ipsilateral hindpaw *(solid lines)* and to the contralateral hindpaw *(dotted lines),* produced by a 20-sec 1 Hz conditioning stimulus at C-fiber strength to the sural nerve at the time shown by the *arrow.* In the **top panel** the excitability increase in a control animal is shown while the **lower panel** shows that when the sural conditioning stimulus is applied to a chronic decerebrate rat 7 days following a turpentine injection, the excitability increase lasts much longer.

CHANGES FOLLOWING CHRONIC INJURY

Although the excitability changes described above are large and are likely to be important for explaining acute postinjury hypersensitivity, their duration is relatively short compared to clinical pain disorders. We have attempted to establish if a chronic inflammatory lesion produces changes which are qualitatively different from those which result from acute injuries. In order to do this the electrophysiological experiments have been performed in chronic decerebrate rats 5 to 8 days following a contact thermal injury or turpentine injection. Preliminary data indicate that in keeping with the behavioral measures of the reflex, there is a fall in the von Frey thresholds of the flexor motoneurons' cutaneous receptive fields. Interestingly, a fall in threshold occurs both if the injury is on the ipsilateral or on the contralateral paw. In single motoneurons ipsilateral to the injury there is also an increase in the duration of the response to a standard pinch, and many units, unlike the control situation, have an after-discharge to cutaneous stimuli lasting up to 2 min (Fig. 4). Unfortunately, it is not possible in these animals to determine the "central" contribution to these changes using a sensory block with anesthetic, because injection of the anesthetic into the inflamed tissue results in a significant systemic uptake, and we have found that low doses of systemic Xylocaine suppress the activity of the

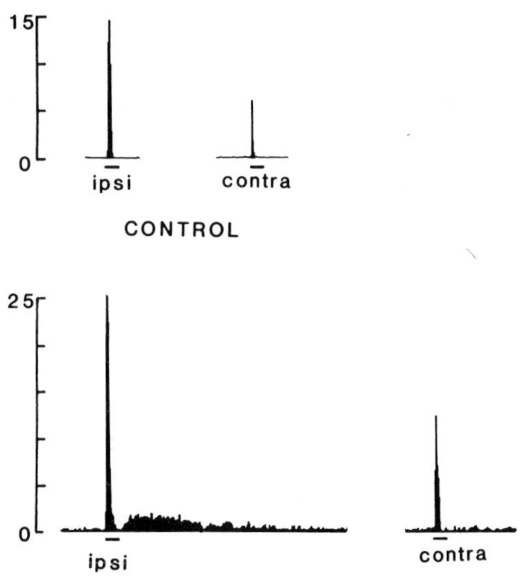

FIG. 4. Ratemeter recordings of the responses of single flexor motoneurons to stimulation of the ipsilateral and contralateral hindpaws with a stand and suprathreshold pinch. In control animals the response consists of a brief high frequency burst of activity with the ipsi input much longer than the contralateral one. In chronic decerebrate rats, 7 days postturpentine injections, the responses are longer and have a distinct afterdischarge (Bin width 200 μsec).

flexor reflex. It is interesting to note that systemic local anesthetics have been used to treat chronic pain in patients (1).

One change that we have found in the decerebrate rats with chronic injuries is that the excitability increase resulting from a sural conditioning stimulus is 4 to 5 times longer than that found in control animals (Fig. 3). A chronic injury results, therefore, in changes in the spinal cord that alter the temporal profile of the effects of a C-fiber input. Whether this effect appears immediately after the injury and whether it is maintained after the inflammation has resolved are questions that we plan to study.

DISCUSSION

On the basis of the results obtained in this series of experiments the term functional plasticity has been introduced to indicate that in the spinal cord the relationship beween noxious stimulus and flexor response is not fixed but is plastic, and that it changes in a way that depends on previous inputs (Fig. 5). Acute and chronic inflammatory lesions and electrical C-fiber inputs have been found to produce prolonged alterations in the excitability of the spinal cord. Whether the same mechanism underlies all these effects has yet to be established. If similar changes occur in neurons projecting to the brain then the degree of pain experienced following injury in man may depend on central mechanisms as well as the number of peripheral nociceptors activated. The answer to the question of whether the prolonged periph-

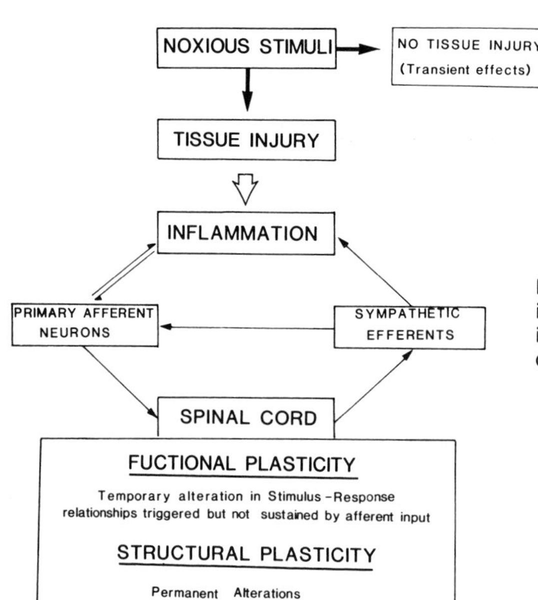

FIG. 5. Schematic model illustrating the changes that peripheral injury can produce in the spinal cord.

eral afferent input resulting from a long-lasting inflammatory lesion can produce "permanent" alterations in the spinal cord, in addition to a short-term functional plasticity, may help to elucidate the physiological basis of chronic pain. However, it is clear that we must examine the performance of the nervous system over a time band from milliseconds to days if we are to understand its response to peripheral tissue injury, and that the outcome of any input will depend on a balance of excitatory and inhibitory influences.

ACKNOWLEDGMENTS

I thank the Medical Research Council and the Wellcome Trust for financial support, and Pat Wall and Steve McMahon with whom some of these experiments were performed.

REFERENCES

1. Linblom, U., and Linström, P. (1984): Analgesic effect of tocainide in neuralgia. *Pain (Suppl.),* 2:S411.
2. Lynn, B. (1977): Cutaneous hyperalgesia. *Br. Med. Bull.,* 33:103–107.
3. McMahon, S. B., and Woolf, C. J. (1984): The effects of peripheral injury on the mechanosensitivity of rat unmyelinated cutaneous afferents. *J. Physiol. (Lond.),* 353:10P.
4. Urban, L., and Randic, M. (1984): Slow excitatory transmission in rat dorsal horn: possible mediation by peptides. *Brain Res.,* 290:336–342.
5. Wall, P. D., and Woolf, C. J. (1984): Muscle but not cutaneous C-afferent input produces prolonged increases in the excitability of the flexion reflex in the rat. *J. Physiol. (Lond.),* 356:443–458.
6. Willer, J. C. (1977): Comparative study of perceived pain and nociceptive flexion reflex in man. *Pain,* 3:69–80.
7. Woolf, C. J. (1983): Evidence for a central component of post-injury pain hypersensitivity. *Nature,* 306:686–688.
8. Woolf, C. J. (1984): Long term alterations in the excitability of the flexion reflex produced by peripheral tissue injury in the chronic decerebrate rat. *Pain,* 18:325–343.
9. Woolf, C. J., and Swett, J. E. (1984): The cutaneous contribution to the hamstring flexor reflex in the rat: an electrophysiological and anatomical study. *Brain Res.,* 303:299–312.

Advances in Pain Research and Therapy, Vol. 9, edited by H. L. Fields et al. Raven Press, New York © 1985.

Transcutaneous Nerve Stimulation Inhibits Spinothalamic Tract Cells

Kyu Ho Lee, Jin Mo Chung, and William D. Willis

Marine Biomedical Institute and Departments of Physiology and Biophysics and Anatomy, University of Texas Medical Branch, Galveston, Texas 77550

Transcutaneous nerve stimulation (TENS) has proven to be a useful non-ablative technique for pain relief (1,3,7,8,12–14,19,20). The way in which TENS produces its analgesic effect is not known, although it seems likely that inhibitory mechanisms in the spinal cord play an important role (15).

Recently, we have found that repetitive stimulation of a mixed peripheral nerve in the hindlimb of the monkey can produce a prolonged inhibition of the responses of spinothalamic tract (STT) cells in the lumbosacral enlargement of the spinal cord (5,6). This inhibition is most effectively evoked by stimulation of $A\delta$ fibers, although there are also contributions from $A\beta$ and C fibers. Some inhibition results from stimulus frequencies as low as 0.5 Hz, and the amount of inhibition increases with stimulus frequency up to at least 20 Hz. The best inhibition was produced when the conditioning stimulation was applied to a peripheral nerve in the same limb as the excitatory receptive field. A similar inhibition has also been seen in recordings from dorsal horn interneurons in the cat (21). These results suggested to us the possibility that the inhibition of STT cells that we observed might have relevance to the analgesia produced by TENS. For this reason, we have examined the effects of stimulating the skin with a commercially available TENS unit to see if we could produce an inhibition comparable to that which results from direct stimulation of a peripheral nerve. The results were affirmative.

METHODS

The experiments were done on 7 monkeys *(Macaca fascicularis)* anesthetized with α-chloralose (60 mg/kg, i.v.) and an infusion of sodium pentobarbital (4 mg/kg/hr, i.v.). The animals were immobilized with gallamine triethiodide and artificially ventilated. End-tidal CO_2 was kept at 3.5 to 4.5%, and temperature was regulated near 37°C.

The extracellular action potentials of STT cells were recorded from the dorsal horn of the lumbosacral enlargement. The STT cells were identified by antidromic activation from the caudal part of the ventral posterior nucleus of the contralateral thalamus (16,18).

The amplified action potentials of STT cells were led to a window discriminator, the output pulses of which were used by a digital computer to compile peristimulus time histograms of the activity evoked by stimulation of a peripheral nerve at an intensity and duration (1 msec) sufficient to activate both A and C fibers. To enhance responses to C fibers by temporal summation, we generally used a train of three stimuli (at 30 Hz). The response to a C-fiber input for one STT cell is shown in Fig. 1A (the part of the histogram indicated by the horizontal bracket). The discharges during the C-fiber response were summed by the computer, and the summed discharge for each response elicited at 10-sec intervals is shown in Fig. 1B as a vertical line. Conditioning stimuli were delivered with a TENS unit (Medtronics, Model 7728) to the skin through carbon rubber electrodes placed in contact with the skin after the hair was clipped. Electrical contact was improved by use of conductive paste. Two modes of stimulation were available: high frequency continuous trains (80 μsec pulses at 85 Hz) and low rate "comfort bursts" (bursts of 7 80-μsec pulses at 85 Hz repeated at 3 bursts/sec). Stimulus intensity could be varied.

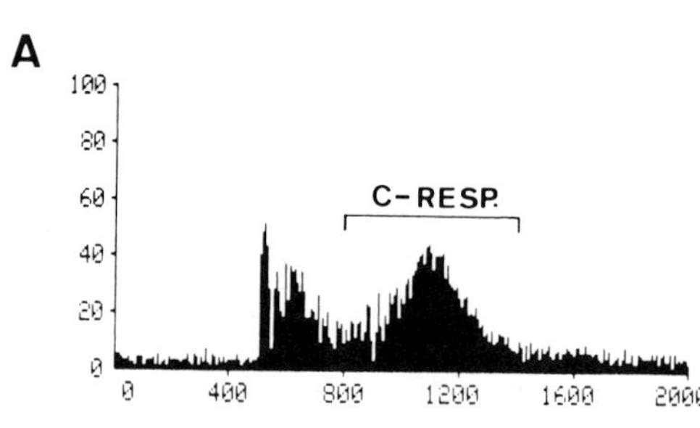

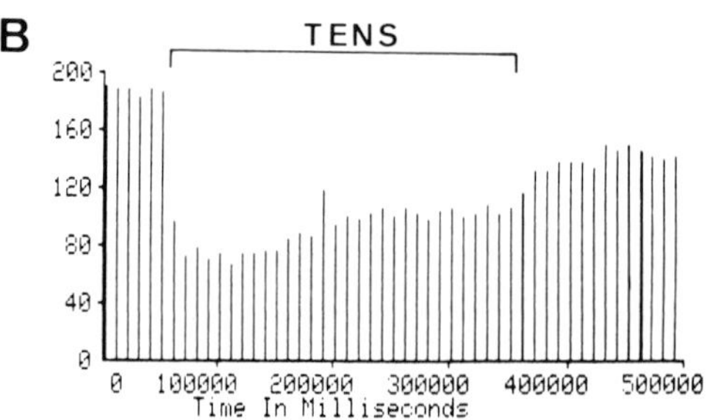

FIG. 1. Response of a primate spinothalamic tract (STT) cell to volleys in the A and C fibers of a peripheral nerve and the inhibitory effect of transcutaneous electrical nerve stimulation (TENS). The peristimulus time histogram in **A** shows the summed responses of an STT cell to 10 consecutive stimulations of the common peroneal nerve. The stimuli were trains of 3 pulses (30 Hz, each 1 msec in duration) at a strength sufficient to activate C fibers. The stimulus train began at a delay of 500 msec. *Horizontal bracket* shows the part of the response attributed to the effects of the C fibers. All of the impulses in this part of the response were counted by computer, and the values of the responses to C volleys evoked at 10-sec intervals were displayed as *vertical lines* in histograms such as that shown in **B** and in later figures. TENS was applied in the excitatory receptive field of the STT cell during the time indicated by the *horizontal bracket* in **B**. The TENS mode used was the "comfort burst" one.

RESULTS

A total of 14 STT cells were investigated. All were classified as wide dynamic range (or multireceptive) cells because they could be excited by both innocuous and noxious mechanical stimuli applied to the skin. The noxious stimuli were more effective than the innocuous ones.

Figure 1B shows the inhibitory effect of TENS on the responses of an STT cell to C-fiber input. The inhibitory effect was apparent within the 10-sec period between the last control response and the first response recorded after the initiation of TENS. The inhibition increased at first with successive trials, but later decreased.

The intensity of TENS was varied to see what strength was most effective. Figure 2 shows the result in one such experiment. The way in which stimulus intensity was related to the nerve fibers that were stimulated was as follows. Electrical stimulation of the Aβ fibers in a cutaneous nerve results in a negative evoked potential (the N1 wave) that can be recorded from the dorsal surface of the spinal cord (10). When Aδ fibers are also activated, we have shown that another, longer-latency, negative evoked potential (called by us the N3 wave) can also be recorded from the cord dorsum in the mon-

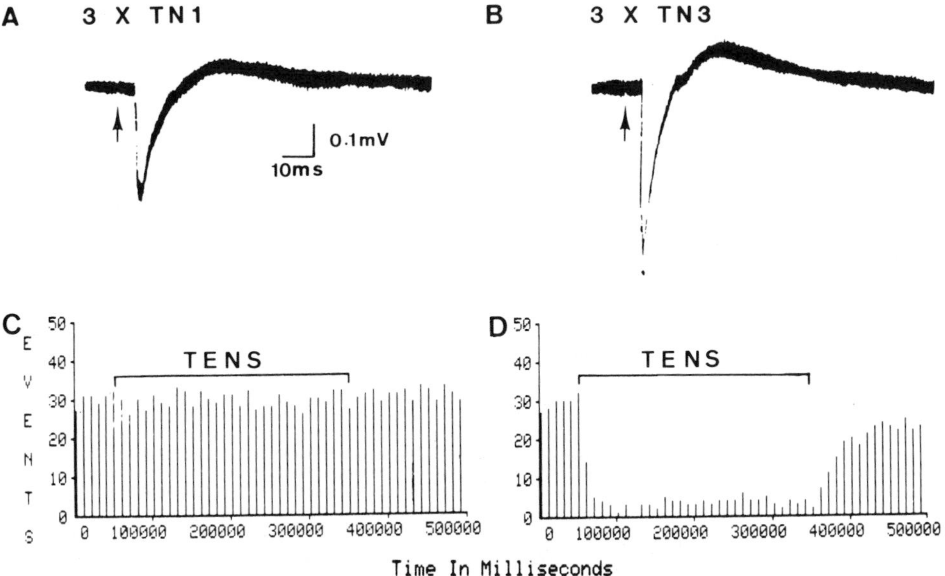

FIG. 2. Effects of changing the strength of the pulses used during TENS on the amount of inhibition of an STT cell. **A** and **B** show the cord dorsum N waves evoked by stimulus pulses of the same strengths that were later used for TENS. The pulse used for A was 3 times threshold for evoking an N1 wave, whereas that in B was 3 times threshold for an N3 wave (see text). In **C**, it is seen that TENS at the lower intensity had no effect on the responses of the STT cell to C-fiber volleys, whereas in **D** it is shown that the stronger intensity TENS produced a profound inhibition. The TENS mode used in C and D was the "comfort burst" one.

key (2). We monitored the development of the N1 and N3 waves in response to graded increases in the strength of the TENS pulses that were applied to the monkey skin. We also measured the stimulus current produced by the TENS unit and used those dial settings for stimulus intensities that were equivalent to 3 times the threshold for the N1 wave and then 3 times threshold for the N3 wave when testing the effects of TENS on the responses of STT cells. The negative cord dorsum potentials produced by these stimulus strengths in one experiment are shown in Fig. 2A and B, respectively. The histograms in Fig. 2C and D show that a stimulus strength confined to that sufficient to activate just Aβ fibers had no inhibitory effect on the C-fiber responses of the STT cell, whereas a stimulus strength that would excite many Aδ fibers produced a powerful inhibition.

The bar graph in Fig. 3 shows a statistical comparison of our results when

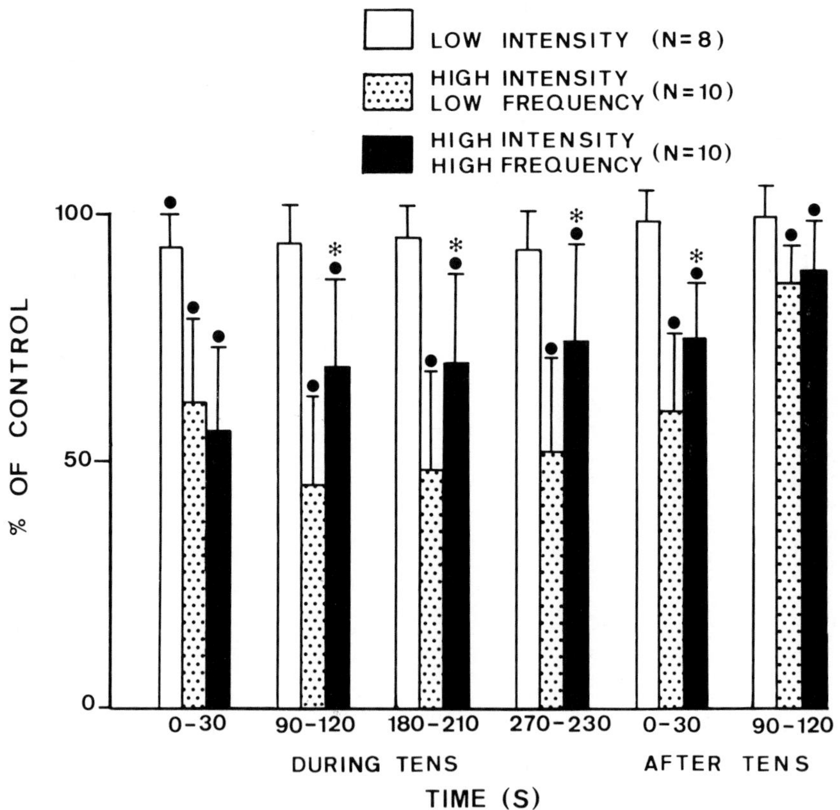

FIG. 3. *Bars* show the responses of a population of STT cells to C-fiber volleys as a percentage of control during and after TENS using several stimulus intensities. *Dots* indicate values significantly different from preTENS control values. *Asterisks* indicate values significantly different from the values obtained using high intensity, low frequency TENS.

using low intensity stimuli (activating just Aβ fibers), high intensity "comfort bursts," or high intensity continuous trains. The measurements were made at several times during and after TENS. There was no significant inhibition when low intensities of stimulation were employed, except during the initial 30 sec of TENS. A significant inhibition was produced by high intensity TENS (activating Aδ fibers), whether the stimulus trains were applied in the "comfort burst" or continuous mode. At most times during TENS, however, the "comfort burst" mode of stimulation was more effective in producing inhibition than was the continuous mode.

It has been shown in human subjects that TENS may involve the release of endogenous opioids, at least when high intensity TENS is used (4,17). The evidence for this is that naloxone, which is an opiate receptor antagonist, can reduce the effectiveness of these forms of TENS. To see whether or not an opioid mechanism might play some role in the inhibition of STT cells that is produced by TENS, we examined the effect of naloxone on the inhibition. The inhibition in Fig. 4A was the result of a period of TENS using the "comfort mode" of stimulation. Naloxone was then administered intravenously in a dose of 0.05 mg/kg, and after 5 min TENS was repeated. There was no change in the amount or time course of the inhibition. Similar results were obtained for the two other STT cells that were tested.

Since there are earlier reports (3,11) suggesting that the inhibitory mechanism of TENS is due to peripheral conduction failure, we checked this possibility by testing the compound action potential in the C fibers of the sural nerve. The results of one such experiment are shown in Fig. 5. The signal averaged compound action potential shown in Fig. 5A was recorded from

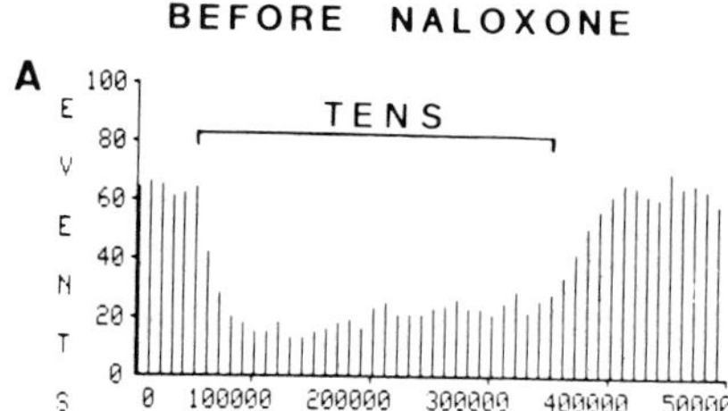

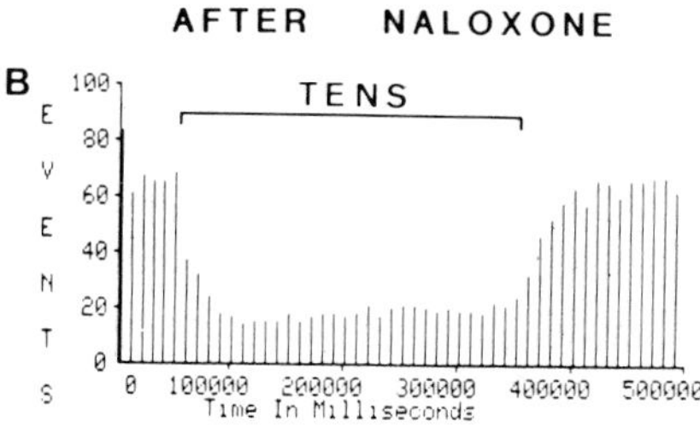

FIG. 4. Naloxone fails to affect the inhibition produced by TENS, using high intensity stimulation and the "comfort burst" mode.

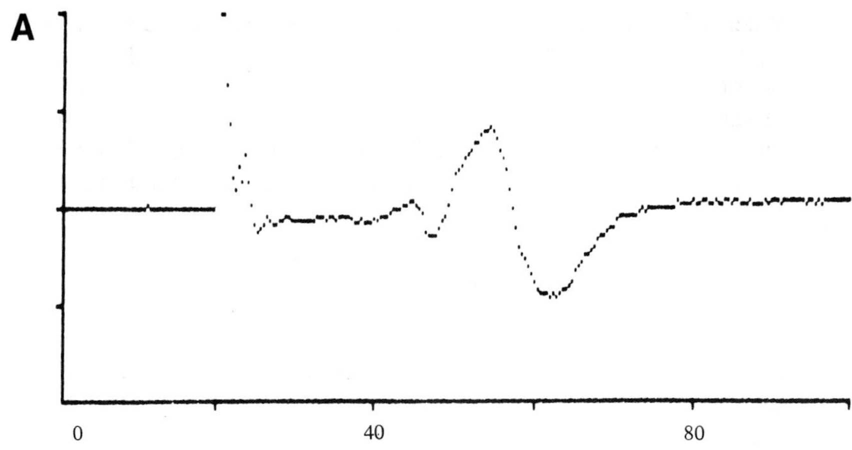

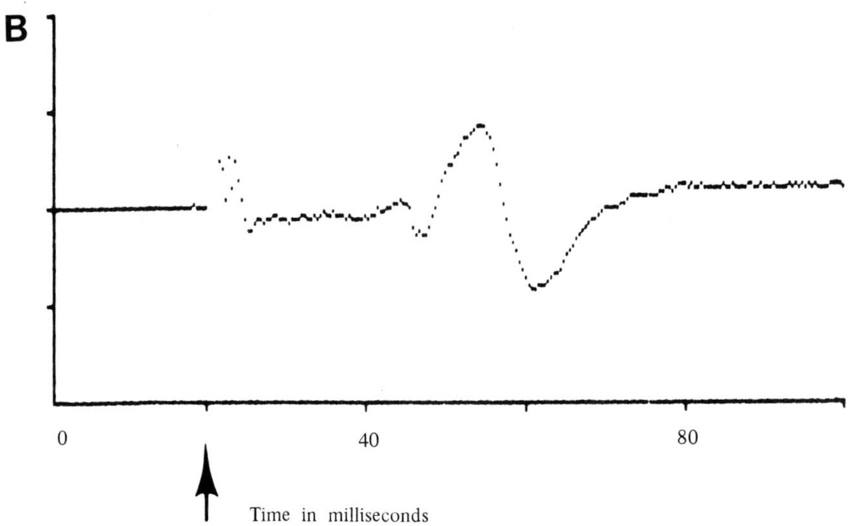

FIG. 5. Signal averaged recordings of the compound action potential in the sural nerve produced by volleys in A and C fibers, showing that TENS failed to alter the C-fiber compound action potential. The signals were averaged from 10 consecutive stimuli. The large wave in **A** represents the compound action potential in C fibers of the sural nerve. **B** was taken immediately after 5 min of TENS. There was no change in the wave.

the sural nerve in response to an electrical shock that was supramaximal for the A and C fibers. The part of the compound action potential due to the A fibers is poorly seen just after the time of stimulation (arrow at bottom), but the wave due to the C fibers is prominent. In Fig. 5B, it can be seen that there is no change in the C-fiber volley recorded after 5 min of TENS. No decrease in size of the C-fiber volley was observed during application of TENS.

DISCUSSION

The experiments described show that primate STT cells can be inhibited by TENS in much the same way as they are inhibited by direct stimulation of a mixed peripheral nerve (5,6). Given that STT cells function as part of the pain transmission system, it seems reasonable to assume that the inhibition of STT cells is part of the mechanism by which TENS produces analgesia. However, there is no reason to suppose that this action constitutes the sole mechanism of TENS analgesia. The observation in our experiments that naloxone has no effect on the inhibition of STT cells by TENS suggests that the interference by naloxone with TENS analgesia in human subjects (4,17) is at another level of the nervous system than the STT. However, it should be noted that not all investigations have demonstrated an interference with TENS analgesia by naloxone (e.g., ref. 9).

It is unlikely that conduction failure of peripheral C fibers was involved in the inhibitory effects of TENS in the present experiments. We were able to demonstrate that there was no reduction of a C-fiber volley recorded from the sural nerve during TENS, even though contrasting results have been previously reported (3,11).

Our results encourage us to believe that TENS analgesia may be in part due to the inhibition of STT cells. It will be important in future experiments to examine the neural pathways and pharmacology of the inhibitory system.

ACKNOWLEDGMENTS

The authors thank H. Willcockson, J. Unbehagen, and G. Gonzales for expert technical assistance, and P. Waldrop for typing the manuscript. The work was supported by National Institutes of Health grants NS 09743, NS 11255, NS 18830, and NS 21266, and by grants from the Moody Foundation and the American Heart Association, Texas Affiliate.

REFERENCES

1. Augustinsson, L. E., Bohlin, P., Bundsen, P., Carlsson, C. A., Forssman, L., Sjöberg, P., and Tyreman, N. O. (1977): Pain relief during delivery by transcutaneous electrical nerve stimulation. *Pain,* 4:59–65.

2. Beall, J. E., Applebaum, A. E., Foreman, R. D., and Willis, W. D. (1977): Spinal cord potentials evoked by cutaneous afferents in the monkey. *J. Neurophysiol.,* 40:199–211.
3. Campbell, J. N., and Taub, A. (1973): Local analgesia from percutaneous electrical stimulation. *Arch. Neurol.,* 28:347–350.
4. Chapman, C. R., and Benedetti, C. (1977): Analgesia following transcutaneous electrical stimulation and its partial reversal by a narcotic antagonist. *Life Sci.,* 21:1645–1648.
5. Chung, J. M., Fang, Z. R., Hori, Y., Lee, K. H., and Willis, W. D. (1984): Prolonged inhibition of primate spinothalamic tract cells by peripheral nerve stimulation. *Pain,* 19:259–275.
6. Chung, J. M., Lee, K. H., Hori, Y., Endo, K., and Willis, W. D. (1984): Factors influencing peripheral nerve stimulation produced inhibition of primate spinothalamic tract cells. *Pain,* 19:277–293.
7. Ericksson, M. B. E., and Sjölund, B. H. (1979): Long term results of peripheral conditioning stimulation as an analgesia measure in chronic pain. *Pain,* 6:335–347.
8. Fox, E. J., and Melzack, R. (1976): Transcutaneous electrical stimulation and acupuncture: comparison of treatment for low-back pain. *Pain,* 2:141–148.
9. Freeman, T. B., Campbell, J. N., and Long, D. M. (1983): Naloxone does not affect pain relief induced by electrical stimulation in man. *Pain,* 17:189–196.
10. Gasser, H. S., and Graham, H. T. (1933): Potentials produced in the spinal cord by stimulation of dorsal roots. *Am. J. Physiol.,* 103:303–320.
11. Ignelzi, R. J., and Nyquist, J. K. (1979): Excitability changes in peripheral nerve fibers after repetitive electrical stimulation. *J. Neurosurg.,* 51:824–833.
12. Loeser, J. D., Black, R. G., and Christman, A. (1975): Relief of pain by transcutaneous stimulation. *J. Neurosurg.,* 42:308–314.
13. Long, D. M., and Hagfors, N. (1975): Electrical stimulation in the nervous system: the current status of electrical stimulation of the nervous system for relief of pain. *Pain,* 1:109–123.
14. Melzack, R. (1975): Prolonged relief of pain by brief, intense transcutaneous somatic stimulation. *Pain,* 1:357–373.
15. Melzack, R., and Wall, P. D. (1965): Pain mechanisms: A new theory. *Science,* 150:971–979.
16. Olszewski, J. (1952): *An Atlas for Use with the Stereotaxic Instrument: The Thalamus of Macaca Mulatta.* Karger, Basel.
17. Sjölund, B. H., and Eriksson, M. B. E. (1979): The influence of naloxone on analgesia produced by peripheral conditioning stimulation. *Brain Res.,* 173:295–301.
18. Trevino, D. L., Coulter, J. D., and Willis, W. D. (1973): Location of cells of origin of spinothalamic tract in lumbar enlargement of the monkey. *J. Neurophysiol.,* 36:750–761.
19. Wall, P. D., and Sweet, W. H. (1967): Temporary abolition of pain in man. *Science,* 155:108–109.
20. Woolf, C. J. (1979): Transcutaneous electrical nerve stimulation and the reaction to experimental pain in human subjects. *Pain,* 7:115–127.
21. Zimmerman, M. (1979): Peripheral and central nervous mechanisms of nociception, pain and pain therapy: facts and hypotheses. In: *Advances in Pain Research and Therapy, Vol. 3,* edited by J. J. Bonica, J. C. Liebeskind, and D. G. Albe-Fessard, pp. 3–32. Raven Press, New York.

Advances in Pain Research and Therapy, Vol. 9, edited by H. L. Fields et al. Raven Press, New York © 1985.

Neural Mechanisms of Trigeminal Pain

Toshikatsu Yokota

Department of Physiology, Medical College of Shiga, Seta, Otsu 520-21, Japan

During the past decade, considerable information has been accumulated on the basic mechanisms of trigeminal pain. This chapter considers recent findings related to central mechanisms of trigeminal pain.

TRIGEMINAL NOCICEPTIVE NEURONS IN CAUDAL MEDULLA OBLONGATA

Trigeminal Tractotomy and Subnucleus Caudalis

The sensory trigeminal nuclear complex within the brainstem receives afferent fibers from the skin and ectodermal mucous membrane of the head by way of the trigeminal nerve. These fibers have their origin in the Gasserian ganglion. On entering the pons, many of them bifurcate into short ascending and long descending branches. The ascending branches terminate in the main sensory nucleus; the descending branches run through the spinal tract and terminate in the spinal trigeminal nucleus. Some of the fibers without bifurcation pass into the spinal tract.

In 1892, Bregmann (6) transected the Gasserian ganglion in the rabbit. Utilizing the Marchi staining, he demonstrated that the spinal tract consists of trigeminal primary afferents. Following this study, Wallenberg (55) described, in 1895, the neurological picture produced by the thrombosis of the posterior inferior cerebellar artery; it is still known as Wallenberg syndrome. Part of the syndrome consists of analgesia and thermal anesthesia with preservation of tactile sensation in the corresponding half of the face. Knowing the work of Bregmann (6), he ascribed this dissociated sensory loss to a lesion of the spinal tract. Wallenberg (56) confirmed this clinical interpretation of the spinal tract by experimental sections in the medulla oblongata of the rabbit. He thus performed the first trigeminal tractotomy. These findings were successfully applied to the treatment of trigeminal neuralgia in 1938 by Sjöqvist (49). He sectioned the spinal tract in the medulla oblongata just below the lowest vagal rootlet which is 8 to 10 mm rostral to the obex. The operation was designed to abolish pain sensation and preserve tactile sensation in the trigeminal nerve territory.

Sjöqvist (49) reported a few postoperative complications, but later operators have had more difficulties. Probably the operation would have been dropped if Grant, in 1939, had not accidentally misplaced the incision 8 mm below the obex. This patient fortunately had complete analgesia in the trigeminal nerve territory. Subsequently, Weinberger and Grant (57) regularly placed the incision from 6 to 8 mm below the obex. From this time on, neurosurgeons adopted Grant's lower modification and obtained complete analgesia in a certain percentage of patients with sections 1 to 7 mm below the obex. These clinical observations suggested that the caudal part of the spinal trigeminal nucleus is concerned with trigeminal pain.

Already, in 1919, Fuse (17), on the basis of his myeloarchitectonic investigation, denied the idea that the spinal trigeminal nucleus is a homogeneous structure extending throughout the medulla oblongata and the caudal part of the pons. He was able to subdivide the human spinal trigeminal nucleus into three parts—spinalis, medullaris, and pontina—arranged in series along the longitudinal axis of the brainstem. On the basis of its cytoarchitectonic structure, Olszewski (41) confirmed Fuse's subdivision, and named these three parts nucleus tractus spinalis trigemini caudalis, nucleus tractus spinalis trigemini interpolaris, and nucleus tractus spinalis trigemini oralis. He concluded that only the nucleus tractus spinalis trigemini caudalis conducts the sensations of pain and temperature. Later, Crosby and Yoss (11) made a phylogenetic study of the spinal trigeminal nucleus, and modified Olszewski's terminology to meet the need for a wider range of terms: They called these three parts subnucleus caudalis, subnucleus interpolaris, and subnucleus oralis, respectively.

Although there have been reports (4,7,51,70) of electrophysiological as well as behavioral studies that not only the subnucleus caudalis but also more rostral subnuclei of the spinal trigeminal nucleus receive nociceptive input and send out this information to the thalamus, investigations carried out in both Dubner's and our laboratories support the classical idea that the subnucleus caudalis is the major component of the spinal trigeminal nucleus concerned with trigeminal nociception (14,22,27,46,58,59,64,67,69).

Morphology of Subnucleus Caudalis

On the basis of cytoarchitectonic structure, Olszewski (41) proposed a subdivision of the trigeminal subnucleus caudalis into three layers. They are now called the marginal layer, substantia gelatinosa, and magnocellular layer. Just above the level of the obex, the subnucleus caudalis makes an abrupt transition to an entirely different structure, subnucleus interpolaris. At the caudal end, the subnucleus caudalis is continuous with the apex of the dorsal horn of the first cervical segment. In the cat, the rostralmost level of the first cervical segment is some 5 mm caudal to the obex.

The primary afferent projection to the subnucleus caudalis includes myelinated and unmyelinated fibers (32). It has long been known that the caliber of individual myelinated fibers in the spinal tract decreases markedly below the level of the obex. Both groups of fibers penetrate the subnucleus caudalis from the spinal tract in a spatially ordered pattern. The larger fibers terminate mainly within the deeper zone of substantia gelatinosa and magnocellular layer (32). Studies on afferent projections from the tooth pulp (3) and cornea (43) showed that small fibers terminate mainly in the marginal layer, substantia gelatinosa, and neck region of the dorsolateral gray matter which is ventromedially adjacent to the subnucleus caudalis.

Marginal Layer

The marginal layer is a narrow strip of neurons and neuropil just beneath and partly within the spinal tract of the trigeminal nerve. The marginal layer contains a row of small, elliptical bundles of axons. A line connecting medial borders of these bundles denotes the medial border of the marginal layer (19). The characteristic neurons of this layer are the marginal neurons, projection neurons, including the marginal neurons of Waldeyer. In the transverse section, most of the marginal neurons are fusiform and some are pear-shaped or polygonal. They are usually located in a narrow band just beneath the spinal tract of the trigeminal nerve where their somata parallel the tract. From these somata, thick, long dendrites emerge to arborize repeatedly and extend around the curvature of the substantia gelatinosa. The marginal neurons are also located in the small islets of neuropil within the spinal tract of the trigeminal nerve (16,19). They are, however, oriented radially in the transverse section (16). Ramon y Cajal (46a) named them interstitial neurons.

The marginal neurons give rise to myelinated axons whose initial segments do not emit axon collaterals in the marginal layer (19). Following injection of horseradish peroxidase (HRP) into the thalamus and midbrain, several groups of investigators have found that the enzyme is retrogradely transported into the somata of marginal neurons (1,8,16,25,36,48).

Substantia Gelatinosa

Substantia gelatinosa has the shape of a horseshoe and is readily recognized owing to its paucity of myelinated axons and the abundance of small neurons. This can be subdivided into outer and inner zones (15,20). In the outer zone, neurons are more densely packed, whereas the inner zone contains more loosely arranged neurons.

In Golgi-stained sections, several different kinds of neurons have been identified in the substantia gelatinosa. One is the limitrophe cell of Ramon y Cajal (46a). Gobel (18) named this neuron "stalked cell." This is found on the border between the marginal layer and the substantia gelatinosa, and is characterized by numerous, short, stalk-like branches of dendrites directing toward the hilus of the horseshoe. Its axon arises either from the soma or one of the basal dendritic branches and crosses into the marginal layer where it arborizes extensively among the dendrites of marginal neurons (20).

The second type of substantia gelatinosa neurons is the islet cell (18) which emits its basal dendritic branches into a more or less common circular area, comprising the "island" of substantia gelatinosa described by Ramon y Cajal (46a). The axon of islet cell, like the islet cell dendritic tree, is confined within the substantia gelatinosa (18).

The third type of substantia gelatinosa neuron is the spiny cell which is named for the numerous, evenly distributed dendritic spines along its secondary and tertiary dendrites (18). Its soma is located in the inner zone of the substantia gelatinosa and its dendrites cross into both the marginal and magnocellular layers. The axon arises from either the soma or one of the primary dendrites, and its terminals distribute in all three layers of the trigeminal subnucleus caudalis, thus representing the sole output of the substantia gelatinosa to the magnocellular layer.

There are two more types of substantia gelatinosa neurons: the arboreal cell and the II-III border cell (20). Both of them are found in the outer zone of the substantia gelatinosa. The islet cell, arboreal cell, and II-III border cell are all Golgi type II neurons (20). Among them, the islet cell is most common. These Golgi type II substantia gelatinosa neurons may function as inhibitory interneurons, while the limitrophe cell is supposed to function as excitatory interneuron transmitting input from primary afferents to marginal neurons (20).

Magnocellular Layer

The magnocellular layer fills the hilus of the horseshoe, and is characterized by large numbers of small- and medium-sized neurons. Only a small fraction of these neurons project to the thalamus (1,8,16,25,36,48). Following HRP injection into the lateral cervical nucleus, however, labeled neurons were found in the magnocellular layer as well as in lamina IV of the spinal cord dorsal horn in the cat (10).

Reticular Formation Surrounding Subnucleus Caudalis

Ventral to the trigeminal subnucleus caudalis is nucleus reticularis medullae oblongatae which is subdivided into subnucleus reticularis dorsalis and subnucleus reticularis ventralis (37). The subnucleus reticularis dorsalis is cytoarchitecturally characterized by a relative abundance of nerve cells and fairly uniform cell density. It contains medium-sized polygonal cells with a fairly uniform structure, short dendrites, large nuclei, and little Nissl substance. Therefore, they appear rather pale in Nissl-stained sections, but accompanying glial cells are richly developed (37). Dorsolaterally, it is bordered by the magnocellular layer of the trigeminal subnucleus caudalis which contains smaller nerve cells. Ventrally, it is bordered by the subnucleus reticularis ventralis, in which nerve cells are scarce and large nerve cells with an abundance of Nissl substance are particularly characteristic (37). Studies using the technique of retrograde axonal transport of HRP from the thalamus and midbrain showed projections from these subnuclei to rostral levels of the brainstem (25,36,48).

Nociceptive Neurons in Trigeminal Subnucleus Caudalis and Surrounding Reticular Formation

In the trigeminal subnucleus caudalis and its nearby reticular formation, there are three general categories of nociceptive neurons which can be activated by noxious stimulation of the skin and ectodermal mucous membrane of the trigeminal nerve territory. They are nociceptive specific (NS) neurons, wide dynamic range (WDR) neurons, and subnucleus reticularis ventralis (SRV) neurons.

Trigeminal Nociceptive Specific Neurons

Trigeminal NS neurons respond exclusively, or nearly exclusively, to noxious mechanical stimuli applied to a restricted area of the oral facial integument. They are concentrated in the marginal layer and also in the outer zone of the substantia gelatinosa (29,40,46,64,67). Some NS neurons in the marginal layer are antidromically invaded by impulses from the nucleus ventralis posterior medialis (VPM) of the contralateral thalamus.

The receptive fields of trigeminal NS neurons in the superficial layers (the marginal layer and the outer zone of the substantia gelatinosa) are related to the mediolateral location of the neuron (64,67) (Fig. 1). Neurons located in the dorsomedial region of the superficial layers have a receptive field in the mandibular division of the trigeminal nerve. Neurons in the lateral region have a receptive field in the ophthalmic division, and those located in between have a receptive field in the maxillary division. The organization is precisely the same as has been reported for primary afferent fibers descending in the spinal tract of the trigeminal nerve (32). There is also a somatotopic pattern along the rostrocaudal axis of the trigeminal subnucleus caudalis (Fig. 1). The nose and mouth are represented near the level of the obex, while the scalp, preauricular skin, and lateral face are found more caudally. There is a concentric shift of receptive field representation between these two levels (64,67). The pattern is in accord with the idea of

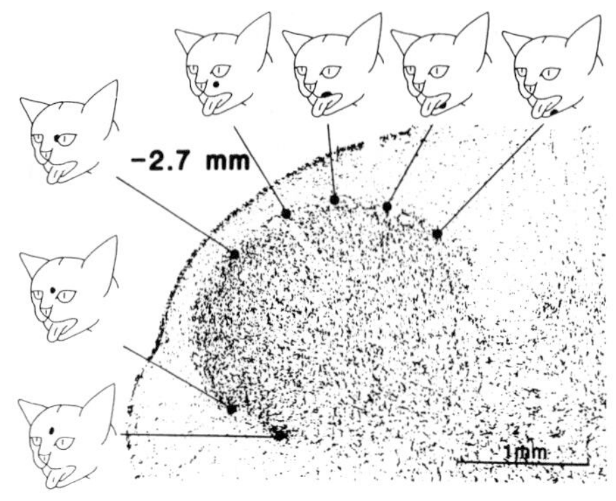

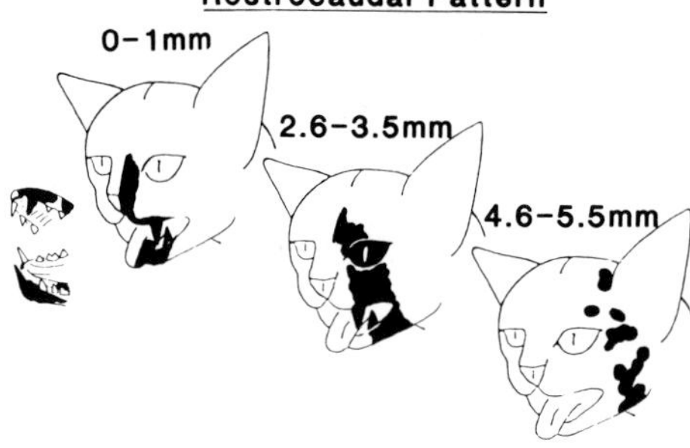

FIG. 1. Somatotopic organization of NS neurons in the superficial layers of the subnucleus caudalis. **Upper:** Locations and receptive fields of marginal layer NS neurons obtained from transverse plane 2.7 mm caudal to the obex. **Lower:** Receptive fields of NS neurons within the superficial layers at various levels of the subnucleus caudalis. There is a concentric shift of receptive field representation along the rostrocaudal axis of the caudal medulla oblongata.

"onion peel segmentation of facial dermatomes" first described by Dejerine (13). Neurons exclusively responsive to electrical stimulation of tooth-pulp afferents are also located in the superficial layers (58,69).

Trigeminal Wide Dynamic Range Neurons

Trigeminal wide dynamic range neurons are activated by both tactile and noxious mechanical stimuli applied to the ipsilateral trigeminal integument (29,63,65). These neurons have a graded response in the center of the receptive field to brush, touch, pressure, and noxious stimuli. Surrounding this relatively small area is an area wherein the neurons respond differentially to pressure and noxious stimuli. This area is, in turn, surrounded by an exclusively nociceptive area. Many also respond to electrical stimulation of the ipsilateral maxillary and/or mandibular tooth-pulp afferents (69). Some of them are antidromically excited by electrical stimulation of the contralateral VPM. Intravenous subconvulsive dose of strychnine causes a marked expansion of the nociceptive part of the receptive field, without affecting the size of the low threshold center of the receptive field (66). In contrast, intravenous subconvulsive dose of picrotoxin causes an expansion of the low threshold center, concomitantly producing marked shrinkage of the nociceptive part of receptive field (68). These pharmacological findings suggest inhibitory influences acting upon WDR neurons.

Trigeminal WDR neurons are concentrated in the narrow neck of the dorsolateral gray matter of the caudal medulla oblongata which corresponds to the lateral part of subnucleus reticularis dorsalis and show a somatotopic organization (64,65) (Fig. 2). In general, WDR neurons having a low threshold center of the receptive field in the mandibular division are located dorsomedially. Trigeminal WDR neurons having a low threshold center in the ophthalmic division are located ventrolaterally. Trigeminal WDR neurons having a low threshold center in the maxillary division fall in between. There is also a rostrocaudal somatotopic organization. Apparently, trigeminal WDR neurons in the lateral part of the subnucleus reticularis dorsalis reticularis dorsalis are place-specific.

Previously, Kunc (35) observed that if the spinal trigeminal tract is completely incised at the rostral pole of the subnucleus caudalis, analgesia over the whole ipsilateral trigeminal nerve territory results. On the other hand, if the tractotomy is performed more caudally, analgesia is incomplete with sensory sparing of the center of the face. With still more caudal sections, this area expands concentrically. He concluded that primary afferent fibers from the center of the face terminate at the highest and those from the

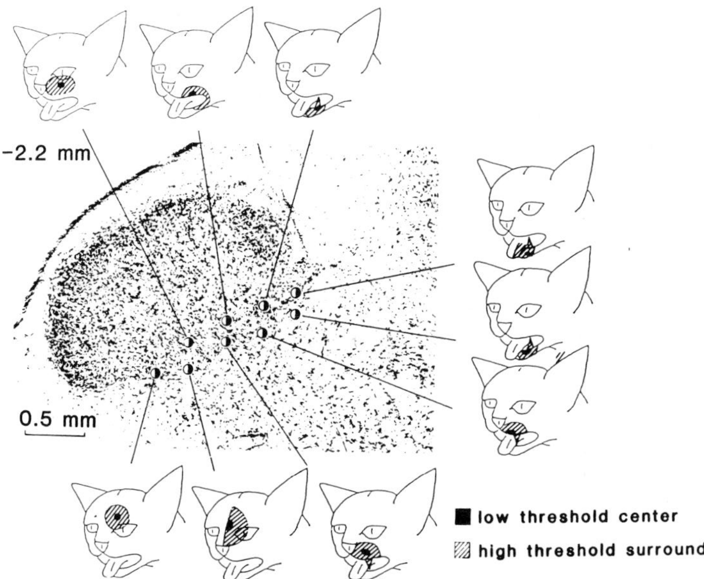

FIG. 2. Locations and receptive fields of trigeminal WDR neurons obtained from transverse plane 2.2 mm caudal to the obex. Trigeminal WDR neurons are located in the lateral part of the subnucleus reticularis dorsalis and show a somatotopic organization.

periphery at the lowest level of the trigeminal subnucleus caudalis. The rostrocaudal somatotopic organization of trigeminal NS and WDR neurons is in good accord with these clinical observations.

Subnucleus Reticularis Ventralis Neurons

The third class of trigeminal nociceptive neurons is located in the dorsolateral part of the subnucleus reticularis ventralis (SRV) (Fig. 3). These SRV neurons are regularly responsive to pressure (> 1 g von Frey force) applied to the ipsi- or bilateral corneal surface. In addition, they are frequently responsive to noxious mechanical stimulation of the ipsi- or bilateral pinna, face, and/or tongue. Tapping of the ipsilateral dorsum of nose sometimes excites them. Some of them are responsive to ipsi- or bilateral tooth-pulp afferents.

Electrical stimulation of the contralateral mesencephalic reticular formation antidromically excites some of these SRV neurons. These projection

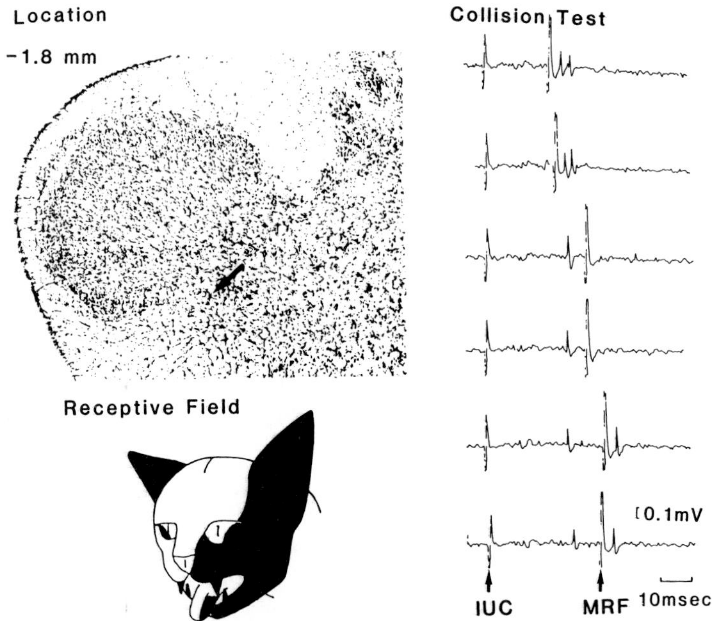

FIG. 3. Location, receptive field, and antidromic responses of a SRV neuron. The neuron was obtained from the subnucleus reticularis ventralis at the level 1.8 mm caudal to the obex. The neuron responded to pressure applied to the bilateral cornea, noxious mechanical stimulation of bilateral pinna, ipsilateral face, and ipsilateral tongue. Electrical stimulation of the bilateral canine tooth pulp afferents was also effective. Collision tests show antidromic responses of the neurons to electrical stimulation of the contralateral midbrain reticular formation (MRF). Orthodromic stimulation was applied to the ipsilateral upper canine tooth pulp (IUC).

neurons may subserve emotional motivational aspects of pain rather than its sensory discriminative aspects.

Responses of Trigeminal Nociceptive Neurons After Trigeminal Tractotomy

After trigeminal tractotomy near the level of the obex, neither low threshold mechanoreceptive (LTM), nor NS, nor WDR neurons are found within the trigeminal subnucleus caudalis and ventromedially adjacent subnucleus reticularis dorsalis, but SRV neurons are still identified (60). Trigeminal input into SRV neurons seems to be relayed via neurons located more rostrally. Hockfield and Gobel (26) found retrogradely labeled neurons in the reticular formation adjacent to the trigeminal subnuclei interpolaris and oralis after a massive HRP injection into the caudal medulla oblongata. They failed to find retrogradely labeled neurons in the same region after a small injection of HRP into the trigeminal subnucleus caudalis. Neurons antidromically excited by electrical stimulation of the subnucleus reticularis ventralis were also found in the same region of the reticular formation (60). They had parts of receptive fields of SRV neurons. Trigeminal inputs into SRV neurons seem to be relayed via neurons located in the reticular formation ventromedially adjacent to the trigeminal subnuclei interpolaris and oralis (60).

It was reported that chronic trigeminal tractotomy in the cat (51) and monkey (70) modified neither conditioned behavior nor nocifensive reactions elicited by tooth-pulp stimulation. Such results were interpreted as showing that the neurophysiological mechanisms involved in dental nociception may differ from those involved in cutaneous facial nociception. After acute trigeminal tractotomy, however, a certain proportion of SRV neurons still respond to electrical stimulation of tooth-pulp afferents (60). These SRV neurons would provide an alternative pathway that could account for an animal's reaction to tooth-pulp stimulation after the trigeminal tractotomy.

Laminar Structure of Dorsolateral Gray Matter of Medulla Oblongata

Previously, there was a lack of uniformity in the terminology used to describe various structures in the caudal medulla oblongata and their relationship to corresponding structures in the spinal cord. Hence, an attempt was made to divide the gray matter of the caudal medulla oblongata into 8 layers comparable to those in the spinal cord (21). The proposed scheme was only tentative, and by no means completely satisfactory. The time now appears to be ripe to consider this matter in some detail, because experimental evidence adduced largely in the past decade renders it possible to analyze the laminar structure in terms of physiological properties of neurons.

Ramon y Cajal (46a) observed that the lower portion of the spinal trigeminal nucleus that is now called the subnucleus caudalis, closely resembles the apex of the dorsal horn of the spinal cord. On passing from the cervical dorsal horn into the trigeminal subnucleus caudalis, there is considerable structural transformation, an increase in size, but, nonetheless, the first four cytoarchitectonic laminae of Rexed (47) can be differentiated: (a) the marginal layer that corresponds to the lamina I, (b) the substantia gelatinosa that corresponds to the lamina II, and (c) the magnocellular layer which, although much expanded, is homologous with laminae III and IV (47).

Rexed (47) concluded that the reticular formation makes its appearance first in the first cervical segment, perhaps as an extension of the lateral zone of lamina V. He considered that laminae V and VI do not extend into the medulla oblongata, but merge with the reticular formation. In the spinal dorsal horn, WDR neurons are mainly located in lamina V (53). In the caudal medulla oblongata, trigeminal WDR neurons are located in the neck region of the dorsolateral gray matter, which is ventromedially adjacent to the magnocellular layer, and is a part of the lateral reticular formation (64,65). According to the terminology of Meessen and Olszewski (37), this region corresponds to the lateral part of the subnucleus reticularis dorsalis. This region may be looked on as the homolog of lamina V.

Deep to subnuclei caudalis and reticularis dorsalis is the subnucleus reticularis ventralis of Meessen and Olszewski (37). In the dorsolateral part of this subnucleus, there are trigeminal nociceptive neurons of special category, i.e., SRV neurons. Neurons with similar receptive field characteristics are also found in lamina VII of the first cervical segment (59). The dorsolateral part of the subnucleus reticularis ventralis may be the homolog of the lamina VII of the spinal cord.

A question has been raised of where the lamina VI equivalent is located in the gray matter of the caudal medulla oblongata. In the spinal cord, lamina VI is characterized by location of neurons having mixed cutaneous and movement receptive fields (53). In the caudal medulla oblongata, neurons receiving tactile as well as low threshold muscle afferents were found in the

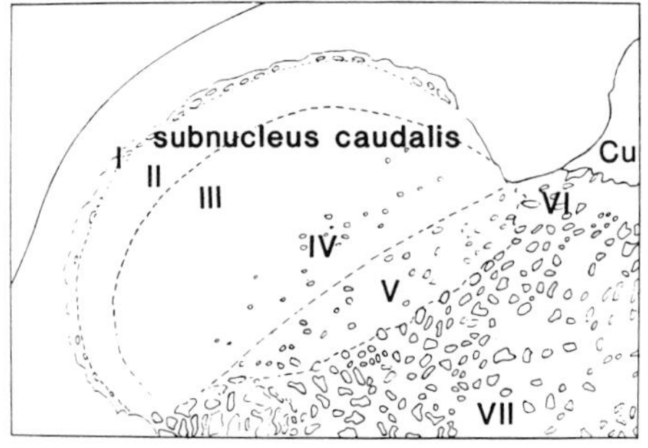

FIG. 4. Laminar structure of the dorsolateral gray matter of the caudal medulla oblongata.

junctional area between the trigeminal subnucleus caudalis and the cuneate nucleus (59). Near the rostral end of the first cervical cord, lamina VI is confined to a small mediobasal part of the dorsal horn which lies ventrolateral to the cuneate nucleus (47). The junctional area is continuous with the lamina VI of the first cervical segment. This area may be the homolog of the lamina VI of the spinal cord. The laminar structure of the dorsolateral gray matter of the caudal medulla oblongata may be summarized as shown in Fig. 4.

Neurons in Caudal Medulla Oblongata Responsive to Mechanical Distortion of Experimentally-Produced Neuroma

If an axon of a peripheral nerve has been interrupted, recovery involves generation of a new axon. During the first week, there is retrograde degeneration for a few millimeters from the cut end, and multiple sprouts (up to 50) appear from the distal end of the intact portion of the axon. In a crush injury, severed fibers succeed in growing a sprout into a distal Schwann cell tube. The sprout then will reinnervate its proper target cells, and surplus sprouts disappear. If a nerve is transected and its continuity is lost, sprouts with their Schwann cells and a developing connective tissue scar may form a tangled mass called a neuroma. This occurs in humans after amputation or after failure of regeneration of a damaged nerve. Sharp, radiating pain may be produced by tapping on a neuroma. The pain may also originate spontaneously from a neuroma, and may be precipitated by cold (50).

Experimentally-produced neuroma sprouts and ganglion cells of their parent axons adopt new physiological and pharmacological properties. They become spontaneously active, and are excited by slight mechanical distortion and by the alpha action of adrenalin (54). Two weeks after section and ligation of the infraorbital nerve in the cat, neurons responsive to mechanical distortion of the neuroma were found in superficial layers of the trigeminal subnucleus caudalis, in the lateral part of the subnucleus reticularis dorsalis, and in the dorsolateral part of the subnucleus reticularis ventralis (Fig. 5). These are areas wherein normally trigeminal nociceptive neurons are located (61). In contrast, the same stimulation failed to excite neurons located in the magnocellular layer wherein normally tactile neurons are located. Seven weeks after the operation, however, neurons responsive to mechanical distortion of the neuroma were also found in the magnocellular layer. These findings suggest that 2 weeks after the operation, nerve impulses spilling off the neuroma were carried by small nerve fibers including nociceptive fibers, whereas 7 weeks after the operation, impulses from the neuroma were also carried by larger nerve fibers.

Höckfelt et al. (24) discovered that substance-P-like immunoreactivity is restricted to small ganglion cells and only thin sensory fibers distributing within the superficial layers of the trigeminal subnucleus caudalis. Cuello et

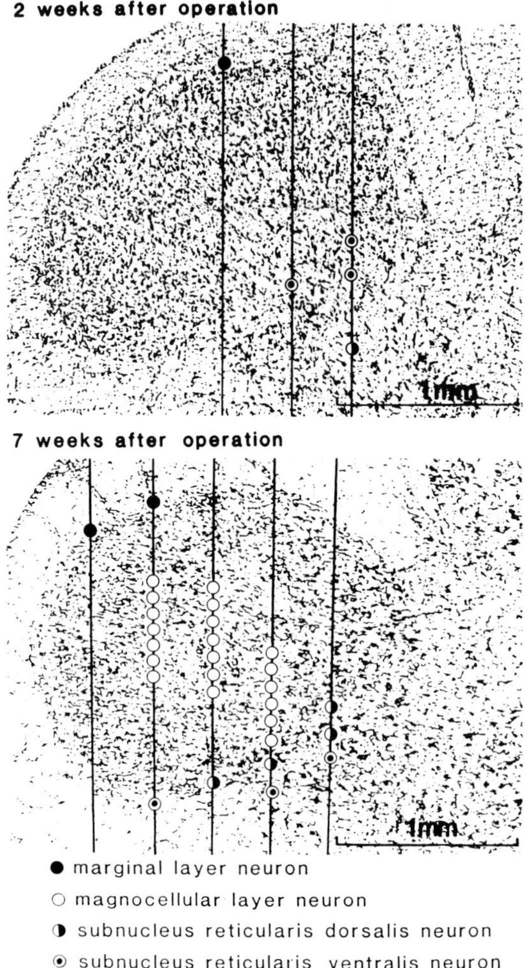

FIG. 5. Locations of neurons responsive to mechanical distortion of an experimentally produced neuroma in the infraorbital nerve. The neuroma was produced by section and ligation of the infraorbital nerve. Two weeks or 7 weeks after the operation, the caudal medulla oblongata was explored for neurons responsive to mechanical distortion of the neuroma.

al. (12) found that substance-P-like immunoreactivity is prominent not only in the superficial layers of the trigeminal subnucleus caudalis, but also in the reticular formation ventromedially adjacent to the trigeminal subnucleus caudalis. Both are areas wherein trigeminal nociceptive neurons exist. Following electrolytic lesion of the Gasserian ganglion and trigeminal rhizotomy, the trigeminal subnucleus caudalis showed a marked depletion of substance-P-like immunoreactivity, and the reticular formation showed a small decrease in the reactivity (12). Henry et al. (23) reported that iontophoretic application of substance P excites only these neurons that respond to noxious cutaneous stimuli. The release of substance P from the rat trigeminal subnucleus caudalis was shown by Jessel and Iversen (30) to be antagonized by opiates. These findings suggest that substance P is a neurotransmitter of small diameter nociceptive afferents.

Unfortunately, other findings indicate such a conclusion may be premature. For instance, 2 weeks after section and ligation of the infraorbital nerve, substance-P-like immunoreactivity disappeared in a highly defined area of the marginal layer and outer zone of the substantia gelatinosa where the terminals of the sectioned nerve are known to exist (Fig. 6). These findings are complementary to the observations made by Barbut et al. (5) in the spinal cord after section and ligation of the sciatic nerve. At this stage, neurons responsive to mechanical distortion of the neuroma were found in the depleted area. Seven weeks after the operation, no sign of depletion, was noted. Namely, substance P reappeared in the depleted area. These findings suggest that substance P is not necessarily required in the synaptic transmission of small nerve fiber impulses in the marginal layer and outer zone of the substantia gelatinosa.

TRIGEMINAL NOCICEPTIVE NEURONS IN THALAMUS

According to Krieg (34), nucleus ventralis posterior consists of four parts, i.e., nucleus arcuatus lateralis, nucleus arcuatus medialis, nucleus posterior lateralis, and nucleus posterior inferior, in the rhesus monkey. In Olszewski's terminology, they are nucleus ventralis posterior medialis (VPM proper), nucleus ventralis posterior medialis parvocellularis (VPMpc), nucleus ventralis posterior lateralis (VPL), and nucleus ventralis posterior inferior (VPI), respectively. The somatosensory part of Krieg's nucleus ventralis posterior is called the ventrobasal (VB) complex, and includes only the VPM proper and VPL. Walker (52) included the VPMpc in his nucleus ventralis posteromedialis, but Olszewski (42) clearly separated it from the VPM proper. Mountcastle and his group (39,44,45) did not include the VPMpc in the VB complex. There is considerable evidence that the VPMpc is a thalamic nucleus for gustation. Ventral to the VPM proper and VPMpc and dorsal to the external medullary lamina lies an area characterized by small, scattered, rather pale cells. This area was designated nucleus ventralis posterior inferior (VPI) of the thalamus by Olszewski (42). Generally, this nucleus is not included in the VB complex. It has been well-established that the VB complex receives specific mechanoreceptive and thermoreceptive input, but whether it also receives nociceptive input was uncertain. Poggio and Mountcastle (44,45) did not find VB neurons preferentially sensitive to noxious stimuli in the cat and monkey. Instead, they found that the majority of neurons recorded in the posterior nuclear complex (PO) of the thalamus were sensitive to noxious stimuli in the cat (46). They proposed that this

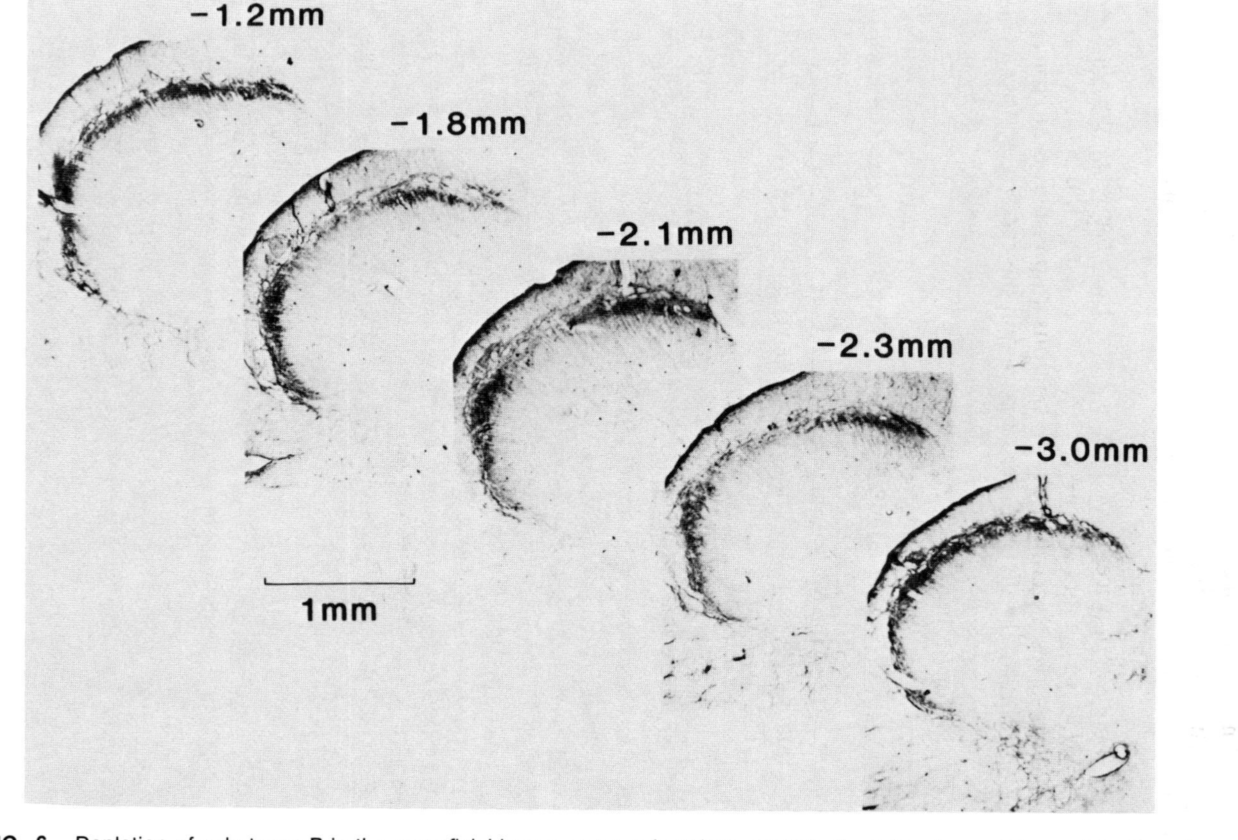

FIG. 6. Depletion of substance P in the superficial layers of the subnucleus caudalis 2 weeks after section and ligation of the infraorbital nerve. Substance P-like immunoreactivity disappeared in a highly defined area of the marginal layer and outer zone of the substantia gelatinosa where the terminals of the sectioned nerve are known to exist.

part of the thalamus plays a major role in the conscious perception of pain. Receptive fields of PO neurons were large, frequently bilateral, and sometimes discontinuous. Furthermore, these neurons did not have a somatotopic organization. Hence, it seemed possible that pain localization depends on a separate population of neurons rather than that responsible for pain sensation.

Recently, however, nociceptive neurons have been found in the shell region of the VPL in the rat (38), cat (28,33), and monkey (31). In the VPM proper which receives trigeminal input, neurons responsive to electrical stimulation of tooth-pulp afferents were reported in the cat (2), and trigeminal NS as well as WDR neurons were discovered in the shell region of the caudal VPM proper of the cat in our laboratory (62,63).

Trigeminal NS Neurons in VPM

In the VPM proper, the trigeminal integument is represented in an orderly topographic manner. A great majority of neurons are low threshold mechanoreceptive (LTM) neurons. They are modality-specific; that is, a given neuron can only be activated by one particular form of stimulation. The neurons are also place-specific and each neuron responds only to stimulation of a restricted area of the contralateral side of the orofacial region. In a perpendicular microelectrode penetration passing through the caudal third of the VPM proper in the cat, trigeminal NS neurons are encountered near the dorsal and/or ventral ends of a column of LTM neurons. The trigeminal NS neurons respond best to high intensity, presumably painful mechanical stimulation such as application of serrated forceps or pinpricks, but do not respond to mechanical stimulation such as hair movement or light pressure. Their receptive fields are circumscribed in the trigeminal integument. Hence, their response characteristics are much the same as those of trigeminal NS neurons in the superficial layers of the trigeminal subnucleus caudalis.

Trigeminal NS neurons in the VPM proper are located at or near the margin of this nucleus except for the area along the border between the VPM proper and the VPL (Fig. 7). That is, they are located in the shell region of the VPM proper. They show a somatotopic organization. In the rostral part of the caudal third of the VPM proper, NS neurons having a receptive field in the ophthalmic division are found dorsolaterally, maxillary NS neurons are found dorsomedially, and mandibular NS neurons are encountered ventromedially along the border between the VPM proper and VPMpc. Near the caudal pole of the VPM proper, maxillary NS neurons are found in the dorsal shell region, whereas mandibular NS neurons are encountered in the ventromedial shell region. Ophthalmic NS neurons are not found at this level. Latency measurements suggest that all the trigeminal NS neurons in the shell region of the VPM proper receive Aδ input.

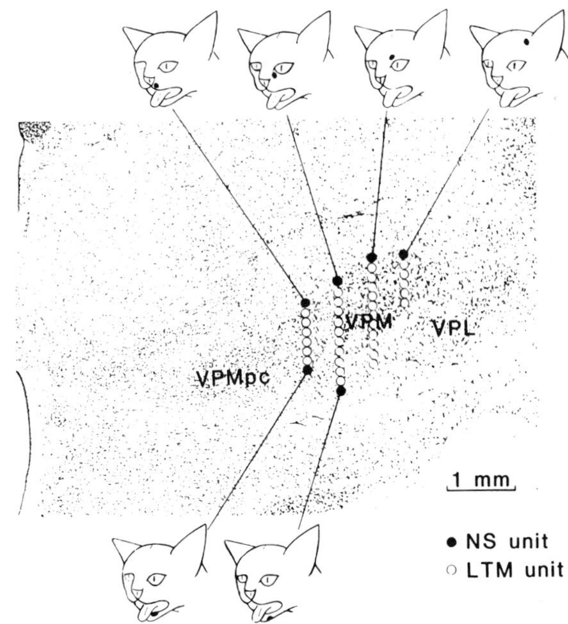

FIG. 7. Somatotopic distribution of trigeminal NS neurons within the shell region of the VPM proper.

Trigeminal WDR Neurons in VPM

Trigeminal WDR neurons in the VPM proper of the cat are located in a narrow band (about 300 μm wide) of the shell region just rostral to the region wherein trigeminal NS neurons are located. They have a graded response in the center of the receptive field to mechanical stimuli such as brush, touch, pressure, and noxious pinch, but respond only to noxious pinch in the periphery of the receptive field. The mechanical threshold shows a gradual increase from the center toward the periphery of the receptive field. The receptive fields are strictly contralateral even in the central structure such as the nose and mouth. These characteristics are much the same as those of trigeminal WDR neurons in the lateral part of the subnucleus reticularis dorsalis. Some of them also respond to electrical stimulation of the contralateral maxillary and/or mandibular tooth-pulp afferents.

As in the case of trigeminal NS neurons located in the shell region of the VPM proper, trigeminal WDR neurons show a somatotopic organization (Fig. 8). That is, trigeminal WDR neurons having a center of the receptive field in the ophthalmic division are found in the lateral part of the dorsal shell region. Those having a center of the receptive field in the maxillary

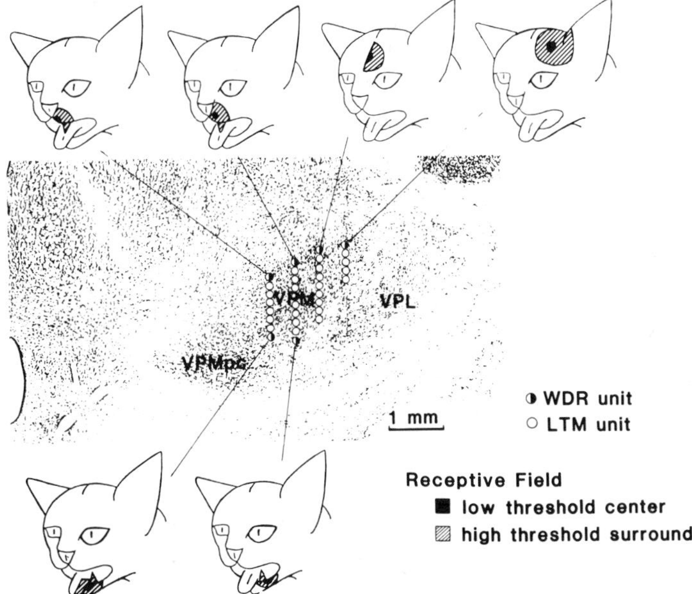

FIG. 8. Somatotopic distribution of trigeminal WDR neurons within the shell region of the VPM proper.

division occur in the medial part of the dorsal shell region and those having a center of the receptive field in the mandibular division are encountered in the ventromedial shell region adjacent to the VPMpc.

Locations of Trigeminal and Spinal Nociceptive Neurons in Shell Region of VB Complex

Neither NS nor WDR neurons have been found in the ventrolateral part of the shell region of the VPM proper which is adjacent to the VPL. There have been reports (28,31,33,38) that the lateral shell region of the VPL contains spinal nociceptive neurons. Taking these results together, nociceptive neurons are located in the shell region surrounding the whole VB complex. Then, a question has been raised if the spatial segregation of NS and WDR neurons found in the VPM proper also exists in the shell region of the VPL. Experiments carried out in our laboratory indicate that this is the case. That is, in the caudal part of the VB complex, trigeminal and spinal NS units are located in the shell region of the VB complex in an orderly topographic manner (Fig. 9). Trigeminal and spinal WDR neurons are located in a narrow band of the shell region just rostral to the region where NS neurons are located. They also show a somatotopic organization.

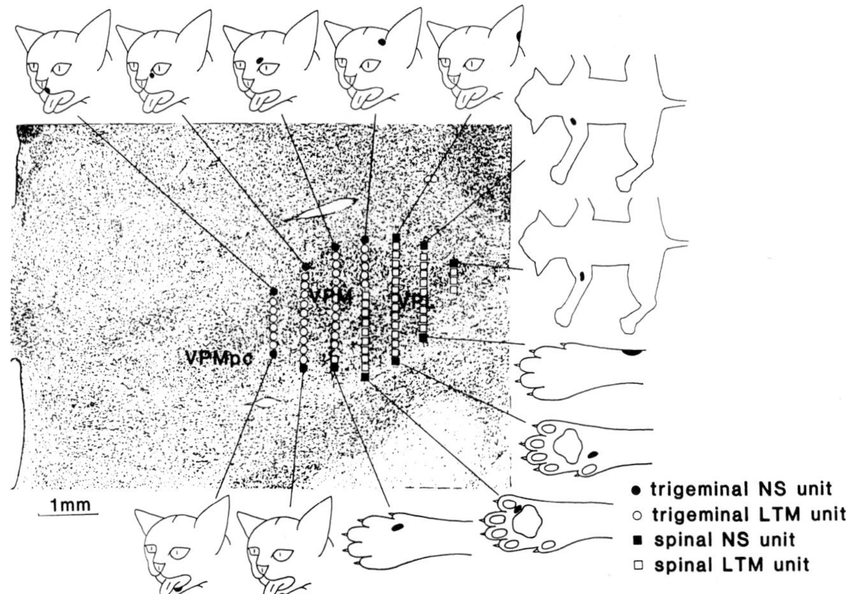

FIG. 9. Somatotopic distribution of trigeminal and spinal NS neurons within the shell region of the ventrobasal complex consisting of the VPM proper and VPL.

Location of Neurons Relaying Trigeminal Nociceptive Input into VPM

Electrical stimulation of the caudal VPM elicits antidromic excitation of trigeminal NS neurons in the marginal layer of the trigeminal subnucleus caudalis and of trigeminal WDR neurons in the lateral part of the subnucleus reticularis dorsalis. These findings suggest that trigeminal nociceptive input into the shell region of the VPM proper is relayed via these neurons. This was further confirmed by cooling experiments and by trigeminal tractotomy (62). After having tested the receptive field properties and responses to electrical stimulation of the cutaneous receptive field of a NS neuron, the contralateral spinal trigeminal tract and subnucleus caudalis were cooled by a thermode positioned on the dorsal surface of the contralateral medulla oblongata caudal to the obex. Ten-minute cooling abolished responses of neurons to noxious mechanical as well as electrical stimulation of the cutaneous receptive field. The response recovered after the cessation of cooling. After interruption of the spinal tract near the level of the obex, responses of NS neurons in the shell region of the VPM proper were irreversibly abolished, but electrical stimulation of the spinal tract at a level caudal to the incision still elicited excitation of these neurons. Similar observations were made on trigeminal WDR neurons in the shell region of the VPM proper.

Nociceptive responses of thalamic NS and WDR neurons appear to depend on the integrity of the caudal medulla oblongata.

SUMMARY AND CONCLUSION

In the subnucleus caudalis and its nearby lateral reticular formation, there are three general categories of trigeminal nociceptive neurons. They are nociceptive specific (NS) neurons, wide dynamic range (WDR) neurons, and subnucleus reticularis ventralis (SRV) neurons. NS neurons are located in the marginal layer and outer zone of the substantia gelatinosa. WDR neurons are located in the lateral part of the subnucleus reticularis dorsalis. SRV neurons are located in the dorsolateral part of the subnucleus reticularis ventralis. Both NS and WDR neurons project to the contralateral VPM, whereas SRV neurons project to the brainstem reticular formation. Both NS and WDR neurons show a somatotopic organization, and their rostrocaudal somatotopic pattern is in accord with the onion peel segmentation of facial dermatomes proposed by Déjerine (13).

In the VPM proper of the thalamus, there are trigeminal NS and WDR neurons. NS neurons are located in the shell region of the caudal third of VPM proper. WDR neurons are located in a narrow band of shell region just rostral to the NS region. Both of them show a somatotopic organization. Hence, they are place-specific. There is a weight of evidence that trigeminal input into NS and WDR neurons in the VPM proper is primarily relayed via NS neurons in the marginal layer of the subnucleus caudalis and WDR neurons in the lateral part of the subnucleus reticularis dorsalis, respectively.

REFERENCES

1. Albe-Fessard, D., Boivie, I., Grant, G., and Levante, A. (1975): Labelling of cells in the medulla oblongata and the spinal cord of the monkey after injection of horseradish peroxidase in the thalamus. *Neurosci. Lett.*, 1:75–80.
2. Albe-Fessard, D., Nashold, B., Pollen, B., and Woda, A. (1977): Thalamic and mid-brain responses to dental pulp afferent messages in awake cats. *J. Physiol. (Paris)*, 73:347–357.
3. Arvidson, J., and Gobel, S. (1981): An HRP study of the central projections of primary trigeminal neurons which innervate tooth pulps in the cat. *Brain Res.*, 210:1–16.
4. Azerad, J., Woda, A., and Albe-Fessard, D. (1982): Physiological properties of neurons in different parts of the cat trigeminal sensory complex. *Brain Res.*, 246:7–21.
5. Barbut, D., Polak, J. M., and Wall, P. D. (1982): Substance P in spinal cord dorsal horn decreases following peripheral nerve injury. *Brain Res.*, 205:289–298.
6. Bregmann, E. (1892): Ueber experimentelle aufsteigende Degeneration motorischer und sensibler Hirnnerven. *Arb. Neurol. Inst. (Wien)*, 1:73–97.
7. Broton, J. G., and Rosenfeld, J. P. (1982): Rostral trigeminal projections singnal perioral facial pain. *Brain Res.*, 243:395–400.
8. Burton, H., and Craig, A. D. (1979): Distribution of trigeminothalamic projection cells in cat and monkey. *Brain Res.*, 161:515–521.
9. Reference deleted.

10. Craig, A. D. (1978): Spinal and medullary input to the lateral cervical nucleus. *J. Comp. Neurol.*, 181:729–744.
11. Crosby, E. C., and Yoss, R. E. (1954): The phylogenetic continuity of neural mechanisms as illustrated by the spinal tract of V and its nucleus. *Res. Assoc. Nerv. Ment. Dis.*, 33:147–208.
12. Cuello, A. C., Fiacco, M. D., and Paxinos, G. (1978): The central and peripheral ends of the substance P-containing sensory neurones in the rat trigeminal system. *Brain Res.*, 152:499–509.
13. Déjerine, J. J. (1914): *Semiologie des Affections du Systême Nerveux.* Masson, Paris.
14. Dubner, R., Hoffman, D. S., and Hayes, R. L. (1981): Neuronal activity in medullary dorsal horn of awake monkeys trained in thermal discrimination task. III. Task-related responses and their functional role. *J. Neurophysiol.*, 46:444–464.
15. Falls, W. M., and Gobel, S. (1979): Golgi and EM studies of the formation of dendritic and axonal arbors: the interneurons of the substantia gelatinosa of Rolando in newborn kittens. *J. Comp. Neurol.*, 187:1–18.
16. Fukushima, T., and Kerr, F. W. L. (1979): Organization of trigeminothalamic tracts and other thalamic afferent systems of the brainstem in the rat: presence of gelatinosa neurons with thalamic connections. *J. Comp. Neurol.*, 183:169–184.
17. Fuse, G. (1919): Beitrage zur normalen Anatomie des der spinalen Trigeminuswurzel angehörigen Graus, vor allem der Substantia gelatinosa Rolando beim Menschen. *Arb. Anat. Inst. Univ. Sendai,* 2:87–189.
18. Gobel, S. (1975): Golgi studies of the substantia gelatinosa neurons in the spinal trigeminal nucleus. *J. Comp. Neurol.*, 162:397–415.
19. Gobel, S. (1978): Golgi studies of the neurons in layer I of the dorsal horn of the medulla (trigeminal nucleus caudalis). *J. Comp. Neurol.*, 180:375–393.
20. Gobel, S. (1978): Golgi studies of the neurons in layer II of the dorsal horn of the medulla (trigeminal nucleus caudalis). *J. Comp. Neurol.*, 180:395–414.
21. Gobel, S., Falls, W. M., and Hockfield, S. (1977): The division of the dorsal and ventral horns of the mammalian caudal medulla into eight layers using anatomical criteria. In: *Pain in the Trigeminal Region,* edited by D. J. Anderson and B. Matthews, pp. 443–453. Elsevier, Amsterdam.
22. Hayes, R. L., Dubner, R., and Hoffman, D. S. (1981): Neuronal activity in medullary dorsal horn of awake monkeys trained in a thermal discrimination task. II. Behavioral modulation of responses to thermal and mechanical stimuli. *J. Neurophysiol.*, 46:428–443.
23. Henry, J. L., Sessle, B. J., Lucier, G. E., and Hu, J. W. (1980): Effects of substance P on nociceptive and nonnociceptive trigeminal brain stem neurons. *Pain,* 8:33–45.
24. Höckfelt, T., Kellerth, J. O., Nilsson, G., and Pernon, B. (1975): Experimental immunohistochemical studies on the localization and distribution of substance P in cat primary sensory neurons. *Brain Res.*, 100:235–252.
25. Hockfield, S., and Gobel, S. (1978): Neurons in and near nucleus caudalis with long ascending projection axons demonstrated by retrograde labeling with horseradish peroxidase. *Brain Res.*, 139:333–339.
26. Hockfield, S., and Gobel, S. (1982): An anatomical demonstration of projections to the medullary dorsal horn (trigeminal nucleus caudalis) from rostral trigeminal nuclei and the contralateral caudal medulla. *Brain Res.*, 252:203–211.
27. Hoffman, D. S., Dubner, R., Hayes, R. L., and Medlin, T. (1981): Neuronal activity in medullary dorsal horn of awake monkeys trained in a thermal discrimination task. I. Responses to innocuous and noxious thermal stimuli. *J. Neurophysiol.*, 46:409–427.
28. Honda, C. N., Mense, S., and Perl, E. R. (1983): Neurons in ventrobasal region of cat thalamus selectively responsive to noxious mechanical stimulation. *J. Neurophysiol.*, 49:662–673.
29. Hu. J. W., Dostrovsky, J. O., and Sessle, B. J. (1981): Functional properties of neurons in cat trigeminal subnucleus caudalis (medullary dorsal horn). I. Responses to oral-facial noxious and nonnoxious stimuli and projections to thalamus and subnucleus oralis. *J. Neurophysiol.*, 45:173–192.
30. Jessel, T. M., and Iversen, L. L. (1977): Opiate analgesics inhibit substance P release from rat trigeminal nucleus. *Nature (Lond.),* 286:540–551.
31. Kenshalo, D. R., Jr., Giesler, G. J., Jr., Leonard, R. B., and Willis, W. D. (1980): Responses

of neurons in primate ventral posterior lateral nucleus to noxious stimuli. *J. Neurophysiol.*, 43:1594–1614.

32. Kerr, F. W. L. (1970): Fine structure and functional characteristics of the primary trigeminal neuron. In: *Trigeminal Neuralgia,* edited by R. Hassler and A. E. Walker, pp. 180–190. Georg Thieme Verlag, Stuttgart.
33. Kniffki, K. D., and Mizumura, K. (1983): Responses of neurons in VPL and VPL-VL region of the cat to algesic action of stimulation of muscle and tendon. *J. Neurophysiol.*, 49:649–661.
34. Krieg, W. J. S. (1948): A reconstruction of the diencephalic nuclei of Macacus rhesus. *J. Comp. Neurol.*, 88:1–51.
35. Kunc, Z. (1970): Significant factors pertaining to the result of trigeminal tractotomy. In: *Trigeminal Neuralgia,* edited by R. Hassler and A. E. Walker, pp. 90–100. Georg Thieme Verlag, Stuttgart.
36. Matsushita, M., Ikeda, M., and Okado, N. (1982): The cells of origin of the trigeminothalamic, trigeminospinal and trigeminocerebellar projections in the cat. *Neuroscience,* 7:1439–1454.
37. Meessen, H., and Olszewski, J. (1949): *A Cytoarchitectonic Atlas of the Rhombencephalon of the Rabbit.* Karger, Basel.
38. Mitchell, D., and Hellon, R. F. (1977): Neuronal and behavioral responses in rats during noxious stimulation of the tail. *Proc. R. Soc. Lond. (Biol.),* 197:169–194.
39. Mountcastle, V. B., and Henneman, E. (1952): The representation of tactile sensibility in the thalamus of the monkey. *J. Comp. Neurol.*, 97:409–439.
40. Mosso, J. A., and Kruger, L. (1973): Receptor cateroris represented in spinal trigeminal nucleus caudalis. *J. Neurophysiol.*, 36:472–488.
41. Olszewski, J. (1950): On the anatomical and functional organization of the spinal trigeminal nucleus. *J. Comp. Neurol.*, 92:401–413.
42. Olszewski, J. (1952): *The Thalamus of the Macacus Mulatta.* Karger, Basel.
43. Panneton, W. M., and Burton, H. (1981): Corneal and pericorneal representation within the trigeminal sensory complex in the cat studied with transganglionic transport of horseradish peroxidase. *J. Comp. Neurol.*, 199:327–344.
44. Poggio, G. F., and Mountcastle, V. B. (1960): A study of the functional contributions of the lemniscal and spinothalamic systems to somatic sensibility. *Bull. Johns Hopkins Hosp.*, 106:266–316.
45. Poggio, G. F., and Mountcastle, V. B. (1963): The functional properties of ventrobasal thalamic neurons studied in unanesthetized monkeys. *J. Neurophysiol.*, 26:775–806.
46. Price, D. D., Dubner, R., and Hu, J. W. (1976): Trigeminothalamic neurons in nucleus caudalis responsive to tactile, thermal, and nociceptive stimulation of monkey's face. *J. Neurophysiol.*, 39:936–953.

46a. Ramon y Cajal, S. (1909): *Histologie du Systéme Nerveux de l'Homme et des Vertébrés, Vol. 1.* Maloine, Paris.

47. Rexed, B. (1954): A cytoarchitectonic atlas of the spinal cord in the cat. *J. Comp. Neurol.*, 100:297–379.
48. Shigenaga, Y., Nadatani, Z., Nishimori, T., Suemune, S., Kuroda, R., and Matano, S. (1983): The cells of origin of trigeminothalamic projections: especially in the caudal medulla. *Brain Res.*, 277:201–222.
49. Sjöqvist, O. (1938): Studies on pain conduction in the trigeminal nerve. *Acta Psychiatr. Neurol. Scand.*, 17(Suppl.):1–139.
50. Sunderland, S. (1978): *Nerves and Nerve Injuries.* Churchill Livingstone, Edinburgh.
51. Vyklicky, L., Keller, O., Jastreboff, P., Vyklicky, L., Jr., and Bulkhuzi, S. M. (1977): Spinal trigeminal tractotomy and nociceptive reactions evoked by tooth pulp stimulation in the cat. *J. Physiol. (Paris),* 73:379–381.
52. Walker, A. E. (1938): *The Primate Thalamus.* University of Chicago Press, Chicago.
53. Wall, P. D. (1967): The laminar organization of dorsal horn and effects of descending impulses. *J. Physiol. (Lond.),* 188:403–423.
54. Wall, P. D., and Gutnick, M. (1974): Ongoing activity in peripheral nerves: The physiology and pharmacology of impulses originating from a neuroma. *Exp. Neurol.*, 43:580–593.
55. Wallenberg, A. (1895): Akute Bulbäraffektion (Embolie der Art cerebellar. post. inf. sinistr. ?). *Arch. Psychiatr.*, 27:504–540.

56. Wallenberg, A. (1896): Zur Physiologie der spinalen Trigeminuswurzel. *Neurol. Zentralbl.* 15:873–876.
57. Weinberger, L. M., and Grant, F. C. (1942): Experiences with intramedullary tractotomy. III. Studies in sensation. *Arch. Neurol. Psychiatr. (Chicago),* 48:355–381.
58. Yokota, T. (1975): Excitation of units in marginal rim of trigeminal subnucleus caudalis elicited by tooth pulp stimulation. *Brain Res.,* 95:154–158.
59. Yokota, T., and Koyama, N. (1982): Responses evoked in the caudal medulla by stimulation of neck muscle afferents. In: *Anatomical, Physiological and Pharmacological Aspects of Trigeminal Pain,* edited by B. Matthews and R. G. Hill, pp. 103–118. Excerpta Medica, Amsterdam.
60. Yokota, T., and Koyama, N. (1983): Identification of neurons relaying trigeminal nociceptive input onto subnucleus reticularis ventralis in the cat. *Neurosci. Lett.,* 36:273–278.
61. Yokota, T., and Koyama, N. (1983): Functional connection of experimentally produced neuroma with neurons within the trigeminal subnucleus caudalis and nearby bulbar lateral reticular formation. In: *Current Topics in Pain Research and Therapy,* edited by T. Yokota and R. Dubner, pp. 57–67. Excerpta Medica, Amsterdam.
62. Yokota, T., and Matsumoto, N. (1983): Somatotopic distribution of trigeminal nociceptive specific neurons within the caudal somatosensory thalamus in the cat. *Neurosci. Lett.,* 39:125–130.
63. Yokota, T., and Matsumoto, N. (1983): Location and functional organization of trigeminal wide dynamic range neurons within the nucleus ventralis posteromedialis of the cat. *Neurosci. Lett.,* 39:231–236.
64. Yokota, T., and Nishikawa, N. (1977): Somatotopic organization of trigeminal neurons within caudal medulla oblongata. In: *Pain in the Trigeminal Region,* edited by D. J. Anderson and B. Matthews, pp. 243–257. Elsevier, Amsterdam.
65. Yokota, T., and Nishikawa, N. (1980): Reappraisal of somatotopic tactile representation within trigeminal subnucleus caudalis. *J. Neurophysiol.,* 43:700–712.
66. Yokota, T., Nishikawa, N., and Nishikawa, Y. (1979): Effects of strychnine upon different classes of trigeminal subnucleus caudalis neurons. *Brain Res.,* 168:430–434.
67. Yokota, T., Nishikawa, N., and Nishikawa, Y. (1979): Trigeminal nociceptive neurons in the trigeminal subnucleus caudalis and bulbar lateral reticular formation. In: *Advances in Pain Research and Therapy, Vol. 3,* edited by J. J. Bonica, J. C. Liebeskind, and D. AlbeFessard, pp. 211–217. Raven Press, New York.
68. Yokota, T., and Nishikawa, Y. (1979): Action of picrotoxin upon trigeminal subnucleus caudalis neurons in the monkey. *Brain Res.,* 171:369–373.
69. Yokota, T., and Nishikawa, Y. (1982): Responses evoked in the cat caudal medulla by stimulation of tooth pulp. In: *Anatomical, Physiological and Pharmacological Aspects of Trigeminal Pain,* edited by B. Matthews and R. G. Hill, pp. 119–135. Excerpta Medica, Amsterdam.
70. Young, R. F., Oleson, T. D., and Perryman, K. (1981): Effect of trigeminal tractotomy on behavioral response to dental pulp stimulation in the monkey. *J. Neurosurg.,* 55:420–430.

Advances in Pain Research and Therapy, Vol. 9, edited by H. L. Fields et al. Raven Press, New York © 1985.

Convergent Inputs to Neurons Responding to Tooth-Pulp Stimulation in the Trigeminal Nuclei of the Rostral Brainstem of the Minimally Traumatized Cat

N. C. Campbell, R. W. Clarke, and B. Matthews

Department of Physiology, University of Bristol, Medical School, Bristol BS8 1TD, United Kingdom

It is often claimed that trigeminal spinal subnucleus caudalis (VSNC) is the only part of the trigeminal nuclear complex of the brainstem that is involved in the transmission of impulses related to pain (see ref. 9). This view is founded on two lines of evidence:

1. In man, destruction of VSNC, or its isolation from peripheral input by tractotomy, results in a loss of pain sensation from the face ipsilateral to the lesion (14,23).
2. In animals, recordings from trigeminal neurons have indicated that only those in VSNC are capable of differentiating nociceptive from nonnociceptive signals (13; for review see ref. 9).

However, data have recently been obtained that indicate that more rostral parts of the trigeminal nuclear complex may be directly involved in pain. For instance, Young and co-workers (26,27) have demonstrated that sectioning of the descending trigeminal tract above the level of VSNC leaves the oral cavity only partially analgesic and appears to have no effect at all on the aversive responses or pain sensations evoked by stimulation of the teeth in monkey and man. In addition, Azerad et al. (1) showed that, in very lightly anesthetized cats, 27% of their sample of neurons in trigeminal sub-

Present address for Dr. Campbell is Department of Physiology, University of Lund, Sölvegatan 19, S 22362, Lund, Sweden.

Present address for Dr. Clarke is Department of Physiology and Environmental Science, University of Nottingham School of Agriculture, Sutton Bonington, Loughborough, LE12 5RD, United Kingdom.

nucleus oralis (VSNO) had nociceptive receptive fields within and around the mouth.

Many workers have reported that some neurons in VSNO, as well as in VSNC, respond to electrical stimulation of tooth-pulp nerves (e.g., refs. 1,2,10,20,21), although the significance of this has been unclear. Stimulation of tooth pulp in man causes pain, but, close to threshold, other sensations are produced (18,19). Some authors have suggested that the responses of VSNO cells to tooth pulp might be an artifact of the highly synchronous volleys evoked by electrical stimuli (e.g., ref. 8), and evidence has been put forward to suggest that thermal stimulation of teeth evokes responses only in VSNC (12).

Recent work in our laboratory, however, has shown that neurons at all levels of the trigeminal brainstem nuclear complex will respond to thermal stimulation of the teeth at temperatures which would be expected to cause pain in man (6).

We believe that the differences between the results obtained in recordings from neurons in VSNO arise from differences in the preparation of the experimental animals. We have recently demonstrated that surgical trauma and other forms of noxious input can cause a profound and prolonged depression of trigeminal responses to tooth-pulp stimulation (4), and the effect is greater in deeply anesthetized than in very lightly anesthetized cats (7). The depression in the excitability of brainstem neurons can be avoided by minimizing trauma immediately prior to brainstem recording (5). Having demonstrated that VSNO and main sensory nucleus (MSN) neurons will respond to thermal stimulation of teeth in cats prepared in this way (6), we carried out the present experiments to determine if they might also respond to other forms of noxious stimulation. A preliminary report on this work has been published (3).

METHODS

Experiments were performed on 19 young adult cats weighing from 2.5 to 5.0 kg. All cats were sedated with ketamine (Vetalar, Parke-Davis; 10 mg/kg, i.m.) after which anesthesia was induced and maintained with either alphaxalone/alphadolone acetate (Saffan, Glaxovet; 5–10 mg/kg/hr, i.v., 8 cats), methohexitone (Brietal, Eli Lilly; 3.7–8 mg/kg/hr, i.v., 10 cats) or α-chloralose/urethane (40/200 mg/kg, i.v., 1 cat). Surgical preparation of each animal was kept to a minimum. The trachea and the femoral vein and artery on one side were cannulated and the animal's head was supported in a stereotaxic frame using shortened, atraumatic ear bars. Skin incisions were made after local infiltration with 2% lignocaine solution and all wounds were covered with 5% lignocaine ointment (Astra) before closing. Arterial blood pressure and end-tidal CO_2 were monitored and core temperature was maintained at 37.5 $\pm$ 0.5° C using a thermostatically controlled blanket. No data were collected if systolic blood pressure fell below 100 mm Hg or if end-tidal CO_2 was outside the range of 3 to 5%. Thirteen cats were paralyzed with pancuronium bromide (Pavulon, Organon; 400 μg/kg initially and supplemented *s.q.*) and artificially ventilated with room air. A bilateral pneumothorax was performed on these animals and their ECG monitored.

The right upper and lower canine teeth were prepared for electrical and thermal stimulation as described previously (15). Two copper wires were inserted into the anterior part of the ipsilateral digastric muscle for recording EMG; this allowed the threshold of the digastric reflex evoked by tooth-pulp stimulation to be monitored, to provide an indication of the excitability of the trigeminal brainstem neurons (5).

Access to the brainstem was obtained through a small craniotomy alongside the lambdoidal ridge and extending up to 10 mm away from the midline. Recordings were made from neurons in and around VSNO and MSN using glass micropipettes filled with 1.5% pontamine sky blue in 0.5 M sodium acetate solution. The electrodes were advanced through the cerebellum at an angle of 30° to the stereotaxic vertical axis. Neurons were sought using a stimulus of 100 μA, 0.1 msec, applied simultaneously to both ipsilateral canine teeth. The majority of neurons identified in this way were then characterized by recording their threshold and latency to electrical stimulation of each tooth separately, and their responses to thermal (16) and mechanical stimulation of the teeth, and to light brushing or rubbing of the facial skin, oral and nasal mucous membranes, and the cornea. Responses to pinching or pricking the face and oral mucous membrane were also determined. Mechanical stimuli were applied to the mucous membrane deep within the nasal cavity and to the cornea, using a smooth, rounded-tipped metal probe (diameter 1.5 mm). Recording sites were marked by iontophoretic deposition of dye (10 μA for 2 min), and located in 80 μm frozen sections stained with neutral red.

Many neurons were also investigated for projections to the contralateral or ipsilateral thalamus. Antidromic responses were sought during electrical stimulation of the medioposterior nucleus of the ventrobasal thalamus (VPM). The stimuli were applied using all combinations of 2 from an array of four electrodes arranged at the corners of a 2 mm square. Each electrode was a 0.076 mm diameter silver wire that was insulated down to its tip and carried in a needle (diameter 0.4 mm) that was not part of the stimulating circuit. Antidromic responses were identified by their short, stable latencies to thalamic stimulation, their ability to follow stimulation at rates of 200 to 300 Hz and by collision with orthodromically evoked responses from the teeth.

RESULTS

Two hundred and seventeen units responding to electrical stimulation of tooth pulp were isolated from within and around VSNO and MSN. We have divided them into four main categories on the basis of their responses to

TABLE 1. *Classification of cells with input from tooth pulp responding to mechanical stimulation of the face and/or mouth*

Cell type	Intensity of stimulation: Low	High	No.
0	−	−	44
1	+	−	65
2	+	+	87
3	−	+	21
Total			217

mechanical stimulation of the face and mouth. The numbers in each of these groups are given in Table 1. The four types are:

Type 0: No oro-facial mechanoreceptive field.
Type 1: Responded maximally to nonnoxious mechanical stimulation of the face, oral mucosa, and/or teeth (periodontal).
Type 2: Fired in response to low intensity mechanical stimulation of these areas but gave maximal responses to noxious pinching or pricking (Fig. 1).
Type 3: Responded only to such intense mechanical stimuli.

Of the 217 units with input from tooth pulp, 173 had mechanoreceptive fields in the mouth or on the skin of the face; and of these, 108 had nociceptive input from these tissues.

Mechanoreceptive fields were mainly localized in the mouth or on the lips and immediately surrounding skin. In addition, 97 out of the 217 units had receptor fields on the nasal mucous membrane and/or the cornea (Table 2). All but two neurons had exclusively ipsilateral fields. These properties are illustrated in Fig. 2, which shows the recording locations and receptive fields of 23 neurons from one cat.

Corneal receptor fields were always ipsilateral and ranged in size from a small strip or quadrant to the whole corneal surface. Thirty-five of 41 units with input from cornea were of type 2, and 70 of 92 units with receptor fields in the nasal mucous membrane were of type 2 or 3. Thus, there was a strong tendency for units with nasal and/or corneal inputs also to have nociceptive inputs from the mouth and face.

Approximately two-thirds of the units tested responded to thermal stimulation of the tip of one or other of the teeth (Table 3). Most of these cells responded to cooling the tooth to 10° C from either 30° or 50° C (Fig. 1), and 3 fired most spikes in response to heating the tooth to 50° C. There was

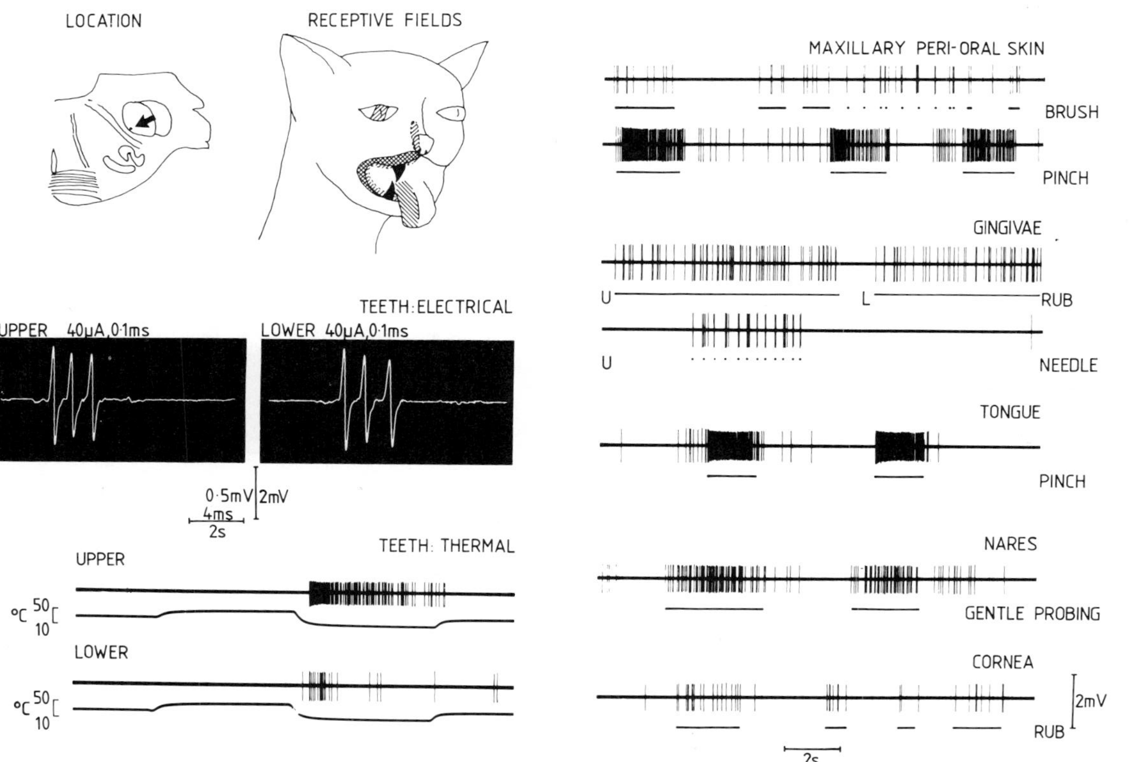

FIG. 1. Receptive field, location, and responses of a type 2 neuron in VSNO. The brainstem section was 7.6 mm rostral to the obex.

TABLE 2. *Distribution of cells responding to stimulation of nasal mucosa and/or cornea*

	Input from				
Cell type	NM[a]	C[a]	NM+C	Neither	Total
0	4	0	0	40	44
1	13	1	5	46	65
2	28	4	31	24	87
3	11	0	0	10	21
Totals	56	5	36	120	217

[a]NM: nasal mucosa; C: cornea.

no clear correlation between a unit's response to thermal stimulation of the teeth and its response to other forms of stimulation. Thermal stimulation of the teeth excited a higher proportion of type 2 units than other cell types, but the difference was not significant (χ^2 test $p > 0.1$). There were similarly no significant differences between the main categories of the units in their thresholds or latencies to electrical stimulation of tooth pulp (Fig. 3).

The recording locations were identified accurately for 159 neurons, of which 107 were in VSNO, 29 in MSN, and 23 in the surrounding reticular formation. The neurons were clustered mainly in the medial parts of the nuclei and those with corneal input tended to lie ventrally. There was no tendency for neurons of a particular type to be segregated in one area.

One hundred and twelve neurons were tested for antidromic invasion from the contralateral VPM and 20 from the ipsilateral VPM. Only 7 neurons were driven from the contralateral and none from the ipsilateral thalamus. Of the neurons projecting to the thalamus, 1 was type 0, 4 were type 1 (Fig. 4), 1 was type 3, and the seventh was not classified. Six units responded with a long (5–12 msec) and unstable latency during stimulation of the contralateral VPM, and one responded similarly from the ipsilateral VPM.

DISCUSSION

Of the pulp-driven VSM/MSN neurons investigated in this study, 50% also responded, exclusively or differentially, to noxious mechanical stimulation of other oral or perio-oral tissues (types 2 and 3). Some of these units also responded to stimulation of the cornea and/or nasal mucous membrane. It is thought that pain is the only sensation which can be evoked from the cornea (for review see ref. 17), and we have found that repeating the mechanical stimulation of the nasal cavity on ourselves causes irritation or pain. Fifty-eight out of the 81 neurons of types 2 and 3 that were tested

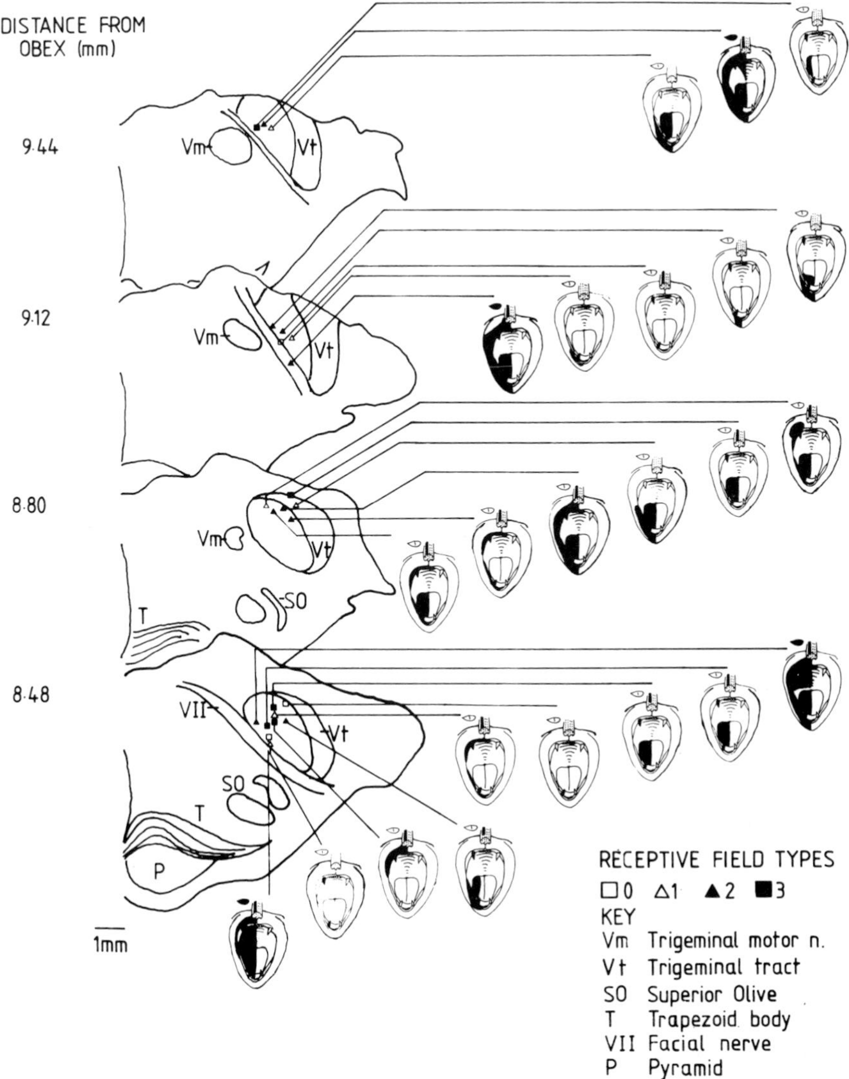

FIG. 2. Receptive field maps and recording locations of 23 neurons in 1 cat.

responded to thermal as well as electrical stimulation of the teeth. These classes of neurons could therefore contribute to nociceptive responses, including pain, although individually they would provide poor spatial localization of the stimulus. They showed characteristics which would be expected of interneurons involved in the jaw-opening reflex (see ref. 24).

Another group of units that may be involved in pain or associated responses is that which appeared to be tooth-pulp specific. Fifteen of 25 such

TABLE 3. *Distribution of cells responding to thermal stimulation of teeth*

Cell type	Input from				Total
	NM[a]	C[a]	NM+C	Neither	
0	1/2	0/0	0/0	14/23	15/25
1	8/11	0/1	2/5	18/31	28/48
2	9/23	2/3	22/27	7/13	50/66
3	6/10	0/0	0/0	2/5	8/15
Totals	34/36	2/4	24/32	41/82	101/154

[a]NM: nasal mucosa; C: cornea.

units responded to thermal as well as electrical stimulation of the teeth but they did not respond to any of the other stimuli investigated.

The fourth category of neuron (type 1) would be classified as low threshold based on their responses to mechanical stimulation of the skin of the face or of oral tissues. However, since all 65 of these units responded to tooth-pulp stimulation (28 to both thermal and electrical) and 19 responded to corneal and/or nasal stimulation, their involvement in nociceptive responses cannot be excluded. Since only neurons with tooth-pulp input were investigated, we have no information on what proportion of neurons in MSN and VSNO would have responded exclusively to non-noxious stimuli in these animals.

Our results confirm the observations of Sessle and Greenwood (21), that neurons in VSNO/MSN with tooth-pulp input have mechanoreceptive fields in and around the mouth, although they found very few units with nociceptive inputs from these other orofacial tissues.

It seems clear that the differences between our findings and those of previous workers (9,13) arise from differences in methodology. It seems that minimizing surgical trauma enhances the excitability of brainstem neurons to tooth-pulp stimulation, and unmasks some inputs to VSNO/MSN. This trauma-induced depression is anesthetic-dependent (7), and the effect would be small in the very lightly anesthetized cats studied by Azerad et al. (1), whose results agree well with those of the present study.

The presence of neurons in VSNO/MSN with input from the cornea is consistent with the results of the anatomical study of Harvey et al. (11) in the rabbit.

Few VSNO/MSN neurons were shown to have projections to contralateral VPM. However Yokota and Koyama (25) have recently shown that neurons in the ventral reticular nucleus (SRV) of the caudal brainstem receive nociceptive trigeminal input from neurons close to VSNO. Furthermore, although few neurons from SRV project to VPM, many more have

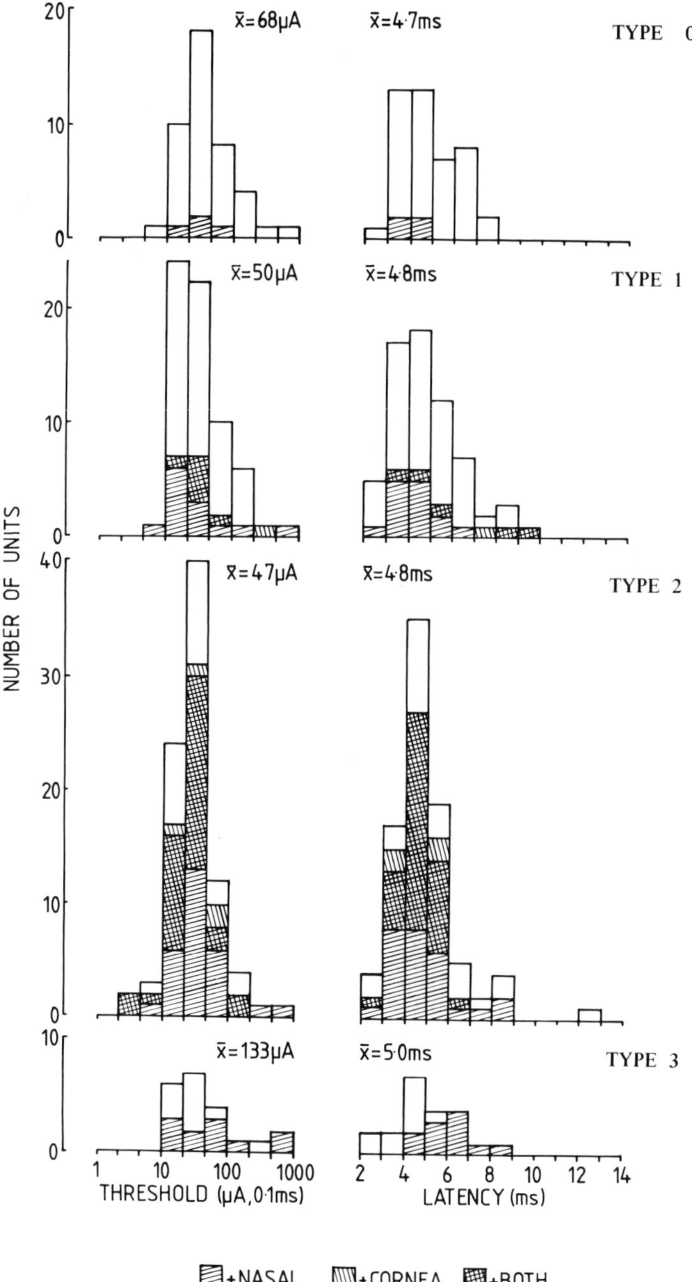

FIG. 3. Frequency distributions of the thresholds and latencies to electrical stimulation of tooth pulp of the 4 types of neurons. Minimum values of threshold and latency have been taken for each unit regardless of the tooth stimulated. The mean value is shown above each histogram, and the proportions of cells receiving input from the nose and cornea are shown by appropriate *shading.* Note that in each case the abscissa of the threshold histogram is plotted on a logarithmic scale.

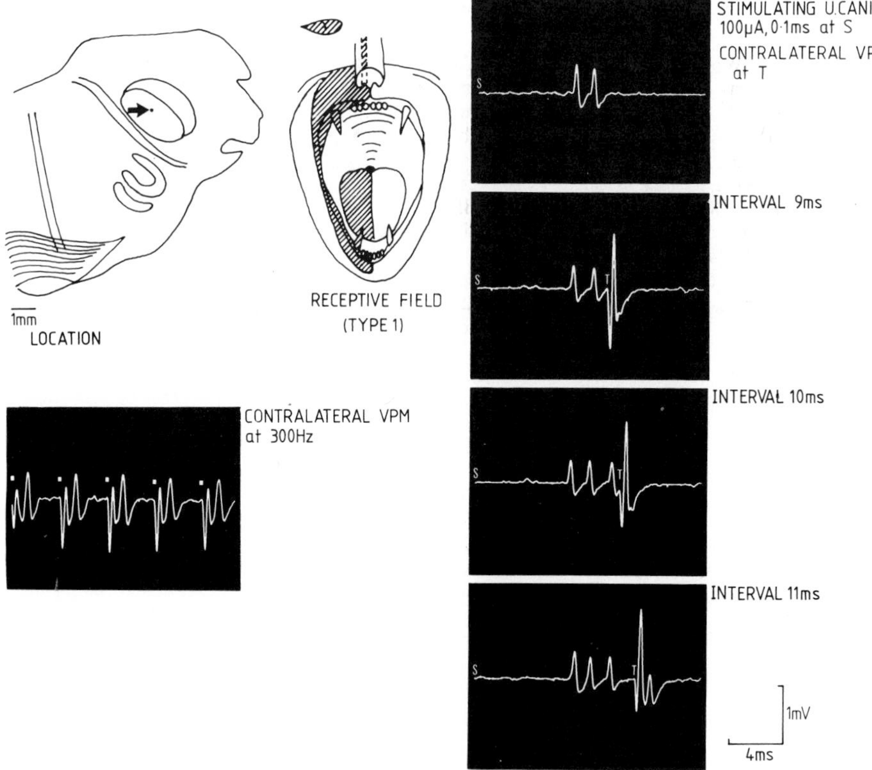

FIG. 4. Responses of a type 1 neuron located in VSNO 7.9 mm rostral to the obex. The neuron was spontaneously active and had a mechanoreceptive field as shown; it also responded to thermal stimulation of the teeth. It could be driven at a short, stable latency by stimulation of the contralateral VPM thalamus and followed stimulation at 300 Hz (**left panel:** *white dots* indicate each stimulus). The **right panel** shows the response of the neuron to electrical stimulation of the upper canine tooth and the collision test confirming antidromic activation from the thalamus.

been shown by histological methods to project to intralaminar and posterior group thalamic nuclei (22). Thus, VSNO neurons might project to the thalamus by an indirect route. VSNO/MSN must relay nociceptive information to higher centers by some route to explain the findings of Young et al. (26,27).

ACKNOWLEDGMENTS

This work was supported by the Medical Research Council. We wish to thank Ian Rogers, Philip Pamplin, Shirley Gorman, Jill Williams, Robin Harris, Perry Robbins, Bridget Parker, and Margaret Clements for their assistance.

REFERENCES

1. Azerad, J., Woda, A., and Albe-Fessard, D. (1982): Physiological properties of neurons in different parts of the cat trigeminal sensory complex. *Brain Res.,* 246:7–21.
2. Cadden, S. W. (1982): Electrical stimulation of cat canine tooth pulp: stimulus intensities required to evoke responses in trigeminal brainstem neurons. In: *Anatomical, Physiological and Pharmacological Aspects of Trigeminal Pain,* edited by B. Matthews and R. G. Hill, pp. 145–181. Excerpta Medica, Amsterdam.
3. Campbell, N. C., and Clarke, R. W. (1985): The properties of neurons in trigeminal sub nucleus oralis responding to tooth-pulp stimulation in the cat. *Philos. Trans. R. Soc. Lond. (Biol.),* 308:424.
4. Clarke, R. W. (1985): The effects on the jaw-opening reflex evoked by tooth-pulp stimulation of surgical trauma, decerebration and destruction of nucleus raphe magnus, periaqueductal grey matter and brainstem reticular formation in the cat. *Brain Res.*, 332:231–236.
5. Clarke, R. W., and Matthews, B. (1983): A comparison of the excitability of trigeminal brainstem neurons in acutely- and chronically-prepared cats. *J. Physiol. (Lond.),* 341:52P.
6. Clarke, R. W., and Matthews, B. (1983): Units in the trigeminal brainstem nuclei responding to thermal stimulation of teeth in the cat. *J. Physiol. (Lond.),* 342:23P.
7. Clarke, R. W., and Matthews, B. (1985): The effects of anaesthetics and remote noxious stimuli on the jaw-opening reflex evoked by tooth-pulp stimulation in the cat. *Brain Res.,* 327:105–111.
8. Dostrovsky, J. O. (1984): An electrophysiological study of canine, premolar and molar tooth pulp afferents and their convergence on medullary trigeminal neurons. *Pain,* 19:1–12.
9. Dubner, R., Sessle, B. J., and Storey, A. T. (1978): *The Neural Basis of Oral and Facial Function.* Plenum Press, New York.
10. Greenwood, L. F. (1973): An electrophysiological study of the central connections of primary afferent nerve fibres from the dental pulp of the cat. *Arch. Oral Biol.* 18:771–781.
11. Harvey, J. A., Land, T., and McMaster, S. E. (1984): Anatomical study of the rabbit's corneal-VIth nerve reflex: connections between cornea, trigeminal sensory complex and the abducens and accessory abducens nuclei. *Brain Res.,* 301:307–321.
12. Hu, J. W., Ball, G. J., and Sessle, B. J. (1981): Comparison of responses of rostral and caudal trigeminal brainstem neurones to electrical and thermal stimulation of tooth-pulp in cats. *Soc. Neurosci. Abstr.,* 7:532.
13. Hu, J. W., Dostrovsky, J. O., and Sessle, B. J. (1981): Functional properties of neurons in cat trigeminal subnucleus caudalis (medullary dorsal horn). I. Responses to oral-facial noxious and non-noxious stimuli and projections to thalamus and subnucleus oralis. *J. Neurophysiol,* 45:173–192.
14. Hun, H. (1897): Analgesia, thermic anaesthesia and ataxia resulting from foci of softening in the medulla oblongata and cerebellum due to occlusion of the left posterior cerebellar artery. *NY Med. J.,* 65:513–519.
15. Kollman, W., and Matthews, B. (1982): Responses of intradental nerves to thermal stimulation of teeth in the cat. In: *Anatomical, Physiological and Pharmacological Aspects of Trigeminal Pain,* edited by B. Matthews and R. G. Hill, pp. 51–65. Excerpta Medica, Amsterdam.
16. Kollman, W., Matthews, B., and Suda, H. (1982): Polymodal receptors in cat teeth? *J. Physiol (Lond.),* 327:9–10*P.*
17. Matthews, B. (1985): Peripheral and central aspects of trigeminal nociceptive systems. *Philos. Trans. R. Soc. Lond. (Biol.),* 308:313–324.
18. Matthews, B., Baxter, J., and Watts, S. (1976): Sensation and reflex responses to tooth pulp stimulation in man. *Brain Res.,* 113:83–94.
19. McGrath, P. A., Gracely, R. H., Dubner, R., and Heft, H. W. (1983): Non-pain and pain sensations evoked by tooth-pulp stimulation. *Pain,* 15:379–388.
20. Nord, S. G. (1976): Responses of neurons in rostral and caudal trigeminal nuclei to tooth pulp stimulation. *Brain Res. Bull.,* 1:489–492.
21. Sessle, B. J., and Greenwood, L. F. (1976): Inputs to trigeminal brainstem neurons from facial, oral, tooth pulp and pharyno-laryngeal tissues. I. Responses to innocuous and noxious stimuli. *Brain Res.,* 117:211–226.

22. Shigenaga, Y., Nakatani, Z., Nishimori, T., Suemune, S., Kuroda, R., and Matano, S. (1983): The cells of origin of cat trigemino-thalamic projections; especially in the caudal medulla. *Brain Res.,* 277:201–222.
23. Sjöquist, O. (1938): Studies on pain conduction in trigeminal nerve contribution to surgical treatment of facial pain. *Arch. Psychiatr. Neurol. (Suppl),* 17:1–139.
24. Sumino, R. (1971): Central neural pathways involved in the jaw-opening reflex in the cat. In: *Oral Facial Sensory and Motor Mechanisms,* edited by R. Dubner and Y. Kawamura, pp. 313–332. Appleton-Century-Crofts, New York.
25. Yokota, T., and Koyama, B. (1983): Identification of neurons relaying trigeminal nociceptive input onto sub nucleus reticularis ventralis in the cat. *Neurosci. Lett.,* 36:273–278.
26. Young, R. F. (1982): Effect of trigeminal tractotomy on dental sensation in humans. *J. Neurosurg.,* 56:812–818.
27. Young, R. F., Oleson, T. D., and Perryman, K. M. (1981): The effect of trigeminal tractotomy on behavioural responses to dental pulp stimulation in the monkey. *J. Neurosurg.,* 55:420–430.

Advances in Pain Research and Therapy, Vol. 9, edited by H. L. Fields et al. Raven Press, New York © 1985.

Thalamocortical Mechanisms of Pain

W. D. Willis

Marine Biomedical Institute, Departments of Physiology and Biophysics and Anatomy, University of Texas Medical Branch, Galveston, Texas 77550-2772

Despite the view expressed by Penfield and Jasper (89) that pain and temperature are sensed at the thalamic, not the cortical, level (see also refs. 55,56), there is increasing evidence that both the thalamus and the cerebral cortex are concerned with pain sensation and also with the motivational-affective aspects of pain (see refs. 1,91,107,120). This should not come as a surprise when one considers that the thalamus is closely coupled to the cerebral cortex through both thalamocortical and corticothalamic connections. Thus, it would be difficult to conceive of the thalamus having a sensory function independent of the cortex.

Some of the evidence concerning the role of the thalamus and cortex in pain can be summarized as follows.

1. Stimulation in the human thalamus during stereotaxic surgery can evoke pain or a burning sensation (47,53,110,111). It is more common to evoke pain by thalamic stimulation when the patient suffers from a chronic pain syndrome of the "deafferentation" type than if the patient has some other disorder (111).
2. Lesions of the thalamus can reduce pain (9,52–54,77,78, 103,105,112,114). The analgesia produced by thalamic lesions can be of different types, depending on where the lesion is placed in the thalamus.
3. A lesion of the thalamus can produce the thalamic syndrome (29) which is characterized by an increased pain threshold with respect to the application of a noxious stimulus, such as pinprick, but by the production of excruciating pain by what would ordinarily be a gentle, tactile stimulus.
4. Stimulation of the somatosensory cerebral cortex in man can sometimes elicit a pain sensation (88). In patients with pain syndromes, pain can also be elicited by stimulation of the parietal association cortex (6,36).
5. Epileptic seizures can have a sensory aura of pain (6,42,73). Albe-Fessard (1) cites evidence from the work of Bancaud and Talairach that such an aura can be extremely well localized, for example to the tip of a digit, and the painful aura can be eliminated in more than 80% of cases by surgical removal of a small zone of cortex at the border of areas 3 and 1.

6. Lesions of the cerebral cortex can result in analgesia (28,33,34, 36,58,72,73,79,102,106,109). If the lesion is in the somatosensory cortex, there can be a long-lasting loss of pain sensation in a localized region of the body with the appropriate somatotopic relationship to the damaged zone of the cortex. On the other hand, if parts of the frontal lobes are damaged, as in prefrontal lobotomy (41,64), a patient may be relieved of the suffering component of pain, and yet the ability to recognize a painful stimulus may be unchanged.

7. A lesion of the cerebral cortex can also produce a pain syndrome that closely resembles the thalamic syndrome of Dejerine and Roussy (29).

From this evidence, it can be safely concluded that both the thalamus and the cerebral cortex have important roles to play in pain. Furthermore, these roles appear to include the processing of different aspects of the pain experience, including both the sensori-discriminative and the motivational-affective components of pain (81,97).

For a more precise understanding of the neural circuitry that underlies the processing of pain information, it is necessary to derive evidence from animal experiments. However, animal work should always be related to what is known from human studies, since animal subjects cannot express in any direct fashion their sensory experience, and since there is considerable evidence for species differences in the organization of the somatosensory system. Several kinds of studies have been done in animals that have advanced our understanding of how the thalamus and cerebral cortex are involved in pain. The emphasis in the review to follow is on evidence from electrophysiological recordings.

RECORDINGS FROM THE CEREBRAL CORTEX

A number of laboratories have now succeeded in recording nociceptive responses from neurons of the cerebral cortex in several different species, including the rat, cat, and monkey. Some of this work is mentioned here, but a more thorough treatment can be found in recent reviews (1,91,120).

Although most investigations of the response properties of neurons in the SI and SII somatosensory regions of the cerebral cortex have emphasized the presence of neurons whose responses are predominantly to innocuous stimulation of the skin or to bending joints, there are reports of some neurons in these cortical zones that behave as though they received an input from nociceptors (3,18,84,119). Recently, increasing emphasis has been placed on the study of nociceptive cortical neurons.

Rat

Lamour et al. (70,71) have succeeded in recording nociceptive responses from the SmI cortex of the rat. Of 292 neurons for which peripheral receptive fields could be demonstrated, 91 units were nociceptive. Of these, 56 received a purely noxious input and 35 responded to both innocuous and noxious stimuli. The neurons with purely nociceptive inputs had large receptive fields that often extended onto the ipsilateral side of the body, whereas the convergent neurons had relatively restricted receptive fields on the contralateral body surface (70). Although the cortical neurons sampled in penetrations normal to the cortex had overlapping receptive fields, it was commonly found that cells at different depths in the cortex responded to different stimulus modalities. Nociceptive cells tended to be located in the infragranular layers, in contrast to the cells with non-noxious inputs, which were found in layers II to V. Furthermore, cells with nociceptive-specific responses tended to be deeper than cells with convergent inputs, being found chiefly in layer VI. Convergent neurons were concentrated in layer Vb.

Cat

Iwamura et al. (59) found 7 neurons in a sample of 123 recorded mainly in area 3a of the cat SI cortex that responded to noxious stimulation of muscle or tendon. Five of these nociceptive neurons were exclusively activated by noxious stimuli and 2 were excited by both innocuous and noxious stimuli.

Monkey

Kenshalo and Isensee (61) encountered 68 neurons in the SI cortex of the monkey that could be classified as nociceptive. Of these, 37 were of the "wide dynamic range" or multireceptive class, and 31 were of the "high threshold" or nociceptive-specific class. Fifty-six of these cells were tested with graded noxious heat stimuli, and 46 responded in a graded fashion. Of these 46 cells, 34 had relatively restricted, contralateral receptive fields. The remaining 12 cells had restricted contralateral fields for innocuous mechanical stimuli, but they could be activated by noxious pinching or heating of the skin anywhere on the body surface. All of the 15 nociceptive cells whose locations were determined by placing lesions at the recording sites were near the junction between area 1 and 3b. Unlike the nociceptive neurons described by Lamour et al. (71) in the rat cortex, the nociceptive cells in the monkey SI cortex were generally located in layer IV. It was suggested that the neurons with relatively restricted receptive fields might play a role in the sensori-discriminative aspects of pain, whereas the neurons with large, bilateral receptive fields might be involved in signaling the intensity of noxious stimuli and also in cortical arousal.

Robinson and Burton have examined the responses of neurons in the SII cortex and adjacent areas in awake, behaving monkeys (99–101). They found only a few nociceptive neurons, and more of these were located in area 7b than in the SII cortex proper (101). However, it may not have been possible to use sufficiently intense stimuli to rule out convergent nociceptive responses for many of the units.

It seems clear from these electrophysiological studies that nociceptive neurons do exist in the somatosensory cortex and that at least some of these cells have properties that suit them for a role in the sensori-discriminative processing of pain.

RECORDINGS FROM THE THALAMUS

As in the case of the somatosensory cortex, there have been a number of reports of nociceptive responses in recordings from neurons within various parts of the thalamus, including the ventrobasal complex (5,43,50, 51,66,83,92), the posterior nuclei (15,19,45,95), and the intralaminar complex (2,19,22,31,86,93,115). Recently, it has been proposed that the nucleus submedius may have a special role to play in pain, since many lamina I spinothalamic tract cells project to this nucleus (25). The nucleus submedius projects to the orbitofrontal cortex (26), suggesting a possible role of this nucleus in the motivational-affective component of pain. The work to be reviewed here emphasizes nociceptive responses that have been recorded in or near the ventrobasal complex.

Rat

Guilbaud et al. (46) and Peschanski et al. (94) found a large population of neurons within the ventral posterior lateral (VPL) nucleus of the rat thalamus that were nociceptive. Of a sample of 163 cells, Guilbaud et al. (46) report that 93 were excited only by noxious stimuli, such as pinch or pinprick. Another 19 neurons were activated by both innocuous and noxious stimuli. Finally, only 51 of the cells were activated exclusively by innocuous mechanical stimuli. The responses to noxious stimuli did not relate to arousal, since electrocorticograms did not show any changes during stimulation. The receptive fields of the nociceptive thalamic neurons were generally larger than those of the cells responding only to innocuous stimuli, and in many cases they were bilateral. Peschanski et al. (94) documented in further detail the responses of nociceptive neurons in the rat VPL nucleus to graded noxious heat stimuli.

Cat

In contrast to the rat, investigations of the cat VPL nucleus reveal very few nociceptive neurons within this nucleus. However, there are two recent reports of nociceptive neurons in the "shell region" that surrounds the VPL nucleus of the cat. Honda et al. (57) found 17 neurons that failed to respond to innocuous mechanical stimuli. Instead, the cells could be activated by noxious stimuli (or by electrically evoked volleys in finely myelinated afferent fibers). Almost all of these units were found in histological reconstructions of the recording sites to be in the "shell region" between the VPL nucleus proper and adjacent structures. In a concurrent investigation to the one by Honda et al. (57), Kniffki and Mizumura (65) found a population of neurons in the cat thalamus that could be activated by noxious stimulation of muscle or tendon. These cells were also located in the "shell region" around the VPL nucleus. Some of the cells appeared to be activated exclusively by musculotendinous nociceptors, while others had a convergent input from cutaneous nociceptors.

Monkey

Casey (19) recorded from units in the posterior complex and in the ventrolateral complex of the squirrel monkey. Some of the units appeared to respond selectively to noxious stimuli when the animals were asleep. However, during quiet wakening, the same units could be activated both by tactile and by noxious stimuli. These observations demonstrate that noxious stimuli can alter the activity of neurons in the somatosensory thalamus in the unanesthetized monkey. Furthermore, they suggest the possibility that thalamic neurons can change their response properties, depending upon behavioral state.

Pollin and Albe-Fessard (96) found a number of units in the VPL nucleus of monkeys with an intact neuraxis that responded to pinprick, as well as to innocuous mechanical stimuli. However, the proportion of such responses was dramatically increased when the dorsal part of the spinal cord was sectioned. In fact, in the lesioned animals, all of the cells found that had hindlimb receptive fields were activated most effectively by pinprick and never just by an innocuous mechanical stimulus. One explanation for this observation might be that the capability of many neurons in the primate VPL nucleus to respond to a noxious stimulus is suppressed when pathways in the dorsal part of the spinal cord are intact, but becomes unmasked after a lesion is made that interrupts these pathways. It is not clear if such an inhibitory action in the intact animal would be the result of activity in pathways that descend or ascend in the spinal cord white matter.

In a recent study, Casey and Morrow (20) were able to find a number of cells in the VPL nucleus of the awake, behaving monkey that responded both to tactile stimuli and to noxious mechanical and thermal stimuli. They have also made some observations of the responses of neurons in the central lateral (CL) nucleus that suggest that these neurons behave quite unlike the nociceptive cells of the VPL nucleus (K. Casey and T. Morrow, *unpublished observations*). Rather than responding in a fashion reflecting sensory stimulation, as do units in the VPL nucleus, cells in the CL nucleus seem to react to the behavioral state of the animal; furthermore, the responses of neurons in the CL nucleus are abolished by small doses of barbiturate, whereas the cells in the VPL nucleus continue to encode sensory information (K. Casey and T. Morrow, *personal communication*).

COMPARISON OF THE RESPONSES OF SPINOTHALAMIC TRACT CELLS AND OF VPL$_c$ NEURONS IN ANESTHETIZED MONKEYS

Our laboratory has been investigating the properties of neurons belonging to the spinothalamic tract (STT) of the monkey. This somatosensory pathway has long been thought to play a key role in transmitting pain (as well as thermal and tactile) information to the thalamus in primates, including humans (37,68,116,117,123). Neurons belonging to the STT in monkeys have been found to respond to several kinds of noxious stimuli (23,39,40,62,82,98,122). Two general types of nociceptive STT neurons that can be recognized are "high threshold" (or "nociceptive-specific") STT cells and "wide dynamic range" (or "multireceptive") STT cells. Both of these kinds of STT cells were found to project to the VPL nucleus (7). This was important to establish, since otherwise it might have been assumed that the well-known projection of the STT to the VPL nucleus in the monkey (8,12,14,63,80) might play a role in touch or in thermal sensation, rather than in pain.

We made a search in the VPL nucleus of the monkey thalamus for units that had response characteristics like those of the STT cells that project to this nucleus. The objective was, in part, to see if nociceptive STT cells excited or inhibited neurons in the VPL nucleus. We were, in fact, able to locate a number of neurons within the VPL nucleus that behaved in a manner quite similar to the wide dynamic range (WDR) and high threshold (HT) cells of the STT (60). Of a total of 54 cells that could be classified, 48 were of the WDR type and 6 of the HT type. An example of a WDR neuron in the VPL nucleus of the monkey is illustrated in Fig. 1. The cell was located in the caudal part of the VPL nucleus [VPL$_c$ of Olszewski (87)], and it had an excitatory receptive field on the skin over the lateral aspect of the leg (Fig. 1A). The neuron responded in a graded fashion to graded intensities of mechanical stimulation (Fig. 1C). It could also be activated by a noxious heat stimulus (Fig. 1D–F). The response to noxious heat was graded, with a threshold of about 47° C and a much larger response to 50° C. Application of a noxious heat stimulus to the tail of the monkey produced no obvious effect during the period of stimulation (not illustrated), suggesting that the response to noxious heating of the receptive field was not likely to be a generalized action, such as might accompany arousal. When the responses of a population of nociceptive VPL neurons to noxious heat were averaged (Fig. 2A), the threshold for the population was found to be about 45° C, which is

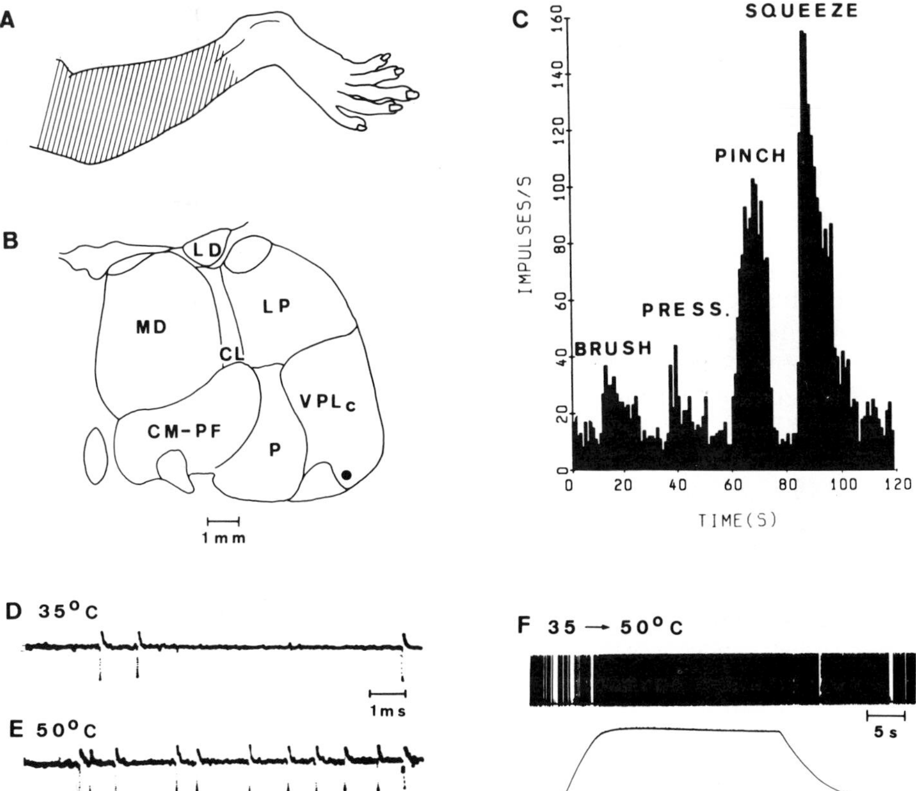

FIG. 1. Response properties of a WDR VPL_c neuron. The receptive field is in **A** and the location of the cell in **B.** The peristimulus time histogram in **C** shows the responses to graded mechanical stimulation of the skin. The records in **D** and **E** show the action potentials photographed from an oscilloscope face before and during a 50° C noxious heat stimulus. The pen writer record in **F** shows window discriminator pulses triggered by the action potentials before, during, and after the same noxious heat stimulus. The *lower trace* is the temperature monitor. (From ref. 60.)

near the human threshold for heat pain (49). The stimulus-response relations for individual units were usually positively accelerating curves (Fig. 2B) that resembled the human psychophysical function relating the intensity of noxious heat stimuli to the severity of noxious heat pain (69).

A role of the STT in the responses of nociceptive VPL neurons was suggested by the observation made in several experiments that the response to noxious heat was largely or entirely dependent on the integrity of the ventrolateral quadrant of the spinal cord on the side ipsilateral to the thalamic unit (contralateral to the receptive field). This is shown in the experiment illustrated in Fig. 3. When the dorsal quadrant of the cord contralateral to

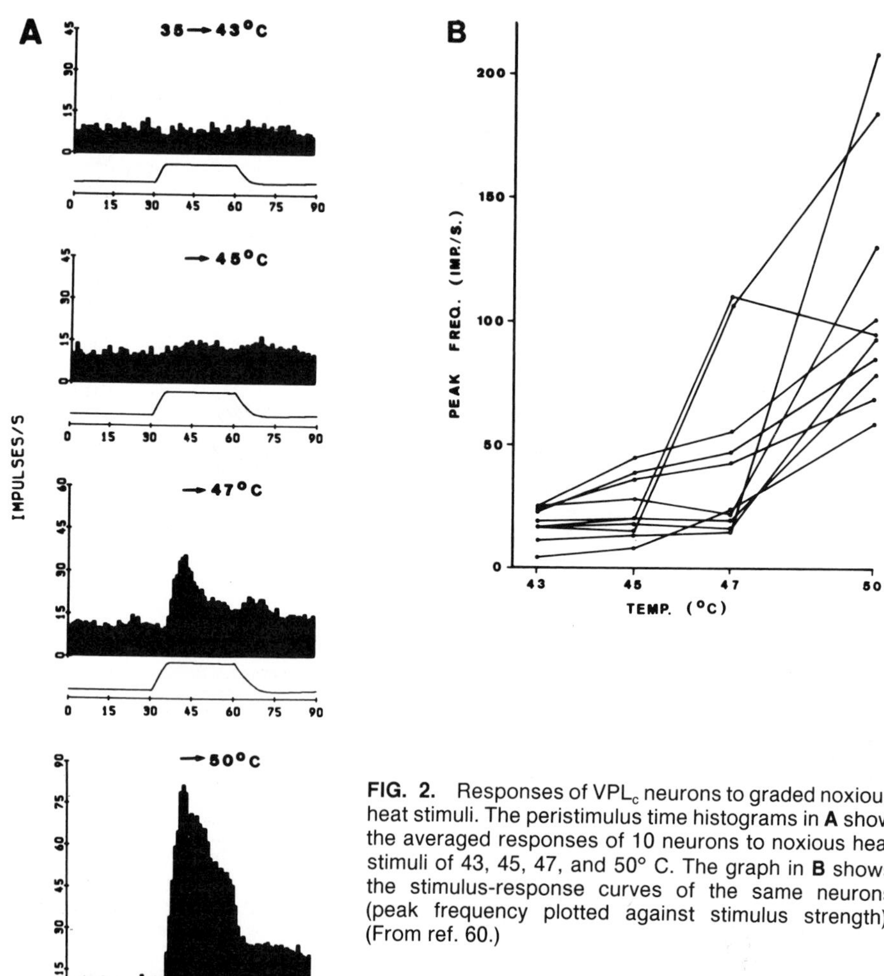

FIG. 2. Responses of VPL_c neurons to graded noxious heat stimuli. The peristimulus time histograms in **A** show the averaged responses of 10 neurons to noxious heat stimuli of 43, 45, 47, and 50° C. The graph in **B** shows the stimulus-response curves of the same neurons (peak frequency plotted against stimulus strength). (From ref. 60.)

the thalamic unit was sectioned, the response to noxious heat remained intact (Fig. 3B), but when the ventrolateral quadrant of the cord was lesioned ipsilaterally to the thalamic unit, the noxious heat response disappeared (Fig. 3C,D).

The locations of the nociceptive units studied were found to be in the somatotopically appropriate region of the VPL_c nucleus. For example, nociceptive cells with receptive fields on the hindlimb were in the lateral part of the nucleus, whereas cells with receptive fields on the forelimb were in the medial part of the nucleus (Fig. 4A).

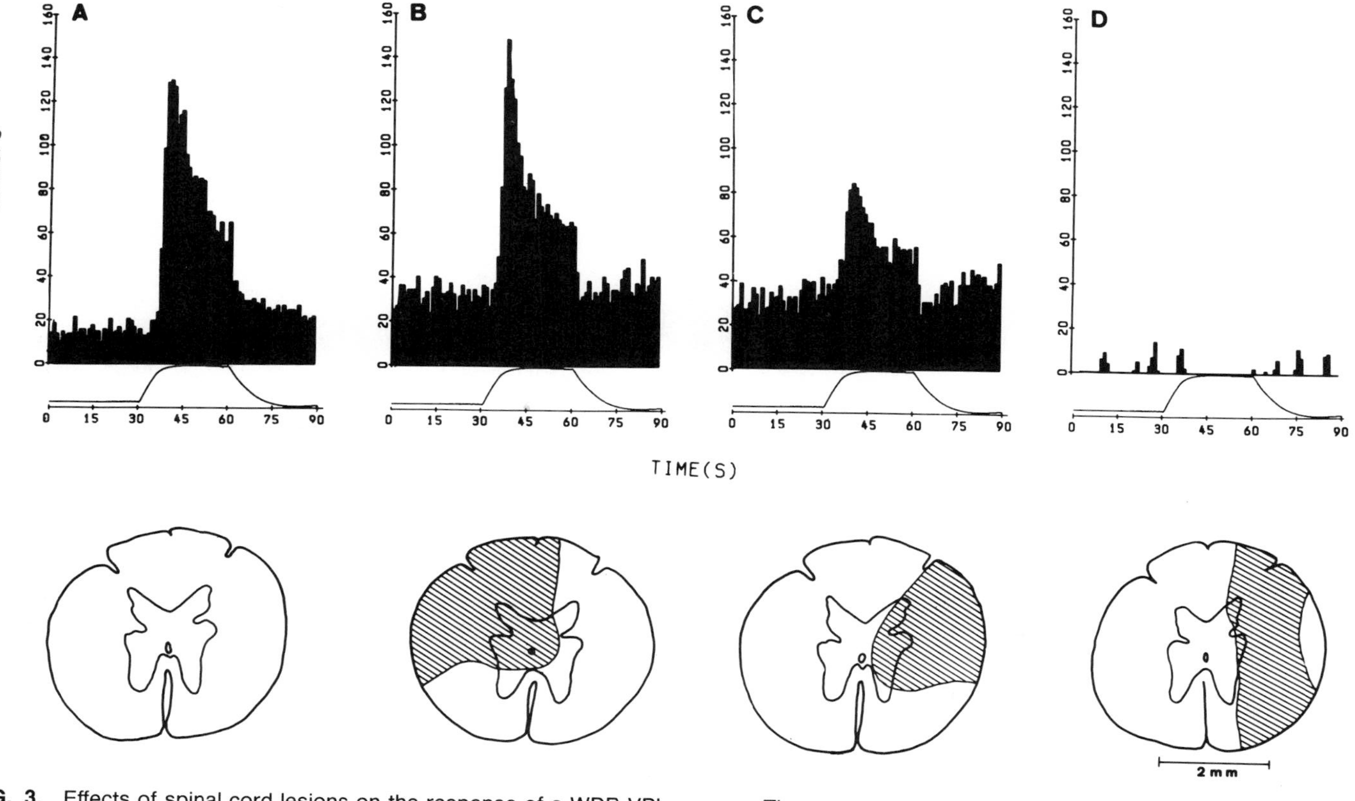

FIG. 3. Effects of spinal cord lesions on the response of a WDR VPL_c neuron. The response to a 50° C noxious heat stimulus is shown in **A** while the spinal cord was still intact. In **B,** the response is unaffected following interruption of the dorsal quadrant of the spinal cord on the side contralateral to the thalamic neuron. In **C,** the response is reduced and in **D** eliminated as successive lesions progressively intrude into the ventrolateral funiculus on the side ipsilateral to the thalamic neuron. (From ref. 60.)

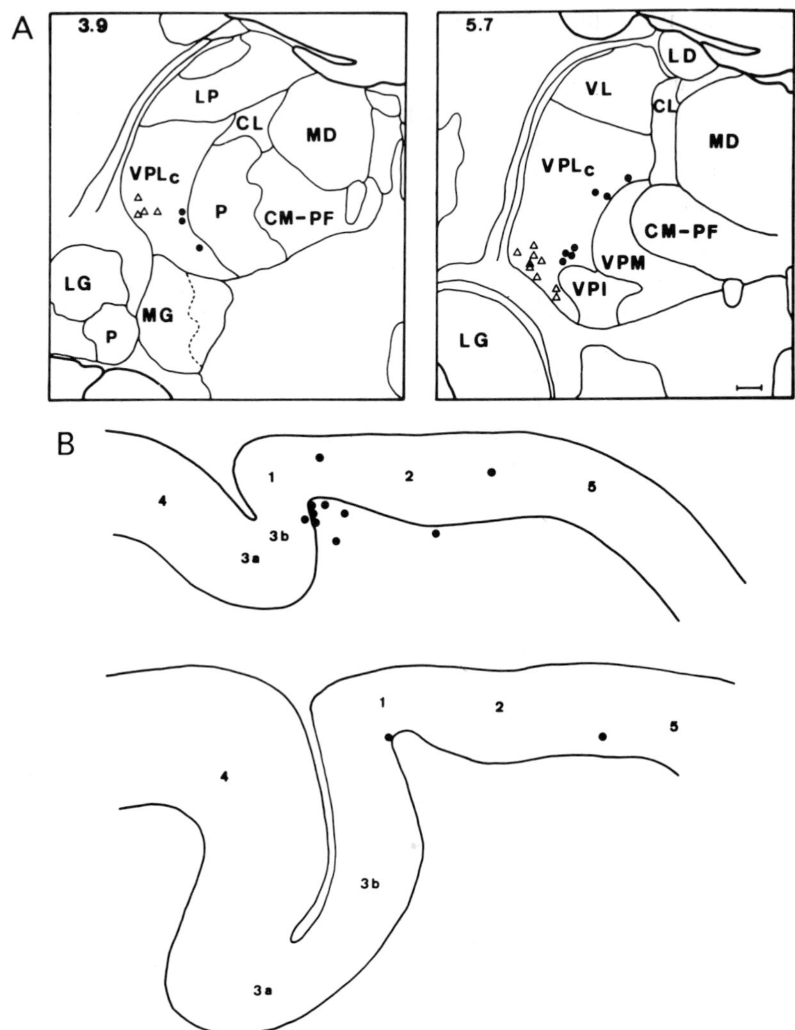

FIG. 4. Somatotopic organization of nociceptive VPL_c neurons and sites in the cerebral cortex from which they can be antidromically activated. **A** shows the locations of nociceptive neurons at two levels in the VPL_c nucleus. Cells with hindlimb receptive fields are shown by *open triangles* and those with forelimb receptive fields by *dots*. **B** shows the stimulus sites in the SI cortex from which nociceptive VPL_c neurons could be antidromically activated. The drawings are of sagittal histological sections through the hindlimb area *(upper)* and the forelimb area *(lower)*. (From ref. 60.)

Most of the nociceptive neurons of the VPL_c nucleus tested could be activated antidromically by stimulation in the SI cortex. The best stimulus site for such antidromic activation was near the border between areas 1 and 3b (Fig. 4B). It should be recalled that this is the same region in which Kenshalo and Isensee (61) have been able to record nociceptive responses from cortical units in the monkey.

There were several striking differences between WDR cells in the VPL_c nucleus and the WDR STT cells that we have studied. The thalamic WDR cells tended to have smaller excitatory receptive fields (although this was not documented systematically), and the responses to noxious heat adapted more slowly. Furthermore, there was often an after-discharge following cessation of a noxious heat response by thalamic WDR neurons, whereas WDR STT cells generally showed no after-discharges and they often showed a reduced discharge rate after a comparable stimulus. It was suggested that the relatively small receptive fields of WDR neurons in the VPL_c nucleus might have resulted from inhibitory interactions in the ascending somatosensory pathways (or possibly from the anesthesia), and that the slower adaptation to heat stimuli might reflect a parallel input from more than one ascending pathway (60).

The method used in the study by Kenshalo et al. (60) for locating nociceptive neurons in the VPL_c nucleus may have favored the isolation of WDR neurons, since the main search stimulus was brisk tapping of the body surface, followed by squeezing the skin when units were detected in the vicinity of the microelectrode. Thus, the high ratio of WDR to HT units may not reflect the true proportions of such cells in the VPL_c nucleus. Furthermore, it is possible that a larger fraction of the cells might have shown nociceptive responses had these been tested. It was assumed that if the cellular activity did not increment when the skin was squeezed, the cell must have been the type of neuron that has been shown in previous work to respond in a selective way to innocuous mechanical stimulation of the skin or to the bending of joints.

NOCICEPTIVE RESPONSES AND MODULATION OF VPL_c NEURONS

Recently, we [Drs. Chung, Lee, Surmeier, Sorkin, Kim, and I; reported in Chung et al. (24)] have reexamined the issue of what proportion of the neurons in the monkey VPL_c nucleus receive a nociceptive input. Recordings were restricted to the hindlimb area of the VPL_c nucleus, and only cells with receptive fields on the distal hindlimb were examined. However, given these restrictions, we examined the responses of all cells whose action potentials could be stably isolated. The search stimulus was electrical stimulation of a peripheral nerve. The primary stimulus employed for classifying the cells was graded innocuous and noxious mechanical stimulation of the skin.

Some neurons had just deep receptive fields, and the responses of such cells have not been included in our analysis. In addition to the responses to graded intensities of mechanical stimulation, for many of the cells we also examined one or more of the following: (a) the responses to noxious heat stimuli; (b) the effects of volleys in various fiber groups in the peripheral nerve supplying the receptive field; (c) the action of volleys in axons of the ventrolateral quadrant ipsilateral to the thalamic unit (contralateral to the receptive field), the contralateral dorsal column and the contralateral dorsolateral funiculus; and (d) in a few experiments the effects of lesions of one or more parts of the spinal cord white matter at a cervical level.

In these experiments, we have recorded the activity of 148 thalamic neurons with hindlimb receptive fields, and we obtained sufficient information about those with cutaneous receptive fields to include 110 cells in our analysis. We are able to reconstruct the locations of 84 of these cells from lesions or Prussian blue marks placed at the recording site or elsewhere in the same or in an adjacent track. Eighty-two of the recording sites were in the VPL_c nucleus (the other two were in the reticular nucleus of the thalamus). The remaining units were likely also to have been in the VPL_c nucleus, since the recordings were made in tracks close to those that were reconstructed, and the depths and the response patterns of the neurons studied and adjacent neurons were identical to those of the units whose locations could be established.

Our initial classification of the units is based on their responses to graded mechanical stimulation of the skin. The response categories include: (a) low threshold (LT) cells; (b) wide dynamic range (WDR) cells; and (c) high threshold (HT) cells. A fourth class of "deep" cells was also recognized, but as mentioned above was not analyzed in detail.

The results of a preliminary analysis of our sample of VPL_c neurons are shown in Table 1. Of 110 cells that could be classified, 56 were judged to be

TABLE 1. *Receptive field properties of neurons in the monkey VPL_c nucleus*

		Mechanical receptive field					Noxious heat threshold			Afferent fiber group		
Class	No.	VS	S	M	L	C	None	<49	>49	$A\alpha\beta$	$A\delta$	A + C
LT	56	21	12	7	11	5	10	3	11	11	16	15
WDR	39	16	6	3	2	9	4	6	18	1	7	20
HT	15	6	2	0	1	5	2	3	6	2	3	7
Total	110							12	35			42

LT = low threshold; WDR = wide dynamic range; HT = high threshold; VS = very small (less than half the surface of the foot); S = small (less than the surface of the foot); M = medium-sized (below the ankle); L = large (extends above the ankle); C = complex (extends beyond contralateral hindlimb).

LT, 39 WDR, and 15 HT. The responses of neurons judged to be typical of each class will now be described.

LT VPL_c Neurons

Most of the LT cells were activated best by brushing the skin with a camel's-hair brush (Fig. 5A,B). Since this stimulus would cause repetitive activation of rapidly adapting mechanoreceptors and since the same neurons could generally also be excited when air was blown over the receptive field (when this was on the hairy skin), we assume that the dominant input to these cells was from such rapidly adapting mechanoreceptors as hair follicle afferents and, in the case of glabrous skin, Meissner's corpuscles (121). Application of arterial clips that served as either a pressure stimulus or as a frankly noxious stimulus had little excitatory effect on these cells (Fig. 5A). In some cases, such stimuli produced an inhibition (Fig. 5B). The other neurons of the LT category were excited best when the arterial clip that served as a pressure stimulus was applied to the skin, but there was a smaller response when a stronger, noxious clip was used or when the skin was squeezed with forceps (Fig. 5C), and sometimes these stronger stimuli caused an inhibition (Fig. 5D). Brushing the skin could be essentially inef-

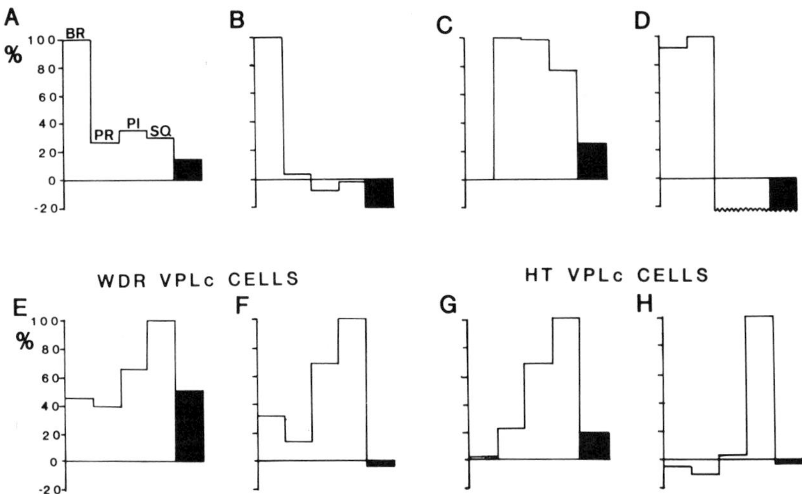

FIG. 5. Graphs showing the different response patterns of neurons that can be recognized in recordings from the monkey VPL_c nucleus. **A** through **D** represent response patterns of low threshold (LT) cells. *Bars* are the normalized responses (as a percentage of the maximum response) produced by brushing (BR), applying pressure (PR), pinching (PI), or squeezing (SQ) the skin in the receptive field. **Solid column** shows the occurrence of an after-discharge (upward) or a reduced discharge (downward) following the squeeze stimulus. Other responses in a downward direction also indicate inhibition. **E** and **F** show the patterns of response of wide dynamic range (WDR) cells and **G** and **H** of high threshold (HT) cells.

fective (Fig. 5C), or was less effective (Fig. 5D) than the pressure stimulus. We presume that cells of this type had a dominant excitatory input from slowly adapting mechanoreceptors. There was sometimes an after-discharge following the strongest stimulus (squeezing the skin) (Fig. 5A,C), although the after-discharge was sometimes minimal. Sometimes there was a reduction in the background discharge rate after the skin was squeezed (Fig. 5B,D).

The receptive fields of LT VPL_c cells were usually either very small (21 cells) or small (12 cells), as shown in Table 1. A few LT cells had larger receptive fields, and in 5 instances the fields were complex.

We did not routinely examine the responses of LT cells to noxious heat in order to minimize the risk of sensitization of the skin (35). However, 14 of the LT cells could be excited by noxious heat stimuli. This suggests that at least some LT cells of the VPL_c nucleus can be affected by a noxious input. Were these cells misclassified?

Table 1 shows the number of LT cells that were excited by different afferent fiber groups in the nerve that supplied the cutaneous receptive field. Eleven of the cells were activated just by $A\alpha\beta$ fibers. These afferent fibers presumably innervated sensitive mechanoreceptors in the skin. Another 16 LT cells appeared to be activated just by $A\delta$ fibers. We presume that they received an input from down hair receptors, which are supplied by $A\delta$ fibers (90). Fifteen LT cells had an input from both A and C fibers. Some of these also showed a response to noxious heat. Given the paucity of C mechanoreceptors in the monkey (67), it is likely that these LT cells had a convergent input from sensitive mechanoreceptors and C polymodal nociceptors.

WDR VPL_c Neurons

Many of the cells in our sample were classified as WDR cells (39 cells; see Table 1) and as LT cells. The criteria on which this classification was based were that the greatest response had to be produced by application of a small arterial clip to the skin or squeezing the skin with forceps, but, in addition, a weak mechanical stimulus, such as brushing (or pressure, in some cases) had to produce a response that was at least 10% of the size of the maximum stimulus. We assume that the increments in the responses to noxious intensities of stimulation were due to the activation of nociceptors and that there was a convergent input from sensitive mechanoreceptors as well. Figure 5E and F show the responses of typical WDR cells in the VPL_c nucleus. Brushing had a substantial effect in most cases, but the hallmark of the responses of WDR cells was the progressively greater discharge that was produced as the stimulus intensity was increased. Some of the cells had an after-discharge following squeezing the skin with forceps (Fig. 5E), and only a few cells showed a reduced discharge rate (Fig. 5F).

The receptive fields of WDR cells in the VPL_c nucleus were often either very small (16 cells) or small (6 cells), as indicated in Table 1. Larger or complex fields were seen in 14 other cases.

We were able to demonstrate that noxious heat stimuli could activate at least 24 of the WDR cells. In 6 cases, the threshold was less than 49° C and we demonstrated a graded response to graded intensities of heat in several of these.

In Table 1 are shown the peripheral nerve fiber groups that could activate WDR VPL_c neurons. In only 1 case did it appear that $A\alpha\beta$ fibers alone could excite a WDR cell. Twenty of the WDR cells had a convergent input from both A and C fibers. The responses to C-fiber volleys could either be synchronous or they could take the form of prolonged trains of discharges.

HT VPL_c Neurons

The third category of cell that we studied in the VPL_c was the HT type. There were 15 of these in our sample (Table 1). The basis for the classification was that the largest response was produced by squeezing the skin, but there was very little (less than 10% of the maximum response) or no effect from brushing (Fig. 5G,H). We assume that all of the responses of these cells can be accounted for on the basis of the activation of nociceptors. Several of these cells showed after-discharges following squeezing of the skin with forceps (Fig. 5G), but others had a reduced discharge (Fig. 5H).

The receptive fields of HT VPL_c cells were usually very small or small (8 cases; Table 1), but large or complex fields were noted in 6 cases.

Noxious heat stimuli could be shown to activate 9 of the HT VPL_c cells. In 2 cases, the threshold was 47° C.

The peripheral nerve fiber groups that activated HT VPL_c cells are indicated in Table 1. In only 2 cases was there an exclusively $A\alpha\beta$ input. Seven of the cells had a convergent input from A and C fibers.

Effects of Stimulation or Lesions of the Spinal Cord White Matter

When electrical stimuli were applied to the ventrolateral funiculus (VLF) on the side of the cord ipsilateral to the thalamic unit or to the dorsal column (DC) or dorsolateral funiculus (DLF) on the contralateral side at a cervical level while recording from a neuron in the VPL_c nucleus with a receptive field on the distal hindlimb, it was often found that a short latency excitation could be produced by volley in more than one of the funiculi. For example, while recording from at least 29 VPL_c cells, we were able to demonstrate a short-latency excitation from 2 or even all 3 funiculi. The latencies of excitation from the dorsal column DC, dorsolateral funiculus DLF or ventrolateral funiculus VLF could all be approximately equal, suggesting that the excitation from DC, for example, was not mediated indirectly by a descending volley that activated neurons of the spinocervical or spinothalamic tracts (17,38). The initial excitation was often followed by inhibition, and there could be additional later periods of excitation and/or inhibition. Sometimes the initial effect of stimulation of 1 or 2 funiculi was an inhibition. These findings suggest that neurons of the VPL_c nucleus receive complex excitatory and inhibitory inputs from several different ascending somatosensory pathways. Thus, the responses of an individual VPL_c neuron may be dependent on an integrative action involving multiple pathways and not on activity conveyed exclusively by a single ascending pathway.

The results of several experiments in which we were able to place one or more lesions in the white matter of the cervical spinal cord, thus interrupting conduction in one or more ascending pathways, support this conclusion.

Furthermore, in some cases the excitatory effect of a noxious heat stimulus could be eliminated by interruption of the ventrolateral quadrant, as in Fig. 3, but in other cases the noxious heat response was apparently mediated by fibers ascending in the dorsal part of the spinal cord. Thus, nociceptive input can reach neurons in the VPL_c nucleus by several routes, including the VLF and also dorsally situated ascending pathways.

DISCUSSION AND CONCLUSIONS

Our initial study of the response properties of neurons in the primate VPL_c nucleus (60) revealed the presence of a population of nociceptive neurons that had properties resembling those of either WDR or HT spinothalamic tract cells. These neurons responded to graded noxious mechanical or heat stimuli in a graded fashion, suggesting that they encode sensory information about the intensity of noxious stimuli. Furthermore, the receptive fields of both types of cell were relatively small, and they were on the side of the body contralateral to the thalamic neurons. The nociceptive VPL_c neurons were located in the somatotopically appropriate region of the VPL_c nucleus, and they projected to the SI somatosensory cortex (to a part of area 1 near its border with area 3b). These observations suggest that nociceptive neurons in the VPL_c nucleus could play a role in coding the intensity, timing, and localization of a noxious stimulus. It remains to be determined what differences there may be in the functions of WDR and HT neurons.

From the recent study by our laboratory of all of the neurons in the hindlimb part of the VPL_c nucleus from which we could make single unit recordings, it appears that a large proportion received at least some input that can be attributed to nociceptors. In addition, most of the cells were excited by sensitive mechanoreceptors. These observations came as a surprise to us, since we had assumed that the overwhelming majority of cells in the VPL_c nucleus of the monkey would be affected only by sensitive mechanoreceptors.

The first possibility to consider is that our impression of a substantial convergent input from both sensitive mechanoreceptors and nociceptors is wrong. Our classification of neurons is based in the first instance on the excitatory effects of graded mechanical stimulation of the skin. The effects of such mechanical stimuli may be misleading, especially when recording from the thalamus in anesthetized animals. It is for this reason that we examined the effect of noxious heat (cf., ref. 60). Of a total of 63 cells on which we tried noxious heat stimuli, 47 were found to be excited (Table 1). The threshold for excitation was often high (above 49° C), but this could have been due to the anesthesia (61). On the other hand, such high thresholds indicate that the noxious heat responses could not have been caused by activity in warm receptors, since these would have ceased firing when the skin temperature was in this range (27). Nor could the responses have been attributed to the paradoxical responses of cold receptors (30,75), in part for the same reason and also because we were unable to activate the VPL_c neurons with cold stimuli of 5 to 10° C below the adapting temperature of 35° C in the 3 cases in which this was tested. It seems to us that the responses that we observed to noxious heat stimuli in VPL_c cells of all categories must indicate an input from nociceptors.

In support of this is our observation that increasing the strength of stimulation of the peripheral nerve that supplied the receptive field to a level that activated C fibers caused an increment in the discharges of at least 42 of the VPL_c neurons in our sample (Table 1). Primates have few C mechanoreceptive afferent fibers in their peripheral nerves (67), and there was no evidence that specific thermoreceptors excited any of the VPL_c neurons in our sample. For this reason, we believe that most of the responses, if not all, produced by C-fiber volleys were due to the action of nociceptors.

Our observation that stimulation of different parts of the spinal cord white matter can produce complex excitatory or inhibitory actions in a given cell of the VPL_c nucleus is consistent with the idea that multiple somatosensory pathways can have access to a given neuron. There is good anatomical evidence that several somatosensory pathways terminate in the VPL_c nucleus of the monkey (8,11–13), but there is a tendency for the endings of different pathways to be on separate clusters of cells (8). However, this observation would not rule out convergence of more than one ascending somatosensory pathway onto individual VPL_c neurons.

The fact that some of the nociceptive responses that we observed in the VPL_c nucleus depended upon the integrity of the VLF, whereas others were mediated by dorsally situated ascending tracts is of interest, especially in view of the tendency of pain reactions to recover with time following cordotomy in monkeys (116) and for pain to return in man months after an initially successful cordotomy (118). The nociceptive input mediated by dorsal pathways may reach the thalamus over the DC, presumably through the postsynaptic dorsal column pathway (4,16,44,76,113), or by way of the spinocervical tract (17,21,48). However, this observation makes the interpretation of why cordotomies are so effective in reducing pain reactions in monkeys (116) and in eliminating pain in humans more difficult (37,117). Perhaps nociceptive inputs mediated by dorsal spinal cord pathways activate thalamic neurons with different cortical projections and different functions than those excited by noxious inputs conveyed by way of the VLF.

Pollin and Albe-Fessard (96) observed that more cells of the VPL_c nucleus of the awake, behaving monkey could be activated by pinprick after the DC and DLF were sectioned than when the neuraxis was intact. Similarly, Whitsel's group (32) commonly found nociceptive neurons in the SI cortex after a lesion of the dorsal somatosensory pathways, but rarely in the intact animal. These observations are consistent with the idea that there are inhibitory, as well as excitatory interactions in the VPL_c nucleus. The implications of inhibitory interactions between ascending tracts in determining the responses of neurons in the thalamus of the human are considerable, since it has been suggested that the explanation for the thalamic syndrome of Dejerine and Roussy is a loss of inhibition (56). Furthermore, the analgesic action of stimulation of the posterior or of the anterior columns in human patients (74,85,104,108) could derive in part from inhibitory interactions at a thalamic level.

ACKNOWLEDGMENTS

The author wishes to thank his colleagues with whom the experiments on the monkey thalamus were done: Drs. J. M. Chung, G. J. Giesler, J. Kim, K. H. Lee, R. B. Leonard, D. R. Kenshalo, Jr., L. S. Sorkin, and D. J. Surmeier. Appreciation is also expressed for the expert technical assistance of Helen Willcockson and Griselda Gonzalez. The manuscript was typed by Phyllis Waldrop. The work was supported by National Institutes of Health grants NS 09743 and NS 11250.

REFERENCES

1. Albe-Fessard, D., Berkley, K. J., Kruger, L., Ralston, H. J. and Willis, W. D. (1985): Diencephalic mechanisms of pain sensation. *Brain Res. Rev. (in press).*
2. Albe-Fessard, D., and Kruger, L. (1962): Duality of unit discharges from cat centrum medianum in response to natural and electrical stimulation. *J. Neurophysiol.,* 25:3–20.
3. Andersson, S. A., and Norrsell, U. (1973): Unit activation in the postcentral gyrus of the monkey via ventral spinal pathways. *Acta Physiol. Scand.,* 87:47A–48A.
4. Angaut-Petit, D. (1975): The dorsal column system. II. Functional properties and bulbar relay of the postsynaptic fibers of the cat's fasciculus gracilis. *Exp. Brain Res.,* 22:471–493.
5. Angel, A., and Clarke, K. A. (1975): An analysis of the representation of the forelimb in the ventrobasal complex of the albino rat. *J. Physiol. (Lond.),* 249:399–423.
6. Angelergues, R., and Hecaen, H. (1958): La douleur au cours des lesions des hemispheres cerebraux. *Journal de Psychologie Normale et Pathologique,* pp. 42–203. Presses Universitaires de France, Paris. (quoted by D. Albe-Fessard et al. in ref. 1.)
7. Applebaum, A. E., Leonard, R. B., Kenshalo, D. R., Jr., Martin, R. F., and Willis, W. D. (1979): Nuclei in which functionally identified spinothalamic tract neurons terminate. *J. Comp. Neurol.,* 188:575–586.

8. Berkley, K. J. (1980): Spatial relationship between the terminations of somatic sensory and motor pathways in the rostral brainstem of cats and monkeys. I. Ascending somatic sensory inputs to lateral diencephalon. *J. Comp. Neurol.*, 193:283–317.
9. Bettag, W., and Yoshida, T. (1960): Über stereotaktische Schmerzoperationen. *Acta Neurochir.*, 8:299–317.
10. Biemond, A. (1956): The conduction of pain above the level of the thalamus opticus. *Arch. Neurol. Psychiatr.*, 75:231–244.
11. Boivie, J. (1978): Anatomical observations on the dorsal column nuclei, their thalamic projection and the cytoarchitecture of some somatosensory thalamic nuclei in the monkey. *J. Comp. Neurol.*, 178:17–48.
12. Boivie, J. (1979): An anatomical reinvestigation of the termination of the spinothalamic tract in the monkey. *J. Comp. Neurol.*, 186:343–370.
13. Boivie, J. (1980): Thalamic projections from lateral cervical nucleus in monkey. *Brain Res.*, 198:13–26.
14. Bowsher, D. (1961): The termination of secondary somatosensory neurons within the thalamus of *Macaca mulatta:* an experimental degeneration study. *J. Comp. Neurol.*, 117:213–227.
15. Brinkhus, H. B., Carstens, E., and Zimmermann, M. (1979): Encoding of graded noxious skin heating by neurons in posterior thalamus and adjacent areas in the cat. *Neurosci. Lett.*, 15:37–42.
16. Brown, A. G., Brown, P. B., Fyffe, R. E. W., and Pubols, L. M. (1983): Receptive field organization and response properties of spinal neurones with axons ascending the dorsal columns in the cat. *J. Physiol. (Lond.)*, 337:575–588.
17. Brown, A. G., and Franz, D. N. (1969): Responses of spinocervical tract neurones to natural stimulation of identified cutaneous receptors. *Exp. Brain Res.*, 7:231–249.
18. Carreras, M., and Andersson, S. A. (1963): Functional properties of neurons of the anterior ectosylvian gyrus of the cat. *J. Neurophysiol.*, 26:100–126.
19. Casey, K. L. (1966): Unit analysis of nociceptive mechanisms in the thalamus of the awake squirrel monkey. *J. Neurophysiol.*, 29:727–750.
20. Casey, K. L., and Morrow, T. J. (1983): Ventral posterior thalamic neurons differentially responsive to noxious stimulation of the awake monkey. *Science*, 221:675–677.
21. Cervero, F., Iggo, A., and Molony, V. (1977): Responses of spinocervical tract neurones to noxious stimulation of the skin. *J. Physiol.*, 267:537–558.
22. Chang, H. T. (1973): Integrative action of thalamus in the process of acupuncture for analgesia. *Sci. Sin.*, 16:25–60.
23. Chung, J. M., Kenshalo, D. R., Jr., Gerhart, K. D. and Willis, W. D. (1979): Excitation of primate spinothalamic neurons by cutaneous C-fiber volleys. *J. Neurophysiol.*, 42:1354–1369.
24. Chung, J. M., Lee, K. H., Surmeier, D. J., Sorkin, L. S., and Willis, W. D. (1984): Nociceptive neurons in the monkey thalamus. *Neurosci. Abstr.*, 1:492.
25. Craig, A. D., and Burton, H. (1981): Spinal and medullary lamina I projection to nucleus submedius in medial thalamus: a possible pain center. *J. Neurophysiol.*, 45:443–466.
26. Craig, A. D., Wiegand, S. J., and Price, J. L. (1982): The thalamocortical projection of the nucelus submedius in the cat. *J. Comp. Neurol.*, 206:28–48.
27. Darian-Smith, I., Johnson, K. O., LaMotte, C., Shigenaga, Y., Kenins, P., and Champness, P. (1979): Warm fibers innervating palmar and digital skin of the monkey: responses to thermal stimuli. *J. Neurophysiol.*, 42:1297–1315.
28. Dejerine, J. and Mouzon, J. (1915): Un nouveau type de syndrome sensitif cortical observe dans un cas de monoplegie corticale dissociée. *Rev. Neurol. (Paris)*, 28:1265–1273.
29. Dejerine, J. and Roussy, G. (1906): Le syndrome thalamique. *Rev. Neurol. (Paris)*, 14:521–532.
30. Dodt, E., and Zotterman, Y. (1952): The discharge of specific cold fibers at high temperatures (the paradoxical cold). *Acta Physiol. Scand.*, 26:358–365.
31. Dong, W. K., Ryu, H., and Wagman, I. H. (1978): Nociceptive responses of neurons in medial thalamus and their relationship to spinothalamic pathways. *J. Neurophysiol.*, 41:1592–1613.
32. Dreyer, D. A., Schneider, R. J., Metz, C. B., and Whitsel, B. L. (1974): Differential con-

tributions of spinal pathways to body representation in postcentral gyrus of *Macaca mulatta. J. Neurophysiol.,* 37:119–145.
33. Echols, D. H., and Cogclough, J. A. (1947): Abolition of painful phantom foot by resection of the sensory cortex. *JAMA,* 134:1476–1477.
34. Erickson, T. C., Bleckwenn, W. J., and Woolsey, C. N. (1952): Observations on the postcentral gyrus in relation to pain. *Trans. Am. Neurol. Assoc.,* 77:57–59.
35. Fitzgerald, M., and Lynn, B. (1977): The sensitization of high threshold mechanoreceptors with myelinated axons by repeated heating. *J. Physiol. (Lond.),* 265:549–563.
36. Foerster, O. (1927): *Die Leitungsbahnen des Schmerzgefuhls und die chirurgische Behandlung der Schmerzzustande.* Urban & Schwarzenberg, Berlin. (Quoted by D. Albe-Fessard et al. in ref. 1.)
37. Foerster, O. and Gagel, O. (1932): Die Vorderseitenstrangdurchscheneidung beim Menschen. Eine klinisch-patho-physiologisch-anatomische Studie. *Z. Neurol. Psychiatr.,* 138:1–92.
38. Foreman, R. D., Beall, J. E., Applebaum, A. E., Coulter, J. D., and Willis, W. D. (1976): Effects of dorsal column stimulation on primate spinothalamic tract neurons. *J. Neurophysiol.,* 39:534–546.
39. Foreman, R. D., Schmidt, R. F., and Willis, W. D. (1979): Effects of mechanical and chemical stimulation of fine muscle afferents upon primate spinothalamic tract cells. *J. Physiol. (Lond.),* 286:125–231.
40. Foreman, R. D., and Weber, R. N. (1980): Responses from neurons of the primate spinothalamic tract to electrical stimulation of afferents from the cardiopulmonary region and somatic structures. *Brain Res.,* 186:463–468.
41. Freeman, W., and Watts, J. W. (1950): *Psychosurgery in the Treatment of Mental Disorders and Intractable Pain.* Thomas, Springfield, Illinois.
42. Garcin, R. (1937): La douleur dans les affections organiques du systems nerveux central. *Rev. Neurol.,* 68:105–153. (Quoted by D. Albe-Fessard et al. in ref 1.)
43. Gaze, R. M. and Gordon, G. (1954): The representation of cutaneous sense in the thalamus of the cat and monkey. *Q. J. Exp. Physiol.,* 39:279–304.
44. Giesler, G. J., Nahin, R. L., and Madsen, A. M. (1984): Postsynaptic dorsal column pathway of the rat. I. Anatomical studies. *J. Neurophysiol.,* 51:260–275.
45. Guilbaud, G., Caille, D., Besson, J. M., and Benelli, G. (1977): Single unit activities in ventral posterior and posterior group thalamic nuclei during nociceptive and non-nociceptive stimulation in the cat. *Arch. Ital. Biol.,* 115:38–56.
46. Guilbaud, G., Peschanski, M., Gautron, M., and Binder, D. (1980): Neurones responding to noxious stimulation in VB complex and caudal adjacent regions in the thalamus of the rat. *Pain,* 8:303–318.
47. Halliday, A. M., and Logue, V. (1972): Painful sensations evoked by electrical stimulation in the thalamus. In: *Neurophysiology Studied in Man,* edited by G. Somjen, pp. 221–230. Exerpta Medica, Amsterdam.
48. Hamann, W. C., Hong, S. K., Kniffki, K. D., and Schmidt, R. F. (1978): Projections of primary afferent fibres from muscle to neurones of the spinocervical tract of the cat. *J. Physiol. (Lond.),* 283:369–378.
49. Hardy, J. D., Wolff, H. G., and Goodell, H. (1952): Pricking pain threshold in different body areas. *Proc. Soc. Exp. Biol. Med.,* 80:425–427.
50. Harris, F. A. (1978): Functional subsets of neurons in somatosensory thalamus of the cat. *Exp. Neurol.,* 58:149–170.
51. Harris, F. A. (1978): Regional variations of somatosensory input convergence in nucleus VPL of cat thalamus. *Exp. Neurol.,* 58:171–189.
52. Hassler, R. (1960): Die zentralen Systeme des Schmerzes. *Acta Neurochir.,* 8:353–423.
53. Hassler, R. (1970): Dichotomy of facial pain conduction in the diencephalon. In: *Trigeminal Neuralgia,* edited by R. Hassler and A. E. Walker, pp. 123–138. Saunders, Philadelphia.
54. Hassler, R., and Riechert, T. (1959): Klinische und anatomische Befunde bei stereotaktischen Schmerzoperationen im Thalamus. *Arch. Psychiatr. Nervenkr.,* 200:93–122.
55. Head, H. (1920): *Studies in Neurology.* Oxford University Press, London.
56. Head, H., and Holmes, G. (1911): Sensory disturbances from cerebral lesions. *Brain,* 34:102–254.

57. Honda, C. N., Mense, S., and Perl, E. R. (1983): Neurons in ventrobasal region of cat thalamus selectively responsive to noxious mechanical stimulation. *J. Neurophysiol.,* 49:662–673.
58. Horrax, G. (1946): Experiences with cortical excisions for the relief of intractable pain in the extremities. *Surgery,* 20:593–602.
59. Iwamura, Y., Kniffki, K. D., Mizumura, K., and Wilberg, K. (1981): Responses of feline SI neurones to noxious stimulation of muscle and tendon. *Pain,* (Suppl 1): S213.
60. Kenshalo, D. R., Jr., Giesler, G. J., Leonard, R. B., and Willis, W. D. (1980): Responses of neurons in primate ventral posterior lateral nucleus to noxious stimuli. *J. Neurophysiol.,* 43:1594–1614.
61. Kenshalo, D. R., Jr., and Isensee, O. (1983): Responses of primate SI cortical neurons to noxious stimuli. *J. Neurophysiol.,* 50:1479–1496.
62. Kenshalo, D. R., Jr., Leonard, R. B., Chung, J. M., and Willis, W. D. (1979): Responses of primate spinothalamic neurons to graded and to repeated noxious heat stimuli. *J. Neurophysiol.,* 42:1370–1389.
63. Kerr, F. W. L. (1975): The ventral spinothalamic tract and other ascending systems of the ventral funiculus of the spinal cord. *J. Comp. Neurol.,* 159:335–356.
64. King, H. E., Clausen, J. and Scarff, J. E. (1950): Cutaneous thresholds for pain before and after unilateral prefrontal lobotomy. *J. Nerv. Ment. Dis.,* 112:93–96.
65. Kniffki, K. D., and Mizumura, K. (1983): Responses of neurons in VPL and VPL-VL region of the cat to algesic stimulation of muscle and tendon. *J. Neurophysiol.,* 49:649–661.
66. Krauthamer, G., McGuiness, C., and Gottesman, L. (1977): Unit responses in the ventrobasal thalamus (VPL) of the cat to bradykinin injected into somatic and visceral arteries. *Brain Res. Bull.,* 2:299–306.
67. Kumazawa, T., and Perl, E. R. (1977): Primate cutaneous sensory units with unmyelinated (C) afferent fibers. *J. Neurophysiol.,* 40:1325–1338.
68. Kuru, M. (1949): *Sensory Paths in the Spinal Cord and Brain Stem of Man.* Sogensya, Tokyo.
69. LaMotte, R. H., and Campbell, J. N. (1978): Comparison of responses of warm and nociceptive C-fiber afferents in monkey with human judgments of thermal pain. *J. Neurophysiol.,* 41:509–528.
70. Lamour, Y., Guilbaud, G., and Willer, J. C. (1983): Rat somatosensory (SmI) cortex: II. Laminar and columnar organization of noxious and non-noxious inputs. *Exp. Brain Res.,* 49:46–54.
71. Lamour, Y., Willer, J. C., and Guilbaud, G. (1983): Rat somatosensory (SmI) cortex: I. Characteristics of neuronal responses to noxious stimulation and comparison with responses to non-noxious stimulation. *Exp. Brain Res.,* 49:35–45.
72. Lende, R. A., Krisch, W. M., and Druckman, R. (1971): Relief of facial pain after combined removal of precentral and postcentral cortex. *J. Neurosurg.,* 34:537–543.
73. Lewin, W., and Phillips, C. G. (1952): Observations on partial removal of the postcentral gyrus for pain. *J. Neurol. Neurosurg. Psychiatr.,* 15:143–147.
74. Long, D. M., and Hagfors, N. (1975): Electrical stimulation in the nervous system: the current status of electrical stimulation of the nervous system for relief of pain. *Pain,* 1:109–123.
75. Long, R. R. (1977): Sensitivity of cutaneous cold fibers to noxious heat: paradoxical cold discharges. *J. Neurophysiol.,* 40:489–502.
76. Lu, G. W., Bennett, G. J., Nishikawa, N., Hoffert, M. J., and Dubner, R. (1983): Extra- and intracellular recordings from dorsal column postsynaptic spinomedullary neurons in the cat. *Exp. Neurol.,* 82:456–477.
77. Mark, V. H., Ervin, F. R., and Hackett, T. P. (1960): Clinical aspects of stereotactic thalamotomy in the human. I. The treatment of severe pain. *Arch. Neurol.,* 3:351–367.
78. Mark, V. H., Ervin, F. R., and Yakovlev, P. I. (1963): Stereotactic thalamotomy. III. The verification of anatomical lesion sites in the human thalamus. *Arch. Neurol.,* 8:528–538.
79. Marshall, J. (1951): Sensory disturbances in cortical wounds with special reference to pain. *J. Neurol. Neurosurg. Psychiatr.,* 14:187–204.
80. Mehler, W. R., Feferman, M. E. and Nauta, W. J. H. (1960): Ascending axon degeneration

following anterolateral cordotomy. An experimental study in the monkey. *Brain,* 83:718–751.

81. Melzack, R., and Casey, K. L. (1968): Sensory, motivational and central control determinants of pain. In: *The Skin Senses,* edited by D. R. Kenshalo, pp. 423–443. Thomas, Springfield, Illinois.
82. Milne, R. J., Foreman, R. D., Giesler, G. J., and Willis, W. D. (1981): Convergence of cutaneous and pelvic visceral nociceptive inputs onto primate spinothalamic neurons. *Pain,* 11:163–183.
83. Mitchell, D., and Hellon, R. F. (1977): Neuronal and behavioural responses in rats during noxious stimulation of the tail. *Proc. R. Soc. (Lond.),* 197:169–194.
84. Mountcastle, V. B., and Powell, T. P. S. (1959): Neural mechanisms subserving cutaneous sensibility, with special reference to the role of afferent inhibition in sensory perception and discrimination. *Bull. Johns Hopkins Hosp.,* 105:201–232.
85. Nashold, B. S., and Friedman, H. (1972): Dorsal column stimulation for control of pain. Preliminary report on 30 patients. *J. Neurosurg.,* 36:590–597.
86. Nyquist, K. K., and Greenhoot, J. H. (1974): Unit analysis of nonspecific thalamic responses to high-intensity cutaneous input in the cat. *Exp. Neurol.,* 42:609–622.
87. Olszewski, J. (1952): *The Thalamus of Macaca Mulatta.* Karger, New York.
88. Penfield, W., and Boldrey, E. (1937): Somatic motor and sensory representation in the cerebral cortex of man as studied by electrical stimulation. *Brain,* 60:389–443.
89. Penfield, W., and Jasper, H. (1954): *Epilepsy and the Functional Anatomy of the Human Brain.* Little, Brown, Boston.
90. Perl, E. R. (1968): Myelinated afferent fibres innervating the primate skin and their response to noxious stimuli. *J. Physiol. (Lond.),* 197:593–615.
91. Perl, E. R. (1984): Pain and nociception. In: *Handbook of Physiology, Section 1, Vol. III, Sensory Processes, Part 2,* edited by I. Darian Smith, pp. 915–975. American Physiological Society, Bethesda.
92. Perl, E. R., and Whitlock, D. G. (1961): Somatic stimuli exciting spinothalamic projections to thalamic neurons in cat and monkey. *Exp. Neurol.,* 3:256–296.
93. Peschanski, M., Guilbaud, G., and Gautron, M. (1981): Posterior intralaminar region in rat: neuronal responses to noxious and nonnoxious cutaneous stimuli. *Exp. Neurol.,* 72:226–238.
94. Peschanski, M., Guilbaud, G., Gautron, M., and Besson, J. M. (1980): Encoding of noxious heat messages in neurons of the ventrobasal thalamic complex of the rat. *Brain Res.,* 197:401–413.
95. Poggio, G. F., and Mountcastle, V. B. (1960): A study of the functional contributions of the lemniscal and spinothalamic systems to somatic sensibility. *Bull. Johns Hopkins Hosp.,* 106:336.
96. Pollin, B., and Albe-Fessard, D. (1979): Organization of somatic thalamus in monkeys with and without section of dorsal spinal tracts. *Brain Res.,* 173:431–449.
97. Price, D. D., and Dubner, R. (1977): Neurons that subserve the sensory discriminative aspects of pain. *Pain,* 3:307–338.
98. Price, D. D., Hayes, R. L., Ruda, M. A., and Dubner, R. (1978): Spatial and temporal transformations of input to spinothalamic tract neurons and their relation to somatic sensations. *J. Neurophysiol.,* 41:933–947.
99. Robinson, C. J., and Burton, H. (1980): Somatotopic organization in the second somatosensory area of *M. fascicularis. J. Comp. Neurol.,* 192:43–67.
100. Robinson, C. J., and Burton, H. (1980): Organization of somatosensory receptive fields in cortical areas 8b, retroinsula, postauditory and granular insula of *M. fascicularis. J. Comp. Neurol.,* 192:69–92.
101. Robinson, C. J., and Burton, H. (1980): Somatic submodality distribution within the second somatosensory (SII), 7b, retroinsula, postauditory, and granular insular cortical areas of *M. fascicularis. J. Comp. Neurol.,* 192:93–108.
102. Russell, W. R. (1945): Transient disturbances following gunshot wounds of the head. *Brain,* 68:79–97.
103. Sano, K., Yoshioka, M., Ogashiwa, M., Ishijima, B., and Ohye, C. (1966): Thalamolaminotomy. *Confin. Neurol.,* 27:63–66.
104. Shealy, C. N., Mortimer, J. T., and Hagfors, N. R. (1970): Dorsal column electroanalgesia. *J. Neurosurg.,* 32:560–564.

105. Spiegel, E. A., Wycis, H. T., Szekely, E. G., and Gildenberg, P. L. (1966): Medial and basal thalamotomy in so-called intractable pain. In: *Pain,* edited by R. S. Knighton and P. R. Dumke, pp. 503–517. Little, Brown, Boston.
106. Stone, T. T. (1950): Phantom limb pain and central pain; relief by ablation of a portion of posterior central cerebral convolution. *Arch. Neurol. Psychiatr.,* 63:739–748.
107. Sweet, W. H. (1981): Cerebral localization of pain. In: *New Perspectives in Cerebral Localization,* edited by R. A. Thompson, pp. 205–240. Raven Press, New York.
108. Sweet, W. H., and Wespic, J. G. (1968): Treatment of chronic pain by stimulation of fibers of primary afferent neuron. *Trans. Am. Neurol. Assoc.,* 93:103–105.
109. Talairach, J., Tournoux, P., and Bancaud, J. (1960): Chirurgie pariétale de la douleur. *Acta Neurochir.,* 8:153–250.
110. Tasker, R. R., Organ, L. W., Rowe, I. H., and Hawrylyshyn, P. (1976): Human spinothalamic tract-stimulation mapping in the spinal cord and brainstem. *Adv. Pain Res. Ther.,* 1:251–257.
111. Tasker, R. R., Tsuda, T. and Hawrylyshyn, P. (1983): Clinical neurophysiological investigation of deafferentation pain. *Adv. Pain Res. Ther.,* 5:713–738.
112. Tsubokawa, T. (1967): The correlation of pain relief, neurological signs, EEG and anatomical lesion sites in pain patients treated by stereotaxic thalamotomy. *Folia Psychiatr. Neurol. Jpn.,* 21:41–51.
113. Uddenberg, N. (1968): Functional organization of long, second-order afferents in the dorsal funiculus. *Exp. Brain Res.,* 4:377–382.
114. Urabe, M., and Tsubokawa, T. (1965): Stereotaxic thalamotomy for the relief of intractable pain- CEM thalamotomy. *Tohoku J. Exp. Med.,* 85:276–298.
115. Urabe, M., Tsubokawa, T., and Watanabe, Y. (1966): Alteration of activity of single neurons in the nucleus centrum medianum following stimulation of the peripheral nerve and application of noxious stimuli. *Jpn. J. Physiol.,* 16:421–435.
116. Vierck, C. J., and Luck, M. M. (1979): Loss and recovery of reactivity to noxious stimuli in monkeys with primary spinothalamic cordotomies, followed by secondary and tertiary lesions of other cord sectors. *Brain,* 102:233–248.
117. White, J. C., and Sweet, W. H. (1955): *Pain, Its Mechanisms and Neurosurgical Control.* Thomas, Springfield, Illinois.
118. White, J. C., and Sweet, W. H. (1969): *Pain and the Neurosurgeon.* Thomas, Springfield, Illinois.
119. Whitsel, B. L., Petrucelli, L. M., and Werner, G. (1969): Symmetry and connectivity in the map of the body surface in somatosensory area II of primates. *J. Neurophysiol.,* 32:170–183.
120. Willis, W. D. (1985): *The Pain System. The Neural Basis of Nociceptive Transmission in the Mammalian Nervous System.* Karger, Basel.
121. Willis, W. D., and Coggeshall, R. E. (1978): *Sensory Mechanisms of the Spinal Cord.* Plenum Press, New York.
122. Willis, W. D., Trevino, D. L., Coulter, J. D., and Maunz, R. A. (1974): Responses of primate spinothalamic tract neurons to natural stimulation of hindlimb. *J. Neurophysiol.,* 37:358–372.
123. Yoss, R. E. (1953): Studies of the spinal cord. 3. Pathways for deep pain within the spinal cord and brain. *Neurology,* 3:163–175.

Advances in Pain Research and Therapy, Vol. 9, edited by H. L. Fields et al. Raven Press, New York © 1985.

Fine Structure of Spinothalamic Tract Axons and Terminals in Rat, Cat, and Monkey Demonstrated by the Orthograde Transport of Lectin Conjugated to Horseradish Peroxidase

*H. J. Ralston, **M. Peschanski, and *D. D. Ralston

**Department of Anatomy, University of California, San Francisco, California 94143; and **INSERM-U161, 75014 Paris, France*

Analysis of degenerating terminals or visualization of terminals labeled with tritiated amino acids after lesion or injection of the dorsal column nuclei, respectively, has allowed the study of the ultrastructural morphology of the lemniscal afferents to the ventrobasal complex (VB) in various species (3,7,8,12). In contrast, the fine structure of axon terminals of the spinothalamic tract (STT) has been difficult to determine because of the difficulty in labeling neurons of the STT with the autoradiographic technique and in finding the scattered degenerated terminals when using experimentally induced degeneration methods.

A recently developed method based upon the orthograde transport of lectin conjugated to horseradish peroxidase (HRP) was used in this study to reveal the morphology of STT axons and terminals, and to compare them with those arising from the dorsal column pathway. This study was undertaken to determine if neuronal impulses elicited by noxious stimulation were conveyed to the thalamus by pathways which terminate in synaptic profiles. Synaptic profiles could be distinguished from those of lemniscal afferents that are primarily involved in the transmission of nonnoxious information. Comparisons of the results obtained in two different areas of projection (lateral thalamus—VB and PO; intralaminar thalamus—centralis lateralis) was done to analyze the morphology of terminals of the two pathways. In addition, the study was performed in three different species (rat, cat, and monkey) in order to determine possible interspecies differences in the neural circuitry of pain pathways.

METHODS

Four rats, 2 cats, and 2 monkeys were anesthetized, and following a laminectomy over 1 to 2 spinal segments, received a slow pressure injection of wheat-germ agglutinin conjugated to HRP (10% in water) into the lumbar or cervical enlargements of the spinal cord.

After a 48- to 96-hr survival time, each animal was reanesthetized and was perfused transcardially with water buffered saline (pH 7.4) followed by a cold phosphate-buffered solution (0.7 M, pH 7.4) of 3% glutaraldehyde, 1% paraformaldehyde, and 4% sucrose. The thalamus was then removed and soaked in 0.1 M phosphate buffer, then cut serially (60 μm-thick sections) in the coronal plane on a Vibratome (Oxford Instruments), and processed for the visualization of HRP at the electron microscopic level by using the following technique:

1. Sections were rinsed rapidly in distilled water, then placed directly in the reaction solution. This solution was made up of 160 μl of acetate buffer (0.01 M, pH 6.0–6.1) containing 200 μg of sodium nitroprusside, 40 μl of alcohol in which 200 μg of benzidine dihydrochloride (BDHC-Sigma) had been previously dissolved at about 60° C, and 0.1 to 0.2 ml of 37% H_2O_2.
2. After 15 to 20 min of reaction, sections were rinsed for a few seconds in acetate buffer then osmicated for 1 hr at 45° C in a solution containing equal parts of 2% OsO_4 and *S*-collidine buffer (0.2 M) containing 26.7 μl 2-4-6 *S*-collidine, 100 mg $CaCl_2$, 200 mg $MgCl_2$, and 131.7 g sucrose/liter, corrected with HCl to a pH of 7.4.

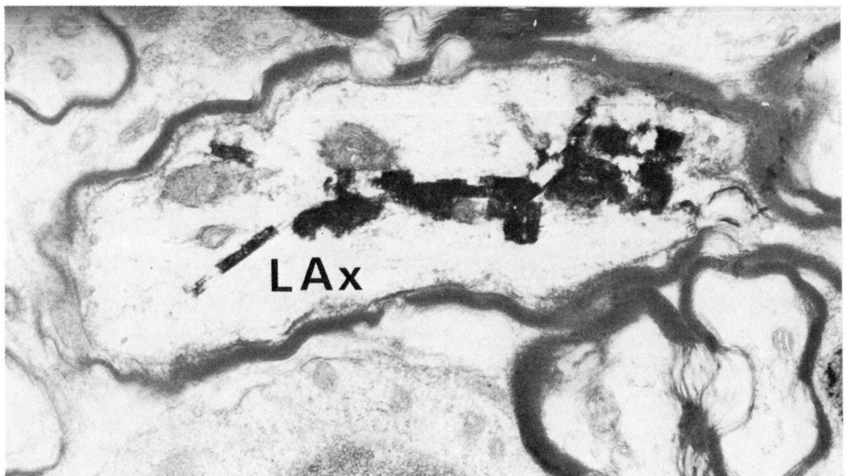

FIG. 1. Electron photomicrograph (× 6,600) showing a large labeled myelinated axon (LAx) in the VB of the rat. The crystalline organization of the BDHC recation product is visible in most of the granules.

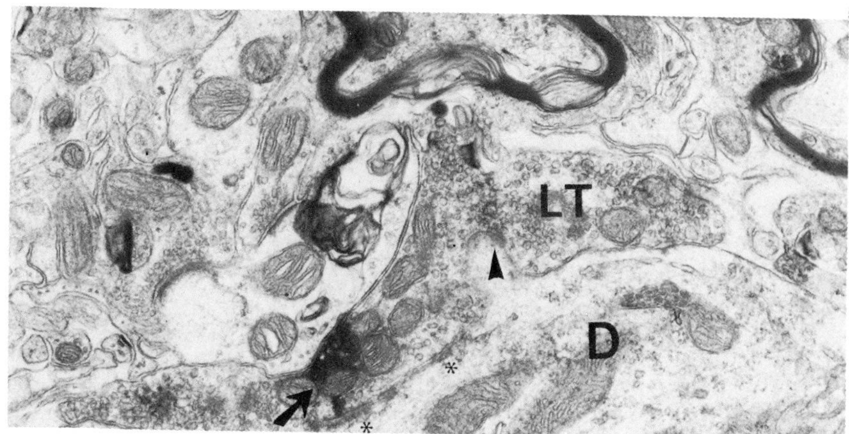

FIG. 2. Electron photomicrograph (× 1,120) showing a labeled terminal (LT) contacting *(arrowhead)* a spine attached to a large dendrite (D) in the VB of the rat. The *arrow* points to BDHC reaction product. *Asterisks* indicate areas of nonsynaptic filamentous contact between the labeled terminals and the dendritic shaft.

3. Osmicated sections were then dehydrated in graded alcohols and embedded flat in a mixture of Epon and Araldite. Once embedded, sections were analyzed using the light microscope and areas of the VB (rat and monkey), POm (cat), and CL of all species which contained reaction product were trimmed out and cut on an ultramicrotome. Thin sections were remounted on single slot Formvar-coated grids and stained with lead citrate (9,13) for observation under the electron microscope.

4. Similar material from other animals which had been studied in regard to the projections of the dorsal column nuclei to the thalamus were available for comparison.

RESULTS

Fine Morphology of Labeled Dendrites

In all the areas and species studied, the STT axons and terminals containing granules of reaction product were similar. Labeled axons (Fig. 1) were 2 to 4 μm in diameter, and were myelinated to within a few microns of termination. The terminals were large, 2 to 6 μm in greatest diameter. They contained numerous round vesicles and several mitochondria. In some cases, these large profiles were indented by dendritic protrusions or spines that they contacted (Fig. 2).

Two kinds of junctions were observed between these profiles and the postsynaptic elements. The first were asymmetrical (Gray type I) synaptic contacts, in which the pre- and postsynaptic membranes showed a thickening

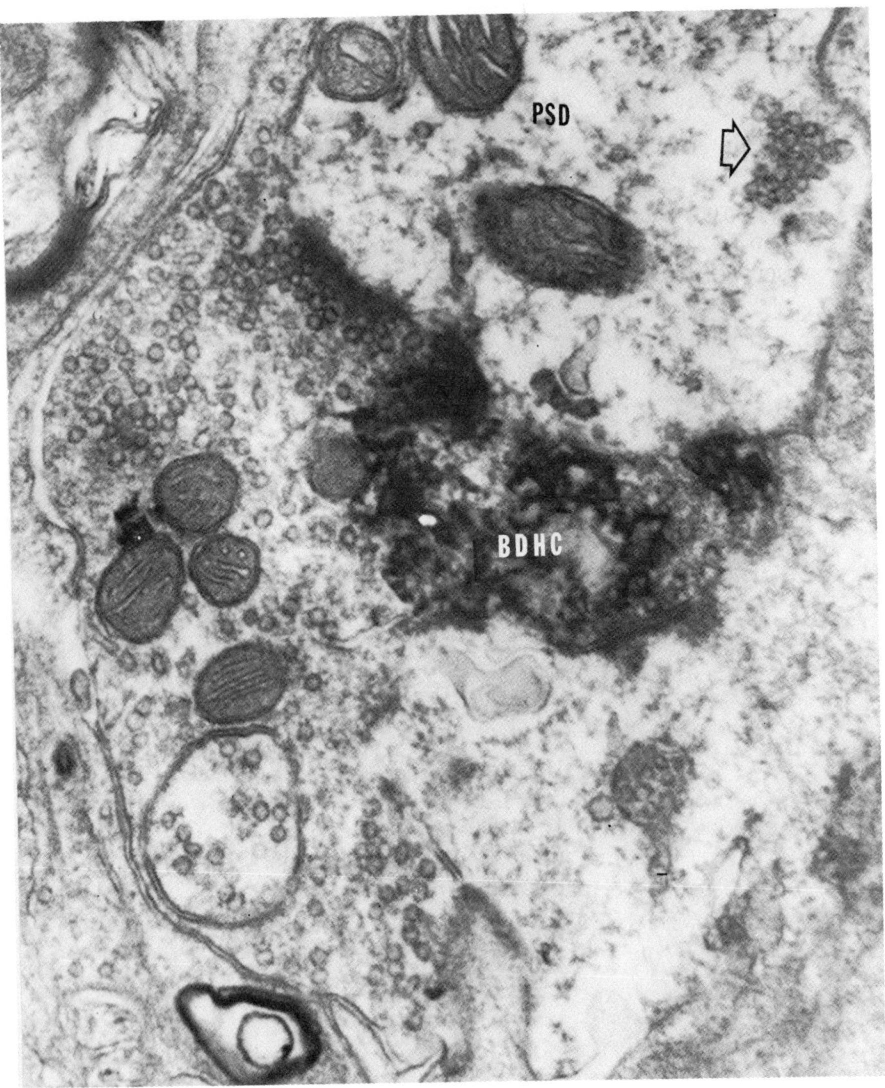

FIG. 3. Electron photomicrograph (× 12,000) of a labeled (BDHC) spinothalamic tract terminal in the POn of the cat which contacts a presynaptic dendrite (PSD) containing a cluster of synaptic vesicles *(arrow)*.

and the synaptic cleft was filled by dense material. Along the presynaptic membrane, numerous vesicles aggregated, and on the postsynaptic side a thick postsynaptic density was visible. The other, nonsynaptic, junctions were observed between the labeled profiles and the dendrites which they contacted, and resembled adhesion plaques in that there was no distinct aggregate of vesicles on the presynaptic side, and there were only symmetrical densities in each profile (Fig. 2).

Synaptic Organization of STT Terminals

In all species and areas studied, most of the synaptic contacts of the STT terminals were with large primary dendrites, either directly on the dendritic shaft or on short spines indenting the terminals. Few axosomatic contacts were observed.

In the cat and in the monkey, an additional type of contact could be observed, involving another synaptic component, a presynaptic dendrite (Fig. 3). In this synaptic complex, which exhibited this "triadic" organization, the STT terminal was presynaptic to a vesicle-containing dendrite which, in turn, synapsed on a large postsynaptic dendrite which could be, in addition, directly contacted by the STT terminal. In both cat and monkey, this kind of organization could be observed both in the lateral and the intralaminar thalamus; in the rat it was not found in any region of the somatosensory thalamus (Fig. 4).

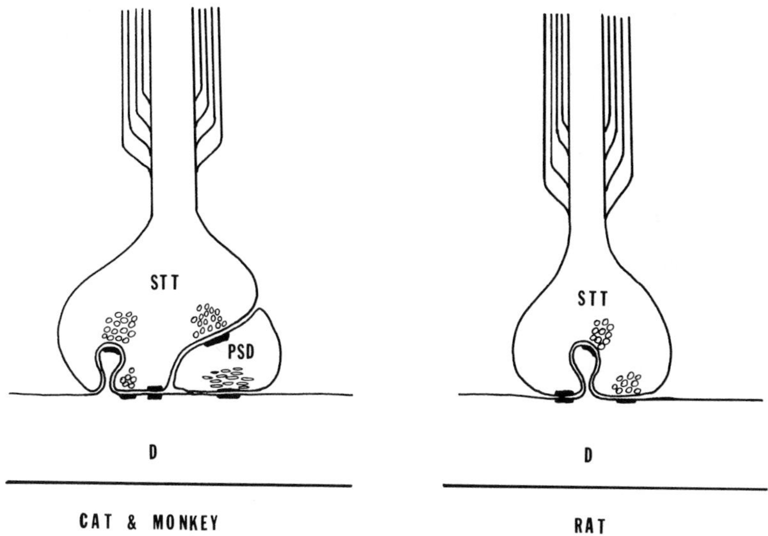

FIG. 4. Diagrams showing the two different types of connections made by spinothalamic terminals (STT) in the cat and monkey **(left)** and in the rat **(right)**. In all species STT terminals originate from large myelinated axons; are large (2–6 μm wide); contain mitochondria and round vesicles. They show nonsynaptic attachments with postsynaptic elements. In the cat and the monkey **(left),** the STT terminal contacts assymetrical synapses either dendritic spines from large dendrites or the dendritic shaft (D) directly, or are involved in a "triadic organization" in which they contact a presynaptic dendrite (PSD) containing pleomorphic vesicles which in turn contacts a large dendrite in a symmetrical synapse. In the rat, there is no triadic organization.

DISCUSSION

The results of the present study indicate that STT terminals in the lateral and intralaminar thalamus exhibit a similar fine-structured morphology, in that they are large profiles with round vesicles, which form asymmetrical synapses. These STT terminals primarily contact large dendrites which are elements of the proximal dendritic tree. All these characteristics are similar to those defined for lemniscal afferents to the lateral thalamus originating from the dorsal column nuclei (3,4,7,8,10,12). This similarity is ever more underlined by the fact that, similar to lemniscal afferents, STT terminals may be involved in "triadic relationships" in the cat and the monkey, but not in the rat.

It can therefore be concluded that the modality properties of STT or lemniscal pathways must be a characteristic of the organization of the neural network, rather than being determined by the structure of single cells or synapses. This conclusion is also supported by our recent demonstration that, in the VB of the rat, noxious and nonnoxious responsive neurons have similar morphologies and are contacted by similar types of terminals (6).

The fact that STT terminals, which would include those involved in pain transmission, are large and make numerous contacts with primary dendrites, indicates that they are capable of influencing strongly the activity of postsynaptic thalamic neurons. Thus, the organization of this pathway, as that of the lemniscal system for nonnoxious inputs, permits the transmission of noxious messages with good synaptic security. Noxious responsive neurons of the VB (2,5) and PO (1) are able to transmit precise information on the intensity of noxious stimuli; and the precise information transmission could be related to this "secure" anatomical organization.

The existence of a "triadic" organization in the VB and POm of monkey and cat has been described in length in the case of lemniscal afferents (7,8). Conclusions drawn from the present study show that this triadic organization also applies to STT terminals. In this relationship, the presynaptic dendrite originates probably from intrinsic local circuit neurons that are thought to be inhibitory (11). The physiological correlates of this structure would thus be successive excitatory-inhibitory actions of STT impulses at the level of this triadic structure. The fact that such a structure seems to appear later in phylogenetic development suggests that it might be a sophistication of the process of thalamic organization in cat and monkey compared to the rat. Its actual role remains to be elucidated in single unit recordings of the responses of thalamic neurons to afferent pathways that exhibit this triadic organization in their terminal synaptic patterns.

REFERENCES

1. Brinklus, H. B., Carskeus, E., and Zimmermann, M. (1979): Encoding of graded noxious skin breaking by neurons in posterior thalamus and adjacent areas in the cat. *Neurosci. Lett.*, 15:37–62.

2. Keushalo, D. R., Giesler, G. J., Leonard, R. B., and Willis, W. D. (1980): Responses of neurons in primate ventral posterior lateral nucleus to noxious stimuli. *J. Neurophysiol.,* 63:1594–1614.
3. Matthews, H. A., and Faciane, C. L. (1977): Electron microscopy of the development of synaptic patterns in the ventrobasal complex of the rat. *Brain Res.,* 135:197–215.
4. McAllister, J. P., and Wells, J. (1981): The structural organization of the ventral posterlateral nucleus in the rat. *J. Comp. Neurol.,* 197:271–301.
5. Peschanski, M., Guilbaud, G., Gautron, M., and Besson, J. M. (1980): Encoding of noxious heat messages in neurons of the ventrobasal thalamic complex in the rat. *Brain Res.,* 197:601–613.
6. Peschanski, M., Lee, C. L., and Ralston, J. H., III (1984): The structural organization of the ventrobasal complex of the rat as revealed by the analysis of physiologically characterized neurons injected intracellularly with horseradish peroxidase. *Brain Res.,* 297:63–74.
7. Ralston, H. J., III (1969): The synaptic organization of lemniscal projections to the ventrobasal thalamus of the cat. *Brain Res.,* 14:99–116.
8. Ralston, H. J., III (1983): The synaptic organization of the ventrobasal thalamus in the rat, cat, and monkey. In: *Somatosensory Integration in the Thalamus,* edited by G. Macchi, A. Rushioui, and R. Spreafico, pp. 241–250. Elsevier/North-Holland, Amsterdam.
9. Reynolds, E. S. (1963): The use of lead citrate at high pH as an electron opaque stain in electron microscopy. *J. Cell. Biol.,* 17:208.
10. Spacek, J., and Lieberman, A. R. (1974): Ultrastructure and three-dimensional organization of synaptic glomeruli in rat somatosensory thalamus. *J. Anat. (Lond).,* 117:487–516.
11. Spreafico, R., Schuechel, D. E., Ellis, L. C., and Rushoui, A. (1983): Cortical relay neurons and interneurons in the n. ventralis ponterolateralis of cats: a horseradish peroxidase, electron microscopic, Golgi and immunocytochemical study. *Neuroscience,* 9:491–509.
12. Tripp, L. N., and Wells, J. (1978): Formation of new synaptic terminals in the somatosensory thalamus of the rat after lesions of the dorsal column nuclei. *Brain Res.,* 155:362–367.
13. Venable, J. H., and Coggeshall, R. E. (1965): A simplified lead citrate stain for use in electron microscopy. *J. Cell. Biol.* 25:407.

Advances in Pain Research and Therapy, Vol. 9, edited by H. L. Fields et al. Raven Press, New York © 1985.

Neuronal Loss in the Ventrobasal Complex of the Rat Thalamus Alters Behavioral Responses to Noxious Stimulation

Valerie Kayser, Marc Peschanski, and Gisele Guilbaud,

Unité de Recherches de Neurophysiologie Pharmacologique, INSERM U 161, 75014 Paris, France

The role of the ventrobasal complex of the thalamus (VB) in the sensory-discriminative aspects of pain has been suggested in the rat by several electrophysiological experiments. It has been demonstrated in particular that VB neuronal responses depended on the location of the stimulus application (4), and its intensity and duration (10). These electrophysiological data were in agreement with the demonstration that, in the same species, spinal dorsal horn neurons projecting to the lateral thalamus and SI cortical neurons which receive inputs from the VB exhibit similar encoding capacities for noxious stimulation (2,3,6).

The present study has therefore been undertaken to reassess systematically the effects of unilateral lesions (8) of the VB on a behavior, tested by using natural noxious stimulation. We have employed a modification of the Randall-Selitto test, which uses a pressure algometer to produce graded localized noxious mechanical stimuli (12,15). It allowed us to analyze simultaneously the threshold of responses to noxious stimulation of a spinal reflex (withdrawal of the limb) on the one hand, and a centrally processed reaction (vocalization) on the other. In addition, we compared the responses to noxious mechanical stimulation applied differentially to each paw.

METHODS

Thirty-five 200-g male Sprague Dawley albino rats were used. They were housed 4 or 5 to a cage and allowed to become adjusted to the laboratory setting for several days before testing.

Surgical and Histological Procedures

Surgery was performed under intraperitoneal chloral hydrate anesthesia (400 mg/kg) on the day following the preliminary testing. The rats received a slow pressure injection of 5 nmoles kainic acid (KA) (in 0.15 μl of water, over 20 min) with the stereotaxic target being just lateral to the external lamina of the thalamus at the level of the rostral VB on one side, in order to assess lateralized effects.

At the end of testing sessions, animals received an overdose of sodium pentobarbital and were perfused transcardially with saline followed by 10% formalin. Serial coronal sections of the brain were cut 100-μm thick and stained with cresyl violet, photographed and drawn using a camera lucida drawing tube, taking care to determine the precise extent of neuronal loss induced by KA in thalamic and other structures.

Testing Procedures

Using the Basile analgesymeter (Apdex), thresholds for withdrawal and vocalization were determined by applying increasing pressure to the paw. For each rat, preliminary threshold determinations were carried out, before the surgery was performed, to obtain two consecutive stable thresholds for each fore- and hindpaw. These preliminary thresholds were of approximately 160 and 180 g for the forepaws and of 200 to 240 g for the hindpaws. This procedure permitted the use of each animal as its own control. In some cases, the threshold of another reaction ("struggle") was noted, but this response, although considered by some authors as reliable (see discussion in ref. 15), is difficult to assess and was therefore not systematically noted. After KA injection, thresholds were determined again after 3 and/or 10 weeks following the same protocol.

RESULTS

Effects of KA Injections

Injections of this neurotoxic agent in the internal capsule or the medial striatum at the level of the rostral VB provoked epileptic seizures beginning less than 1 hr after the end of the injection and lasting 6 to 10 hr. After this period, the animals behaved abnormally for a few days, being aphagic and adipsic, creating a situation which required daily injections of isotonic glucose (10 cc, s.c.) for 5 or 6 days. The weight loss could be as large as 30% at the end of the first week, but the animals then regained their normal weights. After 10 weeks, gross behavioral observation showed them to be indistinguishable from unlesioned rats. The transitory aphagic-adipsic state of the animals prompted us to analyze the responses some time after the injection

(3–10 weeks) to avoid an effect related to the debilitated state of the animal during this period, rather than an effect of the thalamic lesion.

Lesions were quite visible on Nissl-stained sections (Fig. 1) due to the loss of neuronal elements in the area and of the gliosis which persisted up to 10 weeks after the injection. These characteristic features facilitated mapping the extent of the lesions using a camera lucida drawing tube. Though the extent of the lesions was relatively consistent, some were placed in structures unrelated to the VB, due to errors in the stereotaxic placement. This variation permitted the comparison of the effects of these various lesions on the responses to the noxious test. Some animals showing large lesions of the cortex, most likely due to a spread of KA along the needle, were excluded from this study, because a parallel study demonstrated that a lesion of the SI cortex in the rat can, by itself, alter the responses to the noxious test employed here in a way similar to that observed after VB lesions. This phenomenon could have produced a bias in the interpretation of our data in the case of corticothalamic lesions.

Lesions Affecting Structures Other than the VB

In 12 cases, lesions were related to various subcortical structures other than the VB. Some lesions involved a portion of Ammon's Horn, or a pos-

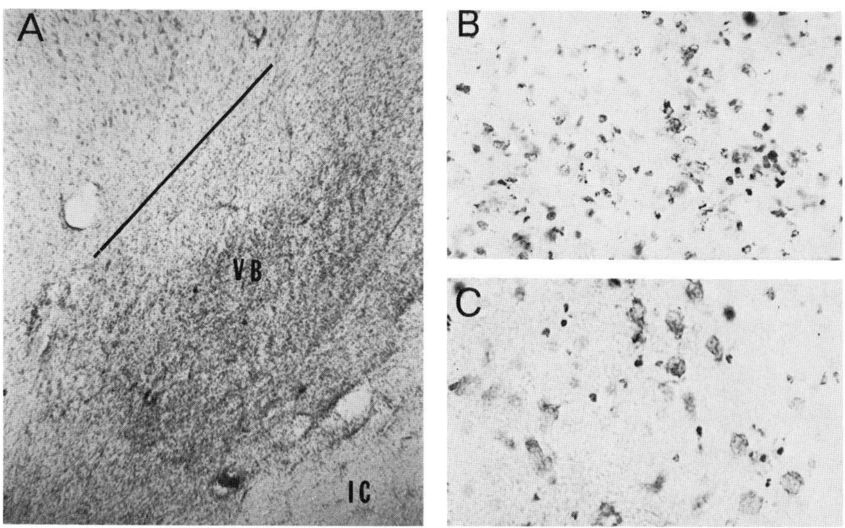

FIG. 1. Photomicrographs showing the effects of an injection of kainic acid. **A:** Low magnification (× 35) of a lesioned area in the VB. The lesioned area is limited laterally by the internal capsule (IC) and its medial border is indicated by the *black line.* **B:** Higher magnification (× 240) of an area of the lesioned VB showing numerous glial elements. **C:** Same magnification of an area of the contralateral unlesioned VB showing larger (neuronal) elements. Cresyl violet staining.

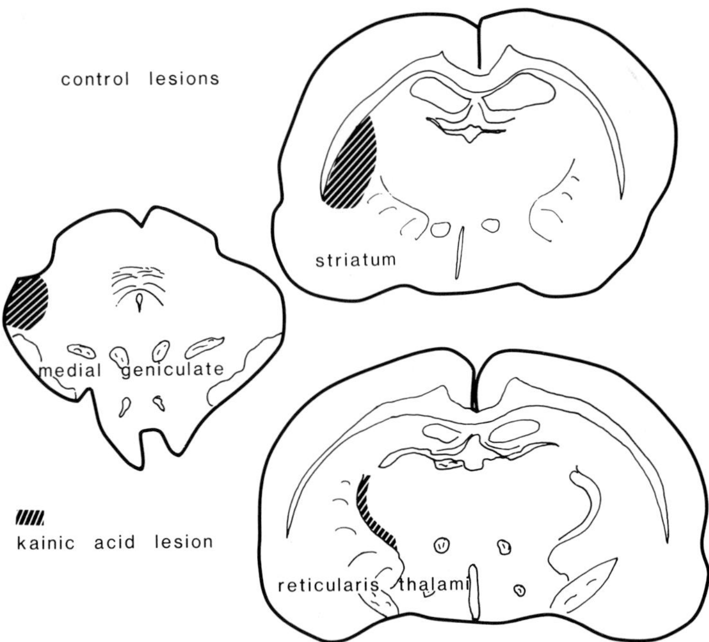

FIG. 2. Camera lucida drawings of three different lesions located outside VB and including parts of the striatum, the medial geniculate body, and the nucleus reticularis thalami. No alteration of the vocalization thresholds was observed in these cases.

teromedial area of the striatum, or the nucleus reticularis thalami or the medial geniculate body (Fig. 2) without affecting the withdrawal or vocalization threshold responses to the test. In 3 of these cases, however, a large lesion of the striatum as well as Ammon's Horn induced a moderate increase of the vocalization threshold (30–40% by comparison with prelesion control values) without affecting the withdrawal threshold. This increase included the responses obtained by pressure on all four paws.

Lesions Affecting the Lateral VB

In 13 cases, the lesion involved the entire extent of lateral VB (i.e., the area of VB receiving afferents from the dorsal column nuclei and the spinal cord; see references in ref. 11). In 3 of these cases, the lesion extended further to medial VB and other thalamic structures (Fig. 3). Three to 10 weeks after the injection of KA, the animals presented no modification of the withdrawal threshold but a major increase (100% and more by comparison with control values) of their vocalization threshold. This dramatic alteration exclusively involved the responses induced by pressure applied to the paws contralateral to the lesion site, and was observed following pressure to the

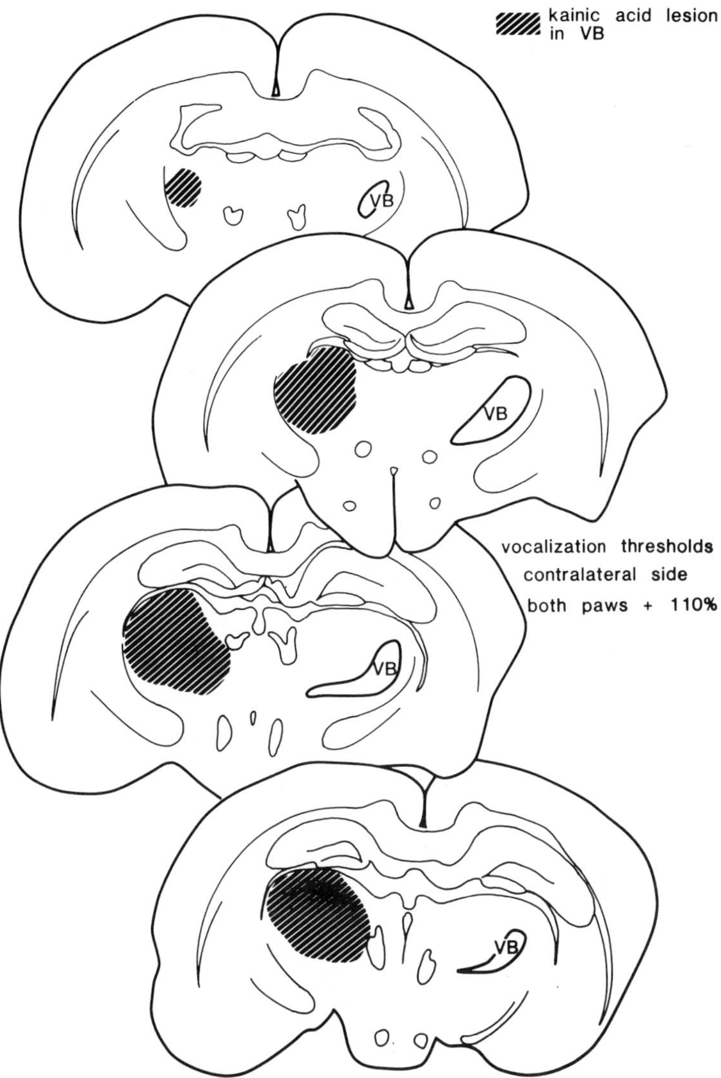

FIG. 3. Camera lucida drawings of successive coronal sections (from *bottom* to *top*, *caudal* to *rostral*) through the VB of an animal with a large lesion and increase of the vocalization threshold for both contralateral fore- and hindpaws. Only the extent of the thalamic lesion is indicated.

fore- as well as the hindpaw. In contrast, vocalization thresholds obtained by pressure of the paws ipsilateral to the lesion site were similar to those obtained before surgery in most cases. In a few cases, a slight increase (30–40%) of this ipsilateral vocalization threshold was observed, probably related to the existence of a large lesion of the striatum (see above).

In addition, it was noted in some cases that the threshold for struggling responses was similar to controls when vocalization threshold was largely increased, which seems to indicate that the two responses do not depend on the same neural mechanisms of pain response.

Lesions Affecting a Portion of the Lateral VB

In 10 cases, the lesion of the VB included only a portion of this nucleus (Fig. 4). In all these cases, the area lesioned was the rostral and lateral VB; that zone which receives afferent projections representing the hindpaw. In these cases, 3 to 10 weeks after the injection, the animals presented no alteration of the withdrawal threshold. In contrast, vocalization threshold was

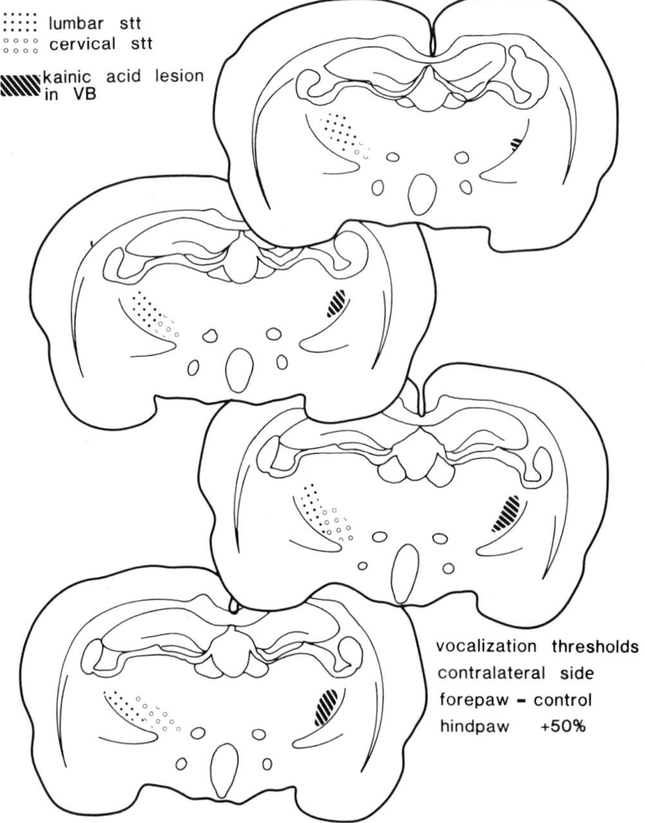

FIG. 4. Camera lucida drawings of successive coronal sections (from *bottom* to *top, caudal* to *rostral*) through the anterior part of the VB of a rat with a lesion limited to rostral and most lateral portions of the VB and increase of the vocalization threshold for the contralateral hindpaw only. Only the extent of the thalamic lesion is indicated. On the *left* part of the drawing are indicated the areas of projection of the spinothalamic tract. (Modified from ref. 11, with permission.)

increased when pressure was applied to the hindpaw, but not to the forepaw, contralateral to the injection site. Increases were less marked than in the previous group of large lesions, ranging between 50 and 80% of the control value. No increase in vocalization threshold was observed for the paws ipsilateral to the injection site.

DISCUSSION

The present results establish the involvement of the VB complex of the rat thalamus in a pathway subserving certain responses to noxious stimulation. Indeed, the neuronal loss in the VB induced by the injection of kainic acid is certainly responsible for the unilateral increase in vocalization threshold observed here, since control experiments demonstrated that this result was obtained only when the lesion encompassed a portion of the VB. This observation is in agreement with the results of clinical studies demonstrating that lesions of the somatosensory thalamus in humans are often accompanied by a diminished sensibility to pain (see references and discussion in ref. 13).

The increase in vocalization following a unilateral VB lesion dealt exclusively with the contralateral part of the body. In addition, the analysis of the alterations induced by limited lesions of the lateral VB showed that there is a topographical arrangement demonstrated by testing the effects of the KA injection. The lesion of the rostral and most lateral VB increased the vocalization threshold with pressure to the hindpaw, without modifying that for pressure applied to the forepaw. These results indicate that the pathway responsible for the transmission of the noxious inputs to the VB is completely crossed and that its projections to the VB are somatotopically organized. On the basis of electrophysiological studies (1) we have demonstrated that VB neurons receive noxious inputs conveyed by the spinothalamic tract. The present behavioral data are in good agreement with these results since the spinothalamic projections are completely crossed in the rat and are somatotopically organized in the VB; the projections originating from the lumbar cord being rostral and lateral to those from the cervical cord as indicated in Fig. 4 (from ref. 11).

In conclusion, the present study demonstrates that, in the rat, the ventrobasal complex of the thalamus is involved in a pathway conveying noxious inputs, which probably includes the spinothalamic tract and the somatosensory SI cortex, since all VB neurons project to this area in the rat (7,14). This pathway clearly subserves some functions necessary for a vocalization response to a localized natural noxious stimulus, as is indicated by the large increase in threshold induced by a lesion of the lateral VB without a change in threshold for the withdrawal response, which is mediated by spinal mechanisms. This result is contradictory to those of some clinical (5,9) and experimental studies (16) that suggested that cortical and/or diencephalic structures were not necessary for pain sensation. It is possible that the use of a localized natural noxious stimulation in the present study (pressure algometer) is the possible explanation for this discrepancy. The fact that, when observed, struggling responses [which are often considered as a "supraspinally integrated" behavior (15)], were not modified in parallel with vocalization seems to indicate that various supraspinal structures can indeed be responsible for different reactions to a noxious stimulation.

ACKNOWLEDGMENTS

The authors are greatly indebted to D. D. Ralston for her editorial work, to E. Dehausse for technical help, and to Dr. J. M. Besson for review of the manuscript. This study was supported by Institute National de la Santé et de la Recherche Medicale (INSERM).

REFERENCES

1. Briand, A., Peschanski, M., and Guilbaud, G. (1984): Spinal pathways conveying noxious inputs to the ventrobasal complex of the rat thalamus. An electrophysiological study. *Pain,* Suppl. 2:S313.
2. Dickenson, A. H., and Le Bars, D. (1983): Diffuse noxious inhibitory controls (DNIC) involve trigeminothalamic and spinothalamic neurones in the rat. *Exp. Brain Res.,* 49:174–180.
3. Giesler, G. J., Menetrey, D., Guilbaud, G., and Besson, J. M. (1976): Lumbar cord neurons at the origin of the spinothalamic tract in the rat. *Brain Res.,* 118:320–324.
4. Guilbaud, G., Peschanski, M., Gautron, M., and Binder, D. (1980): Neurones responding to noxious stimulation in VB complex and caudal adjacent regions in the thalamus of the rat. *Pain,* 8:303–318.
5. Head, H., and Holmes, G. (1911): Sensory disturbances from cerebral lesions. *Brain,* 34: 102–254.
6. Lamour, Y., Guilbaud, G., and Willer, J. C. (1983): Rat somatosensory cortex (SI): I. Characteristics of neuronal responses to noxious stimulation and comparison with responses to nonnoxious stimulation. *Exp. Brain Res.,* 49:39–45.
7. Lee, C. L. (1981): Structural organization of the ventrobasal complex of the thalamus in the rat. *Ph.D. thesis,* University of California, Berkeley.
8. McGeer, E. G., Olney, J. W., and McGeer, P. L. (1978): *Kainic Acid as a Tool in Neurobiology.* Raven Press, New York.
9. Penfield, W., and Boldrey, E. (1937): Somatic motor and sensory representation in the cerebral cortex of man as studied by electrical stimulation. *Brain,* 60:389–443.
10. Peschanski, M., Guilbaud, G., Gautron, M., and Besson, J. M. (1980): Encoding of noxious heat messages in neurons of the ventrobasal thalamic complex in the rat. *Brain Res.,* 197:401–413.
11. Peschanski, M., Mantyh, P. W., and Besson, J. M. (1983): Spinal afferents to the ventrobasal complex of the rat thalamus. An anatomical study using WGA-HRP. *Brain Res.,* 287:240–244.
12. Randall, L. O., and Selitto, J. J. (1957): A method for measurement of analgesic activity on inflamed tissue. *Arch. Pharmacodyn.,* 61:409–419.
13. Riddock, G. (1937): The clinical features of central pain. *Lancet,* 1:1093–1098; 1150–1156.
14. Saporta, S., and Kruger, L. (1977): The organization of thalamocortical relay neurons in the rat ventrobasal complex studied by the retrograde transport of horseradish peroxidase. *J. Comp. Neurol.,* 174:187–208.
15. Winter, C. A., and Flataker, L. (1965): Reaction thresholds to pressure in oedematous hindpaws of rats, responses to analgesic drugs. *J. Pharmacol. Exp. Ther.,* 150:165–171.
16. Woods, J. W. (1964): Behavior of chronic decerebrate rats. *J. Neurophysiol.,* 27:635–644.

Advances in Pain Research and Therapy, Vol. 9, edited by H. L. Fields et al. Raven Press, New York © 1985.

Arousal-Related Changes in the Response of Ventral Posterior Thalamic Neurons to Somatic and Spinothalamic Stimulation in the Awake Monkey

Kenneth L. Casey and Thomas J. Morrow

Neurology Research Laboratories (Neurophysiology), Veterans Administration Medical Center, Ann Arbor, Michigan 48105

Attention to a specific stimulus requires a state of alertness or arousal, the ability to distinguish the stimulus from other ongoing events, and a mechanism for uniquely combining these processes. It is therefore reasonable to expect that the state of arousal should affect the responses of specific sensory neurons in the central nervous system.

Several studies have shown changes in the frequency and pattern of spontaneous, nonevoked neuronal discharge in specific sensory thalamic nuclei, including the ventral posterior (VP) nuclei, during shifts from waking to sleep, and among different stages of sleep (5). In general, the results show an overall reduction in discharge rate and a shift from a nearly random to a bursting pattern of discharge as the animal goes from waking with a desynchronized electroencephalogram (EEG) to sleep with synchronized slow-wave EEG activity.

Arousal-related changes in stimulus-evoked neuronal responses of the VP thalamus have been studied less intensively. Podvoll and Goodman (15) reported marked increases in spontaneous and evoked multiple unit discharge in specific sensory and nonspecific thalamic nuclei when cats shifted from nonarousal to aroused states as defined by EEG and behavioral criteria. Subsequently, Chapin and Woodward (8) showed that the somatosensory responses of SI cortical neurons, which receive VP input, decrease during locomotion, but strongly increase during immobile arousal. Favale et al. (9) also showed arousal-related changes in evoked potentials recorded from the VP thalamus of chronically prepared cats. However, when the sensory responses of single VP neurons have been examined, the evidence for arousal-related changes in responsivness has not been supported. Recordings from the VPL nucleus of awake cats (3) and VPM of awake monkeys (10) have shown changes in spontaneous neuronal discharge associated with shifts between waking and sleep, but no arousal-related changes in the responses of units to somatic stimuli could be detected.

We wished to reexamine this problem at the level of single unit analysis. A major difficulty encountered in experiments of this type is the quantitative analysis of changes in response to controlled, repetitive stimuli while shifts in the level of arousal are either occurring unpredictably or are caused by the stimulus. For our experiments in the awake, partially restrained squirrel monkey, we developed a computer-based method for automatically detecting EEG and behavioral events that defined three levels of arousal within the waking state, and permitted the separate analysis of neuronal responses under each of these behavioral conditions. For stimulus control, we used air puffs of constant intensity and duration as well as single pulse electrical stimulation of the spinal lemniscus (SL). With these techniques, we are able to demonstrate that a significant proportion of VP neurons, including some that respond differentially to noxious stimuli, show arousal-related changes in responsiveness to somatic and to SL stimulation. The results also suggest that the modulating mechanisms act, at least in part, at the thalamic level and, probably, presynaptically.

METHODS

Surgery

Two adult male squirrel monkeys were deeply anesthetized with ketamine (20 mg/kg, i.m.); supplemental doses of 5 to 10 mg/kg were given during surgery as needed to suppress somatic reflexes. Body temperature was maintained at 37° C (rectal) by an automatically controlled heating pad. All surgery was performed under sterile conditions. Under stereotaxic control, two twisted pairs of Teflon® insulated stainless steel wire (254 μm) were inserted through burr holes in the skull so that the bared cut ends rested within the dorsal part of the SL in the lateral midbrain within the trajectory of the spinothalamic tract (6). A silastic-sealed plastic microdrive chamber (13) was placed over a craniotomy located above the VP thalamus and a stainless steel reference electrode was inserted into the underlying parietal cortex. (The microdrive chamber was moved to the opposite side in a second operation for recording from each hemithalamus.) Stainless steel skull screws were used for EEG recording and for securing the recording chamber, connecting plug, and all electrodes to the skull with dental acrylic. Sterile water (30 cc) was given subcutaneously for fluid replacement and penicillin was administered for 1 week postoperatively (150,000 units q.o.d.).

Recording

At least 2 weeks after surgery, the monkeys were adapted to a restraining chair that had a weighted phonograph cartridge mounted on a flexible wand attached to the chair's back. The amplified signal from this device registered all the monkey's movements except for small movements restricted to the hands, feet, or face. An electronic level detector was set to provide a signal to one input of an on-line computer whenever movement was present. Similarly, a specially constructed EEG synchronization detector (T. Morrow, *unpublished observations*) was used to register the presence of three or more consecutive EEG waves of over 50 μV in amplitude, occurring within a frequency range of 5.5 to 15.5 Hz. This device automatically registered the presence of synchronized EEG activity which appeared only when the monkey was quiet and often with eyelids partially closed. Stainless steel microelectrodes, insulated with multiple coats of epoxy resin to an impedance of approximately 10 MΩ (measured at 100 Hz), were inserted through the silastic-sealed craniotomy into the VP thalamus for unit recording by conventional methods. Only well-isolated extracellular action potentials (300–2,000 μV, 1.0 msec or more duration) were used to trigger standard pulses that were led from a window discriminator to an input of the computer. SL stimuli were single pulses (100 to 1,500 μA; 0.1 to 0.2 msec) delivered through bipolar electrodes at 1 to 5 Hz; such stimuli were never observed to elicit any behavioral response. Hand-held brushes and calibrated nylon probes or clips were used to identify the receptive fields and adequate stimuli for single VP neurons. For determining changes in responsiveness to repetitive somatic stimuli, however, we used air puffs of constant intensity and duration applied with the probe nozzle held at a fixed distance from the receptive field. The occurrence of each SL or somatic stimulus was also fed into the computer. In addition, the EEG, movement signal, EEG synchronization detector output, movement detector output, all stimulus signals, and the frequency-to-voltage converted output of the unit window discriminator were recorded on-line on separate channels of a digital chart recorder (Gould TA600).

Data Analysis

The occurrence of each unit discharge, SL, or somatic stimulus, and the presence of movement and synchronized EEG waves were stored in computer disc files. A computer program was developed to allow, for each unit, the off-line construction and analysis of peristimulus time histograms (PSTH) for either SL or somatic stimuli delivered during any of the following defined levels of arousal:

1. EEG desynchronized, movement: awake, moving.
2. EEG desynchronized, no movement: quiet waking.
3. EEG synchronized, no movement: drowsy.

The program computes several statistical parameters that characterize each PSTH, including measures of response variability, so that comparisons can be made between stimulus and arousal conditions.

Histology

Sections of 50 μm were cut with a Vibratome® from the formalin-fixed brain and mounted on slides for staining with cresyl violet. Electrolytic lesions (20 μA DC for 20 sec) made in at least two locations along each microelectrode track were used to identify the sites of unit recording from projected images of the stained brain sections.

RESULTS

Of the 58 units that responded to somatic stimuli, 34 could be examined for arousal-related changes in responsiveness because the monkey's behavioral state shifted among the three levels of arousal during unit recording. Similarly, 16 of the 22 units driven by SL stimulation could be tested for changes in response. Of those tested, 19 (56%) somatically excited and 13 (81%) SL driven units showed arousal-related response changes.

An example of this phenomenon is presented in Fig. 1, which shows several features exhibited by units responding to somatic stimulation. As seen in the sample chart recordings and in the PSTH records, this VP neuron responded maximally to repetitive hair movement (air puff) within its contralateral receptive field when the monkey was in the quiet waking state. The reduced responses to the last two stimuli shown in the sample chart recordings during quiet waking immediately precede the onset of the drowsy condition, an example of which is shown in the middle panel. There, the output of the EEG synchronization (spindle) detector registers the presence of EEG high voltage slow waves and spindles. During this behavioral state, the monkey's eyes remain open. Somatic responses are still present, but are markedly attenuated. Note that the responses promptly return as the EEG shifts from the synchronized to the desynchronized pattern. The responses of this unit were again reduced when the monkey was alert and moving as shown in the right panel of Fig. 1. During this behavioral condition, the stability of the stimulus is maintained by gently restraining the monkey's limb. Of particular interest in this example is the observation that the interstimulus (background) activity of this unit was increased throughout the period of reduced somatosensory responsiveness.

An effect of arousal level on short latency responses elicited by SL stimulation is shown in Fig. 2. This VP neuron was classified as a wide dynamic range (WDR) cell because it responded differentially to pinprick within a receptive field of the contralateral medial thigh (Fig. 2E–G). The monkey did not change arousal level during the testing of this unit's responses to somatic stimuli. During repetitive (1 Hz) SL stimulation, however, the monkey shifted from the quiet waking (Fig. 2A,B) to the drowsy (Fig. 2C,D) state. During quiet waking, all unit discharges occurred within 2 to 3 msec of SL stimulation (Fig. 2B). During drowsiness, the proportion of early

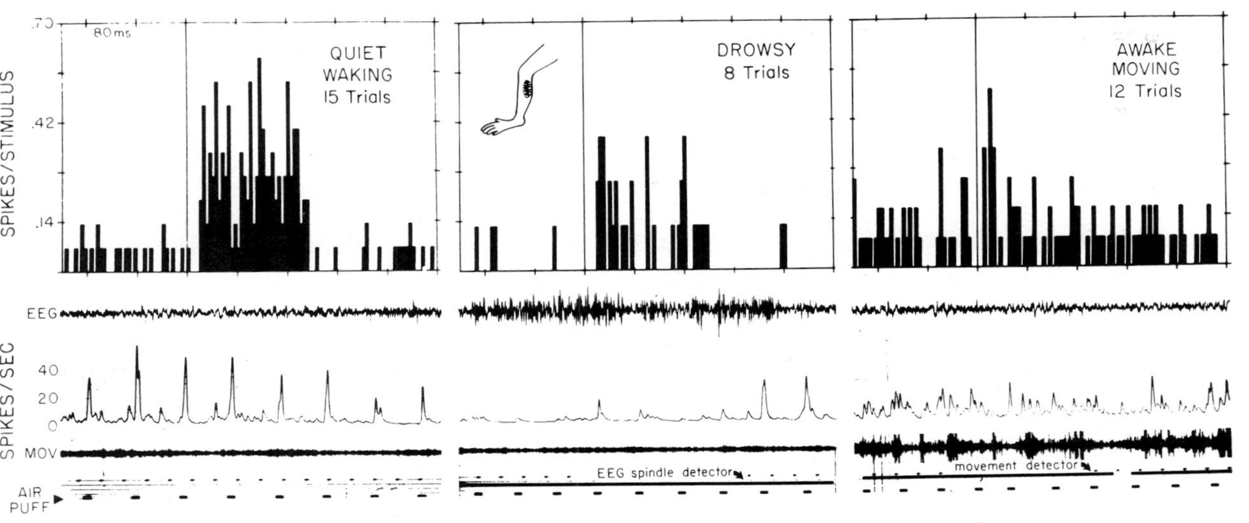

FIG. 1. VP unit responding to hair movement produced by air puffs to the contralateral receptive field shown *(inset)*. Reduction in responsiveness is seen during drowsiness and the awake moving condition. See text for discussion. Time marks above stimulus marker: 1/sec.

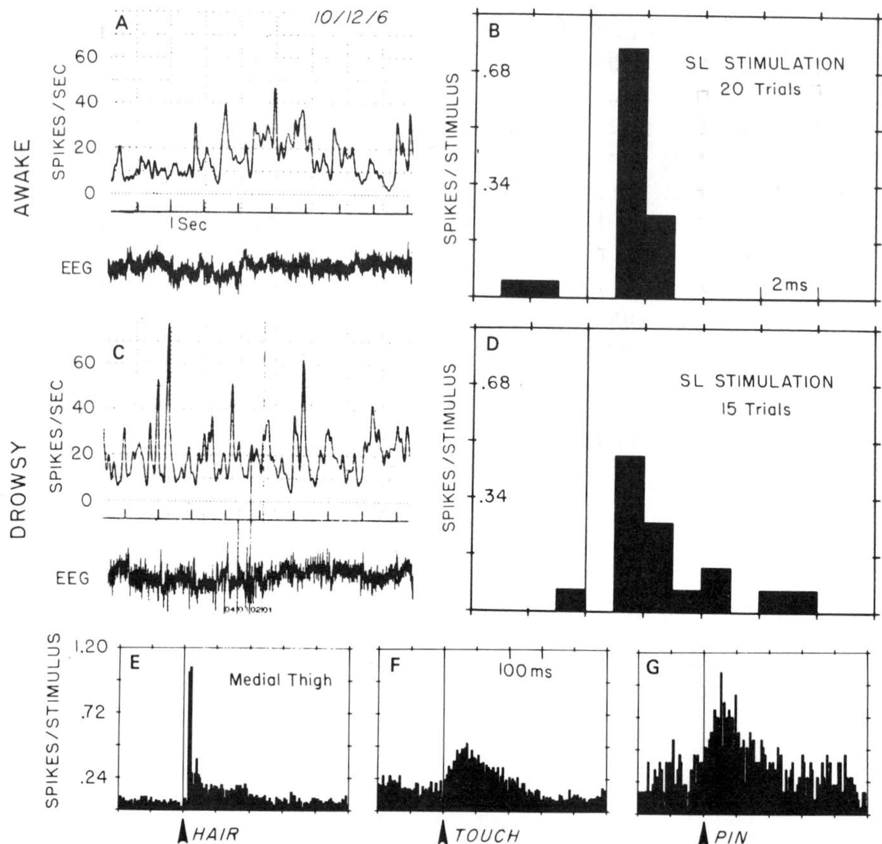

FIG. 2. VP neuron responding differentially to pinprick stimulation on the contralateral medial thigh **(E,F,G)**. Level of ongoing interstimulus activity is shown during quiet waking **(A)** and drowsiness **(C)**. PST histograms show a reduction in the proportion of short latency responses to SL stimuli during drowsiness **(D)** as compared to quiet waking **(B)**. See text for discussion.

responses to the same stimulus is reduced and discharges appear in the 4 to 8 msec poststimulus period (Fig. 2D). Again, it should be noted that this effect took place while overall interstimulus unit activity was slightly increased (Fig. 2A,C). In other units, the response to SL stimulation was nearly eliminated during drowsiness while interstimulus activity was unchanged from the quiet waking state.

It was not possible to test each unit for arousal-related changes in response to both somatic and SL stimulation. However, in the 9 instances in which this was accomplished, the responses to both types of stimuli were affected whenever response modulation could be demonstrated by either stimulus alone.

Although we routinely tested for arousal-related changes in the size of receptive fields, this effect could be demonstrated for only one unit as shown in Fig. 3. During quiet waking, this cell was consistently excited by hair movement within a receptive field on the contralateral tail as diagrammed in Fig. 3A. During drowsiness, markedly reduced responses could be evoked only within the hatched area shown in Fig. 3B.

Table 1 shows the distribution of adequate stimulus modalities among units that did and did not show arousal-related response changes. Although the sample size is too small to draw firm conclusions, the data suggest that VP neurons with cutaneous input are more likely to show arousal-related changes in responsiveness than those responding only to inputs from joints or muscles. Thus, 17 (89%) of the 19 neurons showing modulation were excited by stimulation of hair and/or skin, whereas only 8 (53%) of the 17 unmodulated units had cutaneous inputs. This distribution of properties is nonrandom by Fisher's exact test ($p = 0.02$).

DISCUSSION

A significant proportion of the VP units responding to somatic stimuli show changes in responsiveness associated with changes in the level of arousal as defined by the EEG and behavioral criteria we used. Maximum responsiveness occurred during the quiet waking state when the EEG

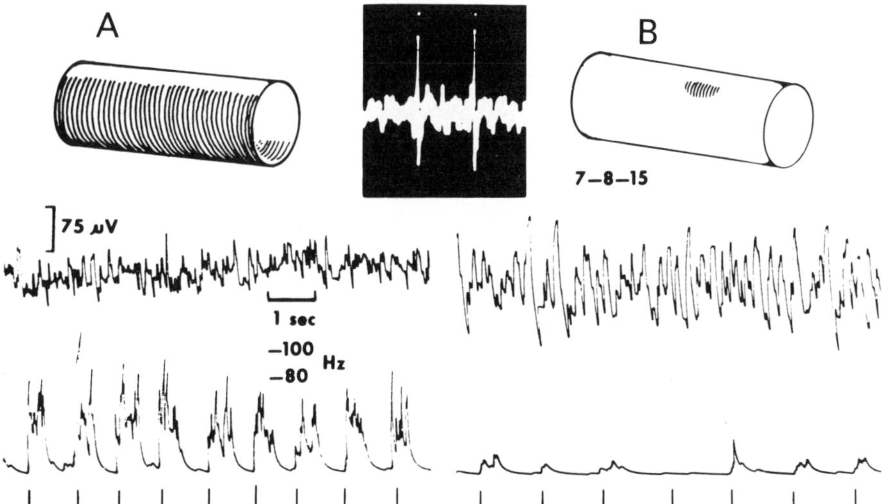

FIG. 3. VP unit *(inset)* responding to hair movements on contralateral tail during quiet waking as shown by shaded area of diagram under **(A).** During drowsiness, receptive field is reduced as shown in **(B).** Chart records show EEG *(upper trace)* and frequency meter output of unit responses *(lower trace).*

TABLE 1. *Categorical distribution of arousal-related response changes and adequate natural stimulus of VP neurons*

	Response changes[a]	
Adequate stimulus	With	Without
Hair	7	2
Touch	4	2
Tap	3	2
WDR	3	2
Muscle	2	4
Joint	0	3
Total	19	15

showed desynchronized, relatively low voltage activity and the monkey was not moving. During either waking movement or drowsiness with synchronized EEG, unit responsiveness decreased.

Why these arousal-related changes were not observed in the studies of Baker (3) or Hayward (10) is not entirely clear since many of the changes are obvious and do not require special analytical or recording procedures. One possible explanation is that we examined neuronal responsiveness during different levels of arousal within the waking state, whereas Baker (3) and Hayward (10) concentrated on changes associated with shifts between waking and sleep. Our monkeys never showed behavioral or EEG manifestations of typical slow-wave or desynchronized sleep. During the drowsy state, the EEG showed runs of 7 to 14 Hz synchronized activity that closely resemble the α-rhythm of humans; the monkey's eyes were open even though the eyelids were sometimes partially closed. It is possible that VP neuronal responsiveness during sleep more closely resembles that seen during quiet waking than during the state we define as drowsy. Furthermore, the decline in responsivness during waking movement might be overlooked if averaged together with the responses during quiet waking. This explanation gains some support from the observation that the amplitude of VP evoked potentials in the cat appeared maximal during sleep and either reduced or enhanced during arousal (9).

Other factors that may account for the contrast between our results and those of Baker (3) and Hayward (10) include the use of central (SL) stimuli, more easily and precisely controlled somatic stimuli, and the development of computer-based data acquisition and analysis procedures that allowed separate and quantitative analysis of responses to stimuli delivered during objectively defined behavioral states.

Our data also show that at least a component of the arousal-related response modulation is mediated by mechanisms acting at the thalamic level. It is most likely that the short latency, single spike responses to SL stimulation involve no more than one or two synaptic delays within the VP thalamus. The arousal-related response modulation of SL driving must therefore occur at or very near the VP thalamus. Additional observations offer some insight into the possible mechanisms of this modulation. Our recordings show, for example, that the interstimulus activity of VP neurons is unchanged or even slightly increased while the response to SL stimulation is either reduced or delayed. This indicates that the attenuated response of the VP neuron to SL input is input-specific and is not attributable to an overall reduction in VP neuronal excitability due to postsynaptic inhibitory influences. This selective modulation could be mediated by mechanisms that are presynaptic to the VP neuron or that postsynaptically block the excitatory effect of SL synapses remote from the spike trigger zone.

Behaviorally related modulation of VP cell responses would be expected on the basis of anatomical and physiological data. Bowsher (7) has presented evidence for direct projections from the midbrain reticular formation to the VP nucleus and the adjacent posterior group of thalamic nuclei. A direct input to the VP from the periaqueductal gray has recently been reported (4). Reticular formation influences may also be mediated via the thalamic reticular nucleus, which is known to receive brainstem reticular formation input (14) and to project to specific thalamic nuclei, including the VP complex (12). The reticular nucleus also mediates corticothalamic influences (12) and has been shown to be largely composed of GABA-containing neurons (11). The role of other descending cortical (18) and brainstem (17) influences on ascending somatosensory pathways has been reviewed, Physiological experiments have shown that all these systems can modulate the transmission of somatosensory inputs through the VP thalamus (1,2,16–19). The mechanisms responsible for the arousal-related modulation of VP neuronal responses we have reported here remain to be determined.

ACKNOWLEDGMENTS

This work was supported by the Veterans Administration and National Institutes of Health grant NS12581. The technical assistance of Avery Gottfried and Bin Yuan is gratefully acknowledged.

REFERENCES

1. Albe-Fessard, D., Condes-Lara, M., Kesar, S., and Sanderson, P. (1983): Tonic cortical controls acting on spontaneous and evoked thalamic activity. In: *Somatosensory Integration in the Thalamus,* edited by G. Macchi, A. Rustioni, and R. Spreafico, pp. 273–285. Elsevier, Amsterdam.
2. Angel, A. (1983): The functional interrelations between the somatosensory cortex and the thalamic reticular nucleus: their role in the control of information transfer across the spe-

cific somatosensory thalamic relay nucleus. In: *Somatosensory Integration in the Thalamus,* edited by G. Macchi, A. Rustioni, and R. Spreafico, pp. 221–239. Elsevier, Amsterdam.

3. Baker, M. A. (1971): Spontaneous and evoked activity of neurones in the somatosensory thalamus of the waking cat. *J. Physiol.,* 217:359–379.
4. Barbaresi, P., Conti, F., and Manzoni, T. (1982): Periaqueductal grey projection to the ventrobasal complex in the cat: a horseradish peroxidase study. *Neurosci. Lett.,* 30:205–210.
5. Benoit, O., and Chataignier, C. (1973): Patterns of spontaneous unitary discharge in thalamic ventrobasal complex during wakefulness and sleep. *Exp. Brain Res.,* 17:348–363.
6. Boivie, J. (1979): An anatomical reinvestigation of the termination of the spinothalamic tract in the monkey. *J. Comp. Neurol.,* 186:343–370.
7. Bowsher, D. (1975): Diencephalic projections from the midbrain reticular formation. *Brain Res.,* 95:211–220.
8. Chapin, J. K., and Woodward, D. J. (1981): Modulation of sensory responsiveness of single somatosensory cortical cells during movement and arousal behaviors. *Exp. Neurol.,* 72:164–178.
9. Favale, E., Loeb, C., Manfredi, M., and Sacco, G. (1965): Somatic afferent transmission and cortical responsiveness during natural sleep and arousal in the cat. *EEG Clin. Neurophysiol.,* 18:354–368.
10. Hayward, J. N. (1975): Response of ventrobasal thalamic cells to hair displacement on the face of the waking monkey. *J. Physiol.,* 250:385–407.
11. Houser, C. R., Vaughn, J. E., Barber, R. P., and Roberts, E. (1980): GABA neurons are the major cell type of the nucleus reticularis thalami. *Brain Res.,* 200:341–354.
12. Jones, E. G. (1975): Some aspects of the organization of the thalamic reticular complex. *J. Comp. Neurol.,* 162:285–308.
13. Morrow, T. J. (1980): An improved technique for recording single unit activity in awake animals. *Brain Res. Bull.,* 5:91–93.
14. Nauta, W. J., and Kuypers, H. G. (1958): Some ascending pathways in the brain stem reticular formation. In: *Reticular Formation of the Brain,* edited by H. H. Jasper and L. D. Proctor, pp. 3–30. Little, Brown, Boston.
15. Podvoll, E. M., and Goodman, S. J. (1967): Averaged neural electrical activity and arousal. *Science,* 155:223–225.
16. Schieppati, M., and Gritti, I. (1983): Influences of locus ceruleus, raphe dorsalis, and periaqueductal gray matter on somatosensory-recipient thalamic nuclei. *Exp. Neurol.,* 82(3):695–705.
17. Sjölund, B., and Björklund (editors) (1982): *Brain-stem Control of Spinal Mechanisms.* Elsevier, Amsterdam.
18. Towe, A. L. (1973): Somatosensory cortex: descending influences on ascending systems. In: *Handbook of Sensory Physiology, Vol. II, Somatosensory System,* edited by A. Iggo, pp. 701–719. Springer-Verlag, Berlin.
19. Yingling, C. D., and Skinner, J. E. (1976): Selective regulation of thalamic sensory relay nuclei by nucleus reticularis thalami. *EEG Clin. Neurophysiol.,* 41:476–482.

Advances in Pain Research and Therapy, Vol. 9, edited by H. L. Fields et al. Raven Press, New York © 1985.

Changes in Responses of Ventrobasal Thalamic Neurons During Carrageenin-Induced Inflammation in the Rat

*,†J. M. Benoist, *V. Kayser, *M. Gautron, and *G. Guilbaud

**Unité de Recherches de Neurophysiologie Pharmacologique, U. 161, 75014 Paris, France; and †Département de Pharmacologie, UER, Cochin Port-Royal Paris, France*

As a step towards elucidation of the mechanisms of clinical pain, a systematic electrophysiological study of various areas of the central nervous system known to be involved in transmission of noxious messages has been undertaken in arthritic rats. Under these pathological conditions, it has been shown that there are dramatic alterations in the responsiveness of the somatosensory neurons recorded in some of these areas (7,8,15,18,19). In these previous studies, the Freund's adjuvant injection into the tail that induced arthritis was performed 3 to 4 weeks before the electrophysiologic investigations. It therefore seemed of interest to attempt a study of possible modifications of neuronal responsiveness during early stages of a painful inflammation. To generate this inflammatory process, we used the local intraplantar injection of carrageenin, a polysaccharide, commonly used to induce inflammation and hyperalgesia in several pharmacological tests of antiinflammatory and analgesic drugs (for references, see refs. 21,23–25). The aim of the present investigation was to record the responsiveness of well-characterized somatosensory neurons in the ventrobasal complex of rats (VB), before and after carrageenin injection. We have previously shown that this nucleus contains many neurons specifically activated by somatic stimuli, known to induce nociceptive reactions in freely moving normal or arthritic animals (7,10).

MATERIAL AND METHODS

Male Sprague Dawley rats weighing 250 to 290 g were used in this study. The surgical preparation, the electrophysiological recordings, and the techniques of peripheral stimulation (mechanical, electrical, thermal) were identical to those used in the studies performed at the thalamic level (10).

Briefly, the recordings (via glass micropipettes filled with NaCl and pontamine sky blue) were carried out in animals immobilized by intravenous injections of gallamine triethiodide (Flaxedil) and artificially ventilated, under a moderate gaseous anesthesia (mixture of ⅓ O_2, ⅔ N_2O-0.5% halothane). This level of anesthesia checked by an electrocorticogram was stable and appeared sufficiently deep, since no sign of suffering or stress could be detected, as previously reported (10). The iontophoretic application of dye at the end of each electrode track allowed the recording sites in the VB complex to be localized by examination of histological sections.

The first study considered 23 VB neurons recorded in 23 rats, driven by nonnoxious (8) or noxious (15) mechanical stimuli applied on receptive fields (RF) including at least a part of the plantar region or of the ankle of the hindpaw contralateral to the recording site.

Once the responsiveness and extent of RF of each neuron had been characterized, control responses (at least 2 from each part of the RF when this extended to another limb or the tail; see below) were recorded with an interval of at least 2.5 min between each stimulation of 15 sec duration.

For the nonnociceptive neurons (NN), the stimulus used was a repetitive brushing (for 4 of them) or a gentle sustained movement (for the others). The RF of these neurons was strictly contralateral to the recording site, and was small, covering either a limited area of the plantar region, or the ankle, or one or several digit joints.

For the nociceptive neurons (N), the stimulus consisted of the application of either a pinch with calibrated forceps, or a hot water bath at 50° C. For these 15 neurons the RF on occasions extended outside the plantar region: towards the tail (N = 10), and/or the other hind limb (N = 8).

After stable control recordings, carrageenin (0.1 ml solution at 1%) was injected subcutaneously in the plantar region. Responses from the various parts of the RF were then tested during a period which lasted from 45 to 120 min after the injection.

For 5 of the 15 N neurons Xylocaine (0.05 ml at 2%) was injected in the inflamed paw after an interval of at least 35 min after carrageenin injection.

A second study was devoted to the measurement of the response threshold of 10 N neurons to thermal stimulation before and after the carrageenin injection. To limit, as much as possible, additional phenomena of sensitization due to repetitive noxious stimuli, the number of stimuli applied were limited to those necessary for the characterization of the neurons. The threshold to thermal stimulation was then measured according to the method previously described (8,20). A paw was plunged for 15 sec into hot water baths of graded temperatures, at 3-min intervals. Temperatures varied from 38° C to the threshold temperature before carregeenin injection and from 35° C to the threshold after the injection. In this series of experiments no suprathreshold stimulus was applied. Simultaneously, we attempted to define the threshold response of the neurons with von Frey hairs [the maximum force applied was 140 mN (about 14 g)].

RESULTS

Responses to Somatic Stimuli After Carrageenin Injection

For the whole neuronal population there was no consistent and systematic modification of the background activity which was usually relatively low in these experimental conditions (0–3 Hz).

For the neurons characterized as non-nociceptive, the carrageenin plantar injection never induced an increase in the responses, nor changes in the RF, at least during the observation period of between 45 and 90 min postinjection.

For the 15 N neurons in this first series of experiments, the responses of the neurons to mechanical and thermal stimulation changed with a delay of 15 to 30 min but in a variable manner. For 12/15 cells there was an increase of 50 to 300% in the responses induced by both mechanical and thermal stimuli applied to the injected paw (Fig. 1). This increase persisted throughout the observation period (45–125 min).

Half of the N neurons with RF initially extending outside the injected paw, exhibited comparable, sometimes greater, increases in responses obtained from these various parts of the RF (Fig. 2). Expansion of the RF was also noticed in some neurons. Responses to pinch or noxious thermal stimuli could be elicited from areas remote to the injured paw from which stimuli were initially inefficient, the other hind limb (6/8), and one or both forelimbs (8/15) (Fig. 3).

When Xylocaine was injected locally in the injured site, there was, with a delay of 5 to 7 min, a decrease or a suppression of the responses evoked not only from this injected paw, but also from the remote areas. Recovery took place 15 to 25 min later.

Threshold Responses to Somatic Stimuli After Carrageenin Injection

In the second series of experiments, there was a dramatic decrease in the threshold response to the thermal stimulation of the injected paw for 8/10 N neurons. It dropped from 44° C $\pm$ 0.65 (N = 10) before, to 40° 30 $\pm$ 1.41 (N = 10) after carrageenin (difference significant at $p < 0.02$). This alteration appeared within 15 min and persisted, unchanged, throughout the observation period (35–105 min). When the RF extended initially to the other hind paw, the threshold response by stimulating this paw with noxious thermal stimulation was 45°14 $\pm$ 0.55 (N = 7) before carrageenin, comparable to that of the opposite site. After the injection, out of 7 neurons studied it was unmodified in 4 cases and decreased in only 1 case (from 45 to 43°). The mean value was not significantly changed, M = 45° $\pm$ 0.80 (N = 5), during the observation period which was at least 35 min.

In the absence of more accurate measurement, it is impossible to state categorically that there were no modifications in the threshold responses to

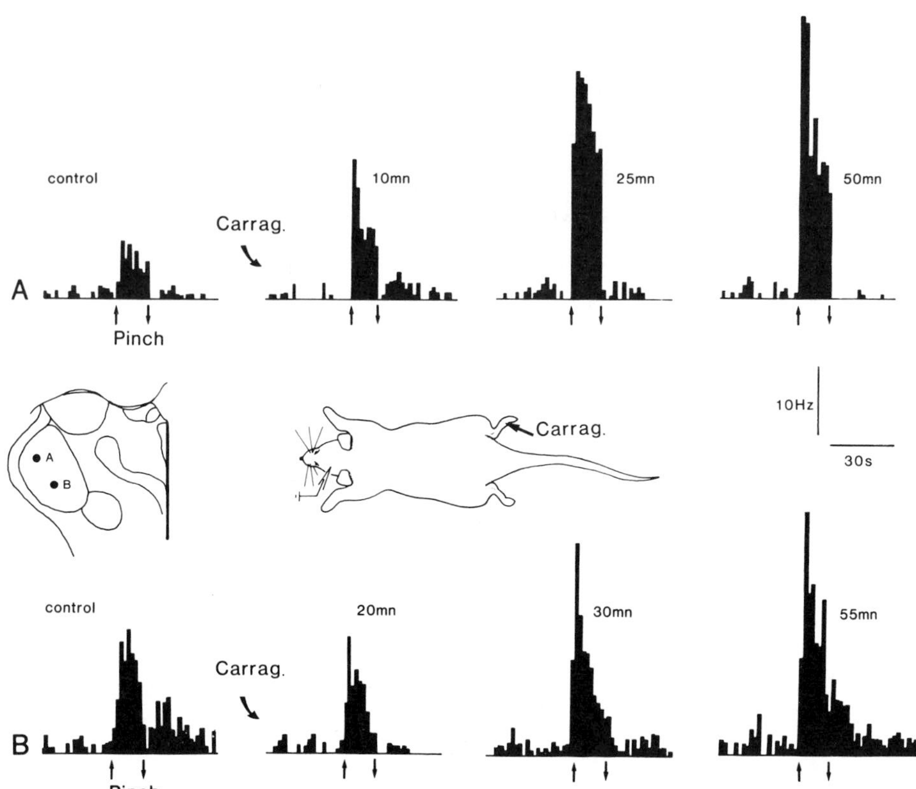

FIG. 1. Responses to pinch of 2 nociceptive neurons **(A,B)** recorded in 2 rats in the left VB before and at various times after the injection of carrageenin (carrag.) in the plantar region of the right hind limb. Duration of the stimulus is indicated by the *arrows.*

mechanical stimuli. However, using calibrated forceps in both series of experiments the threshold was not appreciably lowered since after carrageenin it was always necessary to use a strong stimulus to drive the N neurons; gentle touch with a brush or cotton was always inefficient. The maximum von Frey force which was systematically tested in this second series was always inefficient (as it was before the injection).

DISCUSSION AND CONCLUSION

This study emphasizes that neuronal responses elicited in the VB thalamic complex by somatic non-noxious stimuli are not significantly modified over the course of carrageenin-induced inflammation.

By contrast, responses to noxious stimuli are facilitated in the early stage of this inflammation. These changes appear to be roughly on the same time

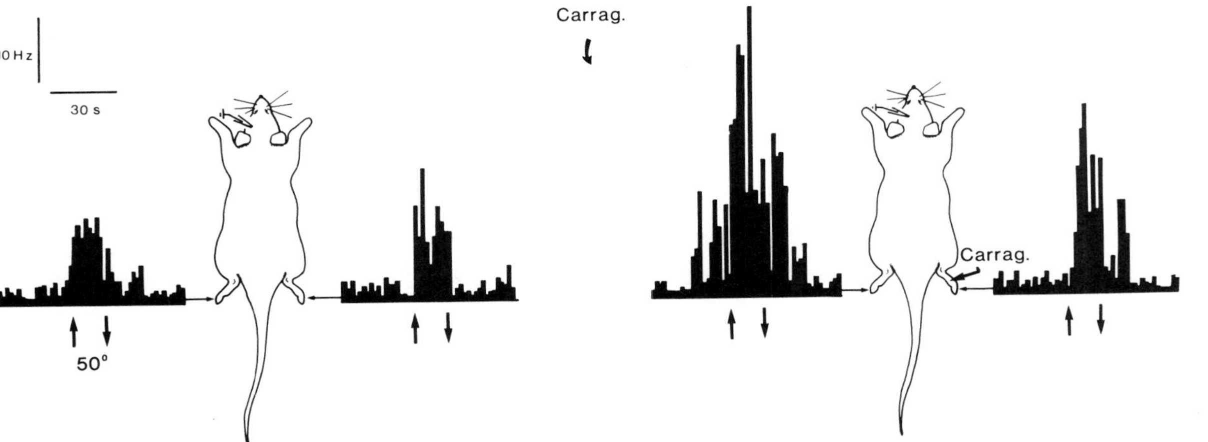

FIG. 2. Responses of a nociceptive neuron recorded in the left VB to 50° before and between 30 and 45 min after carrageenin injection in the right plantar paw. The stimulated areas are indicated by the *thin arrows.* Note the enhancement of responses from both hind limbs which is more pronounced from the left side.

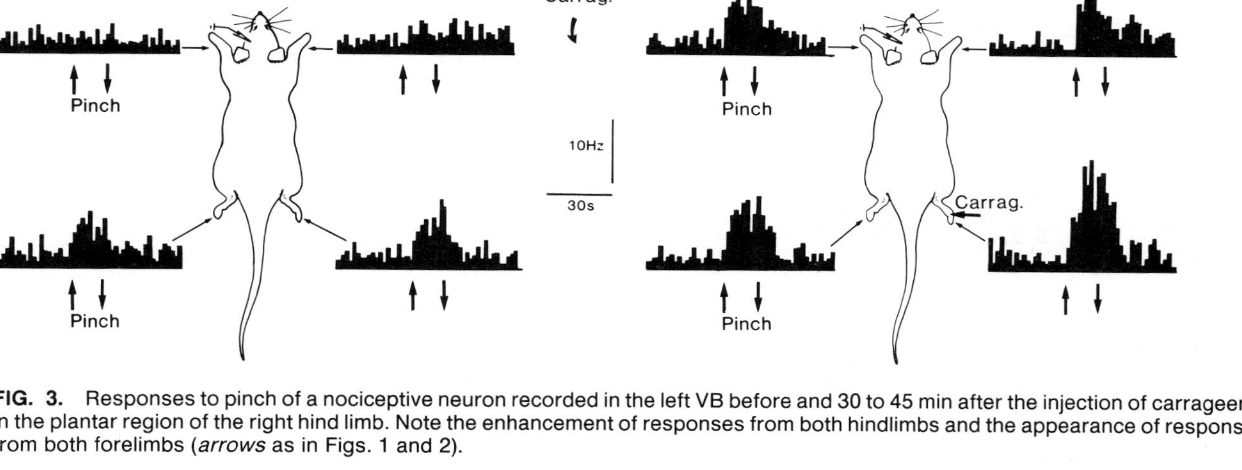

FIG. 3. Responses to pinch of a nociceptive neuron recorded in the left VB before and 30 to 45 min after the injection of carrageenin in the plantar region of the right hind limb. Note the enhancement of responses from both hindlimbs and the appearance of responses from both forelimbs (*arrows* as in Figs. 1 and 2).

scale as the clinical signs of acute inflammation such as edema and hyperalgesia (23–25).

As expected, the enhancement of the responses was mainly of those elicited from the injected paw. This is likely to reflect the peripheral phenomena of sensitization, well demonstrated after heat injury in varous animal species (for recent studies, see refs. 3,6,17) including man (for recent references, see refs. 1,17,22) and induced by the release of substances in the inflammatory exudate. It seems that in carrageenin inflammation these substances are likely to be mainly prostaglandins (PGE_2 and prostacyclin PGI_2), thromboxanes, and leukotrenes (13,14,16). They probably enhance the action of algogenic substances such as bradykinin, also contained in the exudate (for references, see ref. 13). This has been demonstrated electrophysiologically for some peripheral afferents since responses of cutaneous thin afferent fibers to bradykinin and heat are enhanced by prostaglandin (PGE_2) (11).

Recent data demonstrate a clear lowering of the threshold repsonse to mechanical stimuli of thin joint capsule afferents, either in the inflamed ankle of arthritic rats (9) or in the carrageenin-injected knee of cats (4). There is also the very well-known phenomena of hyperalgesia where inflamed areas become very sensitive to light touch. Therefore, since responses of non-nociceptive neurons were not enhanced (see above), a clear shift in the threshold response of nociceptive neurons to mechanical stimulus is likely. Slight modifications in the mechanical threshold cannot be totally excluded but the facts that it was necessary to apply an *intense mechanical stimulus* to drive these N neurons and that a gentle touch with a brush or a cotton was always ineffective (during our observation period) argues for no important change. It is therefore possible that other neurons not activated before inflammation, but relatively easily driven after, could be responsible for the lowered threshold for pain sensation or nociceptive manifestations observed in humans (12,13) and in animals (25) following touch of an inflamed area. Such a suggestion is indirectly supported by previous data obtained from recordings in thalamus and cortex in arthritic animals where we have found numerous neurons easily driven by moderate stimulation of the inflamed paws (7,15,18).

That these recordings were performed under anesthesia may explain the lack of modification of the mechanical threshold, yet the threshold to heat stimulation was lowered by 4° C. Interestingly, the temperature value observed in this study for the response elicited from the injured paw, is similar to that reported to be painful when immersing sunburnt areas in warm water (12,13). In addition, a dissociation between the changes of threshold response to both modalities has also been observed for peripheral fibers after a local injury (2,5). Moreover, the dissociation that we observed at the thalamic level could reflect the wide-range sensitivity of peripheral nociceptors (2) (for recent references, see refs. 1,3,6,17,22) and the fact that their reactivity after an injury is also very variable, some being sensitized, some being depressed or even both (for references, see refs. 1,3,17,22 and ref. 6 for the rat).

Two other unexpected findings of this study were the enhancement of responses elicited from part of the RF remote to the injected site, and the appearance of new responses from distant areas from which it was initially impossible to drive the neurons. This suggests the involvement of facilitatory central mechanisms which could take place at the spinal and/or at the thalamic level. Although participation of some arousal phenomena cannot be totally discarded, arousal was not observed on the ECoG recording which was closely monitored during the study. These phenomena can be related to those reported by Woolf (26) who described an increase in the excitability of a flexion reflex of the hind limb contralaterally to a local injury in the rat. The results also raise the question of distant secondary hyperalgesia studied in humans by Hardy et al. (12) after a local injury produced by prolonged thermal irradiation. They observed that the pain threshold in zones of secondary hyperalgesia was unaltered for both mechanical and thermal stimuli.

The neuronal mechanisms, peripheral and central, that may be responsible for the changes triggered by the local inflammation, require further investigations.

REFERENCES

1. Adriaensen, H., Gybels, J., Handwerker, H. O., and Van Hees, J. (1983): Response properties of thin myelinated (Aδ) fibers in human skin nerves. *J. Neurophysiol.,* 49:111–121.
2. Bessou, P., and Perl, E. R. (1969): Response of cutaneous sensory units with unmyelinated fibers to noxious stimuli. *J. Neurophysiol.,* 32:1025–1043.
3. Campbell, J. N., and Meyer, R. A. (1983): Sensitization of non-myelinated nociceptive afferents in Monkey varies with skin type. *J. Neurophysiol.,* 49:98–110.
4. Coggeshall, R. E., Hong, K. A. P., Langford, L. A., Schaible, H. G., and Schmidt, R. F. (1983): Discharge characteristics of fine medial articular afferents at rest and during passive movements of inflamed knee joints. *Brain Res.,* 224:185–188.
5. Fitzgerald, M., and Lynn, B. (1977): The sensitization of high thresholds mechanoreceptors with myelinated axons by repeated heating. *J. Physiol. (Lond.),* 365:549–563.
6. Fleischer, E., Handwerker, H. O., and Youkhadar, S. (1983): Unmyelinated nociceptive units in two skin areas of the rat. *Brain Res.,* 267:81–92.
7. Gautron, M., and Guilbaud, G. (1982): Somatic responses of ventrobasal thalamic neurones in polyarthritic rats. *Brain Res.,* 237:459–471.
8. Guilbaud, G., Gautron, M., Benoist, J. M., and Kayser, V. (1983): Characteristics of some ventrobasal thalamic neurons in polyarthritic rats. Effects of acute injection of Aspirin in neuronal responses to joint stimulation. In: *Advances in Pain Research and Therapy, Vol. 5,* edited by John J. Bonica et al., pp. 393–400. Raven Press, New York.
9. Guilbaud, G., Iggo, A., and Tegner, R. (1985): Sensory receptors in ankle joint capsule of normal and arthritic rats. *Exp. Brain Res.,* 58:29–40.
10. Guilbaud, G., Peschanski, M., Gautron, M., and Binder, D. (1980): Neurones responding to noxious stimulation in VB complex and caudal adjacent regions in the thalamus of the rat. *Pain,* 8:303–318.
11. Handwerker, H. O. (1976): Influences of algogenic substances and prostaglandins on the discharges of unmyelinated cutaneous nerve fibers identified as nociceptors. In: *Advances in Pain Research and Therapy, Vol. 1,* edited by J. J. Bonica and D. Albe-Fessard, pp. 41–46. Raven Press, New York.
12. Hardy, J. D., Wolff, H. G., and Goodell, H. (1952): *Pain Sensations and Reactions.* Williams & Wilkins, Baltimore.

13. Higgs, G. A., and Moncada, S. (1983): Interactions of Arachidonate products with other pain mediators. In: *Advances in Pain Research and Therapy, Vol. 5,* edited by John J. Bonica et al., pp. 617–626. Raven Press, New York.
14. Higgs, G. A., and Salmon, J. A. (1979): Cyclo-oxygenase products in carrageenin-induced inflammation. *Prostaglandins,* 17:737–746.
15. Kayser, V., and Guilbaud, G. (1984): Further evidence for changes in the responsiveness of somatosensory neurones in arthritic rats: a study of the posterior intralaminar region of the thalamus. *Brain Res.,* 323:144–147.
16. Koshihara, Y., Nagasaki, I., and Murota, S. I. (1981): Reduction of slow reacting substance in rat granulomatous inflammation. *Biochem. Pharmacol.,* 30:1781–1783.
17. Lamotte, R. H., Thalhammer, J. G., and Robinson, C. J. (1983): Peripheral neural correlates and magnitude of cutaneous pain and hyperalgesia: a comparison of neural events in monkey with sensory judgements in human. *J. Neurophysiol.,* 50:1–26.
18. Lamour, Y., Guilbaud, G., and Willer, J. C. (1983): Altered properties and laminar distribution of neuronal responses to peripheral stimulation in the SmI cortex of the arthritic rat. *Brain Res.,* 273:183–187.
19. Menétrey, D., and Besson, J. M. (1982): Electrophysiological characteristics of dorsal horn cells in rats with cutaneous inflammation resulting from chronic arthritis. *Pain,* 13:343–364.
20. Peschanski, M., Guilbaud, G., Gautron, M., and Besson, J. M. (1980): Encoding of noxious heat messages in neurons of the ventrobasal thalamic complex of the rat. *Brain Res.,* 197:401–413.
21. Roch-Arveiller, M., Dunn, C. J., and Giroud, J. P. (1977): Comparaison des propriétés inflammatoires des fractions λ et α de carragénine. *J. Pharmacol. (Paris),* 8:461–476.
22. Torebjörk, H. E., Lamotte, R. H., and Robinson, C. J. (1984): Peripheral neural correlates and magnitude of cutaneous pain and hyperalgesia: simultaneous recordings in human of sensory judgements of pain and evoked responses in nociceptors with C-fibers. *J. Neurophysiol.,* 51:325–339.
23. Vinegar, R., Schreiber, W., and Hugo, R. (1969): Biphasic development of carrageenin oedema in Rat. *J. Pharmacol. Exp. Ther.,* 166:96–103.
24. Willoughby, D. A., and Dieppe, P. (1976): Antiinflammatory models in animals. *Agents Actions,* 6:306–312.
25. Winter, C. A., and Flataker, L. (1965): Reactions thresholds to pressure in oedematous hind paws of rats responses to analgesics drugs. *J. Pharmacol. Exp. Ther.,* 150:165–171.
26. Woolf, C. J. (1983): Evidence for a central component of post-injury pain hypersensitivity. *Nature,* 306:686–688.

Advances in Pain Research and Therapy, Vol. 9, edited by H. L. Fields et al. Raven Press, New York © 1985.

Evoked Cerebral Potential and Pain

Burkhart Bromm

Institute of Physiology, University Hospital Eppendorf, 2000 Hamburg 20, Federal Republic of Germany

One of the most critical aspects in the investigation of pain is its quantitative documentation. Pain is a subjective experience and, on the grounds of its large emotional component, it is quite dependent on the conditions of the person being affected. But, pain is also a consequence of the activation of nociceptive afferent, and neural activity produced by nociceptive stimuli can be measured with the methods commonly applied in sensory physiology. One of these physiological measures is the cerebral potential. The appearance of an evoked cerebral potential gives evidence that the specific sensory system investigated does receive the applied stimulus transmitting the activated peripheral impulse pattern towards the brain. We all are familiar with the clinical usefulness of the visual, the auditory, or the somatosensory evoked cerebral potential especially in the diagnosis of pathological alterations of the sensory channel examined. This chapter deals with new approaches to the assessment of pain by means of evoked cerebral potential measurements.

Evoked cerebral potentials are usually divided into early and late components, which are denoted by their polarity (P:positive; N:negative), and latency (in msec) after stimulus onset. The early components with peak latencies of, e.g., less than 80 msec (depending on the stimulus) are often interpreted as summated postsynaptic potentials of cortical neuron, occurring synchronously with the arrival of the nervous impulse pattern activated by the stimulus (for review, see, e.g., ref. 26). The late potentials can best be recorded over the vertex. They are supposed to coincide with secondary processing of the received information, such as stimulus recognition, magnitude estimation, or the cortical initiation of a movement in response to the event. Therefore, the late components depend on many facts, such as attention and distraction, the vigilance level of the subject investigated, the stimulus expectancy, among many other sources of distortion (for review, see, e.g., refs. 47,67,94). As long as the localization of the generators responsible for these potentials remains uncertain, in the following the more general expression cerebral or brain potential instead of cortical potential is recommended, abbreviated with EP.

In clinical applications of EP measurements, normally only early responses of the fastest conducting myelinated nerve fibers are determined. These Aα and Aβ fibers project information to the brain with conduction velocities for 50 m/sec or more. Thus, the early components are expected to appear with latencies of some 10 msec, depending on the body site stimulated. These components are highly reliable under repeated stimulation with considerably low interindividual variance in healthy subjects (54,75). Pain, in contrast, is transmitted through slowly conducting peripheral axons, Aδ and C fibers. So we can deduce that experimental pain stimuli evoke cerebral potentials with latencies ranging up to several hundred milliseconds or even up to seconds. And here we meet the problem: Pain-related components should emerge in a latency range, in which the late (secondary) cerebral potentials in response to simultaneously coactivated fast-conducting fibers are expected to appear. Therefore, we have to specify several marginal conditions which must be fulfilled in order to conclude that cerebral potentials quantify experimentally induced pain as well as pain relief under analgesic treatments.

This introduction may be concluded with a basic assertion: Experimentally induced pain in a laboratory setting differs fundamentally from pain as seen by the clinician. The experimental pain stimulus can always be discontinued. The subjects are informed about the experimental procedure, and are often interested in the success of the experiment. This leads to a predominantly rational component, so what we measure in the pain laboratory, is the sensory-discriminative component of pain, following the nomenclature of Melzack (88). This component with its clearly lemniscal involvement can well be scaled, and can be correlated with different nociceptive reactions. In contrast, a patient's pain is essentially characterized by an aversive-emotional component which is much more difficult to measure. This differentiation, however, is no restriction in pain research: Most of us are convinced that in most cases the occurrence of pain has a source somewhere in the nociceptive pathways including central centers of pain processing. In other words, clinical pain, with its aversive component, depends on the sensory input. Thus, the two components are not independent. Furthermore, new techniques are being developed which compare chronic pain with experimental test pain by, e.g., multidimensional scaling, by cross-modality matching, or by the measurement of EP modulations (for review, see refs. 6,89).

THE PAIN STIMULUS

The evoked cerebral potential is an assessment of phasic pain as the reaction to a distinct, sharp stimulus event. The onset of nociceptor activation has to be delimited accurately, for example, by sufficiently brief and strong stimuli. Furthermore, the late cerebral potentials exhibit a strong variance from trial to trial in response to each stimulus; repeated measurements are therefore necessary. As such, the experimental pain stimulus should be easily reproducible, certainly painful, but barely noxious in order to avoid severe tissue damage. Heating the skin by long lasting radiation (e.g., refs. 61,113) or by thermodes (e.g., refs. 91,97), the cold pressor test (e.g., refs. 78,117), the tourniquet-exercise method (ischemia pain; e.g., refs. 3,42,87), chemically induced pain (e.g., refs. 83,100), or the application of long-lasting mechanical pressure (e.g., refs. 1,84,118)—none of these stimuli can be applied in the same subject sufficiently often for response averaging. Moreover, the moment of pain onset is rather uncertain. For these reasons, most pain laboratories involved in EP measurements prefer short electrical or mechanical skin stimuli applied to various body sites, electrical tooth-pulp stimulation, or, most recently, short radiant heat pulses emitted by the CO_2 laser.

Figure 1 collects examples of somatosensory evoked potentials in response to all those kinds of stimuli usually applied in pain research. All

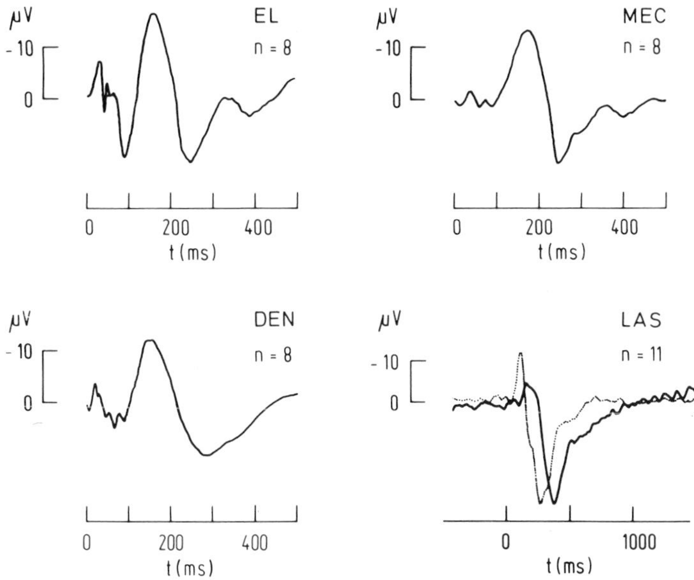

FIG. 1. Evoked cerebral potentials under various pain stimuli (grand means). EPs evoked by 4 stimulus qualities were compared in a sample of subjects (*n*). Stimulus duration was constantly 20 msec, and interstimulus intervals ranged between 20 and 40 sec in all experiments. Different intensities between 0.5- and twofold pain threshold were randomly applied, each intensity 40 times. EPs were recorded from the vertex (Cz) against linked earlobes, and grand means were averaged over all subjects. EL: electrical skin stimuli (left middle finger tip; 2, 4, 6, 8 mA). MEC: mechanical skin stimuli (left middle finger nail; 0.8, 1.6, 2.4, 3.2 Newton, 1.2 mm probe diameter). DEN: electrical tooth-pulp stimuli (upper incisor; electrically insulated electrode; 12, 16, 20, 24 μA). LAS: CO_2 laser skin stimuli (hand back; 13 W, 5.3 mm diameter). (From ref. 7, with permission.)

traces represent grand means, averaged over the numbers of subjects given in the insets; several subjects experienced all four kinds of pain stimuli within the same session. The intensity of each stimulus quality varied in the same way between half- and twofold the mean pain threshold, thus, these grand means reflect comparable degrees of painfulness. Electrical tooth-pulp stimuli have been used, for example, by Spreng and Ichioka (104), Chatrian et al. (39,40), Sano (101), Harkins and Chapman (64), Chapman et al. (33–35,38), Chen et al. (41), Benedetti et al. (4), David et al. (46), and Bromm (7). Cerebral potentials in response to electrical skin stimuli have been investigated in particular by Sitaram et al. (103), Buchsbaum and Davis (19), Buchsbaum et al. (20–22), Bromm and Scharein (12,13), Bromm et al. (10), and Bromm and Meier (9). Mechanically elicited evoked potentials have been reported, for example, by Johnson et al. (73), Stowell (105–107), Pratt et al. (95), and by Bromm and Scharein (12). The CO_2 laser heat pulse has been applied in man especially by Carmon and co-workers (28–31), Kenton et al. (77), and by Bromm and his group (7,11,15; see also below).

There is a remarkable congruence in the grand mean evoked potentials, whether they are elicited by electrical (EL) or mechanical skin stimuli (MEC), or by electrical dental stimuli (DEN). Differences due to the different kinds of stimuli appear in the early components with peak latencies of less than 80 msec, but these early components have not been evaluated systematically in pain research (for review, see ref. 44). All the late potentials can roughly be described by a vertex positivity at approximately 80 msec after stimulus application, the so-called P80, followed by a distinct negativity between 120 and 200 msec (N150), a further positivity between 200 and 400 msec (P250) and, occasionally, a second negativity at the end of the waveform. Whereas mechanical and electrical skin stimuli produce very similar late potentials (12), the EPs due to laser and tooth-pulp stimuli are somewhat delayed. In the case of laser stimuli this delay has been proven to be due to the preferential activation of slowly conducting nerves (see below). It seems interesting that the late EP components in response to dental stimuli are never shifted towards shorter peak latencies, though the conduction distance is much smaller when stimulus site changed from the finger tip to the tooth pulp. With experiments in the same subjects we found no significant latency change of the N150 peak, whereas the positivity at 250 msec under electrical stimuli was shifted to peak latencies of 290 msec in response to dental stimuli. This shift in the late P250, however, can only be observed if the stimulus electrode is electrically well isolated from the surrounding periodontium (cf., refs. 39,85). Obviously the peripheral fiber spectrum activated by tooth-pulp stimuli is different with respect to mean conduction velocity from that mediating electrical skin stimuli.

In the following, data obtained by two stimulus qualities are presented: It is the short noncontact radiant heat pulse, emitted by the CO_2 laser; this stimulus will be described in the last paragraph. The second stimulus is the intracutaneous electrical shock (for detail see ref. 9), which can easily be applied and which elicits highly reliable pain reactions. It is based on the very reproducible electrical skin shock. But the transition resistance between electrode and afferent nerve fiber to be activated is drastically reduced by drilling a small hole into the epidermis under the stimulus electrode in a standardized way. With this skin preparation, the threshold intensities for stimulus detection and pain sensation were lowered by a factor of about 10. The elicited sensation is very different from the paresthesia evoked by conventional skin shocks; it is described as a stabbing hot and sharp pain.

One essential requirement, which was often neglected in algesimetric studies, shall be explained here in more detail: It is the necessity to randomize both the stimulus intervals and stimulus intensities. With intensity randomization, matching unpredictably between nonpain and pain, the arousal state of the subject is kept high and constant (13). Each stimulus is then expected by the subject as potentially painful. The essential influence of the mode of stimulus application on EP form is illustrated by Fig. 2. The subject

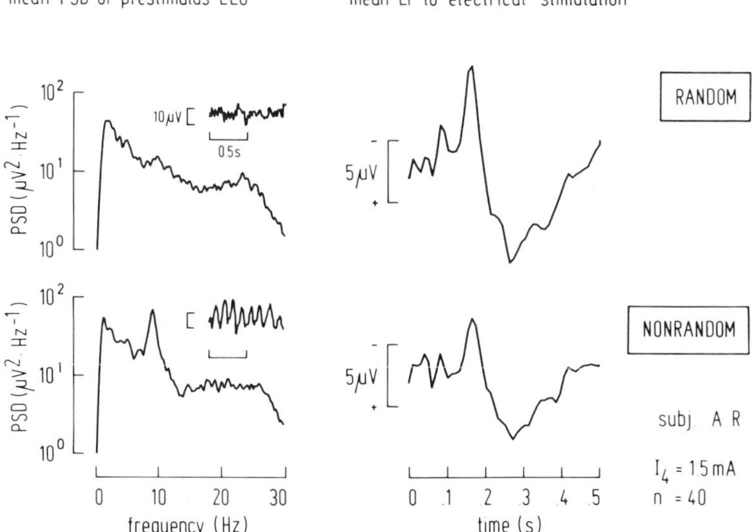

FIG. 2. Effect of intensity randomization upon the evoked cerebral potential. One hundred and sixty intracutaneous stimuli (20 msec; finger tip) were applied with 4 different intensities related to the individual pain threshold Io = 0.46 mA ± 0.03 mA. Each intensity appeared 40 times with randomized interstimulus intervals between 12 and 30 sec. Below intensities were given as a subsequent train: 40 × I1, . . ., 40 × I4. Above intensity itself was randomized, as such the strongest stimuli appeared unpredictably within the total of 160. To the right: evoked potentials averaged over the 40 strongest stimuli I4 = 1.5 mA. To the left: power spectral density functions (Fourier-transformation) of the 5-sec EEG segments immediately before the stimulus was applied. Vertex leads; upward deflection denotes negativity. Subject A. R.; 2 sessions on different days.

had experienced intracutaneous electrical stimuli of 4 intensities; only the results with the strongest intensity are shown. Monotonous stimulation was performed in one session (lower). In another session, the 4 intensities were given in a random order (upper); as such the strongest stimuli appeared 40 times within a total of 160 stimuli of different intensities, alternating unpredictably between prepain and pain.

Though stimulus intensity, number of repetitions, and interstimulus intervals were comparable, the different mode of stimulus application led to very different evoked potential waveforms. The amplitudes of the late potentials were drastically reduced when stimuli were applied in a monotonous intensity sequence. The pain ratings decreased likewise. In the left side of Fig 2, power spectral density functions of the EEG segments preceding each stimulus are given. Under randomized intensities there was a desynchronous EEG with high frequencies and low amplitudes like that shown in the inset (above). In case of monotonous stimulation (below) there was a dominant peak in the 10 Hz frequency range; this means a marked α-rhythm. This experiment proves the essential influence of the mode of stimulus application as well as a possible dependence of late EP amplitudes on prestimulus EEG activity.

For these reasons all our experiments were performed with randomized intensity sequences causing unpredictably nonpain and pain sensations. We prefer 4 intensities, related to the individual pain threshold strength with 2 intensities being below and 2 in the pain range, each intensity appearing 40 times with interstimulus intervals between 15 and 30 sec, each session lasting between 60 and 90 min. The prestimulus EEG is an important means for vigilance control during long-lasting sessions.

MULTIVARIATE STATISTICAL APPROACHES TO PAIN-EVOKED CEREBRAL POTENTIALS

As pointed out, the late cerebral potentials considered in pain research are nonspecific. They are rather similar whether elicited by various somatosensory stimuli (Fig. 1), or by acoustical or visual stimulation (e.g., refs. 57,68). Their amplitudes depend, among other conditions, on stimulus intensity and, therefore, correlate with pain, because of the well-known fact that the stronger the stimulus the greater the probability to produce pain. But, no component of the late EP is pain-specific in the sense that it appears only if pain is felt. Therefore, simply measuring amplitudes or amplitude differences of these late potentials is a heuristic phenomenological approach and does not yield a direct estimate of pain intensity.

One experimental attempt to look for pain-specific alterations in the evoked potential, are investigations in which different kinds of noxious stimuli are applied alternately in the same session (12). Another recent statistical assessment of pain-related components is the application of multivariate procedures, factor analysis, or principal component analysis (PCA). By means of PCA the cerebral potentials are decomposed into a small number of statistically uncorrelated basic waveforms, the principal components (PCs), which account for as much as possible of total variance in the EP recordings. As shown, e.g., by Suter (108), Horst and Donchin (69), or by Johnston and Holcomb (74), principal components in the cerebral potential vary with stimulus conditons. Even changes in the meaning of a word in different context seems to influence single components in the late EPs (16). Comparison of cerebral potentials evoked by painful and nonpainful electrical and mechanical skin stimuli by PCA resulted especially in two principal components (PC2 with a maximum at 150 msec, and PC4 between 260 and 360 msec), the scores of which reflected significantly the degree of painfulness reported by the subject (12). Therefore, these multivariate procedures become of increasing interest in the analysis of pain-induced changes in the electroencephalogram, as well as in attempts to document analgesic effects.

Figure 3 illustrates the procedure with an example of 300 evoked potentials measured with the intracutaneous stimuli in a sample of 15 subjects (above left). The signal was sampled with 100 Hz yielding 50 time points within the 500 msec analysis period. Thus, the data matrix consisted of 300 × 50 elements. From the data matrix, various association matrices can be constructed, by building the cross-products between pairs of columns (above, right), the variances-covariances (below, left), or the correlation coefficients (below, right). The next step in PCA is the solution of the eigenvalue-problem of the association matrices (for detail, see ref. 50), the principal components being proportional to the 50 (not necessarily different) eigenvectors. We preferred the variance-covariance matrix for the further analysis (for detail, see ref. 12). In general, the extraction of 4 to 8 PCs was found to be sufficient for further analysis. In a third step the PCs are rotated to yield simply structured basic waveforms in the time domain (varimax rotation; see ref. 76). In a last step all measured evoked potentials are recalculated from the extracted PCs by determining the degree to which each component is involved in each cerebral potential (component scores).

Meanwhile several investigations dealing with EPs and pain utilized PCA (for review, see ref. 6). Chapman and Jacobson (36), for example, investigated the phenomenon that, with decreasing interstimulus interval correlations between evoked potential amplitudes and pain ratings vanish. The data set, obtained by varying both stimulus intensity and rate of stimulation over trials in a single experiment, was subjected to PCA. Again, this procedure produced a set of components. Regression techniques were employed to determine which components correlated with intensity, and which with rate parameters. Those that were significantly correlated with stimulus intensities were combined, and this combination could be displayed as one waveform, i.e., an intensity waveform. Correspondingly, those components

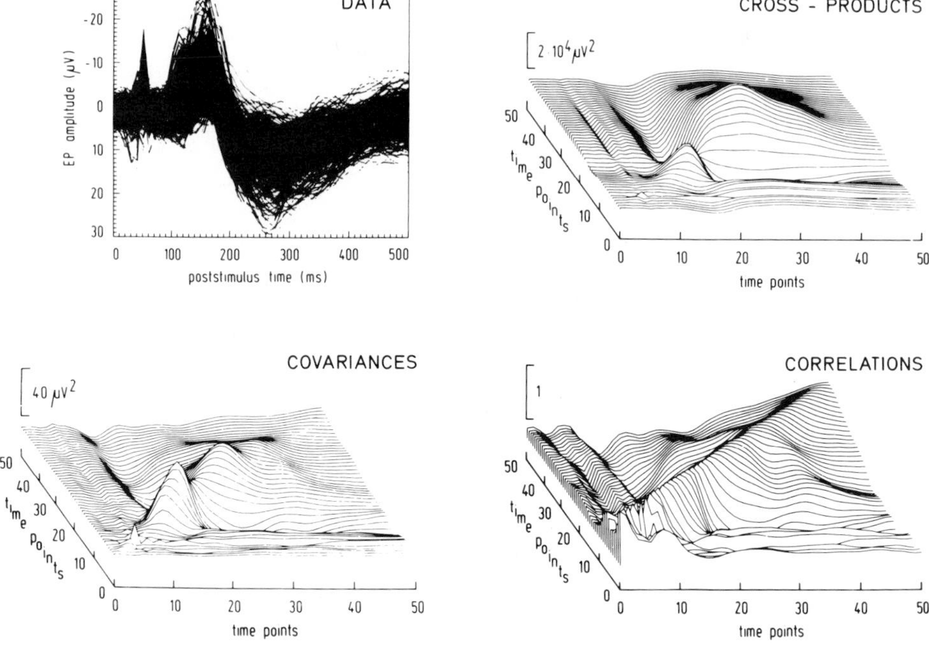

FIG. 3. Data and association matrices of averaged EPs in response to electrical skin stimuli. Data matrix was built from 300 EP measurements (EP averages over 40 stimulus repetitions: 4 intensities, 5 sessions, 15 subjects). Each EP consists of 50 time points in the matrix arranged as a row and plotted as function of time. The 3 most convenient association matrices are calculated, again ordered as function of the 50 time points. The 50 rows are plotted in case of the cross-product matrix **(above right),** the variance-covariance matrix **(below left),** and the correlation matrix **(below right).**

correlating with the stimulus rate were combined to produce a rate waveform. Comparison of the intensity and rate waveforms revealed a small but significant difference in the effects of these two manipulations at the N150 peak, with the stimulus intensity waveform peaking earlier and having a smaller magnitude of effect than the rate waveform (71a). These outcomes were interpreted by the authors that the brain shows a differential response to stimulus intensity and stimulus rate variation.

PCA was furthermore applied to studies dealing with evoked potentials under analgesics. Strong narcotics like pethidine (Dolantin®), or tilidine (Valoron®) have been shown to influence remarkably the scores of the two pain-related components PC2 and PC4. Figure 4 gives one example. Pure tilidine (orally administered, 100 mg) was applied together in different combinations of tilidine and naloxone in a placebo-controlled double-blind study (for detail, see ref. 10). Figure 4 represents (left) the 6 most important

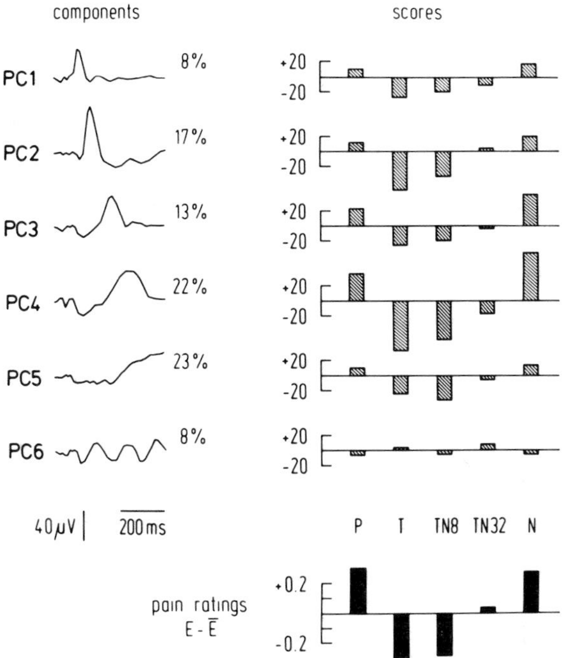

FIG. 4. Principal components and component scores under analgesic treatments. The data matrix (given in Fig. 3) with 300 EPs (averages over 40 stimulus repetitions: 4 intensities, 5 sessions, 15 subjects) was subjected to PCA. The extracted PCs **(left)** ordered with respect to their peak latencies, accounted for about 90% of total variance (as indicated in the *insets*). To the **right** the mean scores of the 6 principal components are built for the different treatments: P, placebo; T, tilidine 100 mg; TN8, tilidine 100 mg + naloxone 8 mg; TN32, tilidine 100 mg + naloxone 32 mg; N, naloxone 32 mg. Below the deviation of pain ratings E from the grand mean values E are given for each treatment. Negative deviations denote decreases in pain. (Modified from ref. 7, with permission.)

PCs which accounted for about 90% of total variance of the whole data set. The bars (right) indicate the component scores averaged over subjects and stimulus intensities, separately for the 5 treatments, describing the degree to which each PC is influenced by the specific drug. In the lowest line the mean pain ratings are given as deviations from the grand mean obtained from all subjects and sessions. As shown in the figure, the component scores varied systematically with the treatments applied. Especially the scores of the components PC2 and PC4 exhibited a significant downward deviation, if the treatment resulted in pain relief (expressed by the downward deflections in the pain ratings, lowest line). As such, replacing simple amplitude measures by PCA may be able to improve the sensitivity and specificity of pharmacological tests by EP measurements.

THE EVOKED CEREBRAL POTENTIAL IN THE FREQUENCY DOMAIN

By definition the evoked cerebral potential is the stimulus-induced change in the electroencephalogram. Thus we have to observe the activity in the ongoing EEG. However, prestimulus-poststimulus relationships are lost if the stimulus-induced changes are averaged, as is usually done to improve the signal-to-noise ratio. Therefore, we prefer the analysis of single trial registrations in the assessment of analgesic effects on pain-related cerebral potentials. Figure 5 illustrates an experiment with the intracutaneous pain stimulus and randomized intensities: 160 single trial EEG records are given, consisting of a prestimulus segment of 500 msec (PRE), followed by the segment immediately after stimulus application (POST1), and 500 msec later (POST2). The stimulus-induced change can clearly be seen in all single trials: the negativity at 150 msec followed by the positivity between 200 msec and 300 msec.

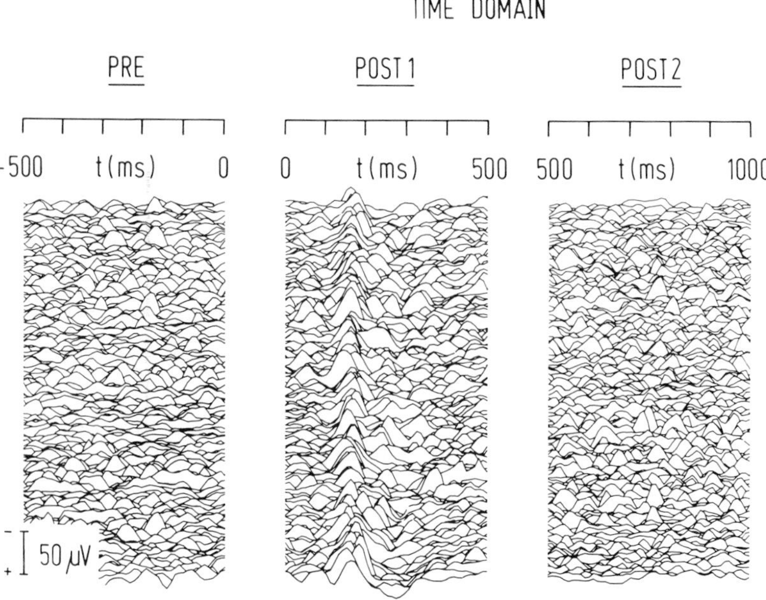

FIG. 5. Single-trial evoked cerebral potentials in the time domain. EEG segments of 500 msec duration before the stimulus **(left:** PRE), immediately after stimulus application (**middle:** POST1), and 500 msec later (**right:** POST2) for 160 stimulus events; records containing artifacts were removed. Read the plots from below upwards. The stimuli followed the randomized sequence described in the text, with two intensities being in the pain range and two below individual pain threshold. In most single trial records distinct evoked potentials can be observed with a negativity at about 150 msec (N150) and a later positivity between 200 and 300 msec (P250) after stimulus onset. There is a remarkable latency jittering between trials. Subject J. T.; vertex versus linked ear lobes. (From B. Bromm and E. Scharein, *unpublished observations.*)

The activity of the spontaneous electroencephalogram is commonly described by the spectral power in the classic frequency bands. Since in evoked potential measurements analysis periods of only 500-msec duration are taken into account, new spectral estimators had to be adapted. The Fourier transformation renders an insufficient frequency resolution for only half-second-lasting EEG segments. Best success has been achieved by utilizing parametric estimators, like the autoregressive (AR) or autoregressive moving average filters (ARIMA), or the maximum entropy method (MEM). These filters yield power density functions by modeling the data generating process. The maximum entropy method enables the investigation of prestimulus-poststimulus-EEG relationships in the frequency domain (for detail, see ref. 102). Figure 6 describes the same segments, transformed into the frequency domain by means of MEM. The ongoing EEG (in the period PRE) exhibits a typical activity with some peaks in the α, β, and δ bands. In the POST1 periods, the stimulus-induced change in EEG activity impresses most of all by an immense increase in the δ-peak, followed by a second peak in the θ range. Though this is the usual nomenclature, it seems questionable

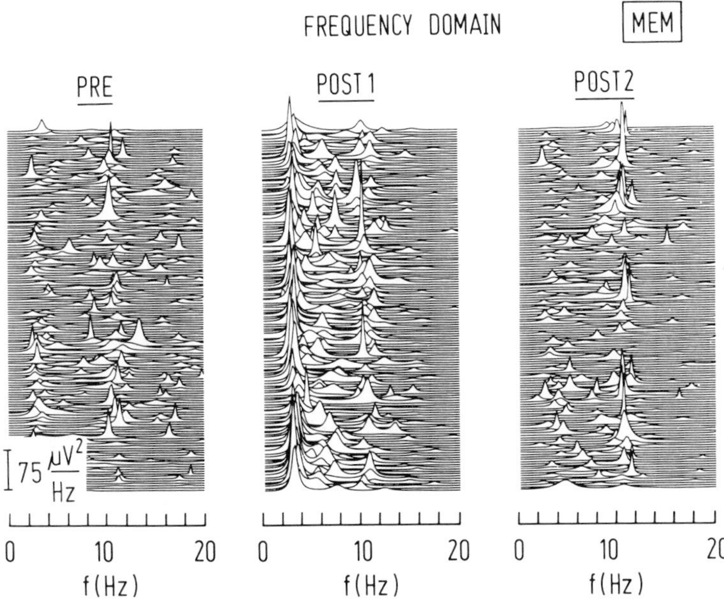

FIG. 6. Single-trial evoked cerebral potentials in the frequency domain, estimated by MEM. Spectra of the above given EEG segments (before stimulus: PRE; immediately after stimulus application: POST1; 500 msec later: POST2) were built for all 160 stimulus events, using the maximum entropy method (MEM) with an order of 20. Read the plots from below upwards. In the prestimulus segments typical EEGs appear with mixed δ-, α-, and β-frequencies. Due to the stimulus a large peak emerges in the δ-band (1–4 Hz), often followed by a second one in the θ-band (4–8 Hz). Furthermore, a considerable synchronization of α waves is seen, which lasts into the POST2-period. Subject J. T.; vertex versus linked ear lobes. (From B. Bromm and E. Scharein, *unpublished observations.*)

to transfer this classification on the spectra of evoked potentials. Sometimes a stimulus-induced α synchronization can be observed, as documented by higher peaks in the 8 to 11 Hz range, even in the later periods POST2.

Whereas the single trial evoked potentials in the time domain (above) exhibit a remarkable latency jittering which modulates the mean values by broadening and amplitude reduction, the stimulus-induced peaks in the frequency domain appear rather constant. Therefore, averaging of the power spectral density functions improves the signal-to-noise ratio more than averaging in the time domain. These methods of evoked potential quantification revealed, for example, that the power in the 2 to 4 Hz frequency range is significantly correlated with the subjective pain ratings, and that it reacts highly sensitively on pain-reducing treatments (B. Bromm and E. Scharein, *unpublished observations*).

Using the intracutaneous electrical stimulus (9) with randomized intensities and interstimulus intervals, and subjecting the single trial registrations to the maximum entropy method, a new aspect to the sometimes controversal arguments about effects of weak analgesics on pain-related EPs could be added. Figure 7 illustrates effects of acetyl salicyclic acid (ASA; Aspirin, 1,000 mg), taken from a placebo-controlled study with analgesic drugs. In the placebo session (left) the stimulus-induced increase of the

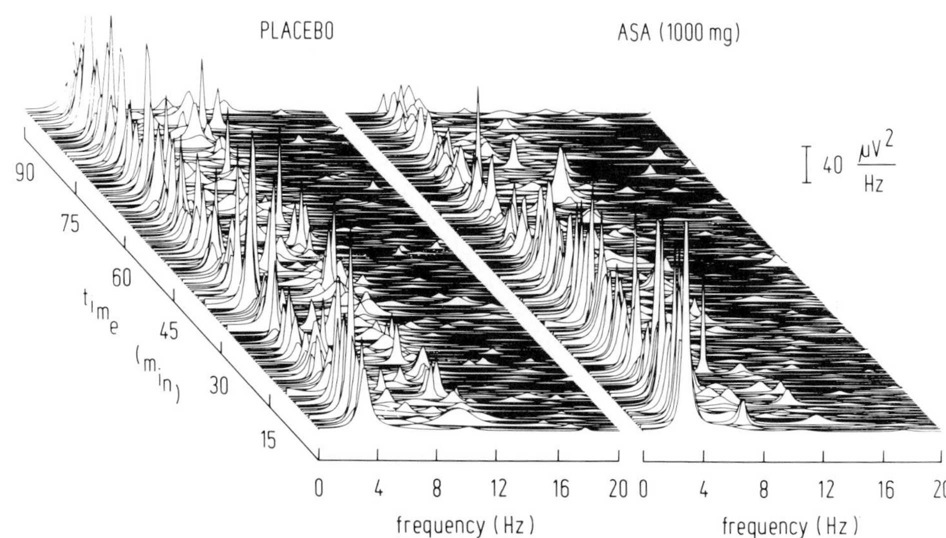

FIG. 7. Effect of acetyl salicylic acid on EP spectra. Data were obtained from a placebo session **(left)** and a session with acetyl salicylic acid (ASA, Aspirin, 1,000 mg; **right**). Drugs were orally applied immediately before data sampling; 240 stimuli were given in randomized order with interstimulus intervals between 12 and 30 sec. Read the graphs from below upwards. The power density functions were calculated by the maximum entropy method (MEM, model order 20). Under placebo, the spectra of the evoked cerebral potentials were remarkably stable during the entire session. In response to the weak analgesic, the power in the 2 to 4 Hz range was drastically reduced. Subject A. R.; vertex versus linked ear lobes. (From B. Bromm, W. Meier, and E. Scharein, *unpublished observations*.).

power in the 2 to 4 Hz frequency range was remarkably constant throughout the entire course of stimulation, proving the reliability of the pain stimulus applied. When looking at the variations of the power spectra in response to the stimuli it may be recalled that intensity was randomized. In contrast, in the presence of ASA (Fig. 7, right) the peaks in the 2 to 4 Hz frequency range decreased significantly in the course of the experiment.

As already mentioned under Fig. 6, the power spectral density functions of the stimulus-induced changes in the EEG can be averaged, proving the clear and significant decrease in the power under ASA. Effects of this magnitude could not be stated with security, when averaging cerebral potentials in the time domain and evaluating amplitudes or amplitude differences of all late evoked potential components. As such, we recommend the experimental and evaluation procedures described here, especially in attempts to document effects of so-called weak analgesics.

MAPPING OF EVOKED CEREBRAL POTENTIALS

Whereas all investigations described above are based on single-electrode recordings from the vertex, in the following some new results using multielectrode recording distributed over the scalp will be reviewed. Such procedures result in a three-dimensional topography of brain sites activated by the painful stimulus. The first attempts to study the distribution of pain-evoked potentials over the scalp were performed by Chatrian and his group (39), using electrical tooth-pulp stimulation by implanted electrodes. These experiments were performed with 20 electrodes fixed at each hemisphere; they verified that the late cerebral potentials are maximal over the vertex consisting of a negative component with latencies between 120 and 160 msec, followed by the positive half-wave with a maximum between 200 and 300 msec after stimulus onset. Since that time the value of examining scalp distributions of cerebral potentials, for the separation of different potential components, the localization of artifact sources, and for clinical applications has been well established (for review, see refs. 18,75).

Multi-lead data, however, are not easily interpreted when presented as multiple raw traces, or quantified and displayed in immense tables. Therefore, many methods have been developed in attempts to visualize the spatial features of quantified recordings, including contour plots of isopotential lines (e.g., refs. 81,82,98,115) spatio-temporal maps (99), and three-dimensional plots (43,58), or number level plots (53). Recent work has presented brain electrical activity maps in color (52), or as dot-density topograms (51).

In order to allow the comparison of scalp distribution maps with data from other techniques to localize cerebral generators, such as the ^{133}Xe blood flow, X-ray transmission tomography scans, or positron emission tomography, Buchsbaum et al. (24) described a laboratory computer system which emphasizes simplicity of data management and a mapping algorithm free of complicated assumptions. For these mappings, Buchsbaum et al. (17,22–24)

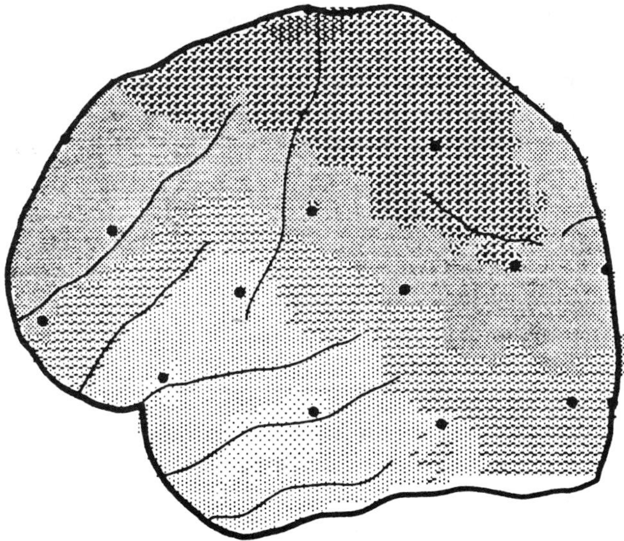

FIG. 8. Grand mean somatosensory N120 EP amplitude map for painful electrical stimuli (16 normal volunteers). Amplitude is displayed as a *light scale* with larger amplitudes as *darker shade.* Note that component is largest over central regions and diminished over frontal, temporal, and occipital regions. (From ref. 17, with permission.)

utilized, in addition to the 12 electrodes normally on the left side (10/20 system) or midline (Fz-Cz-Pz-Oz), 4 additional electrode locations to provide greater resolution of the posterior cortex. The 16 values were then used to interpolate values over the entire scalp area. In the cortical maps, EPs were first detrended using linear regression and were then digitally filtered to remove low (below 4 Hz) and high frequencies (above 30 Hz; for details, see ref. 80). Eye movements and artifacts were monitored, trials exceeding a certain noise threshold were automatically excluded from the further analysis.

Figure 8 shows the group average of scalp distributions of somatosensory evoked potentials from 16 normal volunteers. In this figure only the N120 area integration results are represented in response to electrical painful skin stimuli of 16 mA (for data measurement, see ref. 24). But the N120 and P200 peaks have a similar topographic distribution. As can be seen, the N120 complex is well reflected in the Cz (and C4) leads and its choice in pain studies appears salutary. The geometric outline of the brain is an approximately equal area projection developed from a whole-head cross-sectional atlas (24,45). It has to be noted that the results given in Fig. 8 are approximate, only 16 leads have been used, providing no more than 2 to 5-cm spatial resolution. Nevertheless, the proportional construction of the 10-20 system brings the individual variation of the brain well within this tolerance (17). Recent attempts tend to apply up to 32 leads per hemisphere.

Topographic approaches provide some validating information for EP studies, like the finding of maximal amplitudes and clearest amplitude-gradients over the somatosensory cortex. However, problems in generator localization, spatial aliasing, reference selection, interpolation methodology, anatomic accuracy, and amplitude measurement across waveforms that vary with lead placement, are but some of the technical difficulties yet to be resolved.

Several efforts have been made to determine the sites of generators responsible for the evoked cerebral potential: Measuring the magnetic counterpart of the brain's electrical activity gives additional spatial information. Neuromagnetic recordings of tooth-pulp evoked responses and somatosensory evoked responses have already yielded some interesting new data (62,63). Nuclear spin resonance spectrography promises to allow the quantification of local changes in phosphate and nitrogen metabolism concomitant with repeatedly applied pain stimuli and EP measurements (72). First results correlating EEG and NMR changes under cerebral ischemia in rats have been reported (92). Ingvar and his group investigated microcirculatory changes of the brain's blood flow and recorded the evoked potential at the same time (e.g., refs. 23,70,71).

Positron emission tomography (PET) imaging of fluorodeoxyglucose uptake has the capability of surveying functional activity throughout the brain, and thus bringing the disparate lines of neurochemical and behavioral approaches together. It has adequate resolution to view both individual gyri of the cortex and discrete portions of the basal ganglia and the limbic system (25). The metabolic information from the cortical surface may then be correlated with electrophysiological measures providing collateral localization information, and the temporal information from the EPs can enhance our ability to associate cognitive functions with metabolic increases. In the first such study of patients with visual field lesions, Celesia et al. (32) concluded that the PET-EP combination offered new insights into generator sources. A first report about the cerebral metabolic consequences of painful electrical cutaneous stimulation has appeared recently (22), and in the future these data may be correlated with the corresponding EP maps.

ULTRALATE CEREBRAL POTENTIALS AND PAIN

The EP components discussed up to now refer to analysis periods of 500 msec only. As such they can at best be related to activation of Aδ or even faster conducting nerve fibers. In the following, recent findings are summarized concerning ultralate cerebral potentials which accompany second pain.

For the investigation of delayed second burning pain, noxious thermal stimuli have usually been utilized, for example, the Hardy-Wolff-Goodell radiant heat method (61), or by means of thermodes contacting the skin (97). All of these methods cause a slow increase in cutaneous temperature until the threshold of pain-mediating afferents is reached. In man, these afferents have been determined to be polymodal unmyelinated C-nociceptors, conducting in a range of 0.5 to 2.0 m/sec (e.g., refs. 59,109,110,110a,113,114). However, with those long heat pulses activation of thermosensitive afferents appear with latencies of 250 msec and more, too long and inconstant to achieve time-locking for the early components of the stimulus evoked cerebral potential.

With the introduction of the CO_2 laser in pain research in man, concentration of thermal energy in extremely short time frames became possible (90). Noncontact high power radiant heat pulses of a very few msec duration generates a typical double pain sensation: A first pinprick pain, well localizable, is followed, with a perceivable delay, by a dull burning second component (5,11,28,30). The peripheral and central afferent systems involved in these sensations have just begun to be investigated in animals (48,55,66) and in man (8,14,27,30,77). Roughly it may be said that the first pinprick pain is due largely to activation of myelinated Aδ fibers, whereas the delayed burning pain can be attributed to slowly conducting C fibers.

Figure 9 presents a microelectroneurographic recording from a nociceptive C fiber of the radial nerve at the wrist in an awake subject. The receptive field on the back of the hand was stimulated with a strong and clearly painful radiant heat pulse, which evoked a train of action potentials. Its duration is about 200 msec and the instantaneous discharge rate may be as high as 120 spikes/sec. However, it seems to be the number of spikes evoked by a given stimulus, which correlates best with sensation intensity (8,56,60,111); this may be explained by the fact that temporal summation is necessary especially in the processing of C-fiber input. The recording demonstrates that CO_2 laser stimuli are able to elicit a short duration-high frequency afferent barrage. With conduction velocities of 0.8 m/sec the neuronal impulse pattern may reach the brain not earlier than 1 to 1.5 sec after stimulus onset.

As to the laster-induced EP, only correlates of Aδ fiber-mediated pain have been quantified in the past. Figure 10, first trace, gives an example (see also Fig. 1, LAS). The EPs of one subject are averaged over 40 painful stimuli. A peak latency of about 180 msec for the first vertex negative component was found, and about 400 msec for the main vertex positive one. This waveform has been investigated by Carmon and co-workers as pain-related

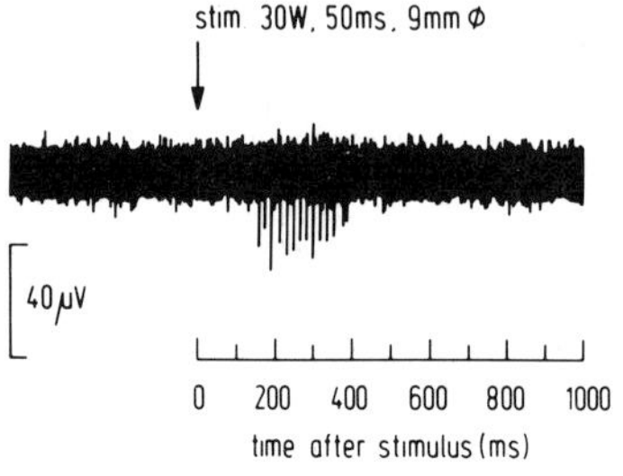

FIG. 9. Response of a single human C-nociceptor to short CO_2 laser pulse. Recordings were made in the awake volunteer, via a microelectrode into the radial nerve at the wrist. The short radiant heat pulse was applied to the corresponding receptive field (hand back), and was felt as marked burning pain. Conduction velocity was measured by electrical test stimuli at 0.83 m/sec. Such experiments indicate that the degree of pain is correlated to the length of nervous impulse train. (From ref. 14, with permission.)

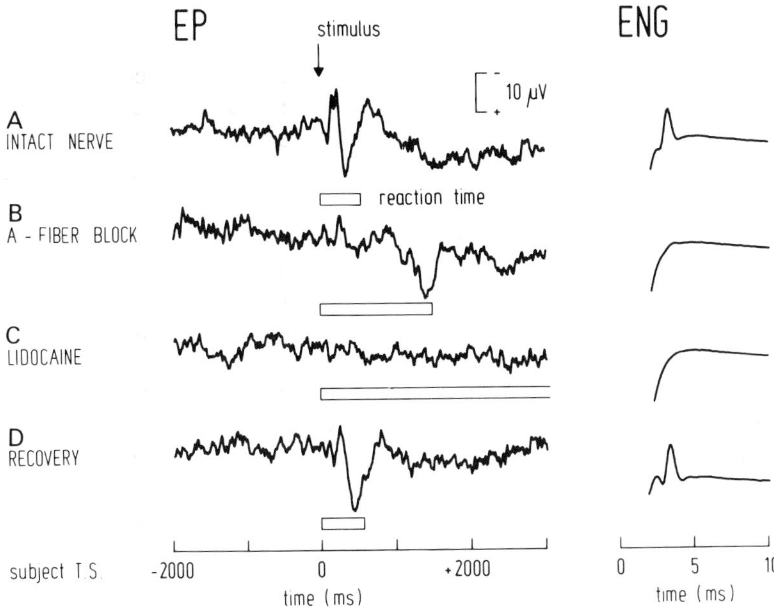

FIG. 10. Ultralate components in response to C-fiber activation, CO_2 activation. CO_2 laser stimuli (20 msec, 8 W) were applied to the hairy skin of the hand. EPs were averaged over 40 stimulus repetitions **(right).** Upward deflection denotes negativity at Cz. The *white bars* under the plots indicate the reaction times RT. **Left:** electroneurography (ENG) from the referred radialis nerve monitors A-fiber activity in response to the electrical stimuli. In **A** a typical laser-induced EP is obtained. After preferential pressure block (64 min) of the radial nerve (**B**) the ENG disappeared, as well as most of the laser EP components, and a distinct positivity at about 1,400 msec emerged. Injections of lidocaine (1%) wiped out all EP components (**C**). Release of the pressure block (**D;** 152 min after block onset) revealed recovery of ENG and EP (and sensation). Subject T. S.; vertex versus linked ear lobes. (Modified from ref. 11, with permission.)

changes in EEG. It clearly is not a C-fiber evoked response but, as shown, e.g., by Kenton et al. (77), induced by Aδ fiber activity. In the second line of Fig. 10 this A-fiber input was blocked by pressure, a commonly used method in neurophysiology (65,79,97). The build-up of the block of myelinated afferents can be monitored by intermittent electroneurography via surface electrodes, by concomitant neurological examination of cutaneous sensitivity, and by evaluation of the subject's reaction time, e.g., to press a button after stimulus perception.

In the experiment shown in Fig. 10, the A-fiber block was complete after 64 min, as can be seen by the absence of the peripheral A-fiber electroneurogram. At this state the subject's reaction time had just increased from 545 ± 16 msec to 1,497 ± 79 msec (40 stimuli). Pain had lost its stinging component, now being described as hot and burning. Under these conditions all evoked potential components, formerly correlated to Aδ fiber activity, vanished and a very late positive component became visible with peak latencies of 1,400 msec, a duration of approximately 400 msec, and a maximum peak amplitude of about 20 μV. Similar ultralate EP components were found under the same experimental conditions in 5 of the 6 volunteers investigated (for detail, see ref. 11). Blocking the remaining conductivity in C fibers by injecting lidocaine around the peripheral nerve, the ultralate potential disappeared, thus proving that these ultralate potentials were triggered by cutaneous afferents. The last trial shows that all of the reported changes were reversible.

C-fiber evoked potentials will, of course, not always be triggered by the same single unmyelinated fiber. Because of their different, slow conduction velocities a considerable latency-jittering has to be expected in C-fiber evoked cerebral potentials. Therefore, the methods of averaging, usually applied to improve the signal-to-noise ratio, cannot be used to elaborate ultralate EP components. We, therefore, again applied single trial analysis. Figure 11 gives examples of single EEG registrations, cut off for a few seconds before and after stimulus application. The two EPs without peripheral pressure block (left) exhibit very similar waveforms, which agree with the averages presented in Fig. 10 or Fig. 1, LAS; the peak latencies are almost identical. As such, an average across single trials is a good estimate for stimulus-induced changes of the electroencephalogram within 500 msec analysis periods. Surprisingly, the shape of the ultralate single trial EPs under A-fiber block (right) are also very similar to each other and, moreover, astonishingly

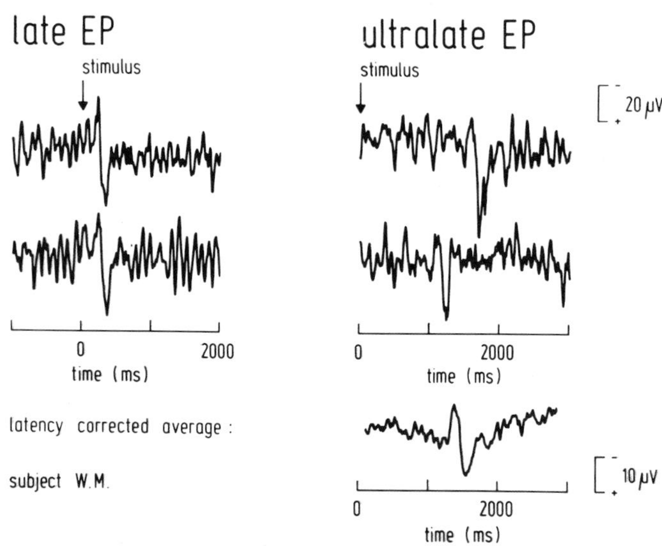

FIG. 11. CO_2 laser-induced EPs in single trials. Segments of 3-sec duration are cut out off the continuous vertex EEG recording. A painful heat pulse of 20 msec was applied to the hand back, causing pricking and burning pain, and the usual late EP components as given to the **left.** The ultralate EP components after peripheral A-fiber block **(right)** are very similar, but exhibit a strong latency jittering. The plot **(below, right)** shows averages of 15 ultralate EPs after De Weerd frequency filtering and Woody latency correction. Subject W. M.; vertex versus linked ear lobes. (From B. Bromm and R.-D. Treede, *unpublished observations.*)

similar to those given to the left. However, their latencies differ by more than the width of the evoked potentials. Thus, conventional averaging is not the appropriate procedure to investigate ultralate cerebral potentials: The single-trial-evoked potentials will then be smeared over a broad interval, as seen in Fig. 10, second line, and may even cancel each other. A better estimate of the ultralate potential waveform may be achieved by a procedure called latency corrected averaging (49,93,119). This was performed in the lowest line of Fig. 11; as a result, the shifted waveforms looked similar to the late cerebral potentials given in Fig. 10, right. As such, we have to strive for more valid evaluation procedures in looking for ultralate cerebral potentials accompanying second pain.

Under certain experimental conditions electrical stimuli are also suitable for eliciting second pain with latencies of more than 1 sec and a burning quality. Using the properties of temporal summation in the C-fiber system, Price (96) demonstrated that in case of repetitive stimulation, with a rate above 0.3 Hz and with blocked myelinated nerve fibers, electrical skin shocks are able to raise second pain, due to wind-up phenomena within the spinal cord, particularly in the dorsal grey matter (see also ref. 97). These experiments were repeated by Harkins et al. (65), who measured cerebral potentials evoked by repeated electrical skin shocks. Though these waves are barely visible in the published records, and the authors stated that they were barely able to measure them reliably, these components fit well with the ultralate EP components observed with laser stimuli.

It seems unlikely that the ultralate EP components reflect the direct arrival of neuronal activity mediated by unmeylinated fibers, in the sense of early nearfield potentials discussed above. Rather, they may more appropriately have been seen as an expression of secondary mechanisms of information processing, triggered now by the slowest conducting afferents. Therefore, these ultralate components should be considered to be a reflection of cognitive processing of sensory input, similar to the late evoked potentials. Then, of course, they are also subject to attention and distraction. This might explain why ultralate potentials have not usually been found, although the laser heat pulses activate C fibers. When stimulating the upper limb, the latency difference between first and second pain is relatively small and both sensations may apparently merge. Myelinated as well as unmyelinated nerve fibers of the nociceptive system may converge at any level of the pain-mediating system, including at the posterior horn of the segment of entry. Therefore, it is conceivable that both fiber systems are triggering the same subcortical generator responsible for the late or ultralate potentials, respectively. However, this is an hypothesis that has to be proven in further experiments.

In conclusion, quantifying C-fiber-mediated second pain is an exceedingly difficult but also important problem. Second pain is usually accompanied by autonomic nervous system reactions, by a considerable feeling of illness, and by vegetative reactions, such as nausea, sweating, and changes in blood flow. It causes an aversive emotional reaction and, in particular, that component of pain most frequently seen and treated by a physician in the clinic. The results reported here are just beginning to open another door to the electrophysiological measurement of C-fiber mediated pain. However, to separate ultralate responses in the cerebral potential from earlier ones elicited by Aβ or Aδ activity, we have to regard all the issues treated above: the ongoing EEG activity, single trial evaluation, multivariate statistical methods, and topographical analysis.

ACKNOWLEDGMENTS

The author wishes to thank Dr. M. S. Buchsbaum, Dr. C. R. Chapman, Dr. G. C. Davis, Dr. S. W. Harkins, E. Scharein, and Dr. R.-D. Treede for very helpful suggestions and criticisms in drawing up this article. This work was supported by the Deutsche Forschungsgemeinschaft (SFB 115).

REFERENCES

1. Anton, F., Kreh, A., Reeh, P. W., and Handwerker, H. O. (1984): Algesimetry using natural stimuli of long duration. In: *Pain Measurement in Man,* edited by B. Bromm, pp. 455–462. Elsevier, Amsterdam.
2. Reference deleted.
3. Beecher, H. K. (1966): Pain: One mystery solved. *Science,* 151:840–841.
4. Benedetti, C., Chapman, C. R., Colpitts, Y. H., and Chen A. C. N. (1982): Effects of nitrous oxide concentration on event-related potentials during painful tooth stimulation. *Anesthesiology,* 56:360–364.
5. Biehl, R., Treede, R.-D., and Bromm, B. (1984): Pain ratings and short radiant heat pulses. In: *Pain Measurement in Man,* edited by B. Bromm, pp. 397–408. Elsevier, Amsterdam.
6. Bromm, B. (editor) (1984): In: *Pain Measurement in Man.* Elsevier, Amsterdam.
7. Bromm, B. (1984): Pain related components in the cerebral potential. Experimental and multivariate statistical approaches. In: *Pain Measurement in Man,* edited by B. Bromm, pp. 257–290. Elsevier, Amsterdam.
8. Bromm, B., Jahnke, M. T., and Treede, R.-D. (1984): Responses of human cutaneous afferents to CO_2 laser stimuli causing pain. *Exp. Brain Res.,* 55:158–166.
9. Bromm, B., and Meier, W. (1984) The intracutaneous stimulus: A new pain model for algesimetric studies. *Methods Findings Exp. Clin. Pharmacol.,* 6(7):405–410.
10. Bromm, B., Meier, W., and Scharein, E. (1983): Antagonism between tilidine and naloxone on cerebral potentials and pain ratings in man. *Eur. J. Pharmacol.,* 87:431–440.
11. Bromm, B., Neitzel, H., Tecklenburg, A., and Treede, R.-D. (1983): Evoked cerebral potential correlates of C fibre activity in man. *Neurosci. Lett.,* 43:109–114.
12. Bromm, B., and Scharein, E. (1982): Principal component analysis of pain related cerebral potentials to mechanical and electrical stimulation in man. *Electroencephalogr. Clin. Neurophysiol.,* 53:94–103.
13. Bromm, B., and Scharein, E. (1982): Response plasticity of pain evoked reactions in man. *Physiol. Behav.,* 28:109–116.
14. Bromm, B., and Treede, R.-D. (1983): CO_2 laser radiant heat pulses activate C nociceptors in man. *Pfluegers Arch.,* 399:155–156.
15. Bromm, B., and Treede, R.-D. (1984): Nerve fibre discharges, cerebral potentials and sensations induced by CO_2 laser stimulation. *Hum. Neurobiol.,* 3:33–40.
16. Brown, W. S., Marsh, J. T., and Smith, J. C. (1979): Principal component analysis of ERP differences related to the meaning of an ambiguous word. *Electroencephalogr. Clin. Neurophysiol.,* 46:709–714.

17. Buchsbaum, M. S. (1984): Quantification of analgesic effects by evoked potentials. In: *Pain Measurement in Man,* editied by B. Bromm, pp. 291–300. Elsevier, Amsterdam.
18. Buchsbaum, M. S. (1985): Brain imaging in psychiatric research *(in press.)*
19. Buchsbaum, M. S., and Davis, G. C. (1979): Application of somatosensory event related potentials to experimental pain and the pharmacology of analgesia. In: *Human Evoked Potentials: Applications and Problems,* edited by D. Lehmann and E. Callaway, pp. 43–54. Plenum Press, New York.
20. Buchsbaum, M. S., Davis, G. C., Coppola, R., and Naber, D. (1981): Opiate pharmacology and individual differences. II. Somatosensory evoked potentials. *Pain,* 10:367–377.
21. Buchsbaum, M. S., Davis, G. C., Goodwin, F. K., Murphy, D. L., and Post, R. M. (1980): Psychophysical pain judgments and somatosensory evoked potentials in patients with affective illness and in normal adults. In: *Clinical Neurophysiological Aspects of Psychopathological Conditions,* edited by C. Perris, L. von Knorring, and D. Kemali, pp. 63–72. Karger, Basel.
22. Buchsbaum, M. S., Holcomb, H. H., Johnson, J., King, A. C., and Kessler, R. (1983): Cerebral metabolic consequences of electrical stimulation in normal individuals. *Hum. Neurobiol.,* 2:35–38.
23. Buchsbaum, M. S., Ingvar, D. H., Kessler, R., Waters, R. N., Cappelletti, J., van Kammen, D. P., King, A. C., Johnson, J., Manning, R. G., Flynn, R. W., Mann, L. S., Bunney, W. E., Jr., and Sokoloff, L. (1982): Cerebral glucography with positron tomography. *Arch. Gen. Psychiatry* 39:251–259.
24. Buchsbaum, M. S., Rigal, F., Coppola, R., Cappelletti, J., King, C., and Johnson, J. (1982): A new system for gray-level surface distribution maps of electrical activity. *Electroencephalogr. Clin. Neurophysiol.,* 53:237–242.
25. Budinger, T. F., Derenzo, S. E., and Huesman, R. H. (1984): Instrumentation for positron emission tomography. *Ann. Neurol.,* 15 (Suppl.):S35–S43.
26. Buser, P. (editor) (1975): Electrical reactions of the brain and complimentary methods of evaluation. In: *Handbook of Electroencephalographic Clinical Neurophysiology, Vol. 8A, Evoked Responses,* edited by A. Rémond. Elsevier, Amsterdam.
27. Campbell, J. N., and LaMotte, R. H. (1983): Latency to detection of first pain. *Brain Res.,* 226:203–208.
28. Carmon, A., Mor, J., and Goldberg, J. (1976): Application of laser to psychophysiological study of pain in man. In: *Advances in Pain Research and Therapy, Vol. 1,* edited by J. J. Bonica and D. Albe-Fessard, pp. 375–380. Raven Press, New York.
29. Carmon, A., Mor, J., and Goldberg, J. (1976): Evoked responses to noxious thermal stimulations. *Exp. Brain Res.,* 25:103–107.
30. Carmon, A., Dotan, Y., and Sarne, Y. (1978): Correlation of subjective pain experience with cerebral evoked responses to noxious thermal stimulations. *Exp. Brain Res.,* 33:445–453.
31. Carmon, A., Friedman, Y., Coger, R., and Kenton, B. (1980): Single trial analysis of evoked potentials to noxious thermal stimulation in man. *Pain,* 8:21–32.
32. Celesia, G. G., Polcyn, R. D., Holden, J. E., Nickles, R. J., Gatley, J. S., and Koeppe, R. A. (1982): Visual evoked potentials and positron emission tomographic mapping of regional cerebral blood flow and cerebral metabolism: Can the neuronal potential generators be visualized? *Electroencephalogr. Clin. Neurophysiol.,* 54:243–256.
33. Chapman, C. R., Benedetti, C., and Butler, C. H. (1977): Cerebral response measures of stimulation-induced and opiate-induced dental analgesia in man: attempted analgesia reversal with narcotic antagonist. In: *Pain in the Trigeminal Region,* edited by D. J. Anderson and B. Matthews, pp. 423–433. Elsevier, Amsterdam.
34. Chapman, C. R., Chen, A. C. N., and Harkins, S. W. (1979): Brain evoked potentials as correlates of laboratory pain: a review and perspective. In: *Advances in Pain Research and Therapy, Vol. 3.* edited by J. J. Bonica, J. C. Liebeskind, and D. G. Albe-Fessard, pp. 791–803. Raven Press, New York.
35. Chapman, C. R., Colpitts, Y. H., Mayeno, J. K., and Gagliardi, G. J. (1981): Rate of stimulus repetition changes evoked potential amplitude: Dental and auditory modalities compared. *Exp. Brain Res.,* 43:246–252.
36. Chapman, C. R., and Jacobson, R. C. (1984): Assessment of analgesic states: can evoked potentials play a role? In: *Pain Measurement in Man,* edited by B. Bromm, pp. 233–256. Elsevier, Amsterdam.

37. Reference deleted.
38. Chapman, C. R., Schimek, F., Gehrig, J. D., Gerlach, R., and Colpitts, Y. H. (1983): Effects of nitrous oxide, transcutaneous electrical stimulation, and their combination on brain potentials elicited by painful stimulation. *Anesthesiology,* 58:250–256.
39. Chatrian, G. E., Canfield, R. C., Knauss, T. A., and Lettich, E. (1975): Cerebral responses to electrical tooth pulp stimulation in man. *Neurology,* 25:745–757.
40. Chatrian, G. E., Fernandes De Lima, V. M., Lettich, E., Canfield, R. C., Miller, R. C., and Sojo, M. J. (1982): Electrical stimulation of tooth pulp in humans. II. Qualities of sensations. *Pain,* 14:233–246.
41. Chen, A. C. N., Chapman, C. R., and Harkins, S. W. (1979): Brain evoked potentials are functional correlates of induced pain in man. *Pain,* 6:365–374.
42. Chen, A. C. N., Treede, R.-D., and Bromm, B. (1984): Modulation of pain evoked cerebral potentials by concurrent subacute pain. In: *Pain Measurement in Man,* edited by B. Bromm, pp. 301–310. Elsevier, Amsterdam.
43. Childers, D. G., Perry Jr., N. W., Halpeny, O. S., and Bourne, J. R. (1972): Spatio-temporal measures of cortical functioning in normal and abnormal vision. *Comput. Biomed. Res.,* 5:114–130.
44. Chudler, E. H., and Dong, W. K. (1983): The assessment of pain by cerebral evoked potentials. *Pain,* 16:221–244.
45. Coppola, R., Buchsbaum, M. S., and Rigal, F. (1982): Computer generation of surface distribution maps of measures of brain activity. *Comput. Biol. Med.,* 12:191–199.
46. David, E., Berlin, J., and Klement, W. (1984): Objective pain registration: the evoked potential in the investigation of pain processing. In: *Pain Measurement in Man,* edited by B. Bromm, pp. 311–316. Elsevier, Amsterdam.
47. Desmedt, J. E. (editor) (1979): Cognitive component in cerebral event-related potentials and selective attention. In: *Progress in Clinical Neurophysiology, Vol. 6.* Karger, Basel.
48. Devor, M., Carmon, A., and Frostig, R. (1982): Primary afferent and spinal sensory neurons that respond to brief pulses of intense infrared radiation: a preliminary survey in rats. *Exp. Neurol.,* 76:483–494.
49. DeWeerd, J. P. C. M. (1981): Facts and fancies about a posteriori "Wiener" filtering. *IEEE Trans. Biomed. Eng.,* BME-28:252–257.
50. Donchin, E., and Heffley, E. F. (1978): Multivariate analysis of event-related potential data: a tutorial review. In *Multidisciplinary Perspectives in Event-Related Brain Potential Research,* EPA-600/9-77-043, edited by D. A. Otto, pp. 555–572. United States Government Printing Office, Washington, D.C.
51. Dubinsky, J., and Barlow, J. S. (1980): A simple dot-density topogram for EEG. *Electroencephalogr. Clin. Neurophysiol.,* 48:473–477.
52. Duffy, F. H., Burchfiel, J. L., and Lombroso, C. T. (1979): Brain electrical activity mapping (BEAM): a method for extending the clinical utility of EEG and evoked potential data. *Ann. Neurol.,* 5:309–321.
53. Estrin, T., and Uzgalis, R. (1969): Computed display of spatiotemporal EEG patterns. *IEEE Trans. Biomed. Eng.,* 16:192–196.
54. Giblin, D. R. (1964): The sensory evoked response in man. *Ann. NY Acad. Sci.,* 112:93–142.
55. Gross-Isseroff, R., Sarne, Y., Carmon, A., and Isseroff, A. (1982): Cortical potentials evoked by innocuous tactile and noxious thermal stimulation in the rat: differences in localization and latency. *Behav. Neurol. Biol.,* 35:294–307.
56. Gybels, J. M., Handwerker, H. O., and Van Hees, J. (1979): A comparison between the discharges of human nociceptive nerve fibres and the subject's ratings of his sensations. *J. Physiol. (Lond.),* 292:193–206.
57. Halliday, A. M. (1978): Clinical applications of evoked potentials. In: *Recent Advances in Clinical Neurology,* editied by W. B. Matthews and G. H. Glaser, Churchill-Livingstone, Edinburgh.
58. Halliday, A. M., Barrett, G., Halliday, E., and Michael, W. F. (1977): The topography of the pattern-evoked potential. In: *Visual Evoked Potentials in Man: New Developments,* edited by J. E. Desmedt, pp. 121–133. Clarendon Press, Oxford.
59. Hallin, R. G. (1984): Human pain mechanisms studied with percutaneous microelectroneurography. In: *Pain Measurement in Man,* edited by B. Bromm, pp. 39–54. Elsevier, Amsterdam.

60. Handwerker, H. O., Adriaensen, H. F. M., Gybels, J. M., and Van Hees, J. (1984): Nociceptor discharges and pain sensations: results and open questions. In: *Pain Measurement in Man,* pp. 55–64. Elsevier, Amsterdam.
61. Hardy, J. D., Wolff, H. G., and Goodell, H. (1952): *Pain Sensations and Reactions.* Williams and Wilkins, Baltimore.
62. Hari, R., Hämäläinen, M., Kaukoranta, E., Reinikainen, K., and Teszner, D. (1983): Neuromagnetic responses from the second somatosensory cortex in man. *Acta Neurol. Scand.,* 68:207–212.
63. Hari, R., Kaukoranta, E., Reinikainen, K., Huopaniemi, T., and Mauno, J. (1983): Neuromagnetic localization of cortical activity evoked by painful dental stimulation in man. *Neurosci. Lett.,* 42:77–82.
64. Harkins, S. W., and Chapman, C. R. (1978): Cerebral evoked potentials to noxious dental stimulation: relationship to subjective pain report. *Psychophysiology,* 15:248–252.
65. Harkins, S. W., Price, D. D., and Katz, M. A. (1983): Are cerebral evoked potentials reliable indices of first and second pain? In: *Advances in Pain Research and Therapy, Vol. 5,* edited by J. J. Bonica et al., pp. 185–191. Raven Press, New York.
66. Heavner, J. E., and Iwazumi, T. (1978): A laser system for stimulating spinal neuron receptive fields. *Brain Res.,* 152:348–352.
67. Hillyard, S. A. (1978): Sensation, perception and attention: Analysis using ERPs. In *Event-Related Brain Potentials in Man,* edited by E. Callaway, P. Tueting and S. H. Koslow, pp. 223–321. Academic Press, New York.
68. Hillyard, S. A., and Woods, D. L. (1978): Electrophysiological analysis of human brain function. In: *Handbook of Behavioral Neurobiology, Vol. 2,* edited by M. S. Gazzaniga, pp. 345–378. Plenum Press, New York.
69. Horst, R. L., and Donchin, E. (1980): Beyond averaging. II. Single-trial classification of exogenous event-related potentials using stepwise discriminant analysis. *Electroencephalogr. Clin. Neurophysiol.,* 48:113–126.
70. Ingvar, D. H., and Franzen, G. (1974): Abnormalities of cerebral blood flow distribution in patients with chronic schizophrenia. *Acta Psychiatr. Scand.,* 50:425–462.
71. Ingvar, D. H., Sjolund, B., and Ardo, A. (1976): Correlation between dominant EEG frequency, cerebral oxygen uptake and blood flow. *Electroencephalogr. Clin. Neurophysiol.,* 41:268–276.
71a. Jacobson, R. C., Chapman, C. R., and Gevlach, R. (1985): Stimulus intensity and interstimulus interval effects on pain-related cerebral potentials. *Electroencephalogr. Clin. Neurophysiol. (in press)*
72. James, A. E., Price, R. R., Rollo, F. D., et al. (1982): Nuclear magnetic resonance imaging: a promising technique. *JAMA,* 247:1331–1334.
73. Johnson, D., Jürgens, R., Kongehl, G., and Kornhuber, H. H. (1975): Somatosensory evoked potentials and magnitude of perception. *Exp. Brain Res.,* 22:331–334.
74. Johnston, V. S., and Holcomb, P. J. (1980): Probability learning and the P3 component of the visual evoked potential in man. *Psychophysiology,* 17:396–400.
75. Jones, S. J. (1982): Somatosensory evoked potentials: The normal waveform. In: *Evoked Potentials in Clinical Testing,* edited by A. M. Halliday, pp. 393–427. Churchill, Livingstone, New York.
76. Kaiser, H. F. (1959): Computer program for various rotation in factor analysis. *Educ. Psychol. Meas.,* 19:413–420.
77. Kenton, B., Coger, R., Crue, B., Pinsky, J., Friedman, Y., and Carmon, A. (1980): Peripheral fibre correlates to noxious thermal stimulation in humans. *Neurosci. Lett.,* 17:301–306.
78. Kunkle, E. C. (1949): Phasic pains induced by cold. *J. Appl. Physiol.,* 1:811–824.
79. LaMotte, R. H., Thalhammer, J. G., Torebjörk, H. E., and Robinson, C. J. (1982): Peripheral neural mechanisms of cutaneous hyperalgesia following mild injury by heat. *J. Neurosci.,* 2:765–781.
80. Lavine, R. A., Buchsbaum, M. S., and Schechter, G. (1980): Human somatosensory evoked responses: effects of attention and distraction on early components. *Physiol. Psychol.,* 8:405–408.
81. Lehmann, D. (1971): Multichannel topography of human alpha EEG fields. *Electroencephalogr. Clin. Neurophysiol.,* 31:439–449.
82. Lehmann, D., and Skrandies, W. (1980): Reference-free identification of components of

checkerboard-evoked multichannel potential fields. *Electroencephalogr. Clin. Neurophysiol.,* 48:609–621.

83. Lim, R. S., and Guzman, F. (1968): Manifestations of pain in analgesic evaluation in animals and man. In: *Pain,* edited by A. Soulairac, J. Cahn and J. Charpentier, pp. 119–152. Academic Press, New York.
84. Lynn, B., and Perl, E. R. (1977): A comparison of four tests for assessing the pain sensitivity of different subjects and test areas. *Pain,* 3:353–365.
85. Martin, R. W., and Chapman, C. R. (1979): Dental dolorimetry for human pain research: Methods Apparatus. *Pain,* 6:349–364.
86. Reference deleted.
87. McGlashan, T. H., Evans, J. J., and Orne, M. T. (1969): The nature of hypnotic analgesic and placebo response to experimental pain. *Psychosom. Med.,* 31:227–246.
88. Melzack, R. (1973): *The Puzzle of Pain.* Basic Books, New York.
89. Melzack, R. (1983, Ed.) *Pain Measurement and Assessment.* Raven Press, New York.
90. Mor, J., and Carmon, A. (1975): Laser emitted radiant heat for pain research. *Pain,* 1:233–247.
91. Mountcastle, V. B. (1980): Pain and temperature sensibilities. In: *Medical Physiology,* edited by V. B. Mountcastle, pp. 391–427. Mosby, St. Louis.
92. Naruse, S., Horikawa, Y., Tanaka, C., Hirakawa, K., Nishikawa, H., and Watari, H. (1984): *In vivo* measurement of energy metabolism and the concomitant monitoring of electroencephalogram in experimental cerebral ischemia. *Brain Res.,* 296:370–372.
93. Peregrin, J., and Valach, M. (1981): Averaging, selective averaging and latency corrected averaging. *Pfluegers Arch. Physiol.,* 391:154–158.
94. Picton, T. W., and Stuss, D. T. (1980): The component structure of the human event-related potentials. In: *Motivation, Motor and Sensory Processes of the Brain,* edited by H. H. Kornhuber and L. Deeke. Elsevier, Amsterdam.
95. Pratt, H., Amlie, R. N., and Starr, A. (1979): Somatosensory potentials in humans evoked by both mechanical stimulation of the skin and electrical stimulation of the nerve. In: *Sensory Functions of the Skin of Humans,* edited by D. R. Kenshalo, pp. 109–129. Plenum Press, New York.
96. Price, D. D. (1972): Characteristics of second pain and flexion reflexes indicative of prolonged central summation. *Exp. Neurol.,* 37:371–387.
97. Price, D. D., Hu, J. W., Dubner, R., and Gracely, R. H. (1977): Peripheral suppression of first pain and central summation of second pain evoked by noxious heat pulses. *Pain,* 3:57–68.
98. Ragot, R. A., and Reymond, A. (1978): EEG field mapping. *Electroencephalogr. Clin. Neurophysiol.,* 45:417–421.
99. Raymond, A., and Offner, F. (1952): A new method for EEG display. *Electroencephalogr. Clin. Neurophysiol.,* 7:453–460.
100. Rodbard, S. (1970): Muscle pain. In: *Pain and Suffering: Selected Aspects,* edited by B. J. Crue, Jr., Thomas, Springfield, Illinois.
101. Sano, H. (1977): Influence of intensity-varied electrical stimulation of a tooth and 30% N_20 premixed gas inhalation on somatosensory evoked potentials (SEPs). *Jpn. J. Dent. Anesthesiol.,* 5:9–21.
102. Scharein, E., Häger, F., and Bromm, B. (1984): Spectral estimators for short EEG segments. In: *Pain Measurement in Man,* edited by B. Bromm, pp. 189-202. Elsevier, Amsterdam.
103. Sitaram, N., Buchsbaum, M. S., and Gillin, J. C. (1977): Physostigmine analgesia and somatosensory evoked responses in man. *Eur. J. Pharmacol.,* 42:285–290.
104. Spreng, M., and Ichioka, M. (1964): Langsame Rindenpotentiale bei Schmerzreizung am menschen. *Pfluegers Arch. Physiol.,* 279:121–132.
105. Stowell, H. (1975): Human evoked responses to potentially noxious stimulation. I. *Activ. Nerv. Sup. (Praha)* 17:1–7.
106. Stowell, H. (1975) Human evoked responses to potentially noxious tactile stimulation. II. *Activ. Nerv. Sup. (Praha),* 17:94–100.
107. Stowell, H. (1977): Cerebral slow waves related to the perception of pain in man. *Brain Res. Bull.,* 2:23–30.

108. Suter, C. (1970): Principal component analysis of average evoked potentials. *Exp. Neurol.,* 29:317–327.
109. Torebjörk, H. E. (1974): Afferent C units responding to mechanical, thermal and chemical stimuli in human non-glabrous skin. *Acta Physiol. Scand.,* 92:374–390.
110. Torebjörk, H. E., and Hallin, R. G. (1976): Skin receptors supplied by unmyelinated (C) fibres in man. In: *Sensory Function of the Skin in Primates,* edited by Y. Zotterman, pp. 475–487. Pergamon Press, Oxford.
110a. Torebjörk, H. E., LaMotte, R. H., Robinson, C. J. (1984): Peripheral neural correlates of the magnitude of cutaneous pain and hyperalgesia: Simultaneous recordings in humans of sensory judgments of pain and evoked responses in nociceptors with C-fibers. *J. Neurophysiol.,* 51:341–355.
111. Treede, R.-D., Jahnke, M. T., and Bromm, B. (1984): Functional properties of CO_2 laser activated nociceptive fibers in an intact human skin nerve. In: *Pain Measurement in Man,* edited by B. Bromm, pp. 65–78. Elsevier, Amsterdam.
112. Vallbo, A. B., Hagbarth, K. E., Torebjörk, H. E., and Wallin, B. G. (1979): Somatosensory, proprioceptive and sympathetic activity in human peripheral nerves. *Physiol. Rev.,* 59:919–957.
113. Van Hees, J. (1976): Human C-fiber input during painful and nonpainful skin stimulation with radiant heat. In: *Advances in Pain Research and Therapy, Vol. 1,* edited by J. J. Bonica and D. Albe-Fessard, pp. 35–40. Raven Press, New York.
114. Van Hees, J., and Gybels, J. M. (1972): Pain related to single afferent C fibres from human skin. *Brain Res.,* 48:397–400.
115. Vaughan, H. G., and Ritter, W. (1970): The sources of auditory evoked responses recorded from the human scalp. *Electroencephalogr. Clin. Neurophysiol.,* 28:360–367.
116. Reference deleted.
117. Wolf, S., and Hardy, J. D. (1941): Studies on pain. Observations on pain due to local cooling and on factors involved in the "cold pressor" effect. *J. Clin. Invest.,* 20:521–533.
118. Wolff, B. B. (1979): Validity of different experimental pain response parameters for human analgesic assays. In: *Advances in Pain Research and Therapy, Vol. 3,* edited by J. J. Bonica, J. C. Liebeskind, and D. G. Albe-Fessard, pp. 831–835. Raven Press, New York.
119. Woody, C. D. (1967): Characterization of an adaptive filter for analysis of variable latency neuroelectric signals. *Med. Biol. Eng.,* 5:539–553.

Advances in Pain Research and Therapy, Vol. 9, edited by H. L. Fields et al. Raven Press, New York © 1985.

Effect of Attention on Tooth-Pulp Evoked Potentials

Massimo Leandri, Jacqueline A. Campbell, and Juan Lahuerta

Pain Relief Foundation, Walton Hospital, Rice Lane, Liverpool L9 1AE, United Kingdom

Tooth-pulp afferents have been traditionally considered to mediate painful sensation. This opinion has been challenged by recent papers presenting evidence that other sensations can be evoked by tooth-pulp stimulation (1,3,12,24,26,27). However, electrical stimulation of the tooth still remains the best method to evoke pain by means of an electrical stimulus, and it has been widely used in the past. Chatrian et al. (18) first showed that scalp responses could be recorded in humans after tooth stimulation; after that, many papers have been published on this topic, claiming that the recorded response would be a correlate of painful perception (6,8,14,21; for a review see ref. 15). In this belief, effects of analgesic drugs or procedures on these potentials have also been studied (2,4,5,7,9,10,13,20,22,25). The scalp potential evoked by tooth stimulation is usually recorded from the vertex, with the reference electrode placed at the inion. It has a multiphasic waveform and the most reliable part of it is a large negative-positive component, whose peaks have been named N2 and P2, or, by their latencies, N150 and P250 (see refs. 7,9,11).

Vertex potentials in this range of latencies can be evoked by other stimulation modalities, e.g., somatosensory, visual, and auditory. It has been demonstrated that attention may influence the amplitude of these potentials (17–19,28), and therefore the biphasic response recorded from the vertex after tooth stimulation could also be influenced by attention.

The aim of this chapter is, therefore, to compare painful with nonpainful somatosensory stimuli and to investigate the effects of attention on them.

Dr. Leandri's present address is Department of Neurology, University of Genoa, 16132 Genoa, Italy.

METHODS

Five healthy volunteers have been studied in four trials of two sessions each. Painful stimuli were delivered to upper incisor teeth. The vestibular surface of two teeth was dried and a small amount of adhesive paste (Bostik Blue-Tack) was placed on them; two holes were made through the paste by means of a wood stick until the enamel was reached; the holes were then filled with conductive jelly and two silver electrodes, connected via small insulated copper wires to the stimulator, were placed into them. More paste was used to seal the electrodes, so that no conductive parts would be in contact with the saliva. A cotton roll was also placed underneath the upper lip to avoid displacement of the electrodes. A constant current stimulator delivered rectangular pulses, 1 msec wide, with intensity set at 1.5 times the sensory threshold (the stimulus was judged painful at the threshold level by all the subjects) that was between 0.2 and 1 mA. Nonpainful stimuli were delivered to the thumb of the nondominant side through two moistened cotton strips wrapped around it. The stimulus width was set at 1 msec and the intensity was 1.5 times the sensory threshold, which ranged between 5 and 10 mA. Each stimulator was independently driven by a random pulse generator, whose window was set between 0.5 and 5 sec. The trigger pulse from each stimulator was sent to a separate channel of a tape recorder, so that separate averaging and comparison of either painful and nonpainful responses within the same session would be possible.

Each trial consisted of two consecutive sessions; the subject always received both stimuli, but he was requested to draw his attention first to one stimulus and then, in the subsequent session, to the other by pressing a button every time he felt it. The results obtained in the two consecutive sessions were then compared (Fig. 1).

The signals were picked up from a vertex-inion derivation, amplified, recorded onto tape, then averaged (usually 32–64 responses) and stored onto computer disks. The latencies of the N150 and P250 peaks were measured; the N150 peak area, defined as the area of the curve above a line drawn between the N150 onset and the P250 peak, was calculated with the aid of a computer. This procedure was considered to be better than the measure of N150-P250 peak-to-peak amplitude because of the broad and ill-defined waveform of these components and of the closer correlation with total neural activity.

RESULTS

Analysis of the combined data obtained by the two consecutive sessions of each trial revealed that when the subject was paying attention to tooth stimuli, the mean latencies ($\pm$ s.d.) of N150 and P250 were 126.69 $\pm$ 20.48 msec and 206.25 $\pm$ 27.63 msec, respectively. These latencies were 129.81

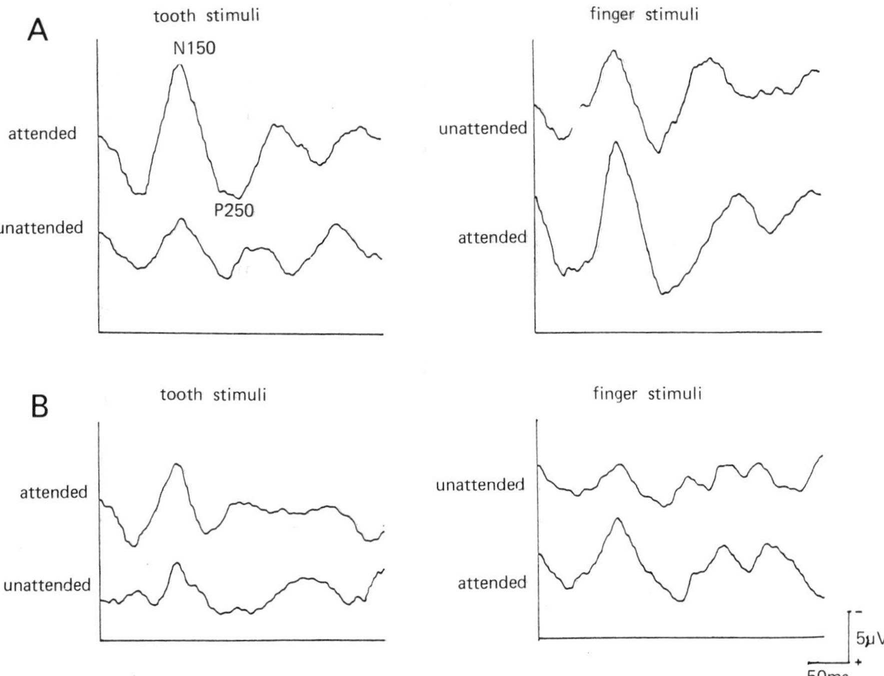

FIG. 1. A: Recordings during the first of two consecutive trials. On the *left* side are the responses to tooth stimuli, occurring in random sequence with finger stimuli, the responses to which are on the *right* side. It is shown that switching of attention affects the amplitude of the responses (in the *upper traces* the subject is attending tooth stimuli and disregarding finger stimuli, while in the *lower traces* the opposite condition occurs). Note that in homologous conditions the responses to tooth and finger stimuli are almost identical. **B:** Recordings during the second trial. Same arrangement of the traces as in A. A process of habituation here takes place and all the responses are smaller than in the first trial; regardless of this, the attention of the subject has a similar effect as during the first trial.

± 30.72 msec and 200.19 ± 46.29 msec, respectively, when the stimuli were not attended. Statistical analysis demonstrated that there was no significant difference in peak latencies (at the 5% level) between these two conditions; the values found were within the range of observations made by previous authors. Finger-evoked N150 and P250 peaks had respective mean latencies of 119.31 ± 21.30 and 187.31 ± 28.33 msec with attention, and 118.5 ± 22.62 msec and 180.87 ± 38.21 msec without attention. Statistical analysis showed that no significant difference existed between the attended and unattended N150 or P250 latencies. Tooth stimuli, when attended, gave rise to a N150 peak area which, measured in arbitrary units, had a mean value of 38.10 ± 18.03, while, when unattended, evoked a smaller deflection, whose mean area was 25.16 ± 17.40. There was a very significant difference between the two areas ($p = 0.0041$). Similarly, attended finger stimulation evoked a wide N150, with a mean peak area of 38.67 ± 19.49, whereas unattended N150 had an area of only 22.81 ± 17.88 with a very significant difference between them (p = 0.0016). Therefore, the area of N150 behaved in the same way with respect to attention regardless of whether it was evoked by tooth or finger stimuli. The areas of the peaks obtained under the same condition of attention were also compared (i. e., attended tooth stimuli versus attended finger stimuli and unattended tooth stimuli versus unattended finger stimuli), and no significant differences (at the 5% level) were found between the two modalities of stimulation.

Comparison between responses obtained in consecutive trials showed that the N150 area underwent some progressive decrease because of habituation. However, statistical analysis revealed that amplitudes of attended responses were not significantly smaller than unattended responses even when cross-comparing the first and the second trial. In fact, mean areas of tooth-evoked N150 in the first trial were 45.33 ± 23.45 (attended) and 28.88 ± 16.37 (unattended), and in the second trial 31.91 ± 9.06 (attended) and 20.66 ± 18.01 (unattended). Finger-evoked N150 had areas of 61.53 ± 9.56 (attended) and 26.06 ± 17.76 (unattended) in the first trial and 30.35 ± 14.39 (attended) and 17.28 ± 13.76 (unattended) in the second trial. The smaller peak areas found with unattended stimuli when compared to those in which the subject was paying attention to the stimuli cannot therefore be attributed to habituation.

DISCUSSION

The data presented show that the late vertex responses to painful tooth stimuli have similar characteristics as the late vertex potentials evoked by nonpainful somatosensory stimuli, and that, like the latter, they are subject to a process which is partially linked with the attention. The resemblance between tooth and finger responses could be extended to potentials evoked by other stimuli, as we know that similar late vertex waves can be evoked also by visual and auditory stimuli. After years of investigation into these potentials it is still debated whether they have a common origin; however, a recent review (23) concluded that they are probably generated in widespread cortical areas. Due to their similarity, the same can be hypothesized about tooth potentials.

A previous comparison between responses from painful and nonpainful stimuli has been performed by Chen and Chapman (13). The auditory shocks used by these authors as nonpainful stimuli evoked potentials whose morphology, amplitude, and latency were different from responses evoked by tooth stimulation; but it should be remarked that they did not monitor the subject's attention. Therefore, this last condition and the different stimulus used do not make a comparison between their results and those of this study possible.

As the tooth evoked potentials are influenced so much by attention of the subject, caution should be used in interpreting experiments about modifications of these waves by analgesic drugs or procedures. The attention of the subject should always be monitored, but should be remembered that the assumption of a correlation between the reported pain and amplitude of the potentials may not be entirely correct, as shown by Cruccu et al. (16), who demonstrated that no correlation between tooth potentials amplitude and verbal reports existed when the subject had foreknowledge of the stimulus.

ACKNOWLEDGMENTS

This research has been supported by Smith and Nephew (M. L.), the Sir Halley Stewart Trust (J. A. C.), and the Cancer Research Campaign, United Kingdom (J. L.).

REFERENCES

1. Azerad, J., and Woda, A. (1977): Sensation evoked by bipolar intrapulpal stimulation. *Pain,* 4:145–152.
2. Butler, S. H., Chapman, C. R., and Colpitts, Y. M. (1980): Opiate antagonist and evoked potentials: Is there a narcotic antagonist placebo effect: *Proceedings: Society for Psychophysiological Research,* Vancouver, British Columbia.
3. Cadden, S. W., Lisney, S. J. W., and Matthews, B. (1982): A beta fibre innervation of tooth pulp in the cat. In: *Anatomical, Physiological and Pharmacological Aspects of Trigeminal Pain,* edited by B. Matthews and R. D. Hill, pp. 41–49. Elsevier, Amsterdam.
4. Chapman, C. R., Benedetti, C., and Butler, S. M. (1977): Cerebral response measures of stimulation-induced and opiate-induced dental analgesia in man: attempted analgesia reversal with narcotic antagonist. In: *Pain in the Trigeminal Region,* edited by D. J. Anderson and B. Matthews, pp. 423–433. Elsevier, Amsterdam.
5. Chapman, C. R., and Benedetti, C. (1979): Nitrous oxide effects on cerebral evoked potentials: partial reversal with a narcotic antagonist. *Anesthesiology,* 51:135–138
6. Chapman, C. R., Chen, A. C. N., and Harkins, S. W. (1979): Cerebral evoked responses as correlates of laboratory pain. In: *Advances in Pain Research and Therapy, Vol. 3,* edited by J. J. Bonica, J. C. Liebeskind, and D. Albe-Fessard, pp. 791–803. Raven Press, New York.
7. Chapman, C. R., Colpitts, Y. M., Benedetti, C., Kitaeff, R., and Gehrig, J. D. (1980): Evoked potential assessments of acupunctural analgesia: attempted reversal with naloxone. *Pain,* 9:183–198.
8. Chapman, C. R., Chen, A. C. N., Colpitts, Y. M., and Martin, R. W. (1981): Sensory decision theory describes evoked potentials in pain discrimination. *Psychophysiology,* 18:114–120.
9. Chapman, C. R., Colpitts, Y. M., Benedetti, C., and Butler, S. (1982): Event-related potential correlates of analgesia: comparison of fentanyl, acupuncture and nitrous oxide. *Pain,* 14:327–337.
10. Chapman, C. R., Schimek, F., Gehrig, J. D., Gerlach, R., and Colpitts, Y. H. (1983): Effects of nitrous oxide, transcutaneous electrical stimulation and their combination on brain potentials elicted by painful stimulation. *Anesthesiology,* 58:250–256.
11. Chatrian, G. E., Canfield, R. C., Knauss, T. A., and Lettich, E. (1975): Cerebral responses to electrical tooth pulp stimulation in man. *Neurology,* 25:745–757.
12. Chatrian, G. E., Fernandes De Lima, V. M., Lettich, E., Canfield, R. C., Miller, R. C., and Sojo, M. J. (1982): Electrical stimulation of tooth pulp in humans. II. Qualities of sensations. *Pain,* 14:233–246.
13. Chen, A. C. N., and Chapman, C. R. (1980): Aspirin and analgesia evaluated by event-related potentials in man: possible central action in brain. *Exp. Brain Res.,* 39:359–364.

14. Chen, A. C. N., Chapman, C. R., and Harkins, S. W. (1979): Brain evoked potentials are functional correlates of induced pain in man. *Pain,* 6:365–374.
15. Chudler, E. H., and Dong, W. K. (1983): The assessment of pain by cerebral evoked potentials. *Pain,* 16:221–244.
16. Cruccu, G., Fornarelli, M., Inghilleri, M., and Manfredi, M. (1983): The limits of tooth pulp evoked potentials for pain quantitation. *Physiol. Behav.,* 31:339–342.
17. Debecker, J. (1967): Contribution a l'étude physiologique chez l'homme de certains mecanismes cerebraux mis en jeu dans la perception sensorielle. *Unpublished Thesis,* Brussels.
18. Desmedt, J. E., and Debecker, J. (1979): Waveform and neural mechanism of the decison P350 elicited without prestimulus CNV or readiness potential in random sequences of near-threshold auditory clicks and finger stimuli. *Electroencephalogr. Clin. Neurophysiol.,* 47:648–670.
19. Desmedt, J. E., and Debecker, J. (1979): Slow potential shifts and decision P350 interactions in tasks with random sequences of near-threshold clicks and finger stimuli delivered at regular intervals. *Electroencephalogr. Clin. Neurophysiol.,* 47:671–679.
20. Gehrig, J. D., Colpitts, Y. H., and Chapman, C. R. (1981): Effects of local anesthetic infiltration on brain potentials evoked by painful dental stimulation. *Anesth. Analg.,* 60:779–782.
21. Harkins, S. W., and Chapman, C. R. (1978): Cerebral evoked potentials to noxious dental stimulation: relationship to subjective pain report. *Psychophysiology,* 15:248–252.
22. Harkins, S. W., Benedetti, C., Colpitts, Y. H., and Chapman, C. R. (1982): Effects of nitrous oxide inhalation of brain potentials evoked by auditory and noxious dental stimulation. *Prog. Neuropsychopharmacol.,* 6:167–174.
23. Hillyard, S. A., and Picton, T. W. (1979): Event-related brain potentials and selective information processing in man. In: *Conscious Perception and Cerebral Event-Related Potentials,* edited by J. E. Desmedt, pp. 1–52. Karger, Basel.
24. Mumford, J. M., and Bowsher, D. (1976): Pain and protopathic sensibility. A review with particular reference to the teeth. *Pain,* 2:223–243.
25. Rohdewald, P. H., Derendorf, G., Drehsen, C. E., Elger, C. E., and Knoll, O. (1982): Changes in cortical evoked potentials as correlates of the efficacy of weak analgesics. *Pain,* 12:329–341.
26. Sessle, B. J. (1979): Is the tooth pulp a "pure" source of noxious input? In: *Advances in Pain Research and Therapy, Vol. 3,* edited by J. J. Bonica, J. C. Liebeskind, and D. Albe-Fessard, pp. 245–260. Raven Press, New York.
27. Shimizu, T. (1964): Tooth pre-pain sensation elicited by electrical stimulation. *J. Dent. Res.,* 43:467–475.
28. Velasco, M., Velasco, F., Machado, J., and Olivera, A. (1973): Effects of novelty, habituation, attention and distraction on the amplitude of the various components of the somatic evoked responses. *Int. J. Neurosci.,* 5:101–111.

Advances in Pain Research and Therapy, Vol. 9, edited by H. L. Fields et al. Raven Press, New York © 1985.

Neuromagnetic Evoked Responses and Acute Laboratory Pain

*R. Hari, *E. Kaukoranta, and **G. Kobal

**Low Temperature Laboratory, Helsinki University of Technology, SF-02150 Espoo, Finland; and **Institute of Pharmacology and Toxicology, University of Erlangen-Nürnberg, D-8520 Erlangen, Federal Republic of Germany*

The generation of purely noxious stimuli and the measurement of pain experience are the main problems of experimental pain research. In this chapter data are presented indicating that neuromagnetic responses elicited by well defined painful stimuli (electric stimulation of the tooth and chemical stimulation of the nasal mucosa) might be helpful in studies of acute experimental pain.

MAGNETOENCEPHALOGRAPHY

The bioelectric currents which generate EEG-deflections of the scalp also give rise to weak magnetic fields which can be measured noninvasively outside the head by sensitive SQUID (superconducting quantum interference device) magnetometers (Fig. 1). Detailed descriptions of the method and of the results obtained so far are available (13–15). In principle, the only contribution to the magnetoencephalography (MEG) is from current sources tangential to the skull. This means that the MEG mainly reflects activity of fissural cortex, where synchronous activation of the parallel-organized pyramidal cells is accompanied by current flow tangential to the skull. Electric inhomogeneities, like skull, liquor spaces, etc., are transparent to magnetic fields. Because MEG is insensitive to radial and deep current sources, the magnetic evoked responses are influenced by more limited sources than the simultaneously measured electric evoked potentials. Thus, it might be easier to find out the activated brain areas on the basis of magnetic fields patterns than electric evoked potentials.

When the measured magnetic field pattern is dipolar, the three-dimensional location of the equivalent current dipole source can be calculated when the radius of curvature of the measurement sphere is known. So far, simple dipole models have been used in the interpretation of neuromagnetic mappings revealing tonotopic, somatotopic, and retinotopic features of the primary projection cortex.

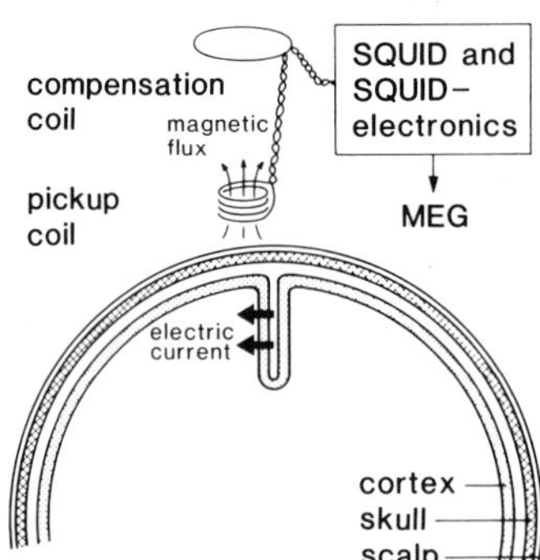

FIG. 1. Schematic presentation of MEG-measurements with a first-order SQUID gradiometer. Only current sources tangenital to the skull give rise to magnetic fields outside the head.

MATERIALS AND METHODS

The recordings were made in the Otaniemi magnetically shielded room (8) with first-order SQUID gradiometers. A 1-channel gradiometer (pickup coil area 1.7 cm^2, sensitivity 26 $fT/\sqrt{Hz}$) was used in the early parts of the dental pain studies. The later dental pain and the nasal mucosa stimulation studies were made with a 4-channel gradiometer (pickup coil area 1.9 cm^2, sensitivity 22 $fT/\sqrt{Hz}$)(5). The axis of the gradiometer was placed perpendicular to the skull to measure the radial component of the field.

Dental Stimulation

Six healthy subjects were studied. The upper central incisor was stimulated through noninvasive electrodes with 10-msec monophasic pulses. The cathode was hand-held against the tooth and the anode was either on the gingiva or on the skin beneath the nose. The interstimulus interval (ISI) was 4 sec.

All single responses were visually checked before averaging to eliminate artifacts. For each measurement location 40 to 56 responses were averaged. The analysis period of 1,024 msec included a prestimulus period of 250 msec.

Chemical Stimulation of the Nasal Mucosa

The nasal mucosa of 5 volunteers was stimulated by 100-msec CO_2 pulses embedded in a continuous airflow (140 ml/sec). The air was humidified and kept at a constant temperature of 36° C (for description of the device, see ref. 9). The concentration of the CO_2 stimuli was 50 to 75%. The risetime of the stimulus was less than 20 msec, and the interstimulus interval was 10 sec. The stimuli were presented asynchronously to respiration. Before the experiment the subjects were trained to breathe through the mouth using velopharyngeal closure to avoid respiratory air flow in the nasal cavity (9). There were neither tactile nor thermal sensations when the zero-stimulus (0% CO_2) was switched on or off.

During the experiment the subjects wore an ear plug in the ear ipsilateral to the magnetometer and an earphone in the contralateral ear. White noise was used to avoid acoustical interference from switching the stimulus on and off (11).

Simultaneously with the magnetic recordings electric evoked potentials were recorded from derivation C_z-A_2, and eye movements from an electrode above the eye referenced to the right ear lobe.

RESULTS

Dental Stimulation

The sensation elicited by dental stimulation was a sharp, well-localized pain in the tooth. The magnetic response to stimulation of the normal tooth peaked at 90 to 100 msec (Fig. 2A). No responses were obtained to stimulation of a devitalized tooth. The field pattern was dipolar at latencies near

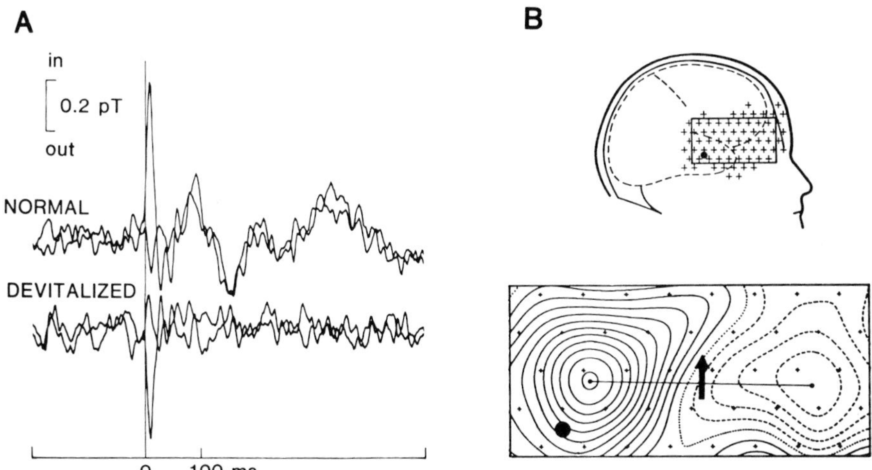

FIG. 2. **A:** Averaged magnetic responses (N = 50) to electric stimulation of a normal and devitalized central incisor. Recordings at the right frontotemporal area (1 cm upwards and 4 cm forwards from T_4 of the 10–20 system). The passband is 0.05 to 50 Hz. Stimulus artifacts can be seen after the zero-time. (From ref. 2, with permission.) **B:** Magnetic field pattern 100 msec after dental stimulation. The curves are separated by 0.04 pT. *Solid lines* indicate flux out of the skull, and *dashed lines* flux into the skull. The interpoint distance is 16 mm, three locations were measured simultaneously. The *dot* indicates the location T_4 and the *arrow* denotes the equivalent current dipole placed to the midpoint of the line connecting the field extrema.

the peak latency (Fig. 2B). The equivalent current dipole explaining the field extremes was calculated to be 3 cm beneath the scalp.

Chemical Stimulation of the Nasal Mucosa

The sensation elicited by CO_2 pulses was a sharp pain deep in the nose; the pain disappeared more slowly than that elicited by dental stimulation. Fig. 3 shows simultaneously measured electric and magnetic responses to CO_2 pulses. The electric response peaked with a vertex-negative deflection at about 370 msec. The magnetic responses were biphasic and the later peak coincided with the electric N370. Both the electric and magnetic responses started simultaneously, about 270 msec after stimulus onset. Although eye blinks can contaminate magnetic evoked responses at the frontotemporal area, it is likely that they have not deteriorated the present responses for the following reasons. Magnetic blink artifacts, which are monophasic (flux out of the skull on the right hemisphere), occur simultaneously with the electrical blinks (1). However, in Fig. 3 the peak of the small reflectory blink does not coincide with the evoked response peaks. Moreover, at the measurement location of Fig. 3 the magnetic blink artifact is not larger than 0.02 pT (i.e., about 5% of the recorded signals) as estimated on the basis of the electric recordings and the data of reference 1.

In 4 out of the 5 subjects the polarities of the main deflections of the magnetic responses were opposite at the anterior and posterior temporal areas. Detailed field mappings are under study.

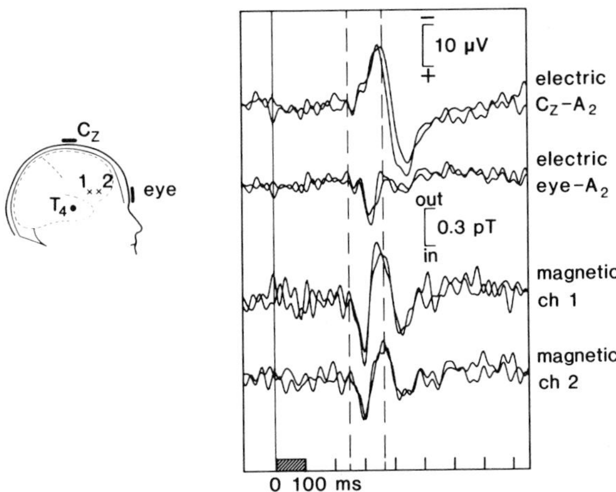

FIG. 3. Simultaneously measured averaged electric and magnetic responses (N = 32) to chemical stimulation of the nasal mucosa. The passband is 0.5 to 30 Hz. The recording locations are indicated in the schematic drawing of the head.

DISCUSSION

Dental Stimulation

The possible extracerebral artifact sources have been extensively discussed earlier (2,4). For example, eye movements and eye blinking can be excluded as sources of the recorded responses on the basis of the field patterns produced by them (1,6). Further, measurements of the magnetic responses at different distances from the scalp support the interpretation that the responses reflect activation of cerebral rather than extracerebral sources.

Tapping of the tooth elicited only minimal evoked responses as compared to responses to electric stimulation at the magnetic field extremes (4). This finding, together with the fact that stimulation of a devitalized tooth in 2 subjects did not elicit any magnetic responses suggests that the responses cannot be transmitted by periodontal fibers.

These magnetic responses are, thus, evidently due to activation of tooth-pulp afferents. The field pattern suggests bilateral activation of brain areas at the rostral end of the Sylvian fissure indicating that the tooth pulp also has a cortical representation in humans. As revealed by extensive neuromagnetic recordings in one subject (Fig. 4), this area seems to be clearly (approximately 3 cm) anterior to the SII area activated by peroneal nerve stimulation and corresponds anatomically to the frontal operculum.

Chemical Stimulation of the Nasal Mucosa

The first report of neuromagnetic responses to painful chemical stimulation of the nasal mucosa is presented. The corresponding electric potentials (EPs) have amplitude maxima at the vertex (10). Fentanyl decreases the amplitude of CO_2-EPs (12) but has little effect on olfactory EPs elicited, e. g., by menthol (G. Kobal et al., *unpublished results*). This finding indicates that CO_2-EPs reflect neural activity underlying central processing of noxious stimuli. The available data do not yet allow determination of the brain areas activated by this kind of stimulus.

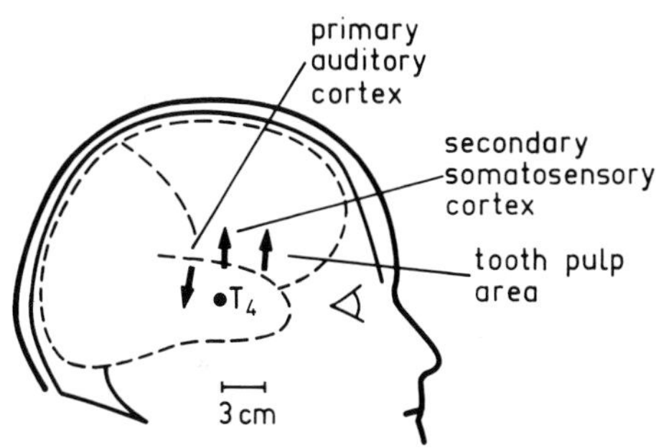

FIG. 4. The approximate locations of the equivalent current dipoles activated by tone pips (3), electric stimulation of the peroneal nerve (7), and electric stimulation of the tooth in 1 subject. The *arrows* have been positioned with reference to T_4; the scale indicates the distance along the scalp.

The present data show that it is possible to record neuromagnetic evoked responses to well defined painful stimuli. These responses provide a means to locate accurately activity of fissural cortex and might be useful in studies of acute experimental pain.

ACKNOWLEDGMENTS

This work has been supported by the Academy of Finland, the Deutsche Forschungsgemeinschaft, Emil Aaltonen Foundation, and by a twinning grant from the European Science Foundation. We thank A. Antervo, M. Hämäläinen, T. Huopaniemi, J. Huttunen, R. Ilmoniemi, J. Mauno, A. Penttinen, H. Pogorzelski, and K. Reinikainen for help in the experiments.

REFERENCES

1. Antervo, A., Hari, R., Katila, T., Ryhänen, T., and Seppänen, M. (1985): Magnetic field pattern produced by eye blinking. In: *Biomagnetism, Applications and Theory,* edited by H. Weinberg, G. Stroink, and T. Katila, pp. 373–377. Pergamon Press, New York.
2. Hari, R., Kaukoranta, E., Reinikainen, K., Huopaniemi, T., and Mauno, J. (1983): Neuromagnetic localization of cortical activity evoked by painful dental stimulation in man. *Neurosci. Lett.,* 42:77–82.
3. Hari, R., Hämäläinen, M., Ilmoniemi, R., Kaukoranta, E., Reinikainen, K., Salminen, J., Alho, K., Näätänen, R., and Sams, M. (1984): Responses of the primary auditory cortex to pitch changes in a sequence of tone pips: Neuromagnetic recordings in man. *Neurosci. Lett.,* 50:127–132.
4. Hari, R., Kaukoranta, E., Reinikainen, K., and Mauno, J. (1985): Neuromagnetic responses to noxious stimulation. In: *Biomagnetism, Applications and Theory,* edited by H. Weinberg, G. Stroink, and T. Katila, pp. 359–363. Pergamon Press, New York.
5. Ilmoniemi, R., Hari, R., and Reinikainen, K. (1984): A four-channel SQUID magnetometer for brain research. *Electroencephalogr. Clin. Neurophysiol.,* 58:467–473.
6. Katila, T., Maniewski, R., Poutanen, T., Varpula, T., and Karp, P. (1981): Magnetic fields produced by the human eye. *J. Appl. Physics,* 52:2565–2571.
7. Kaukoranta, E., Hari, R., and Reinikainen, K. (1985): Magnetic fields evoked by peroneal nerve stimulation. In: *Biomagnetism, Applications and Theory,* edited by H. Weinberg, G. Stroink, and T. Katila, pp. 364–368. Pergamon Press, New York.
8. Kelhä, V. O., Pukki, J. M., Peltonen, R. S., Penttinen, A. A., Ilmoniemi, R. J., and Heino, J. J. (1982): Design, construction and performance of a large volume magnetic shield. *IEEE Trans. Magn.,* MAG-18:260–270.
9. Kobal, G. (1981): *Elektrophysiologische Untersuchungen des menschlichen Geruchsinns.* Georg Thieme Verlag, Stuttgart.
10. Kobal, G. (1984): Pain-related electrical potentials of the human respiratory nasal mucosa elicited by chemical stimuli. In: *Pain Measurement in Man. Neurophysiological Correlates of Pain,* edited by B. Bromm, pp. 463–488. Elsevier, Amsterdam.
11. Kobal, G., and Plattig, K. -H. (1978): Methodische Anmerkungen zur Gewinnung olfaktorischer EEG-Antworten des wachen Menschen (objektive Olfaktometrie). *Z. EEG-EMG,* 9:135–145.
12. Kobal, G., and Müller, G. (1984): Cortical evoked potentials in man elicited by chemical stimulation of the nasal mucosa. *Pain,* Suppl. 2:S167.
13. Okada, Y. C. (1983): Inferences concerning anatomy and physiology of the human brain based on its magnetic field. *Il Nuovo Cimento,* 2D:379–409.
14. Romani, G. L., Williamson, S. J., and Kaufman, L. (1982): Biomagnetic instrumentation. *Rev. Sci. Instrum.,* 53:1815–1845.
15. Williamson, S. J., and Kaufman, L. (1981): Biomagnetism. *J. Magn. Magn. Mat.,* 22:129–202.

Advances in Pain Research and Therapy, Vol. 9, edited by H. L. Fields et al. Raven Press, New York © 1985.

Operant Control of Human Somatosensory Evoked Potentials Alters Experimental Pain Perception

J. P. Rosenfeld, R. Silvia, R. Weitkunat, and Robert Dowman

Departments of Neurobiology/Physiology and Psychology, Northwestern University, Evanston, Illinois 60201

Several studies have shown that animals and humans can voluntarily change the amplitude of discrete evoked potential (EP) components in all modalities in a *non*trivial manner (7,12). (Eye closure would be a trivial way to reduce the amplitude of a photic EP.) Attention turned next to the possible functional significance of these effects: Does the operantly altered amplitude of sensory EPs correlate with altered perception subserved by the EP pathways? The pain modality in rats was chosen first to pursue this issue. So far, it has been shown in two separate studies that both the 30- and 60-msec positive components of the cortical EPs evoked by nonaversive trigeminal tact stimulation can (individually) be changed with operant reinforcement methods (6,10,11). The rats learned to decrease as well as to increase the EP components in separate training phases, and it was further noted that their *sensitivities to thermal facial nociceptive stimulation correlated systematically with conditioned EP amplitude.* Evidence was also obtained that this antinociceptive effect had somatotopic and submodality specificity: Conditioned *left* cortical EPs evoked by right trigeminal tract stimulation were accompanied by *right* facial pain sensitivity changes; smaller changes in the nonexplicitly conditioned right cortex were accompanied by small and nonsignificant changes in left facial pain sensitivity. The reflexive twitch to the nonaversive evoking stimulus—possibly representing the trigeminal throughput of innocuous sensation—was either unchanged in EP conditioning or changed in a manner opposite to that seen with the painful modality. Finally, naloxone antagonized the conditioning-related hypoalgesia.

These results raised the question of whether or not similar operant EP methods might work in humans. Notwithstanding the possible clinical implications of this question, the operant EP approaches may also be of interest to the growing number of workers interested in utilizing EP-pain relations in development of the somatosensory EP as an objective pain index (1–5).

METHODS

Normal humans were recruited from a university employment office. EPs were differentially recorded from vertex referenced to mastoid with the other mastoid grounded. They were evoked in response to bipolar stimulation of the inner, medial forearm (*not* over the ulnar nerve as we wanted to avoid twitches). A stimulus was an isolated 28-msec train of 7 pulses (2 msec on/2 msec off) delivered by a constant current unit. Prior to training, the shock detection (DT) and shock pain tolerance threshold (PT) were determined using an ascending series (1 per 5 sec) of pulse trains; i.e., we recorded the levels at which subjects first became aware of the stimulation (DT) and the level beyond which they would tolerate no further intensity increment (PT). For conditioning, the evoking pulse amplitude was set at 67% of the individually determined pain tolerance threshold, a clearly nonaversive level for all subjects completing the study. On the pretraining day the DT range was 0.18 to 0.22 mA and the PT range was 1.2 to 4.4 mA. Thus, evoking stimuli for conditioning ranged from 0.8 to 2.9 mA. Although PT and DT were repeatedly determined through all training phases as dependent variables of interest, the evoking stimulation level once set remained constant throughout training, regardless of PT changes seen later.

The EPs were amplified 100,000 times and filtered with 3db settings at 3 and 200 Hz. They were conveyed to an 8-bit A/D converter interfaced to a microcomputer programmed by the senior author. The digitization rate was 1 data point every msec for a 500-msec epoch. On one baseline day, 500 EPs were evoked every 5 sec and the average amplitude, latency, and standard deviation of the "P200" component were determined. The tonal beeps, later to be used to signal successful EP responses, were randomly presented on 35% of the trials on this baseline day. The P200 component is the surface positivity typically seen in the somatic sensory vertex EP occurring between 160 and 210 msec (1,14). It has been reported elsewhere to be a pain correlate (1) and is significantly smaller in certain facial pain populations than in normals (9).

Subjects were paid a $3.50/hr flat rate for participation, plus a $1/hr bonus for each session in which the hit rate exceeded the baseline rate by 10% or more. In *uptraining,* P200 had to be 0.35 standard deviations above the baseline mean to satisfy criterion; in *downtraining,* the component had to be 0.35 standard deviations below the baseline mean. The component was defined as the average amplitude of the 10 data points (10 msec) surrounding the peak, referenced to (subtracted from) a 10 msec prestimulus EEG segment. Subjects were told to try to find a state of mind or mood which kept the reinforcement tone beeping as often as possible since each tone meant a hit. They were instructed to minimize eye and other movements, and these were monitored on closed circuit TV and with piezoelectric movement transducers. Bonuses were not paid during high movement density sessions and the sole repeated violator was dropped from the study. Noxious heat reaction latency on the arms and hands was sampled every other day using a resistive heating element which the subjects could remove on pain sensation; it is based on a device we developed for animals (8). Each training phase lasted 15 sessions over 2- to 3-week periods.

RESULTS

As of the present date, 15 subjects have been run, however, only 10 completed most or all phases of training. Among the 5 drop-outs were 4 individuals who, within 2 weeks, became bored with the 4 to 5 sessions/week regimen and 1 who could not desist from making artifact-generating eye movements. One of the remaining 10 subjects failed to show any evidence of EP control (although she did show correlations of her unconditioned P200 amplitude and PT). The other 9 subjects all showed a significantly ($p < 0.05$) larger P200 during uptraining than during downtraining. Individual t-tests on all days of uptraining and downtraining were done because (a) we wanted to identify successful individual subjects, rather than simply test for a group effect (which was also significant for the 10 people completing training), and (b) because of the marked individual differences seen in baseline PTs, and therefore also in levels of stimulation used for conditioning. EP sizes also showed considerable individual variation, and although the highest PT did go with the largest EP, the PT/P200 relationship was not systematic enough in our limited data set to yield a significant correlation overall; (the PT mean for the large EP group was 3.3 mA; it was 2.8 mA for the others).

All 9 subjects who learned uptraining and downtraining showed significant P200/PT correlations (with individual absolute Pearson r-values ranging from 0.5 to 0.8), however, the signs of the correlation coefficients showed a dichotomous grouping: Those 4 subjects with the largest baseline EPs (P200 $\geq$ 4.6 μV) showed positive correlations, whereas the remaining 5 (with baseline P200 $\leq$ 3.0 μV) showed negative correlations. None of the subjects showed significant correlations of DT and P200. These data are seen in Table 1.

These trends are illustrated for one subject (large baseline EP) in Fig. 1, where U indicates uptraining and D downtraining; E, M, and L are early middle and late days of the respective training conditions. The P200/PT relationship is evident; even during the middle downtraining day when the subject's P200 control regressed, the PT followed. DT is flat throughout.

All individually calculated PT/P200 r-values were significant ($p < 0.05$–$p < 0.001$).For the nociceptive heat reaction latencies, parallel effects were

TABLE 1. *Averaged P200, PT, and DT data during the various training phases for the 2 subject groups separated on a post-hoc basis of baseline EP size*[a]

	Large EP group ($N=4$)			Small EP group ($N=5$)		
Measure	Baseline	Uptraining	Downtraining	Baseline	Uptraining	Downtraining
P200 (μV)	4.9 ± 1.6	6.1 ± 2.1	0.16 ± 1.9	1.9 ± 1.1	3.1 ± .91	−0.18 ± 1.4
PT (mA)	2.1 ± 1.1	5.7 ± 3.1	1.3 ± 1.9	1.8 ± 1.4	1.1 ± 2.1	2.9 ± 2.4
DT (mA)	0.21 ± 0.02	0.22 ± 0.1	0.22 ± 0.08	0.19 ± 0.04	0.20 ± 0.02	0.22 ± 0.06

[a]The means are for the last days of training conditions.

observed for the left hand and arm loci (ipsilateral to the evoking stimulation site) in all subjects, reaching significance in 8 of 9 individually tested cases. That is, for the 4 large EP subjects, just as decreased sensitivity (higher shock level tolerated) went with increased P200 amplitude, increased response latency to noxious heat (again, decreased sensitivity) went with increased P200 amplitude. For the small-EP subjects, the reverse relationship was true. For the right hand and arm measures, only 2 of the 6 cases which were measured and tested showed significant correlations of heat reaction latency and P200 amplitude, the correlation signs agreeing with those of the left side correlations.

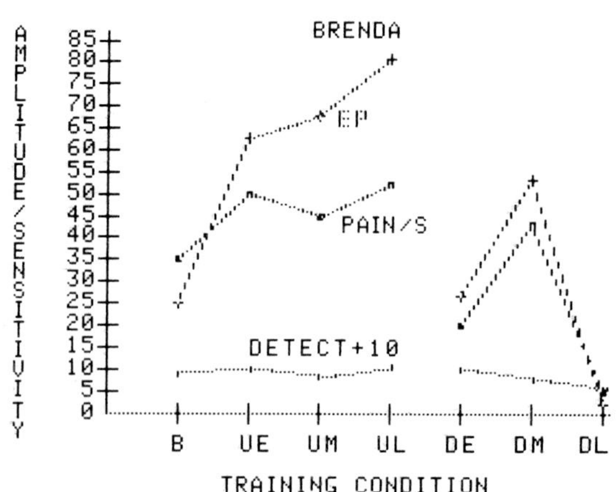

FIG. 1. P200 amplitude (EP) and sensory thresholds as a function of training condition for one subject. EP is computer-coded; difference between EEG prestimulus amplitude and the 10-msec peak average surrounding the criterion component: μV = scale value ÷ 10. *PAIN/S* is the shock pain threshold; mA = scale value ÷ 10. *DETECT* is the shock detection threshold; mA = (scale value −5) ÷ 10. B is last of 4 days of baseline, U and D are uptraining and downtraining, respectively. E is day 2 (early), M is day 7 (middle), and L is day 14 (late) of the particular training phase.

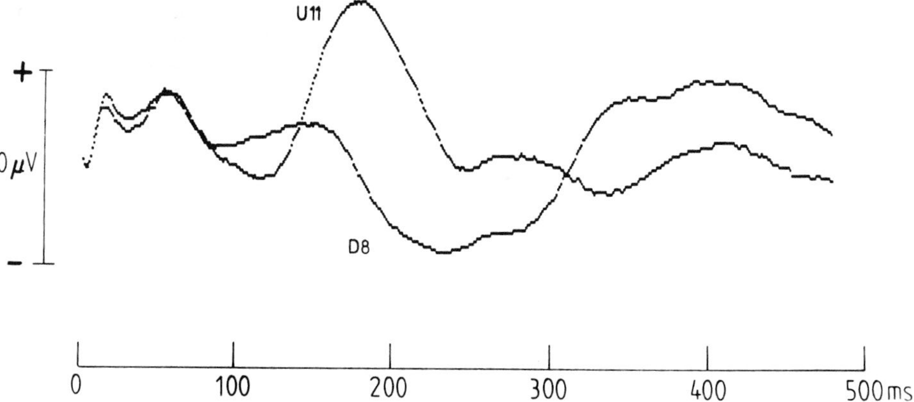

FIG. 2. Two superimposed average EPs of the last 200 trials of uptraining day 11 (U11) and downtraining day 8 (D8) for one subject. Vertex positivity is up.

A representative superimposed pair of averaged EPs from uptraining and downtraining is shown in Fig. 2. For this large EP subject (also the source of Fig. 1 data) it is seen that although the early positive components at about 70 to 80 msec superimpose, other components (besides P200) are notably different between training conditions. This lack of localization was true in 4 other subjects, but was not seen to be related to baseline EP size or PT.

DISCUSSION AND CONCLUSIONS

Human subjects can learn to alter nonaversively evoked somatosensory cortical potentials, as earlier work showed they could do with auditory EPs (13). When aversive sensitivity is probed at the end of a training session, it is seen to vary systematically with the direction of training, and, as seen in rats, this effect appears to show submodality and somatotopic specificity in that (a) more significant correlations were seen on the body side ipsilateral to the evoking stimulation site, and (b) the nonaversive shock detection threshold did not change.

The nature of the EP-pain relationship seemed to vary with baseline EP size: the subjects with large EPs showed a negative correlation of pain sensitivity and EP amplitude; the subjects with small EPs showed a negative relationship. While this EP-based dichotomization was seen on a post-hoc basis and needs replication, two reasons can be given suggesting that the effects seen were not likely to be random fluctuations: (a) In no case where EP control was achieved did we see *no* EP/pain relationship; and (b) all three measures of nociceptive sensitivity—arm shock tolerance, arm heat reaction latency, and hand heat reaction latency—covaried systematically within a subject with EP amplitude.

Since evoking stimulation levels were *individually* set at 67% of baseline pain threshold, a distribution of thresholds was seen. It was not obviously dichotomous, nor did it clearly correspond to the baseline P200 dichotomous distribution. Thus, it would be premature here to suggest evoking stimulus intensity as a key source of variation in P200 amplitude and to then speculate on how evoking stimulus intensity might account for the sign of an EP/pain correlation. More work is needed to obtain closure on the extent to which P200 is predicted by stimulus intensity with the present stimulation parameters; partial relationships have long been known with single-pulse, median nerve stimulation (14).

Although the present results would appear to hold clinical promise, two caveats are appropriate: (a) It is well appreciated that clinical pain, which is often chronic, may be quite different than the acute stimulation effects evoked here. (b) Much work remains to be done in identification of the optimal parameter set for obtaining the operantly conditioned EP effect, as well as the correlated experimental hypoalgesia. We refer here not only to the stimulation parameters, but more particularly to the *conditioning* parameters. It was noted that not all the present subjects changed their EPs in the same way. Some changed mostly the explicitly required P200 amplitude, some changed 2 or 3 other component amplitudes, and some additionally changed peak latencies. As a high-speed microcomputer evaluates each real-time EP, the reinforcement contingency (which was here applied only to P200) could be broadened in future studies to explicitly include or exclude (whichever works best) other EP parameters. Such an extensive parametric program of work would appear to be justified not only in view of the present results, but especially because of the highly specific, robust, and consistent effects seen earlier in rodents (6,10).

ACKNOWLEDGMENTS

This work was supported by United States Public Health Service grants DE05204 and GM23696 awarded to J. P. Rosenfeld.

REFERENCES

1. Buchsbaum, M. S., Davis, G. C., Coppola, R., and Naber, R. (1981): Opiate pharmacology and individual differences. I. Psychophysical pain measurements. *Pain,* 10:357–366.
2. Buchsbaum, M. S., Davis, G. C., Coppola, R., and Naber, R. (1981): Correlation of subjective pain experience with cerebral evoked responses to noxious thermal stimulations. *Exp. Brain Res.,* 33:445–453.
3. Carmon, A., Dotan, Y., and Sarne, Y. (1978): Correlation of subjective pain experience with cerebral evoked responses to noxious thermal stimulations. *Exp. Brain Res.,* 33:445–453.
4. Chapman, R. C., Chen, A. C. N., and Harkins, S. W. (1979): Brain evoked potentials as correlates of laboratory pain: a review and perspective. *Adv. Pain Res. Ther.,* 3:791–803.
5. Chatrian, G. E., Fernandes de Lima, V. M., Lettich, E., Canfield, R. C., Miller, R. C., and

Soso, M. J. (1982): Electrical stimulation of tooth pulp in humans. II. Qualities of sensations. *Pain,* 14:233–246.
6. Dowman, R. J., Rosenfeld, J. P., and Heinricher, M. ((1983): Operant conditioning of trigeminally evoked cortical potentials: Correlated effects on facial nociception. *Brain Res.,* 269:111–118.
7. Rosenfeld, J. P. (1977): Conditioning changes in the evoked response. In: *Biofeedback: Theory and Research,* edited by G. E. Schwartz and J. Beatty, pp. 377–388. Academic Press, New York.
8. Rosenfeld, J. P., Broton, J. G., and Clavier, R. M. (1978): A reliable facial nociception device for unrestrained awake animals. *Physiol. Behav.,* 21:287–290.
9. Rosenfeld, J. P., Diaz-Clark, A., and Olson, R. E. (1983): Response to painful electrical stimulation in MPD Syndrome patients. *J. Dent. Res.,* 62:259.
10. Rosenfeld, J. P., Dowman, R., Heinricher, M., and Silvia, R. (1984): Operantly controlled somatosensory evoked potentials: Specific effects on pain processes. In: *Self-Regulation of the Brain and Behavior,* edited by B. Rockstroh, T. Elbert, W. Lutzenberger, and N. Birbaumer, pp. 164–180. Springer-Verlag, Berlin.
11. Rosenfeld, J. P., Dowman, R., and Silvia, R. (1985): Operant conditioned potentials in pain substrates of rats and humans: Correlated effects on nociception and effects of naloxone. In: *Electroencephalography and Clinical Neurophysiology Supplement, Seventh International Conference on Event Related Potentials Proceedings,* edited by C. McCallum et al. Elsevier, Amsterdam.
12. Rosenfeld, J. P., Hetzler, B. E., Birkel, P., Antoinetti, D., and Kowarch, R. (1976): Operant conditioned potentials, centrally evoked at random intervals. *Behav. Biol.,* 16:305–317.
13. Rosenfeld, J. P., Rudell, A. P., and Fox, S. S. (1969): Operant control of neural events in humans. *Science,* 165:821–823.
14. Uttal, W. R., and Cook, L. (1964): Systematics of the evoked somatosensory cortical potential in man. *Ann. NY Acad. Sci.,* 115:60–80.

Advances in Pain Research and Therapy, Vol. 9, edited by H. L. Fields et al. Raven Press, New York © 1985.

Quality of Pain Sensations Following Local Application of Algogenic Agents on the Exposed Human Tooth Pulp: A Psychophysical and Electrophysiological Study

*Michael L. Ahlquist, **Ove G. Franzén, *Lennart G. A. Edwall, *Uno G. Fors, and *Glenn A. T. Haegerstam

**Department of Endodontics, Karolinska Institutet, 141 04 Stockholm; and*
***Department of Psychology, University of Uppsala, 751 04 Uppsala, Sweden*

AIM OF THE INVESTIGATION

Controversy still lingers regarding interpretation of results from investigations concerned with chemical stimulation of human and cat dental pulp (4,7,11–14,16,22). Inorganic ions (e.g., Na^+, NH_4^+) in hypertonic solutions have been reported to evoke Aδ activity in the feline pulp (24), whereas a highly potent algogenic agent such as bradykinin (internally released after tissue damage) fails to do so after application into cat dentinal cavities, although this agent is known to induce pain when applied to blister base preparation (15) or to lightly abraded skin in man. Furthermore, it has been demonstrated that intra-arterially injected bradykinin sets up unitary activity in heat-sensitive C fibers (6) and that the effect of this substance can be enhanced by the presence of prostaglandins (9,17). Because there is similarity between the skin and the pulp with respect to the types of nociceptive fibers, it is plausible that application of bradykinin on the pulp excites C afferents and thereby gives rise to a feeling of dull pain.

This investigation was undertaken for the purpose of studying the quality of pain sensations elicited by inorganic hypertonic solutions and algogenic substances involved in inflammatory processes. In addition, the electrophysiological technique developed by Ahlquist et al. (1,2) was employed to record intradental nerve activity in man. For comparison and corroboration of the human experiments, the electrical responses of feline pulp to the same solutions and substances were explored.

METHODS

Subjects

This study was carried out on three molars, five premolars, and eight incisors in 1 male and 4 female subjects between 29 and 55 years of age whose teeth were to be extracted for orthodontic or prosthodontic reasons. No clinical signs of pulpitis, sensitivity to thermal stimuli, or tenderness on percussion were observed by the clinician, and no sensation of pain was felt by the subjects before the experimental session began. The project was approved by the medical ethics committee at Huddinge Hospital.

Cavity Preparation and Pulp Stimulation

First the tooth was anesthetized for at least 20 min by means of mepivacain (Carbocain Dental, 30 mg/ml). In order to achieve satisfactory insulation from saliva during the recording and to prevent adjacent teeth and soft tissues from being affected, a rubber dam was placed around the neck of the tooth. One cavity was then prepared on the labial surface of the tooth crown using a manually twirled end-cutting burr, and whenever needed it was rinsed with isotonic sodium chloride. Finally, the pulp was very gently exposed at the bottom of the cavity. The sensitivity of the tooth, vital and intact according to clinical criteria, was tested by means of NH_4 Cl (0.77 M) 60 min after the anesthetic effect had completely subsided. Application of this chemical test stimulus resulted in a sensation of pain in every subject.

Before stimulating the tooth, the fluid in the cavity was carefully soaked up using filter paper. The experiment immediately proceeded, with administration of NaCl (0.77 M), NH_4Cl (0.77 M), histamine (10 mg/ml), or bradykinin (10 μg/ml), and we always made sure that the solution was in full contact with the exposed pulp. Each stimulation was terminated by washing the cavity with physiological saline solution. The pulp was prevented from drying by letting this solution remain in the cavity between stimulations that caused no pain at all. The interval between stimuli was 5 min, and no application exceeded 3 min.

Intradental Nerve Recordings in Cats and Man

Using the procedure described earlier, two cavities were made on the same side of the tooth below the locus of stimulation. In these cavities we implanted electrodes consisting of steel cannulae put in a thin layer of amalgam. The equipment for recording the neural activity was of standard type. For a more detailed description of the experimental procedure, see Ahlquist et al. (2). It is important to point out that in order to achieve optimal stimulating and recording conditions, the cavities have to be of sufficient depth without inflicting any lesion on the pulp itself.

The animal experiments were conducted on adult cats (2–4 kg and 1–3 years old) anesthetized with chloralose (40 mg/kg) and urethane (50 mg/kg). Two cavities were prepared in the canine tooth, one over the pulp horn (coronal cavity) and the other within the gingival part of the crown. The cavities were then filled with saline solution. Platinum-wire electrodes were inserted, and recordings from intradental sensory units were made using the technique described by Edwall and Scott (8). A conventional technique was used to display the signals on a cathode-ray tube and to store the signals on magnetic tape.

Assessment of Pain Quality and Intensity

The pain quality was assessed by the subject's choice of one or more expressions characterizing various aspects of the sensations evoked by the four different chemical stimuli (Fig. 1). The intensity of pain was rated by the subject, who was instructed to select a sensory verbal descriptor that best described the peak sensation following each chemical stimulation. The verbal descriptors covering the full range of pain intensity were as follows: very very weak, very weak, weak, neither strong nor weak, slightly strong, strong, very strong, very very strong, and maximal. During the course of the recording of intradental nerve activity (INA), the intensity of the pain sensation was rated by means of an intermodal scaling procedure called finger span. In this procedure the subject was instructed to adjust the distance between the thumb and the index finger attached to two metal arms that in turn were connected to a linear potentiometer. By doing so we were able to monitor the neural and perceptual output simultaneously.

throbbing(bultande)	*dull pain(dov smärta)*
quivering(dallrande)	*sharp pain(skarp smärta)*
pounding(dunkande)	*shooting pains(ilning)*
pulsing(pulserande)	*itching(kliande)*
vibrating(vibrerande)	*smarting(svidande)*
aching(molande)	*tooth-ache(tandvärk)*
pricking(stickade)	*burning(brännande)*
dental burr-drill(tandläkarborr)	*hot(varmt)*
splitting(blixtrande)	*biting cool(isande)*
penetrating(genomträngande)	*cold(kallt)*
bursting(sprängande)	*slightly aching(malande)*
radiating(strålande)	*feeling of pressure(tryckande)*
stinging(bitande)	*pulling feeling(som ett drag)*
attack of cramp(som kramp)	*swelling pulp(svällande pulpa)*
pinching(nypande)	

FIG. 1. List of qualitative expressions characterizing dental pain presented to the subject after each chemical tooth-pulp stimulation.

RESULTS

Phenomenology of Pain

It was a consistent finding in all subjects that the number of reports of dull pain increased going from NH_4Cl over NaCl and histamine to bradykinin (Fig. 2). Conversely, the response to the inorganic ions was in most cases that of sharp pain. In addition to dichotomizing the nociceptive sensations into sharp and dull, the subjects observed that sharp pain was usually associated with such feelings as pricking, pounding, smarting, pinching, and shooting pains and that dull pain was felt as throbbing toothache. Successive stimulations with histamine and bradykinin produced an increasing erythema, a phenomenon correlated with a gradually decreasing responsiveness of the pulp. In contrast, the inorganic ions produced over and over again perceptions of nearly the same magnitude irrespective of the number of administrations. Despite the fact that histamine and bradykinin ultimately induced no pain after repeated applications, the responses to ammonium and sodium chloride were unaffected. For this reason, the hypertonic inorganic ion solutions were employed as positive controls and the isotonic NaCl as negative control between administrations of the experimental substances.

Collapsing the quality judgments into a two-by-two matrix (Fig. 3) brings out a conspicuous trend in the data, namely, that the subjects experienced sharp pain in 34 of 41 trials when stimulated with inorganic ions; on the

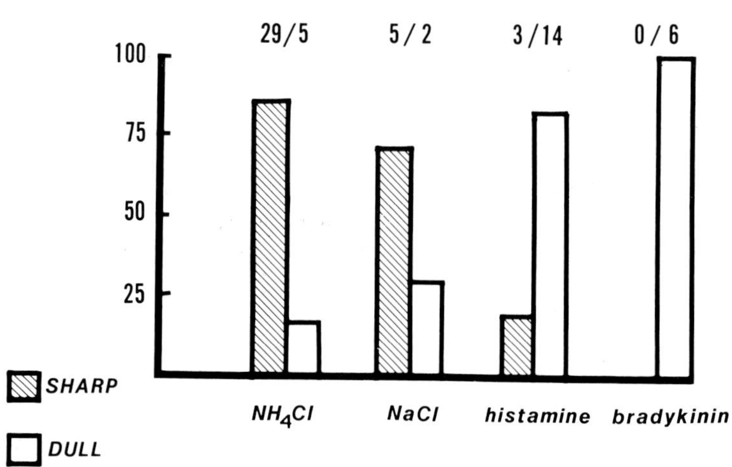

FIG. 2. Columns represent percentages of sharp and dull pains following chemical stimulation of tooth pulp with inorganic ions (NaCl and NH_4Cl) and vasoactive endogenous substances (histamine and bradykinin).

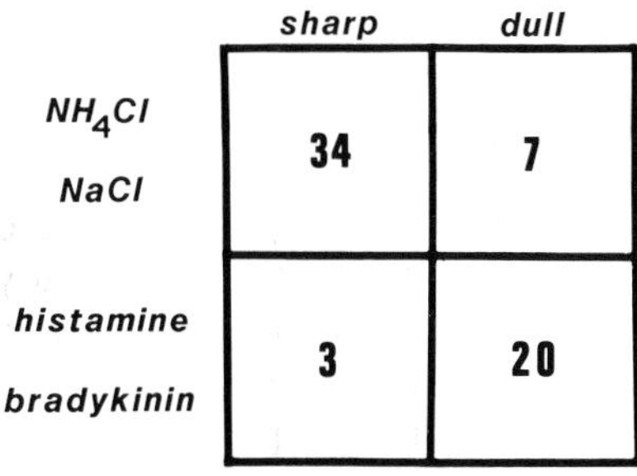

FIG. 3. Distribution of sharp and dull dental pains as a result of applying either hypertonic solutions or vasoactive substances on the exposed pulp tissue. A chi square test provides a p value < 0.001.

other hand, vasoactive endogenous substances such as histamine and bradykinin produced a sensation of dull pain in 20 of 23 exposures.

Pulpal Electrophysiology

Vigorous impulse discharges were elicited in the cat pulp after stimulation with 0.76 M (9%) sodium chloride (Fig. 4a). This observation was contrasted by the consistent failure of bradykinin to induce neural activity that could be recorded from deep cavities with intact dentinal layer (Fig. 4b).

Testing bradykinin in a human tooth pulp confirmed the experimental outcome of the cat study. We were unable to record INA in the human tooth when this substance was applied in the cavity as illustrated in Fig. 5a. The sensation produced by bradykinin was a dull pounding pain that remained almost constant for several minutes, which is shown by the subject's finger-span setting in Fig. 5a. On the sensory descriptor scale the peak intensity was judged by the subject as strong. Figure 5b shows that electrical activity was set up in the intradental sensory units after application of histamine on the same pulp as before, and this event could be recorded by our present technique (2). There was substantial discrepancy, however, between the neural and perceptual responses, in that the subject still felt pain long after the INA had returned to the noise level. The pain sensation was rated as slightly strong, and it had a dull and pulsing quality.

DISCUSSION

All the chemical substances employed in the present study induced pain, but the qualities of the pain sensations differed significantly when evoked by agents classified as inorganic ions (NH_4Cl and NaCl) and those classified as vasoactive endogenous substances (histamine and bradykinin), the latter assumed to be intimately involved as intermediaries in inflammatory reactions.

The feline tooth and the human tooth are innervated by two groups of sensory fibers that belong to the Aδ and C types (5,10,11,16,19,20). How-

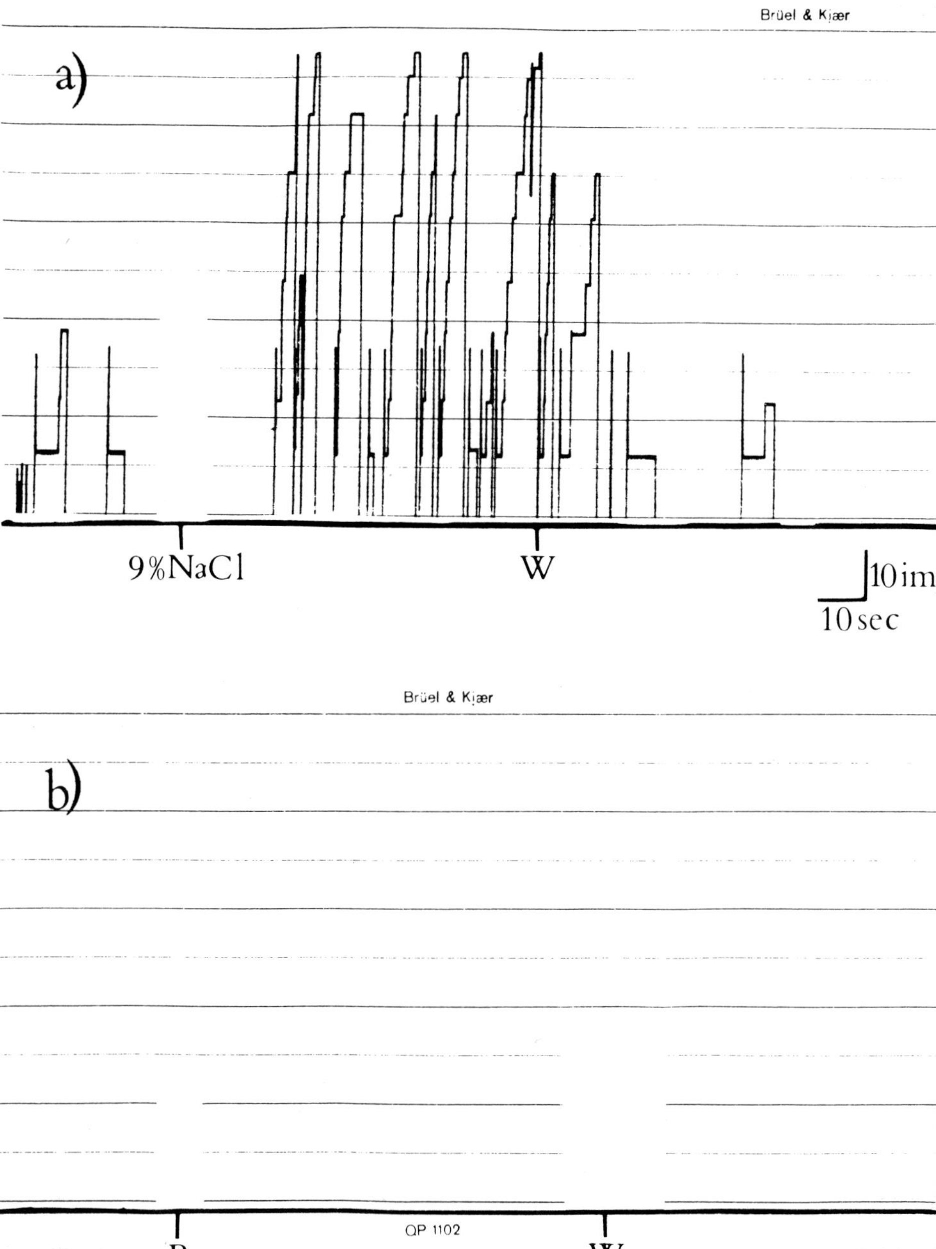

FIG. 4. Graph from a recording of INA in the tooth pulp of the cat. A solution of 9% (0.76 M) sodium chloride applied to a deep dentinal cavity (without pulp exposure) induced nerve activity. This activity was terminated by washing the cavity with 0.9% NaCl (W). INA could not be recorded after application of bradykinin (10 mg/ml)(B), despite the high concentration.

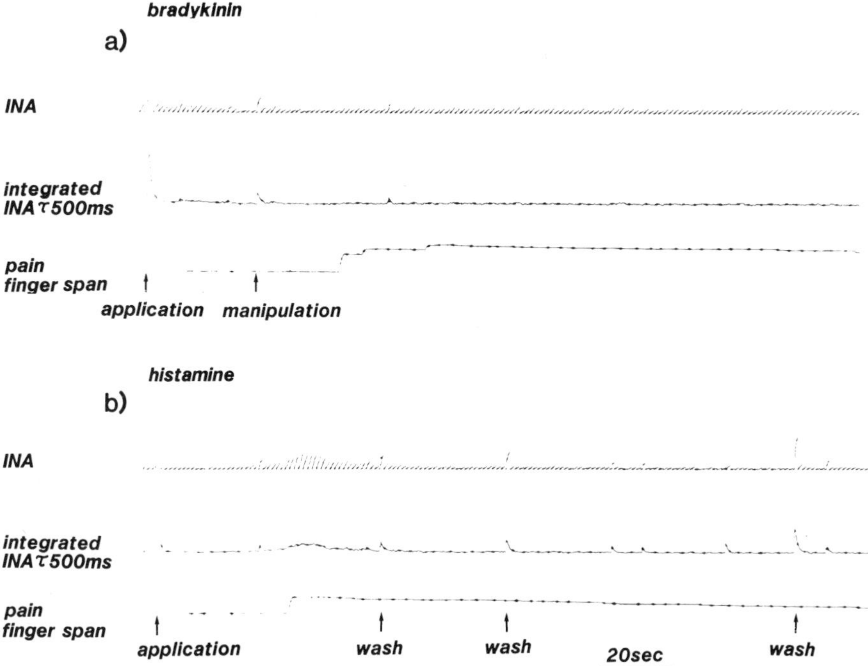

FIG. 5. INA recorded from human tooth pulp after chemical stimulation in a deep dentinal cavity (without pulp exposure) using bradykinin (a) and histamine (b).

ever, our method for recording INA can solely pick up activity in pulpal axons in the Aδ range (2,12). It is generally agreed that sharp, crisp, and distinct pain in the skin is due to activation of sensory myelinated fibers in the Aδ range and that dull and poorly localized pain is the result of excitation of C fibers (26). Having this information at hand, one would be inclined to interpret the response matrix in Fig. 3 in such a fashion that NH_4Cl and NaCl predominantly excite Aδ axons and that bradykinin and histamine mainly activate C fibers. Hypertonic NaCl solutions are said to increase the extracellular sodium concentration in the immediate neighborhood of the nerve, which thereby causes a depolarization of the Aδ axons (14,23). If that is the case, it cannot be excluded that other classes of neural units in the pulp, such as the C fibers, are excited by a hypertonic NaCl solution; that is to say, both types of pulpal axons may be triggered by the presence of this solution in the extracellular space. Because NH_4^+ has some properties in common with Na^+ and K^+, it is not unlikely that NH_4^+ has an effect on the nonmyelinated fibers similar to that of Na^+ and K^+. The significant number of reports of sharp pain after stimulation with NH_4Cl and NaCl may be explained by the masking of the C fiber activity by the Aδ flux that also occurs on the skin after sustained heat or electrical stimulation (26,27).

Bradykinin did not produce any signs of electrical activity in the feline or human pulp (Figs. 4b and 5a, respectively), although it is evident from Fig. 5a that the subject experienced dull pain for as long as she was exposed to the substance. These observations taken together are fully consistent with the fact that bradykinin applied on the exposed cat pulp evoked neural activity only in C fibers classified according to the conduction velocities ($\leq$ 2 m/sec)(21).

With respect to the ability of histamine to trigger neural tissue, the picture is somewhat more complex, because some tissue damage may be a necessary antecedent condition for this substance to become an algogenic agent (15). There are some indications in the literature that histamine under certain conditions gives rise to a dual response (25). The neurophysiological and psychophysical responses in Fig. 5b definitely suggest that both the Aδ and C afferents are activated, because the subject continued to perceive pain despite cessation of the Aδ activities. One case in point is an experiment by Olgart (23) in which he made applications of warm guttapercha to the cat tooth surface. This treatment resulted presumably in pathological changes in the morphology of the pulp (18), and as a consequence Olgart was able to record intradental Aδ activity following histamine stimulation. We conclude, therefore, that the response pattern obtained in Fig. 5b provides us with indirect evidence of an actual pulp inflammation that is interestingly at variance with the diagnosis made by the clinician. It is our intention to come back to this particular problem in an investigation concerned with analysis of INA evoked by heat stimulation of the tooth (3).

In light of the experimental data presented in this study, the controversy referred to at the outset may simply be a manifestation of the shortcoming and limitation of the one-sided use of either a psychophysical or a neurophysiological approach to an understanding of the mechanisms of pulpal pain.

ACKNOWLEDGMENTS

This study was supported by the Swedish Medical Research Council (24X-816), the Swedish Dental Association, Praktikertjänst AB, and the School of Dentistry, Karolinska Institutet, Stockholm, Sweden.

REFERENCES

1. Ahlquist, M., Edwall, L., Franzén, O., and Haegerstam, G. (1980): Pain perception related to intradental nerve activity in man. *J. Dent. Res.,* 59:1904 (abstract).
2. Ahlquist, M., Edwall, L., Franzén, O., and Haegerstam, G. (1984): Perception of pulpal pain as a function of intradental nerve activity. *Pain,* 19:353–366.
3. Ahlquist, M., Franzén, O., Edwall, L., Fors, U., and Haegerstam, G. (1985): The relation-

ship between the intradental nerve activity and pulpal pain after heat stimulation. *(in press).*
4. Anderson, D. J., and Naylor, M. N. (1962): Chemical excitants of pain in human dentine and dental pulp. *Arch. Oral Biol.,* 7:413–415.
5. Beasley, W. L., and Holland, G. R. (1978): A quantitative analysis of the innervation of the pulp of the cat's canine tooth. *J. Comp. Neurol.* 178:487–494.
6. Beck, P. W., and Handwerker, P. O. (1974): Bradykinin and serotonin effects on various types of cutaneous nerve fibres. *Pfluegers Arch.,* 11:209–222.
7. Dellow, P. G., and Roberts, M. L. (1966): Bradykinin application to dentine: A study of sensory receptor mechanism. *Aust. Dent. J.,* 11:384–387.
8. Edwall, L., and Scott, D., Jr. (1971): Influence of changes in the microcirculation on the excitability of the sensory unit in the tooth of the cat. *Acta Physiol. Scand.,* 82:555–566.
9. Ferreira, S. H., Moncada, S., and Vane, J. R. (1973): Prostaglandins and the mechanism of analgesia produced by aspirin-like drugs. *Br. J. Pharmacol.* 47:629–630.
10. Fried, K. (1982): Development, degeneration and regeneration of nerve fibres in the feline inferior alveolar nerve and mandibular incisor pulps. *Acta Physiol. Scand.* [*Suppl. 504.*]
11. Haegerstam, G. (1976): A pharmacological study on intradental sensory nerve endings in cat. Thesis, Karolinska Institutet, Stockholm.
12. Haegerstam, G. (1976): The origin of impulses recorded from dentinal cavities in the tooth of the cat. *Acta Physiol. Scand.,* 97:121–128.
13. Horiuchi, H., and Matthews, B. (1973): In vitro observations on fluid flow through human dentin caused by pain-producing stimuli. *Arch. Oral Biol.,* 18:275–294.
14. Horiuchi, H., and Matthews, B. (1976): Responses of intradental nerves to chemical and osmotic stimulation of dentin in the cat. *Pain,* 2:49–59.
15. Keele, C. A., and Armstrong, D. (1964): *Substances Producing Pain and Itch.* Edward Arnold, London.
16. Matthews, B. (1977): Responses of intradental nerves to electrical and thermal stimulation of teeth in dogs. *J. Physiol. (Lond.),* 264:641–664.
17. Moncada, S., Ferriera, S. H., and Vane, I. R. (1975): Inhibition of prostaglandin biosynthesis as the mechanism of analgesia of aspirin-like drugs in the dog knee joint. *Eur. J. Pharmacol.,* 31:250–260.
18. Nyborg, H., and Brännström, M. (1968): Pulp reaction to heat. *J. Pros. Dent.,* 19:605–612.
19. Närhi, M., Virtanen, A., Huopaniemi, T., and Hirvonen, T. (1982): Conduction velocities of single pulp nerve fibre units in the cat. *Acta Physiol. Scand.,* 116:209–213.
20. Närhi, M., Jyvasjärvi, E., Hirvonen, T., and Huopaniemi, T. (1982): Activation of heat-sensitive nerve fibres in the dental pulp of the cat. *Pain,* 14:317–326.
21. Närhi, M., Jyvasjärvi, E., Huopaniemi, T., and Hirvonen, T. (1984): Functional differenses in intradental A- and C-nerve units in the cat. *Pain* [*Suppl. 2*], 242.
22. Olgart, L. (1974): Excitation of intradental sensory units by pharmacological agents. *Acta Physiol. Scand.,* 92:48–55.
23. Olgart, L. (1974): Pharmacological analysis of intradental sensory nerve excitability. An experimental study in the cat. Thesis, Karolinska Institutet, Stockholm.
24. Panopoulos, P., Mejáre, B., and Edwall, L. (1983): Effects of ammonia and organic acids on the intradental sensory nerve activity. *Acta Odont. Scand.,* 41:209–215.
25. Rosenthal, S. R. (1968): Histamine as the chemical mediator for referred pain. In: *The Skin Senses,* edited by D. R. Kenshalo, pp. 480–498. Charles C Thomas, Springfield, Ill.
26. Vierck, C. J., Jr., Cooper, B. Y., Franzén, O. G., Ritz, L. A., and Greenspan, J. D. (1983): Behavioral analysis of the CNS pathways and transmitter system involved in conduction and inhibition of pain sensations and reactions in primates. In: *Progress in Psychobiological and Physiological Psychology,* edited by J. M. Sprague and A. N. Epstein, pp. 113–165. Academic Press, New York.
27. Vierk, C. J., Jr., Cooper, B. Y., Cohen, R. H., Yeomans, D. C., and Franzén, O. G. (1984): Effects of systemic morphine on monkeys and man: Generalized suppression of behavior and preferential inhibition of pain elicited by unmyelinated nociceptors. In: *Somatosensory Mechanisms,* edited by C. V. Euler, O. Franzén, U. Lindblom, and D. Ottoson, pp. 309–323. Macmillan, London.

Advances in Pain Research and Therapy, Vol. 9, edited by H. L. Fields et al. Raven Press, New York © 1985.

A Quantitative Study of Flexion Reflex in Man: Relevance to Pain Research

Christina W. Y. Chan and Henry H. Y. Tsang

School of Physical and Occupational Therapy, McGill University, Montreal H3G 1Y5, Quebec, Canada

Several investigators showed that transcutaneous electrical stimulation of the sural nerve or its distal receptive field in man evoked two distinct components in the electromyographic (EMG) response of the lower-limb flexors (13,17,21,23). The early low-threshold component appeared at some 40 to 60 msec and was termed the RA II response (13). The late high-threshold component appeared at a latency of 70 to 150 msec and was called the RA III component. These responses were so named because of their similarity to the two components of the flexion reflex (FR) that Lloyd (18) had observed in cats, the first being mediated by group II fibers and the second by group III fibers. On the basis of conduction velocity measurements (13) and Willer's finding (23) that ischemic block of the large-diameter fibers in the sural nerve decreased the RA II response but not the RA III response, the two components of the human FR are now generally thought to be mediated by fiber types similar to those found in cat experiments.

Behavioral studies of the FR have further revealed that whereas the RA II response is closely related to tactile sensation, the RA III response is highly correlated to the subjective report of pain (6,13,23). In fact, evidence is accumulating to show that the latter component of the FR probably provides a good measure of nociception. This belief is based on the following findings regarding the RA III reflex: (a) It is elicited by noxious stimulation and has been viewed as a reflex of protection equivalent to the flexor withdrawal described by Sherrington (22). (b) It is transmitted by the same (group III) fibers (18) as those mediating fast pain (20). (c) It has the same threshold as that of pain sensation (13,23). (d) Its amplitude is modulated in parallel with that of subjective pain sensation by the same conditioning stimuli (25). (e) It is selectively reduced by morphine (1), just as pain is. Hence, the FR has increasingly been used in studies related to the understanding of pain mechanisms (24,26) and pain modulation techniques in human (14) as well as animal (5) experiments. In this respect, it is important to develop methods for providing quantitative measurements of the human

FR that will be reproducible on repeated testing, will remain stable over the duration of the experiment, and will be sensitive to afferent modification. These issues are particularly pertinent because the FR is very prone to habituation during repetitive stimulation. This report describes a stimulus-triggered averaging technique of recording the FR during a constant tonic background contraction of the relevant muscles that fully fulfills these criteria.

METHODS

Altogether, 10 normal subjects between the ages of 20 and 27 years were studied. Six subjects participated in the series to monitor the stability of the FR over a 1-hr period by measuring the FR every 10 min, as will be described later. Five subjects took part in the series to map the FR as a function of stimulus intensity.

During the experimental session, which lasted from 2 to 3 hr, the subject reclined comfortably in the semi-inclined position illustrated in Fig. 1. The right knee and ankle articulations were fixated by partial casts in a relatively extended position to enhance FR excitability (3). The cathode (a Hewlett-Packard 14445A skin electrode) was strapped under pressure over the median arch of the right foot, and the anode (a silver plate) was located slightly proximal to the ankle joint. The FR was elicited by stimulating the median arch of the foot with a 200-Hz train of 6 × 1-msec square pulses, delivered over 30 msec from a Grass S88 stimulator via a stimulus isolation unit (Grass SIU5) and a constant-current unit (Grass CCU1). Except for the series that studied the FR as a function of stimulus intensity, the intensity was adjusted to the maximum level that the subject would tolerate, usually three to four times the sensory threshold.

To avoid habituation of the FR, the stimulation was applied with an interstimulus interval varying between 10 and 20 sec (9), as well as during a tonic background contraction of the relevant muscles (7,16). It should be noted that the latter procedure has also been shown to enhance the FR (15). Subjects were instructed to maintain a constant tonic background contraction of the biceps femoris (BF), the tibialis anterior (TA), and occasionally the hip flexors (HF) at 10, 20, and 10% of the respective maximum voluntary contraction, aided by the display of the filtered and smoothed EMG on an oscilloscope (Tektronix 2213). Because we felt it important to monitor the same type of motoneurons [in terms of size (12)], on-line computer control via a PDP 11/23 plus microprocessor ensured that the stimuli were delivered only when the subject's tonic EMG activity reached 10 to 15% of the desired level for 1 to 2 sec.

Raw EMG activities from the BF and TA, and in 2 subjects also the HF, were recorded bipolarly with surface electrodes (Graphic Control Med 1801) placed on scratched and degreased skin over the respective motor points (2), with a common ground electrode located over the tibia. These signals were

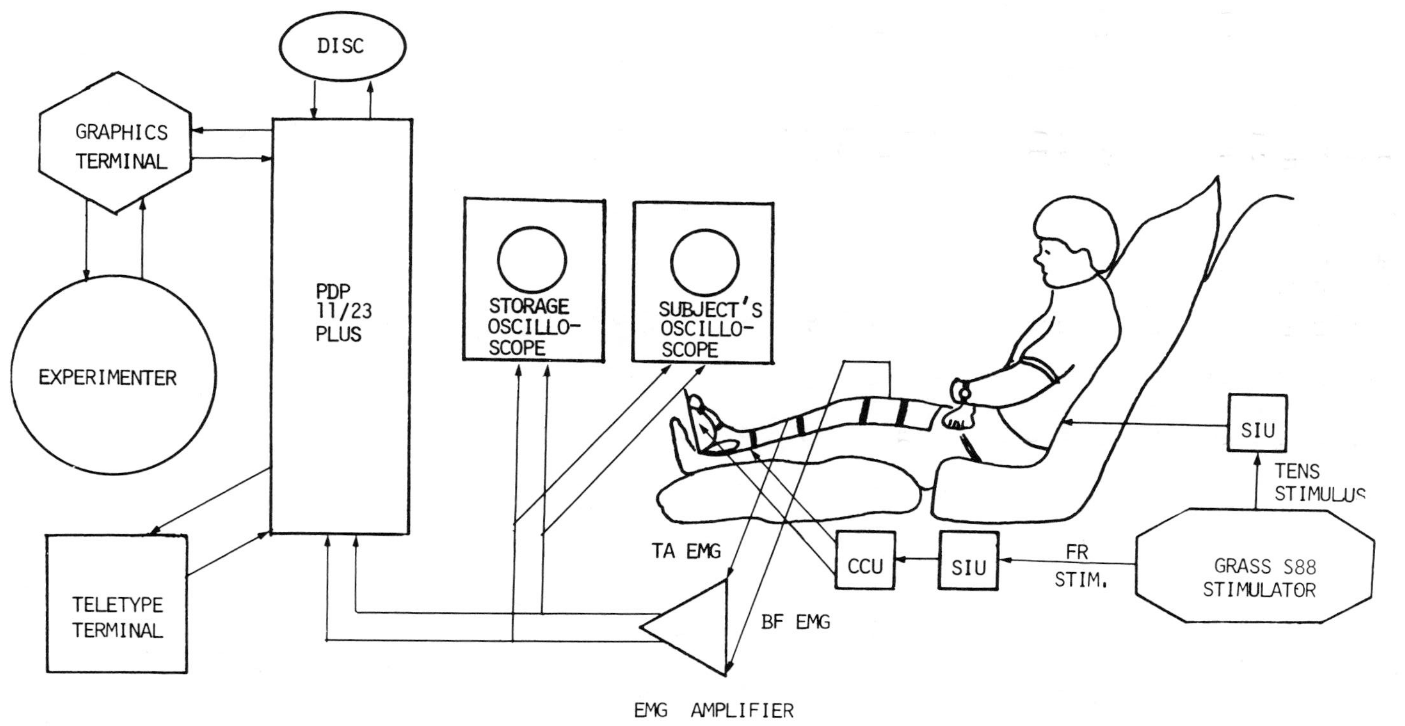

FIG. 1. Experimental setup.

amplified with a gain of 10,000 and were band-pass filtered (10–500 Hz) with EMG amplifiers (Disa 15 C 01). They were then fed into a storage oscilloscope (Tektronix 5111A) for the purpose of cross-checking the data simultaneously processed by the PDP 11/23 plus microprocessor (Fig. 1).

For averaging purpose, 20 responses of the FR were collected. The EMG signals were sampled at a rate of 1.25 kHz for 100 msec prior to and 200 msec after the FR stimuli. They were rectified and smoothed with a low-pass filter having a cutoff frequency at 75 Hz. An averaging technique was applied on-line to extract the mean and standard deviation (SD) of (a) the peak–peak amplitude of the RA III component and (b) the area value of the ensemble FR response over a time window from 40 to 150 msec, once these values exceeded 2 SD of the base line. All the data were printed out on a teletype terminal (Digital LA 120) and were also stored on a Winchester disc (Tranduction DSD 880D/30-Lll-A) to be spooled off to diskettes (Memorex 3201-3104) later for off-line plots or further data analysis.

RESULTS

Figure 2 shows the response patterns for the FR thus elicited by a maximally tolerable stimulus in the BF in 4 subjects. Each trace represents the mean $\pm$ 1 SD for 20 responses of the rectified and smoothed EMG signal. In the majority of subjects the FR typically consisted of an RA III component at a latency of 70 to 80 msec without an RA II response, as illustrated by the top two records. The amplitude of the RA III response varied between 44 and 184 μV from subject to subject, with a mean value of 107.9 $\pm$ 50.8 μV. In contrast, the RA II response was found to be present in only 2 of the 10 subjects. Its amplitude was typically small, and it tended to be fused with the RA III component (bottom two records). In a few subjects, components later than that of the RA III could be observed beyond 120 msec, as illustrated in record TO001. The most remarkable finding was the consistency of the FR responses, demonstrated by the small standard deviations in the four records. In fact, small standard deviations within 10 to 15% of the mean FR value were observed in the majority (61.3%) of subjects under our experimental paradigm. We observed that this phenomenon was largely due to a "constant" level of tonic background contraction being ensured by on-line control.

In spite of slight variability of FR values between subjects, the EMG response pattern was found to be reproducible in a given subject tested on different occasions. Figure 3 illustrates the similarity of the FR values recorded from the BF of subject SW on four different occasions. The response consisted typically only of an RA III component appearing at some 75 msec and lasting until approximately 115 msec. Understandably, its amplitude varied somewhat, between 78 and 113 μV, from day to day.

Habituation has been known to occur frequently with repeated elicitation

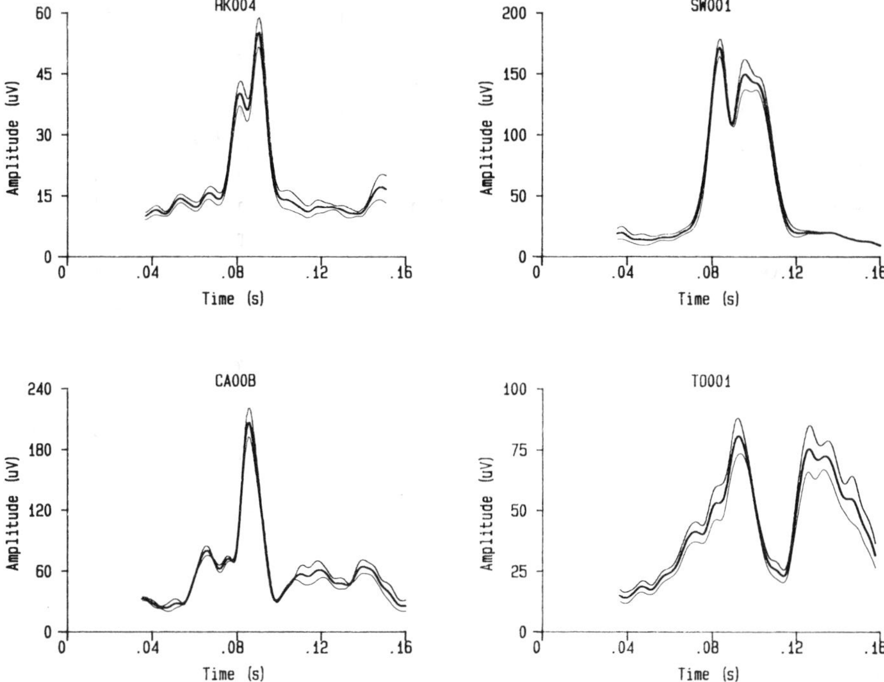

FIG. 2. EMG response patterns of the FR in the BF in 4 subjects. Each trace represents the mean *(thick line)* ± 1 SD *(thin lines)* for 20 responses of the rectified and smoothed EMG signal. The train of electrical pulses occurs between 0 and 0.04 sec on the time scale, but is blanked off here for the sake of clarity. Note the presence of the early RA II response in the bottom two records, but not in the top two records representing the majority of the subjects, in which an RA III response was typically found alone. The consistency of the FR was marked by the very small standard deviations ranging from 10 to 15% in most subjects.

of the FR. To investigate whether or not our experimental paradigm had overcome this problem, 20 responses of the FR were recorded at 10-min intervals for 60 min. Figure 4 demonstrates the stability of the responses evoked in the BF (left column) and the TA (right column) over the time period measured. The peak–peak amplitudes of the RA responses (top records) and the area values of the FR (bottom records) are expressed as percentages of the control data obtained at time zero. Each data point represents the mean ± 1 SD for 20 responses obtained separately from 6 subjects. A one-way analysis of variance failed to show any significant differences among these values for all the three muscles ($p > 0.01$).

The behavior of the FR was then measured as a function of the stimulus intensity to determine its sensitivity to afferent modification. As illustrated in Fig. 5, both the amplitudes (top records) and area values (bottom records) increased linearly with increasing stimulus intensity, all the values being

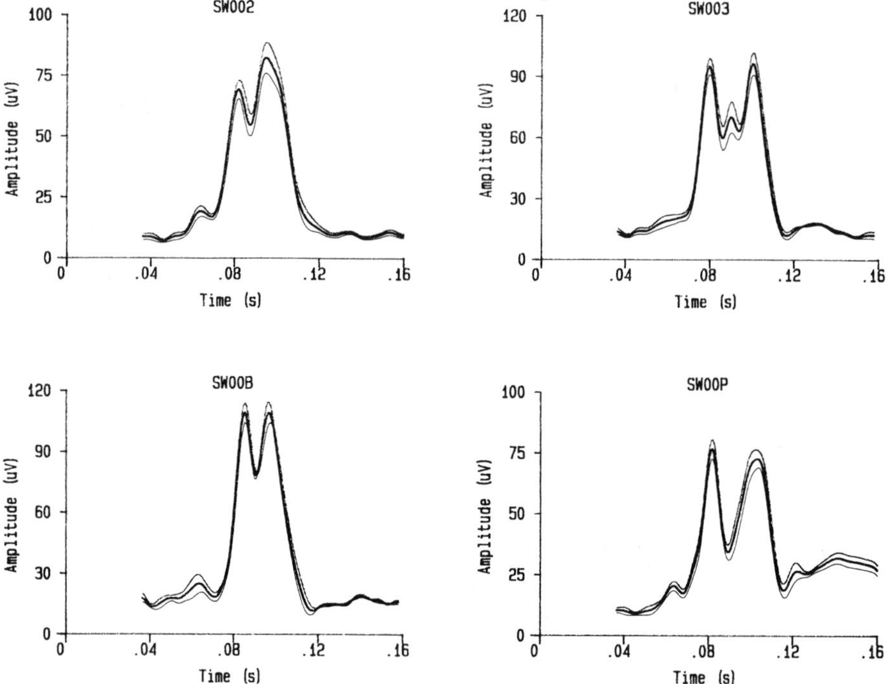

FIG. 3. Similarity of EMG response patterns for the FR evoked in the BF of a given subject on four separate sessions.

expressed as percentages of the maximum (=100%). Each data point represents the mean for 20 responses obtained from the BF in 5 subjects (left column) and from the TA in 4 subjects (right column). For the BF, the correlation coefficient (*r*) of the linear-regression lines drawn through the data points was 0.82 for amplitude and 0.87 for area. For the TA, the *r* values were 0.86 and 0.85, respectively, for amplitude and area; for the HF, the values were 0.88 and 0.91, respectively (not shown).

DISCUSSION

In contrast to the findings with electrical stimulation of the sural nerve itself (8,10,13,21), we found that stimulation of its distal receptive field (the median arch of the foot) produced the characteristic RA III response without an RA II component in the majority of our subjects (see top two records of Fig. 2). Such an observation has also been reported by Willer (23). It is probably due to the more superficial location of group III and IV fibers versus the deeper location of group II fibers in the distal receptive field of the sural nerve (23).

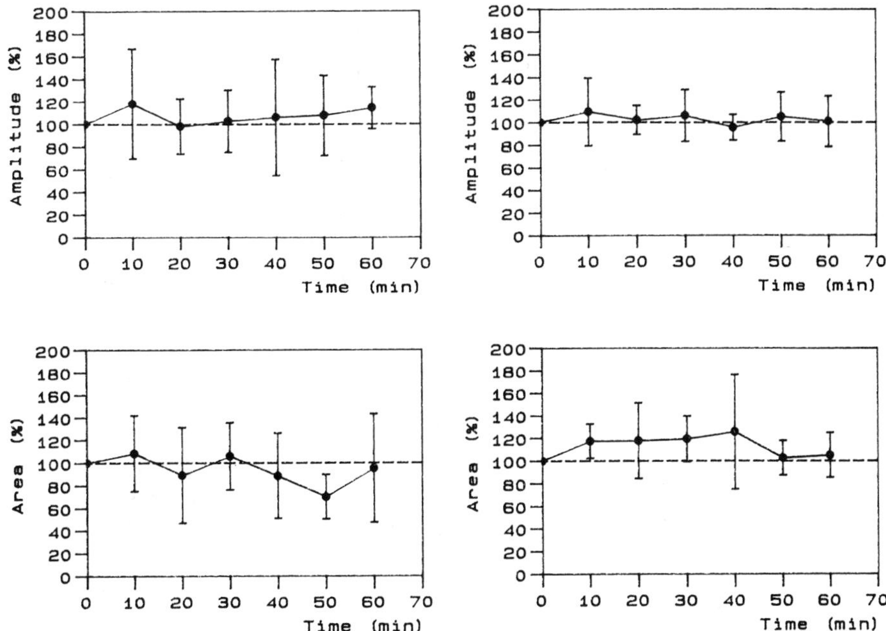

FIG. 4. Stability of the FR evoked in the BF **(left column)** and TA **(right column)** over time (60 min). The amplitudes of the RA III components **(top records)** and the area values of the FR **(bottom records)** are expressed as percentages of the control data obtained at time zero. Each data point represents the mean ± 1 SD for 20 responses obtained separately from 6 subjects. A one-way analysis of variance failed to show any significant difference among these values ($p > 0.01$).

By maintaining the muscles at a constant level of tonic background contraction, it was thought that motoneurons of similar sizes (12) could be brought to similar levels of excitability. Indeed, the FR thus elicited was found to be remarkably consistent in time (latency and duration) as well as amplitude, as revealed by the small standard deviations (10–15%) of the mean values shown in Figs. 2 and 3. Equally remarkable was the finding that the FR was reproducible in a given subject when tested on different occasions. In spite of small changes in the locations of the stimulating and recording electrodes that were bound to occur from day to day, the EMG response patterns remained extremely similar in both their temporal and spatial profiles, although there were minor fluctuations in amplitude (Fig. 3).

We also observed that when the electrical stimulation was applied with a variable interstimulus interval, and the motoneurons were maintained at a similar excitability level through a tonic background contraction in the relevant muscles, the well-known habituation of the FR did not occur. This is illustrated in Fig. 4, which shows the stability of the amplitude and area

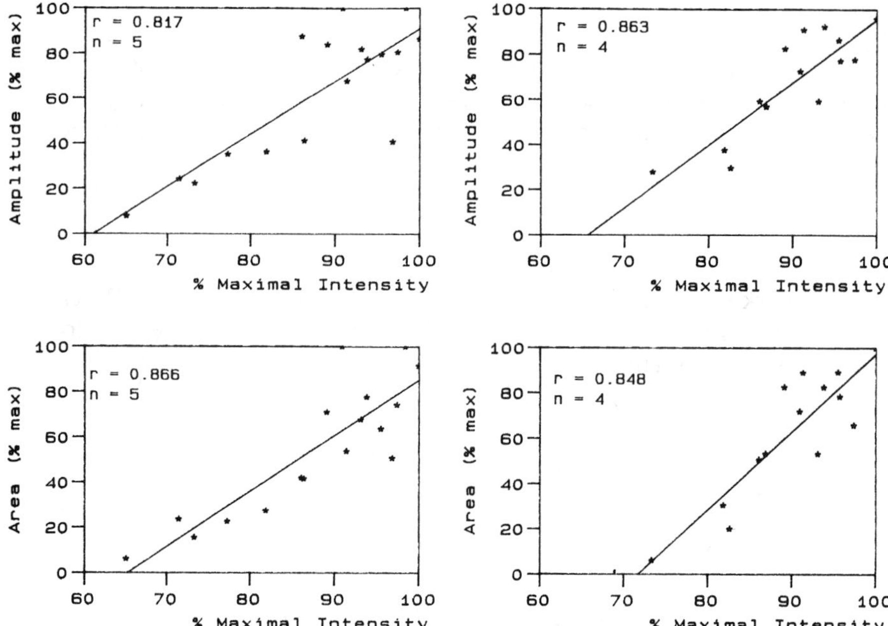

FIG. 5. Behavior of the FR evoked in the BF **(left column)** and TA **(right column)** as a function of stimulus intensity. The amplitudes of the RA III responses **(top records)** and the area values of the FR **(bottom records)** are expressed as percentages of the maximum values (= 100%); the same holds for the stimulus intensity. Each data point denotes the mean of 20 responses obtained from 4 to 5 subjects. Note that the linear-regression lines drawn through the data points all have a correlation coefficient (*r*) greater than 0.8.

values of the FR over a 1-hr period, in spite of repeated testing. In this regard, the influence of voluntary contraction on habituation has also been demonstrated by Desmedt and Godaux (7), and is probably due to enhanced gain in the interneuronal pathway.

Our last finding was that the amplitude and area of the FR increased linearly with increasing stimulus intensity (Fig. 5, $r > 0.8$ in all cases). The influence of stimulus intensity on the FR was documented as early as 1910 by Sherrington (22) in cat experiments. Therefore, a systematic relationship between input (stimulus intensity) and output (FR parameters) is not totally unexpected. Certainly several investigators have reported a decrease in FR latency with increasing intensity (13,21).

Since the human FR was first studied with EMG techniques, it has advanced from single or multiple sweeps of recording (11) to computerized averaging of rectified and smoothed signals (4,19), which provides better and more accurate quantitative data as in our experiments. In addition, our stimulus-triggered averaging technique of recording the FR in various human lower-limb flexors during a constant level of tonic background contraction is able to provide consistent, reproducible, and stable data over time that are also very sensitive to afferent modulation. Among other applications, this methodology will be particularly attractive in studying the influence of pain relief procedures such as transcutaneous electrical nerve stimulation.

ACKNOWLEDGMENTS

This work was financed indirectly by a grant from the Medical Research Council of Canada. Sincere thanks are due to S. Lafontaine, who developed the computer programs for on-line control, data analysis, and off-line plots.

REFERENCES

1. Barton, C., Basbaum, A. I., and Fields, H. L. (1980): Dissociation of supraspinal and spinal actions of morphine: A quantitative evaluation. *Brain Res.,* 188:487–498.
2. Basmajian, J. V., and Blumenstein, R. (1980): *Electrode Placement in EMG Biofeedback.* Williams & Wilkins, Baltimore.
3. Baxendale, R. H., and Ferrell, W. F. (1980): Modulation of transmission in flexion reflex pathways by knee joint afferent discharge in the decerebrate cat. *Brain Res.,* 202:497–500.
4. Bromm, B., and Treede, R. D. (1980): Withdrawal reflex, skin resistance reaction and pain ratings due to electrical stimuli in man. *Pain,* 9:339–354.
5. Chung, J. M., Fang, Z. R., Cargill, C. L., and Willis, W. D. (1983): Prolonged, naloxone-reversible inhibition of the flexion reflex in the cat. *Pain,* 15:35–53.
6. Collins, W. F., Nulsen, F. E., and Randt, C. T. (1960): Relation of peripheral nerve size and sensation in man. *Arch. Neurol.,* 3:381–385.
7. Desmedt, J. E., and Godaux, E. (1976): Habituation of exteroceptive suppression and of exteroceptive reflexes in man as influenced by voluntary contraction. *Brain Res.,* 106:21–29.
8. Dimitrijevic, M. R. (1973): Withdrawal reflexes. In: *New Developments in Electromyography and Clinical Neurophysiology,* Vol. III, edited by J. E. Desmedt, pp. 744–750. Karger, Basel.
9. Dimitrijevic, M. R., Faganel, J., Gregoric, M., Nathan, P. W., and Trontelj, J. K. (1972): Habituation: Effects of regular and stochastic stimulation. *J. Neurol. Neurosurg. Psychiatry,* 35:234–242.
10. Faganel, J. (1973): Electromyographic analysis of human flexion reflex components. In: *New Developments in Electromyography and Clinical Neurophysiology,* Vol. III, edited by J. E. Desmedt, pp. 730–733. Karger, Basel.
11. Hagbarth, K. E. (1960): Spinal withdrawal reflexes in the human lower limbs. *J. Neurol. Neurosurg. Psychiatry,* 23:222–227.
12. Henneman, E., Somjen, G., and Carpenter, D. O. (1965): Excitability and inhibitibility of motoneurons of different sizes. *J. Neurophysiol.,* 28:599–620.
13. Hugon, M. (1973): Exteroceptive reflexes to stimulation of the sural nerve in normal man. In: *New Developments in Electromyography and Clinical Neurophysiology,* Vol. III, edited by J. E. Desmedt, pp. 713–729. Karger, Basel.
14. Janko, M., and Trontelj, J. V. (1983): Flexion withdrawal reflex as recorded from single human biceps femoris motor neurons. *Pain,* 15:167–176.
15. Jenner, J. R., and Stephens, J. A. (1982): Cutaneous reflex responses and their central nervous pathways studied in man. *J. Physiol. (Lond.),* 333:405–419.
16. Kearney, R. E., and Chan, C. W. Y. (1979): Reflex response of human arm muscles to cutaneous stimulation of the foot. *Brain Res.,* 170:214–217.
17. Kugelberg, E. (1948): Demonstration of A and C fibre components in the Babinski plantar response and the pathological flexion reflex. *Brain,* 71:304–319.

18. Lloyd, D. P. C. (1943): Neuron patterns controlling transmission of ipsilateral hindlimb reflexes. *J. Neurophysiol.,* 6:293–315.
19. Meinck, H. M., Piesiur-Strehlow, B., and Koehler, W. (1981): Some principles of flexor reflex generation in human leg muscles. *Electroencephalogr. Clin. Neurophysiol.,* 52:140–150.
20. Perl, E. R. (1969): Somatic sensation: Transfer and processing of information. I. Peripheral receptors. *Electroencephalogr. Clin. Neurophysiol.,* 27:650–654.
21. Shahani, B. T., and Young, R. R. (1971): Human flexor reflexes. *J. Neurol. Neurosurg. Psychiatry,* 34:616–627.
22. Sherrington, C. S. (1910): Flexion-reflex of the limb, crossed-extension reflex and reflex stepping and standing. *J. Physiol. (Lond.),* 40:28–121.
23. Willer, J. C. (1977): Comparative study of perceived pain and nociceptive flexion reflex in man. *Pain,* 3:69–80.
24. Willer, J. C., and Albe-Fessard, D. (1980): Electrophysiological evidence for a release of endogenous opiates in stress-induced "analgesia" in man. *Brain Res.,* 198:419–426.
25. Willer, J. C., Boureau, F., and Albe-Fessard, D. (1980): Human nociceptive reactions: Effects of spatial summation of afferent input from relatively large diameter fibers. *Brain Res.,* 201:465–470.
26. Willer, J. C., and Bussel, B. (1980): Evidence for a direct spinal mechanism in morphine-induced inhibition of nociceptive reflexes in humans. *Brain Res.,* 187:212–215.

Advances in Pain Research and Therapy, Vol. 9, edited by H. L. Fields et al. Raven Press, New York © 1985.

Measurement of Pain: Comparison Between Visual Analog Scale and Analog Chromatic Continuous Scale

E. Grossi, C. Borghi, and M. Montanari

Medical Department, CIBA-GEIGY S.p.A., 21040 Origgio (VA), Italy

The visual analog scale (VAS) was introduced principally to overcome the limits of descriptive rating scales for measurement of feelings (1,2). Although four-point and five-point scales of pain have been widely employed because they are easy to use and require minimal instructions, they oblige patients to choose only few words to describe their pain.

The 100-mm standard VAS (4) has the advantage of providing theoretically infinite choices. The data obtained by VAS are usually measured to the nearest millimeter, and so they can be considered parametric variables and therefore suitable for parametric statistical methods. However, the VAS requires careful explanation of its meaning (some patients do not readily understand how to use it properly) (5), as well as good visual perception and muscular coordination. In addition, it is difficult for a patient to use the VAS, probably because there are no guides for assessment other than the endpoints. For example, it has recently been reported that among 98 consecutive patients participating in a study, 26 were unable to complete an absolute VAS (6).

The analog chromatic continuous scale (ACCS) was developed in an attempt to improve the VAS. In this scale the line is substituted by a colored stripe 100 mm long and 2.5 cm wide, in which color gradually shades from pale pink (no pain) to dark red (unbearable pain). The stripe lies on one face of a double-sided device. The opposite face contains a 100-mm scale on which the points 0 and 100 mm correspond exactly to the ends of the ACCS (no pain and unbearable pain, respectively). Instead of marking the scale with a pen, the patient has to set a transparent double-sided slider, containing a narrow line perpendicular to the colored stripe, at a point corresponding to the pain intensity felt. Simply by turning over the device the physician can read the corresponding value in millimeters. The color graduation is particularly useful in guiding the rating of the patient between the two endpoints and in improving the sensitivity of the scale (3). Moreover, the special features of the ACCS should offer practical advantages in painful conditions in which psychomotor functions are impaired, as in postoperative status.

The aim of this study was to compare the reliabilities of ACCS and VAS in early postoperative status and the sensitivities of the two scales for assessment of a standardized acute experimental pain.

METHODS

One hundred female patients (ages 18–73 years; ASA stage 1–2) scheduled for gynecological surgery were asked, before preanesthetic medication, to evaluate the pain induced by a standardized stimulus (cannulation of the cubital vein) and to assess the severity of postsurgical pain 1, 3, and 6 hrs after peritoneum stitching, using both ACCS and VAS presented in a randomized order. The cubital vein cannulation was performed always by the same physician, with a standard venous catheter. The technical procedure of venous cannulation was kept carefully homogeneous in all patients. With the ACCS for pain assessment, the patient had to set the transparent slider according to her pain, and the physician quantified it simply by turning over the rule and by reading the corresponding value in millimeters. The 100-mm VAS was printed on paper and used horizontally. Both scales were presented to the patients lying in bed.

RESULTS

Comparison of the Two Scales in Standardized Pain

The patients asked to rate their pain intensity caused by cannulation of a vein gave an assessment range of 2 to 83 mm with VAS and 4 to 65 mm with ACCS. A good correlation ($r = 0.202$; $p < 0.05$) existed between the values recorded with the two scales. The regression line and its confidence limits are shown in Fig. 1. Figures 2 and 3 show the VAS and ACCS value distributions, respectively. The differences between the theoretical normal distribution and the observed distribution of pain values were significant for both scales (VAS, $\chi^2 = 92.0$; $p \ll 0.001$; ACCS, $\chi^2 = 18.16$; $p = 0.006$). However, ACCS values tended to have a more "normal" distribution than VAS values (0.52 vs. 0.73, respectively), as well as a lower skewness (0.704 vs. 2.48, respectively) and a lower kurtosis (3.19 vs. 12.54, respectively).

Applicability of the Two Scales in the Early Postoperative Period

The applicability of the two scales in postoperative status was studied by evaluating the ability of patients to use the two scales. All patients were able to give well-defined (measurable) pain assessments with ACCS in each visit scheduled by the protocol.

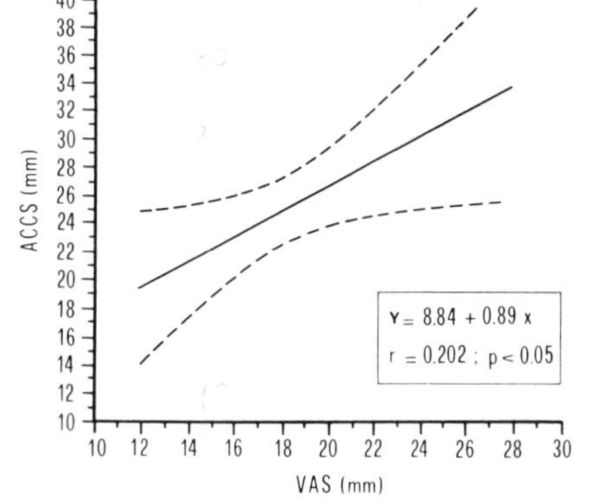

FIG. 1. Regression line and confidence limits for ACCS values plotted against VAS values in standardized pain assessment.

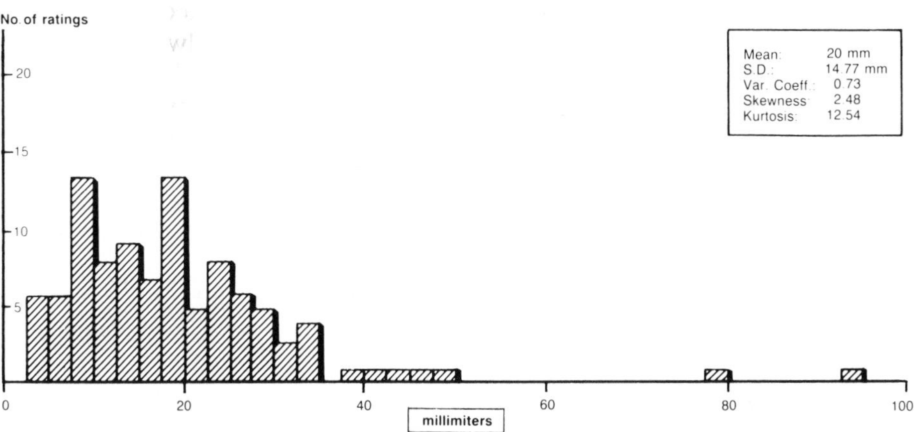

FIG. 2. Frequency distribution of VAS values.

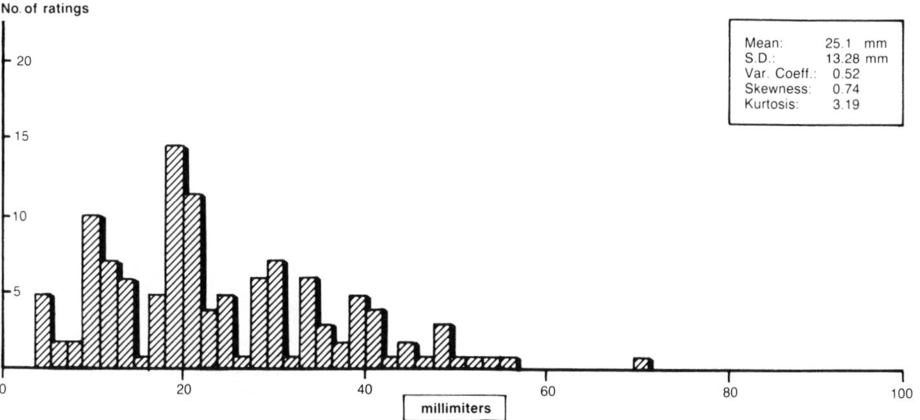

FIG. 3. Frequency distribution of ACCS values.

Use of the 100-mm VAS by patients lying in bed has involved a few problems in exactly defining patients' assessments. We classified these problems as follows:

1. Doubtful definition of VAS value: when two independent observers gave two slightly different readings for a given patient's mark on VAS.
2. Imprecise definition of VAS value: when a patient's mark was measurable, even if the variation of two subsequent measurements could be ± 5 mm.
3. Impossible definition: when the rating was completely unreliable, e.g., because of motor incoordination.

As shown in Table 1, 43% of the ratings made after surgery were considered as doubtful assessment, 15% were not precisely measurable, and 4% were not measurable at all. Seventy-six percent of patients gave at least one doubtful assessment. The highest incidence of unreliable ratings occurred 1 hr after surgery. Most of the unreliable ratings were due to physical problems such as impairment of sight or motor incoordination. A few examples of type 3 ratings are shown in Fig. 4.

DISCUSSION

In clinical trials on postoperative pain, pain measurement is necessary to evaluate the efficacy of analgesic regimens. In patients awakening after anesthesia, pain assessment is often difficult because of postanesthetic impairment of mental and neurological functions. This is probably one of the reasons why the simple descriptive scales are preferred in trials on postoperative pain. Actually, these scales require far less instruction than the VAS.

TABLE 1. *Reliability of 100-mm VAS in the early postoperative period*

	Unreliable ratings							
	1 hr		3 hr		6 hr		Total	
Category	No.	(%)	No.	(%)	No.	(%)	No.	(%)
Type 1	43	(43)	39	(43)	37	(43)	119	(43)
Type 2	17	(17)	9	(10)	6	(7)	32	(12)
Type 3	3	(3)	5	(5)	4	(5)	12	(4)
Total number of ratings	100	(100)	91	(100)	87	(100)	278	(100)

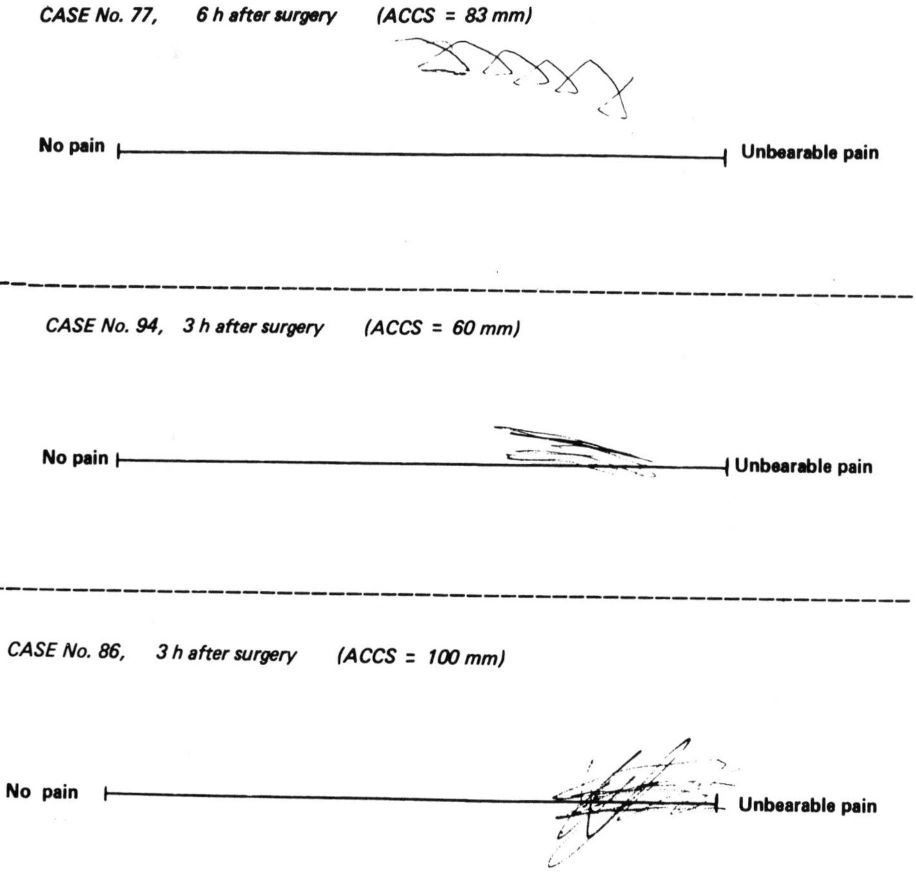

CASE No. 77, 6 h after surgery (ACCS = 83 mm)

No pain ⊢——⊣ **Unbearable pain**

CASE No. 94, 3 h after surgery (ACCS = 60 mm)

No pain ⊢——⊣ **Unbearable pain**

CASE No. 86, 3 h after surgery (ACCS = 100 mm)

No pain ⊢——⊣ **Unbearable pain**

FIG. 4. Typical examples of unmeasurable ratings with VAS in the early postoperative phase.

The most frequently adopted method of pain scoring, the 100-mm VAS, in spite of its high sensitivity, is seldom used in postoperative pain, probably owing to the fact that it requires, in addition to full consciousness, good vision and muscular coordination. These latter functions may also be impaired in the early postoperative period. A method of pain assessment to overcome these problems, without losing the advantages of the VAS, would represent real progress in pain assessment. The evidence coming from this study seems to confirm that the ACCS is at least comparable to the 100-mm VAS as far as sensitivity, accuracy, and reproducibility are concerned.

In a previous study (3) it was shown that the ACCS is more sensitive than the 100-mm VAS in pain assessment. However, the two scales were tested in patients suffering from pain of different origins.

In this study we tried to minimize the between-patient variability of pain intensity by submitting the patients to a standardized painful stimulus very common in the hospital setting: cannulation of cubital vein. Because the stimuli were as homogeneous as possible, the data distribution should be normal, even if the magnitude of this kind of induced pain cannot be known in absolute terms.

ACCS values were found to be more normally distributed than VAS values. The lower skewness, the lower kurtosis, and the lower coefficient of variation for the ACCS value distribution should mean, respectively, higher accuracy, sensitivity, and reproducibility.

As far as the applicability features of the new scale in postoperative pain are concerned, the evidence seems to be more consistent. In fact, the ACCS seems to overcome the clear deficiency in reliability of the VAS in the early postoperative phase. The ACCS can be used even by patients forced to remain in bed with postanesthetic incoordination, who therefore are unable to use a pen.

SUMMARY

A new pain rating scale, the ACCS, was compared with the 100-mm VAS in 100 female patients scheduled for gynecological surgery.

As far as applicability is concerned, the ACCS method has special features that make it a good alternative to the VAS for pain measurement in patients with psychomotor handicaps like those seen in the early postoperative phase. In fact, 76% of patients gave at least one doubtful rating with the VAS, whereas all patients gave measurable ratings with the ACCS.

REFERENCES

1. Aitken, R. C. B. (1969): Measurement of feeling using visual analogue scales. *Proc. R. Soc. Med.,* 62:989–993.
2. Aitken, R. C. B., and Zealley, A. K. (1970): Measurement of moods. *Br. J. Hosp. Med.,* 4:215–224.
3. Grossi, E., Borghi, C., Cerchiari, E. L., Della Puppa, T., and Francucci, B. (1983): Analogue chromatic continuous scale (ACCS): A new method for pain assessment. *Clin. Exp. Rheumatol.,* 1:337–340.
4. Huskisson, E. C. (1974): Measurement of pain. *Lancet,* 2:1127–1131.
5. Kremer, E., Atkinson, J. H., and Ignelzi, R. J. (1981): Measurement of pain: Patient preference does not confound pain measurement. *Pain,* 10:241–249.
6. Walsh, T. D. (1984): Letter to the editor. *Pain,* 19:96–97.

Advances in Pain Research and Therapy, Vol. 9, edited by H. L. Fields et al. Raven Press, New York © 1985.

Simple Rating System for Assessing Treatment Outcome in Chronic Pain Patients

P. J. D. Evans

Charing Cross Hospital, London W6 8RF, England

Management of chronic pain remains a perplexing problem. Frequently the origin of symptoms is obscure, often clouded by the subjective qualities of pain sensation. For many physicians there persists a dichotomy: Is the pain functional, or is it organic? This can significantly influence the treatment patients receive and may lead to bias in assessment. Measurement of pain also poses problems because the majority of observations relate to subjective qualities recorded by the physician or involve the use of self-assessment techniques by the patient. Frequently sequential measurements taken over short periods of time, such as 4 or 6 hr, have little relevance to the progress of patients in whom the pain intensity may be changing during the day (3) and from day to day (2). However, some measure of progress is essential if effective management of patients is to occur.

The average pain clinic may offer 50 or more differing treatment modalities (4), many of which may not have been validated to scientific standards. This may not be the fault of the treatment so much as the difficulty in producing "blind" control groups for therapies such as acupuncture or transcutaneous electrical stimulation or the ethics of using a control group in the case of destructive procedures such as percutaneous cordotomy. These problems have led many physicians to rely on an anecdotal approach to assessing progress. This will inevitably be biased in favor of positive responses, and failure to document therapy may well mask occurrences of treatment failure, as when prescribed medication is not used or side effects develop.

Thus, some simple outcome measure is required that can be applied to all patients at each attendance at the pain clinic. Such a method has now been adopted at Charing Cross Hospital, and this chapter outlines its role and limitations.

TABLE 1. *Rating system*

0 = Worse
1 = No relief
2 = Diagnostic
3 = Short gain (48 hr)
4 = Mod. gain (2 weeks)
5 = Long gain (2 months)
6 = Cure

METHODS

A microcomputer-based data base was used to record relevant information on patients attending the clinic. Basic demography and symptoms were recorded from a questionnaire similar in design to the McGill-Melzack pain questionnaire (8). In addition, at each attendance by the patient, further information was obtained regarding progress. A simple scale was used (Table 1). Measurements were recorded by the physician following direct questioning of the patient. The scale was qualitative, and no attempt was made to produce a quantitative response. It included a diagnostic category to take account of patients receiving techniques such as differential spinal blocks or intravenous morphine challenges. Only the "cure" category was specific and referred to those patients who on return to the clinic were completely relieved of their symptoms or were so able to control their pain that they felt further intervention then or in the future was unnecessary.

Patients were asked, on every attendance at the pain clinic, to indicate whether the treatment they had last received or were still receiving had made their pain better or worse. The duration of any improvement was recorded.

The data base was regularly updated so that no patient could rate more than one response during the period of a single treatment. However, patients returning for repeat procedures such as a second epidural injection or a further course of acupuncture were reentered as a separate treatment. A "treatment session" was defined as a single item of therapy, such as the prescription of a drug, an injection, a course of hypnotherapy, or the use of a transcutaneous nerve stimulator.

RESULTS

This study reports the results for 556 patients who attended the pain clinic over a period of 18 months. It covers a total of 1,906 treatment sessions, although only 1,465 are included in the analysis. The remainder were excluded because of incomplete data or because attendances were for consultation.

TABLE 2. *Range of conditions treated*

Condition	%	Sex ratio (F:M)	Duration of symptoms (mean years)	Mean age (years)
Chronic back pain	22	2.2:1	9.5	68
Malignancy	10	0.9:1	0.8	62
Postherpetic	10	1.5:1	4.8	75
Posttraumatic	10	1.3:1	4.6	50
Degenerative disease (including "frozen joints")	9	1.7:1	6.2	68
Peripheral nerve neuralgias	6	1.7:1	3.9	66
Autonomic neuralgias (including causalgia)	6	1.1:1	5.6	65
Facial pain	5	1.9:1	3.8	55
Cervical spondylitis	3	1.1:1	6.8	59
Peripheral vascular disease	3	0.8:1	3.1	74
Trigeminal neuralgia	2	1.4:1	3.3	61
All others	14	—	—	—

A wide variety of pain syndromes were treated (Table 2). There was a predominance of female patients, and with the exception of cancer-related pain the duration of symptoms was long. The range of therapy provided was extensive, but showed a high incidence of injection techniques (Table 3). The narcotic-analgesic category included the use of pure agonists like morphine as well as mixed-action compounds like buprenorphine. Injection techniques frequently included administration of depot steroid preparations as well as local anesthetic solutions. The percentages for each type of therapy are indicated for the first 9 months and for the second 9 months of the study.

The results were poor. Only 42 patients (7%) obtained sustained benefit and were discharged: 31 women and 11 men. The range of conditions and the types of successful treatments are shown in Table 4. All patients had received previous treatments at the clinic (mean 6.7 ± 4.5). The remaining patients received and continue to receive a variety of treatments, many of which have had limited effect (Table 5). Benefit lasting longer than 2 months was observed in 17%, and benefit for at least 2 weeks was seen in 23%. These values are not mutually exclusive, and there is no definite relationship between successful treatment on one occasion and a similar response on a subsequent occasion.

Transcutaneous electrical nerve stimulation (TENS) was the most effective form of therapy. However, invasive techniques such as cryoanalgesia and phenol and alcohol neurolysis were also effective, but had appreciable incidences of complications (Table 6). The relative benefits of all the common treatments are indicated in Table 7.

The treatments provided at the clinic were also stratified according to the types of problems observed. The scores for chronic back pain and cancer-

TABLE 3. *Range of therapies provided*[a]

Therapy	*N*	9 months (%)	18 months (%)
Consultation/advice	342	18	19
Epidural injections	287	15	15
Acupuncture	189	10	11
Peripheral LA blocks	182	10	10
Trigger-point LA	148	8	7
Narcotic-analgesics	106	6	7
Relaxation/hypnosis	100	5	5
Neurolysis	98	5	3
TENS	93	5	4
Sympathetic blocks	75	4	2
Antidepressants	60	3	3
Cryotherapy	57	3	4
Guanethidine blocks	36	2	2
Facet joint injections	34	2	2
All other therapy	99	—	—
Total	1,906		

[a]Range of treatments provided for the 556 patients, including the percentages for each type of therapy at the end of 9 months and at the end of 18 months.
LA = local anesthetic.

related pain are presented in Table 8. None of the treatments provided was highly effective for any of the conditions observed.

The results were also stratified according to the number of previous treatments that the patient had received. There was no significant difference in the results where few or many had been tried (Table 9).

TABLE 4. *Successful treatment*[a]

Treatment	*N*	Patients	*N*
Local anesthetic and/or steroid injections	15	Chronic back pain	9
Relaxation/hypnosis	9	Frozen joints/arthritis	9
TENS	6	Posttraumatic neuralgia	5
Acupuncture	5	Peripheral nerve neuralgia	12
Drugs	4	Causalgia	2
Neurolysis	2	Postherpetic neuralgia	3
Cryoanalgesia	1	Trigeminal neuralgia	2
Total	42		42

[a]Types of treatments and spectrum of conditions for 42 patients who obtained sustained benefit following treatment at the pain clinic.

TABLE 5. *Overall results (1983–1984) for recorded treatment sessions*[a]

Result		N	%
Long gain	(5)	222	17
Moderate gain	(4)	298	23
Short gain	(3)	286	22
Diagnostic	(2)	96	7
No change	(1)	333	25
Worse	(0)	35	3
Total		1,270	

[a]Ratings for the 1,312 fully documented treatment sessions, excluding the 42 treatments that provided sustained relief. Percentages refer to total treatments, not the numbers of patients.

DISCUSSION

It is often argued that the proliferation of scales for measurement of treatment success leads more to confusion than to validation of the various forms of therapy being assessed. Certainly the rating scale described may have severe limitations and may not easily be transcribed. But the principle that continuous records should be kept of the progress of all patients is paramount. In practice, unless a very simple scale is used, compliance in its use will be low.

This scale was developed to provide a guide for both the range of treatment being offered and the relative benefit of one form of treatment compared with another. In addition, it was hoped that it would provide a pointer toward successful forms of therapy and indicate areas where more specific studies could be undertaken. It was not intended as a substitute for comprehensive measures such as the McGill pain questionnaire or the MMPI (1),

TABLE 6. *Relative benefits of therapy*[a]

Long gain	%	Pain worse/complications	%
TENS	33	Cryoanalgesia	14
Cryoanalgesia	26	Antidepressants	8
Neurolysis	21	Neurolysis	4
Relaxation	19	Narcotic-analgesics	3
Acupuncture	14	LA injections	3

[a]Percentages of those treatments that produced either the greatest number of "long gains" or had the greatest incidence of "complications."

LA = local anesthetic.

TABLE 7. *Percentage value for each therapy according to group*[a]

Therapy	*N*	Relief index: Long (5) (%)	Mod. (4) (%)	Short (3) (%)	None (1) (%)	Worse (0) (%)
TENS	93	33	10	9	21	—
Cryoanalgesia	57	26	14	16	14	14
Neurolysis	98	21	14	11	13	4
Relaxation/hypnosis	100	19	13	13	32	—
Narcotic-analgesic	106	18	17	8	25	3
Sedative/antidepressant	60	15	2	2	30	8
Acupuncture	189	14	25	23	25	—
Trigger-point LA	148	12	30	22	12	3
Epidural injection	287	9	21	14	20	1
Peripheral nerve LA	182	8	23	34	13	2
Sympathetic block	75	5	16	23	31	1

[a]Results for principal treatments offered at the pain clinic: total number in each category and percentages for each treatment within the subsections.

Mod. = moderate; LA = local anesthetic.

TABLE 8. *Ratings stratified according to most frequently provided treatments for chronic back pain and pain of cancer*

Treatment	Relief index: Cure (6)	Long (5)	Mod. (4)	None (1)	Worse (0)
Rating for chronic back pain					
Relaxation/hypnosis	2	5	2	9	
TENS	4	8	3	3	
Acupuncture	1	5	7	6	
Epidural injection	1	9	39	27	
Facet joint injection	1	1	4	6	1
Trigger-point LA		3	4	4	
Narcotic-analgesic		1	5	13	
Rating for cancer-related pain					
Neurolysis	2	12	6	7	2
Opiates		9	2	2	1
TENS				1	
Peripheral LA block			2		
Epidural injection				2	
Antidepressants		2		1	

Mod. = moderate; LA = local anesthetic.

TABLE 9. *Influence of sequential therapy*

No. treatments	Relief index					
	Cure (6)	Long (5)	Mod. (4)	Short (3)	None (1)	Worse (0)
≤4	25	177	26	211	238	31
5	5	12	17	15	25	—
6	4	6	19	12	12	1
7	2	6	12	13	10	2
≥8	6	21	21	33	49	1

Figures represent scores for each category.
Mod. = moderate.

but as a complementary measure if time and staff did not permit their use. The word "gain" was used to register the fact that any progress made by the patient was important and that complete relief was not a prerequisite for recording success. For instance, when behavioral methods were used to treat patients, the only result that may have been achieved was that the patient felt better able to cope with the situation. The use of an ordinal scale might not have registered this response. Only crude estimations of duration of effect were recorded, and these were based on the likely responses expected from treatment. For instance, the 48-hr period covered the maximum period of analgesia that could result from a local anesthetic injection. The 2-week period covered the average interval before patients overcame or started to experience significant side effects from the use of drugs. The interval of 2 months was chosen to conform to the logistics of the pain clinic, where patients were frequently seen at intervals of 6 to 8 weeks. This would downgrade the value of those treatments providing longer benefit.

This rating scale was open to bias because of the direct questioning of patients and because it was possible for the physician to weight the results positively or negatively. However, by avoiding the use of a quantitative scale, it was hoped that this could be minimized. It should be stressed that in contrast to the classic methods of recording changes in pain intensity reviewed by Houde (5) and Huskisson (6), this scale instead attempted to assess the progress of patients and frequently ignored the absolute pain intensity. Because self-assessment was used, the results were open to the many variables that distort self-reports (7). However, even though these factors were not controlled, this simple outcome analysis was of value in managing patients attending the pain clinic.

The spectrum of patients treated was typical of United Kingdom pain clinics; the predominance of female patients has been noted elsewhere (9). The range of therapies provided showed a bias toward invasive procedures and injection techniques and reflected the "anesthetic" background of the physicians. In the second 9 months of the study period, a positive effort was made to increase the use of noninvasive techniques, as preliminary analysis had indicated that they might be more effective. The results show that at the end of 18 months this had not been achieved.

The poor results achieved at the clinic, with only 7% of patients "cured" and only 17% of treatments providing a "gain" in excess of 2 months, require some explanation. Lack of sensitivity of the scale as well as poor technique and poor selection of patients could be blamed. Yet many of the treatments were standard procedures that were easily reproduced, and the approaches to management were those generally adopted at other centers. Lack of sensitivity cannot be excluded until the scale has been validated in other groups of patients where more predictable results are observed. Probably these results are a true reflection of a group of patients with long-standing symptoms, frequently attending for changes in therapy and often considered "untreatable" by conventional methods. Even for the few patients gaining "cures" there was no discernible pattern in either the conditions likely to respond or the types of therapy likely to produce that result.

Transcutaneous electrical nerve stimulation proved the most effective form of treatment, whereas acupuncture, hypnosis, and relaxation therapy produced acceptable results. Although it appeared that cryoanalgesia and nerve neurolysis were more effective than the latter two, both had side effects that for nerve neurolysis were severe and for cryoanalgesia led to a marked increase in patients' pain. All the treatments offered were characterized by a high failure rate and a high frequency for producing short-term gains that could be of no real benefit for the patients.

The results were stratified according to the various symptom diagnoses. Even with the present size of the data base it was frequently impossible to make valid comparisons, because the large number of conditions and wide range of treatments available made the numbers in subsections small. It appeared that for chronic back pain the noninvasive forms of therapy rated well, whereas for cancer-related pain, neurolytic injections had a significant role. This merely confirmed previous reported studies (10,11).

The results were stratified according to the number of treatments provided. A patient was as likely to obtain a "long gain" after the first treatment as after the eighth. In addition, it was noted that treatment successful on one occasion could not always be reproduced in the same patient on a later occasion. Unfortunately, insufficient data were available to analyze more completely the factors relevant to treatment success. Perhaps the frequency, the sequence, and the combinations of treatments may prove important factors.

In conclusion, the use of this scale has proved a useful adjunct in providing information on the range of patients and treatments offered, as well as providing a baseline to assess overall patient progress. However, a much larger data base will be required before comprehensive comparisons can be made.

REFERENCES

1. Dahlstrom, W. G., Welsh, G. S., and Dahlstrom, L. E. (1972): *An MMPI Handbook. Vol. 1. Clinical Interpretation.* University of Minnesota Press, Minneapolis.
2. Evans, P. J. D., Carroll, D., McQuay, H. J., Bullingham, R. E. S., Moore, R. A., and Lloyd, J. W. (1982): *Royal Society of Medicine International Congress and Symposium Series,* 52:29–38.
3. Glynn, C. J., Lloyd, J. W., and Folkhard, S. (1981): Ventilatory responses to intractable pain. *Pain,* 11:201–211.
4. Hannington-Kiff, J. G. (1974): *Pain Relief.* Heinemann Medical, London.
5. Houde, R. W. (1982): Methods for measuring clinical pain in humans. *Acta Anaesth. Scand.* [*Suppl.*], 74:25–29.
6. Huskisson, E. C. (1974): Measurement of pain. *Lancet,* 2:1127–1131.
7. Kremer, E. F., Block, A., and Hampton Atkinson, J. (1983): Assessment of pain behaviour: Factors that distort self-report. In: *Pain Measurement and Assessment,* edited by R. Melzack, pp. 119–127. Raven Press, New York.
8. Melzack, R. (1983): The McGill pain questionnaire. In: *Pain Measurement and Assessment,* edited by R. Melzack, pp. 41–48. Raven Press, New York.
9. McQuay, H. J., Rogers, L., Evans, P. J. D., Moore, R. A., Lloyd, J. W., and Bullingham, R. E. S. (1985): Chronic non-malignant pain. A population prevalence study. *Practitioner (in press).*
10. Prithvi Raj, P., McLennon, J. E., and Phero, J. C. (1982): Assessment and management planning of chronic low back pain. In: *Chronic Low Back Pain,* edited by M. Stanton-Hicks and R. A. Boas, pp. 71–99. Raven Press, New York.
11. Wood, K. M. (1978): The use of phenol as a neurolytic agent. *Pain,* 5:205–229.

Advances in Pain Research and Therapy, Vol. 9, edited by H. L. Fields et al. Raven Press, New York © 1985.

Multidimensional Pain Assessment in Children

*Patricia A. McGrath, *L. L. de Veber, and **Margaret T. Hearn

**Department of Pediatrics, Faculty of Medicine, The University of Western Ontario, War Memorial Children's Hospital; and **Psychology Department, University Hospital, London, Ontario, Canada N6B 1B8*

Although observational (1,3,9), behavioral (6,8,10), projective (13–15,19), and direct-report (5,8,17) techniques are available for assessing distress and pain in children, the majority of research on evaluating the reliability and validity of pain measures has been focused on adults. Consequently, there is a lack of objective and practical information on methods to directly measure the strength or unpleasantness of pain in children. Cross-modality matching procedures have been used both as reliable pain measures for adults (12) and as measures for other sensory modalities with children (2,16,18,20). Children can describe their perception of one stimulus in terms of another; that is, they can adjust the length of a line to match the loudness of different tones so that their line-length responses become, in essence, measures for their auditory perception (18).

Therefore, the purpose of this research study was to evaluate two cross-modality matching procedures, brightness matching and visual analog scales, as measures of children's pain. Several questions were addressed concerning the feasibility, reliability, and validity of these methods for assessing the intensity and unpleasantness of pain in children.

Can children use brightness and visual analog scales in a reliable and valid manner?

METHOD

This first question concerned the feasibility of using cross-modality matching procedures across a group of children varying in age, sex, and pain experience. Are children's responses consistent over time, and do their responses accurately reflect perceptual changes that are related systematically to changes in the stimulus we are measuring? It is possible to determine

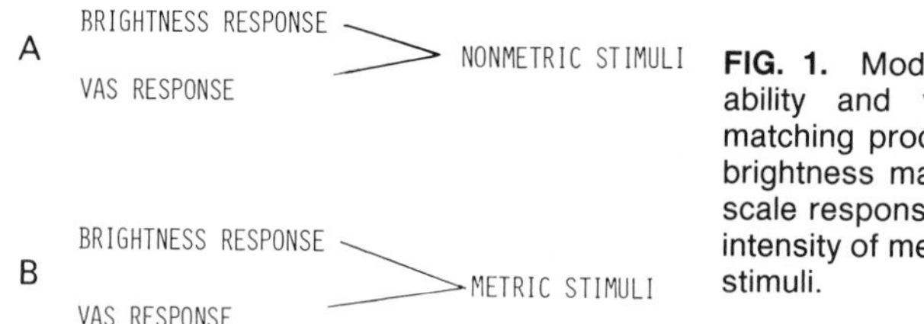

FIG. 1. Model for determining the reliability and validity of cross-modal matching procedures in children. Both brightness matches and visual analog scale responses were used to rate the intensity of metric (**A**) and nonmetric (**B**) stimuli.

the reliability and validity of a pain measure in adult studies by correlating a subject's pain responses to controlled changes in the intensity of a noxious stimulus. However, because ethical reasons preclude the use of experimental pain in children, another validation model was used (Fig. 1A).

Forty children (20 boys and 20 girls, 3–15 years, mean age 8.7; 20 healthy and 20 oncology patients) participated in two psychophysical sessions, approximately 2 weeks apart, in order to evaluate method reliability and validity by sex, age, health status, and between-sessions. Children used both brightness matching and visual analog scales (VAS) to rate the heaviness of five metric stimuli. These five identically appearing containers varied in weight from 75 to 275 g, in 50-g steps. Children were asked to "make the light as bright as the container is heavy" and, in separate trials, to "make the line as long as the container is heavy." The VAS consisted of a 150-mm line. The left endpoint was designated verbally as "not heavy." The right endpoint was designated as "heaviest sensation imaginable." The brightness box had a visual screen, 10 cm^2, that varied in intensity from 0 to 1,200 candelas/m^2. Children adjusted the brightness by turning a simple dimmer switch. Stimulus and response orders were randomized within and across sessions.

RESULTS

Seven children, with a mean age of 4.7 years, were not able to complete the study, either because they could not comprehend the method or because they were unwilling to participate in both sessions. All other children easily completed the scaling procedures.

Figure 2 shows the results of the metric scaling averaged over all the children. Log brightness responses and visual analog scale responses are plotted as functions of stimulus intensity. The slopes obtained for the two response procedures are almost identical: brightness 2.06; visual analog scales 2.12. There were no significant differences in how the children used these measures as a function of their sex, health status, or age, although between-session reliability improved with age. The median between-session correlation coefficient for the youngest children, 5 and 6 years old, was $r = 0.70$, which increased to a value of $r = 0.99$ for those 13 to 15 years old.

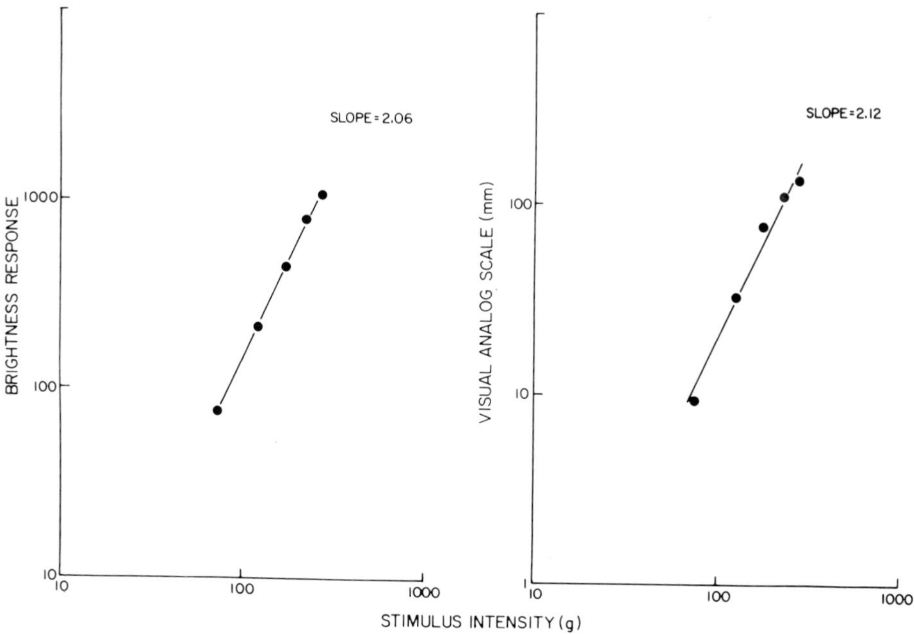

FIG. 2. Log brightness and log visual analog responses of perceived heaviness are plotted as functions of stimulus intensity. Each point represents the geometric mean of 132 responses (4 trials per child) averaged over 33 children. The solid line drawn through the points represents the linear regression obtained with an exponent 2.06 for brightness responses and 2.12 for visual analog responses.

Can children use brightness and visual analog scales to quantify a scale of unpleasantness or affective magnitude that can be used to measure the affective dimension of their pain?

METHOD

An interval scale consisting of nine faces varying in emotional expression (Fig. 3) was selected on the basis of a previous pilot study. Although nonmetric (that is, not physically measurable) scales are often assumed to have equal intervals between stimuli, so that distances between stimuli or faces represent equal perceptual distances, the actual value of affect depicted by each face was determined from the children's own perspectives. The model used (Fig. 1B) was similar to that used by previous investigators for determining the magnitude associated with different nonmetric stimuli, such as verbal pain descriptors (4). Children used the same two cross-modality matching responses, brightness matching and visual analog scales, to rate the magnitude of negative or positive affect depicted by each face. The left

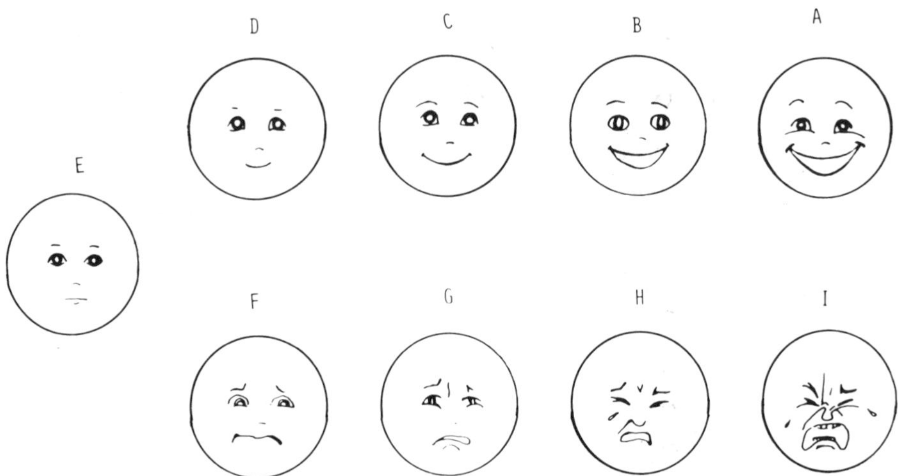

FIG. 3. Nine-face interval scale developed in a pilot study as a measure for pain affect. Faces **A–D** represent varying magnitudes of positive affect; faces **F–I** represent varying magnitudes of negative affect. Face **E** was initially assumed to represent a neutral face.

and right endpoints of the visual analog scale were verbally designated as the saddest and happiest faces imaginable.

If the relationship between children's brightness and visual analog scale responses for these nonmetric stimuli was consistent with the relationship that was obtained previously when children used the same two methods to assess the intensity of the metric stimuli, then the assumption could be made that children were using the methods consistently and that their brightness and visual analog scale values accurately reflected their perceptions of the nonmetric stimuli. Each face was presented four times in random order; brightness and visual analog responses were made in separate trials.

RESULTS

Children were able to use the cross-modality matching procedures consistently. There were no significant differences in children's values by sex, age, or health status. Consequently, children's responses were averaged to obtain a mean affective value for each face. The obtained numerical values were transformed so that a maximum negative value corresponded to 1 (indicating the most unpleasant feeling) and the maximum positive value corresponded to 0 (indicating the most pleasant feeling). The units of affective magnitude represented by each face are shown in Fig. 4. Although the intervals between faces were approximately equal for the positive faces (A–E), the intervals between negative faces were not equal (Fig. 5). In fact, the intended neutral face (face E) had a value of 0.60, indicating that children

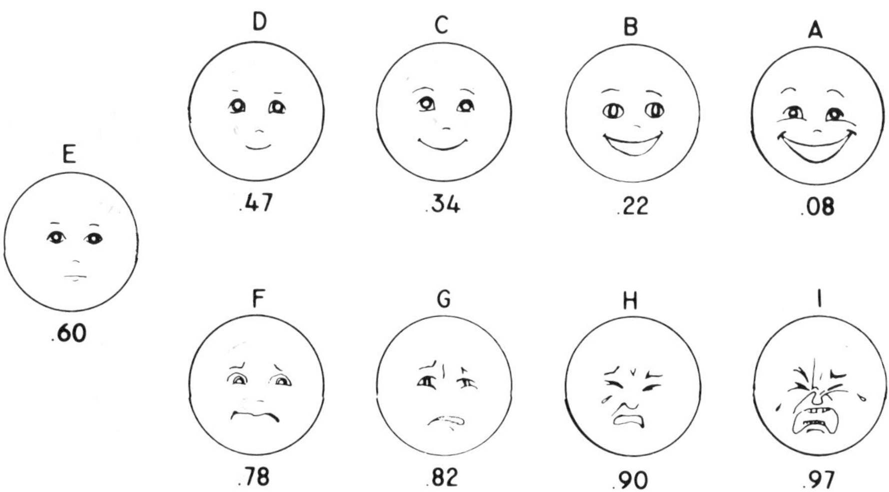

FIG. 4. Facial scale with the mean affective magnitude for each face determined from children's direct scaling using brightness matching and visual analog scales. Each value represents the geometric mean of 132 responses (4 trials per child) averaged over 33 children. The mean values were then transformed to a 0–1 scale on which the maximum negative affective value equals 1 and the maximum positive affective value equals 0.

perceived it as unpleasant (a value of 0.50 would represent a true neutral point). Because the intervals were not all equal, it was necessary to use the children's scaled numerical estimates as measures of affect. Since this study, visual analog scaling of the affective magnitude of these faces has been completed by a larger group of children and adults. Results indicate that it is possible to use the values shown in Fig. 4 as units of affective magnitude.

How do children use visual analog scales and an affective interval scale to measure their own pain?

METHOD

All children with cancer used both visual analog and facial scales to evaluate the pain produced by necessary medical procedures, such as checkups,

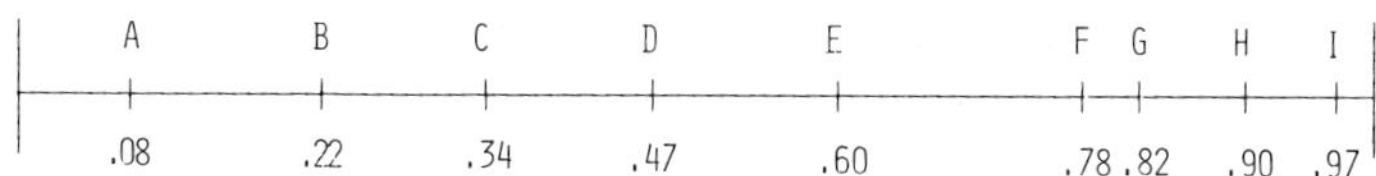

FIG. 5. Affective magnitudes depicted for the 9 faces (**A–I**, Figs. 3 and 4) are represented along the visual analog scale. The values of affective magnitude were determined from children's direct scaling using their brightness matches and visual analog responses. Each value represents the geometric mean of 132 responses (4 trials per child) averaged over 33 children. The values were transformed to a 0–1 scale, on which the maximum negative affective value equals 1 and the maximum positive affective value equals 0.

finger pricks, intravenous injections, lumbar punctures, and bone marrow aspirations. Behavioral distress scales were also completed for each procedure by a nurse, physician, and trained observer.

RESULTS

Results from children's self-report measures showed that there were consistent differences in the pain associated with different medical procedures, regardless of the age or sex of the child. Group mean pain intensity and affective values for four procedures are listed in Table 1.

DISCUSSION

Direct reports of pain using visual analog scales and affective facial scales were shown to be reliable methods for measuring pain in children. Although children's distress behaviors (crying, stalling, refusing treatment) were frequently correlated with their pain rating, children who were not afraid or anxious did not always demonstrate behavioral distress even though they reported pain. Consequently, observations of distress behavior alone were not sufficient as measures of a child's pain. Children's self-reports were shown in a previous study to be both reliable and valid measures of the pain associated with different medical procedures and also valid indices of the efficacy of a pain control program for children with cancer (11).

More recently, 25 healthy children used pain logs, consisting of visual analog and affective face scales, for 1 month to describe any pain that they experienced during their normal activities. Normative data for acute childhood pain are being collected in the same manner as those collected for the acute pain associated with cancer procedures. Initial results indicate that the visual analog and facial scales are valid methods for discriminating among natural pain experiences.

In conclusion, several questions about the use of cross-modality matching procedures for assessing pain intensity and pain affect in children have been

TABLE 1. *Mean pain intensity (visual analog scale) and affect (affective facial scale) associated with oncology procedures*

Procedures	Pain intensity	Affect
Checkup	2.3	0.28
Finger prick	6.3	0.34
Injection	13.4	0.40
Lumbar puncture		
All children	31.7	0.74
With sedation	80.2	0.83
Without sedation	51.3	0.79
Pilot sample, in pain control program	16.0	0.61

addressed. Children above 5 years of age can use visual analog scales and an affective interval face scale to describe their pain in a meaningful way. These direct scaling techniques enable us to more precisely assess pain in children and more precisely evaluate the efficacy of different pain relief programs.

ACKNOWLEDGMENTS

This study was supported by a National Health Research and Development Award (project 6606-2244-04). Dr. McGrath is supported as a Career Scientist by the Ontario Ministry of Health, Health Research Personnel Development Program.

REFERENCES

1. Apley, J. (1976): Pain in childhood. *J. Psychosom. Res.,* 20:383–389.
2. Bond, B., and Stevens, S. S. (1969): Cross-modality matching of brightness to loudness by 5 year olds. *Perception and Psychophysics,* 6:337–339.
3. Eland, J. M., and Anderson, J. E. (1977): The experience of pain in children. In: *Pain: A Source Book for Nurses and Other Health Professionals,* edited by A. K. Jacox, pp. 453–471. Little, Brown, Boston.
4. Gracely, R. H., McGrath, P. A., and Dubner, R. (1978): Ratio scales of sensory and affective verbal pain descriptors. *Pain,* 5:5–18.
5. Hester, N. K. (1979): The preoperational child's reaction to immunization. *Nurs. Res.,* 28:250.
6. Jay, S. M., Ozolins, M., Elliott, C. H., and Caldwell, S. (1983): Assessment of children's distress during painful medical procedures. *Health Psychology,* 2:133–147.
7. Jeans, M. E. (1983): The measurement of pain in children. In: *Pain Measurement and Assessment,* edited by R. Melzack, pp. 183–189. Raven Press, New York.
8. Katz, E. R., Sharp, B., Kellerman, J., Marston, A. R., Hershman, J. M., and Siegel, S. E. (1982): β-endorphin immunoreactivity and acute behavioural distress in children with leukaemia. *J. Nerv. Ment. Dis.,* 170:72–77.
9. Lollar, D. J., Smits, S. J., and Patterson, D. L. (1982): Assessment of paediatric pain: An empirical perspective. *J. Pediatr. Psychol.,* 7:267–277.
10. Melamed, B. C., and Siegel, L. (1975): Reduction of anxiety in children facing hospitalization and surgery by use of filmed modelling. *J. Consult. Clin. Psychol.,* 43:511–521.
11. McGrath, P. A., de Veber, L. L., and Hearn, M. T. (1983): Modulation of acute pain and anxiety for pediatric oncology patients. *Abstracts of the American Pain Society,* 106:93.
12. Price, D. D., McGrath, P. A., Rafii, A., and Buckingham, B. (1983): The validation of visual analogue scales as ratio measures of experimental and chronic pain. *Pain,* 17:45–56.
13. Savedra, M., Gibbons, P., Tesler, M., Ward, J., and Wegner, C. (1982): How do children describe pain? A tentative assessment. *Pain,* 14:95–104.
14. Scott, R. (1978): It hurts red: A preliminary study of children's perception of pain. *Percept. Mot. Skills,* 47:787–791.
15. Shultz, N. (1971): How children perceive pain. *Nurs. Outlook,* 19:670–693.
16. Siegel, A. W., and McBurney, D. H. (1970): Estimation of line length and number: A developmental study. *J. Exp. Child Psychol.,* 10:170–180.
17. Stewart, M. L. (1977): Measurement of clinical pain. In: *Pain: A Source Book for Nurses and Other Health Professionals,* edited by A. K. Jacox, pp. 107–137. Little, Brown, Boston.
18. Teghtsoonian, M. (1980): Children's scales of length and loudness: A developmental application of cross-modal matching. *J. Exp. Child Psychol.,* 30:290–307.
19. Unruh, A., McGrath, P. J., Cunningham, S. J., and Humphreys, P. (1983): Children's drawings of their pain. *Pain,* 17:385–392.
20. Zwislocki, J. J., and Goodman, D. A. (1980): Absolute scaling of sensory magnitudes: A validation. *Perception and Psychophysics,* 28:28–38.

Advances in Pain Research and Therapy, Vol. 9, edited by H. L. Fields et al. Raven Press, New York © 1985.

CHEOPS: A Behavioral Scale for Rating Postoperative Pain in Children

*Patrick J. McGrath, **Garry Johnson, *John T. Goodman, †John Schillinger, ‡Jennifer Dunn, and §Jo-Anne Chapman

*Departments of *Psychology and **Anaesthesia, and †Urology Service, Children's Hospital of Eastern Ontario, Ottawa K1H 8L1, Ontario, Canada; ‡Department of Psychology, University of Windsor, Windsor, Ontario, Canada; and §Department of Psychology, Carleton University, Ottawa, Ontario, Canada*

One of the more difficult challenges health professionals and clinical researchers face is assessment and measurement of pain in children. With children, the problems are confounded by their changing, but relatively limited, cognitive ability to understand measurement instructions and articulate descriptions of their pain (6).

Investigations into measurements of postoperative pain in children have been virtually nonexistent, and this dearth of research may have contributed to the well-documented undermedication of children for postoperative pain (1,3).

Pain can be conceptualized as an event that has several components or aspects. Each component of pain is only one way of approaching the entire phenomenon. The three most frequently considered aspects of pain are the cognitive or phenomenological component, the behavioral component, and the physiological component. Not only are there multiple components of pain, but for each component there may be several different measurement strategies.

The cognitive component of pain in children has been measured by verbal scales, numerical rating scales, colors, drawings, and projective tests. However, because of their verbal limitations, very young children and children emerging from anesthetic are unable to report their pain with any of these cognitive measuring techniques.

Physiological measures of pain in children have included heart rate, respiration, PO_2, sweating, and endorphins. Each is of some utility, but none has gained widespread use or has been thoroughly evaluated. As with all measures of pain, it is not always possible to completely distinguish between pain and other forms of distress. Some researchers have preferred to use the term *stress* or *distress* to describe the reaction to noxious stimuli as measured by behavioral or physiological indices (7). However, there is legitimacy in calling what appears to be pain, pain, even if no self-report is available.

Perhaps the most obvious pain behavior in children that can be measured by observation is crying. The presence or absence of crying is the most common way that parents and health professionals judge a young child's pain. Although crying may be indicative of a number of different states, Wasz-Hockert et al. (10) have demonstrated that the pain cry can be electronically differentiated from the hunger or birth cry and that these differences can be detected by experienced health professionals.

In order to quantify the behavioral aspect of pain, experienced adults can rate the amount of pain they perceive that a child is suffering. Visual analog scales (VAS) (4), for example, have been used by nurses to rate the amount of pain that children appear to experience (9). However, care must be taken to ensure that the anchors used are clear. Martin (9) used such a scale to measure the effectiveness of two approaches to pain relief following circumcision. Unfortunately, the two anchors of the scale were "unconscious" at one end and "screaming" at the other, with the midpoint reserved for a rating of an alert and calm child. Consequently, two pairs of children, one pair consisting of an unconscious child and a screaming child, and one pair consisting of two alert, calm children, would both receive the same ratings. No research on the reliability and validity of VAS used in this way has been published.

Izard's research group (5) described the facial expressions of infants who were receiving injections or having blood taken. The clinical utility of these expressions as measures of pain intensity has not been explored.

Other researchers have developed behavioral rating scales for use in assessing pain in young children undergoing discrete painful medical procedures. Katz et al. (7) compiled a list of behaviors that children exhibit before, during, and after bone marrow aspirations (BMA) from their observations of children aged 8 months to 17 years 9 months. Of the 25 behaviors originally selected, 13 discriminated between children who were rated by nurses as highly distressed and children rated as less distressed. These 13 items comprise the Procedure Behavior Rating Scale. The scale demonstrated inter-rater reliability above 0.85 and good evidence of validity. However, several of the items are peculiar to the BMA procedure and would not be of use in rating pain or distress in other situations.

In a similar study, Craig et al. (2) developed a scale to measure pain expression in children aged 2 to 24 months who were undergoing immunization. Items in the scale included crying, pain vocalization, distortion of face, and rigidity of torso. The scale demonstrated inter-rater reliability for some of the items and some evidence of validity.

The lack of any well-validated measure that was appropriate for measuring postoperative pain in young children undergoing surgery led to the development of the Children's Hospital of Eastern Ontario Pain Scale (CHEOPS).

METHODS AND RESULTS

Development of the Scale

Meetings were held with experienced recovery room nurses who were queried as to what behaviors they most frequently observe to determine if a child is in pain. Descriptions of these behaviors were developed, and children were observed to determine if the descriptions reflected behavior in the recovery room. As a result, a preliminary version of CHEOPS was developed in which six behaviors were defined. Two observers used the preliminary version of the scale to simultaneously, but independently, rate 7 children. Five seconds of observation were followed by 25 sec to record the rating. Differences and difficulties in ratings were discussed to clarify the definitions of each category and to develop the final version of CHEOPS, which is presented in Table 1.

Inter-rater Reliability of CHEOPS

Inter-rater reliability for raw data collection was determined by having two raters, previously trained to use CHEOPS, independently and simultaneously observe 26 children, aged 1 to 5 years, emerging from anesthesia following a variety of surgical procedures, including hernia repair, tonsillectomy, circumcision, and hypospadias repair. As can be seen from Table 2, which summarizes the inter-rater reliability data, the average percentage agreement by patient was excellent, ranging from 90 to 99.5%.

Scoring of CHEOPS

A scoring method was devised for CHEOPS in order to transform the nominal descriptive information afforded by the raw data into ordinal data that would be more amenable to statistical analysis. Each behavior of the raw data form of CHEOPS was assigned a value according to the following criteria: 0 = behavior that is the antithesis of pain; 1 = behavior that is not indicative of pain and is not the antithesis of pain; 2 = behavior indicating mild or moderate pain; 3 = behavior indicative of severe pain. Table 1 contains the values for each behavior in CHEOPS. Using this scoring method, the range of the total score on CHEOPS is 4 to 13 for each time period sampled.

TABLE 1. *Behavioral definitions and scoring of CHEOPS*

Item	Behavior	Score	Definition
Cry	No cry	1	Child is not crying.
	Moaning	2	Child is moaning or quietly vocalizing, silent cry.
	Crying	2	Child is crying, but the cry is gentle or whimpering.
	Scream	3	Child is in a full-lunged cry; sobbing; may be scored with complaint or without complaint.
Facial	Composed	1	Neutral facial expression.
	Grimace	2	Score only if definite negative facial expression.
	Smiling	0	Score only if definite positive facial expression.
Child verbal	None	1	Child not talking.
	Other complaints	1	Child complains, but not about pain, e.g., "I want to see mommy" or "I am thirsty."
	Pain complaints	2	Child complains about pain.
	Both complaints	2	Child complains about pain and about other things, e.g., "It hurts; I want mommy."
	Positive	0	Child makes any positive statement or talks about other things without complaint.
Torso	Neutral	1	Body (not limbs) is at rest; torso is inactive.
	Shifting	2	Body is in motion in a shifting or serpentine fashion.
	Tense	2	Body is arched or rigid.
	Shivering	2	Body is shuddering or shaking involuntarily.
	Upright	2	Child is in a vertical or upright position.
	Restrained	2	Body is restrained.
Touch	Not touching	1	Child is not touching or grabbing at wound.
	Reach	2	Child is reaching for but not touching wound.
	Touch	2	Child is gently touching wound or wound area.
	Grab	2	Child is grabbing vigorously at wound.
	Restrained	2	Child's arms are restrained.
Legs	Neutral	1	Legs may be in any position but are relaxed; includes gentle swimming or serpentine-like movements.
	Squirming/kicking	2	Definitive uneasy or restless movements in the legs and/or striking out with foot or feet.
	Drawn up/tensed	2	Legs tensed and/or pulled up tightly to body and kept there.
	Standing	2	Standing, crouching, or kneeling.
	Restrained	2	Child's legs are being held down.

TABLE 2. *Inter-rater reliability for CHEOPS categories*

Item	No. of cases	No. of observations	Range of inter-rater agreement (%)	Average inter-rater agreement (%)
Cry	26	1,152	76–100	93.2
Facial	26	1,143	61–100	90
Child verbal	26	1,152	95–100	99.5
Torso	26	1,140	76–100	90.6
Touch	26	1,150	87–100	99.2
Legs	26	1,152	76–100	92

Validity of CHEOPS

The validity of CHEOPS was determined by measuring the internal correlation of the scale, by comparing the scale with other measures of pain, by measuring changes in the scale as a result of intravenous narcotic, and by social validation.

Internal Correlation and Correlation with Other Pain Measures

CHEOPS was used to measure pain behavior in 30 children aged 1 to 7 years in the hour following surgery for circumcision. Pearson correlations of the CHEOPS items (Table 3) indicate significant correlations between each pair of items, indicating that the scale is measuring a single construct "pain."

In order to establish the relationship between CHEOPS and another pain measure, children were rated by recovery room nurses using a horizontal VAS 100 mm long. The two anchors were "no pain" and "pain as severe as possible." Rating was done immediately following an incident of nursing care to the patient in the recovery room. The nurses were blinded to the

TABLE 3. *Pearson intercorrelations among CHEOPS items (N = 127)*

Item	Cry	Facial	Torso	Touch	Legs	Total score
Cry	—	0.81	0.46	0.40	0.54	0.90
Facial		—	0.48	0.36	0.45	0.87
Torso			—	0.35	0.42	0.70
Touch				—	0.37	0.56
Legs					—	0.72

No instances of verbal behavior occurred.

TABLE 4. *Pearson intercorrelations between CHEOPS items and VAS ratings (N = 127)*

	Nurse's rating	Observer's rating	Cry	Facial	Torso	Touch	Legs	Total score
Nurse's rating	—	0.91	0.76	0.64	0.52	0.55	0.63	0.81
Observer's rating		—	0.77	0.69	0.53	0.50	0.75	0.86

CHEOPS ratings given for that time period. A second VAS was independently completed by the research assistant. A total of 127 sets of ratings were collected on 30 patients. It should be noted that the research assistant, although blind to the nurses' ratings, was not blinded to the CHEOPS score. Table 4 contains the correlations between the nurses' ratings and the research assistant's ratings and the individual item and total scores on CHEOPS. As can be seen, the two VAS ratings correlated highly (0.91). Correlations between the individual and total scores of CHEOPS and the VAS ranged from 0.50 to 0.86, with the total score correlating most highly. These data indicate close correspondence between the nurses' ratings and the CHEOPS score.

Changes in Response to Narcotic-Analgesics

If CHEOPS is a measure of pain, analgesic medication given to children in pain should be reflected in declines in CHEOPS scores. Figure 1 plots the average pain scores for 20 children from 3 min prior to administration of fentanyl for pain relief to 3 min following injection of fentanyl. The high levels of pain immediately prior to injection, as measured by CHEOPS (9.9), showed a dramatic reduction to 6.3 at 3 min following the intravenous narcotic. Unfortunately, ratings were not blinded.

Social Validation

The final method of assessing the validity of CHEOPS was to subject the scale to social validation. Social validation (8) is a method of determining if a measurement of behavior is measuring the construct for which it was intended. Although social validation has not been used in pain measurement, it provides an ideal method of assessing whether or not specific behaviors (in this case, items on CHEOPS) relate to the construct of pain.

Eighty-eight teachers viewed 14 5-sec video clips of children in the recovery room and rated each clip on a horizontal VAS with anchors of "no pain" and "pain as severe as possible." In addition, each video clip was rated by a trained rater on CHEOPS. The correlation for the total score on CHEOPS and the VAS scores of the teachers was $r = 0.85$, $p < 0.05$. Similarly, the

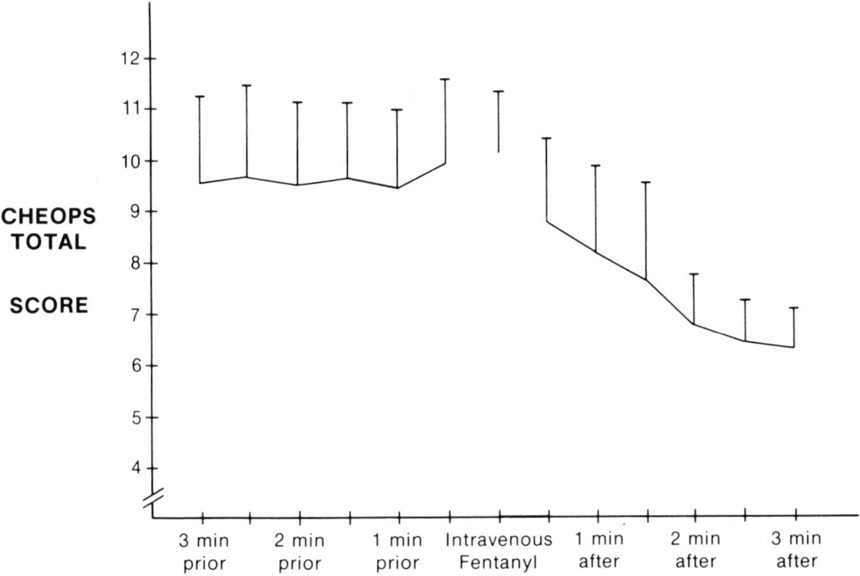

FIG. 1. Mean CHEOPS scores and standard deviations for 3 min prior to and following intravenous fentanyl.

correlations for the subcategories were as follows: Cry ($r = 0.83$, $p < 0.05$); Facial ($r = 0.69$, $p < 0.05$); Torso ($r = 0.79$, $p < 0.05$); Legs ($r = 0.55$, $p < 0.05$). The clips used did not contain any instances of verbal or touching behavior, and consequently no correlations were available for these subscales.

CONCLUSIONS

CHEOPS, a time-sampling behavioral pain scale, has been shown to have excellent inter-rater reliability and good evidence of validity when used for young children following surgery. The simple scoring method appears to be effective. Comparison of the scale with nurses' ratings also provides support for the validity of nurses' ratings of children's pain using VAS. Use of CHEOPS for measurement of postoperative pain could lead to an increase in the development and evaluation of analgesic strategies for children undergoing surgery.

ACKNOWLEDGMENTS

The authors wish to acknowledge the financial assistance of Sterling Drugs (Canada) and the Children's Hospital of Eastern Ontario Foundation and the contributions of M. Lascelles, C. Heick, N. Somers, S. J. Cunningham, and the staff of the recovery room. Dr. McGrath is supported by a Career Scientist Award from the Ontario Ministry of Health.

REFERENCES

1. Beyer, J., DeGood, D. E., Ashley, L. C., and Russell, G. A. (1983): Patterns of postoperative analgesic use with adults and children following cardiac surgery. *Pain,* 17:71–81.
2. Craig, K. D., McMahon, R. J., Morison, J. D., and Zaskow, C. (1984): Developmental changes in infant pain expression during immunization injections. *Soc. Sci. Med.,* 19(12):1331–1337.
3. Eland, J. M., and Anderson, J. E. (1977): The experience of pain in children. In: *Pain: A Source Book for Nurses and Other Health Professionals,* edited by A. K. Jacox, pp. 453–473. Little, Brown, Boston.
4. Huskisson, E. C. (1983): Visual analogue scales. In: *Pain Measurement and Assessment,* edited by R. Melzack, pp. 33–37. Raven Press, New York.
5. Izard, C. E., Huebner, R. R., Resser, D., McGiness, G. C., and Dougherty, L. M. (1980): The infant's ability to produce discrete emotional expressions. *Dev. Psychol.,* 16:132–140.
6. Jeans, M. E. (1983): Pain in children: A neglected area. In: *Advances in Behavioral Medicine for Children and Adolescents,* edited by P. Firestone, P. McGrath, and W. Feldman, pp. 23–37. Erlbaum, Hillsdale, N.J.
7. Katz, E. R., Kellerman, J., and Seigel, S. E. (1980): Distress behavior in children with cancer undergoing medical procedures: Developmental considerations. *J. Consult. Clin. Psychol.,* 48:356–365.
8. Kazdin, A. E. (1977): Assessing the clinical or applied importance of behavior change through social validation. *Behavior Modification,* 1:427–449.
9. Martin, L. V. H. (1982): Postoperative analgesia after circumcision in children. *Br. J. Anaesth.,* 54:1263–1266.
10. Wasz-Hockert, O., Lind, J., Vuorenkoski, V., Partanen, T., and Valanne, E. (1968): The infant cry: A spectographic and auditory analysis. *Clin. Dev. Med.,* 29:9–42.

Advances in Pain Research and Therapy, Vol. 9, edited by H. L. Fields et al. Raven Press, New York © 1985.

Liquid-Crystal Thermography: A Noninvasive Technique to Document Treatment Results in Patients with Low Back Syndrome

*P. Sebastian Thomas, *Lido Chen, **Bruce E. Frederickson, **Hansen A. Yuan, *Linda C. Stehling, and *Howard L. Zauder

*Departments of *Anesthesiology and **Orthopedics, State University of New York, Upstate Medical Center, Syracuse, New York 13210*

Pain is a subjective phenomenon that cannot be documented objectively. Chronic pain is complex and involves both central and peripheral mechanisms. This is especially true in patients with low back pain syndrome. Epidural steroid injections have been used successfully in recent years, especially in patients with radiculopathy who are not candidates for surgery.

Liquid-crystal thermography (LCT) is a technique that uses cholesterol crystals that change color in response to variations in surface temperature (2). In patients with nerve root irritation these temperature changes follow the affected dermatome because of sympathetic hyperactivity in the affected nerve root (2). The purpose of this study was to document objectively the effectiveness of epidural steroid injections in patients with radiculopathy symptoms due to discogenic disease who were not candidates for surgical intervention, as well as to examine the relationship between pain and the physical findings.

METHODS

Twenty-five patients with the diagnosis of radiculopathy made by the referring orthopedic surgeon, based on physical examination and CT myelogram, were included in the study. LCT was performed in all patients. The thermographic changes in the affected dermatomes correlated in all patients with the CT myelogram and physical findings. A difference of 1.5°C between the extremities was considered abnormal. A series of one to three epidural injections of 0.25% bupivacaine and 80 mg Depo-Medrol was performed in all patients at 2-week intervals. Immediate pain relief and the efficacy of the block were assessed by a visual pain analog (VPA) scale and thermography. All patients showed increased temperatures in the extremities immediately following the procedure, indicating a successful block. Two weeks after cessation of the series of epidural blocks, LCT and physical examination were repeated, and the pain was assessed using VPA. Postblock data were compared with the preblock findings. A Student paired *t*-test was used to evaluate the results.

There were 20 females and 5 males. Ages varied from 31 to 62 years, with a mean of 43 years. The duration of pain varied from 3 to 52 months (Table 1). Seven patients had had previous laminectomy. Seventeen patients had positive straight leg raising (SLR) and the remaining were negative. In 16 of 25 patients the herniated disc was at L5,S1 (Table 2). In 9 of 25 patients it varied between lumbar and sacral segments. In 18 of 25 patients the clinical diagnosis was discogenic disease, and in 7 of 25 the diagnosis was postlaminectomy syndrome with radiculopathy.

TABLE 1.

Patient	Age	Sex	Duration (months)
1	31	F	7
2	46	M	24
3	37	F	6
4	53	F	23
5	48	F	9
6	55	F	24
7	42	F	5
8	47	F	7
9	41	F	48
10	62	F	24
11	27	F	6
12	54	M	3
13	30	F	8
14	36	F	4
15	40	F	4
16	35	F	3
17	29	F	4
18	48	M	3
19	50	F	3
20	31	F	3.5
21	27	M	8
22	43	M	1
23	55	F	12
24	54	F	8
25	54	F	9
Mean	43		13.5

TABLE 2. *Thermography findings*

Patient	Dermatome level	Temperature difference between extremities at affected dermatome (°C)	
		Pre-injection	Post-injection
1	L3,4	1.5	0.7
2	S1,2	1.7	0.7
3	S1	1.5	0
4	L5,S1,	1.5	0
5	L5	2	1.4
6	L3,4	2	0.8
7	S1,2	2.5	0
8	S1	2.4	1.4
9	S1	2.5	1.5
10	L5,S1	3.2	0
11	L5,S1	3	0
12	S1	1.8	1.1
13	L5,L4	1.9	0
14	L5,S1	1.83	0
15	L4	2	0
16	S1	2.25	0
17	S1	2.5	0
18	L5,S1	2.1	0
19	L5,S1	2.73	1.76
20	S1	1.8	0
21	S1	2.15	1.3
22	L5	1.8	0.3
23	L5	1.8	0.9
24	L5	2.7	0
25	L5	2.7	1.7

RESULTS

All patients had positive thermography before institution of epidural steroid therapy. At the end of 8 weeks, 2 weeks after cessation of the series of blocks, 21 of 25 patients demonstrated negative results on thermography. Two of 4 patients who had positive thermography results did not have any pain relief (Table 3).

Twenty-one of 25 patients (84%) had negative thermography results post block, indicating absence of nerve root irritation (Table 3). Two of these 21 patients reported no relief of pain by VPA scale.

Two of 4 patients who reported no relief of pain post block had negative thermography results. It is postulated that either their pain was centralized or their pain threshold was low. Two of 21 patients who reported relief of pain post block had persistent positive thermography results even though their patterns of radiculopathy actually improved, as the temperature dif-

TABLE 3.

	Total no. patients	No. patients with negative results	No. patients with positive results
Patients with pain relief by VPA	21	19 (90.48%)	2 (9.52%)
Patients without pain relief by VPA	4	2 (50%)	2 (50%)

ference between two extremities was considerably less than before the block, even though it was still greater than 1.5°C.

Negative thermography results post block correlated with excellent to moderate pain relief in 76.2% of patients (Fig. 1).

Positive thermography results post block correlated significantly ($p <$

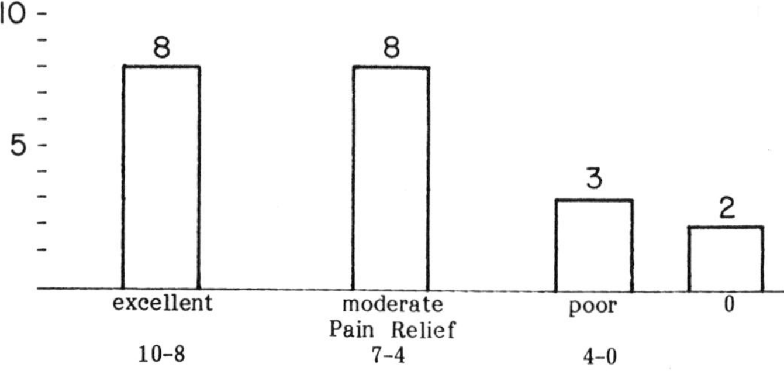

FIG. 1. Negative thermography results post block in 21 patients.

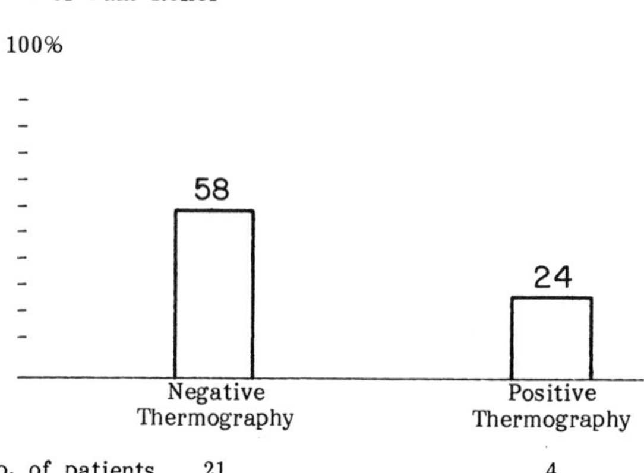

FIG. 2. Progress assessed by thermography.

0.10) with poor pain relief. Thermography provides objective assessment of the patient's symptoms and the progress of the disease (Fig. 2).

CONCLUSION

Our findings suggest that LCT is an effective device to monitor and document responses to therapy. LCT is a simple, noninvasive technique that can complement physical examination and CT myelography. It can also effectively differentiate organic pain syndromes from psychogenic pain or malingering. LCT provides objective and reproducible evidence of the disease state and the result of therapy.

REFERENCES

1. Pochacezevsky, R. (1982): Liquid crystal thermography of the spine and extremities. *J. Neurosurg.,* 56:386–395.
2. Uematus, S. (1976): *Medical Thermography: Theory and Clinical Applications.* Brentwood Publishing, Los Angeles.

Advances in Pain Research and Therapy, Vol. 9, edited by H. L. Fields et al. Raven Press, New York © 1985.

Assessment of Abnormal Evoked Pain in Neurological Pain Patients and Its Relation to Spontaneous Pain: A Descriptive and Conceptual Model with Some Analytical Results

Ulf Lindblom

Department of Neurology, Karolinska Hospital, S-104 01 Stockholm, Sweden

There were several reasons for selecting the topic of abnormal evoked pain for this chapter on pain assessment: (a) Although assessment of spontaneous pain has been the subject of several recent studies and reviews, little attention has been paid to assessment of evoked pain in patients, especially abnormal painful sensations. (b) Abnormal evoked pain is an important part of many pain syndromes and causes suffering to the patient either by itself or in addition to the spontaneous pain. (c) Analysis of evoked pain will be relevant for understanding the mechanisms of both evoked and ongoing pain if there is a common basis. That this may be the case is suggested by the fact that the two types of pain often occur together. (d) Evoked pain can be assessed more objectively than spontaneous pain by means of precise stimulation and psychophysical quantification. Assessment of evoked pain might be used as an index of ongoing pain if a correlation can be shown. Clinically there is a well-recognized need for supplementary diagnostic criteria for ongoing pain, especially in chronic pain patients.

Clinical evoked pain differs from experimental evoked pain in several respects. It is caused by an occasional injury or disease and has much greater variability in location and character and probably also in pathophysiology. Furthermore, it is often superimposed on a state of ongoing pain and emotional distress. In neurological pain patients, sensation is often disturbed in the pain region where the stimulus is applied, which means that the baseline conditions for stimulation may be abnormal. These various circumstances necessitate special selection and design of procedures for testing clinical evoked pain. Techniques that have been developed for experimental pain may be inadequate or may need modification. Furthermore, it is uncertain if the psychophysical laws that have been worked out in experiments on healthy subjects with unaffected nervous systems (6) will be valid for clinical evoked pain, although a few examples suggest that abnormal sensations associated with the pain condition fit power functions (11). What is clear is that the pain taxonomy derived from normal subjects is insufficient. Clinical pain often has a peculiar character for which words are lacking, and it may be mixed with sensory phenomena other than pain.

To overcome these difficulties inherent in assessment of evoked pain in patients, our laboratory design has been adapted to clinical conditions as much as possible. We have tried to select patients with defined lesions and to standardize the examination procedures. Yet the variable phenomenology and pathogenesis will require large samples to demonstrate any systematic relations or differences.

This chapter, which represents an extension of previous work (5,11,14), will first describe our methodological and conceptual approach to the problem of quantification and classification of abnormal evoked pain in neurological pain patients. It is hoped that the same or a similar approach may be applicable, as well, in other types of patients with chronic pain. This chapter will also describe some individual patient records and statistical results to illustrate the various types of abnormal evoked pain and the effects of pain-relieving procedures. In the material thus far analyzed, cold allodynia occurs more frequently than expected and is relatively resistant to therapy. Differential effects of treatment on various painful responses were common. A simple relation between spontaneous and evoked pain might exist but is not apparent.

PATIENTS AND METHODS

Patients

There were 18 female and 12 male patients between 21 and 71 years of age (median 47 years). All patients suffered from sustained pain (mean duration 5 years, range 0.8–17 years) and had evidence of a peripheral nerve lesion of traumatic or entrapment origin. Surgical trauma was the most common type of lesion ($N = 10$). The pain regions were face, hand, abdomen, knee, lower leg, foot, or other, without obvious preponderance for any location. The most common dominating character of the ongoing pain was aching and/or burning.

Sensibility Screening

Sensory screening was carried out with conventional bedside techniques using a camel-hair brush for touch, figure writing for tactile discrimination, pinprick or pressure for mechanically evoked pain, and two metallic rollers kept at 20°C and 40°C, respectively, for cold and warmth. Skin temperature was measured with a thermocouple instrument (Ellab) or an infrared thermometer (Thermophil type M 202). Only patients with distinct sensory abnormalities on screening were accepted for further analysis. The spatial distribution of sensibility disturbances agreed reasonably well with the innervation territory of one or more peripheral nerves in 2/3 of the cases, but was wider, although still regional, in 1/3 of the cases, suggesting an additional central dysfunction that expanded the sensory abnormality.

Quantitative Sensory Testing

Tactile threshold measurements and magnitude estimations were performed with von Frey hairs and in some cases with pulses from a mechanical stimulator (10). The threshold for mechanically evoked pain was estimated with a forceps algometer for superficial pain (12) and with a pressure algometer similar to Cattell's for deep pain (19). The Marstock method (4), which provides selective thermal stimulation, was used to determine warm and cold thresholds, expressed as the warm–cold difference limen, as well as heat and cold pain thresholds. Reaction times were determined by means of tactile and thermal pulses (5). Series of pulsed stimuli were sometimes applied for tentative observations of abnormal summation or habituation.

The characters of each evoked sensation were recorded and classified according to stimulus modality and the proposed taxonomy scheme *(vide infra).* The intensity and duration of sensation were recorded by means of diode-ramp visual analog, which was monitored by the patient by turning a circular potentiometer connected to a potentiometric recorder. Aftersensations were usually estimated with a stopwatch. The spontaneous pain was rated on an ordinary visual analog scale (VAS).

Treatment

All patients were given one or more treatments with conditioning stimulation or pharmacological agents. In 20 cases the best treatment blocked the pain totally or to less than 10% on VAS: dorsal column stimulation in 10 cases, transcutaneous electrical nerve stimulation (TENS) in 1 case, heat stimulation in 2 cases, other stimulation in 2 cases, guanethidine block in 2 cases, and systemic medication in 3 cases.

Data Processing

A data base was established for the various quantitative and categorical data. This was done in collaboration with Dr. Alexander Beric, Department of Clinical Neurophysiology, TIRR, Houston, Texas, with the intention that it also should be applicable in the large material of spinal cord injuries at this center. Statistical analysis was made by means of STATPAC, designed by the Department of Medical Information Processing at the Karolinska Institute using a Nord 100 computer.

RESULTS

Quantification and Categorization of Abnormal Evoked Pain and Other Sensory Abnormalities

Quantitative changes measurable as altered perception threshold or magnitude of sensation are illustrated diagrammatically in Fig. 1, where the left box represents normal threshold (lower border) and magnitude (upper border). The second box depicts hypoesthesia as an elevated threshold level with reduced magnitude of sensation on suprathreshold stimulation. Hyperesthesia is the opposite, i.e., lowered threshold or increased magnitude, or both (third box in Fig. 1). The right-hand box depicts the common combination of an elevated threshold and increased magnitude of sensation. This hypo-hyperesthesia is a typical part of the syndrome of sensory abnormalities known as hyperpathia (3,24). Hypoalgesia and hyperalgesia constitute a subclass of quantitative abnormalities pertaining to stimuli that normally are painful (mechanical, thermal, or chemical). All quantitative abnormalities can be assessed numerically for each sensory modality by combining selective stimulation with conventional psychophysical methodology.

The qualitative, spatial, and temporal abnormalities are listed in Table 1. Allodynia occurs when normally nonpainful stimuli such as touch, light pressure, or moderate temperatures (20°C–40°C) produce pain (17). Dysesthesia occurs when the patient judges the sensation not as painful, but as abnormally unpleasant. Paresthesia is broadly defined as an abnormal sensation (18), but will in the present context be restricted to mean an altered quality of sensation other than allodynia and dysesthesia. It is usually difficult to describe paresthetic sensations, because specific words are lacking, and the patient uses metaphorical expressions like "crawling," "running water," "tingling," "tightness," etc., or simply states "different from normal" (26). The three qualitative alterations will later be illustrated with different screens (Figs. 4–6).

The categorization of the qualitative changes of sensation is obviously dependent on the wording of the examiner's instruction and on the criteria set by the patient. The spatial and temporal abnormalities (Table 1), on the other hand, may all be quantified in some way. Radiation and faulty local-

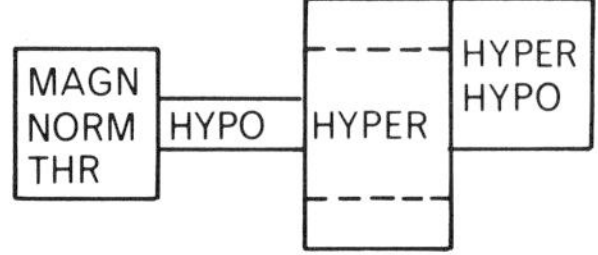

FIG. 1. Schematic illustration of quantitative sensory changes in terms of altered threshold and/or magnitude of sensation.

TABLE 1. *Qualitative, spatial, and temporal sensory abnormalities*

Qualitative	Spatial	Temporal
Allodynia	Abnormal radiation	Abnormal latency
Dysesthesia	Poor localization	Abnormal aftersensation
Paresthesia	Impaired discrimination	Abnormal summation
		Abnormal adaptation
		Abnormal habituation

ization of the stimulus can be estimated by distance, and impaired spatial discrimination by testing figure writing (graphesthesia), directional sensitivity, or two-point resolution. Abnormal latency can be recorded with reaction-time measurements. Aftersensation can be measured in seconds or minutes, and altered adaptation and abnormal summation or habituation by means of sustained or repeated pulsed stimuli.

Figures 2 and 3 illustrate some sensory abnormalities, including the two principal types of abnormal evoked pain: allodynia and hyperalgesia. Figure 2 shows an abnormally low pain threshold for pressure and aftersensation. Conventionally, this would be described as tenderness or hyperalgesia, but the new term *allodynia* may also be used, because a pressure of only 20 g/mm^2 with a blunt object does not normally evoke pain, at least not in this skin region (foot sole).

In Fig. 3, the records from thermal stimulation of a patient with meralgia

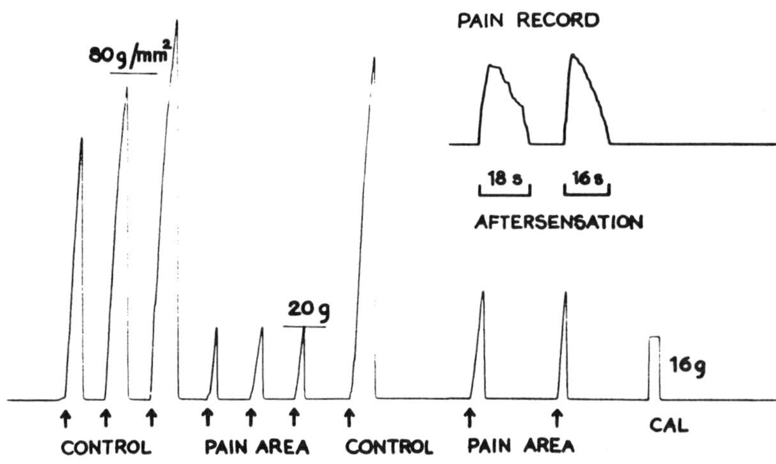

FIG. 2. Potentiometric recordings of pain thresholds and aftersensations in a patient with sciatic nerve causalgia. A blunt-ended pressure algometer was applied in the pain area (foot sole), where pain was elicited at an abnormally low pressure, 20 g/mm^2, compared with 80 g in the normal homologous region contralaterally. About 30 g pressure in the pain area evoked rather intense pain, with 16 to 18 sec of aftersensation.

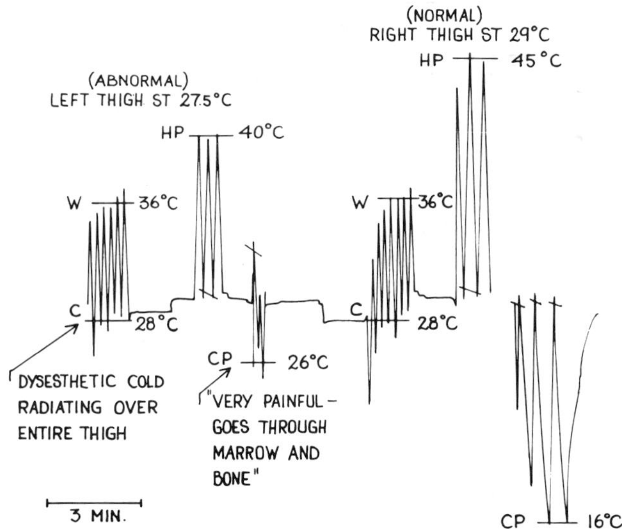

FIG. 3. Potentiometric recordings of thresholds for warm (W), cold (C), heat pain (HP), and cold pain (CP) with the Marstock method in a patient with meralgia paresthetica. ST, skin temperature.

paresthetica are reproduced. The record to the left was obtained from the center of the pain area. The perception thresholds for warm and cold were normal, but the cold sensation was unpleasant and radiating. The cold pain and heat pain thresholds were both abnormal, as appears from comparison with the record (Fig. 3, right), which was obtained from the normal contralateral side. In the pain area there was only a 2°C range between the thresholds for cold and cold pain, which appeared by 26°C. It seems appropriate to call this abnormal pain response cold allodynia, because such a high temperature is normally never painful on the thigh. In this particular patient the cold pain threshold was about 16°C on the control side. Heat pain occurred at 40°C on the pain side, which was significantly lower than contralaterally. Hyperalgesia may be a better term than allodynia in this case, because heat pain may occur normally at 40°C. This temperature may also produce some discharge in normal heat nociceptors. In the patient illustrated in Fig. 3, the heat pain threshold of the pain area varied between 40°C and 45°C on different occasions, and it may be speculated that such slightly lowered heat pain thresholds were due to central facilitation and perhaps a less complicated mechanism than the allodynic responses.

Spontaneous Pain Versus Evoked Sensations

To explore the possibility of a close correlation between spontaneous pain, on the one hand, and evoked pain or any other sensory changes, on

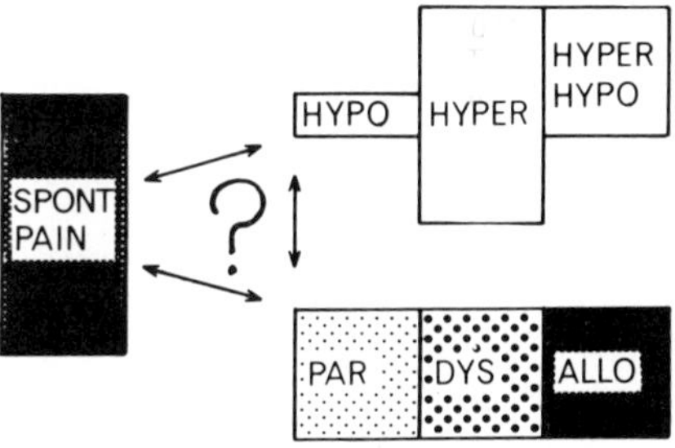

FIG. 4. Schematic illustration of the three principal sets of studied data: spontaneous pain and quantitative and qualitative alterations of evoked sensations including abnormal painful responses.

the other hand (Fig. 4), repeated measurements were performed before and after treatment that abolished or significantly reduced the spontaneous pain. The most commonly effective treatment in our patients thus far studied was dorsal column stimulation (DCS), and, thanks to close collaboration with Dr. Björn Meyerson at the Department of Neurosurgery, a number of such patients were available for study. In some patients pain relief was achieved by other types of conditioning stimulation or pharmacological means *(vide supra).*

As could be expected from previous general experience with bedside testing, significant changes in evoked responses were encountered after treatment, but the results were quite different from case to case. Figure 5 illustrates diagrammatically the results of tactile and cold stimulations in another patient with meralgia paresthetica before and after treatment with

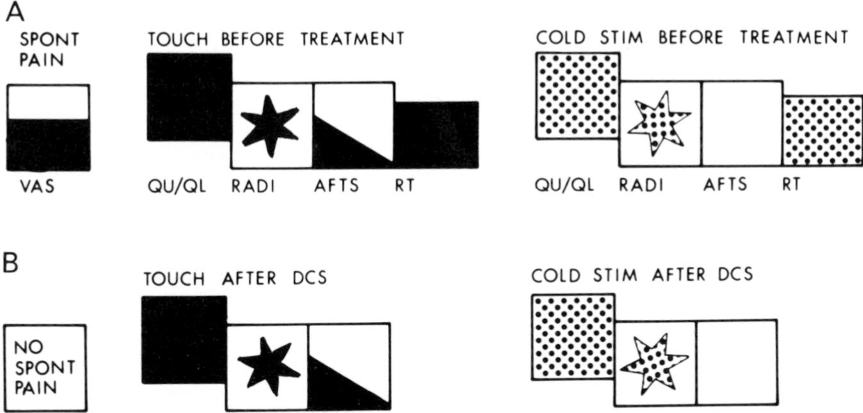

FIG. 5. Spontaneous pain and sensations evoked by tactile and cold stimulation before (**A**) and after (**B**) treatment with DCS in a 47-year-old female patient with meralgia after assumed entrapment and neurolysis of nervus cutaneous femoris lateralis; 70% ongoing pain on VAS before and none after treatment. QU/QL shows type of quantitative and qualitative abnormality of evoked sensation with the symbols given in Figs. 1 and 4. Abnormal radiation (RADI) is indicated by a star, and aftersensation (AFTS) by a slanted screen. Reaction time (RT) indicates slightly reduced delay of sensation as compared with normal.

DCS. The base-line spontaneous pain before treatment was estimated to 70% on VAS (left-hand block in A). The elevated position of the second block indicates both raised threshold and increased magnitude of sensation on tactile stimulation, and solid block indicates that the type of response was allodynia (see Fig. 4). The sensation was pure pain without any concomitant tactile sensation. The star in the next block in Fig. 5 denotes that the sensation radiated, and the slanted screen in the following block indicates that there was a painful aftersensation. The last block represents the reaction time, which was slightly reduced, suggesting a central facilitation. The response to cold stimulation was similar, but the sensation was unpleasant rather than painful, and there was no aftersensation. Figure 5B shows the situation after DCS when the spontaneous pain was totally blocked. The patient was pleased and did not even complain of tactile hypersensitivity in the pain region. This subjective report was misleading, however, because a repeated sensory test revealed that the tactile allodynia persisted, only with a somewhat higher threshold, and so did the cold dysesthesia.

In another patient, ongoing pain and evoked responses were affected together, as illustrated in Fig. 6. This patient suffered from ulnar nerve causalgia and displayed a similar picture of tactile and cold allodynia as the preceding patient before treatment, although the tactile response was without aftersensation, and the reaction time to cold was prolonged instead of reduced. Following pain relief, which in this case was obtained by means of a guanethidine block, the tactile allodynia was replaced by a paresthetic, hypoesthetic, radiating tactile sensation without pain (Fig. 6B). The response to cold was slightly altered. A radiating paresthetic cold sensation appeared at threshold. The aftersensation was reduced from approximately 30 sec to a few seconds. Slightly above threshold, the sensation again

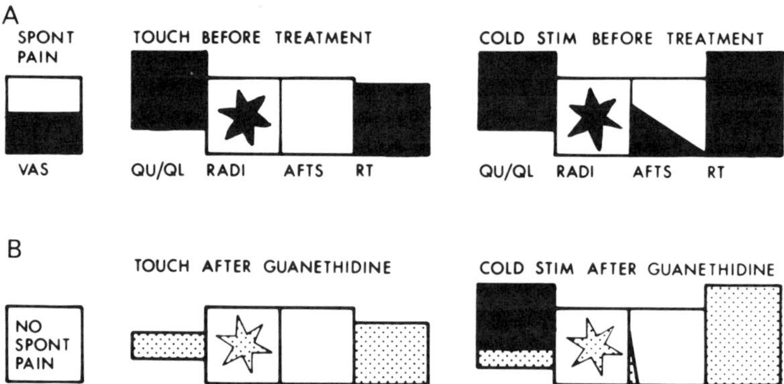

FIG. 6. Spontaneous pain and evoked responses before (**A**) and after (**B**) guanethidine block in a 38-year-old patient with ulnar nerve neuralgia after penetrating trauma to the lower arm (exploding carboy) and surgical repair with a sural nerve graft. Symbols as in Figs. 1, 4, and 5.

became painful as before the treatment. Thus, whereas the tactile allodynia was relieved, cold allodynia persisted.

Other patients displayed similar differential effects or covariation of spontaneous pain and allodynia, but it is too early to tell if any type of effect may be treatment-specific or related to other clinical parameters. In the material thus far analyzed, cold allodynia was as conspicuous as tactile allodynia and more consistent. This was confirmed by statistical analysis, as illustrated in Fig. 7, which shows the average thresholds for warm (W), cold (C), heat pain (HP), and cold pain (CP) in the patients (N = 13) with complete data before and after effective pain relief. The cold pain threshold was significantly ($p < 0.01$) "reduced" from 16.1°C (SD 7.7°C) on the control side to 23.7°C (SD 6.8°C) in the pain area. After treatment, CP dropped to 21.4°C (SD 6.0°C) ($p < 0.05$), but CP remained significantly abnormal. Thus, even if cold allodynia can be reduced by treatment, it persists in the absence of spontaneous pain. Tactile allodynia was also relatively resistant, but a statistical analysis has not yet been performed. Allodynia on the warm side (pain below 40°C) was less common than both cold and tactile allodynia, but a slight reduction in heat pain (hyperalgesia) was observed in several cases. Statistically, the heat pain threshold was not significantly different from the control side, and there was no average change after treatment (Fig. 7). Likewise, there were no significant changes of the W-C difference limen (DL) in this patient group. In the whole group with complete thermal records (N = 25), the DL was significantly wider in the pain area, 10.1°C (SD 9.8°C) versus 4.7°C (SD 4.3°C) in the control area ($p < 0.01$).

Even when the averaged data were unremarkable, as with HP and DL in Fig. 7, notable changes were seen in some patients after treatment. This is

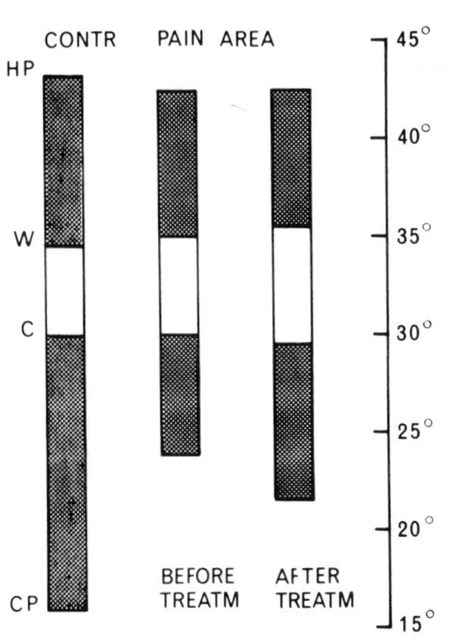

FIG. 7. Mean thermal thresholds in 13 patients in the control area (left column), and in the pain area before and after treatment that relieved spontaneous pain. Cold pain was significantly abnormal in the pain area both before and after treatment. HP, heat pain; W, warmth; C, cold; CP, cold pain.

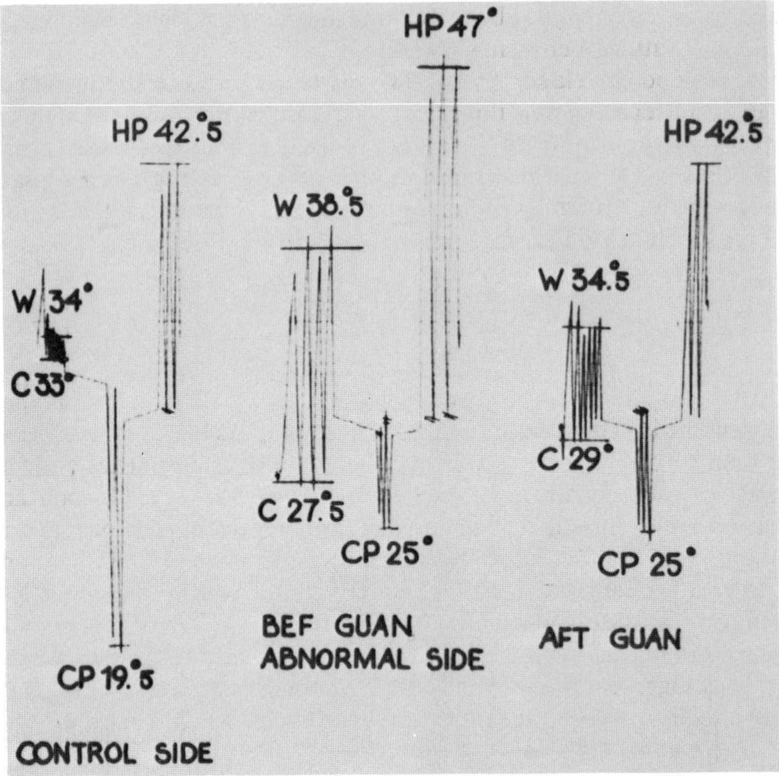

FIG. 8. Thermal record from same patient as in Fig. 6 illustrating improved sensibility in pain area in terms of recovered heat pain threshold and reduced W-C difference limen, after treatment with guanethidine. The abnormal cold pain threshold did not change.

illustrated in Fig. 8, which is the thermal record from the patient with the nerve graft (Fig. 6). Although cold allodynia appeared at the same temperature before and after treatment, DL was reduced from 11°C to 5.5°C and HP from 47°C to 42.5°C. Hence, the pain relief was accompanied by a normalization of the heat pain threshold and a reduced thermohypesthesia.

Miscellaneous Observations

Reduced thresholds for pain evoked by pinch or pressure were recorded in 18 patients before treatment and 9 patients after treatment. The relation between this type of abnormal evoked pain and the other sensory abnormalities, or the spontaneous pain, has not yet been analyzed. The relation between spontaneous pain and evoked thermal pain was tested by correlating the VAS values with the cold and heat pain levels. There were no correlations, either when these levels were expressed directly in degrees centigrade or as ratios between abnormal and control sides. Furthermore, there were no correlations between VAS and DL or tactile thresholds. However, there was a good correlation ($r = 0.68$) between DL and touch threshold. A very good correlation was noted between tactile threshold measurement with von Frey hairs and with mechanical pulses ($r = 0.95$). This strengthens the value of the former, old and simple, way of quantitating tactile sensation and agrees with the correlation between force and indentation thresholds of the tactile receptors (9).

DISCUSSION

Assessment of Hyperpathia

The present investigation confirmed that it is feasible to collect quantitative data to describe the abnormal evoked painful responses and most other sensory abnormalities in neurological pain patients. The application of quantitative techniques (12) is the main difference between ours and earlier studies. Among these, the bedside analysis and semantic discussion of Noordenbos (21) remains classic. The analyzed phenomena are basically the same in our work, but a different approach is taken to the terminology and taxonomy on the basis of the aquired knowledge of psychophysics and basic neurophysiology. The taxonomy is the same as proposed before (11), but the categorization of the qualitative changes now includes the new term *allodynia,* which allows hyperalgesia to be referred to the group of quantitative abnormalities and restricted to responses to normally painful stimuli. In most cases the separation of allodynia and hyperalgesia is obvious, but there will always be borderline cases with slightly lowered thresholds for pain that will require operational definitions. For example, in the present study it was reasonable to set the borders between thermal allodynia and hyperalgesia at 40°C and 20°C on the heat and cold sides, respectively.

A main question during the investigation was whether or not a correlation exists between spontaneous pain and any kind of abnormal evoked pain or other sensory abnormality in chronic pain patients. No close relation was apparent and larger samples will be required to answer this question. The statistical analysis confirmed that the covariation of pain and hyperpathia is only relative, because the threshold for cold pain in the pain area remained significantly abnormal when the ongoing pain was relieved. In our previous smaller sample (13), the dominance of cold allodynia in this type of patient was canceled out by the alternate occurrence of hypoalgesia. Enkvist et al. (2) demonstrated a similar cold hypersensitivity in amputees.

Besides cold and tactile allodynia, lowered thresholds for pain evoked by pinch or pressure were encountered in several patients. These thresholds responded differently to treatment. They recovered during pain relief in some patients, as reported earlier (13), but remained abnormal in others.

Various hyperpathic phenomena may thus exist in isolation, without ongoing pain, in neurological pain patients. The same dissociation occurs during nerve regeneration, and is not uncommon in patients with neuropathies of metabolic or other origin. In experimental pain, allodynia or hyperalgesia may also occur without spontaneous pain. It remains to be studied if the opposite may occur, i.e., if other therapeutic manipulations may relieve abnormal evoked pain but not ongoing pain.

Pathophysiology

Several observations suggest that the sensory dysfunction in neurological pain patients reflects a profound physiological disturbance that is not restricted to the site of lesion in the peripheral nerve, but extends to the central nervous system. One such observation is the rather common spread of the sensory dysfunction outside the borders of the injured nerve. Reaction-time measurements indicate that allodynia, at least in some cases, is generated centrally (5,14). Concomitant thermal or tactile hyperesthesia (11) is best explained by central facilitation. Further arguments and evidence of central changes have been discussed, for example, by Sunderland (23) and quite recently by Wall (24). Dr. Campbell has provided evidence in this volume that experimental tactile allodynia may also be of central origin. It may be mentioned here that Hardy et al. (8) originally suggested a central mechanism for secondary hyperalgesia.

Although several peripheral pain-producing factors have been clarified by ingenious experiments during recent years (25), central mechanisms of both evoked and ongoing pain are still obscure. We do not even know if or when a particular level of the nervous system is more or less responsible. Dysfunction at segmental spinal levels seems plausible because of the regional and multimodal character of the clinical signs and symptoms. It is easy to imagine that disintegration of the intricate circuitry and interactive biochemistry of the dorsal horn could produce a variety of clinical phenomena. For example, it has been speculated that excitatory spread to the subliminal fringe may explain radiation of sensation and that allodynia is due to loss of funneling and selective inhibition of low-threshold input to convergent interneurons.

Focusing future studies on the pathophysiology of the various phenomena associated with chronic pain appears to be the best way to improve therapy, which currently is largely empirical. The pathophysiology is obviously more complex than ectopic impulse formation in nociceptive neurons at the site of injury, and therefore simple measures like neurolytic blocks often fail. Noordenbos and Wall (22) excised and grafted the damaged segment of the nerve in causalgia patients. The fascinating result was that the whole hyperpathic syndrome recurred after regeneration, which indicates a centrally imprinted dysfunction. Our patient with an ulnar nerve graft (Figs. 6 and 8) was similar, although the graft was made soon after the injury without a preexisting pain condition. This case is also interesting because of the combination of residual allodynia and improved sensibility after the guanethidine block that relieved the spontaneous pain. Guanethidine is taken to act peripherally by depleting the norepinephrine stores of sympathetic terminals (7). Loh et al. (15) reported a series of patients in whom both pain and hyperpathia were relieved immediately after the block. The persistent cold allodynia in our case would be explained either by a peripheral mechanism that is different from monoaminergic hypersensitivity or by a central disturbance. Other modes of action of guanethidine should also be taken into account, as discussed by Loh et al. (15), who found variable effects on pain, hyperpathia, and vasomotor activity. We delayed the postinjection test a few days to let the acute effect wear off, and yet see perhaps even more dissociated effects (S. Arnér and U. Lindblom, *unpublished observations*).

Functional Sensory Loss

It is a general firsthand belief among clinicians that hypesthesia in patients with documented or suspected peripheral nerve lesions is due to fiber loss at the lesion site. However, there are reasons to consider other mechanisms, especially in pain patients. Several years ago Nathan (20) reported improvement of sensibility in such patients after the pain had been removed by treatment. Such observations suggest that the pain may have a reversible blocking effect on sensory transmission that may be restored after pain relief. The recovery of the heat pain threshold and the reduction of thermal hypoesthesia in the patient illustrated in Fig. 8 may be an example of such a block. The residual hypesthesia after the pain relief would then reflect a structural sensory loss due to incomplete reinnervation through the graft. Callaghan et al. (1) demonstrated that impaired two-point discrimination and perception of heat and electrical shocks in chronically painful limbs improved during TENS. This might be another example of functional somatosensory blockade in a pain state. It is also of interest that discrimination may improve after pain relief in myofascial pain (16).

SUMMARY

Abnormal evoked pain and other sensory abnormalities were studied in 30 patients with traumatic or entrapment neuralgia. The spontaneous pain was rated with VAS. The evoked sensations were categorized and quantified psychophysically by means of modality-selective and graded sensory stimulation of the pain area.

Tactile and cold allodynia were the most conspicuous types of abnormal evoked pain. Cold allodynia was statistically the most consistent change of the perception thresholds. Alterations of heat pain were more variable. On mechanical stimulation with pinch or pressure, reduced pain threshold and excessive pain intensity were frequently recorded.

Following treatment that relieved the spontaneous pain, the hyperpathic phenomena behaved differently. Tactile and cold allodynia were relatively persistent. Modality differential effects were not uncommon. Larger patient samples will be required to demonstrate if such effects are correlated to mode of treatment and if the spontaneous pain is more closely related to any particular type of abnormal evoked pain.

The pathophysiology of the various phenomena of altered sensation and pain is currently speculative, but indirect evidence is accumulating that they largely reflect a central neurophysiological disturbance that is precipitated by peripheral lesions in certain individuals or under certain circumstances.

ACKNOWLEDGMENTS

This study was supported by the Folksam Research Foundation and by the Vivian L. Smith Foundation for Restorative Neurology. Berit Lindblom is acknowledged for skillful technical assistance and considerate patient care.

REFERENCES

1. Callaghan, M., Sternbach, R. A., Nyquist, J. K., and Timmermans, G. (1978): Changes in somatic sensitivity during transcutaneous eletrical analgesia. *Pain,* 5:115–127.
2. Enkvist, O., Wahren, L. K., Wallin, G., Torebjörk, E., and Nyström, B. (1985): Effects of regional intravenous guanethidine block in posttraumatic cold intolerance in hand amputees. *J. Hand. Surg., (in press)*
3. Foerster, O. (1927): *Die Leitungsbahnen des Schmerzegefuhle.* Urban & Schwartzenberg, Vienna.
4. Fruhstrofer, H., Lindblom, U., and Schmidt, W. G. (1976): Method for quantitative estimation of thermal thresholds in patients. *J. Neurol. Neurosurg. Psychiatry,* 39:1071–1075.
5. Fruhstorfer, H., and Lindblom, U. (1984): Sensibility abnormalities in neuralgic patients studied by thermal and tactile pulse stimulation. In: *Somatosensory Mechanisms,* edited by C. von Euler, O. Franzén, U. Lindblom, and D. Ottoson, pp. 353–361. Macmillan, London.
6. Gescheider, G. A. (1976): *Psychophysics. Methods and Theory.* Lawrence Erlbaum Associates, New York.
7. Hannington-Kiff, J. G. (1974): *Pain Relief.* Heinemann, London.
8. Hardy, J. D., Wolff, H. G., and Goodell, H. (1950): Experimental evidence on the nature of cutaneous hyperalgesia. *J. Clin. Invest.,* 29:115–140.
9. Johansson, R. S., Vallbo, Å. B., and Westling, G. (1980): Thresholds of mechanosensitive afferents in the human hand as measured with von Frey hairs. *Brain Res.,* 184:343–351.
10. Lindblom, U. (1974): Touch perception threshold in human glabrous skin in terms of displacement amplitude on stimulation with single mechanical pulses. *Brain Res.,* 82:205–210.
11. Lindblom, U. (1979): Sensory abnormalities in neuralgia. In: *Advances in Pain Research and Therapy,* Vol. 3, edited by J. J. Bonica et al., pp. 111–120, Raven Press, New York.
12. Lindblom, U. (1981): Quantitative testing of sensibility including pain. In: *Clinical Neurophysiology, Neurology 1,* edited by E. Stålberg and R. R. Young, pp. 168–190. Butterworth, London.

13. Lindblom, U., and Meyerson, B. A. (1975): Influence on touch, vibration and cutaneous pain of dorsal column stimulation in man. *Pain,* 1:257–270.
14. Lindblom, U., and Verrillo, R. T. (1979): Sensory functions in chronic neuralgia. *J. Neurol. Neurosurg. Psychiatry,* 42:422–435.
15. Loh, L., Nathan, P. W., Schott, G. D., and Wilson, P. G. (1980): Effects of regional guanethidine infusion in certain painful states. *J. Neurol. Neurosurg. Psychiatry,* 43:446–451.
16. Malow, R. M., and Olson, R. E. (1981): Changes in pain perception after treatment for chronic pain. *Pain,* 11:65–72.
17. Merskey, H. (1979): Pain terms: A list of definitions and notes on usage. *Pain,* 6:249–252.
18. Merskey, H. (1982): Pain terms: A supplementary note. *Pain,* 14:205–206.
19. Merskey, H., and Spear, F. G. (1964): The reliability of the pressure algometer. *Br. J. Soc. Clin. Psychol.,* 3:130–136.
20. Nathan, P. W. (1960): Improvement in cutaneous sensibility associated with relief of pain. *J. Neurol. Neurosurg. Psychiatry,* 23:202–206.
21. Noordenbos, W. (1959): *Pain.* Elsevier, Amsterdam.
22. Noordenbos, W., and Wall, P. D. (1981): Implications of the failure of nerve resection and graft to cure chronic pain produced by nerve lesions. *J. Neurol. Neurosurg. Psychiatry,* 44:1068–1073.
23. Sunderland, S. (1976): Pain mechanism in causalgia. *J. Neurol. Neurosurg. Psychiatry,* 39:471–480.
24. Wall, P. D. (1984): The hyperpathic syndrome: A challenge to specificity theory. In: *Somatosensory Mechanisms,* edited by C. von Euler, O. Franzén, U. Lindblom, and D. Ottoson, pp. 327–337. Macmillan, London.
25. Wall, P. D., and Melzack, R. (1984): *Textbook of Pain.* Livingstone, London.
26. Wilson Kinnier, S. A. (1928): Dysaesthesiae and their neural correlates. In: *Modern Problems in Neurology,* pp. 297–331. Edward Arnold, London.

Advances in Pain Research and Therapy, Vol. 9, edited by H. L. Fields et al. Raven Press, New York © 1985.

Phantom Limb Phenomena in Amputees Seven Years After Limb Amputation

*Børge Krebs, **Troels S. Jensen, *Karsten Krøner, *Jørn Nielsen, and *Hans S. Jørgensen

*Departments of *Orthopaedic Surgery and **Neurology, Aarhus University Hospital, DK-8000 Aarhus C, Denmark*

Immediately after amputation of a limb, most amputees report a feeling of the missing limb—a phenomenon known as phantom limb (3,4,10). Phantom limb sensations have a wide range, from short-lasting tingling sensations in the phantom to a constant vivid experience of the missing limb (6,10). Occasionally the phantom becomes the site of painful sensations, known as phantom pain. The incidence and temporal course of phantom pain are not settled, but it is generally assumed to be persistent in less than 5 to 10% of cases (1,4,9). This rate of phantom pain is in sharp contrast to that reported in some recent studies (2,5,8,12,13). For example, in a prospective study of mainly nontraumatic amputees (5,8) we found that phantom pain occurred in more than 60% of patients during the first 2 years after limb amputation. To determine if this high rate of phantom pain was due to a relatively short time span elapsed between amputation and follow-up, we recorded phantom pain and related phenomena in another group of patients amputated more than 5 years earlier. Because of the high mortality among amputees with underlying peripheral vascular disease causing limb amputation, this study was carried out as a retrospective investigation.

MATERIALS AND METHODS

Subjects. In two orthopedic surgical departments in the Aarhus area, 624 consecutive patients had limb amputations during a 7-year period from 1970 to 1977. At follow-up in 1983, 95 patients (15%) were alive. Nine patients were excluded from the study because of dementia; therefore 86 patients participated in the study. The median age at the time of amputation was 60.0 years (1st quartile 47.6 years, 3rd quartile 68.2 years). The median

Dr. Krebs' present address is Ludvig Holbergsvej 27, DK-8230 Åbyhøj, Denmark.

follow-up period was 7.2 years (1st quartile 6.2 years, 3rd quartile 8.4 years). The reasons for amputation were peripheral vascular disease in 59 patients, trauma in 20 patients, and various other diseases such as tumors or chronic osteomyelitis in 7 patients. Eleven patients had multiple amputations on the same limb. Eighteen patients had amputations on the contralateral side, but among these patients only the first amputation during the study period was considered.

Procedure. The 86 amputees were interviewed personally by one of the authors in their family surroundings by means of a standard questionnaire regarding phantom limb sensation, phantom pain, and stump pain. The procedure and questionnaire were the same as previously described (5).

RESULTS

Site of amputation. There were 3 upper-limb amputations and 83 lower-limb amputations (4 transmetatarsally, 46 between knee and foot, and 33 above the knee); 47 (54.7%) of the amputations were right-sided.

Phantom Limb Phenomena

Sensations. Phantom limb sensations occurred in 66 patients (76.7%), but varied considerably among individual patients with regard to character, intensity, and frequency. In some patients the phantom limb experience was limited to a short-lasting pricking sensation; in others, the phantom limb perception included a clear feeling of the entire missing limb. In 55% of patients the phantom was felt as an existing part of the body, as evidenced by a clear feeling of length, volume, and/or other spatial sensation; 30% of these patients noted a shortening (telescoping) of the phantom. The distribution of phantom limb sensations is shown in Table 1. As previously noted, distal parts of the phantom were the most prominent parts felt (7).

Movements. Thirty-nine patients with phantom limb sensations experienced associated phantom movements of the phantom limb. Of these, 26 patients (66.7%) reported voluntary movements, 9 patients (14%) involun-

TABLE 1. *Distributions of phantom limb sensations and phantom pain in patients with either*

Part of the extremity	Phantom limb (N = 66)	Phantom pain (N = 45)
Total limb	42	18
Proximal limb	2	4
Distal limb	56	78

tary movements, and 4 patients (6%) both voluntary and involuntary movements. In 25 patients (38%), phantom limb movements were associated with visible muscle contractions in the stump.

Aggravating factors. Phantom limb sensations could be provoked by various internal and external stimuli such as concentration or anxiety (21%), touching the stump (23%), and various other factors in another 21% of patients.

Use of prosthesis. The use of a prosthesis induced or increased phantom limb sensations in 11% of patients, whereas 6% noted attenuation of the phantom limb feeling with use of a prosthesis (Table 2). In 64% of patients with phantom limb sensations there was no relation between the phantom limb sensation and the use of a prosthesis.

Phantom Limb Pain

The incidence of phantom limb pain was 52.3% (45 patients). The distribution of phantom limb pain is shown in Table 1. As in the case of nonpainful phantom limb sensations, phantom pain was most common in the distal parts of the phantom limb.

Character of pain. Phantom pains varied considerably in intensity, frequency of attacks, and the experienced quality. The most frequently reported pain was a knifelike type of pain, which occurred in 65% of patients, whereas burning and squeezing types of pain were reported by 25% of patients.

Aggravating factors. Touching the stump, movements, cold, and rest could provoke or aggravate phantom pains in 13 to 29% of patients. Another 53% of patients stated that cough, anxiety, heat, and other factors could increase their phantom pains. In many patients, several environmental stimuli could provoke attacks of phantom pain.

Relieving factors. Touching and moving the stump reduced phantom pains in 30 and 18%, respectively. Heat relieved the pain in 9%, and 20% of patients noted various other ameliorating factors for their pains.

TABLE 2. *Relationships between phantom limb phenomena and use of a prosthesis*

Relationship	Phantom limb (*N* = 66)	Phantom pain (*N* = 45)
Better	6	2
Worse	11	29
Independent	64	58
Unknown	19	11

Percentage of patients with the phantom phenomenon.

Use of prosthesis. Most of the patients with phantom pain did not report any relation between the use of a prosthesis and the experience of phantom pain (Table 2); 30% stated that their phantom pains increased, and only 2% were relieved of their phantom pains by using a prosthesis.

Stump Pain

The incidence of stump pain was 23.3% (20 patients), among which 60% stated that their pains had been unchanged since the time of amputation.

Aggravating factors. Rest, movements, and touching the stump increased stump pains in 25, 15, and 10% of patients, respectively. A variety of internal and external stimuli could likewise increase stump pains in another 30% of patients.

Relieving factors. Firm pressure around the stump decreased stump pains in 5 patients (25%). Various movements or elevation of the stump above the horizontal level relieved stump pains in 20%, and 35% of patients noted other ameliorating factors.

Use of prosthesis. The use of a prosthesis increased stump pains in 9 patients (45%), whereas 10 patients (50%) did not report any relation between their stump pains and the use of a prosthesis.

DISCUSSION

This study shows that 7 years after limb amputation, approximately 75% of patients still have a feeling of the missing limb, and in more than 50% of patients this phantom limb feeling involves complex kinesthetic sensations, as evidenced by feelings of length, volume, or other spatial sensations. In addition, our study shows that phantom pain is seen in more than 50% of amputees several years after limb amputation. This figure for phantom pain is close to the rate reported in a similar group of mainly old people with peripheral vascular diseases followed for the first 2 years after amputation (8). Neither age nor the reason for amputation seemed to play any role in the present high rate of phantom pain. Sherman et al. (12,13) recently found among American veterans who had amputations at a mean age of 25 years, mainly because of combat injuries or accidents, that more than 75% of amputees complained of phantom pain 20 to 30 years later. On the basis of these findings we conclude that persistent phantom limb pain is a more common problem than is usually assumed. As previously noted (11), few patients seek treatments for their phantom pains or discuss their problems with their physicians. Amputees with the worst phantom pains tend to seek treatment, which may in part explain why pain-relieving treatments have generally failed to work. Our study and previous reports (13) clearly emphasize the need for carefully conducted double-blind control trials with systematic follow-up assessment.

ACKNOWLEDGMENTS

We wish to thank the patients who participated in this study. This work was supported by the Danish Medical Research Council (82-4174), the Knud Højgaards Foundation, and the Foundation for Experimental Research in Neurology.

REFERENCES

1. Abramson, A. S., and Feibel, A. (1981): The phantom phenomenon, its use and disuse. *Bull. N.Y. Acad. Med.,* 57:99–112.
2. Carlen, P. L., Wall, P. D., Nadvorna, H., and Steinbach, T. (1978): Phantom limbs and related phenomena in recent traumatic amputations. *Neurology (Minneap.),* 28:211–217.
3. Cronholm, B. (1951): Phantom limb in amputees. *Acta Psychiatr. Neurol. Scand.* [*Suppl.*], 72:1–310.
4. Henderson, W. R., and Smyth, G. E. (1948): Phantom limbs. *J. Neurol. Neurosurg. Psychiatry,* 11:88–112.
5. Jensen, T. S., Krebs, B., Nielsen, J., and Rasmussen, P. (1983): Phantom limb, phantom pain and stump pain in amputees during the first 6 months following limb amputation. *Pain,* 17:243–256.
6. Jensen, T. S., and Rasmussen, P. (1984): Amputation. In: *Textbook of Pain,* edited by P. D. Wall and R. Melzack, pp. 402–412. Churchill Livingstone, Edinburgh.
7. Jensen, T. S., Krebs, B., Nielsen, J., and Rasmussen, P. (1984): Non-painful phantom limb phenomena in amputees: Incidence, clinical characteristics and temporal course. *Acta Neurol. Scand.,* 70:407–414.
8. Jensen, T. S., Krebs, B., Nielsen, J., and Rasmussen, P. (1985): Immediate and long-term phantom limb pain in amputees: Incidence, clinical characteristics and relationship to preamputation limb pain. *Pain,* 21:267–278.
9. Melzack, R. (1971): Phantom limb pain: Implications for treatment of pathological pain. *Anesthesiology,* 35:409–419.
10. Riddoch, G. (1941): Phantom limbs and body shape. *Brain,* 64:197–222.
11. Sherman, R. A., Sherman, C. J., and Gall, N. G. (1980): A survey of current phantom limb pain treatment in the United States. *Pain,* 8:85–99.
12. Sherman, R. A., and Sherman, C. J. (1983): Prevalence and characteristics of chronic phantom limb pain among American veterans. *Am. J. Phys. Med.,* 62:227–238.
13. Sherman, R. A., Sherman, C. J., and Parker, L. (1984): Chronic phantom and stump pain among American veterans: Results of a survey. *Pain,* 18:83–95.

Advances in Pain Research and Therapy, Vol. 9, edited by H. L. Fields et al. Raven Press, New York © 1985.

Mechanisms of Neuropathic Pain: Cumulative Observations, New Experiments, and Further Speculation

*José L. Ochoa, **Erik Torebjörk, *Paolo Marchettini, and †Mark Sivak

**Department of Neurology, University of Wisconsin Medical School, Madison, Wisconsin 53792; **Department of Clinical Neurophysiology, Academic Hospital, Uppsala, Sweden; and †Department of Neurology, Mt. Sinai Medical Center, New York, New York 10029*

Everyone knows that nerves hurt when molested and that sick nerves hurt even more and may hurt spontaneously. For example, if a patient with chronic spontaneous pain and allodynia[1] has a lump at the site of an old nerve injury, gently tapping on that neuroma will evoke a further painful sensation projected down to the territory of the nerve in the hand (sign of Tinel). Concomitantly, one can pick up ascending volleys of unitary nerve impulses using a Vallbo-Hagbarth intraneural electrode placed at a distance in the same nerve (52). Clearly, that sick nerve hurts because it transmits "painful messages" up to the brain. But one does not need an intraneural recording to reach such a conclusion; that is obvious to anyone who knows that the pain is felt in the "fingers" of the brain rather than in the fingers of the hand. The real questions then are the following: (a) What in the nature of those "messages" makes them painful? (b) Why may such abnormal painful sensation occur spontaneously in the absence of any stimulation, or inappropriately in response to non-noxious stimulation?

A logical approach to these questions about pain as a symptom of neuropathy is to study them in the light of what we know about pain as a normal somatosensory submodality. But is it legitimate to export, to neuropathic pain, knowledge about pain as a normal response to natural stimulation with adequate noxious stimuli? That generalization would be legitimate if neuropathic pain were expressed through the same system as normal pain, rather than being a new submodality emerging from disturbed sensory

[1]Allodynia is defined as pain due to a non-noxious stimulus.

mechanisms. Let us adopt the working hypothesis that these two kinds of pain are expressions of a single subjective submodality. Let us then divide the task of analyzing neuropathic pain into three themes:

1. What is known in man about the subjective attributes of the submodality pain as an adequate response to natural stimulation with noxious stimuli?
2. Why and when is there pain as an inadequate response in neuropathy?
3. What is the role of the sympathetic system in neuropathic pain?

DETERMINANTS OF THE SUBJECTIVE SUBMODALITY (PAIN) AS A PHYSIOLOGICAL RESPONSE TO STIMULATION OF PRIMARY SENSORY UNITS

Stated in the simplest terms, if one applies, via receptors, a stimulus that causes pain, special nociceptor units become activated. However, by the time those nociceptors reach the threshold for discharge, other sensory units (mechanoreceptors or thermoreceptors) have already been activated by the noxious stimulus, as reviewed elsewhere (64) (see chapter by E. R. Perl, *this volume*). Thus, normal pain naturally occurs in the context of coactivation of different kinds of primary sensory units. Therefore, it may be asked whether the prerequisite for pain to occur is (a) central interactions of the complex coactivated input, (b) a special coded pattern of discharge initiated in no matter what kind of sensory unit (59), or (c) sufficient activation of nociceptor units regardless of (a) coactivation of other unit types or (b) pattern of discharge.

To test these alternatives it is necessary to perform experiments, in awake human subjects, in which coactivation can be controlled and in which the pattern of discharge can be manipulated in identified kinds of sensory units. These goals are achieved through an experimental strategy that combines *microneurography* (18,70,71) with *intraneural microstimulation* (23,50,57,66,69). Indeed, by allowing either selective activation of primary sensory units or coactivation of various kinds of them, the combined strategy reveals that qualitatively pure subjective somatosensory submodalities can be evoked in the absence of coactivation. Pain is no exception (49,50,57,66). By allowing either monotonous or patterned activation of primary sensory units, the combined strategy reveals that the quality of a somatic sensation is not dependent on any pattern of discharge. Again, pain is no exception (51,66). By allowing selective activation of primary sensory units that can be identified by receptor location and can be classified by electrophysiological characteristics of the receptor response, the combined strategy reveals that the quality of a somatic sensation is associated with the kind of sensory unit transmitting the afferent messages (50,66,69). Pain is no exception; pain occurs in humans when either A or C nociceptor units are activated (49,66). Further, pain can normally be decomposed into varieties: (a) a sharp pain, with a fast reaction time, from skin that is evoked by activation of Aδ nociceptors, (b) a dull pain, with a slow reaction time, that is evoked by activation of skin C nociceptors, and (c) a cramp-like muscle pain whose neural apparatus remains unknown in humans and that may characteristically be referred to remote regions in the body (49,66,68).

In conclusion, what normally determines that a sensation evoked by excitation of primary sensory units be qualitatively distinct is not in the pattern of the afferent message, it is in the destination of the "messenger"; for pain, specific nociceptor pathways must be activated by adequate noxious stimuli. Having accepted that, we are now bound to explain why in neuropathy there may be pain from natural stimulation with non-noxious stimuli (allodynia) or without any natural stimulus at all.

MECHANISMS AND CAUSES OF NEUROPATHIC PAIN

If one assumes that the normal sensation *pain* results from activation of nociceptor pathways by impulses initiated in their primary sensory units, when adequately excited via receptors, one becomes liable to take for granted pain as a symptom of neuropathy. Indeed, neuropathic pain may be assumed to reflect activation of those very same nociceptor pathways, but here the impulses would be initiated abnormally in primary nociceptor units now responding inadequately to non-noxious natural stimuli, or would be initiated abnormally in nonreceptor sites along nociceptor fibers, or would converge aberrantly to nociceptor pathways after adequate initiation in non-nociceptors.

This assumption may encounter resistance on the grounds of differences experienced in the subjective qualities of some neuropathic pains as compared with physiological pain. We believe some of the perverted subjective attributes of neuropathic pains can be explained on the same basis as those of paresthesias due to nerve impulse generation at nonreceptor sites (48,67). In brief, the distorted qualities would not reflect new submodalities emerging from new afferent patterns; they would simply reflect pure elementary sensations that are unfamiliar because they can be experienced only when particular kinds of afferent fibers are selectively recruited intraneurally. These elementary sensations are to be contrasted with the normal blended sensations that result from recruitment of multiple afferent pathways via natural coactivation of receptors (51,52). In addition, characteristic neuropathic *partial* blends, like burning pain, can be explained by abnormal selective coactivation of specific C warm units plus specific C nociceptor units, both of which utilize unmyelinated nerve fibers, possibly intermixed closely within nerve fascicles (46).

In the following we shall present scattered evidence that supports the assumption that neuropathic pain is due to inadequate activation of conventional, specific nociceptor pathways. We shall then discuss possible mechanisms of pathological activation of sensory fibers at nonreceptor sites, and finally we shall list painful primary disorders of the peripheral nervous system.

Neuropathic Pain Coded Via Specific Nociceptor Pathways

There exists a clear-cut example in which pain as a response to natural stimulation with non-noxious stimuli is associated with, and accepted as being due to, pathological activation of sensitized primary A or C nociceptor units. This aberration is exemplified by allodynia (primary hyperalgesia) following thermal skin injury (35,65). Although in a sense this case of sensitization of receptors represents an ultraperipheral form of neuropathy and is a valid example of pain from disease of the nociceptors themselves, it seems clear that allodynia from the more usual forms of polyneuropathy or mononeuropathy is not due to a similar mechanism (6,16,26,45). We shall come back to this later. The painful sign of Tinel, in cases like the neuroma discussed earlier, emerges as an example of neuropathic pain due to initiation of afferent impulses in nonreceptor sites. Nevertheless, the nature of the pertinent "messenger" remains unknown, because in neuromas there is limited access to unit classification by receptor characteristics (52). The painful signs of Lasègue and Spurling, during straight leg raising or neck positioning in spinal root compression, also suggest initiation of afferent impulses at nonreceptor sites. Here, too, ectopically generated nerve impulses have been recorded in man as the electrical correlate, but again the nature of the generator units remains unknown (44).

Reproduction of clinical neuropathic pain by experimental activation of nociceptor fibers should constitute valid evidence toward the idea that the symptom utilizes the specific physiological apparatus for expression. But practical difficulties can be anticipated in certifying the degree of selectivity in experimental fiber nociceptor activation, particularly when subpopulations of receptors are denervated or reinnervated, thus blurring classification by receptor characteristics. Nevertheless, symptomatic pain from neuropathy has been reproduced by intraneural microstimulation in patients. For example, in Dr. W. S., intraneural microstimulation of an ulnar nerve fascicle supplying hypothenar muscles reproduced faithfully his symptomatic cramp-like pain, projected to hypothenar muscles and also referred segmentally to precordial regions (P. Marchettini, J. Ochoa, and E. Torebjork, *unpublished data*). This is a striking parallel to the observation that also in normal subjects, pain evoked by intraneural stimulation of nerve fascicles supplying striated muscle has a cramp-like quality and is projected to the appropriate muscle and often, in addition, is referred segmentally to remote locations (49,66,68). Thus, both the symptomatic pain and the experimentally reproduced pain in the patient were identical to the pain produced by similar means in normal subjects.

These examples support the idea that pain from disease of nerves may be due to abnormal activation of ultimately physiological nociceptor pathways. However, the concept seems challenged by the fact that in allodynia, as a symptom of neurological disease, pain can be evoked by non-noxious natural stimuli. Such allodynia could be construed as pain from activation of non-nociceptors in a critical pattern so as to create that sensation, but the conflict is only apparent and will be reconciled with our running hypothesis later. Be that as it may, definitive evidence is yet to come for the claim that pain from disease of nerves (rather than disease of sensory endings) is due to activation of nociceptor fibers along the pathway. The awaited evidence should include documentation of impulse activity initiated at nonreceptor sites in identified nociceptor units from patients experiencing neuropathic pain.

Abnormal Activation of Sensory Pathways at Nonreceptor Sites

Several mechanisms, established or presumed, might abnormally activate a neural pathway.

Ectopic Impulse Generation

The experimental evidence for ectopic activation of nerve fibers at nonreceptor sites is vast and vintage and will not be reviewed here again (8). Significant news relevant to pain, contributed in the 1980s, includes the following:

1. The demonstration that ectopic impulse generation from sensory units can be documented via microneurography in man and that the subjective correlates of such ectopic activity are paresthetic sensations (44,48,51,52,67).
2. The demonstration by Blumberg and Jänig (4) that C afferent fibers in damaged animal nerves are indeed capable of engaging in spontaneous and mechanosensitive ectopic discharges, and probably in ephaptic cross-talk. This is particularly significant in the context of pain symptomatic of neuropathy and might become documented in human neuropathy in the future.
3. A rationalization of possible biophysical derangements leading to spontaneous ectopic impulse generation from nerve fibers (7,13).

Ephapses

Electrical cross-talk was shown as a short-term animal phenomenon in mechanically injured nerves by Granit et al. (17). They proposed that the aberration could explain some forms of neuropathic pain in humans, but the concept somehow became discredited, and then Wall and Devor (75) were unable to confirm ephapses in long-term injured nerves. But Seltzer and Devor (58) did, and Rasminsky (53,54) already had, and most elegantly, in an animal model of nontraumatic disease of nerve fibers in sensory roots. Thus, the ephapse is rehabilitated. Moreover, it has recently been detected unambiguously in human sick nerves displaying obvious clinical manifestations of inadequate activation of nerve fibers within nerve trunks. However, this example, hemifacial spasm, involves motor nerve fibers, and its clever documentation was possible only by using double electromyography (40,41,42). Comparable documentation of ephapses in human sensory nerves, via double microneurography, seems only remotely possible. Nevertheless, in the context of neuropathic pain, an ephaptic mechanism could well explain some forms of stimulus-induced allodynia and some forms of sympathetic-dependent pain.

Central Transfer

But neither ectopic generation of impulses from within primary nociceptor units nor electrical cross-talk from non-nociceptor to nociceptor pathways can explain certain forms of pain as a symptom of disease of the primary sensory unit. An explicit example is root avulsion, a disaster so often complicated by spontaneous pains (80). This condition implies abolition of all input from the damaged sensory units, because their centrally directed branch in the amputated nerve roots degenerates and cannot emerge as a generator. Proposed explanations for this kind of deafferentation pain imply spontaneous pathological activation of central nociceptor neurons, with development of denervation hypersensitivity or suppression of tonic inhibition, as reviewed elsewhere (45). A striking electrophysiological correlate in an experimental model of root avulsion consists of paroxysmal activity in CNS somatosensory centers and cortex (31,32). Such activity could not be readily documented in human patients, but it probably is one cause of spontaneous central pain and suggests that only therapies directed to the CNS will be of value.

Stimulus-induced allodynia may accompany spontaneous deafferentation pain. Here it must be central reorganization that allows the transfer of activation to central nociceptor neurons from primary afferent input of the wrong kind, even when initiated by natural stimuli given outside the deafferented territory. Thus, a follow-up explanation can be offered for allodynia from disease of the primary sensory unit that is not in conflict with the running hypothesis that neuropathic pain is ultimately expressed through physiological nociceptor systems. Campbell et al. (6) currently propose that *secondary* hyperalgesia (allodynia) following cutaneous thermal injury is due in part to central changes leading to excitation by low-threshold mechanoreceptor afferents of CNS neurons that subserve pain sensation. In this context, an irresistible parallel can be drawn with idiopathic hyperhidrosis. In this congenital disorder, a nonthermal mechanical stimulus inappropriately causes reflex sweating by exciting afferent impulses from dynamic low-threshold mechanoreceptors. The autonomic response is resolved mostly at the segmental level bilaterally. It selectively recruits sudomotor outflow. In the context of allodynia this emphasizes that connections between low-threshold mechanoreceptor afferents and other systems may preexist in a nonfunctional state in the spinal cord, to become unmasked in pathological states (33). Wall (74) has emphasized the same idea, but in relation to the establishment of new connectivity in the spinal cord following nerve injury.

The subject of allodynia will be pursued later in the context of sympathetic-dependent pain.

Primary Disorders of the Peripheral Nervous System Often Accompanied by Pain

Leaving aside patients with headaches, angina, arthritis, dysmenorrhea, etc., who suffer the straightforward consequences of ongoing or recurrent adequate activation of nociceptors, very many other patients suffer chronic pain in the absence of adequate stimuli. The vast majority of those have pain as a symptom of disease of the nervous system. Within this group, most have active disease of the primary sensory unit or its sequela; they have neuropathies or radiculopathies.

Mononeuropathies and radiculopathies are by far the commonest causes of neuropathic pain and are very highly prevalent causes of chronic pain. Because the subject of pain in local nerve lesions has been reviewed recently (45), only an updated summary will be given here. Chronic spontaneous pain as a sequel of acute nerve injury has been postulated to be due to (a) release of nociceptor activity due to predominant damage to large-diameter afferents [fiber dissociation theory (43), gate control theory (34,73)], (b) electrical (ephapses) or chemical nerve fiber cross-talk, (c) ectopic generation in primary nociceptors, or (d) secondary central changes.

Although direct demonstration is still lacking for any of these possibilities in man, the immature regenerating nerve sprouts from small-diameter afferents remain potential substrates for ectopic impulse generation and neuropathic pain (1,2,47,75,77). The idea of fiber dissociation is not consistent with revised morphometric studies (45,47) and is not consistent with neurophysiological evidence gathered by microneurography; there is normally no ongoing activity in human nociceptors to be disinhibited (63).

Distinct from chronic pain as a sequel of acute nerve injury, chronic nerve entrapment usually leads to a type of chronic pain that we believe to have a separate mechanism of production. These tend to be recurrent pains that are stimulus-induced rather than truly spontaneous. The stimulus is inadequate in that it does not act via receptors; it is direct mechanical trauma to the nerve trunk, with excitation of nociceptor fibers within the nerve fascicles causing the pain. The abnormal quality of the recurrent pain in entrapment has been interpreted as due to activation of an afferent fiber spectrum abnormally depopulated of large-caliber axons (45). How much of the pain that may eventually develop from local nerve entrapment is pain due to adequate activation of nociceptors by natural mechanical noxious stimuli acting locally on the nervi nervorum of the nerve sheath? This is difficult to evaluate retrospectively, but it is a pertinent consideration (1,62). An important differentiating feature should be the localization of the pain; the pain from sheath nociceptors should be projected locally to the site of mechanical injury on the nerve, whereas the pain from nerve fiber activation within the nerve trunk is projected to the innervation territory, or appropriately referred remotely (49,68). Nervi nervorum pain has been proposed for pain localized on infarcted, inflamed, or neoplastic nerve trunks in mononeuropathy (1,62). It is probably of relatively minor clinical significance.

Pain in radiculopathy may be regarded as a form of local nerve pain, although special ground rules seem to govern it, such as the liability for deafferentation change in root injury, and the low threshold of the dorsal root ganglion cells for ectopic impulse generation (22,76). Human nerve roots are relatively inaccessible to scientific study; their histopathology is practically unknown, but insights into their potential role as ectopic impulse generators are already available by means of antidromic microneurography (44; J. Ochoa, P. Marchettini, and M. Sivak, *unpublished data*). This is an area requiring much future investment of research effort.

Thomas's review of polyneuropathies (62) remains up to date and could only be done disservice by attempting to summarize it. The reader is encouraged to consult the original.

ROLE OF THE SYMPATHETIC SYSTEM IN NEUROPATHIC PAIN

Efferent and Not Self-Sufficient

Anyone who claims to understand how the sympathetic system influences pain is probably mistaken or has chosen to explain only some aspects of a complex issue. This is a fascinating, vague field. If Bonica, Noordenbos, Nathan, Sunderland, and Sweet have doubts, there is little hope for the rest of us. A role for the sympathetic system in triggering or perpetuating pain from nerve disease is unambiguous in its existence but not in its prevalence or its mechanism. Suppression of the sympathetic innervation to a limb by surgical sympathectomy (24,60), by local anesthetic sympathetic blocks (5,25,27), or by regional pharmacological block (19,20,29) might abolish neuropathic pain for various lengths of time. But, in terms of the pain, is the role of the sympathetic afferent or efferent? From World War II experience, Nathan (38) concluded that no somatic sensation is conveyed by the sympathetic. Then, in 1948, Walker and Nulsen (72) briefly reported that after upper thoracic sympathectomy, stimulation of the distal stump reproduced the pain in 3 patients with causalgia, but not in controls. Thus, after the 1940s, the centrifugal role of the sympathetic in relation to pain became generally accepted, with notable exceptions (43). More recently, the beneficial effects on neuropathic pain of regional pharmacological blocks, which suppress peripheral adrenergic neurotransmission, have clinched the efferent role.

From classic descriptions of clinical signs sometimes indicating regionally exaggerated autonomic cutaneous effector responses of patients with sympathetic-dependent pain, there is a tendency to assume that in this condition the neural sympathetic outflow to skin must be exaggerated and that an exaggerated outflow might be enough to cause the painful consequence. Neither is the case. Chronically exaggerated sympathetic activity of normal character in itself is not sufficient to produce pain. For example, patients with idiopathic hyperhidrosis, shown to be due to pathologically increased autonomic sudomotor (cholinergic) outflow to skin, do not complain of spontaneous pain (33). Clearly an associated neurological lesion involving sensory pathways, more commonly at the periphery, is required for the painful sympathetic-dependent syndrome to develop. Besides, if the neural lesion involves significant C fiber loss, the distal neurogenic deficit will feature signs of diminished sympathetic function, and nevertheless sympathetic-dependent pain might be present. This means that if the presumed sympathetic-to-afferent interaction occurs peripherally, that is, distal to the level of nerve injury and axonal dropout, the interaction may be effective even at low levels of neural sympathetic output. On the other hand, if the sympathetic outflow is not diminished by axonal loss, sympathetic effector signs may indeed be regionally exaggerated in neuropathy. The mechanism of this hyperactivity is far from elucidated, and one cannot exclude theoretical possibilities such as (a) ectopic impulse generation within sympathetic efferents, (b) an abnormal neural cross-talk in reverse, in which sympathetic efferents are the receiving pathway, or (c) abnormal spinal reflex sympathetic drive. Denervation hypersensitivity can be ruled out in those instances in which the hyperactivity is abolished by blocking or ablating sympathetic neural outflow or neurotransmission (rather than by blocking receptors in the effector organs). However, we have observed signs of exaggerated autonomic effector response (i.e., regional vasoconstriction matching sensory loss) in areas shown to be denervated. Obviously this situation is sympathetic-dependent but should not be sympathectomy-dependent. From the foregoing it can be concluded that regional sympathetic neural outflow need not be exaggerated in patients with sympathetic-dependent pain and that when ostensibly exaggerated it is not necessarily the cause of pain; it might be just another positive phenomenon consequent to the neural lesion.

Predicting Sympathetic-Dependent Muscle Pain

Thus far, the measure of sympathetic function in the painful region has taken into account cutaneous effects. It has been largely ignored that the sympathetic outflow, at least to human limbs, is differentially compartmentalized in muscle versus skin fascicles (78) and that muscle nerve fascicles do contain afferents that evoke pain (49,66,68) and that muscle nerve fascicles may be selectively injured in patients. If the key ingredients for sympathetic dependent pain are a sympathetic outflow (of nerve impulses and/or neurotransmitters) and a damaged afferent system accessible to such outflow, then the required formula is intrinsically available in the human innervation of muscle. *We propose that sympathetic-dependent muscle pain must exist but is not recognized because of our clinical bias toward cutaneous dysautonomic manifestations and because of the deep cramplike, rather than superficial burning, quality of the anticipated pain.*

Level and Nature of Sympathetic Action in Determining Pain

Since it became accepted that the role of the sympathetic in neuropathic pain is centrifugal, it has been more or less implicit that the abnormality involves an interaction with nociceptor fibers within peripheral nerves. Initially, Doupe et al. (14) proposed electrical ephapses between nerve fibers of the two systems at the site of neural injury, and Nathan (38) supported the idea. This explanation seemed satisfactory until Hannington-Kiff (19) showed that neuropathic pain can be abolished by pharmacological depletion of neurotransmitter in adrenergic sympathetic endings. Thus, the abnormal interaction would not be electrical but chemical, a view strongly supported by animal experiments started by Wall and Gutnick (77) and continued by Scadding (55,56) and Devor and associates (11) showing ectopic alpha-adrenergic chemosensitivity in neuromas. Further, because these regional guanethidine blocks remain effective even when the site of injury of the nervous system is situated proximal to the ischemic cuff, the presumed site of abnormal interaction must be shifted distally (29,39) and possibly as far as the nerve terminals themselves, because iontophoretic application of norepinephrine to previously symptomatic skin, in 4 successfully sympathectomized patients, transiently resuscitated spontaneous pain (79). Loh and Nathan (29), seemingly unaware at the time of the experimental results and conclusions of Wallin et al. (79), proposed that the afferent limbs in these abnormal loops were large-diameter fibers from low-threshold tactile mechanoreceptors. Such presumed input would be responsible for both the spontaneous pain and the hyperalgesia through hypothetical central disinhibition caused by "constant firing." Wallin et al. (79) had not imposed a common afferent limb to explain both the resuscitated pain and the hyperalgesia (allodynia). They had confined their interpretation to the hyperalgesia and tentatively incriminated myelinated nociceptors with small-diameter Aδ fibers as the afferent carriers.

Devor and associates (11) have strengthened the chemical theory for sympathetic-dependent pain with the weight of their animal experiments, but they have rescued the presumed site of sympathetic-somatic interaction back to the level of the nerve injury, which is not surprising, because their material was amputation neuromas. Devor (11) does not reconsider the argument that necessarily had shifted, to begin with, the presumed site of interaction in human sympathetic-dependent pain to the periphery. Devor discusses the human experiments of Wallin et al. (79) in the context of hyperalgesia and accepts for it a chemical interaction at skin level between sympathetic and nociceptor afferents, but he does not discuss the observation that spontaneous pain was as well resuscitated as was the hyperalgesia by application of norepinephrine to the skin, which also implies a peripheral interaction for the spontaneous pain. Recently, coupling of action-potential activity between unmyelinated fibers in skin of normal monkeys has been discovered, and its potential significance in pathological sympathetic-nociceptor interaction has been stressed (36).

In the context of sympathetic-dependent pain, the idea of postganglionic sympathetic effect is often narrowly locked to the idea of adrenergic effect, for which, as stated earlier, there is experimental support. Nevertheless, it should be kept in mind that there is a cholinergic component in the (sudomotor) sympathetic postganglionic outflow and that although the recent literature focuses mostly on ectopic alpha-adrenergic chemosensitivity, it was shown in the 1950s that regenerating nerves discharge ectopically in the presence of acetylcholine (12). Of course, in the hypothetical case of selective ectopic cholinergic chemosensitivity, blocking the neural sympathetic outflow with local anesthetics would be expected to suppress the pain, whereas the use of guanethidine or reserpine probably would not.

From the foregoing it can be accepted that the sympathetic system may excite afferent fibers that have become abnormally receptive to sympathetic events at the periphery. One may point out that for the abnormal interaction, which need not be electrical, but chemical, the transmitters need not necessarily be locally neurosecreted; they might be circulating. Therapeutic manipulations such as (a) blockade of transmitter binding at ectopic receptors, (b) selective pharmacological abolition of neurosecretion, or (c) suppression of sympathetic nerve impulses that trigger neurosecretion should abolish the abnormal interaction. However, as will be discussed later, these maneuvers are largely directed to the periphery, and if similar abnormal interactions occurred centrally, a therapeutic failure would not deny sympathetic dependence of the pain.

Associated Hyperalgesia (Allodynia)

The hyperalgesia (allodynia) that may associate with sympathetic-dependent pain is the most puzzling issue in this area, particularly because it is reported as being in itself sympathetic-dependent (29,79). Wallin et al. (79) and Devor (11) have seen it as part and parcel of the ectopic alpha-adrenergic chemosensitivity phenomenon. One can envisage how nociceptor endings could become sensitized, as they would incorporate an additional depolarizing conductance and would fire with lowered threshold to natural mechanical stimuli. But it is hard to explain why these excitability changes should take place remotely peripheral to the site of neural damage and with a time course sometimes incompatible with the regrowth of chemosensitive sprouts from the injury down to sensory endings. Unless it is postulated that the receptors of intact distal nociceptor units have developed adrenergic chemosensitivity (which seems far-fetched but can be tested in humans), the explanation for sympathetic-dependent hyperalgesia must find a secondary abnormality in distal nociceptor fibers that escaped the primary injury. Otherwise, observation or theory is wrong, and the afferent limbs for the hyperalgesia are intact low-threshold mechanoreceptors, with large myelinated fibers, responding adequately to non-noxious stimuli but transferring proximally to nociceptor pathways—which leaves the sympathetic dependence unexplained. Of course, secondary abnormalities do occur in originally intact fibers distal to nerve injury. Collateral sprouting is one possible change, but even if such sprouts might be abnormally excitable, what we need to explain is the change in excitability of receptors rather than nerve fibers. Another possible change is the secondary demyelination and axonal atrophy well described in surviving fibers distal to a constriction. But, again, could these changes result in alpha-adrenergic-determined receptor sensitization?

The fact that the hyperalgesia (allodynia) associated with sympathetic-dependent pain may be related not to mechanical but to thermal stimuli calls for further elaboration of these ideas. The Aδ nociceptor endings, brought into this context by Wallin et al. (79), may have become sensitized not to their adequate mechanical stimulus (as a consequence of the development of alpha-adrenergic chemosensitivity that would lower the receptor threshold), but rather may have become polysensitive (polymodal). Alternatively, the afferent limbs for thermal allodynia are intact specific thermoreceptor units responding adequately to non-noxious stimuli but transferring proximally to nociceptor pathways. Again, sympathetic dependence remains unexplained.

An unusually well documented clinical case of sympathetic-dependent pain and mechanical allodynia is most relevant to this discussion. Hoffert et al. (21) have documented clearly separate mechanisms for the spontaneous pain that was sympathetic-dependent and for the allodynia that was decidedly not relieved by sympathectomy.

The Burning Quality of Some Neuropathic Pains

Such quality was emphasized by S. W. Mitchell (37) in his description of causalgia (burning pain) following peripheral nerve trauma, but of course it is not exclusive for traumatic mononeuropathies. Burning pain may develop in radiculopathies, in polyneuropathies, and in diseases of the CNS. Burning pain is sometimes assumed to be necessarily associated with sympathetic dependence, which need not be so. Conversely, sympathetic-dependent pain need not be burning in quality.

In normal individuals, intraneural microstimulation (INMS) will elicit burning dull pain when the stimuli are given in fascicles to skin, provided the intraneural probe is obviously close to C unmyelinated fibers and the stimulus intensity is high enough to coactivate many fibers. Such burning quality is interpreted as reflecting coactivation of specific warm C fibers together with specific C nociceptors. The burning quality of the blended pain induced by INMS is present mostly when fascicles to hairy skin rather than to glabrous skin are stimulated. Burning is not a component of pain induced by INMS from nerve fascicles supplying striated muscle. This is probably a function of the relative contents of specific warm afferents in the different kinds of fascicles. Spontaneous neuropathic burning pain presumably reflects abnormal coactivation of specific warm plus specific nociceptor pathways at nonreceptor sites. If the sympathetic were involved in triggering at nerve trunk level the events leading to the painful burning sensations, an obvious level for interaction would be nerve fascicles destined to skin where all three kinds of C fibers coexist, probably in close spatial proximity (46; E. Torebjörk and J. Ochoa, *unpublished observations*).

CNS Events in Sympathetic Dependent Pain

Thus far we have simple-mindedly managed to more or less rationalize sympathetic-dependent pain (and the associated allodynia) by just inserting ectopic chemosensitivity in nociceptor afferents affected by primary or secondary nerve fiber abnormalities. In this way, a normal, or even a diminished, neural outflow might innocently trigger the painful response. But there are clinical and experimental observations that justify the proposal that the sympathetic system exerts an active pathogenetic role in sympathetic-dependent syndromes. Inappropriate sympathetic outflow has been thought to be capable of damaging tissues, to cause "dystrophy," as assiduously discussed in the context of Sudeck's atrophy and "reflex sympathetic dystrophy," conditions in which tissues undergo trophic decay that may recover following suppression of sympathetic function (10,15,20,28,61). One of the multiple enigmas that plague this subject is the nature of whatever triggers the abnormal autonomic response. Such response may occur in the absence of detectable damage to the nerves supplying the dystrophic territory and therefore is unlikely to reflect primary dysfunction of autonomic efferent nerve fibers, and for that reason it is thought to be determined via a spinal reflex. The afferent limb primarily responsible for such a lethal reflex would be somatic sensory fibers, and the precipitating stimulus might be a trivial phlebitis or a small fracture, only mildly painful, and not necessarily an injury to the nervous system. An experimental animal model has been produced recently by Blumberg and Jänig (3) in which, secondary to primary afferent damage, the sympathetic reflex outflow becomes qualitatively abnormal. However, dystrophic effects have not been reproduced. But fascinating abnormal sympathetic reflexes triggered by somatic afferents may occur naturally in man. In hyperhidrosis, for example, as described earlier, gently stroking the skin of one hand to excite rapidly adapting low-threshold mechanoreceptors elicits reflex sweating on both sides, with a corresponding increase in the neural sudomotor outflow shown by microneurography (33). In this constitutional anomaly of connectivity in the spinal cord, dormant somatic-sympathetic hookups are thought to be disinhibited, and in our group the idea keeps coming up that a comparable appropriate anomaly might predispose to reflex sympathetic dystrophy. Thus, a vicarious reflex recruitment of the autonomic nervous system in response to normal or abnormal afferent input, as well as dystrophic consequences, at tissue level, of the inappropriate output, seem established phenomena. However, the connection between those events and pain remains loose for those cases in which the precipitating afferent event does not appear to involve pain afferents, and we should reopen our minds to the possibility that abnormal sympathetic outflow, triggered from somatic afferents, may damage the nociceptors and render them abnormally receptive to sympathetic events: the vicious circle of Livingston (28).

The fact that primary lesions of the CNS may be complicated by pain and sympathetic dystrophy underlines the concept that the pathological process can fully develop starting from the efferent limb; that is, a primary disorder of sensory nerve fibers is not *sine qua non.* Surprisingly, the predjudice that, in these cases, therapeutic manipulations directed to the periphery must fail is wrong. Perhaps in the patients of Loh et al. (30) and Hannington-Kiff (20), treated by sympathetic block or guanethidine block, the therapeutic success was due to breaking the vicious circle whereby the abnormal sympathetic outflow secondarily damaged and excited nociceptors. But it is also possible that in these painful CNS syndromes associated with peripheral changes of sympathetic dystrophy, the pain and the sympathetic phenomena might not be linked at the periphery but centrally, or they might be unlinked, totally independent expressions of central dysfunctions of two systems. Either case might explain failure of therapies directed to the periphery. As to the possible central linkage between pain and sympathetic dysfunction, we identify no rational constraint against the thought that damaged afferents could well develop abnormal receptiveness to sympathetic events, within the CNS, as shown for the periphery.

Thermography in the Study of Neuropathic Pain

We are currently convinced that despite a potential for misuse of thermography as a lucrative noninvasive diagnostic procedure, the technique has a perfectly well defined useful application in the workup of patients with sensory disorders of primary neurological origin. Often the cutaneous territory affected by sensory symptoms exhibits matching abnormality of skin temperature indicative of sympathetic vasomotor imbalance. These changes are important to detect because they may constitute the only objective document of neurological dysfunction. This is certainly the case in patients with pure sensory manifestations, because there are no truly objective clinical signs for the negative symptom (sensory loss) or the positive symptoms (pain and paresthesias). Although electrophysiological testing will detect nerve conduction deficit if the disorder involves hypoactivity in large-diameter afferent pathways, the function of small-diameter fibers escapes routine electrophysiology. Moreover, no routine test reliably documents the overactivity that obviously underlies positive sensory phenomena such as paresthesias and pains.

In addition to its application in the study of autonomic disorders evolving in parallel with sensory disorders of peripheral nervous system origin, thermography can be useful in revealing abnormalities in patients with primary disorders of the CNS associated with pain, such as reflex sympathetic dystrophy following stroke, syringomyelia, CNS tumors, etc.

In summary:

1. It is very clear from the results of animal experimentation that an abnormal chemical interaction can occur at nerve trunk level between alpha-

adrenergic agonists (neurosecreted locally or circulating) and damaged nerve fibers.

2. It is fairly clear from human observations that sympathetic-dependent pain may involve an adrenergic-to-afferent interaction that may take place in tissues peripheral to the site of neurological damage. Similar interactions can be envisaged within the CNS.
3. The indirect evidence incriminating a particular type of afferents in conveying the sympathetic-dependent "painful" signals to the CNS is conflicting.
4. The burning quality (and also the cold quality) is common but not exclusive for sympathetic painful syndromes. It can be explained by coactivation of afferents subserving temperature and pain.
5. The association of sympathetic-dependent pain and hyperalgesia is common but not obligatory. This hyperalgesia is not necessarily sympathectomy-dependent itself. The mechanisms responsible are the obscurest.
6. Hyperalgesia associated with sympathetic-dependent pain need not be related exclusively to mechanical stimuli. It may relate selectively to thermal stimuli (warm or cold allodynia) (16).
7. A role for abnormal transfer of electrical nerve signals from non-nociceptor to nociceptor pathways, rather than sensitization of receptors, cannot be ruled out in these hyperalgesias associated with sympathetic-dependent pain.
8. Certain clinical and neurophysiological observations indicate that in sympathetic-dependent pain and dystrophy, the inappropriate autonomic outflow might be regarded as (a) reflexly recruited and (b) actively responsible for tissue damage, inclusive of sensory units.

ACKNOWLEDGMENTS

This work was supported in part by the National Institutes of Health, the Muscular Dystrophy Association of America and the Medical Research Council of Sweden.

REFERENCES

1. Asbury, A. K., and Fields, H. L. (1984): Pain due to peripheral nerve damage: A hypothesis. *Neurology (Minneap.),* 34:1587–1590.
2. Blumberg, H., and Jänig, W. (1981): Neurophysiological analysis of efferent sympathetic and afferent fibers in skin nerves with experimental produced neuromata. In: *Phantom and Stump Pain,* edited by J. Siegfried and M. Zimmerman, pp. 15–31. Springer-Verlag, Berlin.
3. Blumberg, H., and Jänig, W. (1983): Changes of reflexes in vasoconstrictor neurons supplying the cat hindlimb following chronic nerve lesions: A model for studying mechanisms of reflex sympathetic dystrophy? *J. Auton. Nerv. Syst.,* 7:399–411.
4. Blumberg, H., and Jänig, W. (1984): Discharge patterns of afferent fibers from a neuroma. *Pain,* 20(4):335–353.

5. Bonica, J. J. (1979): Causalgia and other reflex sympathetic dystrophies. In: *Advances in Pain Research and Therapy,* Vol. 3, edited by J. J. Bonica, J. C. Liebeskind, and D. G. Albe-Fessard, pp. 141–166. Raven Press, New York.
6. Campbell, J. N., Meyer, R. A., and Raja, S. N. (1984): Hyperalgesia: New insights. *Pain* [*Suppl.*], 2:S3.
7. Culp, W. J. (1983): Abnormal impulse generation. In: *Neuromuscular Diseases,* edited by G. Serratrice, D. Cros, C. Desnuelle, J. L. Gastaut, J. F. Pelissier, J. Pouget, and A. Schiano, pp. 303–308. Raven Press, New York.
8. Culp, W. J., and Ochoa, J. (1982): *Abnormal Nerves and Muscles as Impulse Generators.* Oxford University Press, New York.
9. Culp, W. J., Ochoa, J., Torebjörk, E. K. (1983): Positive phenomena from dysfunction of the human sensory unit. In: *Clinical and Biological Aspects of the Peripheral Nervous System Diseases,* edited by L. Battistin, G. Hashin, and A. Lajtha, pp. 335–347. Alan Liss, New York.
10. de Takats, G. (1937): Reflex dystrophy of the extremities. *Arch. Surg.,* 34:939–956.
11. Devor, M. (1983): Nerve pathophysiology and mechanisms of pain in causalgia. *J. Auton. Nerv. Syst.,* 7:371–384.
12. Diamond, J. (1959): The effect of injecting acetylcholine into normal and regenerating nerves. *J. Physiol. (Lond.),* 145:611–629.
13. Diamond, J., Ochoa, J., and Culp, W. J. (1982): An introduction to abnormal nerves and muscles as impulse generators. In: *Abnormal Nerves and Muscles as Impulse Generators,* edited by W. J. Culp and J. Ochoa, pp. 3–24. Oxford University Press, New York.
14. Doupe J., Cullen, C. H., and Chance, G. Q. (1944): Post traumatic pain and causalgic syndrome. *J. Neurol. Neurosurg. Psychiatry,* 7:33–48.
15. Evans, J. A. (1946): Sympathectomy for reflex sympathetic dystrophy. *J.A.M.A.,* 16:620–623.
16. Fruhstorfer, H., and Lindblom, U. (1984): Sensibility abnormalities in neuralgic patients studied by thermal and tactile pulse stimulation. In: *Somatosensory Mechanisms,* edited by K. von Euler, O. Franzén, U. Lindblom, and D. Ottoson, pp. 353–361. Macmillan, London.
17. Granit, R., Leksell, L., and Skoglund, C. R. (1944): Fiber interaction in injured or compressed region of nerve. *Brain,* 67:125–140.
18. Hagbarth, K. E., and Vallbo, A. B. (1967): Afferent response to mechanical stimulation of muscle receptors in man. *Acta Soc. Med. Upsal.,* 72:102–104.
19. Hannington-Kiff, J. G. (1974): Intravenous regional sympathetic block with guanethidine. *Lancet,* 1:1019–1020.
20. Hannington-Kiff, J. G. (1982): Hyperadrenergic-effected limb causalgia: Relief by pharmacologic norepinephrine blockade. *Am. Heart J.,* 103:152–153.
21. Hoffert, M. J., Greenburg, R. P., Wolskee, P. J., Gracely, R. H., Wirdzek, P. R., Vinayakon, K., and Dubner, R. (1984): Abnormal and collateral innervations of sympathetic and peripheral sensory fields associated with a case of causalgia. *Pain,* 20:1–12.
22. Howe, J. F., Loeser, J. D., and Calvin, W. H. (1977): Mechanosensitivity of dorsal root ganglia and chronically injured axons: A physiological basis for the radicular pain of nerve root compression. *Pain,* 3:25–41.
23. Konietzny, F., Perl, E. R., Trevino, D., Light, A., and Hensel, H. (1981): Sensory experiences in man evoked by intraneural electrical stimulation of intact cutaneous afferent fibers. *Exp. Brain Res.,* 42:219–222.
24. Leriche, R. (1916): De la causalgie envisagée comme une nevrite du sympathique et son traitement par la denudation et l'excision des plexus nerveux peri-arteriels. *Presse Med.,* 24:178–180.
25. Leriche, R., and Fontaine, R. (1934): L'anésthèsie isolée du ganglion étoile. *Presse Med.,* 41:849–850.
26. Lindblom, U., and Verrillo, R. T. (1979): Sensory functions in chronic neuralgia. *J. Neurol. Neurosurg. Psychiatry,* 42:422–435.
27. Livingston, K. (1938): Fantom limb pain; report of 10 cases in which it was treated by injections of procaine hydrochloride near thoracic sympathetic ganglions. *Arch. Surg.,* 37:353–370.

28. Livingston, W. K. (1948): The vicious circle in causalgia. *Ann. N.Y. Acad. Sci.*, 50:247–258.
29. Loh, L., and Nathan, P. W. (1978): Painful peripheral states and sympathetic blocks. *J. Neurol. Neurosurg. Psychiatry,* 41:664–671.
30. Loh, L., Nathan, P. W., and Schott, G. D. (1981): Pain due to the lesions of central nervous system removed by sympathetic block. *Br. Med. J.,* 282:1026–1028.
31. Lombard, M. C., Jarlet, M. A., and Daheb, S. (1984): Correlation between deafferentation, self mutilation, neuronal rhythmical activity and sleep disturbance in the rat. *Pain* [*Suppl.*], 2:S445.
32. Lombard, M. C., Lariah, Y., and Albe-Fessard, D. (1981): Electrophysiological study of cervical dorsal horn cells in partially deafferented rats. *Pain* [*Suppl.*], 1:S129.
33. Marchettini, P., Torebjörk, H. E., Culp, W., and Ochoa, J. (1983): Pathological disinhibition of somatosensory-sympathetic reflex in individuals with idiopathic hyperhidrosis. *Abstracts Society Neuroscience 13th Annual Meeting,* Boston, 265(1):903.
34. Melzack, R., and Wall, P. D. (1965): Pain mechanisms: A new theory. *Science,* 150:971–979.
35. Meyer, R. A., and Campbell, J. N. (1981): Myelinated nociceptive afferents account for the hyperalgesia that follows a burn to the hand. *Science,* 213:1527–1529.
36. Meyer, R. A., Campbell, J. N., and Raja, S. N. (1984): Coupling of action potential activity between unmyelinated fibers in the normal peripheral nerve of monkey. *Pain* [*Suppl.*], 2:S8.
37. Mitchell, S. W. (1872): *Injuries of Nerves and Their Consequences.* J. B. Lippincott, Philadelphia.
38. Nathan, P. W. (1947): On pathogenesis of causalgia in peripheral nerve injuries. *Brain,* 70:145–170.
39. Nathan, P. W. (1983): Pain and the sympathetic system. *J. Auton. Nerv. Syst.,* 7:363–370.
40. Nielsen, V. K. (1984): Pathophysiology of hemifacial spasm: I. Ephaptic transmission and ectopic excitations. *Neurology (Minneap.),* 34:418–426.
41. Nielsen, V. K. (1984): Pathophysiology of hemifacial spasm: II. Lateral spread of the supraorbital nerve reflex. *Neurology (Minneap.),* 34:427–431.
42. Nielsen, V. K., and Jannetta, P. J. (1984): Pathophysiology of hemifacial spasm: III. Effects of facial nerve decompression. *Neurology (Minneap.),* 34:891–897.
43. Noordenbos, W. (1959): *Pain.* Elsevier, Amsterdam.
44. Nordin, M., Nyström, B., Wallin, U., and Hagbarth, K. E. (1984): Ectopic sensory discharges and paresthesiae in patients with disorders of peripheral nerves, dorsal roots and dorsal columns. *Pain,* 20:231–245.
45. Ochoa, J. (1982): Pain in local nerve lesions. In: *Abnormal Nerves and Muscles as Impulse Generators,* edited by W. J. Culp and J. Ochoa, pp. 568–587. Oxford University Press, New York.
46. Ochoa, J. (1984): Peripheral unmyelinated units in man: Structure, function, disorder and role in sensation. In: *Advances in Pain Research and Therapy,* Vol. 6, *Neural Mechanisms of Pain,* edited by L. Kruger and J. C. Liebeskind, pp. 53–68. Raven Press, New York.
47. Ochoa, J., and Noordenbos, W. (1979): Pathology and disordered sensation in local nerve lesions: An attempt at correlation. In: *Advances in Pain Research and Therapy,* Vol. 3, edited by J. J. Bonica, J. C. Liebeskind, and D. G. Albe-Fessard, pp. 67–90. Raven Press, New York.
48. Ochoa, J., and Torebjörk, H. E. (1980): Paraesthesiae from ectopic impulse generation in human sensory nerves. *Brain,* 103:835–853.
49. Ochoa, J. L., and Torebjörk, E. K. (1981): Pain from skin and muscle. *Pain* [*Suppl.*], 1:S87.
50. Ochoa, J. L., and Torebjörk, H. E. (1983): Sensations evoked by intraneural microstimulation of single mechanoreceptor units innervating the human hand. *J. Physiol. (Lond.),* 342:633–654.
51. Ochoa, J., Torebjörk, E., and Culp, W. (1984): Determinants of subjective attributes of normal cutaneous sensation and of paraesthesiae from ectopic nerve impulse generation. In: *Somatosensory Mechanisms,* edited by K. von Euler, O. Franzén, U. Lindblom, and D. Ottoson, pp. 377–387. Macmillan, London.
52. Ochoa, J. L., Torebjörk, H. E., Culp, W. J., and Schady, W. (1982): Abnormal spontaneous activity in single nerve fibers in humans. *Muscle and Nerve,* 5:S74–S77.

53. Rasminsky, M. (1978): Ectopic generation of impulses and cross talk in spinal nerve roots of "dystrophic" mice. *Ann. Neurol.,* 3:351–357.
54. Rasminsky, M. (1982): Ectopic excitation, ephaptic excitation and autoexcitation in peripheral nerve fibers of mutant mice. In: *Abnormal Nerves and Muscles as Impulse Generators,* edited by W. J. Culp and J. L. Ochoa, pp. 344–362. Oxford University Press, New York.
55. Scadding, J. W. (1981): Development of ongoing activity, mechanosensitivity and adrenaline sensitivity in severed peripheral nerve axons. *Exp. Neurol.,* 73:345–364.
56. Scadding, J. W. (1982): Ectopic impulse generation in experimental neuromas: Behavioral, physiological and anatomical correlates. In: *Abnormal Nerves and Muscles as Impulse Generators,* edited by W. J. Culp and J. Ochoa, pp. 533–552. Oxford University Press, New York.
57. Schady, W. J. L., Torebjörk, H. E., and Ochoa, J. L. (1983): Cerebral localization function from the input of single mechanoreceptive units in man. *Acta Physiol. Scand.,* 119:277–285.
58. Seltzer, Z., and Devor, M. (1979): Ephaptic transmission in chronically damaged peripheral nerves. *Neurology (Minneap.),* 29:1061–1064.
59. Sinclair, D. C. (1955): Cutaneous sensation and the doctrine of specific energy. *Brain,* 78:584–614.
60. Spurling, R. G. (1930): Causalgia of upper extremity; treatment by dorsal sympathetic ganglionectomy. *Arch. Neur. Psychiatry,* 23:784–788.
61. Sudeck, P. (1931): Die trophische Extremitatenstorung durch periphere (infektiose und traumatische) Reize. *Deutsche Ztschr. Chir.,* 234:596–612.
62. Thomas, P. K. (1982): Pain in peripheral neuropathy: Clinical and morphological aspects. In: *Abnormal Nerves and Muscles as Impulse Generators,* edited by W. J. Culp and J. Ochoa, pp. 553–562. Oxford University Press, New York.
63. Torebjörk, H. E. (1974): *Single Unit Activity in Afferent and Sympathetic C Fibres Recorded from Intact Human Skin Nerves.* Ph.D. Thesis. Acta Universitatis Upsaliensis Almqvist & Wiksell, Stockholm.
64. Torebjörk, H. E. (1985): Nociceptor activation and pain. *Philos. Trans. R. Soc. Lond. [Biol.],* 308:227–234.
65. Torebjörk, H. E., LaMotte, R. H., and Robinson, C. J. (1984): Peripheral neural correlates of magnitude of cutaneous pain and hyperalgesia: Simultaneous recordings in humans of sensory judgments of pain and evoked responses in nociceptors with C-fibers. *J. Neurophysiol.,* 51:325–339.
66. Torebjörk, H. E., and Ochoa, J. L. (1980): Specific sensations evoked by activity in single identified sensory units in man. *Acta Physiol. Scand.,* 110:445–447.
67. Torebjörk, H. E., Ochoa, J., and McCann, F. V. (1979): Paraesthesiae: Abnormal impulse generation in sensory nerve fibers in man. *Acta Physiol. Scand.,* 105:518–520.
68. Torebjörk, H. E., Ochoa, J. L., and Schady, W. (1984): Referred pain from intraneural stimulation of muscle fascicles in the median nerve. *Pain,* 18:145–156.
69. Vallbo, A. B. (1981): Sensations evoked from the glabrous skin of the human hand by electrical stimulation on unitary mechanosensitive afferents. *Brain Res.,* 215:359–363.
70. Vallbo, A. B., and Hagbarth, K. E. (1968): Activity from skin mechanoreceptors recorded percutaneously in awake human subjects. *Exp. Neurol.,* 21:270–289.
71. Vallbo, A. B., Hagbarth, K. E., Torebjörk, H. E., and Wallin, B. G. (1979): Somatosensory, proprioceptive and sympathetic activity in human peripheral nerves. *Physiol. Rev.,* 59:919–957.
72. Walker, A. E., and Nulsen, F. (1948): Electrical stimulation of the upper thoracic portion of the sympathetic chain in man. *Arch. Neurol. Psychiatry,* 59:559–560.
73. Wall, P. D. (1978): The gate control theory of pain mechanisms: A re-examination and a re-statement. *Brain,* 101:1–18.
74. Wall, P. D. (1984): Mechanisms of acute and chronic pain. In: *Advances in Pain Research and Therapy,* Vol. 6, *Neural Mechanisms of Pain,* edited by L. Kruger and J. C. Liebeskind, pp. 85–104. Raven Press, New York.
75. Wall, P. D., and Devor, M. (1978): Physiology of sensation after peripheral nerve injury, regeneration and neuroma formation. In: *Physiology and Pathology of Axons,* edited by S. G. Waxman, pp. 377–378. Raven Press, New York.

76. Wall, P. D., and Devor, M. (1983): Sensory afferent impulses originate from dorsal root ganglia as well as from the periphery in normal and nerve injured rats. *Pain,* 17:321–339.
77. Wall, P. D., and Gutnick, M. (1974): Properties of afferent nerve impulses originating from a neuroma. *Nature,* 248:740–743.
78. Wallin, B. G. (1981): New aspects of sympathetic function in man. In: *Neurology,* Vol. 1, *Clinical Neurophysiology,* edited by E. Stålberg and R. R. Young, pp. 145–167. Butterworth, London.
79. Wallin, G., Torebjörk, E., and Hallin, R. (1976): Preliminary observations on the pathophysiology of hyperalgesia in the causalgic pain syndrome. In: *Sensory Function of the Skin,* edited by Y. Zotterman, 489–502. Pergamon Press, Oxford.
80. Wynn Parry, C. B. (1980): Pain in avulsion lesions of the brachial plexus. *Pain,* 9:41–53.

Advances in Pain Research and Therapy, Vol. 9, edited by H. L. Fields et al. Raven Press, New York © 1985.

Corticosteroids Reduce Neuroma Hyperexcitability

Marshall Devor, Ruth Govrin-Lippmann, and Pnina Raber

Life Sciences Institute, Hebrew University of Jerusalem, Jerusalem 91904, Israel

Systemic and locally applied corticosteroids are widely used, highly effective agents for relief of somatosensory symptoms (especially itch and pain) in a broad range of dermatologic, rheumatologic, and neurologic conditions (1,5). The rationale generally given is that the primary therapeutic action of these drugs is antiinflammatory. Reduction in inflammation presumably reduces the concentrations of algesic substances in joints and skin and consequently the excitation of sensory endings. However, clinical reports suggest the possibility of a direct corticosteroid action on abnormally excitable damaged nerve fibers. For example, there have been occasional reports of effective pain relief produced by injection of corticosteroids directly into amputation stump neuromas (7,13). A related use is direct injection of depot corticosteroids into the tender spots along nerves supplying painful joints. Pybus (10,11) has recently claimed impressive control of pain in osteoarthritis using this approach, in contrast to the generally unsatisfactory results obtained from intrasynovial injection of corticosteroids. In this study we examined the effects of soluble and depot forms of corticosteroids when applied directly to experimental nerve-end neuromas. This treatment produces a rapid and prolonged suppression of the hyperexcitability normally seen in damaged neuroma fibers, and under conditions that suggest that the suppression is not secondary to reduced inflammation. A full report of this study is available elsewhere (4).

METHODS

Adult male rats of the Wistar-derived Sabra strain underwent an initial operation in which one or both sciatic nerves were tightly ligated with 5/0 silk and then cut distally. In some of the rats the acutely cut nerve stump was treated with one of three commercially available glucocorticoid preparations [triamcinolone hexacetonide suspension 20 mg/ml (Lederspan, Lederle); triamcinolone diacetate suspension 20 mg/ml (Ledercort Forte diluted with saline, Lederle); or dexamethasone 4 mg/ml (Dexacort, Ikapharm)] or one of two control solutions [saline or the aqueous suspension vehicle of Lederspan that contained 0.4% polysorbate 80, 0.4% benzyl alcohol, and 50% sorbitol solution (USP)]. The remaining rats were operated a second time 1 to 10 days after the first operation. On that occasion one or both of the previously sectioned nerves were reexposed and treated with one of the corticosteroids or controls. The treatment regimen was either (a) infiltration of the nerve stump with 100 to 125 μl of the corticosteroid or control preparation or (b) gentle application of drug-soaked Gelfoam pads to the intact perineurium for 10 min.

A terminal electrophysiological preparation was carried out either (a) immediately after the corticosteroid or control treatment or (b) 1 to 14 days later, which was 5 to 14 days after the original nerve section. In these experiments we measured the percentage incidence of spontaneous impulse discharge generated in the sciatic nerve-end neuroma using a method described in detail elsewhere (3). Briefly, we counted the number of spontaneously active axons in fine nerve filaments dissected in continuity with the neuroma and divided this value by the total fiber content of the filament determined by electrically stimulating the neuroma at gradually increasing current strength while counting the number of all-or-none units recruited. Overall, we sampled 144 $\pm$ 37 (mean $\pm$ SD) A fibers per rat. Statistical comparisons are based on two-tailed t-tests.

RESULTS

Single doses of all three corticosteroid preparations substantially reduced ($p < 0.01$) the incidence of spontaneous discharge in neuroma A fibers as compared with the saline controls or with a larger series of untreated neuromas from earlier studies. This was observed when the drugs were applied to the acutely cut nerve, in which case intense ectopic discharge failed to develop, or when the drugs were applied to already active neuromas, in which case the intensity of the discharge was reduced (Fig. 1). There was no significant difference between the two routes of administration: infiltration and perineural application ($p > 0.1$). Similarly, we found no significant differences in effectiveness among the three corticosteroid preparations ($p > 0.2$). At the end of many of the experiments we applied stimuli that are known to be excitatory in untreated neuromas (2,15), including mechanical probing, systemic injection of epinephrine (1 μg), and asphyxia. In every case in which spontaneous discharge had been suppressed by corticosteroid treatment, response to these stimuli was also eliminated.

In 2 control rats with 5-day-old neuromas, 2.5 mg of triamcinolone hexacetonide was injected intraperitoneally (7.4 mg/kg). This had no effect on spontaneous discharge ($p > 0.2$) measured the following day. Application of the steroid to the contralateral nerve (two experiments) also had no effect on chronic (3- and 7-day) neuromas.

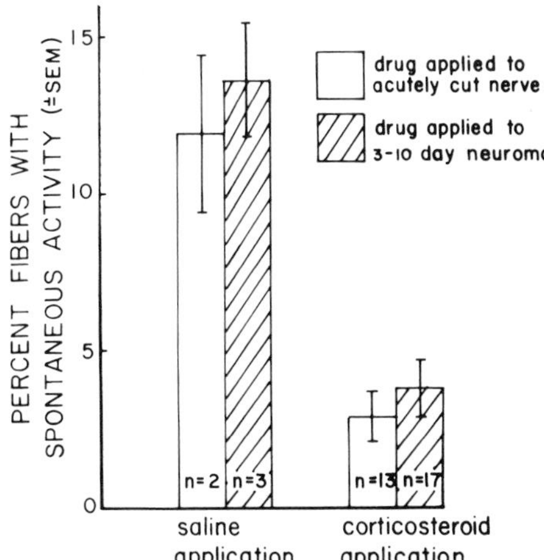

FIG. 1. Suppression of spontaneous ectopic discharge in nerve-end neuromas by local corticosteroid application. Triamcinolone hexacetonide was used in 20 experiments, triamcinolone diacetate was used in 6, and dexamethasone was used in 4.

Discharge suppression following local corticosteroid treatment came on rapidly (minutes to hours) (4) and lasted at least 14 days for acutely cut nerves. Indeed, comparing the activities in neuromas tested at various times after triamcinolone hexacetonide treatment, the inhibition increased with time: 4.2 ± 2.2% of fibers 1 to 2 days posttreatment (N = 6 rats), 2.9 ± 1.3% at 5 to 7 days (N = 6), and 2.0 ± 0.7% after 8 to 14 days (N = 8). Because the incidence of spontaneous activity in A fibers normally falls off strongly early in the third postoperative week (6), we do not know how long a single corticosteroid dose can remain effective after 14 days.

Conduction velocities of the fibers studied fell within the Aβ and Aδ range. We reported in previous studies that C fibers rarely have spontaneous discharge in neuromas of only 1 to 14 days standing (3,6), and this was confirmed in the control experiments of the present study. Corticosteroid treatment did not elicit activity in this fiber population, but in view of the very low background discharge level, we can make no comments on possible inhibitory effects.

DISCUSSION

Injury causes peripheral afferent fibers to undergo dramatic alterations in electrical excitability (2,15). Frequently, a prolonged spontaneous impulse discharge is generated at the site of injury and it becomes abnormally sensitive to various physical and chemical stimuli. The ectopic afferent barrage thus produced is believed to contribute to the neuralgic pains and paresthesias often associated with nerve injury. We have shown that local application of three corticosteroids (triamcinolone hexacetonide, triamcinolone diacetate, and dexamethasone) largely prevents the development of spontaneous ectopic discharge in freshly cut nerves and substantially reduces the incidence of ectopic discharge generated in nerve-end neuromas that are already active. This effect began rapidly and persisted for as long as our model system permitted us to follow it (14 days). In fact, the degree of suppression increased rather than decreased during this period (tested for triamcinolone hexacetonide only). It is likely that for the depot-form corticosteroids triamcinolone hexacetonide and triamcinolone diacetate the drug effect is present throughout the sustained-release period of the preparations, which is given nominally by the manufacturer as several weeks to several months.

We believe that the corticosteroids act locally on the damaged nerve end, on the grounds that an equivalent drug dose administered systemically or applied to the contralateral nerve had no significant effect on ongoing neuroma discharge. Furthermore, discharge suppression began within minutes of application in some cases. The mechanism of action is more difficult to specify. The rapid onset and the fact that neuroma formation is not associated with pronounced inflammation (14) suggest that ectopic discharge suppression is not secondary to reduced tissue inflammation. A number of well-known actions of corticosteroids, such as immunosuppression and antimitotic activity (1,5), are similarly ruled out, at least as primary causes. A more likely possibility is that corticosteroids affect the impulse-generating mechanism in the damaged neuroma fibers by directly or indirectly changing membrane conductances or other membrane properties (8,9,12,16). There is also evidence that corticosteroids hyperpolarize nerve cells by activating an electrogenic Na^+ pump (9).

If indeed corticosteroid compounds act directly on electrogenic properties of sensory nerve fibers, this constitutes an alternative to the common presumption that intralesion and topical cutaneous corticosteroid treatment reduces pain and itch as a consequence of the drug's antiinflammatory effects. Furthermore, these data encourage the use of local depot corticosteroid infiltration at sites of ectopic impulse generation (e.g., tender spots) in the treatment of pains and paresthesias associated with nerve injury.

SUMMARY

Local application of three corticosteroids, triamcinolone hexacetonide (Lederspan), triamcinolone diacetate (Ledercort), and dexamethasone (Dexacort), substantially reduced the incidence of spontaneous ectopic impulse discharge generated in experimental nerve-end neuromas in rats and prevented later development of ectopic discharge when applied to freshly cut nerves. A local action on the injured fibers within the neuroma is indicated. It is suggested that direct perineural or intraneural steroid application may be useful in the management of paresthesias and pain associated with peripheral nerve injury.

ACKNOWLEDGMENTS

This work was supported by a grant from the United States–Israel Binational Science Foundation. We thank P. Pybus for suggesting this line of research to us.

REFERENCES

1. Bowman, W. C., and Rand, M. J. (1980): *Textbook of Pharmacology,* ed. 2. Blackwell, Oxford.
2. Devor, M. (1984): The pathophysiology and anatomy of damaged nerve. In: *Textbook of Pain,* edited by P. D. Wall and R. Melzack, Churchill Livingstone, London.
3. Devor, M., and Govrin-Lippmann, R. (1983): Axoplasmic transport block reduces ectopic impulse generation in injured peripheral nerves. *Pain,* 16:73–86.
4. Devor, M., Govrin-Lippmann, R., and Raber, P. (1985): Corticosteroids suppress ectopic neural discharge originating in experimental neuromas (in press).
5. Goodman, L. S., and Gilman, G. (editors) (1975): *The Pharmacological Basis of Therapeutics,* ed. 5. Macmillan, New York.
6. Govrin-Lippmann, R., and Devor, M. (1978): Ongoing activity in severed nerves: Source and variation with time. *Brain Res.,* 159:406–410.
7. Kohnlein, K.-E., Ocker, K., Seitz, H. D., and Schwanst, K. H. (1980): Experimental trials to inhibit neuroma formation. *Chir. Plastica (Berl.),* 5:207–212.
8. Hall, E. D. (1982): Acute effects of intravenous glucocorticoid on cat spinal motor neuron electrical properties. *Brain Res.,* 240:186–190.
9. Hall, E. D. (1982): Glucocorticoid effects on central nervous excitability and synaptic transmission. *Int. Rev. Neurobiol.,* 23:165–195.
10. Pybus, P. K. (1980): Osteoarthritis of the knee. *Practitioner,* 224:928–930.
11. Pybus, P. K. (1984): Osteoarthritis: a new neurological method of pain control. *Med. Hypoth.,* 14:413–422.
12. Seeman, P. M. (1966): Membrane stabilization by drugs: Tranquillizers, steroids and anesthetics. *Int. Rev. Neurobiol.,* 9:145–169.
13. Smith, J. R., and Gomez, N. H. (1970): Local injection therapy of neuromata of the hand with triamcinolone acetonide. *J. Bone Joint Surg.,* 52A:71–83.
14. Spencer, P. S. (1974): The traumatic neuroma and proximal stump. *Bull. Hosp. Joint Dis.,* 35:85–102.
15. Wall, P., and Gutnick, M. (1974): Ongoing activity in peripheral nerves: The physiology and pharmacology of impulses originating from a neuroma. *Exp. Neurol.,* 43:580–593.
16. Wilson, R. W., Ward, M. D., and Johns, T. R. (1974): Corticosteroids: A direct effect at the neuromuscular junction. *Neurology (Minneap.),* 24:1091–1095.

Advances in Pain Research and Therapy, Vol. 9, edited by H. L. Fields et al. Raven Press, New York © 1985.

Do Herniated Disks Produce Pain?

Hubert L. Rosomoff

The Comprehensive Pain Center, Department of Neurological Surgery, University of Miami School of Medicine, Miami, Florida 33101

Low back pain is a condition experienced by 80% of the world's population, ranking first among all health problems in frequency of occurrence. Its costs, on the basis of lost earnings, worker compensation, and disability payments and expenses for medical care, exceed those for any other single health disorder. Its frequency and impact are expected to increase over the next decades as longevity and the average age of the work force increase (1). The symptom complex of back pain extending into the leg, sciatica, is traditionally conceived as being presumptively due to a herniated disk; i.e., "pinching" or compression of one or more spinal nerve roots. By best estimates, some 200,000 to 450,000 operations are performed annually for this presumed condition (12,13). Physiological studies, however, demonstrate that, except for transient pain when first impacted, sustained nerve root compression or pinching does not produce further pain (19). There may be numbness or loss of function, e.g., as when one's leg falls asleep when sitting too long, but it is not a painful event. Therefore, other causes must be considered as the agents giving rise to pain. It follows that successful definition of such, with appropriate treatment, may result in relief or prevention of pain and disability, without resorting to surgery with its attendant risks and failures.

From simple inspection of human anatomy it is inescapably clear that all low back injuries must have associated soft-tissue abnormalities, because the protective covering offered by the muscle represents the bulk of the anatomy affected. Even if the forces applied reach sufficient strength to herniate or rupture an intervertebral disk, these forces must be transmitted first through the overlying soft tissue that binds the spine together as a functional unit. These tissues, when injured, undergo breakdown of the cell membranes to arachidonic acid, from which biosynthesis of chemicals like prostaglandins and associated products ensues. One important issue to this process is the induction of a state of hyperalgesia, following which a pain signal will evolve, when excessive mechanical stimulation occurs or when compounds of the reaction to injury, like histamine or bradykinin, are produced (18). The nerve, itself, does not originate the pain signal. Nociceptors are stimulated to originate the transmission of the signal. Whether or not sensory neurotransmitters like substance P, somatostatin, or other substances are mediators is another problem for investigation (20).

It is the thesis of this presentation that the disordered musculoskeletal system is responsible for initiating these phenomena. These structures are extraspinal in the surrounding paraspinal muscles, buttocks, hips, and legs. These peripheral sites and syndromes are treatable, and when treatment is successful, function is restored and pain is alleviated without the need to correct any number of intraspinal pathological entities that have traditionally been designated as being competent causes for the production of pain and neurologic deficit.

Is there clinical support for this thesis? There is: One basic clinical observation is that when individuals are operated on under local anesthesia, the nerve root that is distorted by the herniated disk is quite irritable on manipulation and stimulation. This is productive of a painful state, but this is primarily a dysesthetic type of response. If the nerve immediately above or below the pathological root is manipulated; there is no painful sensation (10,16). It follows, then, that the pathological root is undergoing an irritative phenomenon, rendering the system hyperalgesic. These pathological axons respond to algesic chemicals that excite the nociceptive nerve endings, whereas normal axons do not. The algesic chemicals derive from the injured soft tissues (9).

Cell membranes of the injured soft tissues break down to arachidonic acid, which then is biosynthesized into prostaglandins, thromboxane, monohydroxy fatty acids, and leukotrienes (5,8,11). These, individually and collectively, are involved in the reactions to injury, producing hyperalgesia, vascular instability, and an inflammatory reaction, with loss of function (7). The symptoms produced depend on the relative proportions of these substances at the site of injury. For example, prostaglandins produce vasodilatation, and the part feels warm. Thromboxane produces vasoconstriction, and the part feels cold. The leukotrienes produce inflammation leading to the development of the focal trigger points. These substances, when interacted with polypeptides like bradykinin and histamine, or in the presence of excessive mechanical stimulation, go on to evolve a nociceptive impulse to be accepted by the receptor for transmission onward to the central nervous system (4). These reactions are inhibited by steroids, aspirin, and related products, effects that then provide a rationale for pharmacological treatment (6). However, even more interesting is the reversal of these same phenomena by focal physical forms of therapy such as application of ice, which, parenthetically, has been well established as a method for limiting or averting tissue reaction to injury (14). Vigorous activation of the musculoskeletal system also limits the reaction to injury, as enkephalin is released at two to three times base-line levels; this serves as an endogenous pain control system (3). It follows, then, that therapeutic application of these basic principles should lead one to prescribe the use of ice and vigorous exercise, rather than the traditional weeks of bed rest, analgesics, and muscle relaxants.

Neurophysiologically speaking, the sudden onset of pain in the primary afferent system is caused by stimulation of the terminals that are sensitive to pressure, temperature, and chemicals, thereon transmitted as an electrical signal by stimulation of the axon's ending, but resulting in axonal block (19). Pressure applied to the axon, as with a herniated disk, does produce nerve distortion when the membrane is stretched. This produces depolarization and an action potential that is transient, followed by accommodation and a decrease in the current density. Axonal block occurs after this initial mechanical distortion from disinhibition of the central structures. A further clinical observation is that after the immediate injury, there is a quiescent period with little or no discomfort and then a crescendo of secondary delayed pain. This is over a period of several hours. This is ascribed to a sensitization process from repeated stimulation, lowering of thresholds, giving rise to hyperesthesia. The delay also allows the reaction to injury to proceed, and inflammation results, in which there now is found prostaglandin hyperalgesia, chemical mediation of pain signals by bradykinin and histamine, and further spread of this process through the surrounding adjacent tissues. There further ensues a number of secondary effects like muscle contraction, referred pain, autonomic reflex change, and antidromic impulses. These represent themselves as clear-cut clinical phenomena on physical examination, typically represented as trigger points and myofascial pain syndromes seen in the trochanteric, ischial tuberosity, and sacroiliac areas (17).

The muscle contraction produces restricted ranges of motion, which create further pain. This is not a reflex muscle contraction, as previously thought. It is, in fact, a chemical phenomenon wherein the traumatized muscle releases calcium ions, which combine with ATP for an uncontrolled contraction, with pain, tenderness, vasoconstriction, decreased blood supply, and an energy-deficit contracture. It is this inflammatory reaction and accompanying decreased muscle length that produce the restricted range of joint movement and tendon and fascial shortening. The result is functional disability (2). It is of further clinical interest that immobilization, a traditional mode of treatment, and emotional tension are prime contributors to the production of disability, whence the conclusion that treatment programs should avoid immobilization but should incorporate relaxation and behavioral modification techniques to eliminate tension and stress.

The outstanding symptom of low back disorders is pain. Full examination of the patient finds only 3 to 25% of these individuals with bona fide neurologic deficits. These syndromes include referred pain patterns primarily involving the sciatic nerve. The nidus for the reference points includes the soft-tissue injuries and inflammation, particularly in the area of the low back and hip, giving rise to sciatica.

Further confirmation of these principles is provided by our clinical experience of the past 5 years in more than 1,000 patients, for whom studious attention to the correction of peripheral musculoskeletal disorders alone, without surgical correction of demonstrated intraspinal compressive lesions like herniated disks or bony stenosis, has led to restoration of functional capacities and major relief or abolition of the painful state. The central space-occupying lesions have been left *in situ,* without surgical removal. The peripheral mechanisms have been treated, and restoration of function has occurred and has been sustained in long-term follow-up studies up to 7 years (15).

Clinicians must be willing to revise traditional clinical tenets when presented with laboratory investigative data that support new methods of treatment. As just presented, surgery for low back pain disorders has been virtually eliminated, even when all the classic clinical and traditional indications for surgery have existed. Herniated disks with chronic nerve root compression, per se, do not directly produce pain.

REFERENCES

1. Bonica, J. J. (1980): Pain research and therapy: Past and current status and future needs. In: *Pain, Discomfort, Humanitarian Care,* edited by J. J. Bonica and L. K. Ng, pp. 1–46. Elsevier/North Holland, Amsterdam.
2. Calliet, R. (1980): *Soft Tissue Pain and Disability.* F. A. Davis, Philadelphia.
3. Carr, D. B., Bullen, B. A., Skrinar, G. S., Arnold, M., Rosenblatt, M., Beitens, I. Z., Martin, J. B., and McArthur, J. W. (1981): Physical conditioning facilities the exercise-induced secretion of beta-endorphin and beta-hypoprotein in women. *N. Engl. J. Med.,* 305:560–563.
4. Ferreira, S. H. (1983): Prostaglandins: Peripheral and central analgesia. In: *Advances in Pain Research and Therapy,* Vol. 5, edited by J. J. Bonica, U. Lindblom, and A. Iggo, pp. 597–603. Raven Press, New York.
5. Granström, E. (1983): Biochemistry of the prostaglandins, thromboxanes, and leukotrienes. In: *Advances in Pain Research and Therapy,* Vol. 5, edited by J. J. Bonica, U. Lindblom, and A. Iggo, pp. 605–615. Raven Press, New York.
6. Higgs, G. A., Flower, R. J., and Vane, J. R. (1977): A new approach to anti-inflammatory drugs. *Biochem. Pharmacol.,* 28:1959–1961.
7. Higgs, G. A., and Moncada, S. (1983): Interactions of arachionate products with other pain mediators. In: *Advances in Pain Research and Therapy,* Vol. 5, edited by J. J. Bonica, U. Lindblom, and A. Iggo, pp. 617–626. Raven Press, New York.
8. Juan, H. (1978): Prostaglandins as modulators of pain. *Gen. Pharmacol.,* 9:403–409.
9. Koschorke, G. M., and Zimmerman, M. (1985): Responses to algesic substances of nonmyelinated fibers in normal and chronically damaged cutaneus nerves of the cat. In: *Advances in Pain Research and Therapy,* Vol. 8, edited by K. M. Foley and C. Inturissi. *(in press)*
10. MacNab, I. (1972): The Mechanisms of Spondylogenic Pain. In: *Cervical Pain,* edited by C. Hirsch and Y. Zotterman, pp. 89–95. Pergamon Press, New York.
11. Moncada, S., Ferreira, S. H., and Vane, J. R. (1978): Pain and inflammatory mediators. In: *Inflammation Handbook of Experimental Pharmacology,* Vol. 50, edited by J. R. Vane and S. H. Ferreira, pp. 588–616. Springer-Verlag, Berlin.
12. Nordby, C. J. (1981): Epidemiology and diagnosis in low-back injury. *Occup. Health and Safety,* 50:38–42.
13. Pheasant, H. C. (1977): Backache—its nature, incidence and cost. *West. J. Med.,* 126:330–332.
14. Rosomoff, H. L., Clasen, R. A., Harstock, R., and Bebin, J. (1965): Brain reaction to experimental injury after hypothermia. *Arch. Neurol.,* 13:337–345.

15. Rosomoff, H. L., Green, C., Silbret, M., and Steele, R. (1981): Pain and low back rehabilitation program at the University of Miami School of Medicine, new approaches to treatment of chronic pain. In: *A Review of Multidisciplinary Pain Clinics and Pain Centers,* NIDA Research Monograph 36, edited by L. K. Y. Ng, pp. 92–111.
16. Smyth, M. J., and Wright, V. (1958): Sciatica and the intervertebral disc. An experimental study. *J. Bone Joint Surg.,* 40A:1401–1418.
17. Travell, J., and Rinzler, S. H. (1952): The myofascial genesis of pain. *Postgrad. Med.,* 11:425–434.
18. Vane, J. R. (1983): Pain of inflammation: An introduction. In: *Advances in Pain Research and Therapy,* Vol. 5, edited by J. J. Bonica, U. Lindblom, and A. Iggo, pp. 597–603. Raven Press, New York.
19. Wall, P. D. (1974): Physiological mechanisms involved in the production and relief of pain. In: *Recent Advances on Pain: Pathophysiology and Clinical Aspects,* edited by J. J. Bonica, P. Procacci, and C. A. Pagni, pp. 36–63. Charles C Thomas, Springfield, Ill.
20. Wall, P. (1980): The role of substantia gelantinosa as a gate control. In: *Pain,* edited by J. J. Bonica, pp. 205–231. Raven Press, New York.

Advances in Pain Research and Therapy, Vol. 9, edited by H. L. Fields et al. Raven Press, New York © 1985.

Families of Opioid Peptides and Classes of Opioid Receptors

L. Terenius

Department of Pharmacology, University of Uppsala, S-751 24 Uppsala, Sweden

Even after the existence of endogenous opioids was no longer hypothetical it was difficult to foresee that there was in fact a whole family of endogenous substances with such activity (18,40). However, the first report on the chemical identity of such substances had already indicated structural diversity. Two related pentapeptides, Leu- and Met-enkephalin, were described (19), and it was also found that the Met-enkephalin sequence was contained within the previously known pituitary hormone beta-lipotropin (Li 1964). Altogether, more than 20 individual opioid peptides have been identified (4). However, thus far, every opioid peptide of neuronal origin possesses the same N-terminal tetrapeptide sequence as the enkephalins. Cross-species comparisons have shown remarkable conservation from molluscs to man.

Preceding the discovery of opioid peptides was the notion of multiple opioid receptors, as reviewed by Martin et al. (27). The discovery of the endogenous opioid peptides (endorphins) stimulated further interest in receptor multiplicity, and attempts were made to establish the relationship between various opioid peptide systems and particular receptors.

An exciting new phase of research commenced in 1979 with the discovery that a protein, a so-called prohormone, serves as the precursor to beta-endorphin (30). The same prohormone is also the precursor of ACTH, a peptide of indisputable physiologic importance, and of melanocyte stimulatory hormones (MSH). The prohormone was named proopiomelanocortin. This is just one illustration of the close connection between the neuropeptide and endocrine systems. With developments in recombinant DNA technology, it has now been established that there are three different prohormones for opioid peptides (Fig. 1). Thus, it is possible to establish generic relationships between individual opioid peptides and their respective precursors. Each of these systems is pluripotent and capable of releasing several opioid peptides. It seems as if one cell expresses only one prohormone system.

The aim of this chapter is to summarize basic biochemical and molecular aspects of the opioid peptide systems and their receptors. Much of the rel-

PROOPIOMELANOCORTIN

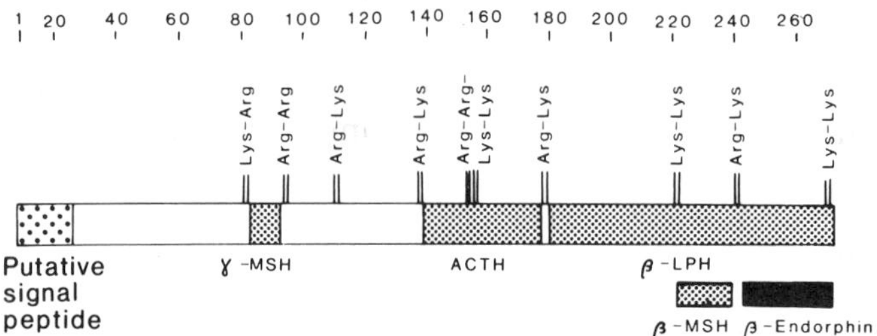

PROENKEPHALIN A

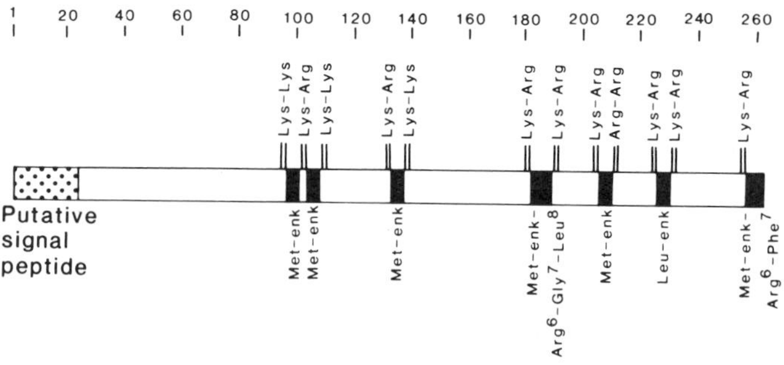

PROENKEPHALIN B

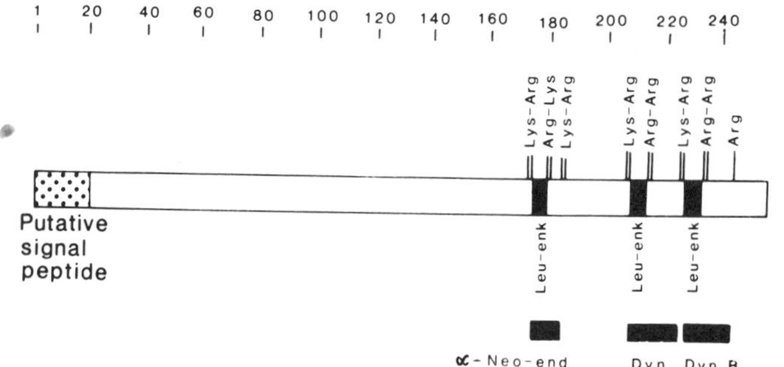

FIG. 1. Schematic representation of the prohormones for opioid peptides. Each prohormone is a protein of 240 to 260 amino acids. Dyn = dynorphin; end = endorphin; enk = enkephalin.

evant literature is probably not readily available to the pain physiologist or the clinician with interest in pain. The author is of the opinion, however, that the use of techniques of molecular biology and genetics to study these systems will illuminate some of the functional characteristics of pain modulation. Understanding of such basic mechanisms may also ultimately lead to better understanding of clinical conditions with hyperalgesia involving dysfunction in endogenous pain modulation. Explanations of how opioids exert their effects on receptors and how phenomena like tolerance develop may also be found.

OPIOID PEPTIDES: THEIR BIOSYNTHESIS AND DEGRADATION

Schematically, the biosynthesis and degradation of opioid peptides can be summarized as follows (Table 1). It should be emphasized that the same basic principles are valid for neuronal and nonneuronal (endocrine) tissues. However, the processing of the prohormone to the various endorphin fragments is at least partly tissue-specific.

Genes and Control of Transcription

The opioid peptide genes have been mapped in several species, including man. They show the characteristics of eukaryotic genes in general, including splicing, meaning that certain segments (introns) are not transcribed. The overall structures of the three genes of the known systems show similarities (17). Sequences toward the 5′ end of exon (transcribed region) 1 are probably important for control of the expression of the gene, i.e., the rate of transcription. Thus, glucocorticoid hormones increase the expression of proenkephalin A and decrease expression of proopiomelanocortin, probably through an action on this control region (7). Nonallelic multiple genes for

TABLE 1. *Schematic representation of biosynthesis and degradation of opioid peptides (and peptides in general)*

Transformation	Process name	Molecular events
		DNA
1	Transcription	↓
		mRNA
2	Translation	↓
		Protein
3	Processing	↓
		Peptide
4	Metabolism	↓
		Peptide fragment

proopiomelanocortin have been described in the rat, which has two genes, whereas the pig has one (32). Whether or not multiplicity exists for the other genes is unknown. Restriction fragment length polymorphism of the pro-opiomelanocortin gene has been detected in man (11) and other species. The importance of this polymorphism is not known, but it is conceivable that it can affect the control region of the gene and thereby ultimately its expression. Techniques are becoming available to analyze for "pathologic" DNA sequences, e.g., in patients with congenital insensitivity to pain or in patients with hyperalgesias. It can be foreseen that such technology will be used to investigate patients with genetically abnormal pain sensitivity.

Transcription of DNA leads to formation of messenger-RNA (mRNA), containing the nucleotide sequence necessary for translation to prohormone, but also for a signal peptide (Fig. 1) that serves as a "postal code" marker. Very recent data suggest that mRNA for proenkephalin A, the prohormone for the enkephalins, is present in about the same concentration in CNS areas that are rich in enkephalin, such as striatum or hypothalamus, as in the cerebellum, which is low in enkephalins (38). Apparently, there must be other processes farther downstream (Table 1) that are not brought into action in the cerebellum.

Prohormones

The prohormones in the three opioid systems are very similar in size (Fig. 1). Each contains several hormonal messages: in the case of proenkephalin A, no less than seven enkephalin sequences; in proenkephalin B, three sequences. The enkephalin sequences in proenkephalin A and B are flanked by pairs of basic amino acids. This is a characteristic found in many other prohormones, such as proinsulin, progastrin, etc. The paired basic amino acids serve as signals for proteolytic cleavage, so-called processing. Cleavage occurs mainly at the bond between the basic amino acids, leaving one basic amino acid with the enkephalin peptide. Trimming of this basic amino acid occurs with a carboxypeptidase (6). This scheme is probably quite general and also to some extent statistical. More recent studies have indicated exceptions to this rule. The main products of proenkephalin B are peptides longer than Leu-enkephalin, i.e., alpha-neoendorphin, dynorphin, and dynorphin B (Table 2). Other mechanisms of posttranslational modification are also known. Acetylation of the N-terminal Tyr residue may occur, a pathway leading to loss of opioid activity; this reaction is prominent in the pituitary (6). C-terminal modification by amide formation has also recently been described in the opioid peptide family (42). This reaction requires a glycine-*X* sequence, where *X* is lysine or arginine, i.e., the processing signal; this sequence is uniquely found in a proenkephalin A segment, being the immediate precursor of methorphamide (Table 2). Such posttranslationally modified peptides are potentially of importance, because this modification produces certain metabolic resistance.

TABLE 2. *Generic relationships between opioid peptides and their respective precursors (prohormones)*

Prohormone	Peptides	Structures
Proopiomelanocortin	Beta-endorphin	Tyr-Gly-Gly-Phe-Met-Thr-Ser-Glu-Lys-Ser-Gln-Thr-Pro-Leu-Val-Thr-Leu-Phe-Lys-Asn-Ala-Ile-Ile-Lys-Asn-Ala-His-Lys-Lys-Gly-Gln
	Gamma-endorphin (= beta-endorphin$_{1-17}$)	Tyr-Gly-Gly-Phe-Met-Thr-Ser-Glu-Lys-Ser-Gln-Thr-Pro-Leu-Val-Thr-Leu$_{17}$
Proenkephalin A	Leu-enkephalin	Tyr-Gly-Gly-Phe-Leu
	Met-enkephalin	Tyr-Gly-Gly-Phe-Met
	Heptapeptide	Tyr-Gly-Gly-Phe-Met-Arg-Phe
	Methorphamide	Tyr-Gly-Gly-Phe-Met-Arg-Arg-Val-NH_2
Proenkephalin B	Dynorphin	Tyr-Gly-Gly-Phe-Leu-Arg-Arg-Ile-Arg-Pro-Lys-Leu-Lys-Trp-Asp-Asn-Gln
	Dynorphin$_{1-8}$	Try-Gly-Gly-Phe-Leu-Arg-Arg-Ile
	α-Neoendorphin	Tyr-Gly-Gly-Phe-Leu-Arg-Lys-Tyr-Pro-Lys
	Dynorphin B	Tyr-Gly-Gly-Phe-Leu-Arg-Arg-Gln-Phe-Lys-Val-Val-Thr

The table shows only major peptide species. Processing of proenkephalin B apparently does not progress substantially toward Leu-enkephalin, indicating a specificity of enzymes involved.

Active Peptides

If all opioid peptides had essentially the same properties, it would be rather trivial which peptide is released from any one system. However, the different peptides differ markedly with regard to metabolic stability and, as will be discussed later, to receptor profile (42,43). Low-molecular-weight peptides such as the enkephalins are metabolized more rapidly than longer peptides such as beta-endorphin. It is possible that, depending on past and present activity in the opioid peptide neuron, different products will be released. Table 2 summarizes the major products from each opioid peptide system. However, it is known that there are additional peptides representing different stages in the processing of the prohormone. Measurement of opioid peptides is usually by radioimmunoassay; such assays are sequence-specific, usually encompassing a 4- to 7-amino-acid sequence at the C terminus. For instance, an antiserum for dynorphin would normally show negligible cross-reaction with dynorphin B, beta-endorphin, or the enkephalins. This means, indirectly, that there may exist important peptide species that have not been identified. An alternative approach is therefore to use a receptor assay capable of recognizing the pool of opioid peptides. Using this approach, we have observed a whole range of components from the opioid peptide systems in human body fluids, some of which cannot be attributed to previously described peptides (31). Receptor assay has been used to study patients with chronic pain syndromes, as will be discussed later. More recently, we have introduced an alternative approach, as detailed in Table 3. The principle is

TABLE 3. *Basis of a general procedure for assigning generic relationships between any isolated opioid peptide and the three opioid prohormones*

Prohormone	Trypsin degradation products	
	Structure	Copies per prohormone
Proopiomelanocortin	Met-enkephalin-Thr^6-Ser^7-Glu^8	1
Proenkephalin A	Met-enkephalin-Lys^6	3
	Met-enkephalin-Arg^6	3
	Leu-enkephalin-Lys^6	1
Proenkephalin B	Leu-enkephalin-Arg^6	3

The products formed are measured by specific radioimmunoassay.

to use the enzyme trypsin, which cuts protein and peptides indiscriminantly to the C-terminal side of a basic amino acid, in the sequence. Because opioid peptide sequences are flanked by basic amino acids (Fig. 1), defined peptide species will be generated that can be measured by specific radioimmunoassays and attributed to the proper opioid peptide systems.

Metabolic Fragmentation of Opioid Peptides

As already indicated, the enkephalins are relatively unstable in the circulation or in CNS tissue. Removal of only one amino acid will reduce opioid activity by at least 99%. Several enzymes have been found to degrade enkephalins, including angiotensin-converting enzyme and "enkephalinase." The latter enzyme was initially thought to be relatively specific for enkephalin degradation (36), but it has been found to be a fairly ubiquitous enzyme that also degrades other neuropeptides, including substance P (28), a peptide associated with pain afferents. Certain drugs and experimental substances selectively block these enzymes: captopril, angiotensin-converting enzyme, and thiorphan enkephalinase. Thiorphan introduced intracerebrally has been found to produce analgesia that can be reversed by naloxone (34). Dynorphin is metabolically split by a specific enzyme that has very recently been characterized (9). The product, dynorphin$_{1-8}$, retains opioid activity, but its receptor selectivity has shifted from kappa to delta preference *(vide infra).* Removal of the N-terminal tyrosine in any of the opioid peptides will produce complete loss in opioid activity. This is probably an important route of inactivation, but it is not known whether it involves enzymes with specificity for the opioid peptides or general aminopeptidases. The importance of this route of inactivation is particularly clear in pharmacologic experiments. To study the biologic effects of opioid peptides, it is common to introduce an amino acid with unnatural configuration, such as D-alanine following the N-terminal tyrosine (29). Such analogs of, for instance, the enkephalins have greater metabolic stability. This modification does not seem to alter the receptor selectivity.

Metabolic fragmentation is the likely mode of inactivation of neuropeptides. For those having a local role only in the CNS, metabolism has to be more efficient than, for instance, in endocrine systems, where the peptide should survive blood transport. Studies on the metabolism of opioid peptides therefore have a central role in this area of research.

PEPTIDE NEURON: BASIC CHARACTERISTICS

It is only recently that it has been realized that many neurons in the CNS express specific neuropeptides in addition to a classic neurotransmitter. In fact, it is conceivable that this so-called coexistence between the neurotransmitter and neuropeptide is the common situation (26). It may be useful to point out some principal differences between neurotransmitters and neuropeptides with regard to the dynamics of their biosynthesis and release. The neurotransmitter or its precursor is taken up by the nerve terminal, where biosynthesis or recycling is a fast process. The whole process, uptake and biosynthesis, is fast, and newly synthesized transmitter may be released after only seconds or minutes from the nerve terminal. The neuropeptide, on the other hand, is a product of a complicated biosynthetic pathway originating in the nerve cell body (which often is at considerable distance from the nerve terminal) with synthesis of prohormone. The prohormone is secreted from the Golgi apparatus, packed into secretory granules, and transported via fast axonal transport. During transport, processing of the prohormone to active peptide is likely to occur, and the vesicles near the nerve terminal are assumed to contain the active peptide. Clearly, this whole sequence, biosynthesis of prohormone, axonal transport, and processing, is relatively slow, and the whole cycle may require hours or even days. This also suggests functional specialization. In a neuron with a coexisting neurotransmitter and neuropeptide, the former may be responsible for immediate effects and the latter for long-term modulatory effects. Thus, the neurotransmitter may be giving the electrophysiologically recorded spike, whereas the neuropeptide has a "permissive" role (5). This model could also accommodate partial neuroendocrine functions of a neuropeptide, as is suggested by the endocrine function of biosynthetically identical opioid peptide systems outside of the CNS. Neuroendocrine mechanisms might explain phenomena such as the diurnal variation in pain sensitivity (39).

OPIOID RECEPTORS

For a long while, compounds having morphine-like properties were named opiates, even if their chemical structures were quite different from that of morphine. Since the opioid peptides were discovered and it has become obvious that they are the natural ligands of these receptors, the more general terms *opioid* and *opioid receptor* have been introduced. The term *opioid receptor* tends to become too wide if not coupled to an additional criterion: sensitivity to blockade or antagonism by naloxone.

Evolution of Terminology

The early conceptualization of the opiate receptor was the negative image of the classic opiates such as morphine (3). Because morphine has a rigid structure, it also defines a receptor surface quite well, and through structure-activity analysis it has been possible to deduce the dimensions and points of binding of the receptors quite accurately. Such analysis has shown that thousands of compounds with morphine-like properties can be fitted into one receptor. However, Martin and his group (27) recognized that certain benzomorphan analogs showed activities that were qualitatively different from those of morphine-like substances, and they introduced two more receptors. They were designated with Greek letters for their respective indicator drugs: mu (for morphine) being the classic opiate receptor, *k* (for ketocyclazocine), and sigma (for SKF 10,047). Typical actions elicited through these receptors are summarized in Table 4. The opioid peptides did not fit into this system entirely. The action profile of the enkephalins required introduction of a delta receptor (25), and there have been suggestions of other receptors, including an epsilon receptor with selectivity for beta-endorphin (35). Pharmacologic characterization of the opioid peptides has been carried out extensively in *in vitro* systems. There are several reasons for this: (a) The peptides are metabolically unstable in plasma and are restricted by the blood-brain barrier, making systemic administration impractical. (b) After intracerebral administration, metabolism is considerable. (c) Access and cost of peptides are also limiting factors. However, sev-

TABLE 4. *Opiate receptor classification stemming from studies in spinal dogs*

Organ/effect	Receptor		
	μ	κ	σ
Pupil	Miosis	Miosis	Mydriasis
Respiratory rate	Stimulation, then depression	No change	Stimulation
Heart rate	Bradycardia	No change	Tachycardia
Body temperature	Hypothermia	No change	No change
Affect	Indifference	Sedation	Delirium
Nociceptive flexor reflexes	Decrease	Decrease	Modest decrease

From Iwamoto and Martin (21), with permission.

eral classic pharmacologic preparations are sensitive to opiates. Interestingly, but thus far never explained in physiologic terms, there are considerable species differences in peptide sensitivities, which in turn can be ascribed to different kinds and proportions of receptors in the different tissues. Binding analysis using more or less purified synaptic membrane preparations from brain or spinal cord has become the *in vitro* substitute for *in vivo* testing on the CNS. These techniques are now becoming sophisticated. By computer modeling, the simultaneous presence of different binding sites (often assumed to equate with receptors) and the relative affinities of a test compound for these receptors can be calculated and evaluated by statistical methods.

Correspondence Between Opioid Peptide System and Receptor Subtype

A tentative classification of the opioid receptors and their natural ligands is given in Table 5. It also lists the naloxone sensitivity of each receptor and the typical *in vitro* system used for testing. It should be pointed out that these peptides show considerable overlap between receptors. The enkephalins, for instance, also bind to mu receptors. Until recently, no peptide with selectivity for mu receptors was known. Now, methorphamide is known to have such properties, but it seems to be a minor species from the proenkephalin A system (42). Dynorphin and related molecules, dynorphin B, and alpha-neoendorphin all have predominantly kappa-receptor selectivity (44). However, shorter fragments such as dynorphin$_{1-8}$ become more enkephalin-like (mixed mu/delta receptor profile). On the other hand, prestages to enkephalin in the proenkephalin A system have kappa-receptor selectivity. Therefore, the degree of peptide prohormone processing will define not only the magnitude of receptor occupation but also which receptors will be preferentially occupied. This indicates that there is no simple relationship between activity in a particular opioid precursor system and activation of a particular receptor subtype. The sigma receptor has uncertain status in the table. This receptor is apparently not sensitive to naloxone, and therefore it

TABLE 5. *Opioid receptors, principal natural ligands, sensitivities of receptors to naloxone reversal, and principal in vitro test systems*

Receptor	Natural ligand/prohormone	Naloxone sensitivity	*In vitro* test system
μ	Methorphamide/proENK A	Strong	Guinea pig ileum
κ	Dynorphin/proENK B	Intermediate	Rabbit vas deferens
σ	?	None?	
δ	Enkephalin/proENK A	Weak	Mouse vas deferens
ϵ	β-Endorphin/POMC	Weak	Rat vas deferens

ENK = enkephalin; POMC = proopiomelanocortin.

probably should not be considered among opioid receptors. Certain psychotomimetic drugs such as PCP (33) may act through this receptor, which also may explain psychotomimetic effects seen clinically with certain antagonist analgesics such as pentazocine.

Recent developments in autoradiography have made it possible to show a differential distribution of different opioid receptors in brain and spinal cord. The mu receptor is abundant in central areas for pain control, in periaqueductal gray matter, in brainstem and dorsal spinal cord, and also in the limbic system. The kappa receptor is present in these areas as well, but also in deeper layers of the cerebral cortex, whereas delta receptors are quite generally distributed. Differences in cytoarchitecture observed with different ligands provide compelling evidence for the existence of multiple opioid receptors in the CNS (16). Recently, mu receptors were visualized in the human brain by positron-emission tomography (13).

OPIOID PEPTIDES AND CLINICAL PAIN

The powerful analgesic action of the classic opiates is a strong indication of the intrinsic capacity of the opioid receptors. The frank analgesia is probably mainly mediated via mu receptors, except in the spinal cord, where activation of delta (45) and kappa (15) receptors has been found to induce antinociception. The plethora of opioid peptide neurons at all levels of the neuroaxis should provide the potential for efficient pain modulation. Indeed, several opioid peptides, including beta-endorphin and the enkephalin analog metkephamide (12), are clinically effective. It therefore seems paradoxical that the physiological role of opioid peptides in pain modulation remains equivocal (39). One possible explanation is that opioid peptide systems usually require major trauma to become activated. Such trauma would be unethical to induce experimentally and equally unethical to probe with drugs such as naloxone or by invasive sampling techniques in patients. It may also be, however, that the questions that have been asked in the past have been based on assumptions that do not exist naturally. If naloxone only marginally increases clinical pain (23), it may be because the opioid peptide circuitry is very complex, and the net pharmacologic effect becomes very small. Neurochemical measurements, on the other hand, may not have been directed to the right variable. It is beyond the scope of this review to cover the vast literature in this area. Only the question whether or not opioid peptides are involved in chronic pain syndromes will be discussed.

OPIOID PEPTIDES AND CHRONIC PAIN

Chronic pain is by definition a therapeutic failure, and globally it is a major therapeutic problem. Drugs that are effective for acute pain often are not acceptable, because of their dependence liability, or are ineffective, because of tolerance development or for unknown reasons. Surgical techniques for intervention have diminished in importance because of the risk of relapse. Recent years, however, have witnessed a revival of paramedical techniques for treatment and increased interest in techniques such as acupuncture and electric stimulation. It must seem ironic to the pain therapist who wants to act rationally that a revival of old, prescientific medical treatment occurs at the same time as an increasingly more sophisticated view of endogenous systems for pain modulation is developing. It seems important at this stage to arrive at new working models that might explain the failures of the old techniques and the value of new ones proposed. Thus, the neurochemical basis for acupuncture as studied in animals and in man was recently reviewed, concluding not unexpectedly that the effects on the CNS are very complex (14).

Chronic pain (and pain in general) in human beings certainly has dimensions beyond those in experimental animals. Therefore, several important aspects of painful diseases must be studied in patients. We have asked ourselves if neurochemical studies may contribute to an understanding of chronic pain syndromes. The work has been based on measurements of opioid peptides in the cerebrospinal fluid (CSF) of patients with chronic pain (2,39). A wide group of patients were the subjects, the inclusion criterion being pain of at least 6 months' duration, and the exclusion criteria being organic brain disease or drug or alcohol abuse. The patients were carefully examined both with regard to somatic illness and by structured interviews and psychologic ratings. Based on the results of these examinations, which were done blind to the results of chemical analysis, three major diagnostic groups were identified: neuralgic pain (earlier named neurogenic) with verified nerve lesions, nociceptive pain (earlier named somatic) with somatic illness such as ischemia or malignancy, and idiopathic pain (earlier named psychogenic) with no objective evidence for somatic lesions. For comparison, a group of healthy volunteers and a group of patients with major depressive disorders are also shown (Table 6). The CSF in these

TABLE 6. *Fraction I in CSF in healthy volunteers and patients with chronic pain syndromes*

	<0.6	0.6–1.2	>1.2 pmol/ml[a]
Healthy volunteers	3	12	4
Neuralgic pain	29	2	2
Nociceptive pain	2	3	3
Idiopathic pain	3	9	10
Depressive disorders	—	3	12

[a]Measured as Met-enkephalin equivalents.
Data from Almay et al. (2) and von Knorring et al. (22).

patients was measured for opioid activity in a chromatographically identified fraction, called fraction I (41). This fraction contains a pool of opioid peptides that are chemically rich in basic amino acids (31) and are in the molecular-weight range of 1,000 to 1,500. It appears that this rather simple assay gives a surprisingly conclusive result: Patients with chronic neuralgic pain have very low fraction I levels; patients with idiopathic pain have high fraction I levels; patients with nociceptive pain have intermediate levels, essentially as in the controls. Patients with idiopathic pain show some parallel with patients with depressive disorder, which is of clinical interest because of the commonalities between these syndromes (37).

Apparently, certain kinds of chronic pain syndromes are accompanied by generalized changes in opioid peptide concentrations in CSF in a characteristic manner. The low CSF levels of opioid activity in neuralgic pain suggest that endorphinergic tonus is subnormal, whatever the mechanistic explanations may be. Strong afferent stimulation, by acupuncture or transcutaneous nerve stimulation (TNS), is known to cause endorphin release (14) and to provide pain relief in certain clinical cases. In a series of chronic pain patients, Eriksson et al. (10) reported particularly high clinical responses in patients with neuralgic pain (87%, $N = 92$), moderate responses in nociceptive pain (44%, $N = 16$), and poor responses in idiopathic pain (24%, $N = 17$). Thus, patients with neuralgic pain who seem to have subnormal endorphinergic tonus show the best response. In a more recent study, we found that daily treatment for 1 week with TNS in neuralgic pain patients produced increases in fraction I endorphins. This effect was particularly clear in the best responders (1). These patients may therefore benefit from restitution of endorphinergic tonus induced by the TNS treatment.

CONCLUDING REMARKS

There are several apparently unique features of central opioid systems.

There is a variety of partly homologous peptides deriving from three separate prohormones. The products of these prohormones are not well-defined, each prohormone being pluripotent. In terms of measurement of activity in the different systems, this multitude gives rise to methodological problems.

The three opioid peptide systems are present in wide areas of the CNS, and they are richly represented throughout the CNS networks engaged in pain transmission. Despite their wide distribution, most observations suggest that the tonic activity in these systems is low. However, if activity is below a certain physiological level, there may be pathophysiological consequences, as suggested by observations of low CSF levels of opioid activity in patients with neuralgic pain.

Somatic stimulation may require induction of muscular activity in order to be an effective mode of activation. In clinical pain, techniques such as acupuncture and TNS give focal stimulation of these systems.

The multitude of opioid receptors suggests that there is functional subspecialization. However, all three major subclasses, mu, delta, and kappa, appear to be potential mediators of antinociceptive effects and may therefore be involved in pain modulation. The classic opiates act mainly via the mu receptor. Current drug development therefore focuses on the other receptors and may lead to more acceptable centrally acting analgesics.

ACKNOWLEDGMENT

Work from this laboratory is supported by the Swedish Medical Research Council.

REFERENCES

1. Almay, B. G. L., Johansson, F., von Knorring, L., Sakurada, T., and Terenius, L. (1985): Long-term high frequency transcutaneous electrical nerve stimulation (hi-TNS) in chronic pain. Clinical response and effects on CSF-endorphins, monoamine metabolites, substance P-like immunoreactivity (SPLI) and pain measures. *Psychosom. Res., (in press).*
2. Almay, B. G. L., Johansson, F., von Knorring, L., Terenius, L., and Wahlström, A. (1978): Endorphins in chronic pain. I. Differences in CSF endorphin levels between organic and psychogenic pain syndromes. *Pain,* 5:153–162.
3. Beckett, A. H., and Casy, A. F. (1953): Synthetic analgesics: Stereochemical considerations. *J. Pharm. Pharmacol.,* 6:986–999.
4. Bloom, F. E. (1983): The Endorphins: A growing family of pharmacologically pertinent peptides. *Annu. Rev. Pharmacol. Toxicol.,* 23:151–170.
5. Bloom, F. E. (1984): The functional significance of neurotransmitter diversity. *Am. J. Physiol.,* 246:C184–C194.
6. Brownstein, M. J. (1982): Post-translational processing of neuropeptide precursors. *Trends Neurosci.,* 5:318–320.
7. Civelli, O., Birnberg, N., Comb, M., Douglass, J., Lissitzky, J. C., Uhler, M., and Herbert, E. (1983): Regulation of opioid gene expression. *Peptides,* 4:651–656.
8. Corbett, A. D., Paterson, S. J., McKnight, A. T., Magnan, J., and Kosterlitz, H. W. (1982): Dynorphin$_{1-8}$ and dynorphin$_{1-9}$ are ligands for the *K*-subtype of opiate receptor. *Nature,* 299:79–81.
9. Devi, L., and Goldstein, A. (1983): Dynorphin converting enzyme with unusual specificity from rat brain. *Proc. Natl. Acad. Sci. U.S.A.,* 81:1892–1896.
10. Eriksson, M. B. E., Sjölund, B. H., and Nielzén, S. (1979): Long term results of peripheral conditioning stimulation as an analgesic measure in chronic pain. *Pain,* 6:335–347.
11. Feder, J., Migone, N., Chang, A. C. Y., Cochet, M., Cohen, S. N., Cann, H., and Cavalli-Sforza, L. L. (1983): A DNA polymorphism in close physical linkage with the proopiomelanocortin gene. *Am. J. Hum. Genet.,* 35:1090–1096.
12. Frederickson, R. C. A., Smithwick, E. L., Shuman, R., and Bemis, K. G. (1981): Metkephamid, a systemically active analog of methionine enkephalin with potent opioid δ-receptor activity. *Science,* 211:603–605.
13. Frost, J. J., Wagner, H. N., Dannals, R. F., et al. (1984): Imaging opiate receptors in the human brain by positron tomography. *Nature, (in press).*
14. Han, J. S., and Terenius, L. (1982): Neurochemical basis of acupuncture analgesia. *Annu. Rev. Pharmacol. Toxicol.,* 22:193–220.
15. Han, J. S., Xie, G.-X., and Goldstein, A. (1984): Analgesia induced by intrathecal injection of dynorphin B in the rat. *Life Sci.,* 34:1573–1579.
16. Herkenham, M., and Pert, C. B. (1982): Light microscopic localization of brain opiate receptors: A general autoradiographic method which preserves tissue quality. *J. Neurosci.,* 2:1129–1149.
17. Horikawa, S., Takai, T., Toyosato, M., Takahashi, H., Noda, M., Kakidani, H., Kubo, T., Hirose, T., Inayama, S., Hayashida, H., Miyata, T., and Numa, S. (1983): Isolation and structural organization of the human pre-proenkephalin B gene. *Nature,* 306:611–614.

18. Hughes, J. (1975): Isolation of an endogenous compound from the brain with pharmacological properties similar to morphine. *Brain Res.,* 88:295–308.
19. Hughes, J., Smith, T. W., Kosterlitz, H. W., Fothergill, L. A., Morgan, B. A., and Morris, H. R. (1975): Identification of two related pentapeptides from the brain with potent opiate agonist activity. *Nature,* 258:577–579.
20. Hökfelt, T., Skirboll, L., and Lundberg, J. (1983): Neuropeptides and pain pathways. In: *Advances in Pain Research and Therapy,* Vol. 5, edited by J. J. Bonica, U. Lindblom, and A. Iggo, pp. 227–246. Raven Press, New York.
21. Iwamoto, E. T., and Martin, W. R. (1981): Multiple opioid receptors. *Medicinal Res. Rev.,* 1:411–440.
22. Knorring, L. von, Terenius, L., and Wahlström, A. (1983): Fraction I endorphin in cerebrospinal fluid. In: *Neurobiology of Cerebrospinal Fluid,* Vol. 2, edited by J. H. Wood, pp. 80–86. Plenum, New York.
23. Levine, J. D., Gordon, N. C., Jones, R. T., and Fields, H. L. (1978): The narcotic antagonist naloxone enhances clinical pain. *Nature,* 272:826–827.
24. Li, C. H. (1964): Lipotropin, a new active peptide from pituitary glands. *Nature,* 201:924.
25. Lord, J. A. H., Waterfield, A. A., Hughes, J., and Kosterlitz, H. W. (1977): Endogenous opioid peptides: Multiple agonists and receptors. *Nature,* 267:495–499.
26. Lundberg, J. M., and Hökfelt, T. (1983): Coexistence of peptides and classical neurotransmitters. *Trends Neurosci.,* 6:325–333.
27. Martin, W. R., Eades, C. G., Thompson, J. A., Huppler, R. E., and Gilbert, P. E. (1976): The effects of morphine- and nalorphine-like drugs in the nondependent and morphine-dependent chronic spinal dog. *J. Pharmacol. Exp. Ther.,* 197:517–532.
28. Matsas, R., Fulcher, I. S., Kenny, A. J., and Turner, A. J. (1983): Substance P and Leu-enkephalin are hydrolyzed by an enzyme in pig caudate synaptic membranes that is identical with the endopeptidase of kidney microvilli. *Proc. Natl. Acad. Sci. U.S.A.,* 80:3111–3115.
29. Morley, J. S. (1980): Structure-activity relationships of enkephalin-like peptides. *Annu. Rev. Pharmacol. Toxicol.,* 20:81–110.
30. Nakanishi, S., Inoue, A., Kita, T., Nakamura, M., Chang, A. C. Y., Cohen, S. N., and Numa, S. (1979): Nucleotide sequence of cloned cDNA for bovine corticotropin-beta-lipotropin precursor. *Nature,* 278:423–427.
31. Nyberg, F., Wahlström, A., Sjölund, B., and Terenius, L. (1983): Characterization of electrophoretically separable endorphins in human CSF. *Brain Res.,* 259:267–274.
32. Oates, E., and Herbert, E. (1984): 5′ sequence of porcine and rat proopiomelanocortin mRNA. *J. Biol. Chem.,* 259:7421–7425.
33. Quirion, R., Hammer, R., Herkenham, M., and Pert, C. B. (1981): Phencyclidine/sigma opiate receptor; its visualization by tritium sensitive film. *Proc. Natl. Acad. Sci. U.S.A.,* 78:5881–5885.
34. Roques, B. P., Fournié-Zaluski, M. C., Soroca, E., Lecomte, J. M., Malfroy, B., Llorens, C., and Schwartz, J.-C. (1980): The enkephalinase inhibitor thiorphan shows antinociceptive activity in mice. *Nature,* 288:286–288.
35. Schulz, R., Wüster, M., and Herz, A. (1981): Pharmacological characterization of the epsilon-opiate receptor. *J. Pharmacol. Exp. Ther.,* 216:604–606.
36. Schwartz, J.-C., Malfroy, B., and De La Baume, S. (1981): Biological inactivation of enkephalins and the role of enkephalin-dipeptidyl-carboxypeptidase ('enkephalinase') as neuropeptidase. *Life Sci.,* 29:1715–1740.
37. Sternbach, R. A. (1974): *Pain Patients, Traits and Treatments.* Academic Press, New York.
38. Tang, F., Costa, E., and Schwartz, J. P. (1983): Increase of proenkephalin mRNA and enkephalin content of rat striatum after daily injection of haloperidol for 2 to 3 weeks. *Proc. Natl. Acad. Sci. U.S.A.,* 80:3841–3844.
39. Terenius, L. (1981): Endorphins and pain. *Front. Horm. Res.,* 8:162–177.
40. Terenius, L., and Wahlström, A. (1975): Search for an endogenous ligand for the opiate receptor. *Acta Physiol. Scand.,* 94:74–81.
41. Terenius, L., and Wahlström, A. (1975): Morphine-like ligand for opiate receptors in human CSF. *Life Sci.,* 16:1759–1764.
42. Weber, E., Esch, F. S., Böhlen, P., Paterson, S., Corbett, A. D., McKnight, A. T., Kosterlitz, H. W., Barchas, J. D., and Evans, C. J. (1983): Metorphamide: Isolation, structure, and

biologic activity of an amidated opioid octapeptide from bovine brain. *Proc. Natl. Acad. Sci. U.S.A.,* 80:7362–7366.

43. Weber, E., Evans, C. J., and Barchas, J. (1983): Multiple endogenous ligands for opioid receptors. *Trends Neurosci.,* 6:333–336.
44. Wüster, M., Rubini, P., and Schultz, R. (1981): The preference of putative pro-enkephalins for different types of opiate receptors. *Life Sci.,* 29:1219–1227.
45. Yaksh, T. L. (1983): *In vivo* studies on opiate receptor systems mediating antinociception. I. Mu and delta receptor profiles in the primate. *J. Pharmacol. Exp. Ther.,* 226:303–316.

Advances in Pain Research and Therapy, Vol. 9, edited by H. L. Fields et al. Raven Press, New York © 1985.

Neural Mechanisms of Opiate Analgesia

Howard L. Fields

Departments of Neurology and Physiology, University of California San Francisco, San Francisco, California 94143

Opiate agonists such as morphine are the most potent analgesic drugs in present use. Although it is generally accepted that opiates produce analgesia by an action on the central nervous system (CNS), it is only in the past two decades that details of the neuronal mechanisms of this effect have come to light. This chapter will review some of the most relevant findings.

One of the first questions to be addressed was where in the CNS opiates act to produce analgesia. The morphine microinjection technique was used to systematically map CNS sites that produce analgesia (49,55,57). Early studies concentrated on the brainstem and revealed that opiate-sensitive sites are limited to small well-defined regions in the midbrain and medullary tegmentum. There is now general agreement that antinociceptive effects are elicited by local injection of opiates at these midbrain sites (15,21,27), suggesting that anatomically discrete groups of brainstem neurons contribute to the analgesic action of systemically administered opiates. Subsequent research has confirmed this idea and greatly expanded our understanding of the neural networks that underlie morphine analgesia.

Over the past decade there has been a remarkable advance in our understanding of the networks that modulate nociceptive transmission. The best-described network has links in the midbrain periaqueductal gray (PAG), rostral ventral medulla (RVM), and spinal cord dorsal horn (9,10,35). Microinjection of morphine into either the PAG (21,28,57) or the RVM (1,5,17) produces behavioral analgesia. The PAG and RVM are reciprocally connected (13,33), and the RVM projects to the trigeminal nucleus caudalis and via the dorsolateral funiculus (DLF) to the spinal cord dorsal horn (8). Cells in RVM are an important relay for the control by PAG of nociceptive transmission at the spinal cord (12,50). Raphe-spinal cells are excited by PAG stimulation (18), and lesions of RVM block the inhibitory actions of PAG on the spinal cord (12,22). Yaksh and Rudy pointed out that the midbrain sites most sensitive to the analgesic effect of morphine are located in the caudal and ventrolateral PAG, which is known to have a large projection to RVM. Heinricher and colleagues (23) have recently shown that microinjection of morphine into ventrolateral PAG affects the firing of a significant number of RVM cells.

Description of the network linking PAG, RVM, and spinal cord led to the proposal that systemic opiates activate it and thus selectively inhibit nociceptive transmission. This proposal is supported by the observation that spinalization reduces systemic morphine's suppression of spinal nocifensor reflexes (26). A similar reduction is seen following lesions of the RVM (47) or of its spinal projection through the DLF (7). However, Yaksh and Rudy (56) observed that morphine has an analgesic effect when applied directly to the spinal cord, a finding that has been amply confirmed by subsequent clinical studies (for review, see chapter by P. R. Bromage, *this volume*). This spinal action indicates that activation of descending pathways does not completely explain systemic morphine's analgesic effect. Yaksh and Rudy (55) suggested that opiates might have both direct and indirect (i.e., supraspinal) actions on nociceptive transmission at the cord.

Although there is no doubt that morphine microinjection into the brainstem can produce analgesia, the dose required produces local tissue concentrations that are at least an order of magnitude higher than those produced by analgesic doses of systemically administered morphine (15,24). Thus, the mechanism of the analgesia produced by local application of morphine is not necessarily the same as that of the analgesia produced by systemic administration.

Resolution of these problems of the relative spinal and supraspinal contributions to systemic morphine analgesia and of the requirement of a high local tissue concentration for microinjected morphine began with the studies of Yeung and Rudy (58). They confirmed that although antinociceptive effects are produced by injection of morphine into either the lumbar intrathecal space or the third ventricle, the tissue concentrations produced by morphine microinjections sufficient for analgesia are higher than would be achieved by systemic administration of an analgesic dose of morphine. However, they found that analgesia could be produced by microinjection of much lower doses of morphine provided that injections of the lower doses were made *concurrently* at spinal and supraspinal sites. In fact, there was an apparent multiplicative analgesic effect when morphine was concurrently injected at these two anatomically separate sites, an observation that has recently been confirmed (48). This multiplicative action suggests that systemic morphine produces analgesia by acting simultaneously on neurons at multiple anatomically separate but interconnected sites. This concept is strongly supported by observations that analgesia produced by systemic injection of morphine can be blocked by microinjection of naloxone into PAG (27,28,49), RVM (5), or spinal cord (56).

What properties do these analgesia-producing opiate-sensitive CNS sites have in common? By definition, PAG, RVM, and spinal cord should all have opiate binding sites (receptor). In fact, high-affinity opiate binding has been demonstrated by autoradiography in PAG (46) and in the superficial layers of the dorsal horn (4). Furthermore, all three sites have dense concentrations of one or more of the endogenous opioid peptides (10). Enkephalins, for example, are present in PAG, RVM, and the superficial dorsal horn, and beta-endorphin is present in PAG. Beta-endorphin and metabolically stable analogs of enkephalin produce analgesia when injected intracerebrally.

It is important to point out that the opiate receptor was originally defined using the rank order of potency for clinical analgesia of a series of opiate-like drugs. It is also significant that the characterization of the opiate receptor was a crucial step in isolating the enkephalins (25). Thus, the close anatomical association between the endorphins and the components of the analgesia network supports the notion that the proposed nociceptive modulatory network has physiological significance. A corollary of this idea is that modulation of nociceptive transmission is an important physiological function of the endorphins. Furthermore, although they are found elsewhere in the CNS, the presence of endorphins in high concentration at sites at which morphine microinjection produces analgesia suggests that exogenous opiates may act, in part, by mimicking the action of endorphins at opiate receptors in the analgesia network.

ACTIONS OF OPIATES ON NEURONS OF THE NOCICEPTIVE MODULATORY CIRCUIT

In order to further analyze the mechanism of opiate analgesia, it is necessary to determine what effects opiates have on the neurons that have been proposed to modulate pain transmission. In the brainstem components of the network, electrical stimulation and microinjection of glutamate and of opiate agonists all inhibit spinal nociceptive transmission. Because glutamate and electrical stimulation directly excite all neural elements, the net effect of locally injected morphine must be to excite the inhibitory output neurons that project from PAG to RVM or from RVM to spinal cord (10,55). Although there were reports that systemic, iontophoretic, or PAG-microinjected opiates had a predominantly excitatory effect on neurons in the medullary reticular formation, these early studies were inconclusive, because inhibition or no effect was also observed (18,21,39,40). One possible reason for the inconsistent results is that the neurons in the PAG and RVM represent functionally heterogeneous populations. In fact, recent studies in our laboratory have shown that opiates have more consistent actions on physiologically defined subpopulations of brainstem neurons.

We recorded the activity of neurons in RVM during application of noxious heat to the tail. Rats were lightly anesthetized so that they could still flick their tails, and the degree to which cell firing was correlated with the heat stimulus or with the tail flick was determined. We found a class of neuron, the off-cell, that was inhibited by noxious stimuli over most of the body surface and that paused just before the tail flick occurred (19). We demonstrated that these off-cells are excited by PAG stimulation (50) and that a significant proportion project to the spinal cord (51). We propose that these spinally projecting off-cells are the crucial elements in RVM that inhibit nociceptive transmission. Thus, electrical stimulation of RVM blocks nociceptive transmission by preventing off-cells from pausing. Consistent with this idea is our observation (20) that systemic morphine in analgesic doses increases the mean "spontaneous" discharge frequency and blocks the pause of off-cells. The pause would otherwise permit the tail flick to occur. Morphine microinjected into the PAG has the same effect (23). Other classes of cells in RVM are not affected in the same way. One can tentatively conclude that opiates have an excitatory action on the RVM off-cells that we have proposed project to and inhibit nociceptive transmission neurons in the spinal cord.

Cellular Mechanisms

The studies described earlier using extracellular recording cannot reveal whether or not the excitatory action of morphine on the off-cells is direct. In fact, inhibition seems to be the most common effect of opiates on neurons (42,43), but also see Gebhart (21), and studies to date of direct cellular actions of opiates using *in vitro* methods have revealed only inhibitory actions (38). Opiates inhibit acetylcholine release in the sympathetic ganglion (14,31) and substance P release from dorsal root ganglion cells (29,41). The latter effect apparently is the result of reducing a voltage-dependent inward Ca^{2+} current (41,52). In mouse dorsal root ganglion cells there is some evidence that opiates increase K^+ conductance. This could secondarily reduce a voltage-dependent Ca^{2+} current (53) and explain the opiate-induced reduction of transmitter release (32). Such a presynaptic action on the terminals of primary afferent nociceptors could contribute to the analgesic effect that is observed when opiates are applied directly to the spinal cord.

In addition, opiates act postsynaptically, hyperpolarizing myenteric plexus neurons (44), dorsal horn interneurons (37,59), and norepinephrine-containing cells in the locus ceruleus (54). Each of these effects is apparently the result of increased K^+ conductance.

Thus, there is abundant evidence for both presynaptic and postsynaptic inhibitory actions of opiates. There is as yet no evidence for a direct excitatory effect of opiates on nerve cells, although the possibility has not been ruled out. This observed lack of any direct excitatory action of opiates *in vitro* has to be reconciled with the evidence discussed earlier that, *in vivo,* systemic or microinjected opiates have a net excitatory action on putative nociceptive modulating neurons. One possibility is that the excitation of off-cells may result from inhibiting an inhibitory input (55). In fact, Nicoll and colleagues (42) have demonstrated that enkephalin blocks several forms of inhibition in the CNS. For example, hippocampal pyramidal cells are strongly excited by enkephalin. This action results from inhibiting an inhibitory GABA-containing interneuron. They proposed that disinhibition may be a common action of opiates in the CNS. More direct evidence for disinhibition in PAG or RVM is necessary.

Possible Analgesic Actions of Morphine at Rostral Sites

Thus far, this discussion has focused on the contribution of the well-described descending pathways to morphine analgesia. It may be that these descending systems are sufficient to completely account for morphine analgesia, but it is also possible that other opiate actions contribute to analgesia.

Although there has been little documentation, some authors have stated that opiates have a disproportionately powerful action on what Beecher (11) called the "reactive" component of pain. Obviously, the descending pathways, by reducing activity in ascending pathways, could reduce the perceived intensity of and therefore the reaction to a noxious stimulus. However, the emotional or "affective-motivational" component of the pain experience may represent activity in forebrain structures that are anatomically distinct from those underlying the purely sensory functions (36).

Early studies on animals demonstrated that escape or avoidance behavior can be elicited by electrical stimulation of diencephalic (45) and limbic cortical structures (16). Barber has reviewed data on patients treated for intractable pain by frontal lobotomy or cingulumotomy (6). These patients became apathetic and complained less about their pain. The most striking observation was that when questioned, most of the patients said their pain was still present, though they showed little anxiety. Interestingly, when standard experimental methods were used, many of these patients reported pain thresholds that were unchanged or *even lower* after surgery that appeared to relieve their pain. Beecher has remarked on the similarity between the effect of morphine and that of lobotomy (11, p. 117).

Opiates could inhibit the reactive component of pain by a direct action on forebrain structures activated by nociceptive input. In fact, opiates have been shown to inhibit cortical neurons (61). However, another possibility is that opiates activate an ascending modulatory pathway. In fact, both PAG (34) and RVM (60) project rostrally to medial and intralaminar thalamus and hypothalamus, which in turn project to limbic structures. Electrical stimulation of dorsal raphe inhibits intralaminar nociceptive neurons in rats (2). The inhibition is blocked by the serotonergic neurotoxin 5,7-dihydroxytryptamine and mimicked by local iontophoresis of 5-HT (3). Morphine microinjected into PAG inhibits neurons in ventrobasal thalamus (30). These effects, however, could all be explained by a descending inhibition of spinal or brainstem inputs to these thalamic regions. Thus, any analgesic effect of morphine other than by activating descending pathways is little more than conjecture at this point.

In summary, current evidence indicates that systemic morphine produces analgesia by activating an intrinisic endorphin-mediated analgesia network. It acts concurrently at multiple widely separated sites in brainstem and spinal cord. Part of its action depends on disinhibiting brainstem neurons that project to and inhibit spinal nociceptive transmission cells.

ACKNOWLEDGMENTS

Mary Heinricher made valuable suggestions on the text, and Steve Guinn provided editorial assistance. Research support was provided by USPHS grants DA-01949 and NS-07442 and by the National Migraine Foundation.

REFERENCES

1. Akaike, A., Shibata, T., Satoh, M., and Takagi, H. (1978): Analgesia induced by microinjection of morphine into and electrical stimulation of nucleus reticularis paragigantocellularis of the rat medulla oblongata. *Neuropharmacology,* 17:775–778.
2. Andersen, E., and Dafny, N. (1982): An ascending serotonergic pain modulation pathway from the dorsal raphe nucleus to the parafascicularis nucleus of the thalamus. *Brain Res.,* 269:57–67.
3. Andersen, E., and Dafny, N. (1983): Microiontophoretically applied 5-HT reduces responses to noxious stimulation in the thalamus. *Brain Res.,* 241:176–178.
4. Atweh, S. F., and Kuhar, M. J. (1977): Autoradiographic localization of opiate receptors in rat brain. I. Spinal cord and lower medulla. *Brain Res.,* 124:53–67.
5. Azami, J., Llewelyn, M. B., and Roberts, M. H. T. (1982): The contribution of nucleus reticularis paragigantocellularis and nucleus raphe magnus to the analgesia produced by systemically administered morphine, investigated with the microinjection technique. *Pain,* 12:229–246.
6. Barber, T. X. (1959): Toward a theory of pain: Relief of chronic pain by prefrontal leucotomy, opiates, placebos, and hypnosis. *Psychol. Bull,* 56:430–460.
7. Barton, C., Basbaum, A. I., and Fields, H. L. (1980): Dissociation of supraspinal and spinal actions of morphine: A quantitative evaluation. *Brain Res.,* 188:487–498.
8. Basbaum, A. I., Clanton, C. H., and Fields, H. L. (1977): Three bulbospinal pathways from the rostral medulla of the cat. An autoradiographic study of pain modulating systems. *J. Comp. Neurol.,* 178:209–224.
9. Basbaum, A. I., and Fields, H. L. (1978): Endogenous pain control mechanisms: Review and hypothesis. *Ann. Neurol.,* 4:451–462.
10. Basbaum, A. I., and Fields, H. L. (1984): Endogenous pain control systems: Brainstem spinal pathways and endorphin circuitry. *Annu. Rev. Neurosci.,* 7:309–338.
11. Beecher, H. K. (1959): *Measurement of Subjective Responses: Quantitative Effects of Drugs.* Oxford University Press, New York.
12. Behbehani, M. M., and Fields, H. L. (1979): Evidence that an excitatory connection between the periaqueductal gray and nucleus raphe magnus mediates stimulation produced analgesia. *Brain Res.,* 170:85–93.
13. Beitz, A. J. (1982): The organization of afferent projections to the midbrain periaqueductal grey of the rat. *Neuroscience,* 7:133–159.
14. Bornstein, J. C., and Fields, H. L. (1979): Morphine presynaptically inhibits a ganglionic cholinergic synapse. *Neurosci. Lett.,* 15:77–82.
15. Clark, S. L., Edeson, R. O., and Ryall, R. W. (1983): The relative significance of spinal and supraspinal actions in the antinociceptive effect of morphine in the dorsal horn: An evaluation of the microinjection technique. *Br. J. Pharmacol.,* 79:807–818.

16. Delgado, J. M. R. (1955): Cerebral structures involved in transmission and elaboration of noxious stimulation. *J. Neurophysiol.,* 18:261–275.
17. Dickenson, A. H., Oliveras, J. L., and Besson, J. M. (1979): Role of the nucleus raphe magnus in opiate analgesia as studied by the microinjection technique in the rat. *Brain Res.,* 170:95–111.
18. Fields, H. L., and Anderson, S. D. (1978): Evidence that raphespinal neurons mediate opiate and midbrain stimulation produced analgesia. *Pain,* 5:333–349.
19. Fields, H. L., Bry, J., Hentall, I. D., and Zorman, G. (1983): The activity of neurons in the rostral medulla of the rat during withdrawal from noxious heat. *J. Neurosci.,* 3:2545–2552.
20. Fields, H. L., Vanegas, H., Hentall, I. D., and Zorman, G. (1983b): Evidence that disinhibition of brain stem neurones contributes to morphine analgesia. *Nature,* 306:684–686.
21. Gebhart, G. F. (1982): Opiate and opioid peptide effects on brain stem neurons: Relevance to nociception and antinociceptive mechanisms. *Pain,* 12:93–140.
22. Gebhart, G. F., Sandkuhler, J., Thalhammer, J. G., and Zimmerman, M. (1983): Inhibition of spinal nociceptive information by stimulation in midbrain of the cat is blocked by lidocaine microinjected in nucleus raphe magnus and medullary reticular formation. *J. Neurophysiol.,* 50:1446–1459.
23. Heinricher, M. M., Cheng, Z.-F., and Fields, H. L. (1984): Differential effect of microinjection of morphine into the periaqueductal gray on activity of two classes of neurons in the rostral ventromedial medulla. *Soc. Neurosci. Abstr.,* 10:100.
24. Herz, A., and Teschemacher, H.-J. (1971): Activities and sites of antinociceptive action of morphine-like analgesics and kinetics of distribution following intravenous, intracerebral and intraventricular application. *Adv. Drug Res.,* 6:79–119.
25. Hughes, J., Smith, T. W., Kosterlitz, H. W., Fothergill, L. A., Morgan, B. A., and Morris, H. R. (1975): Identification of two related pentapeptides from the brain with potent opiate agonist activity. *Nature,* 258:577–579.
26. Irwin, S., Houde, R. W., Bennett, D. R., Hendershot, L. C., and Seevers, M. H. (1950): The effects of morphine, methadone and meperidine on some reflex reponses of spinal animals to nociceptive stimulation. *J. Pharmacol. Exp. Ther.,* 101:132–143.
27. Jacquet, Y. F., and Lajtha, A. (1973): Morphine action at central nervous sites in the rat: Analgesia or hyperalgesia depending on site and dose. *Science,* 182:490–492.
28. Jacquet, Y. F., and Lajtha, A. (1976): The periaqueductal gray: Site of morphine analgesia and tolerance as shown by 2-way cross tolerance between systemic and intracerebral injections. *Brain Res.,* 103:501–513.
29. Jessell, T. M., and Iversen, L. L. (1977): Opiate analgesics inhibit substance P release from rat trigeminal nucleus. *Nature,* 268:549–551.
30. Kayser, V., Benoist, J.-M., and Guilbaud, G. (1983): Low dose of morphine microinjected in the ventral periaqueductal gray matter of the rat depresses responses of nociceptive ventrobasal thalamic neurons. *Neurosci. Lett.,* 37:193–198.
31. Konishi, S., Tsunoo, A., and Otsuka, M. (1979): Enkephalins presynaptically inhibit cholinergic transmission in sympathetic ganglia. *Nature,* 282:515–516.
32. MacDonald, R. L., and Nelson, P. G. (1978): Specific-opiate-induced depression of transmitter release from dorsal root ganglion cells in culture. *Science,* 199:1449–1450.
33. Mantyh, P. W. (1982): The ascending input to the midbrain periaqueductal gray of the primate. *J. Comp. Neurol.,* 211:50–64.
34. Mantyh, P. W. (1983): The connections of the midbrain periaqueductal gray in the monkey. I. The ascending efferent projections. *J. Neurophysiol.,* 49:567–581.
35. Mayer, D. J., and Price, D. D. (1976): Central nervous system mechanisms of analgesia. *Pain,* 2:379–404.
36. Melzack, R., and Casey, K. L. (1968): Sensory, motivational, and central control determinants of pain. In: *International Symposium on the Skin Senses,* edited by D. R. Kenshalo, pp. 423–439. Charles C Thomas, Springfield, Ill.
37. Miletic, V., and Randic, M. (1982): Neonatal rat spinal cord slice preparation: Postsynaptic effects of neuropeptides on dorsal horn neurons. *Dev. Brain Res.,* 2:432–438.
38. Miller, R. (1984): How do opiates act? *Trends Neurosci.,* 7:184–185.
39. Mohrland, J. S., and Gebhart, G. F. (1980): Effects of focal electrical stimulation and morphine microinjection in the periaqueductal gray of the rat mesencephalon on neuronal activity in the medullary reticular formation. *Brain Res.,* 201:23–37.
40. Mohrland, J. S., and Gebhart, G. F. (1981): Effect of morphine administered in the peria-

queductal gray and at the recording locus on nociresponsive neurons in the medullary reticular formation. *Brain Res.,* 225:401–412.
41. Mudge, A. W., Leeman, S. E., and Fischbach, G. D. (1979): Enkephalin inhibits release of substance P from sensory neurons in culture and decreases action potential duration. *Proc. Natl. Acad. Sci. U.S.A.,* 76:526–530.
42. Nicoll, R. A., Alger, B. E., and Jahr, C. E. (1980): Enkephalin blocks inhibitory pathways in the vertebrate CNS. *Nature,* 287:22–25.
43. North, R. A. (1979): Opiates, opioid peptides and single neurones. *Life Sci.,* 24:1527–1546.
44. North, R. A., Katayama, Y., and Williams, J. T. (1979): On the mechanism and site of action of enkephalin on single myenteric neurons. *Brain Res.,* 165:67–77.
45. Olds, M. E., and Olds, J. (1963): Approach-avoidance analysis of rat diencephalon. *J. Comp. Neurol.,* 120:259–295.
46. Pert, C. B., Kuhar, M. J., and Snyder, S. H. (1976): Opiate receptor: Autoradiographic localization in rat brain. *Proc. Natl. Acad. Sci. U.S.A.,* 73:3729–3733.
47. Proudfit, H. K., and Anderson, E. G. (1975): Morphine analgesia: Blockade by raphe magnus lesions. *Brain Res.,* 98:612–618.
48. Roerig, S. C., O'Brien, S. H., Fujimoto, J. M., and Wilcox, G. L. (1984): Tolerance to morphine analgesia: Decreased multiplicative interaction between spinal and supraspinal sites. *Brain Res.,* 308:360–363.
49. Tsou, K., and Jang, C. S. (1964): Studies on the site of analgesic action of morphine by intracerebral microinjections. *Sci. Sin.,* 13:1099–1109.
50. Vanegas, H., Barbaro, N. M., and Fields, H. L. (1984): Midbrain stimulation inhibits tail-flick only at currents sufficient to excite rostral medullary neurons. *Brain Res.,* 321:127–133.
51. Vanegas, H., Barbaro, N. M., and Fields, H. L. (1984): Tail-flick related activity in medullospinal neurons. *Brain Res.,* 321:135–141.
52. Werz, M. A., and MacDonald, R. L. (1982): Opioid peptides decrease calcium-dependent action potential duration of mouse dorsal root ganglion neurons in cell culture. *Brain Res.,* 239:315–321.
53. Werz, M. A., and MacDonald, R. L. (1983): Opioid peptides selective for mu- and delta-opiate receptors reduce calcium-dependent action potential duration by increasing potassium conductance. *Neurosci. Lett.,* 42:173–178.
54. Williams, J. T., Egan, T. M., and North, R. A. (1982): Enkephalin opens potassium channels on mammalian central neurones. *Nature,* 299:74–77.
55. Yaksh, T. L., and Rudy, T. A. (1978): Narcotic analgesics: CNS sites and mechanisms of action as revealed by intracerebral injection techniques. *Pain,* 4:299–359.
56. Yaksh, T. L., and Rudy, T. A. (1977): Studies on the direct spinal action of narcotics in the production of analgesia in the rat. *J. Pharmacol. Exp. Ther.,* 202:411–428.
57. Yaksh, T. L., Yeung, J. C., and Rudy, T. A. (1976): Systemic examination in the rat of brain sites sensitive to the direct application of morphine: Observation of differential effects within the periaqueductal gray. *Brain Res.,* 114:83–103.
58. Yeung, J. C., and Rudy, T. (1980): Multiplicative interaction between narcotic agonisms expressed at spinal and supraspinal sites of antinociceptive action as revealed by concurrent intrathecal and intracerebroventricular injections of morphine. *J. Pharmacol. Exp. Ther.,* 215:633–642.
59. Yoshimura, M., and North, R. A. (1983): Substantia gelatinosa neurones hyperpolarized *in vitro* by enkephalin. *Nature,* 305:529–530.
60. Zemlan, F. P., Behbehani, M. M., and Beckstead, R. M. (1984): Ascending and descending projections from nucleus reticularis magnocellularis and nucleus reticularis gigantocellularis: An autoradiographic and horseradish peroxidase study in the rat. *Brain Res.,* 292:207–220.
61. Zieglgansberger, W., Fry, J. P., Herz, A., Moroder, L., and Wunsch, E. (1976): Enkephalin-induced inhibition of cortical neurones and the lack of this effect in morphine tolerant/dependent rats. *Brain Res.,* 115:160–164.

Advances in Pain Research and Therapy, Vol. 9, edited by H. L. Fields et al. Raven Press, New York © 1985.

Activation of Dorsal Hypothalamus-Spinal Dorsal Horn Descending Inhibitory System by Cyclazocine, an Analgesic Drug

Masamichi Satoh, Shin-ich Kawajiri, and Hiroshi Takagi

Department of Pharmacology, Faculty of Pharmaceutical Sciences, Kyoto University, Sakyo-ku, Kyoto 606, Japan

Electrical and chemical stimulation of the periaqueductal gray (PAG) and rostral ventromedial medulla including the nucleus raphe magnus (NRM) and nucleus reticularis paragigantocellularis (NRPG) is known to produce behavioral analgesia and inhibition of spinal pain transmission neurons (3). Behavioral studies have shown that analgesia is also produced by electrical stimulation of more rostral structures (8). Recently, Carstens (1) reported that electrical stimulation of the medial hypothalamus of the cat reduced the responses of single lumbar dorsal horn neurons to noxious radiant heating of footpad skin. In a preliminary study, we observed a dose-dependent analgesic effect of cyclazocine, a potent agonist-antagonist analgesic, microinjected into the dorsal hypothalamic area of the rat, in the bradykinin (BK)-induced flexor reflex test (S. Kawajiri and M. Satoh, *unpublished data*). Kawajiri and Satoh (5) showed that systemic cyclazocine depressed the activity of dorsal horn neurons induced by intra-arterial injection of BK (painful stimulation) by facilitating descending inhibitory systems which originate from supraspinal structures. These observations prompted us to examine whether or not microinjection of cyclazocine into, and electrical stimulation of, the dorsal hypothalamic area inhibits the BK-induced responses of single dorsal horn neurons.

METHODS

Experiments were performed on ether-anesthetized, male albino rabbits (2.5–3.2 kg) that were fixed on a stereotaxic apparatus, immobilized with gallamine triethiodide, and artificially respired. All wound edges and pressure points were infiltrated with lidocaine throughout the experiments. Microinjections of cyclazocine (10 μg/1.0 μl/rabbit for 80–120 sec) into the dorsal hypothalamic area were coordinately given by means of an injection cannula (0.3 mm o.d.) according to the atlas of Sawyer et al. (10); A:2 ~ P:2, L:0.5 ~ 2.0, H:+1 ~ −3.

Electrical stimulation (pulse duration; 0.5 msec, 200–400 μA, 10 pulses of 200 Hz/sec for 3–4 min) of the same area was delivered through a bipolar stainless-steel electrode inserted stereotaxically. Tungsten microelectrodes were used for extracellular recording of unitary activity of the lamina-V-type neurons at the L6 level of the spinal cord which was exposed by lumbar laminectomy. The neuron was stimulated peripherally by single injections of BK (Protein Research Foundation, Mino, Japan; 0.5–5.0 μg) into the femoral artery, at a fixed interval of 5 or 10 min. In the present experiments, we selected only those neurons that showed evidence of excitation due to intra-arterial injection of BK. The difference between the numbers of spikes during the 64-sec period before and after each BK injection was regarded as BK-induced activity. The 95% confidence limits were calculated using three or more values of BK-induced activity obtained before the microinjection of cyclazocine or electrical stimulation. When the BK-induced activity was below the confidence limits after such treatments, the effect was regarded as being inhibitory. Each rabbit was used only once. At the end of each experiment, the site of microinjection or electrical stimulation was histologically verified.

The drugs used were cyclazocine (a gift from Torii, Tokyo, Japan) and naloxone HCl (a gift from Endo Laboratories, Garden City, New York). The former was dissolved in physiological saline containing 0.5% lactate and the latter in physiological saline.

RESULTS

The effects of microinjections of cyclazocine into various sites in the dorsal hypothalamic area were examined on 21 lamina-V-type neurons of the lumbar dorsal horn (21 rabbits). As shown in Fig. 1, cyclazocine (10 μg) microinjected into the site just dorsal to the nucleus paraventricularis (PV) (AP:0, L:0.8, H:−1; see inset of Fig. 1) significantly inhibited the BK-induced excitatory response. This inhibition appeared within 3 min after the microinjection and lasted for 80 min or more; it was reversed by intravenous naloxone (0.3 mg/kg), indicating the involvement of specific opioid receptors. Similar effects of cyclazocine were obtained following microinjections of the drug into the area surrounding the PV and dorsal part of medial preoptic area at the levels of A:1 ~ AP:0 (Fig. 2). Such levels correspond to those of the rostral part of arcuate nucleus. However, the other sites examined were not effective in depressing BK-induced responses of lumbar lamina-V-type neurons. Spontaneous activity was increased by microinjections of cyclazocine in the dorsal hypothalamic area in 6 of 21 lumbar lamina-V-type neurons examined, but activity was unaffected in the other neurons. In

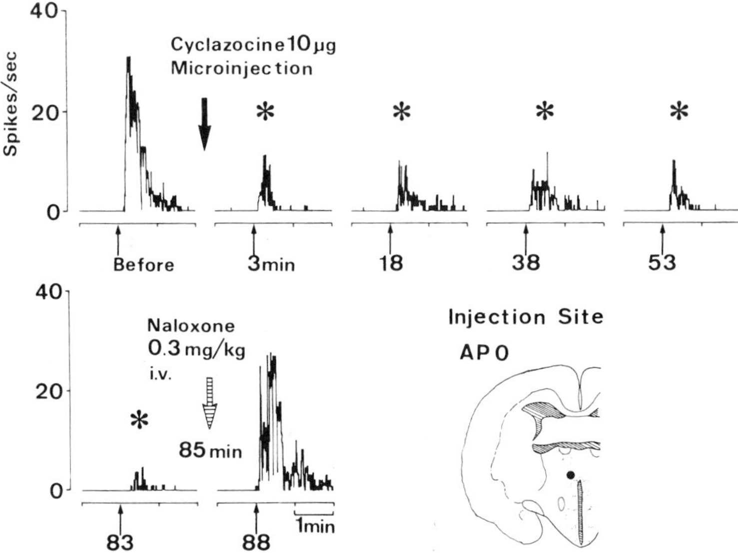

FIG. 1. Inhibitory effect of cyclazocine (10 μg/rabbit) microinjected into a site in the dorsal hypothalamic area on the BK-induced response of a lumbar lamina-V-type neuron and its reversal by naloxone (0.3 mg/kg, i.v.). At *upward arrows* BK was injected into the femoral artery in an interval of 5 min. *Asterisk* indicates a significant inhibition. Before microinjection of cyclazocine the BK-induced responses were observed three times. Note: all BK-induced responses are not represented. *Filled circle* in the inset [APO plane of the atlas of Sawyer et al. (10)] shows the microinjection site.

2 out of 6 neurons tested, the BK-induced responses were suppressed by cyclazocine. Thus, there was no consistent correlation between the effects of cyclazocine microinjected into the dorsal hypothalamic area on BK-induced and spontaneous activities of lumbar lamina-V-type neurons. Further, such microinjections did not produce any notable changes in blood pressure and heart rate. The vehicle alone in a volume of 1.0 μl did not significantly affect the spinal unitary activities, blood pressure, and heart rate.

Electrical stimulation of the region at which microinjections of cyclazocine were effective suppressed the BK-induced responses of the lumbar lamina-V-type neurons without affecting spontaneous activities in all of 3 rabbits tested.

DISCUSSION

Systemic cyclazocine has been reported to produce a dose-dependent and potent antinociceptive effect in the BK-induced flexor reflex test (9) but not in the tail-flick and the hot-plate methods (4). Furthermore, intraveous cyclazocine (0.5 mg/kg) inhibited the BK-induced activity of lumbar lamina-V-type neurons in the intact preparation, but this inhibition was tem-

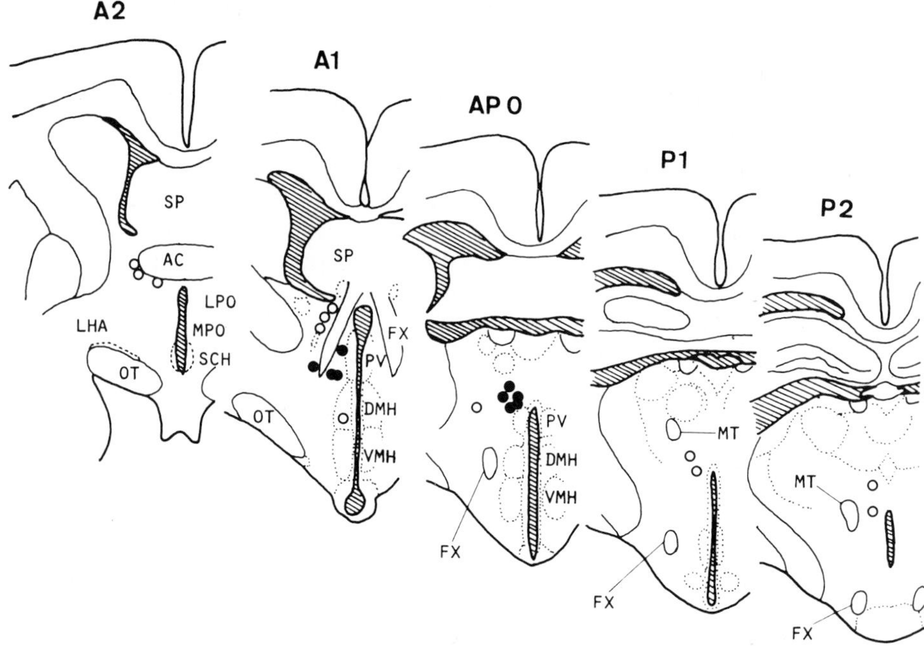

FIG. 2. Sites of microinjections of cyclazocine (10 μg/rabbit) plotted on the planes from A2 to P2 of the atlas of Sawyer et al. (10). *Filled circles* show sites where the microinjections produced an inhibition of the BK-induced responses of lamina-V-type neurons. *Open circles* indicate sites where similar microinjections did not produce such an inhibition. AC, anterior commissure; DMH, n. dorsomedial hypothalami; FX, fornix; LHA, lateral hypothalamic area; LPO, lateral preoptic area; MPO, medial preoptic area; MT, mammillothalamic tract; OT, optic tract; PV, n. paraventricularis; SCH, n. suprachiasmatics; SP, septum pellucidum; VMH, n. ventromedialis hypothalami.

porarily reversed during transient spinalization by cold block (5). The results obtained in the present experiments provided the first evidence that the medial part of the dorsal hypothalamic area at the level of the rostral part of the arcuate nucleus is one of the primary target sites of an analgesic cyclazocine for suppressing nociceptive information at the spinal dorsal horn. Such a mechanism probably underlies the analgesic action of cyclazocine. Electrical stimulation of that region inhibited the BK-induced response of lumbar lamina-V-type neurons. On the other hand, discrete electrolytic lesions of the dorsal part of the medial hypothalamus of the rat, corresponding to the site of action of cyclazocine revealed in this study using rabbits, has been shown to induce clear-cut hyperalgesia (13). These observations suggest that the medial part of the dorsal hypothalamic area plays an important role in the production of antinociception.

Carstens (1) showed that, in the cat, the most effective sites at which electrical stimulation inhibited dorsal horn unit heat-evoked responses were in the periventricular gray region at posterior through anterior hypothalamic levels. Such a region seems to include the cyclazocine sensitive sites shown in the present experiments, but the latter are localized in a rather limited region, possibly because of the distribution of the opioid receptors with high affinity to cyclazocine. Moreover, noxious stimuli employed were different with Carstens (heating the skin) and us (intraarterial injection of BK). In this context, it was recently found in our laboratory that different neuropeptides, substance P and somatostatin, in the primary afferents are separately involved in the transmission of different modalities of pains produced by noxious pinching and heating, respectively (6). Although the neurotransmitter(s) in the primary afferents mediating BK-induced pain is not known, the nociceptive information resulting from different noxious stimuli may be differentially regulated by various descending and/or propriospinal neuronal systems in the spinal dorsal horn.

Concerning the descending systems mediating the inhibition of spinal nociceptive transmission by medial hypothalamic stimulation, Carstens et al. (2) suggested an involvement of the serotonergic systems. On the other hand, anatomical studies have established that the PV neurons containing vasopressin or oxytocin project not only to the neurohypophysis but also to the spinal cord (11,12). Further, electrical stimulation of the PV of the rat has been demonstrated to yield increased amounts of immunoreactive vasopressin and oxytocin in the spinal perfusates (7). Preliminarily, we observed an analgesic effect of oxytocin intrathecally injected (M. Yasui et al., *unpublished data*). Thus, the direct descending pathway from the PV to the spinal dorsal horn might be mediating the inhibition of nociceptive transmission in the spinal dorsal horn following stimulation of the dorsal hypothalamus. The mechanisms of descending inhibitory influence of cyclazocine microinjected into the dorsal hypothalamic area remain to be elucidated.

In conclusion, microinjection of cyclazocine into, and electrical stimulation of, the medial part of the dorsal hypothalamic area inhibited the BK-induced responses of the lumbar lamina-V-type neurons. Such a descending inhibition probably underlies the analgesic action of cyclazocine.

ACKNOWLEDGMENTS

We thank M. Ohara for reading the manuscript. Part of this study was supported by a grant-in-aid for scientific research (58480404) from the Ministry of Education, Science and Culture of Japan.

REFERENCES

1. Carstens, E. (1982): Inhibition of spinal dorsal horn neuronal responses to noxious skin heating by medial hypothalamic stimulation in the cat. *J. Neurophysiol.*, 48:808–822.
2. Carstens, E., MacKinnon, J. D., and Guinan, M. J. (1983): Serotonin involvement in

descending inhibition of spinal nociceptive transmission produced by stimulation of medial diencephalon and basal forebrain. *J. Neurosci.,* 3:2112–2120.
3. Fields, H. L. (1984): Brainstem mechanisms of pain modulation. In: *Advances in Pain Research and Therapy,* Vol. 6, edited by L. Kruger and J. C. Liebeskind, pp. 241–252. Raven Press, New York.
4. Harris, L. S., and Pierson, A. K. (1964): Some narcotic antagonists in the benzomorphan series. *J. Pharmacol. Exp. Ther.,* 143:141–148.
5. Kawajiri, S., and Satoh, M. (1982): Temporary spinalization reverses the inhibitory effect of cyclazocine on the nociceptive response of rabbit spinal dorsal horn lamina V-type neurons. *Eur. J. Pharmacol.,* 78:237–240.
6. Kuraishi, Y., Hirota, N., Sato, Y., Hino, Y., Satoh, M., and Takagi, H. (1985): Evidence that substance P and somatostatin transmit separate information related to pain in the spinal dorsal horn. *Brain Res.,* 325:294–298.
7. Pittman, Q. J., Riphagen, C. L., and Lederis, K. (1984): Release of immunoassayable neurohypophyseal peptides from rat spinal cord, in vivo. *Brain Res.,* 300:321–326.
8. Rhodes, D. L., and Liebeskind, J. C. (1978): Analgesia from rostral brain stem stimulation in the rat. *Brain Res.,* 143:521–532.
9. Satoh, M., Kawajiri, S., Yamamoto, M., Foong, F.-W., and Masuda, C. (1979): Analgesic action of cyclazocine: blocking nociceptive responses induced by intra-arterial bradykinin-injection and tooth pulp stimulation. *Arch. Int. Pharmacodyn.,* 241:300–305.
10. Sawyer, C. H., Everett, J. W., and Green, J. D. (1954): The rabbit diencephalon in stereotaxic coordinates. *J. Comp. Neurol.,* 101:801–824.
11. Swanson, L. W., and McKellar, S. (1979): The distribution of oxytocin- and neurophysin-stained fibers in the spinal cord of the rat and monkey. *J. Comp. Neurol.,* 188:87–106.
12. Swanson, L. W., Sawchenko, P. E., Wiegand, S. J., and Price, J. L. (1980): Separate neurons in the paraventricular nucleus project to the median eminence and to the medulla or spinal cord. *Brain Res.,* 198:190–195.
13. Vidal, C., and Jacob, J. (1980): The effect of medial hypothalamus lesions on pain control. *Brain Res.,* 199:89–100.

Advances in Pain Research and Therapy, Vol. 9, edited by H. L. Fields et al. Raven Press, New York © 1985.

Midbrain Stimulation-Induced Antinociception in the Rat: Characterization of Role of Brain β-Endorphin

Maria H. Millan, Mark J. Millan, and Albert Herz

Department of Neuropharmacology, Max-Planck-Institut für Psychiatrie, D-8033 Planegg-Martinsried, Federal Republic of Germany

It is well-established that electrical stimulation of certain regions of the midbrain or brainstem reliably elicits antinociception both in experimental animals and in man (1,3,6,7,10,15,19). Particularly well-studied has been the periaqueductal gray and adjacent regions of the midbrain as regards a possible role of opioids in the mediation of stimulation-induced antinociception (SIA). Though midbrain SIA shows tolerance and cross-tolerance to morphine, studies in rats have yielded contradictory data concerning the effect of naloxone, with SIA being either refractory to, or susceptible to, attenuation by this opioid antagonist (see refs. 7,10,15). Recent studies indicate that the precise location of the stimulating electrode may be a critical variable underlying these discrepancies with sites in and around the dorsal raphe and ventral to the aqueduct yielding an SIA highly sensitive to blockade by opioid antagonists (1,15). Although endogenous opioids appear to participate in SIA, the particular opioid(s) responsible remains unidentified.

The following points suggest that β-endorphin (β-EP) could be a possible candidate.

Firstly, β-EP-containing fibers that originate from perikarya in the mediobasal arcuate hypothalamus are present in this region of the midbrain (4,13).

Secondly, administration of β-EP into the brain (or directly into the PAG) leads to a profound antinociception readily reversible by naloxone (7,8,16).

Thirdly, in man, midbrain electrical stimulation produces both a naloxone-sensitive antinociception and an increased level of immunoreactive (ir)-β-EP in the CSF (6,7).

Fourthly, there is evidence suggestive of a role of central β-EP in the determination of basal nociceptive thresholds and in the mediation of the antinociception elicited by either acute stress or acupuncture in the rat (17,18).

We have, thus, evaluated the influence of either naloxone or destruction of central β-EP-containing neurons on midbrain SIA in the rat.

METHODS

Male Sprague-Dawley rats were stereotaxically implanted under pentobarbitol anesthesia with single, bipolar, twisted stainless-steel electrodes (diameter 125μm). These were aimed at the dorsal raphe and adjacent tissue lying ventral to the aqueduct and including the tegmental part of the dorsal lateral fasciculus. Seven days were allowed for recovery prior to testing, during which time the rats were adapted to handling and to the test procedures. Stimulation of freely moving animals comprised 5 min of constant-current (pulse duration 50 μsec, pulse delay 10 μsec, train duration 425 msec). Extensive preliminary experiments showed that 200 to 250 μsec of current was sufficient to reliably induce a significant rise in nociceptive thresholds and 225 μA was employed in these studies. Tail-flick latencies to noxious heat were read as previously with a mean of 4 readings at each time-point taken. Intensity was adjusted to give basal values of 3.5 to 4.0 sec and a cut-off of 8 sec was enforced. For the naloxone study, latencies were read, rats injected with naloxone (2 mg/kg, 4.0 ml/kg, i.p.) or saline, allowed to rest for 10 min, latencies re-read, stimulated for 5 min, and latencies read immediately poststimulation. The experimenter did not know whether the rats had received naloxone or saline.

An independent group of rats were subjected to bilateral radiofrequency lesions of the mediobasal arcuate hypothalamus (electrode tip at 55° C for 25 sec) or sham operations (unheated electrode) as described previously (11). While still under anesthetic, the stimulating electrode was implanted. On testing, latencies were determined, rats stimulated for 5 min, and latencies immediately re-read.

Two days after the evaluation of stimulation antinociception, rats were decapitated and electrode positions evaluated in frontal sections stained with toluidine blue. In the case of the lesioned rats, the hypothalamus and septum were also taken and levels of ir-β-EP determined as described previously (11).

RESULTS

Histological examination of brains revealed that the electrodes were invariably well below the aqueduct and located in and around the dorsal raphe and tegmental part of the dorsal longitudinal fasciciulus. No differences were apparent between the various groups of rats as regards the location of the electrodes.

As shown in Fig. 1, saline-injected rats displayed a clear rise in tail-flick latencies following 5 min stimulation. It is also apparent that naloxone

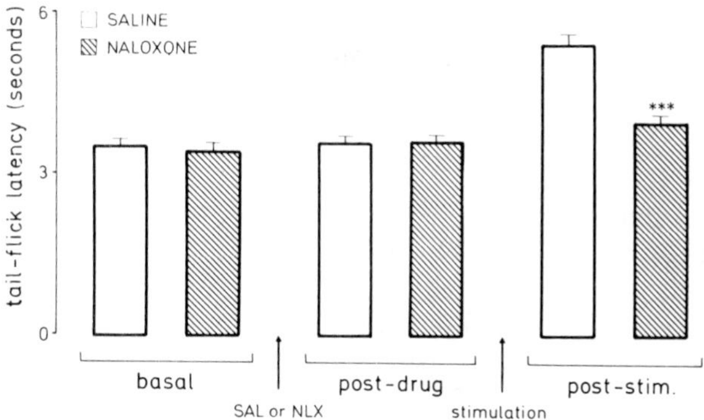

FIG. 1. Influence of the opioid antagonist, naloxone, on midbrain stimulation-elicited antinociception in the rat. Mean ± SEM shown: saline, = 8; naloxone, = 9. Significance of naloxone versus values indicated. ***, $p < 0.001$ (Student's two-tailed t-test).

strongly attenuated this antinociception. The stimulation was accompanied by an ipsilateral head turning reaction and by rotation of the body, but naloxone did not affect these motor responses (not shown in Fig. 1). No stereotypic actions such as gnawing and no aversive effects of stimulation were seen (in saline- or naloxone-treated rats) during or following stimulation.

The lesions of the arcuate hypothalamus greatly depleted ir-β-EP from the septum which indicates substantial damage to the central network of β-EP-containing neurons (Fig. 2). These lesions did not influence basal thresholds, but greatly moderated the antinociception produced by midbrain stimula-

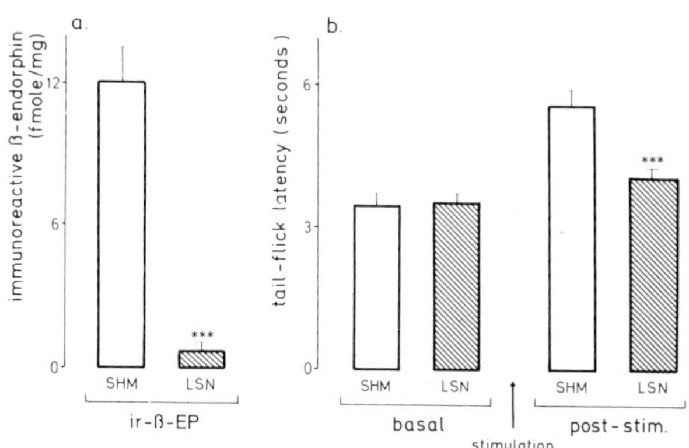

FIG. 2. Influence of lesions of the mediobasal arcuate hypothalamus on (a) levels of immunoreactive β-endorphin in the septum, and (b) stimulation-evoked antinociception in the rat. Mean ± SEM shown: sham (SHM), = 9; lesion (LSN), = 13. Significance of lesion versus sham values indicated. ***, $p < 0.001$ (Student's two-tailed t-test).

tion (Fig. 2). No effect of the lesions on the motor effects of stimulation was seen (not shown).

DISCUSSION

The present data corroborated previous studies in the rat demonstrating that electrical stimulation of the dorsal raphe and adjacent tissue leads to a rise in thresholds for response to noxious heat which is strongly attenuated by a moderate dose of naloxone (Fig. 1) (7,15). In addition, we have demonstrated the sensitivity of this mode of SIA to naloxone in freely moving animals. Indeed, the use of completely unrestrained rats also allowed for a confirmation of the very recent contention by Fardin et al. (3) that stimulation in this region at intensities leading to antinociception is accompanied by motor effects which cease abruptly poststimulation and appear to cause the animals no distress. As these proved unaffected by naloxone (see results), opioids may not mediate these motor changes.

Since by the use of systemic naloxone it is not possible to identify the particular opioids underlying SIA, we examined the effects of elimination of central β-EP. Thus, lesions of the mediobasal arcuate hypothalamus, the site of synthesis of the β-EP-containing neurons projecting to the midbrain (4,13), strongly attenuated the SIA (Fig. 2). Evidently, the mediobasal arcuate hypothalamus is essential for the manifestation of this mode of SIA, an observation that coincides with previous indications for a significance of this region in nociceptive processes (11). However, it is reasonable to question whether the effects of the lesions simply reflect loss of central β-EP. In fact, we recently observed that similar lesions also affect pools of ir-dynorphin (DYN) in the midbrain (9). However, this reduction was minor in comparison to that of ir-β-EP. Further, DYN appears to exert its actions via κ-receptors, which are largely insensitive to naloxone (2,5,14), whereas SIA is strongly moderated by even low doses of this antagonist (1). Moreover, there are no indications that either DYN or other (synthetic) κ-agonists can produce antinociception against noxious neat via an action in the brain (5). Thus, an action on DYN is unlikely to relate to the lesion-produced reduction in SIA. Further, these lesions do not affect pools of Met-enkephalin in the midbrain (9).

It must be pointed that an involvement of β-EP in this SIA would not necessarily exclude a role of other opioids. Indeed, it has recently been shown that intrathecally applied naloxone attenuates the antinociception elicited by β-EP injected into the brain (16). Further, that stimulation of brain tissue can affect spinal pools of opioids is revealed by the finding that antinociception evoked by stimulation of the ventromedial medulla is attenuated by intrathecal naloxone (19). Moreover, it is possible that the lesions interfere with nonopioid mechanisms indispensible for the expression of SPA.

Nevertheless, the most reasonable hypothesis to be derived from the data and the evidence summarized above concerning a possible antinociceptive role is that β-EP is an opioid underlying a major component of this SIA.

It is of interest to compare the present data to those acquired with the antinociception evoked by the environmental stimulus of stress. Duration of exposure is a critical variable as concerns stress-antinociception, and in contrast to longer term stressors, short-term stressors produce an antinociception largely refractory to opioid antagonists (10,12,18). Indeed, we found a 5-min noxious foot-shock stress to produce a rise in thresholds to noxious heat resistant to low doses of naloxone, non-cross-tolerant to morphine, and only marginally influenced by lesions of β-EP neurons (11,12). In contrast, in the present study naloxone or such lesions strongly antagonized SIA. These differences suggest a proportionately greater contribution of opioids and, possibly, β-EP to SIA as compared to noxious stress-antinociception of a comparable duration.

In conclusion, the present study demonstrates a major participation of opioids in the generation of antinociception by stimulation of the dorsal raphe region of the midbrain in the rat. The data also indicate that β-EP may be the opioid underlying this phenomenon. Further studies, for example involving treatment with selective antibodies against β-EP, should be undertaken in order to evaluate further this possibility.

SUMMARY

Electrical stimulation of the ventral midbrain in or adjacent to the dorsal raphe in freely moving rats increased the withdrawal latency in the tail-flick test. The opioid antagonist, naloxone, strongly attenuated this stimulation-induced antinociception (SIA) without affecting basal prestimulation thresholds. Bilateral lesions of the mediobasal arcuate hypothalamus greatly depleted β-endorphin from the brain and strongly moderated the stimulation-elicited antinociception without affecting basal thresholds.

It is concluded that endogenous opioids mediate a major component of this mode of SIA. Further, the data show that the integrity of the mediobasal arcuate hypothalamus is essential for this midbrain SIA and suggest a role of central β-endorphin in its mediation in the rat.

ACKNOWLEDGMENTS

We thank Drs. B. Sutor and W. Zieglgänsberger for advice. M. J. Millan was supported by the Deutsche Forschungsgemeinschaft.

REFERENCES

1. Cannon, J. T., Prieto, G. J., Lee, A., and Liebeskind, J. C. (1982): Evidence for opioid and non-opioid forms of stimulation-produced analgesia in the rat. *Brain Res.*, 243:315–321.

2. Chavkin, C., James, I. F., and Goldstein, A. (1982): Dynorphin is a selective endogenous ligand of the κ-opiate receptor. *Science,* 215:413–415.
3. Fardin, V., Oliveras, J. L., and Besson, J.-M. (1984): A re-investigation of the analgesic effect induced by stimulation of the periacqueductal gray matter in the rat. I. The production of behavioural side effects together with analgesia. *Brain Res.* 306:105–123.
4. Finley, J. C., Lindström, P., and Petrusz, P. (1981): Immunocytochemical localization of β -endorphin-containing neurons in the rat brain. *Neuroendocrinology,* 33:28–42.
5. Hayes, A. G., Skingle, M., and Tyers, M. B. (1983): Antinociceptive profile of dynorphin in the rat. *Life Sci.* 33 (Suppl. 33):657–660.
6. Hosobuchi, Y., Adams, J. E., and Linchitz, R. (1977): Pain relief by electrical stimulation of the central gray matter in humans and its reversal by naloxone. *Science,* 197:183–186.
7. Hosobuchi, Y., and Bloom, F. E. (1983): Analgesia induced by brain stimulation in man: Its effect on release of β-endorphin and adrenocorticotropin into CSF. In: *Neurobiology of Cerebrospinal Fluid,* edited by J. H. Wood, pp. 97–105. Plenum Press, New York.
8. Jacquet, Y. (1978): Opiate effects after adrenocorticotropin or β-endorphin injection in the periacqueductal gray matter of rats. *Science,* 201:1032–1034.
9. Millan, M. H., Millan, M. J., and Przewlocki, R. (1984): Lesions of the hypothalamic arcuate nucleus modify discrete brain and pituitary pools of dynorphin in addition to β-endorphin in the rat. *Neurosci. Lett.,* 48:149–154.
10. Millan, M. J. (1982): Endorphins and nociception: an overview. *Methods Findings Exp. Clin. Pharmacol.,* 4:445–462.
11. Millan, M. J., Gramsch, C., Przewlocki, R., Höllt, V., and Herz, A. (1980): Lesions of the hypothalamic arcuate nucleus produce a temporary hyperalgesia and attentuate stress-evoked analgesia. *Life Sci.* 27:1513–1523.
12. Millan, M. J., Przewlocki, R., Jerlicz, M., Gramsch, C., Höllt, V., and Herz, A. (1981): Stress-induced release of brain and pituitary β-endorphin: major role of endorphins in generation of hperthermia not analgesia. *Brain Res.,* 308:325–338.
13. Romagnano, M. A., and Joseph, S. A. (1983): Immunocytochemical localization of $ACTH_{1-39}$ in the brainstem of the rat. *Brain Res.,* 276:1–16.
14. Schulz, R., Wüster, M., and Herz, A. (1982): Endogenous ligands for κ-opiate receptors. *Peptides,* 3:973–976.
15. Swajkowski, A. R., Mayer, D. J., and Johnson, J. H. (1980): Blockade by naltrexone of analgesia produced by stimulation of the dorsal raphe nucleus. *Pharmacol. Biochem. Behav.,* 15:419–423.
16. Tseng, L-F., and Fujimoto, M. (1984): Evidence that spinal endorphin mediates intraventricular β-endorphin-induced tail-flick inhibition and catalepsy. *Brain Res.,* 302:231–237.
17. Xie, G. X., Han, J. S., and Höllt, V. (1983): Electroacupuncture analgesia blocked by microinjection of anti-beta-endorphin antiserum into periacqueductal gray of the rabbit. *Int. J. Neurosci.,* 18:287–292.
18. Watkins, L. R., and Mayer, D. J. (1982): Organization of endogenous opiate and non-opiate pain control systems. *Science,* 216:1185–1192.
19. Zorman, G., Belcher, G., Adams, J. E., and Fields, H. L. (1982): Lumbar intrathecal naloxone blocks analgesia produced by microstimulation of the ventromedial medulla in the rat. *Brain Res.,* 236:77–84.

Advances in Pain Research and Therapy, Vol. 9, edited by H. L. Fields et al. Raven Press, New York © 1985.

Pharmacology of Central Pain-Modulating Networks (Biogenic Amines and Nonopioid Analgesics)

Donna L. Hammond

Department of Biological Research, G. D. Searle Research and Development, Skokie, Illinois 60077

Antinociception can be produced by electrical or chemical activation of neurons of the somatosensory cortex, hypothalamus, thalamus, periaqueductal gray, mesencephalic reticular formation, and medullary reticular formation (see ref. 24 for review). The mechanism of this stimulation-produced decrease in pain sensitivity is thought to be an inhibition of the response of dorsal horn neurons to noxious stimuli (19,24,77). Although the transmission of nociceptive information can also be inhibited at supraspinal sites, the dorsal horn of the spinal cord represents the first central site in the afferent pain pathway at which the transmission of nociceptive information can be selectively interrupted or attenuated to produce antinociception (80). Because of this fact and because of the relative ease with which the spinal cord can be accessed, numerous investigators have focused their attention on the spinal actions of the neurons of the pain-modulating nuclei. In addressing the pharmacology of the endogenous pain-modulating network, this chapter emphasizes the descending projections of its component neurons and the neurotransmitters whose release from the spinal terminals of these neurons mediates the production of antinociception.

ANATOMY OF THE ENDOGENOUS PAIN-MODULATING NETWORK

An extensive body of literature describes the efferent projections of neurons of the pain-modulating nuclei, particularly with respect to their termination in the spinal cord. Briefly summarized, many neurons of somatosensory cortex (2), hypothalamus (32,71), periaqueductal gray, mesencephalic reticular formation (15,50), locus coeruleus, nucleus raphe magnus, and nucleus reticularis paragigantocellularis (4,74) project directly to the spinal cord. Neurons of these nuclei also project to nuclei of the mesencephalic and medullary reticular formation known to project to the spinal cord (1,23,78). Thus, neurons of the pain-modulating nuclei may influence the transmission of nociceptive information in the spinal cord either directly or indirectly. In view of the paucity of thalamic projections to the spinal cord, it has been postulated that the thalamic influence on spinal function is mediated by antidromic activation of spinothalamic tract collaterals to the periaqueductal gray and medullary reticular formation (21). The efferent projections of these neurons to the spinal cord and reticular formation are described in greater detail in several recent reviews (24,43,73).

PHARMACOLOGY OF THE CENTRAL PAIN-MODULATING NETWORK

The neurotransmitters whose release in the spinal cord mediates the actions of the network of pain-modulating nuclei remain to be unequivocally identified. However, a number of candidate neurotransmitters have been proposed. In general, studies of the pharmacology of the pain-modulating nuclei have utilized three approaches: (a) neuroanatomical, (b) neuropharmacological, and (c) neurochemical.

Neuroanatomical: Localization of Candidate Neurotransmitters

The existence of a substance within neurons of a pathway fulfills one criterion for its identification as the neurotransmitter of that neuronal pathway. The neurotransmitters contained within perikarya of the pain-modulating nuclei have been visualized and identified using immunohistochemical and immunocytochemical techniques. Table 1 presents a brief

TABLE 1. *Neurotransmitters contained within neurons of the endogenous pain-modulating nuclei*

Nucleus	5HT	NE	ENK	DYN	SP	CCK	VP	OT	NT	ST	VIP	TRH
Hypothalamus			17	41	47		**53**	**53**	36	18		44
Periaqueductal gray	**11**		17	41	**69**	**69**			36	18	68	
Raphe dorsalis	**11**		17		47				36		68	
Mesencephalic reticular formation	**11**			41	47							
Raphe magnus	**11**		**31**		**12**	**49**						**12**
Reticularis paragigantocellularis	**11**		**31**		**12**	**49**				18		
Locus coeruleus	70	**75**	17						36			

This list is not intended to be inclusive, but rather to indicate the large number of neurotransmitters that may mediate the actions of the endogenous pain-modulating nuclei. Note that no one neurotransmitter is unique to any nucleus. Furthermore, this listing makes no attempt to identify those nuclei in which subpopulations of the neurons contain more than one neurotransmitter. Each number corresponds to a representative reference. Numbers in *boldface* indicate that neurons containing the neurotransmitter have been demonstrated to project to the spinal cord.

5HT, serotonin; NE, norepinephrine; ENK, enkephalin; DYN, dynorphin; SP, substance P; VIP, vasoactive intestinal polypeptide; OT, oxytocin; VP, vasopressin; ST, somatostatin; NT, neurotensin; CCK, cholecystokinin; TRH, thyrotropin-releasing hormone.

list of these neurotransmitters and indicates those neurotransmitters contained within neurons that project to the spinal cord. Until proven otherwise, each neurotransmitter is a candidate to mediate the spinal actions of the nucleus within which it is contained. Furthermore, certain neurons of these nuclei contain more than one neurotransmitter (16,22,29,38,45,69). The large number of candidate neurotransmitters and the coexistence of more than one neurotransmitter within certain neurons of these nuclei are two major factors contributing to the complex pharmacology of the pain-modulating network. The probable involvement of peptidergic neurons of the spinal cord as interneurons in the bulbospinal pathways is a third contributing factor (5,30). Of all the candidate neurotransmitters, serotonin and norepinephrine have thus far proven the most amenable to pharmacological manipulation. Since their role in the modulation of pain sensitivity has been studied more extensively than that of the peptides, the remainder of this chapter focuses on the involvement of these two monoamines.

Neuropharmacological: Exogenously Applied Neurotransmitters

The neuropharmacological approach utilized in studies of the endogenous pain-modulating network is actually twofold. The first aspect involves demonstrating that exogenous application of the candidate neurotransmitter will mimic the effect of activating the endogenous system. For example, activation of the pain-modulating nuclei inhibits the responses of dorsal horn neurons to noxious stimuli (19,24,77). If the release of serotonin or norepinephrine from the spinal terminals of these nuclei mediates the inhibition, then one would expect that the responses of dorsal horn neurons would similarly be inhibited by iontophoretic application of these monoamines. Numerous investigators have demonstrated that iontophoretic application of either serotonin or norepinephrine to dorsal horn neurons inhibits their responses to noxious stimuli in a manner similar to that produced by activation of the pain-modulating nuclei (8,28,40,57,76). In addition, stimulation of or microinjection of drugs in these nuclei produces antinociception (see ref. 24 for review). This antinociception can be mimicked by intrathecal administration of serotonin (34,67,83) or norepinephrine (33,35,42,58). These studies provide support for the proposal that serotonin and norepinephrine mediate the spinal actions of the endogenous pain-modulating network.

Recent studies have examined the receptor subtypes that mediate the antinociceptive effect of intrathecally administered serotonin and norepinephrine. The results of these studies have direct application to studies of the pharmacology of the endogenous pain-modulating network. Of the three serotonin receptors postulated to exist in the central nervous system (52), the antinociceptive effect of intrathecally administered serotonin appears to be mediated predominantly by a $5HT_1$ receptor (67). This conclusion is based on several observations: (a) ketanserin, a selective $5HT_2$ antagonist (46), was the least potent antagonist of serotonin's effect (67), (b) spiroperidol, frequently used to characterize the $5HT_2$ binding site (55), blocked the effect of serotonin only at a dose that by itself decreased response threshold (67), and (c) the spinal cord does not contain an appreciable number of $5HT_2$ receptors (9,51). In contrast, the antinociceptive effect of intrathecally administered norepinephrine appears to be mediated by both α_1- and α_2-receptors (33,58). However, yohimbine, an α_2-antagonist, is a more potent antagonist of the antinociceptive effect of norepinephrine than is prazosin, an α_1-antagonist (35). This observation suggests that the α_2-receptor plays a predominant role in the antinociceptive effect of norepinephrine. Sagen and Proudfit (62) have similarly concluded from their study of the hyperalgesia produced by intrathecally injected noradrenergic antagonists that the antinociceptive effect of the tonically active bulbospinal noradrenergic system is mediated by an α_2-receptor. The results of radioligand binding and autoradiographic localization studies of noradrenergic receptors in the spinal cord support this interpretation. Thus, the spinal cord contains both α_1- and α_2-receptors (39). However, unlike the α_1-receptors which are homogeneously distributed throughout the gray matter, α_2-receptors are preferentially concentrated in the substantia gelatinosa of the spinal cord (72,86). North and Yoshimura (54) have recently determined that the hyperpolarization of substantia gelatinosa neurons produced by norepinephrine is mediated by α_2-receptors while the excitatory effect is mediated by α_1-receptors. Barbaro et al. (3) have recently reported that the antinociception produced by stimulation of medullary pain-modulating nuclei is attenuated by intrathecally administered yohimbine. This report is consistent with the proposal that α_2-receptors mediate the noradrenergic component of antinociception.

Neuropharmacological: Effects of Antagonism or Depletion

The second aspect of the neuropharmacological approach utilized in studies of the endogenous pathways involves demonstrating that the actions of the endogenous pain-modulating neurons can be antagonized by either (a) administration of an appropriate antagonist or (b) depletion of the neurotransmitter itself. Thus, if release of serotonin from the spinal terminals of an endogenous pathway mediates the production of antinociception, then intrathecal administration of a serotonin antagonist such as methysergide or depletion of serotonin in the spinal cord should antagonize or attenuate the antinociception.

Carstens et al. (13,14) have recently begun to characterize the pharmacology of the spinal influence exerted by nuclei of the medial and lateral hypothalamus and the basal forebrain. They have demonstrated that systemic administration of the serotonergic antagonist methysergide antagonizes the inhibition of dorsal horn neurons produced by stimulation of the medial diencephalon and basal forebrain (14) and of the lateral hypothalamus (13).

In addition, depletion of serotonin in the central nervous system by systemic administration of *p*-chlorophenylalanine also attenuates the effects of stimulation in these nuclei (14). These results suggest that the inhibitory effects produced by stimulation of these nuclei are mediated by serotonin. However, they offer no insight as to the involvement of a serotonergic synapse in the spinal cord because (a) the antagonist was administered systemically rather than intrathecally, and (b) the depletion of serotonin was widespread, rather than limited to the spinal cord. Because direct, serotonergic hypothalamospinal or diencephalospinal projections have not been identified (11), it has been proposed that the serotonergically mediated actions of these diencephalic nuclei result from subsequent activation of the spinally projecting serotonergic relay nuclei to which they project (e.g., n. raphe magnus, n. reticularis paragigantocellularis, periaqueductal gray, or n. raphe dorsalis) (13,14). The involvement of norepinephrine in mediating the spinal actions of these nuclei has not yet been examined.

In contrast to studies of the pharmacology of the diencephalic nuclei, studies of the mesencephalic and medullary pain-modulating nuclei have focused on the involvement of both serotonin and norepinephrine. In these studies the site of action of the antagonists was restricted to the spinal cord by administering them intrathecally (81). Consequently, these studies have been able to selectively examine the extent to which activation of spinally projecting serotonergic and noradrenergic neurons mediates the antinociception produced by stimulation of these nuclei. Using this technique, Yaksh has demonstrated that the antinociception produced by microinjection of morphine (79) or of glutamate (37) in the periaqueductal gray is antagonized by intrathecal administration of methysergide or of phentolamine, a noradrenergic antagonist. Although the blockade produced by either antagonist when administered alone was partial, coadministration of both methysergide and phentolamine totally antagonized the antinociception (79). These results indicate that the antinociception produced by stimulation of the periaqueductal gray is mediated by the release of both serotonin and norepinephrine in the spinal cord. However, this antinociception cannot be attributed to activation of serotonergic and noradrenergic neurons of the periaqueductal gray that project to the spinal cord because: (a) serotonergic neurons of this nucleus project only to the cervical level of the spinal cord (11) whereas the action of methysergide was principally confined to the lumbar level, and (b) this nucleus does not contain noradrenergic perikarya that project to the spinal cord (75). Rather, like the diencephalic nuclei, it is likely that the serotonergically mediated actions of the periaqueductal gray are mediated through a relay with spinally projecting serotonergic neurons of the medulla (4,5). Similarly, the noradrenergically mediated actions of the periaqueductal gray are likely to be mediated by its projections to noradrenergic nuclei such as the locus coeruleus and A7 and A5 catecholamine nuclei that project to the spinal cord (75).

Recent evidence suggests that the serotonergic contribution to the antinociception produced by periaqueductal gray activation is not mediated entirely by spinally projecting serotonergic neurons of the nucleus raphe magnus and nucleus reticularis paragigantocellularis. Thus, a portion of the periaqueductal gray projection to the nucleus raphe magnus and nucleus reticularis paragigantocellularis is composed of serotonergic neurons (7,84). In addition, microinjection of serotonin in the nucleus raphe magnus has been shown to produce antinociception (48). Thus, this serotonergic synapse on raphe-spinal and reticulospinal neurons (not necessarily serotonergic) represents another site, in addition to the spinal cord, at which systemically administered serotonergic antagonists could act to block the antinociception produced by activating the periaqueductal gray (85).

The antinociception produced by activation of the nucleus raphe magnus and nucleus reticularis paragigantocellularis in the medulla is postulated to be mediated by activation of serotonergic and noradrenergic neurons that project to the spinal cord. Thus, the antinociception produced by electrical stimulation or microinjection of morphine, glutamate, or noradrenergic antagonists in the nucleus raphe magnus and adjacent nucleus reticularis paragigantocellularis is antagonized by intrathecal administration of methysergide or phentolamine (25,26,37,60,66) or by depletion of serotonin or norepinephrine in the spinal cord (63). Interestingly enough, the majority of these studies failed to examine the effects of more than one type of intrathecally administered antagonist at any one stimulation site. This weakness in experimental design has contributed to an overly simplified view that the effects of activation of the nucleus raphe magnus and nucleus reticularis paragigantocellularis are mediated by serotonin and norepinephrine, respectively (see refs. 65,66). Yet, the blockade produced by depletion or by antagonism of either neurotransmitter alone has frequently been merely partial. Furthermore, the large number of neurotransmitters contained within spinally projecting neurons of the nucleus raphe magnus and nucleus reticularis paragigantocellularis (see Table 1) would argue that more than one neurotransmitter is likely to mediate their actions. We examined this issue in a recent study in which the effects of intrathecally administered methysergide and phentolamine were evaluated on the antinociception produced by stimulation of the same medullary sites (25). In that study, the antinociception produced by stimulation of sites in the nucleus raphe magnus and nucleus reticularis paragigantocellularis was attenuated by intrathecal injection of either methysergide or phentolamine. Furthermore, the blockade produced by either antagonist was partial, not complete. We therefore concluded that the antinociception produced by activation of the nucleus raphe magnus and nucleus reticularis paragigantocellularis was mediated by *coactivation* of bulbospinal serotonergic and noradrenergic neurons. Although the nucleus raphe magnus and nucleus reticularis paragigantocellularis contain serotonergic neurons that project to the spinal cord (11), they do not contain noradrenergic perikarya (75). It has, therefore, been proposed that the noradrenergically mediated effects of stimulation in these nuclei are mediated by activation of afferent projections to noradrenergic nuclei that, in turn, project to the spinal cord (25,60,61,63).

Neurochemical: Spinal Release of Endogenous Monoamines

In identifying a substance as the neurotransmitter of a neuronal system it is critical to demonstrate that the substance is released on activation of the system. Therefore, the third and final approach utilized in studies of the pharmacology of the endogenous pain-modulating network has frequently been neurochemical. It is perhaps the most difficult of all three approaches because (a) the sensitivity of methods for measurement of the endogenous neurotransmitter and its metabolites must be in the picomolar and femtomolar range, and (b) most regions of the central nervous system are not easily accessed for measurement of neurotransmitter efflux. However, until specific antagonists for the peptidergic neurotransmitters are introduced, this approach will become increasingly important as investigators attempt to establish a role for these substances as neurotransmitters of the endogenous pain-modulating network.

Studies utilizing the neurochemical approach have attempted to correlate behavioral alterations in nociceptive threshold with alterations in the efflux of the endogenous neurotransmitter from various regions of the spinal cord. Yaksh has used this technique extensively in his studies of the pharmacology of the monoaminergic bulbospinal pain-modulating pathways. Thus, he has demonstrated that microinjection of morphine in the periaqueductal gray increased the release of endogenous serotonin into *in vivo* superfusates of the spinal cord as measured by HPLC with electrochemical detection (82). These results are complemented by those of a previous neuropharmacological study in which intrathecal injection of methysergide attenuated the antinociception produced by microinjection of morphine in the periaqueductal gray (79). Taken together, these results provide very strong evidence that the antinociceptive action of periaqueductal gray activation is mediated by a release of serotonin in the spinal cord.

Several investigators have utilized a neurochemical approach to obtain evidence in support of the proposal that the antinociception produced by activation of the nucleus raphe magnus and nucleus reticularis paragigantocellularis is mediated by serotonin in the spinal cord. Thus, Bourgoin et al. (10) have reported that stimulation of the nucleus raphe magnus increased the synthesis of serotonin in the spinal cord as measured by the accumulation of 5-hydroxytryptophan. More recently, Rivot et al. (59) arrived at a similar conclusion using differential *in vivo* pulse voltametry to measure undefined 5-hydroxyindoles in the dorsal horn. Neither study addressed the involvement of norepinephrine in mediating the actions of these nuclei. This was particularly unfortunate because in each study the stimulation-produced increase in serotonin synthesis was small, on the order of 40% (10,59). This observation and the results of our neuropharmacological study with the monoaminergic antagonists suggested to us that a release of serotonin in the spinal cord could not be totally responsible for the antinociceptive effects of these nuclei. We therefore examined the effects of nucleus raphe magnus and nucleus reticularis paragigantocellularis stimulation on the efflux of both endogenous serotonin and norepinephrine into *in vivo* superfusates of the rat spinal cord (27). In this study, electrical stimulation of the nucleus raphe magnus and nucleus reticularis paragigantocellularis with current strengths sufficient to produce antinociception resulted in an increase in the efflux of endogenous serotonin and norepinephrine. Importantly, the efflux of *both* serotonin and norepinephrine was increased by such stimulation providing additional support for the proposal that the antinociceptive effects of these nuclei are mediated by coactivation of bulbospinal serotonergic and noradrenergic neurons.

SUMMARY

Neurons of the pain-modulating network may regulate afferent transmission of nociceptive information at the level of the spinal cord either directly, by means of projections to the dorsal horn (e.g., nucleus raphe magnus and nucleus reticularis paragigantocellularis), or indirectly, via their projections to spinally projecting neurons of the medulla and mesencephalon (e.g., hypothalamus and periaqueductal gray) (6,20,56,64). The pharmacology of these neurons is made particularly complex by the large number of neurotransmitters contained within these neurons, the coexistence of neurotransmitters within one neuron and the probable existence of interneurons in the pathways to the spinal cord. With the exception of endogenous opioid peptides (see H. L. Fields, *this volume*), evidence for the involvement of the different peptidergic neurotransmitters is sparse. This fact does not so much reflect a lack of involvement as it does the lack of specific antagonists and methods of quantitation. In contrast, there is strong evidence that both serotonin and norepinephrine mediate the actions of pain-modulating neurons at the level of the spinal cord. This evidence includes the findings that (a) exogenous application of serotonin or norepinephrine in the spinal cord mimics the actions of the endogenous pathways (see above); (b) these two neurotransmitters are contained within neurons of the endogenous pain-modulating nuclei that project to the spinal cord (see Table 1); (c) intrathecal administration of monoaminergic antagonists or depletion of spinal monoamine content antagonizes the actions of the endogenous pathways; and (d) activation of pain-modulating nuclei results in a release of endogenous serotonin and norepinephrine from the spinal cord.

ACKNOWLEDGMENT

I thank H. K. Proudfit for his helpful comments on an earlier version of this manuscript and acknowledge the support of G. D. Searle & Co.

REFERENCES

1. Abols, I. A., and Basbaum, A. I. (1981): Afferent connections of the rostral medulla of the cat: a neural substrate for midbrain medullary interactions in the modulation of pain. *J. Comp. Neurol.,* 201:285–297.
2. Armand, J. (1982): The origin, course and terminations of corticospinal fibers in various mammals. *Prog. Brain Res.,* 57:329–360.
3. Barbaro, N., Hammond, D. L., and Fields, H. L. (1983): Antagonism of micro-stimulation produced analgesia by intrathecal injection of methysergide and yohimbine. *Neurosci. Abstr.,* 9:791.
4. Basbaum, A. I., and Fields, H. L. (1979): The origin of descending pathways in the dorsolateral funiculus of the spinal cord of the cat and rat: Further studies on the anatomy of pain modulation. *J. Comp. Neurol.,* 187:513–532.
5. Basbaum, A. I., and Fields, H. L. (1984): Endogenous pain control systems: brainstem spinal pathways and endorphin circuitry. *Annu. Rev. Neurosci.,* 7:309–338.
6. Behbehani, M. M., and Fields, H. L. (1979): Evidence that an excitatory connection between the periaqueductal gray and nucleus raphe magnus mediates stimulation-produced analgesia. *Brain Res.,* 170:85–93.
7. Beitz, A. J., Shepard, R. D., and Wells, W. E. (1983): The periaqueductal gray-raphe magnus projection contains somatostatin, neurotensin and serotonin, but not cholecystokinin. *Brain Res.,* 261:132–137.
8. Belcher, G., Ryall, R. W., and Schaffner, R. (1978): The differential effects of 5-hydroxytryptamine, noradrenaline and raphe stimulation on nociceptive and non-nociceptive dorsal horn interneurones in the cat. *Brain Res.,* 151:307–321.
9. Blackshear, M. A., Steranka, L.R., and Sanders-Bush, E. (1981): Multiple serotonin receptors: regional distribution and effect of raphe lesions. *Eur. J. Pharmacol.,* 76:325–334.
10. Bourgoin, S., Oliveras, J. L., Bruxelle, J., Hamon, M., and Besson, J. M. (1980): Electrical stimulation of the nucleus raphe magnus in the rat. Effects on 5-HT metabolism in the spinal cord. *Brain Res.,* 194:377–389.
11. Bowker, R. M., Westlund, K. N., Sullivan, M. C., and Coulter, J. D. (1982): Organization of descending serotonergic projections to the spinal cord. *Prog. Brain Res.,* 57:239–265.
12. Bowker, R. M., Westlund, K. N., Sullivan, M. C., Wilber, J. F., and Coulter, J. D. (1983): Descending serotonergic, peptidergic and cholinergic pathways from the raphe nuclei: a multiple transmitter complex. *Brain Res.,* 288:33–48.
13. Carstens, E., Fraunhoffer, M., and Suberg, S. N. (1983): Inhibition of spinal dorsal horn neuronal responses to noxious skin heating by lateral hypothalamus stimulation in the cat. *J. Neurophysiol.,* 50:192–204.
14. Carstens, E., MacKinnon, J. D., and Guinan, M. J. (1983): Serotonin involvement in descending inhibition of spinal nociceptive transmission produced by stimulation of medial diencephalon and basal forebrain. *J. Neurosci.,* 3:2112–2120.
15. Castiglioni, A. J., Gallaway, M. C., and Coulter, J. D. (1978): Spinal projections from the midbrain in monkey. *J. Comp. Neurol.,* 178:329–346.
16. Chan-Palay, V. (1979): Combined immunocytochemistry and autoradiography after *in vivo* injections of monoclonal antibody to substance P and ^{3}H-serotonin: coexistence of two putative transmitters in single raphe cells and fiber plexuses. *Anat. Embryol. (Berl.),* 156:241–255.
17. Finley, J. C. W., Maderdrut, J. L., and Petrusz, P. (1981): The immunocytochemical localization of enkephalin in the central nervous system of the rat. *J. Comp. Neurol.,* 198:541–565.
18. Finley, J. C. W., Maderdrut, J. L., Roger, L. F., and Petrusz, P. (1981): The immunocyto-

chemical localization of somatostatin-containing neurons in the rat central nervous system. *Neuroscience,* 6:2173–2192.

19. Gebhart, G. (1985): Modulatory effects of descending systems on dorsal horn neurons. In: *Functional Organization of Spinal Afferent Processing,* edited by T. L. Yaksh. Plenum Press, New York.
20. Gebhart, G. F., Sandkuhler, J. G., Thalhammer, J. G., and Zimmerman, M. (1983): Inhibition of spinal nociceptive information by stimulation in midbrain of the cat is blocked by lidocaine microinjected in nucleus raphe magnus and medullary reticular formation. *J. Neurophysiol.,* 50:1446–1459.
21. Gerhart, K. D., Yezierski, R. P., Fang, Z. R., and Willis, W. D. (1983): Inhibition of primate spinothalamic tract neurons by stimulation in ventral posterior lateral (VPL_c) thalamic nucleus: possible mechanisms. *J. Neurophysiol.,* 49:406–423.
22. Glazer, E. J., Steinbusch, H., Verhofstad, A., and Basbaum, A. I. (1981): Serotonin neurons in nucleus raphe dorsalis and paragigantocellularis of the cat contain enkephalin. *J. Physiol. (Paris),* 77:241–245.
23. Grofova, I., Ottersen, O. P., and Rinvik, E. (1978): Mesencephalic and diencephalic afferents to the superior colliculus and periaqueductal gray substance demonstrated by retrograde axonal transport of horseradish peroxidase in the cat. *Brain Res.,* 146:205–220.
24. Hammond, D. L. (1985): Control systems for nociceptive afferent processing: the descending inhibitory pathways. In: *Functional Organization of Spinal Afferent Processing,* edited by T. L. Yaksh. Plenum Press, New York.
25. Hammond, D. L., and Yaksh, T. L. (1984): Antagonism of stimulation-produced antinociception by intrathecal administration of methysergide or phentolamine. *Brain Res.,* 298:329–337.
26. Hammond, D. L., Levy, R. A., and Proudfit, H. K. (1980): Hypoalgesia induced by microinjection of a norepinephrine antagonist in the nucleus raphe magnus: reversal by intrathecal administration of a serotonin antagonist. *Brain Res.,* 201:475–479.
27. Hammond, D. L., Tyce, G. M., and Yaksh, T. L. (1985): Efflux of serotonin and noradrenaline into spinal cord superfusates during stimulation of the cat ventromedial medulla. *J. Physiol. (Lond.)* 359:151–162.
28. Headley, P. M., Duggan, A. W., and Griersmith, B. T. (1978): Selective reduction by noradrenaline and 5-hydroxytryptamine of nociceptive responses of cat dorsal horn neurones. *Brain Res.,* 145:185–189.
29. Hokfelt, T., Ljungdahl, A., Steinbusch, H., Verhofstad, A., Nilsson, G., Brodin, E., Pernow, B., and Goldstein, M. (1978): Immunohistochemical evidence of substance P-like immunoreactivity in some 5-hydroxytryptamine containing neurons in the rat central nervous system. *Neuroscience,* 3:517–538.
30. Hokfelt, T., Skirboll, L., Lundberg, J. M., Dolsgaard, C.-J., Johansson, O., Pernow, B., and Jancso, G. (1983): Neuropeptides and pain pathways. In: *Advances in Pain Research and Therapy, Vol. 5,* edited by J. J. Bonica, U. Lindblom, and A. Iggo, pp. 227–246. Raven Press, New York.
31. Hokfelt, T., Terenius, L., Kuypers, H. G. J. M., and Dann, O. (1979): Evidence for enkephalin immunoreactive neurons in the medulla oblongata projecting to the spinal cord. *Neurosci. Lett.,* 14:55–60.
32. Hosoya, Y. (1980): The distribution of spinal projection neurons in the hypothalamus of the rat, studied with the HRP method. *Exp. Brain Res.,* 40:79–87.
33. Howe, J. R., Wang, J.-Y., and Yaksh, T. L. (1983): Selective antagonism of the antinociceptive effect of intrathecally applied alpha adrenergic agonists by intrathecal prazosin and intrathecal yohimbine. *J. Pharmacol. Exp. Ther.,* 224:552–558.
34. Hylden, J. L. K., and Wilcox, G. L. (1983): Intrathecal serotonin in mice: analgesia and inhibition of a spinal action of substance P. *Life Sci.,* 33:789–795.
35. Hylden, J. L. K., and Wilcox, G. L. (1983): Pharmacological characterization of substance P-induced nociception in mice: modulation by opioid and noradrenergic agonists at the spinal level. *J. Pharmacol. Exp. Ther.,* 226:398–404.
36. Jennes, L., Stumpf, W. E., and Kalivas, P. W. (1982): Neurotensin: topographical distribution in rat brain by immunohistochemistry. *J. Comp. Neurol.,* 210:211–224.
37. Jensen, T., and Yaksh, T. L. (1985): Spinal monoamine and opiate systems partly mediate

the antinociceptive effects of glutamate microinjected at brain stem sites. *Brain Res.,* 321:287–297.

38. Johansson, O., Hokfelt, T., Pernow, B., Jeffcoate, S. L., White, N., Steinbusch, H. W. M., Verhofstad, A. A. J., Emson, P. C., and Spindel, E. (1981): Immunohistochemical support for three putative transmitters in one neuron: coexistence of 5-hydroxytryptamine, substance P- and thyrotropin releasing hormone-like immunoreactivity in medullary neurons projecting to the spinal cord. *Neuroscience,* 6:1857–1881.
39. Jones, D. J., Kendall, D. E., and Enna, S. J. (1982): Adrenergic receptors in rat spinal cord. *Neuropharmacology,* 21:367–370.
40. Jordan, L. M., Kenshalo, D. R., Jr., Martin, R. F., Haber, L. H., and Willis, W. D. (1978): Depression of primate spinothalamic tract neurons by iontophoretic application of 5-hydroxytryptamine. *Pain,* 5:135–142.
41. Khachaturian, H., Watson, S. J., Lewis, M. E., Coy, D., Goldstein, A., and Akil, H. (1982): Dynorphin immunocytochemistry in the rat central nervous system. *Peptides,* 3:941–954.
42. Kuraishi, Y., Harada, Y., and Takagi, H. (1979): Noradrenaline regulation of pain transmission in the spinal cord mediated by α-adrenoceptors. *Brain Res.,* 174:333–336.
43. Kuypers, H. J. G. M., and Huisman, A. M. (1982): The new anatomy of the descending brain pathways. In: *Brain Stem Control of Spinal Mechanisms,* edited by B. Sjolund and A. Bjorklund, pp. 29–54. Elsevier, Amsterdam.
44. Lechan, R. M., Molitch, M. E., and Jackson, I. M. D. (1983): Distribution of immunoreactive human growth hormone-like material and thyrotropin-releasing hormone in the rat central nervous system: evidence for their coexistence in the same neurons. *Endocrinology,* 112:877–884.
45. Leger, L., Charnay, Y., Chayvialle, J. A., Berod, A., Dray, F., Pujol, J. F., Jouvet, M., and Dubois, P. M. (1983): Localization of substance P- and enkephalin-like immunoreactivity in relation to catecholamine-containing cell bodies in the cat dorsolateral pontine tegmentum: an immunofluorescence study. *Neuroscience,* 8:525–546.
46. Leysen, J. E., Awouters, F., Kennis, L., Laduron, P. M., Vandenberk, J., and Jenssen, P. A. J. (1981): Receptor binding profile of R41 468, a novel antagonist at $5HT_2$ receptors. *Life Sci.,* 28:1015–1022.
47. Ljungdahl, A., Hokfelt, T., and Nilsson, G. (1978): Distribution of substance P-like immunoreactivity in the central nervous system of the rat. I. Cell bodies and nerve terminals. *Neuroscience,* 3:861–943.
48. Llewelyn, M. B., Azami, J., and Roberts, M. H. T. (1983): Effects of 5-hydroxytryptamine applied into nucleus raphe magnus on nociceptive thresholds and neuronal firing rate. *Brain Res.,* 258:59–68.
49. Mantyh, P. W., and Hunt, S. P. (1984): Evidence for cholecystokinin-like immunoreactive neurons in the rat medulla oblongata which project to the spinal cord. *Brain Res.,* 291:49–54.
50. Mantyh, P. W., and Peschanski, M. (1982): Spinal projections from the periaqueductal grey and dorsal raphe in the rat, cat and monkey. *Neuroscience,* 7:2769–2776.
51. Monroe, P. T., and Smith, D. J. (1983): Characterization of multiple [^{3}H]5-hydroxytryptamine binding sites in rat spinal cord tissue. *J. Neurochem.,* 41:349–355.
52. Nelson, D. L. (1982): Central serotonergic receptors: evidence for heterogeneity and characterization by ligand-binding. *Neurosci. Biobehav. Rev.,* 6:499–502.
53. Nilaver, G., Zimmerman, E. A., Wilkins, J., Michaels, J., Hoffman, D., and Silverman, A. J. (1980): Magnocellular hypothalamic projections to the lower brain stem and spinal cord of the rat. *Neuroendrocrinology,* 30:150–158.
54. North, R. A., and Yoshimura, M. (1984): The actions of noradrenaline on neurones of the rat substantia gelatinosa *in vitro. J. Physiol. (Lond.),* 349:43–55.
55. Peroutka, S. J., and Snyder, S. J. (1981): Two distinct serotonin receptors: regional variations in receptor binding in mammalian brain. *Brain Res.,* 208:339–347.
56. Prieto, G. J., Cannon, J. T., and Liebeskind, J. C. (1983): N. raphe magnus lesions disrupt stimulation-produced analgesia from ventral but not dorsal midbrain areas in the rat. *Brain Res.,* 261:53–57.
57. Randic, M., and Yu, H. H. (1976): Effects of 5-hydroxytryptamine and bradykinin on cat dorsal horn neurones activated by noxious stimuli. *Brain Res.,* 111:197–203.

58. Reddy, S. V. R., Maderdrut, J. L., and Yaksh, T. L. (1980): Spinal cord pharmacology of adrenergic agonist-mediated antinociception. *J. Pharmacol. Exp. Ther.*, 213:525–533.
59. Rivot, J. P., Chiang, C. Y., and Besson, J. M. (1982): Increase of serotonin metabolism within the dorsal horn of the spinal cord during nucleus raphe magnus stimulation as revealed by *in vivo* electrochemical detection. *Brain Res.* 238:117–126.
60. Sagen, J., and Proudfit, H. K. (1981): Hypoalgesia induced by blockade of noradrenergic projections to the raphe magnus: reversal by blockade of noradrenergic projections to the spinal cord. *Brain Res.*, 223:391–396.
61. Sagen, J., and Proudfit, H. K. (1983): The role of the A7 catecholamine group in the modulation of pain perception. *Neurosci. Abstr.* 9:785.
62. Sagen, J., and Proudfit, H. K. (1985): Effect of intrathecally administered noradrenergic antagonists on nociception in the rat. *Brain Res.*, 310:295–301.
63. Sagen, J., Winker, M. A., and Proudfit, H. K. (1983): Hypoalgesia induced by the local injection of phentolamine in the nucleus raphe magnus: blockade by depletion of spinal cord monoamines. *Pain*, 16:253–263.
64. Sandkuhler, J., and Gebhart, G. F. (1984): Relative contributions of the nucleus raphe magnus and adjacent medullary reticular formation to the inhibition by stimulation in the periaqueductal gray of a spinal nociceptive reflex in the pentobarbital-anesthetized rat. *Brain Res.*, 305:77–87.
65. Satoh, M., Akaike, A., Nakazawa, T., and Takagi, H. (1980): Evidence for involvement of separate mechanism in the production of analgesia by electrical stimulation of the nucleus reticularis paragigantocellularis and nucleus raphe magnus in the rat. *Brain Res.*, 194:525–529.
66. Satoh, M., Oku, R., and Akaike, A. (1983): Analgesia produced by microinjection of L-glutamate into the rostral ventromedial bulbar nuclei of the rat and its inhibition by intrathecal α-adrenergic blocking agents. *Brain Res.*, 261:361–364.
67. Schmauss, C., Hammond, D. L., Ochi, J. W., and Yaksh, T. L. (1983): Pharmacological antagonism of the antinociceptive effects of serotonin in the rat spinal cord. *Eur. J. Pharmacol.*, 90:349–357.
68. Sims, K. B., Hoffman, D. L., Said, S. I., and Zimmerman, E. A. (1980): Vasoactive intestinal polypeptide (VIP) in mouse and rat brain: an immunocytochemical study. *Brain Res.*, 186:165–183.
69. Skirboll, L., Hokfelt, T., Dockray, G., Rehfeld, J., Brownstein, M., and Cuello, A. C. (1983): Evidence for periaqueductal cholecystokinin-substance P neurons projecting to the spinal cord. *J. Neurosci.*, 3:1151–1157.
70. Steinbusch, H. W. M. (1981): Distribution of serotonin-immunoreactivity in the central nervous system of the rat. Cell bodies and terminals. *Neuroscience*, 6:557–618.
71. Swanson, L. W., and Kuypers, H. G. J. M. (1980): The paraventricular nucleus of the hypothalamus: cytoarchitectonic subdivisions and organization of projections to the pituitary, dorsal vagal complex, and spinal cord as demonstrated by retrograde fluorescence double-labeling methods. *J. Comp. Neurol.*, 194:555–570.
72. Unnerstall, J. R., Kopojtic, T. A., and Kuhar, M. J. (1984): Distribution of α_2 agonist binding sites in the rat and human central nervous system: analysis of some functional anatomic correlates of the pharmacologic effects of clonidine and related adrenergic agents. *Brain Res. Rev.*, 7:69–101.
73. Walberg, F. (1982): Paths descending from the brain stem—an overview. In: *Brain Stem Control of Spinal Mechanisms*, edited by B. Sjolund and A. Bjorklund, pp. 1–27. Elsevier, Amsterdam.
74. Watkins, L. R., Griffin, G., Leichnetz, G. P., and Mayer, D. J. (1981): Identification and somatotopic organization of nuclei projecting via the dorsolateral funiculus in rats: a retrograde tracing study using HRP slow-release gels. *Brain Res.*, 223:237–255.
75. Westlund, K. N., Bowker, R. M., Ziegler, M. G., and Coulter, J. D. (1982): Descending noradrenergic projections and their spinal terminations. *Prog. Brain Res.*, 57:219–238.
76. Willcockson, W. S., Chung, J. M., Hori, Y., Lee, K. H., and Willis, W. D. (1984): Effects of iontophoretically released amino acids and amines on primate spinothalamic tract cells. *J. Neurosci.*, 4:732–740.
77. Willis, W. D. (1982): Control of nociceptive transmission in the spinal cord. In: *Progress*

in Sensory Physiology, edited by H. Autrum, D. O. Ottoson, E. R. Perl, and R. F. Schmidt, pp. 76–111. Springer-Verlag, Berlin.

78. Wise, S. P., and Jones, E. G. (1977): Cells of origin and terminal distribution of descending projections of the rat somatic sensory cortex. *J. Comp. Neurol.,* 175:129–158.
79. Yaksh, T. L. (1979): Direct evidence that spinal serotonin and noradrenaline terminals mediate the spinal antinociceptive effects of morphine in the periaqueductal gray. *Brain Res.,* 160:180–185.
80. Yaksh, T. L., and Hammond, D. L. (1982): Peripheral and central substrates involved in the rostrad transmission of nociceptive information. *Pain,* 13:1–85.
81. Yaksh, T. L., and Rudy, T. A. (1976): Chronic catheterization of the spinal subarachnoid space. *Physiol. Behav.,* 17:1031–1036.
82. Yaksh, T. L., and Tyce, G. M. (1979): Microinjection of morphine into the periaqueductal gray evokes the release of serotonin from spinal cord. *Brain Res.,* 171:176–181.
83. Yaksh, T. L., and Wilson, P. R. (1979): Spinal serotonin terminal system mediates antinociception. *J. Pharmacol. Exp. Ther.,* 208:446–453.
84. Yezierski, R. P., Bowker, R. M., Kevetter, G. A., Westlund, K. N., Coulter, J. D., and Willis, W. D. (1982): Serotonergic projections to the caudal brain stem: a double label study using horseradish peroxidase and serotonin immunoreactivity. *Brain Res.,* 239:258–264.
85. Yezierski, R. P., Wilcox, T. K., and Willis, W. D. (1982): The effects of serotonin antagonists on the inhibition of primate spinothalamic tract cells produced by stimulation in nucleus raphe magnus or periaqueductal gray. *J. Pharmacol. Exp. Ther.,* 220:226–277.
86. Young, W. S., and Kuhar, M. J. (1980): Noradrenergic $\alpha 1$ and $\alpha 2$ receptors: light microscopic autoradiographic localization. *Proc. Natl. Acad. Sci. USA,* 77:1696–1700.

Advances in Pain Research and Therapy, Vol. 9, edited by H. L. Fields et al. Raven Press, New York © 1985.

Glutamate-Induced Analgesia: Effects of Spinal Serotonin, Norepinephrine, and Opioid Antagonists

Troels S. Jensen and Tony L. Yaksh

Department of Neurosurgical Research, Mayo Clinic, Rochester, Minnesota 55905

Studies on the analgesic effect of electrical stimulation or microinjection of opioid agonists into discrete brainstem loci have led to the suggestion that a neural system originating in the periaqueductal gray matter (PAG) via an intermediary link in the rostral medulla may modulate spinal nociceptive transmission (for review, see refs. 3,14). Recent studies with the excitatory substance glutamate administered into either the PAG (2,11) or the raphe complex (10), including the nucleus raphe magnus (NRM) and the nucleus reticularis paragigantocellularis (NRPGC), support the notion that direct excitation of neuronal populations within the PAG or the NRM/NRPGC may activate a descending inhibitory system. In addition to exerting an inhibitory effect on spinal reflexes, this descending system activated by supraspinal manipulations is also assumed to reduce nociceptive transmission from the cord to the brain (12).

Ample evidence exists to indicate that spinopetal serotonergic and noradrenergic systems (15) and possibly also a spinal opioid synapse (8,16) may be involved in mediating the analgesic effects of opioids and electrical stimulation at brainstem sites. It is therefore conceivable that these systems also contribute to the antinociceptive effect produced by the focal excitation of glutamate in discrete brainstem loci.

We studied the ability of spinal-acting serotonergic, noradrenergic, and opioid antagonists to counteract the analgesic effect of glutamate administered into the PAG or the NRM/NRPGC on both a spinal- and a supraspinal-mediated nociceptive response. Some of the present findings are published elsewhere (5).

Dr. Jensen's present address is Department of Neuromedicine, University of Copenhagen, KAS Gentofte, DK-2900 Hellerup, Denmark.

MATERIALS AND METHODS

In male Sprague-Dawley rats the antinociceptive action was evaluated by the spinal mediated tail-flick (TF) and the supraspinal organized hot-plate (HP) response latencies. In the TF test the latency of a rat to withdraw its tail from a radiant heat source was measured. The intensity of radiant heat focused to the tail was sufficient to produce a tail twitch in a spinal transected animal (6). In the HP test the latency of a rat to lick its hindpaw following placement on a 52.5° C metal surface was recorded. The cut-off times in the absence of a response on the TF and HP responses were 6 and 60 sec, respectively.

One week before an experiment rats were stereotaxically implanted with a microinjection cannula above the PAG or the NRM/NRPGC and a spinal intrathecal (i.t.) catheter. TF and HP response latencies were measured both before as well as 1, 3, 5, and 10 min after an intracerebral injection of 30 nmoles monosodium glutamate given in a volume of 0.5 μl. Drugs used for i.t. injection were methysergide, phentolamine, and naxolone, which were all given in a volume of 10 μl followed by an injection of 10 μl saline. After completion of the experimental series, intracerebral injection sites were identified histologically and transferred to corresponding plates of the Pellegrino atlas (9).

RESULTS

Glutamate administered into either the PAG or the NRM/NRPGC produced a short-lasting increase in TF and HP response latencies (Figs. 1 and 2). As shown in Fig. 1 the maximal elevation of nociceptive threshold was seen immediately after glutamate injection and with a return to baseline levels within 10 min. Whereas the increase in TF and HP response latencies were seen when the glutamate injection fell within the borders of the PAG or the raphe complex, glutamate usually failed to influence TF and HP measures when administered outside these brainstem loci. Although some motor rigidity occurred when glutamate was injected into PAG sites and, to a lesser extent, when injected into the NRM/NRPGC complex, basic nonnociceptive reflexes were preserved during the period of elevated TF and HP response latencies.

One week after the first glutamate injection rats received a second glutamate injection (30 nmoles/0.5 μl) into sites previously shown to be glutamate-responsive. Before the second glutamate injection rats were randomly pretreated with either saline; the serotonergic antagonist, methysergide; the noradrenergic antagonist, phentolamine; or the opioid antagonist, naloxone. As shown in Fig. 3 and Fig. 4, none of the pretreatments influenced baseline nociceptive threshold. Within the PAG (Fig. 3) pretreatments significantly influenced the elevated TF responses ($F = 8.40$, df:3/23, $p < 0.001$) due to

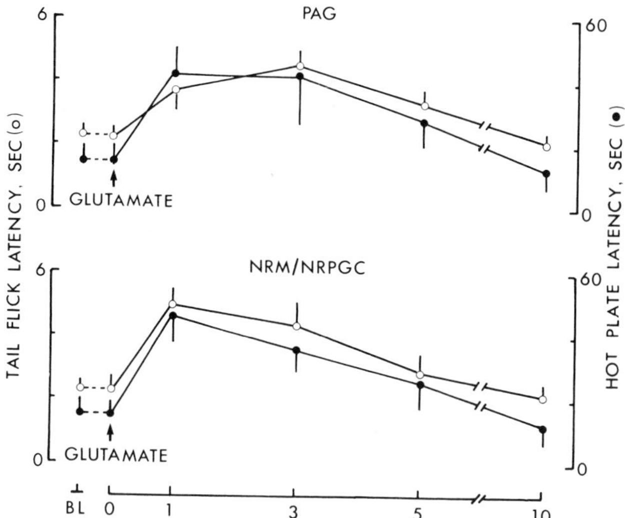

FIG. 1. Magnitude and time course of elevated tail-flick *(open circles)* and hot-plate *(closed circles)* response latencies following a microinjection of glutamate (30 nmoles/0.5 μl) into 9 brainstem sites within the periaqueductal gray (PAG) and 9 brainstem sites within the nucleus raphe magnus (NRM) or the nucleus reticularis paragigantocellularis (NRPGC). Values reprsent mean ± SE

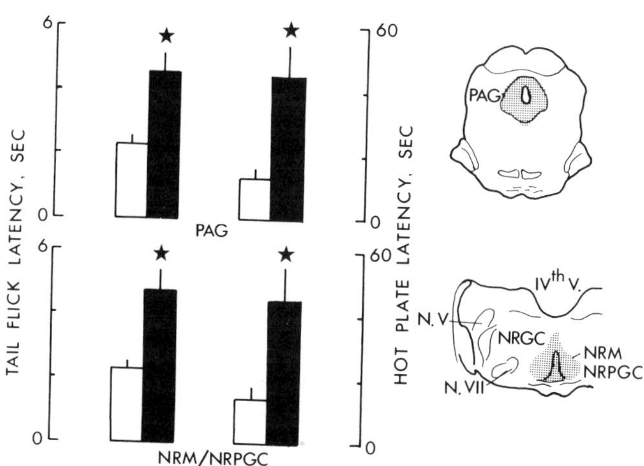

FIG. 2. Tail-flick **(left)** and hot-plate **(right)** response latencies before *(open bars)* and 1 min after *(closed bars)* an intracerebral injection of glutamate (30 nmoles/0.5 μl) into 27 sites within the PAG and 26 sites within the NRM/NRPGC. Values represent mean ± SE. *Stars* indicate significant difference from corresponding baseline values by *t*-tests, $p < 0.01$.

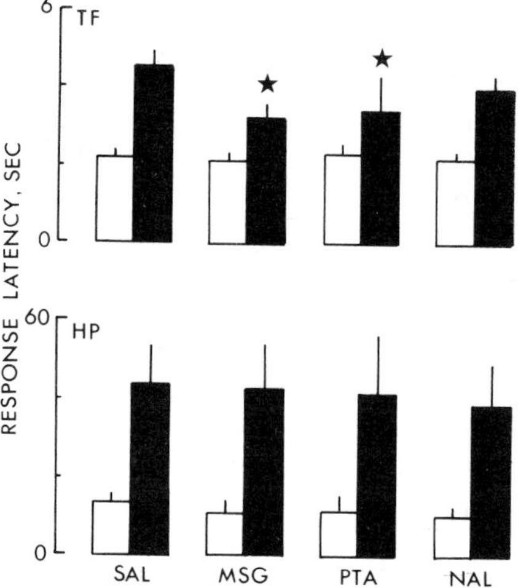

FIG. 3. Effects of intrathecal pretreatments on the elevation of tail-flick (TF) and hot-plate (HP) response latencies produced by glutamate (30 nmoles/0.5 μl) injected into the PAG. Rats were pretreated intrathecally with either saline (SAL), methysergide (MSG), phentolamine (PTA), or naloxone (NAL), and TF and HP response latencies were measured 10 to 15 min after pretreatments *(open bars)* and 1 min after *(closed bars)* intracerebral glutamate. Values represent mean ± SE of 6 to 9 rats. *Stars* indicate significant difference from corresponding saline value, $p < 0.01$.

a significant reduction by methysergide and phentolamine. On the other hand, pretreatments did not interfere with the elevated HP response latencies produced by PAG glutamate (F = 0.17, df:3/23, NS). Within the NRM/NRPGC (Fig. 4) pretreatment with either methysergide, phentolamine, or naloxone significantly reduced the elevation of TF, but not HP response latencies (F = 13,37, df:3/22, $p < 0.001$, and F = 1.25, df:3/22, NS, respectively).

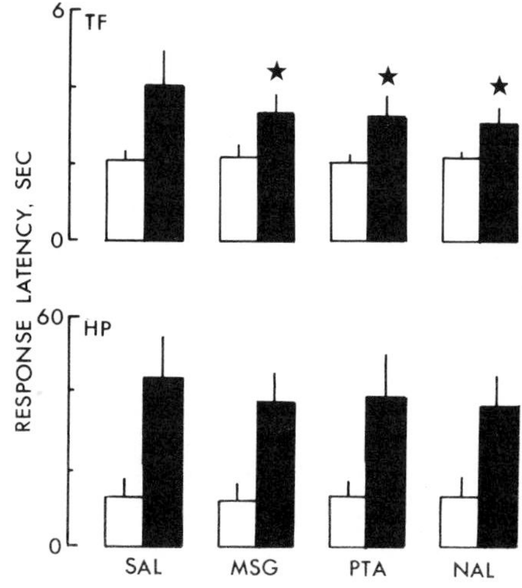

FIG. 4. Effects of intrathecal pretreatments on the elevation of tail-flick and hot-plate response latencies produced by glutamate (30 nmoles/0.5 μl) into the NRM/NRPGC. Text otherwise as described in Fig. 3.

DISCUSSION

This study confirms previous observations that direct excitation of discrete cell populations in the brainstem can alter spinal reflex activity via a spinopetal system (2,11). Since the behavioral end-point of the TF reflex is a motor response, inhibition of the segmental reflex may either be the consequence of an effect on dorsal horn nociceptive processing, on flexor/extensor motor activity, or a combination of such mechanisms. However, it is unlikely that the segmental reflex inhibition produced by intracerebral glutamate is due to a pure motor blockade since glutamate also attenuated the supraspinally organized HP response.

The observation that serotonergic and noradrenergic antagonists with an action limited to the spinal cord reduced the effects of brainstem glutamate on spinal cord function suggests that brainstem glutamate receptor activation results in the excitation of spinopetal monoaminergic pathways which modulates spinal reflex activity. Further studies have indicated that the pharmacological properties of the spinal receptor systems which mediate the effects of intracerebral glutamate can not be distinguished from those produced by electrical stimulation or opioids at brainstem sites (1,4,7,13). This suggests that spinopetal monoaminergic fiber systems may represent a common inhibitory system recruited by supraspinal manipulations. A spinal opioid synapse also appears to be involved in mediating the segmental reflex inhibition produced by activation of cells within the NRM/NRPGC, but not in the PAG. Thus, spinopetal inhibition may either recruit or bypass a spinal opioid link depending on the site of focal brainstem excitation.

Intrathecally administered antagonists failed to counteract the effects of intracerebral glutamate on the supraspinally organized HP response. These findings are at variance from those reported by Satoh et al. (10). This discrepancy may, in part, be due to differences in methods used for assessing antinociception. We have used a thermal evoked response, whereas Satoh et al. (10) have used a biting response to strong tail pressure. The failure of i.t.-administered antagonists to reverse the effect of intracerebral glutamate on the supraspinally mediated HP response as compared to the spinally mediated TF response suggests that brainstem systems produce antinociception by means other than a simple blockade of ascending nociceptive traffic to the brain. One possibility could be that supraspinal manipulations such as electrical stimulation, microinjection of morphine or glutamate exerts a direct effect on supraspinal structures involved in the processing of nociceptive information to the brain.

ACKNOWLEDGMENTS

We would like to thank Ms. Gail Harty and Ms. Margareth Mourning for technical assistance. This work was supported by funds from NS 16541,

Mayo Foundation, DMRC 12-3561, 82-4174, and Knud Hojgaard's Foundation.

REFERENCES

1. Azami, J., Llewelyn, M. B., and Roberts, M. H. T. (1982): The contribution of nucleus reticularis paragigantocellularis and nucleus raphe magnus to the analgesia produced by systemically administered morphine investigated with the microinjection technique. *Pain,* 12:229–246.
2. Behbehani, M. M., and Fields, H. L. (1979): Evidence that an excitatory connection between the PAG and nucleus raphe magnus mediates SPA. *Brain Res.,* 170:85–93.
3. Gebhart, G. F. (1982): Opiate and opioid peptide effects on brain stem neurons: Relevance to nociception and antinociceptive mechanisms. *Pain,* 12:93–140.
4. Hammond, D. L., and Yaksh, T. L. (1982): Intrathecal methysergide and phentolamine antagonize stimulation-produced analgesia from the nucleus raphe magnus. *Soc. Neurosci.,* 8:769.
5. Jensen, T. S., and Yaksh, T. L. (1984): Spinal monoamine and opiate systems partly mediates the antinociceptive effects produced by glutamate at brainstem sites. *Brain Res.,* 321:287–297.
6. Jensen, T. S., and Yaksh, T. L. (1985): I. Comparison of antinociceptive action of morphine in the periaqueductal gray, medial and paramedial medulla in rat. *Brain Res. (in press).*
7. Jensen, T. S., and Yaksh, T. L. (1985): II. Examination of spinal monoamine receptors through which brain stem opiate sensitive systems act in the rat. *Brain Res. (in press).*
8. Levine, J. D., Lane, S. R., Gordon, N. C., and Fields, H. L. (1982): A spinal opioid synapse mediates the interaction of spinal and brain stem sites in morphine analgesia. *Brain Res.,* 236:85–91.
9. Pellegrino, L. J., Pellegrino, A. S., and Cushman, A. J. (1979): *A Stereotaxic Atlas of the Rat Brain.* Plenum Press, New York.
10. Satoh, M., Oku, R., and Akaike, A. (1983): Analgesia produced by microinjection of L-glutamate into the rostral ventromedial bulbar nuclei of the rat and its inhibition by intrathecal α-adrenergic blocking agents. *Brain Res.,* 261:361–364.
11. Urca, G., Nahin, R. L., and Liebeskind, J. C. (1980): Glutamate-induced analgesia: Blockade and potentiation by naloxone. *Brain Res.,* 192:523–530.
12. Willis, W. D., Haber, L. H., and Martin, R. F. (1977): Inhibition of spinothalamic tract cells and interneurons by brainstem stimulation in the monkey. *J. Neurophysiol.,* 50:968–981.
13. Yaksh, T. L. (1978): Direct evidence that spinal serotonin and noradrenalin terminals mediate the spinal antinociceptive effects of morphine in the periaqueductal gray. *Brain Res.,* 160:180–185.
14. Yaksh, T. L., and Rudy, T. A. (1978): Narcotic analgetics: CNS dites and mechanisms of action as revealed by intracerebral injection techniques. *Pain,* 4:299–359.
15. Yaksh, T. L., Hammond, D. L., and Tyce, G. M. (1981): Functional aspects of bulbospinal monoaminergic projections in modulating processing of somatosensory information. *Fed. Proc.,* 40:2786–2794.
16. Zorman, G., Belcher, G., Adams, J. E., and Fields, H. L. (1982): Lumbar intrathecal naloxone blocks analgesia produced by microstimulation of the ventromedial medulla in the rat. *Brain Res.,* 236:77–84.

Advances in Pain Research and Therapy, Vol. 9, edited by H. L. Fields et al. Raven Press, New York © 1985.

Acupuncture-Like Transcutaneous Electrical Nerve Stimulation Analgesia Is Influenced by Spinal Cord Endorphins but Not Serotonin: An Intrathecal Pharmacological Study

J. M. Peets and B. Pomeranz

Department of Zoology, University of Toronto, Toronto, Ontario, Canada M5S 1A1

Changes in nociceptive threshold can be produced by a variety of peripheral somatic stimuli. Transcutaneous electrical nerve stimulation (TENS) and electroacupuncture (EA) use innocuous patterned stimulation of various frequencies to produce an analgesic effect that significantly outlasts the actual conditioning stimulus. Previous studies on TENS and EA, using systemic drug administrations, have demonstrated that at low frequencies of stimulation (4 Hz), the analgesic effect appears to be mediated by endorphinergic pathways (1,12,14–16,19,21). High frequency TENS and EA, on the other hand, appear to be mediated by serotonergic pathways (see ref. 20). These systemic pharmacological studies do not give any indication as to where in the neuraxis the stimulation is acting.

Using the technique of intrathecal cannulation developed by Yaksh and Rudy (23), we investigated the behavioral pharmacology of TENS at the spinal level. Drugs enhancing endorphinergic pathways (the dipeptides L-tyrosyl glycine and L-tyrosyl alanine) (4) and drugs blocking opiate receptors (naloxone hydrochloride) were administered intrathecally to determine the contribution of spinal endorphins to TENS analgesia. Similarly, cinanserin (a serotonin receptor blocker) and zimelidine (a serotonin reuptake inhibitor) were used to study the role of spinal serotonin.

Our results indicate that, at the spinal level, low frequency TENS (4 Hz) is mediated by endorphins, while high frequency TENS (200 Hz) is mediated by neither endorphins nor serotonin.

MATERIALS AND METHODS

Male Wistar rats, 300 to 350 g, were anesthetized using Nembutal (40 mg/kg) and placed in a stereotaxic holder. The dura on the dorsal atlanto-occipital junction was exposed, cut, and a PE10 polyethylene cannula (Intramedic) was then inserted into the lumbar subarachnoid space. The rostral end of the cannula was brought forward under the scalp and through the skin on top of the head. After the cannula had been flushed with 15 μl of artificial cerebrospinal fluid (CSF), the exposed tip was heat sealed. This procedure was based on that reported by Yaksh and Rudy (23).

Following a 1- to 2-week recovery, rats were observed for any signs of neurological damage; if such damage was observed the animal was removed from this study. Rats were lightly restrained in clear Plexiglas holders for the behavioral testing. Small silver surface electrodes covered with EKG gel were taped to the lateral aspect of both heels. The rats were then allowed roughly 10 min to acclimatize to the holders.

Thresholds to noxious stimuli were determined by means of a semiautomated tailflick apparatus that we constructed. The rat's tail was placed over a slit above a photoresistor, and a circuit actuated that turned on a heat lamp above the tail and started a timer. Any significant movement of the tail exposed the photoresistor, causing a cutoff of the heat lamp and stopping the timer. A 1-cm band of tail 3 cm from the tip was blackened and placed directly under the heat lamp. The cutoff time for exposure to the heat lamp was 10 sec. No tissue damage to the tail was ever observed among the rats used in this study.

Determinations of tail-flick latency (2) were made at intervals of 2 min. Initial baseline latency values were determined as the average of 3 trials at 2-min intervals following the acclimatization period. Drugs were then administered intrathecally in a 5-μl volume of artificial CSF. The drugs were followed by a 10-μl artificial CSF flush. Each rat received only one intrathecal injection.

TENS was given following the drug injection, using a pair of Grass SD9 stimulators. Low frequency TENS consisted of trains of biphasic pulses. Trains were of 70 msec duration, had an internal frequency of 100 Hz, and were delivered at a rate of 4 Hz. The pulses within the trains were of 0.1 msec duration. The stimulating voltage was gradually increased until a movement of the foot was noticed. Currents used ranged from 1.4 to 2.0 mA. At these voltages, the rats never vocalized and showed no signs of overt discomfort related to the stimulus (i.e., struggling, defecation). The TENS was given for 30 min, during which the voltage of the stimulus was titrated (usually upwards) to maintain the same degree of foot movement. Increasing the voltage a further 10 to 20% would cause rats to vocalize, and this was carefully avoided in the experimental animals to minimize stress. Immediately after cessation of the TENS, a tail-flick latency determination was made. Subsequent readings were made at 10 min intervals for the next 50 min.

As a measure of the analgesic effect of TENS we calculated the percent increase over baseline in the latency to tail flick. Comparisons of drug and control group means were made using a multivariate analysis of variance (MANOVA), and group effects were deemed significant at $p < 0.05$. The MANOVA was used on data points betwen the 30- and 50-min samples since preliminary studies showed a peak TENS effect at these times. Use of the MANOVA allowed us to analyze between-group differences while avoiding repeated *t*-tests. Each drug group consisted of 15 rats, with the exception of the low frequency TENS serotonin study, which used a group size of 13. Each animal was used only once in this study.

RESULTS

Figure 1 shows the effect of intrathecal naloxone on the analgesic effects of low frequency TENS. The vehicle control group demonstrated a clear analgesic effect that reached a peak at approximately 30 min post-TENS and lasted beyond the time window of our study. A statistically significant ($p < 0.001$) blockade of this effect is seen in the naloxone-injected group.

The effect of the intrathecal dipeptides is demonstrated in Fig. 2. The upper dipeptide group represents the animals receiving both TENS and dipeptide. The vehicle group received artificial CSF and TENS. There is a small but statistically significant ($p < 0.05$) difference between these 2 groups, suggesting that the dipeptides somewhat potentiated the analgesic effect of the low frequency TENS. The lower line, labeled dipeptide, in Fig.

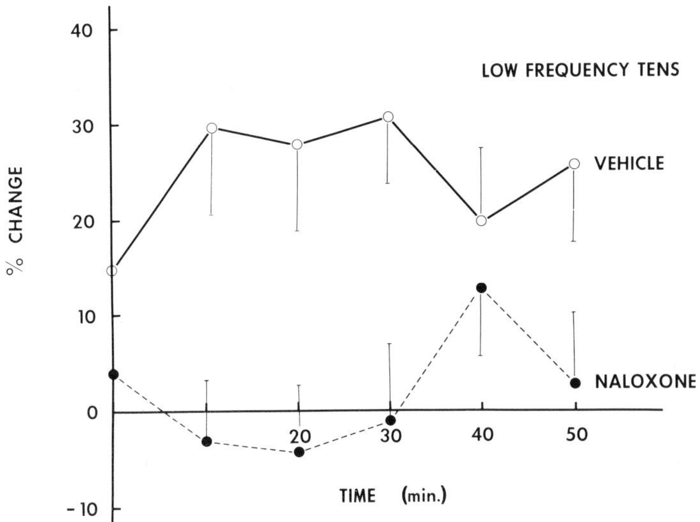

FIG. 1. Effect of intrathecal naloxone on the analgesia from low-frequency TENS. Percent change in latency to tail flick from control baseline values is plotted against time after cessation of the TENS. *Solid line:* intrathecal injection of CSF vehicle; *Broken line:* intrathecal naloxone (5 μg).

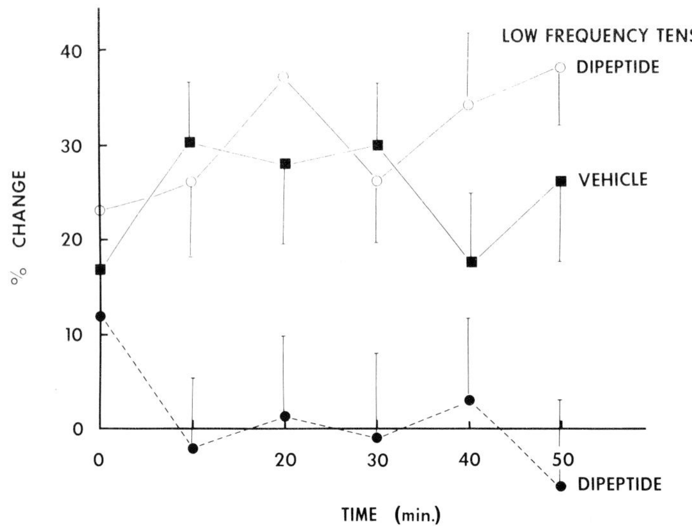

FIG. 2. Effect of intrathecal dipeptide. *Lower line,* labeled dipeptide, represents a group-administered intrathecal dipeptide (10 μg) but not given TENS. *Upper line,* labeled dipeptide, represents the group given both TENS and intrathecal dipeptide. *Solid line,* labeled vehicle, represents the TENS + CSF group.

2 represents a control group receiving intrathecal dipeptide but no TENS. No change in latencies was observed as a result of the dipeptides alone.

Cinanserin and zimelidine were without effect on low frequency TENS analgesia ($p > 0.05$).

Cinanserin had no significant effect on the analgesia from high frequency TENS ($p > 0.05$). Similarly, there was no effect of naloxone on high frequency TENS ($p > 0.05$). Figure 3 summarizes the findings of this study.

DISCUSSION

Innocuous stimulation causing analgesia includes electroacupuncture and transcutaneous nerve stimulation. Both techniques cause alterations in pain sensitivity at body sites remote from the conditioning site, involve the excitation of comparatively low threshold cutaneous afferents, have a similar frequency dependence, and similar pharmacological properties (1,3,12,14–16,19,21). At low stimulation frequencies (2–4 Hz), both TENS and EA cause a naloxone-reversible analgesia, while stimulation at higher frequencies causes an analgesia that appears to be mediated by serotoninergic synapses. Noxious stimulation has also been reported to decrease pain sensitivity, but this effect can readily be distinguished from TENS or EA analgesia in that the former shows a much shorter time course and faster onset. For example, LeBars et al. reported that noxious mechanical stimuli caused a short-duration, immediate onset analgesic effect that he termed diffuse nox-

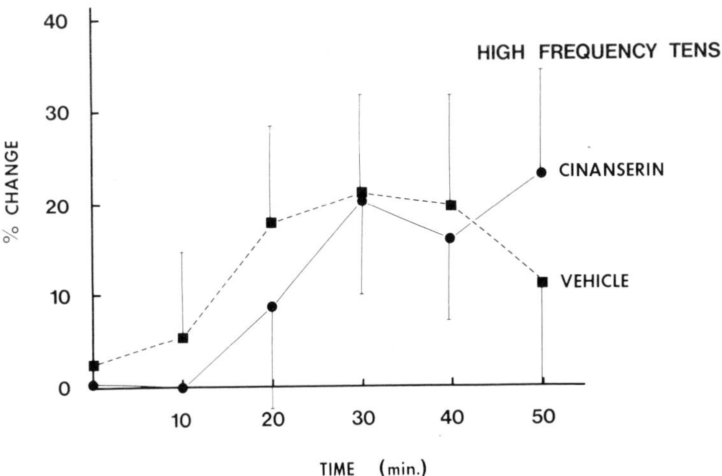

FIG. 3. Summary of results. Drug/treatment combinations are tabulated showing effects of intrathecally administered endorphinergic modifiers on low-frequency TENS analgesia. Other drug/treatment combinations showed no effect.

ious inhibitory controls (DNIC) (9). This contrasts sharply with the time course of EA and TENS where the onset typically requires 20 to 30 min, and effects may last beyond 90 min (indeed, several hours in the case of clinical reports). There are numerous reports in the literature of short-term inhibition of neuronal responses to noxious inputs following both noxious and non-noxious conditioning stimuli. Invariably, though, the duration of inhibition does not exceed a few hundred milliseconds. Recordings of single second-order neurons and excitability testing of primary afferent terminals have demonstrated a significant but extremely short-lived effect of conditioning somatic stimuli, possibly mediated by depolarization of the primary afferent terminals (e.g., ref. 6). These studies, however, cannot be related to the behavioral analgesia reported here, primarily because of the marked discrepancy in time course. It is interesting to note that a single conditioning stimulus causes a very brief blockage of nociceptive inputs, whereas repetition of the stimulus induces a much longer-lasting effect that appears to be mediated by different neurotransmitter/neuromodulator systems. In fact, the underlying systems seem also to be determined by the pattern in which the conditioning stimuli are presented (as exemplified by the endorphin involvement in low- but not high-frequency TENS and EA). The present study demonstrates, in agreement with numerous previous reports, that low-frequency conditioning stimuli cause an analgesic effect mediated by a naloxone-sensitive-link. It further demonstrates that at least one component of this naloxone-sensitive link is located within the spinal cord. The presence of opiate receptors and endorphins in the spinal cord of the rat has been frequently described. The analgesic effect of opiates and endorphins when injected directly onto the cord has also been well documented in studies by Yaksh and his colleagues, as well as others. Furthermore, it has been shown by a number of investigators that endorphins are released into the CSF of man, cat, and rat as a result of somatic stimulation (21,25,26). Numerous clinical reports of pain relief following TENS and EA demonstrate that a correlation may exist between the observations of endorphin release and analgesia as a result of somatic conditioning stimuli.

Another form of environmental stimulus resulting in analgesia is "stress" (e.g., refs. 2,10,11,22). Most studies reporting stress analgesia rely on frankly painful stimuli (i.e., limb breakage, cold water immersion, footshock, etc.) to produce an observable effect. The time course of the analgesic effect more closely resembles that of TENS and EA, sometimes lasting hours. Some forms of stress analgesia are naloxone reversible as well (2,10,22). We doubt that analgesia due to immobilization stress was a significant factor in our study, since preliminary experiments in which the rats were kept in their holders and stimulated at 0.2 Hz showed no analgesic effect. Since the group of rats receiving high-frequency TENS did not demonstrate a naloxone-reversible analgesia, it seems unlikely that the naloxone-reversible analgesia from low-frequency TENS is identical to footshock (stress)-induced opiate analgesia.

The absence of a cinanserin effect suggests that serotonin did not mediate the low-frequency analgesia, while it has been reported to mediate some forms of stress analgesia. Serotonin does act directly at the cord level as an analgesic agent (8,13,24), but may not play a role in some forms of analgesic manipulation such as stimulation of some midbrain sites (5,7; but see also ref. 18). Another possible candidate for mediating high-frequency TENS at the spinal level is norepinephrene (17).

In summary, our intrathecal studies suggest that low-frequency TENS analgesia in the rat is probably mediated by a spinal endorphinergic link. Spinal serotonin does not appear to be involved. High-frequency TENS analgesia does not appear to be mediated by a spinal endorphinergic or serotonergic link. This finding does not rule out a role for serotonin at higher centers in the CNS.

ACKNOWLEDGMENTS

This study was funded by the Natural Sciences and Engineering Research Council of Canada. We thank Endo Laboratories for the naloxone hydrochloride, Squibb Canada for the cinanserin, and Astra Pharmaceuticals of Canada for the zimelidine. For his invaluable assistance with this study, many sincere thanks to J. Phelan.

REFERENCES

1. Chapman, C. R., and Benedetti, C. (1977): Analgesia following transcutaneous electrical stimulation and its partial reversal by a narcotic antagonist. *Life Sci.,* 21:1645–1648.

2. Coderre, T. J., and Rollman, G. B. (1983): Naloxone hyperalgesia and stress-induced analgesia in rats. *Life Sci.*, 32:2139–2146.
3. D'Amour, F. E., and Smith, D. L. (1941): A method for determining loss of pain sensation. *J. Pharmacol. Exp. Ther.*, 72:74–79.
4. Gorenstein, C., and Snyder, S. H., (1980): Enkephalinases. *Proc. R. Soc. Lond. (Biol.)*, 210:123–132.
5. Griersmith, B. T., Duggan, A. W., and North, R. A. (1981): Methysergide and supraspinal inhibition of the spinal transmission of nociceptive information in the anesthetized cat. *Brain Res.*, 204:147–158.
6. Hentall, I. D., and Fields, H. L. (1979): Segmental and descending influences on intraspinal thresholds of single C-fibers. *J. Neurophysiol.*, 42:1527–1536.
7. Johannessen, J. N., Watkins, L. R., Carlton, S. M., and Mayer, D. J. (1982): Failure of spinal cord serotonin depletion to alter analgesia elicited from the periaqueductal grey. *Brain Res.*, 237:373–386.
8. Jordan, L. M., Kenshalo, D. R., Jr., Martin, R. F., Haber, L. H., and Willis, W. D. (1978): Depression of the primate spinothalamic tract neurones by iontophoretic application of 5-Ht. *Pain,* 5:135–142.
9. Le Bars, D., Dickenson, A. H., and Besson, J.-M. (1976): Diffuse noxious inhibitory controls (DNIC). I. Effects on dorsal horn convergent neurones in the rat. *Pain,* 6:283–304.
10. Lewis, J. W., Cannon, J. T., and Liebeskind, J. C. (1980): Opioid and non-opioid mechanisms of stress analgesia. *Science,* 208:623–625.
11. Maier, S. F., Drugan, R. C., and Grau, J. W. (1982): Controllability, coping behaviour and stress-induced analgesia in the rat. *Pain,* 12:47–56.
12. Mayer, D. J., Price, D. D., and Rafii, A. (1977): Antagonism of acupuncture analgesia by the narcotic antagonist naloxone. *Brain Res.,* 121:368–372.
13. Messing, R. B., and Lytle, L. D. (1977): Serotonin-containing neurons: their possible role in pain and analgesia. *Pain,* 4:1–21.
14. Pert, A., Dionne, R., Ng., L., Bragin, E., Moody, T. W., and Pert, C. B. (1981): Alterations in rat central nervous system endorphins following transauricular electroacupuncture. *Brain Res.,* 224:83–93.
15. Pomeranz, B., and Chiu, D. (1976): Naloxone blockade of acupuncture analgesia: endorphins implicated. *Life Sci.,* 19:1757–1762.
16. Pomeranz, B., and Cheng, R. (1979): Supression of noxious responses in single neurons of cat spinal cord by electroacupuncture and its reversal by the opiate antagonist naloxone. *Exp. Neurol.,* 64:327–341.
17. Reddy, S. V. R., and Yaksh, T. L. (1980): Spinal noradrenergic terminal system mediates antinociception. *Brain Res.,* 189:391–401.
18. Rivot, J. P., Chaouch, A., and Besson, J. M. (1980): Nucleus raphe magnus modulation of the response of rat dorsal horn neurones to unmyelinated fiber inputs: partial involvement of serotonergic pathways. *J. Neurophysiol.,* 44:1039–1057.
19. Sjolund, B. H., and Eriksson, M. B. E. (1979): The influence of naloxone on analgesia produced by peripheral conditioning stimuli. *Brain Res.,* 173:295–301.
20. Sjolund, B. H., and Erikkson, M. B. E. (1980): Stimulation techniques in the management of pain. In: *Pain and Society,* edited by H. W. Kosterlitz and L. Y. Terenius, pp. 415–430. Dahlem Konferenzen, Weinheim: Verlag Chemie GmbH.
21. Sjolund, B. H., Terenius, L., and Eriksson, M. (1977): Increased cerebrospinal fluid levels of endorphins after electroacupuncture. *Acta Physiol. Scand.,* 100:382–384.
22. Watkins, L. R., and Mayer, D. J. (1982): Organization of endogenous opiate and nonopiate pain control systems. *Science,* 216:1185–1192.
23. Yaksh, T. L., and Rudy, T. A. (1976): Chronic catheterization of the spinal subarachnoid space. *Physiol. Behav.,* 17:1031–1036.
24. Yaksh, T. L., and Wilson, P. R. (1980): Spinal serotonin terminal system mediates antinociception. *J. Pharmacol. Exp. Ther.,* 208:446–453.
25. Yaksh, T. L., and Elde, R. P. (1980): Release of methionine-enkephalin immunoreactivity from the rat spinal cord *in vivo. Eur. J. Pharmacol.,* 69:359–362.
26. Yaksh, T. L., Terenius, L., Nyberg, F., Jhamandas, K., and Wong, J. Y. (1983): Studies on the release by somatic stimulation from rat and cat spinal cord of active materials which displace dihydromorphine in an opiate binding assay. *Brain Res.,* 268:119–128.

Advances in Pain Research and Therapy, Vol. 9, edited by H. L. Fields et al. Raven Press, New York © 1985.

Spinal and Supraspinal Actions of Pro-Enkephalin A Fragments on Gastrointestinal Transit and Reflex Urinary Bladder Contractions

F. Porreca, T. F. Burks, and A. Dray

Department of Pharmacology, College of Medicine, University of Arizona Health Sciences Center, Tucson, Arizona 85724

Three precursor molecules, pro-opiomelanocortin, pro-enkephalin A, and pro-enkephalin B are the source of all known mammalian opioid peptides (6). These parent peptide molecules can be cleaved by proteolytic enzyme activity *in vivo* into intermediate length peptides. For pro-enkephalin A, these include peptide E, BAM 22P, BAM 20P, BAM 12P, Met^5-enkephalin-Arg^6-Phe^7(MEAP), Met^5-enkephalin-Arg^6-Gly^7-Leu^8(MEAGL), Met- and Leu-enkephalin, and peptide F (6). These intermediate peptides were found originally in the adrenal medulla but are also found to be unevenly distributed in the mammalian brain and spinal cord (for references, see refs. 6 and 8).

At present, little is known of the biological activity of these fragments or of their physiological significance. The possibility arises that the actions attributed to larger fragments may result from degradation to smaller fragments. Also, enzymatic modifications may produce fragments with differing biological properties. Preliminary reports show that the pro-enkephalin A fragments possess analgesic activity (7), and *in vitro* receptor binding studies suggest these substances interact with several opioid receptor subtypes (4,5,11,12). We now further report on the *in vivo* activity of the pro-enkephalin A fragments and show that these substances produce potent centrally mediated inhibition of gastrointestinal transit and of reflex urinary bladder contractions. These effects are consistent with the activation of central opioid receptors (2,3,9,10).

METHODS

Gastrointestinal transit was evaluated as previously described (9). Male, ICR mice (20–25 g), fasted overnight, received graded intracerebroventricular (i.c.v.) or intrathecal (i.t.) doses of peptide or saline concurrently with an oral, radiolabeled marker (^{51}CR as sodium chromate/saline solution, 0.2 ml/mouse). After 35 min the mice were killed, the stomach and the small intestine were excised, placed on a ruled template, and divided into 10 equal portions. Each intestinal segment was then placed into individual and consecutive culture tubes and the radioactivity in each tube was determined by γ-counting for a 1-min period. Gastrointestinal transit was expressed as the geometric center, a sensitive index of the relative distribution of radioactivity along the bowel. The geometric center was calculated as the sum of the fraction of radioactive ^{51}Cr marker in each segment of bowel $\times$ segment number. Lower geometric centers indicated inhibition of gastrointestinal transit.

Reflex urinary bladder contractions were studied in female Sprague-Dawley rats (200–220 g) anesthetized with urethane (1.2 g/kg, i.p.) and anesthesia supplemented as necessary. Body temperature was maintained at 37° C by means of a warm-water blanket. The urinary bladder was catheterized via the urethra and intravesicular pressure was measured using a physiological pressure transducer and displayed continuously on a chart recorder. The bladder was filled via the recording catheter until spontaneous contractions occurred as a result of central reflex activity (intravesicular pressure 5–13 cm of water). Contractions were then recorded isometrically and occurred rhythmically and reproducibly for many hours.

Injections (i.c.v.) were made stereotaxically into a lateral ventricle via a burr hole in the skull (coordinates 2 mm posterior to Bregma, 2 mm lateral to midline, and 4 mm deep from skull surface). Substances were administered i.t. by direct injection between the intervertebral space (L_2–L_5). Microinjections of physiological saline were used as control. All substances were administered in a volume of 1to 4 μl using a Hamilton syringe and 26-gauge needle. For potency comparisons only one dose of each substance was tested per animal to avoid the possibility of tachyphylaxis or cross-tolerance from repeated drug administrations. In other tests (for example, threshold dose determinations) approximately 60 min was allowed between recovery from the effects of one dose and the administration of another. All the peptides were obtained from Peninsula Laboratories (Belmont, California).

RESULTS

Gastrointestinal studies in mice revealed that i.c.v. microinjections of peptide E, BAM 22P, and the highest dose of MET-enkephalin produced dose-related inhibition of transit of the orally administered marker. No significant effects were observed with any of the other pro-enkephalin A fragments tested (Table 1). Following i.t. administration, all of the fragments produced dose-related inhibition of transit (Table 1). The effects of peptide E and BAM 22P appeared somewhat more potent following i.t. than i.c.v. administration (Table 1).

TABLE 1. *Effect of intracerebroventricular and intrathecal pro-enkephalin A fragments on gastrointestinal transit in mice.*

	Intracerebroventricular		Intrathecal	
Peptide	Dose	Geometric center	Dose	Geometric center
Saline		6.9 ± 0.8		
Peptide E	3 (1.0)	5.3 ± 0.7	3 (1.0)	2.2 ± 0.3[a]
	10 (3.2)	2.7 ± 0.3[a]	10 (3.2)	1.9 ± 0.5[a]
	20 (6.3)	2.9 ± 0.6[a]	20 (6.3)	1.6 ± 0.3[a]
BAM 22P	1 (0.4)	4.8 ± 0.8	1 (0.4)	4.9 ± 0.5
	3 (1.1)	4.3 ± 0.6	3 (1.1)	2.6 ± 0.5[a]
	10 (3.5)	3.2 ± 0.5[a]	10 (3.5)	2.3 ± 0.5[a]
	20 (7.0)	2.9 ± 0.4[a]		
	40 (14.0)	2.8 ± 0.3[a]		
BAM 12P	1 (0.7)	5.8 ± 0.4		
	3 (2.1)	5.4 ± 0.5		
	10 (7.0)	6.0 ± 0.5	10 (7.0)	2.9 ± 0.4[a]
	20 (14.0)	5.1 ± 0.1	30 (21.0)	4.1 ± 0.3[a]
	100 (70.2)	4.1 ± 0.9	60 (42.0)	1.8 ± 0.2[a]
Peptide F	1 (0.3)	5.7 ± 0.5		
	3 (0.8)	5.9 ± 0.2	3 (0.8)	5.2 ± 0.5
	10 (2.6)	6.4 ± 0.6	10 (2.6)	3.2 ± 0.5[a]
	20 (5.2)	4.4 ± 0.5		
	40 (10.4)	3.6 ± 0.9	40 (10.4)	2.4 ± 0.4[a]
MEAP	10 (11)	6.6 ± 0.5	10 (11)	6.2 ± 0.4
	30 (34)	6.0 ± 0.2	30 (34)	5.8 ± 0.4
	60 (68)	5.7 ± 0.5	60 (68)	3.6 ± 0.6[a]
	100 (114)	3.7 ± 0.4	100 (114)	2.4 ± 0.2[a]
	200 (228)	4.0 ± 0.9	200 (228)	2.2 ± 0.3[a]
MEAGL	30 (33)	5.2 ± 0.5	30 (33)	5.1 ± 0.6
	100 (111)	4.8 ± 0.4	100 (111)	4.5 ± 0.5
	200 (222)	4.7 ± 0.4	200 (222)	3.1 ± 0.5[a]
Metenkephalin	100 (170)	5.5 ± 0.3		
	200 (350)	5.6 ± 0.3		
	400 (690)	3.4 ± 0.4[a]		

Doses are expressed in μg (nmoles) per animal. Lower geometric centers indicate inhibition of transit. All data are mean ± SE (N = 5–8 animals per dose).

[a] $p < 0.05$ compared to saline. Data were compared by analysis of variance (ANOVA) and where significance was indicated were analyzed further using Student's *t*-test.

Spontaneous reflex bladder contractions were inhibited by each of the pro-enkepahlin A fragments following i.c.v. or i.t. administration (Table 2). Effects on bladder activity occurred rapidly (20–90 sec) and, at threshold doses, were characterized by a gradual reduction in the rate and amplitude of contractions (Fig. 1). This pattern of activity either culminated in complete cessation of bladder contractions or, at suprathreshold doses, contractions ceased abruptly following the microinjection (Fig. 1). The period of bladder quiescence provided an easily measured index of peptide activity and in this respect the effects of each substance was dose-related (Table 2). Peptide E, BAM 22P, and peptide F were the most potent of the fragments

TABLE 2. *Inhibition of reflex contractions of the urinary bladder in the anesthetized rat by intracerebroventricular and intrathecal pro-enkephalin A fragments*

	Intracerebroventricular		Intrathecal	
Peptide	Dose	Time (min)	Dose	Time (min)
Saline		0		0
Peptide E	5 (1.6)	21 ± 8	2 (0.6)	9 ± 2
	10 (3.2)	42 ± 12	4 (1.2)	20 ± 6
	20 (6.3)	62 ± 8	8 (2.4)	41 ± 9
BAM 22P	5 (1.8)	17 ± 7	2 (0.7)	17 ± 3
	10 (3.5)	32 ± 4	4 (1.4)	39 ± 12
	20 (7.0)	55 ± 19	8 (2.8)	89 ± 19
BAM 12P	10 (7.0)	9 ± 3	5 (3.5)	14 ± 4
	20 (14.0)	13 ± 2	10 (7.0)	24 ± 6
	40 (28.1)	20 ± 4	20 (14.0)	46 ± 8
Peptide F	2 (0.5)	13 ± 6	2 (0.5)	8 ± 3
	4 (1.0)	25 ± 6	4 (1.0)	26 ± 9
	8 (2.0)	39 ± 10	8 (2.0)	64 ± 9
MEAP	20 (22)	9 ± 2	20 (22)	15 ± 3
	40 (44)	15 ± 3	40 (44)	34 ± 5
	80 (88)	28 ± 6	80 (88)	60 ± 10
MEAGL	50 (52)	9 ± 2	12.5 (13)	10 ± 3
	100 (104)	15 ± 4	25 (26)	18 ± 3
	200 (208)	21 ± 5	50 (52)	43 ± 12
Metenkephalin	100 (170)	8 ± 2	10 (17)	11 ± 4
	200 (350)	13 ± 3	20 (35)	18 ± 4
	400 (690)	34 ± 7	40 (69)	36 ± 11

Doses are expressed in μg (nmoles) administered i.c.v. or i.t. in each animal. Inhibition of bladder contractions is expressed as the time (min) for complete suppression of isometric contractions. All data are mean ± SE (*N* = 5–6 animals per dose).

tested either by the i.c.v. or i.t. route, and Met-enkephalin was the least potent. Interestingly, each substance appeared to produce more prolonged inhibition of bladder contractions when administered by the i.t. route.

DISCUSSION

A number of the pro-enkephalin A fragments produced centrally mediated inhibition of gastrointestinal transit or inhibited reflex bladder contractions when administered i.c.v. or by i.t. microinjection. At present, it is not clear if the effects of the peptide fragments were due to enzymatic cleavage *in vivo* into active substances. It is also unclear whether the ineffectiveness of some fragments (gastrointestinal transit studies) and the apparent changes in activity of smaller fragments (compare peptide E fragments on bladder activity) were also due to metabolism to inactive peptides or peptides with differing pharmacological properties. The rapid time

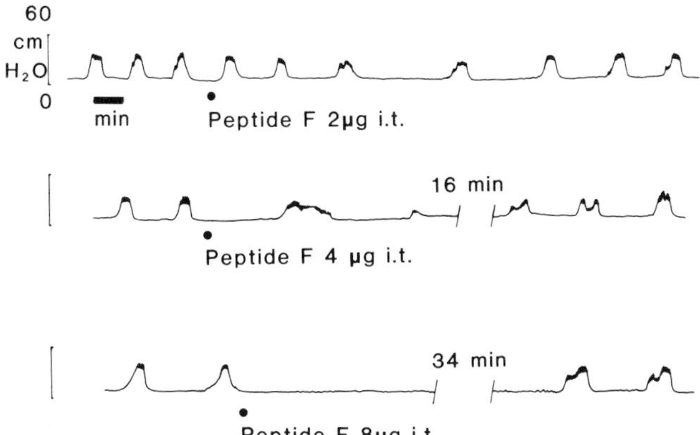

FIG. 1. Inhibition of reflex urinary bladder contractions by intrathecal (i.t.) administrations of peptide F. **Top trace** shows a reduction in the rate and amplitude of contractions at a threshold dose (2 μg, i.t.). **Middle** and **bottom traces** show complete cessation of bladder contractions. The duration of this was dose-related. Length of the break in the records is indicated above. All records were taken from the same animal. *Calibration bars* are 60 cm of water and 1 min.

course, however, of the inhibition of reflex bladder contractions following peptide microinjections would favor the possibility that the effects were, at least in part, mediated by the microinjected substance. Peptide E, for example, is known to be centrally processed to BAM 22P, BAM12P, and Met-enkephalin (1); however, its prolonged half-life determined *in vitro* (1) strongly suggests that the activity observed in the present experiments was, in fact, due to peptide E. Information on the biological half-life of other pro-enkephalin A fragments is not available at present, although the low potency and brief activity of Met-enkephalin can be readily explained by peptidase inactivation.

The reason for the apparent difference in the activity of compounds administered i.c.v. or i.t. is uncertain. These may have resulted from differences in spinal and supraspinal distribution of the peptide, or from differences in proteolytic enzyme activity in these regions.

It seems likely, however, that the central effects observed in the two animal models were due to the opioid properties of the pro-enkephalin A fragments. κ-Opioid receptors, accessible by i.c.v. or i.t. microinjection, do not appear to be involved in either the inhibition of gastrointestinal transit or bladder contractions. The inhibition of gastrointestinal transit appears, however, to be mediated supraspinally by μ-opioid receptors and spinally by μ and δ-opioid receptors (9,10). In addition, the inhibition of reflex bladder contractions is mediated by both μ- and δ-receptors at spinal and supraspinal sites (2,3). Therefore the inhibition of gastrointestinal transit by i.c.v. peptide E, BAM 22P, and high doses of Met-enkephalin would be compatible with μ-receptor activity. On the other hand, the activity exhibited by each of the fragments administered i.t. would suggest additional δ-opioid receptor properties. These conclusions are broadly supported by the observed i.c.v. and i.t. effectiveness of each of the fragments in inhibiting reflex bladder contractions. In addition, preliminary data suggest that low i.c.v. or i.t. doses of naloxone (1–2 μg) which readily antagonize μ-receptor ligands such as morphine and [D-Ala^2, Me-Phe^4, Gly (ol)^5]enkephalin (DAGO) (2,3) also attenuate the actions of peptide E, and to a certain extent those of BAM 22P and BAM 12P (1). Higher doses of naloxone (10–12 μg) are required to antagonize the effects of MEAGL, MEAP, and peptide F. Receptor binding studies indicate that peptide E, BAM 22P, and BAM 12P have predominantly μ and κ activity with some degree of δ activity. On the other hand, MEAGL, MEAP, Met-enkephalin, and peptide F appear as predominantly δ-agonist with some additional μ- and κ-receptor properties (4,5,11,12).

In conclusion, the pro-enkephalin A fragments possess central opioid receptor activity *in vivo* revealed by the inhibition of gastrointestinal transit in the mouse and reflex urinary bladder contractions in the rat. These effects may be mediated by μ- and δ-opioid receptor activity. The physiological significance of these peptide fragments is unclear, but the present studies suggest their involvement in central regulation of visceral function in addition to postulated roles in nociception (7).

REFERENCES

1. Davis, T. P., Porreca, F., and Dray, A. (1984): The pro-enkephalin A derivative, peptide E, is centrally processed to active fragments. *Proc. West. Pharmacol. Soc.,* 27:577–581.
2. Dray, A., and Metsch, R. (1984): Opioids and central inhibition of urinary bladder motility. *Eur. J. Pharmacol.,* 98:155–156.
3. Dray, A., and Metsch, R. (1984): Spinal opioid receptors and inhibition of urinary bladder motility *in vivo. Neurosci. Lett.,* 47:81–84.
4. Garzon, J., Sanchez-Blazquez, P., Hollt, V., Lee, N. M., and Loh, H. H. (1983): Endogenous opioid peptides: comparative evaluation of their receptor affinities in the mouse brain. *Life Sci.,* 33 (Suppl. 1):291–294.
5. Goldstein, A., and James, I. F. (1984): Site-directed alkylation of multiple opioid receptors II. Pharmacological selectivity. *Mol. Pharmacol.,* 25:343–348.
6. Hollt, V. (1983): Multiple endogenous opioid peptides. *Trends Neurosci.,* 6:24–26.
7. Hollt, V., Cankat Tulunay, F., Wood, S. K., Loh, H. H., and Herz, A. (1982): Opioid peptides derived from proenkephalin A but not from proenkephalin B are substantial analgesics after administration into brain of mice. *Eur. J. Pharmacol.,* 85:355–356.
8. Pittius, C. W., Seizinger, B. R., Pasi, A., Mehraein, P., and Herz, A. (1984): Distribution and characterization of opioid peptides derived from proenkephalin A in human and rat central nervous system. *Brain Res.,* 304:127–136.
9. Porreca, F., and Burks, T. F. (1983): The spinal cord as a site of opioid effects on gastrointestinal transit in the mouse. *J. Pharmacol. Exp. Ther.,* 227:22–27.
10. Porreca, F., Mosberg, H. I., Hurst, R., Hruby, V. J., and Burks, T. F. (1984): The roles of mu, delta and kappa opioid receptors in spinal and supraspinal mediation of gastrointestinal transit effects and analgesia in the mouse. *J. Pharmacol. Exp. Ther.,* 230:341–348.
11. Rezvani, A., Hollt, V., and Way, E. L. (1983): K-receptor activities of the three opioid peptide families. *Life Sci.,* 33 (Suppl. 1):271–274.
12. Quirion, R., and Weiss, A. S. (1983): Peptide E and other proenkephalin-derived peptides are potent kappa opiate receptor agonists. *Peptides,* 4:445–449.

Advances in Pain Research and Therapy, Vol. 9, edited by H. L. Fields et al. Raven Press, New York © 1985.

Potentiation of the Effects of Intrathecal Methionine-Enkephalin by Aminopeptidase Inhibition

R. Noueihed and T.L. Yaksh

Section of Neurosurgical Research, Mayo Clinic, Rochester, Minnesota 55905

Opiates with an action limited to the spinal cord will produce a powerful analgesia mediated by one of several subpopulations of opioid receptors (8,10). The pentapeptide enkephalins located in the spinal cord represent presumed agonists for these sites. The intrathecal administration of the enkephalin pentapeptides will, however, produce only a mild elevation in the nociceptive response latencies (12). This limited effect has been presumed to occur because of the rapid metabolism of these short-chained peptides. The half-life of these two pentapeptides *in vivo* and *in vitro* is in the order of 1 min. As the whole pentapeptide sequence is necessary for efficiency of the opiate receptor, this rapid metabolism is thought to, in part, account for the low level of opioid activity following the injections of these pentapeptides.

In the present studies, we sought to examine the effects of antagonizing peptidase activity by the use of an aminopeptidase inhibitor, amastatin (2), on the antinociceptive effects and pharmacology of methionine-enkephalin in the spinal cord.

MATERIALS AND METHODS

Animal Preparation

Male Sprague-Dawley rats were implanted with intrathecal catheters as described by Yaksh and Rudy (13). Briefly, polyethylene (PE-10) tubing is inserted through a slit in the atlanto-occipital membrane and passed 7.5 to 8.5 cm caudal to the rostral limit of the lumbar enlargement. Rats were examined 5 to 7 days following recovery.

Drug Administration and Drugs

Drugs were given in a volume of 10 μl followed by an injection of 10 μl saline to flush the catheter. Drugs administered were methionine-enkephalin (Sigma), and amastatin was a generous gift from Dr. H. Umezawa.

Nociceptive Tests

To measure the behavioral response to noxious stimuli two tests were employed: (a) the spinal-mediated, thermal-evoked tail-flick response, and (b) the thermal-evoked hot-plate response. The tail flick was produced by placing the tail over a slit through which a 300 W quartz projection bulb was focused and the time to tail withdrawal was recorded. The hot-plate response was assessed by placing the rats on a metal surface maintained at 52.5° C. The end-point was taken as the time when the rat licked the hindpaw. To prevent tissue damage, tests were terminated after 6 and 60 sec on the tail flick and hot plate, respectively.

Behavioral Tests

In rats, the degree of rigidity, catalepsy, the ability to descend in a coordinated fashion a 60° inclined wire mesh ramp, the presence or absence of placing and righting reflexes were systematically noted.

RESULTS

Effect of Intrathecal Amastatin Alone

The intrathecal administration of amastatin(3–10 μg) has no significant effect on the hot-plate and tail-flick response latency. Amastatin, in the doses employed in these experiments, displayed no evident signs of toxicity. No detectable effect on motor function or on simple reflex activity such as placing, stepping, or righting reflexes were observed. Motor tone as evidenced by the ability of the animal to withdraw the hindpaw upon stretching, was not detectably altered. The ability of the animal to negotiate a 60° inclined wire mesh surface was likewise unaffected.

Time Effect Curves of Intrathecal Methionine-Enkephalin and Amastatin

Figure 1 shows that intrathecal methionine-enkephalin (200 μg; 300 nM) on the hot-plate and tail-flick response can alone produce a significant but transient elevation in the response latency. This effect is significantly facilitated both in magnitude and duration of action by the concomitant intrathecal administration of amastatin (10 μg; 30 nM). Comparable effects are seen on both the hot plate and tail flick.

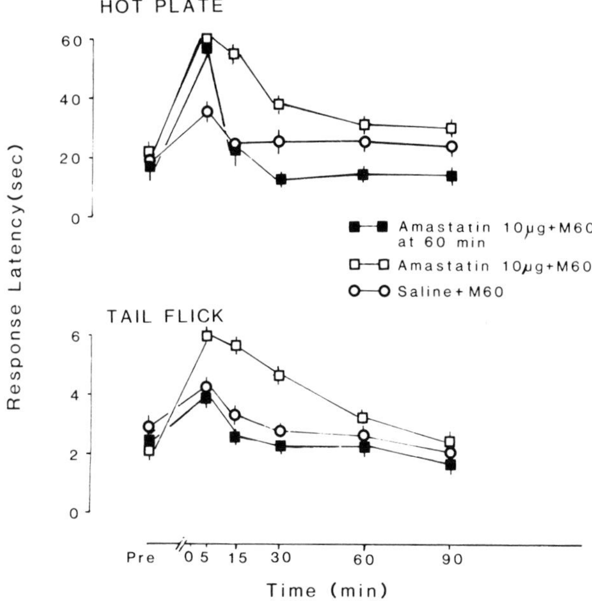

FIG. 1. Effect on hot-plate and tail-flick response latencies of the intrathecal administration of Met^5-enkephalin 200 μg (M200) alone, M200 and amastatin 10 μg (A10), A10 1 hr prior to intrathecal M200. Each curve presents the mean and SE of 4 rats.

Pretreatment with the aminopeptidase inhibitor 1 hr prior to injection of the peptide showed a surprisingly brief effect on the hot-plate response latency, but little effect on the tail flick.

Dose-Response Curves of Intrathecal Methionine-Enkephalin and Amastatin

Figure 2 represents dose-response effect of intrathecal Met^5-enkephalin (60 μg) carried out in the presence of 0.3, 1, 3, or 10 μg amastatin on the hot plate and tail flick. As can be seen, doses as low as 3 μg (9 nM) significantly potentiate the effects of intrathecal Met^5-enkephalin. Similar data are obtained in the presence of leucine-enkephalin (data not shown).

Figure 3 presents the degree of potentiation of 6, 20, 60, 200 μg of methionine-enkephalin the presence of a fixed dose of amastatin. As can be seen, concomitant injection of amastatin resulted in a significant increase in the slope of the intrathecal methionine-enkephalin dose-response curve.

Amastatin and Morphine

The intrathecal administration of morphine sulfate (4 μg) resulted in a MPE of 61.5 $\pm$ 8.9 and 48.4 $\pm$ 3.8 on the hot plate and tail flick, respec-

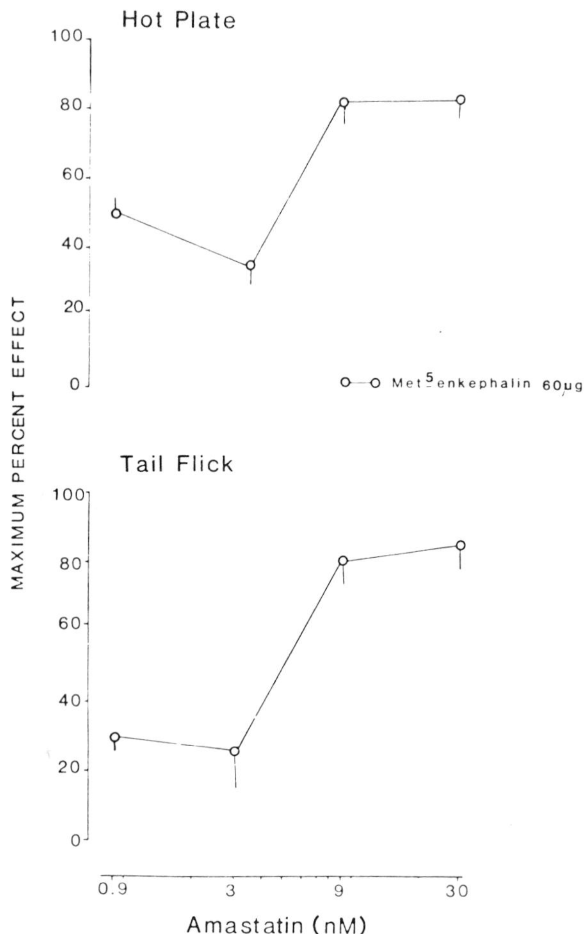

FIG. 2. Dose-response curve on the hot plate and tail flick of intrathecally administered amastatin 0.3, 1, 3, 10 μg concurrently injected with 60 μg Met^5-enkephalin. Each point presents the mean and SE of 4 to 6 rats.

tively. The concomitant administration of 10 μg amastatin had no effect on the antinociceptive potency of morphine.

Naloxone Antagonism

The effects of intrathecal methionine-enkephalin (60 μg) + amastatin (10 μg) were returned to normal by the subcutaneous (1 mg/kg) or intrathecal (10 μg) of naloxone.

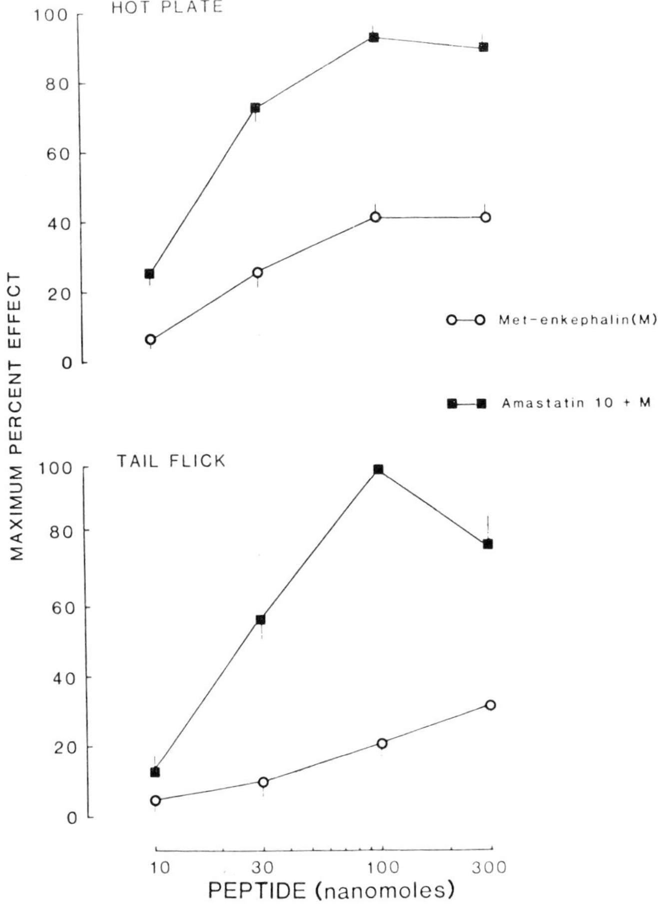

FIG. 3. Dose-response curves of intrathecal Met[5]-enkephalin alone in doses of 6, 20, 60, 200 μg and with the concomitant administration of amastatin 10 μg. Each point presents the mean and SE of 4 to 6 rats.

DISCUSSION

Our results suggest that aminopeptidase inhibition potentiates the effects of exogenously administered methionine-enkephalin at doses of amastatin, which alone produce no effects. Intrathecally administered amastatin in doses of 10 μg or less, had no significant effects on either the hot plate, tail flick, or animal behavior. The resulting potentiation of the effects of intrathecal methionine-enkephalin were manifested not only in terms of an increased duration of action, but a shift in the dose-response curve. The facilitated effects of spinally administered methionine-enkephalin and amastatin were uniformly antagonized by naloxone.

Amastatin is a low molecular weight tetrapeptide isolated by Umezawa and co-workers in an effort to discover inhibitors of therapeutically important enzymes (9). *In vitro* studies shows that it inhibits aminopeptidase A (AP-A), leucine AP and AP-M (6) in a competitive fashion. Amastatin is more potent than bestatin, another aminopeptidase currently used in pharmacologic studies, but probably metabolized as rapidly (9). This short half-life is consistent with our observation that pretreatment with amastatin at 1 hr before injection of the enkephalin fails to result in a facilitation of the enkephalin activity.

These studies demonstrate the importance of an amastatin-sensitive peptidase in controlling the activity of exogenously administered methionine-enkephalin in spinal cord, but do not exclude a role for other enzyme systems. We have, for example, earlier demonstrated the relevance of spinal dipeptidyl carboxypeptidase (commonly designated as enkephalinase) systems. Thus, the effects of intrathecal D-Ala^2-Met^5-enkephalin (DAME) are significantly potentiated by thiorphan (11), whereas captopril, an angiotensin-converting enzyme inhibitor, was inactive, suggesting the irrelevance of such a system to degradation of DAME.

A variety of investigations now indeed indicate that both aminopeptidase and carboxypeptidase systems participate in the degradation of endogenous enkephalins (1–3).

Whether such a potentiation as observed in these studies has clinical relevance remains to be seen. In any case it must be remembered that for a peptidase inhibitor to produce a physiological effect, the peptide first must be sensitive to the appropriate enzyme and, second, it must be released—where there is no "enkephalin" tone, there will be no effect. The present experiments suggest that under the stimulus conditions of the hot plate or tail flick, an endogenous opioid activity, destroyed by an amastatin-sensitive enzyme, does not exist in spinal cord.

ACKNOWLEDGMENTS

We would like to thank Ms. Gail Harty and Ms. Ann Rockafellow for their assistance. This work was supported by funds from DA-02110 and TW-03188.

REFERENCES

1. Bouboutou, R., Waksman, G., Devin, J., Fournié-Zaluski, M., and Roques, B. (1984): Bidentate peptides: highly potent new inhibitors of enkephalin degrading enzymes. *Life Sci.,* 35:1023–1030.
2. Chaillet, P., Marcaiscollado, H., Costentin, J., Yi, C. C., De Labaume, S., and Schwartz, J. C. (1983): Inhibition of enkephalin metabolism by, and antinociceptive activity of, Bestatin, an aminopeptidase inhibitor. *Eur. J. Pharmacol.,* 86:329–336.
3. De Labaume, S., Yi, C. C., Schwartz, J. C., Chaillet, P., Maracais-Collado, H., and Costentin, J. (1983): Participation of enkephalinase and aminopeptidase activities in the metabolism of endogenous enkephalins. *Neuroscience,* 8:143–145.

4. Elde, R., Hökfelt, T., Johansson, O., and Terenius, L. (1976): Immunohistochemical studies using antibodies to leucine enkephalin: Initial observations on the nervous system of the rat. *Neuroscience,* 5:349–351.
5. Hughes, J., Kosterlitz, W., Mcknight, A. T., Sasa, R., Lord, J., and Waterfield, A. A. (1978): Pharmacological and biochemical aspects of the enkephalins. In: *Centrally Acting Peptides,* edited by J. Hughes, pp. 179–193. University Park Press, Baltimore.
6. Rich, O., Moon, B. J., and Harbeson, S. (1984): Inhibition of aminopeptidases by Amastatin and Bestatin derivatives. Effect of inhibitor structure on slow binding processes. *J. Med. Chem.,* 27:160–166.
7. Sar, M., Stumpf, W., Miller, R., Chang, K. -J., and Cuatrecasas, P. (1978): Immunohistochemical localization of enkephalin in rat brain and spinal cord. *J. Comp. Neur.,* 182:17–38.
8. Schmauss, C., and Yaksh, T. L. (1983): *In vivo* studies on spinal opiate receptor systems mediating antinociception. II. Pharmacological profiles suggesting a differential association of mu, delta and kappa receptors with visceral chemical and cutaneous thermal stimuli in the rat. *J. Pharmacol. Exp. Ther.,* 228:1–12.
9. Umezawa, H. (1982): Low molecular-weight enzyme inhibitors of microbial origin. *Annu. Rev. Microbiol.,* 36:75–99.
10. Yaksh, T. L. (1983): *In vivo* studies on spinal opiate receptor systems mediating antinociception. I. Mu and delta receptor profiles in the primate. *J. Pharmacol. Exp. Ther.,* 226:303–316.
11. Yaksh, T. L., and Harty, G. (1982): Effects of thiorphan on the antinociceptive actions of intrathecal [D-Ala^2-Met^5]-enkephalin. *Eur. J. Pharmacol.,* 79:293–300.
12. Yaksh, T. L., Huang, S. P., Rudy, T. A., and Frederickson, R. C. A. (1977): The direct and specific opiate-like effect of Met^5-enkephalin and analogues on the spinal cord. *Neuroscience,* 2:593–596.
13. Yaksh, T. L., and Rudy, T. A. (1976): Chronic catheterization of the spinal subarachnoid space. *Physiol. Behav.,* 17:1031.

Advances in Pain Research and Therapy, Vol. 9, edited by H. L. Fields et al. Raven Press, New York © 1985.

Behavioral and Electrophysiological Investigations of Opiate/Cholecystokinin Interactions

S. N. Suberg, E. S. Culhane, E. Carstens, and L. R. Watkins

Department of Animal Physiology, University of California, Davis, California 95616

The distribution of cholecystokinin (CCK) in the central nervous system (CNS) has been well defined (3,18) and observed to exist in high concentrations in areas also containing endogenous opiates (33). Many of these CCK-containing CNS loci are areas previously implicated in pain modulation (i.e., periaqueductal gray, spinal cord dorsal horn, dorsal raphe) and, recently, Skirbol and co-workers found CCK-containing neurons projecting from the periaqueductal gray to the spinal cord (31). The anatomical overlap of CCK and opiate systems suggests that a functional interaction may occur as well. Indeed, under certain conditions the physiological actions of CCK are opposite those of opiates (9,24–26,32). Also, CCK has been found to antagonize analgesia produced by morphine and the release of endogenous opiates (13) as well as by administration of β-endorphin (20). These findings indicate that CCK may be modulating the antinociceptive effects of opiates leading to the hypothesis that CCK may act as a physiological endogenous opiate antagonist (13).

CCK may be modulating opiates through a negative feedback mechanism such that the presence of opiates triggers the release of endogenous CCK, thereby returning the animal toward a state of basal pain sensitivity (13,38). If this occurs, preventing endogenous CCK from interacting with opiates may prolong the action of opiates. This hypothesis has recently been tested and supported using proglumide, a putative competitive CCK receptor antagonist (16,27). Though a recent study suggests that proglumide does not bind to cortical CCK receptors (6), there is overwhelming behavioral and electrophysiological evidence that proglumide blocks the effects of CCK in the CNS (5,14,21,34,36,39,40). Although there is a discrepancy between the receptor studies and electrophysiological/behavioral studies, all the *in vivo* studies clearly show that proglumide does selectively and profoundly block CCK in the CNS. Thus, proglumide appears to be the best currently available means to study the effect of CCK blockage on analgesia.

Regarding the effect of proglumide on analgesia, proglumide has been observed to potentiate the onset, peak, and duration of opiate analgesia (38,39) as measured by the tail-flick test. Potentiation was observed when proglumide was combined with either intrathecal (IT) morphine or endogenous opiates [IT D-alanine methionine enkephalinamide (DALA)] or induced release by forepaw foot shock. Importantly, proglumide neither produced analgesia when injected in the absence of opiates nor potentiated various forms of nonopiate analgesia, implying that proglumide is selectively interacting with opiate systems in order to produce these effects.

To date, the ability of proglumide to potentiate opiate analgesia in rats has been limited to behavioral assessments using the tail-flick test. Knowing that different pain tests assess different types of pain and that various types of pain are modulated by neurochemically distinct pain suppressive systems (1,2,10), we raised the question as to whether the potentiation noted by Watkins et al. (38) could be specific to the radiant-heat pain stimulus used.

Thus, the aim of the present series of experiments was twofold: firstly, to extend the initial findings by behaviorally examining the effect of proglumide on opiate analgesia as assessed by a variety of behavioral tests; and, secondly, to electrophysiologically examine the effect of proglumide on opiate-induced suppression of responses from single dorsal horn neurons to noxious stimuli placed in their receptive fields. The results from these studies should provide an extended understanding of the interaction between CCK and opiate systems at both a cellular and behavioral level.

EXPERIMENT 1: BEHAVIORAL ASSESSMENT OF DALA AND PROGLUMIDE INTERACTION

Methods

Adult male Sprague-Dawley rats (450–455 g, Simonsen Laboratories, singly housed with 12-hr light cycle, food and water *ad libitum*) were used in all experiments. Animals were implanted with IT catheters (37) while under sodium pentobarbital anesthesia. Two to 3 weeks after surgery animals were habituated to Plexiglas restraining cylinders (5 daily sessions lasting 1 hr each) which would be used during test sessions. After being randomly assigned to drug groups, rats were injected IT with either proglumide (PROG; 0, 0.005, 0.01, or 0.02 μg) or equivolume saline (0.5 μl) at 10 min and again just before DALA (0, 3.0, 4.5, 6.0, or 9.0 μg in 0.5 μl saline). DALA was chosen based on previous behavioral studies (40) showing that proglumide was most effective in potentiating analgesia produced by this opiate. Behavioral testing was then performed blind with respect to the drug received. The behavioral assessments used in this investigation were modifications of the tail-flick (8), hot-plate (41), formalin (11), tail-shock vocalization (4), and tail-pinch (7) tests. For the tail-flick and formalin tests, rats were repeatedly assessed through 1 hr after IT injection. For the hot-plate, tail-shock vocalization, and tail-pinch tests, rats were tested 30 to 40 min post-IT drug; that is, at the time that maximal DALA analgesia was observed for both the tail-flick and formalin tests. The test responses of each rat (except for those assessed using the formalin test) were expressed as a percent of maximum possible effect (% MPE), using the following general equation (32):

$$\% \text{ MPE} = [(\text{TR} - \text{BR})/(\text{CO} - \text{BR})] \times 100$$

where TR is the test response recorded after drug injection, BR is the baseline response recorded prior to drug injection, and CO is the appropriate cut-off value chosen for each test to prevent tissue damage. Since for the formalin test a % MPE formula is not appropriate, the number of leg flinches occurring every other 5-min interval was recorded. For all tests, statistical comparisons between drug groups were made using analyses of variance (ANOVA) to determine main effects.

RESULTS

Tail-Flick Test

PROG (0.01 μg) was found to markedly enhance onset, peak, and duration of DALA analgesia (3.0 μg) in the tail-flick test, in accordance with previous results (38,40). PROG alone had no effect on responsivity (Fig. 1).

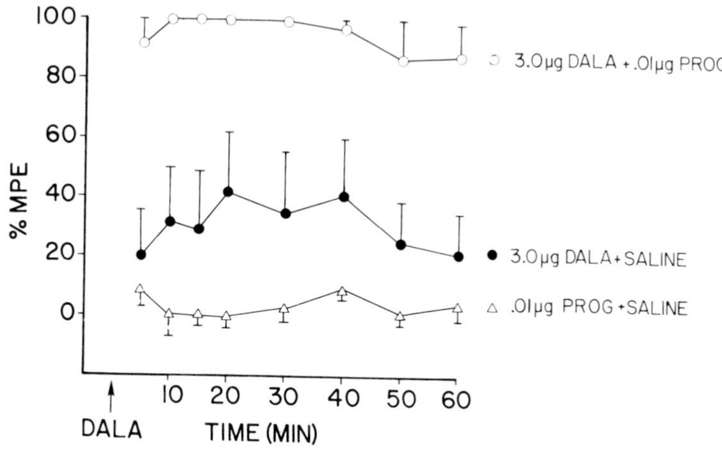

FIG. 1. Potentiation of DALA analgesia by proglumide (PROG) in the tail-flick test. PROG significantly ($p < 0.001$) potentiates DALA analgesia in the tail-flick test. Graph shows mean percent of maximal effect ± SE, across time, after 3.0 μg DALA IT (*Closed circles, N* = 7), 3.0 μg DALA + 0.01 μg PROG IT (*open circles, N* = 7) or 0.01 μg PROG IT (*triangles, N* = 5).

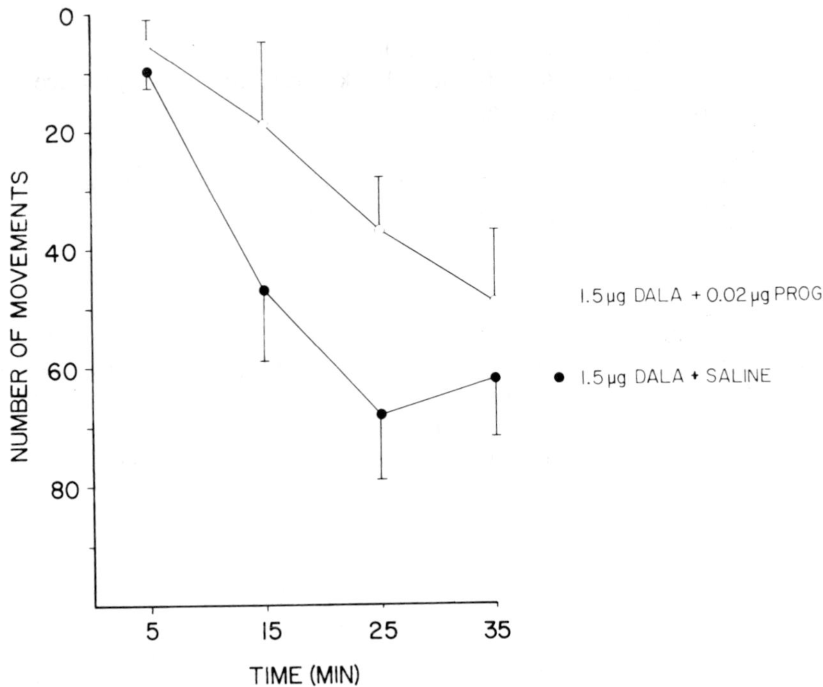

FIG. 2. Increase in DALA analgesia by proglumide (PROG) in the formalin test. This graph plots the number of leg flinches across time, after 1.5 μg DALA IT (*closed circles, N* = 14) or 1.5 μg DALA + 0.02 μg PROG IT (*open circles, N* = 5). PROG significantly ($p < 0.005$) increased the degree of DALA analgesia in the formalin test as compared to analgesia produced by DALA alone.

Results from this test indicate that maximal DALA analgesia occurred at approximately 30 min after IT injection of DALA.

Formalin Test

DALA produced an increasing degree of analgesia with increasing dosage (0, 1.5, and 3 μg). From our testing procedure using either 0, 0.005, 0.01 or 0.02 μg PROG and 0, 1.5 or 3.0 μg DALA, we found that PROG (0.02 μg) was capable of potentiating the analgesic effects of DALA (1.5 μg) (Fig. 2). Although PROG can potentiate DALA analgesia at certain dose combinations, a complex dose response relationship is present and similar to that previously seen using the tail flick test (38); that is, various doses of PROG can either potentiate, have no effect on, or antagonize opiate analgesia.

Hot-Plate, Tail-Shock Vocalization, and Tail-Pinch Tests

Using various doses of DALA (0, 3.0, 4.5, 6.0, and 9.0 μg) no clear dose-response relationship was observed for these tests (Fig. 3). Furthermore, when proglumide was administered along with DALA, no potentiation of the analgesic effects of DALA was evident. In fact, addition of 0.01 μg PROG with 9.0 μg DALA in the tail-shock vocalization test produced an attenuation of DALA analgesia.

EXPERIMENT 2: ELECTROPHYSIOLOGICAL ASSESSMENT OF MORPHINE AND PROGLUMIDE INTERACTION

Methods

As in the behavioral experiments, adult male Sprague-Dawley rats were used in the electrophysiological investigations. The jugular vein was cannulated for continual maintenance of anesthesia (sodium pentobarbital, 10 mg/hr) and the femoral vein was cannulated for systemic injection of naloxone (10 mg/kg). The lumbosacral spinal cord was exposed by laminectomy. A pool formed by agar (Bacto-Agar, DIFCO Laboratories) was constructed surrounding the exposed cord to allow for the placement of drugs directly onto the spinal cord (17) in a fashion similar to that of intrathecal injection techniques used in experiment 1. Tungsten microelectrodes were used to record the responses of single dorsal horn neurons to noxious radiant heating (50–54° C, 10 sec, 2–3 min intervals) applied to the ventral surface of the rat's hindfoot. Following determination of baseline (pre-drug) responsivity, recordings of heat-responsive dorsal horn neurons were made to determine each cell's response, over time, to the spinal application of morphine (MOR, 0.1 μg in 0.1 ml saline), proglumide (PROG, 0.04 ng in 0.1 ml saline) and combined application of MOR and PROG (0.1 μg MOR and 0.04 ng PROG in 0.1 ml saline). MOR remained on the cord until the response level was 50% of baseline or for 30 min if less than 50% inhibition occurred. PROG was left on the cord for 40 min. The combined application of MOR and PROG remained on the cord between 30 to 60 min, dependent on the cell's prior response to morphine. Between each drug application the cord was rinsed with saline and the cell's responsivity was required to return to baseline. Comparisons between drug effects were made as a percentage of baseline responses.

Results

In all cells studied to date (N = 10), responses observed after the application of PROG either remained within ± 10% of baseline levels or showed an excitation (20% increase over baseline). Upon application of 0.1 μg MOR, cells responded to heating either: (a) with no MOR-induced inhibition (N = 2) or (b) with MOR-induced inhibition (N = 5). In cells showing no MOR-induced inhibition, there was a marked inhibition of the cell's response following the combined application of MOR and PROG (Fig. 4). In cells showing MOR-induced inhibition, combined application of MOR

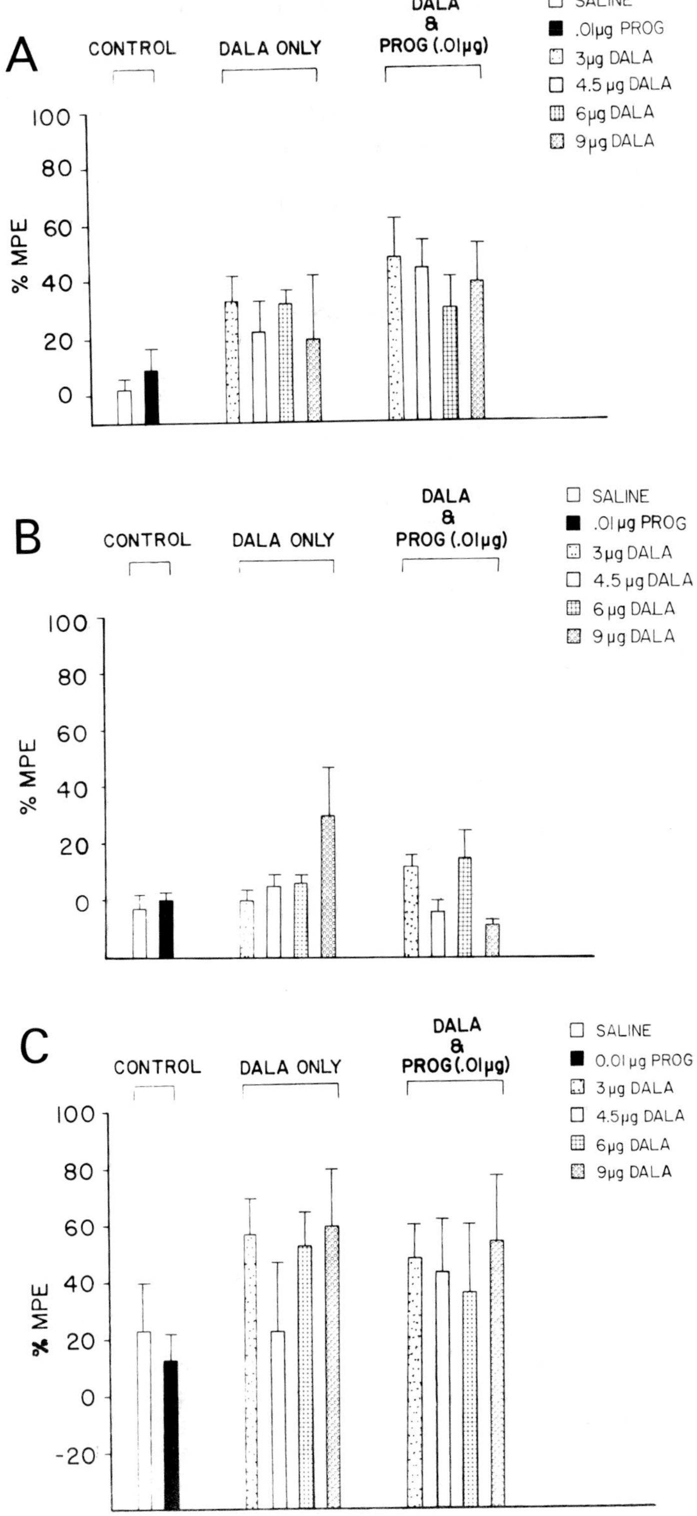

A
CONTROL
DALA ONLY
DALA & PROG (.01µg)
SALINE
.01µg PROG
3µg DALA
4.5 µg DALA
6µg DALA
9µg DALA
% MPE
100
80
60
40
20
0
B
CONTROL
DALA ONLY
DALA & PROG (.01µg)
SALINE
.01 µg PROG
3µg DALA
4.5 µg DALA
6 µg DALA
9 µg DALA
% MPE
100
80
60
40
20
0
C
CONTROL
DALA ONLY
DALA & PROG (.01µg)
SALINE
0.01 µg PROG
3 µg DALA
4.5µg DALA
6µg DALA
9µg DALA
% MPE
100
80
60
40
20
0
-20

and PROG produced a far greater inhibition than with MOR alone; specifically, there was an enhancement of the onset and degree of inhibition. In all cells the inhibition caused by MOR and PROG was totally reversed by systemic naloxone (10 mg/kg, i.v.) within 1 to 5 min. The cell's responses either returned to baseline or showed a slight (< 20%) hyperexcitability to the noxious heat stimulus.

Discussion

The present series of behavioral and electrophysiological experiments provide strong evidence that endogenous CCK can antagonize the pain inhibitory effects of opiates. Spinal application of proglumide, a putative CCK receptor antagonist (5,8,16,36,38; cf. ref. 6), does not elicit analgesia by itself though when combined with opiates is capable of potentiating both their analgesic effects and suppression of spinal transmission. However, it is important to emphasize that potentiation of opiate effects occurred only in tests where increasing opiate doses produced progressive increases in pain inhibition (i.e., the tail-flick and formalin tests of the behavioral series of studies and, using radiant heating, in the electrophysiological study).

BEHAVIORAL ASSESSMENTS

As noted above, increasing dosages of DALA produced an increasing degree of analgesia in the behavioral experiments for the tail-flick (21) and formalin tests. A potentiation of DALA analgesia by proglumide occurred only in these same tests. Possible explanations for the discrepancy between tests where DALA produces does-dependent analgesia (tail-flick and formalin tests) and those where DALA does not (hot-plate, tail-shock vocalization, and pinch tests) could be as follows:

1. In tests where DALA produced a dose-dependent "analgesia" (tail flick and formalin) the lack of a behavioral response could have been due to generalized motor suppression. This possibility is negated in that normal righting reflexes, placing and grasping reflexes of the hindpaws, postural adjustments, and locomotion were observed in every rat tested. Also, in

←

FIG. 3. Effect of DALA (3.0, 4.5, 6.0, or 9.0 μg, N = 10 for each dose) combined either with saline or proglumide (PROG, 0.01 μg, N = 10 with each dose) expressed as mean percent of maximum effect ± SE on 3 pain tests. **A:** Hot-plate test: No clear dose-response relationship occurred with increasing doses of DALA and there was no signficant potentiation of DALA analgesia with PROG. **B:**Tail-shock vocalization test: No clear dose-response relationship occurred with increasing doses of DALA, though with 9.0 μg there was a significant (p < 0.005) increase in DALA analgesia. PROG produced no significant potentiation of DALA analgesia and at 9.0 μg DALA + 0.01 μg PROG there was an attenuation of DALA analgesia. **C:**Tail-pinch test: No dose-response relationship occurred with increasing doses of DALA and there was no significant potentiation of DALA analgesia with PROG.

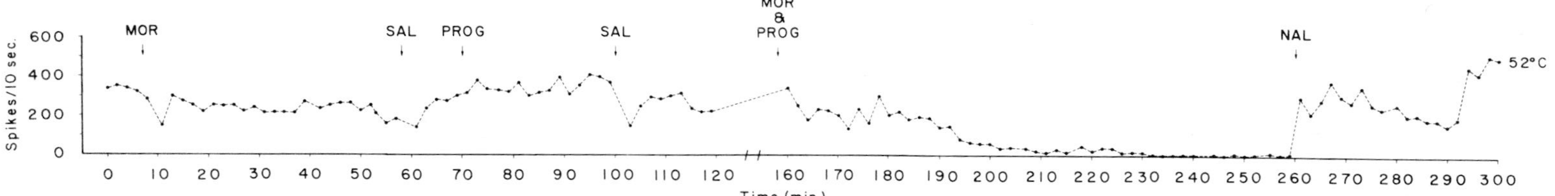

FIG. 4. Proglumide markedly potentiates morphine-induced inhibition of spinal nociceptive transmission. Time course of effect of morphine (MOR, 0.1 μg) and proglumide (PROG, 0.04 ng) applied directly onto the spinal cord, and of systemic naloxone (NAL, 10 mg/kg, i.v.), during noxious heating of the rat's hindfoot pad. Graph plots the number of action potentials recorded from a single unit during the 10-sec heat period, against time. A 50% reduction in the units response to 52° C was not observed until 50 min after application of morphine, with the units firing rate remaining within 10% of predrug level after application of PROG alone. Following application of MOR + PROG, the units' firing rate was more rapidly reduced to 50% at 26 min, and to 97% at 100 min postdrug application. Naloxone immediately reversed the reduced firing rate to predrug levels.

animals judged analgesic following spinal injection of drugs there was no struggling, orientation, or vocalization indicative of rostral transmission of pain.

2. DALA may be suppressing spinally mediated reflexes and not supraspinally mediated behaviors. Initially, such a hypothesis may seem plausible since DALA did not cause dose-dependent analgesia in the hot-plate or tail-shock vocalization tests where supraspinally mediated responses (and, therefore, rostral transmission of pain) are clearly required. Additionally, the tail-flick test is a spinally mediated reflex (19) and DALA did produce analgesia on this test in a dose-dependent manner. However, we believe that our data clearly show that the effects of DALA are not due simply to generalized suppression of spinal reflexes, since as noted above, impairment of diverse motoric reflexes was never observed. Importantly, a dose-dependent analgesia was also observed in the formalin test. Since leg-flinch behaviors are not observed in spinalized animals in response to subcutaneous formalin injection (S. Suberg et al., *unpublished observations*) the response to formalin cannot be reflexive and must be a supraspinally mediated behavior like that required by the hot-plate and tail-shock vocalization tests. Therefore, there is no clear delineation between those tests in which DALA produced a dose-dependent relationship on the basis of whether the behaviors are supra- or intraspinally mediated.
3. In tests where DALA did not produce dose-dependent analgesia, DALA may not be the appropriate opiate for blocking the noxious stimuli associated with those tests. This third possibility arises from earlier observations that various types of pain may be modulated by different neural systems (1,2,10). Concurrent with the work of Schmauss and co-workers (29,30), our laboratory recognized the possibility that different opiate receptors modulate different pain modalities. Our data extend the observations by Schmauss et al. (29,30) and suggest that stimuli arising from the hot-plate, tail-shock vocalization, and pinch tests may be modulated by different neural opiate systems than those of the tail-flick and formalin tests. Multiple opiate receptor types (23) have been found in the rat spinal cord (35), thus supporting this possibility. The reason that DALA does not produce dose-dependent analgesia in the hot-plate, tail-shock vocalization, and pinch tests may be because DALA is not specific for the neural modulating systems involved.

Knowing that DALA is a δ- and/or μ-receptor agonist (22), it appears that δ- and/or μ-receptors are involved in modulating painful stimuli arising during the tail-flick and formalin tests. Since proglumide can potentiate these DALA analgesias, proglumide can apparently interact with δ- and/or μ-receptors. However, in the formalin test, a complex dose-response relationship between DALA and proglumide was noted. If the dose of DALA remained constant while increasing the dose of proglumide, a greater potentiation of DALA analgesia did not occur. Increasing the dose of proglumide while also increasing the dose of DALA also did not result in a greater potentiation of analgesia. This could possibly be due to an improper ratio of proglumide to DALA. It was also noted for the formalin test that when proglumide was administered alone, the 0.01 μg dose of proglumide significantly reduced the number of leg flinches as compared to saline within the first 35 min. Since proglumide was not observed to exert analgesic effects on an acute pain test (tail flick) (38), these data indicate that there might be a release of endogenous opiates in response to tonic pain and that proglumide is interacting with these released opiates.

Both opiates and CCK have been localized in the spinal cord dorsal horn, though the exact neurochemistry of opiate/CCK interactions has not been clearly demonstrated. Furthermore, whether proglumide even binds to CCK (or opiate) receptors in the spinal cord also has yet to be investigated. Since proglumide can potentiate the effects of both morphine (38) and DALA on certain behavioral tests, the specificity of proglumide may be determined by the effective opiate modulating the incoming pain stimuli. The interaction that is occurring to produce the potentiation may be occurring indirectly via an allosteric interaction between CCK and opiate receptors, as has been previously suggested (28).

ELECTROPHYSIOLOGICAL ASSESSMENT

In the electrophysiological assessment, proglumide markedly potentiated the morphine-induced suppression of nociceptive transmission in a naloxone reversible manner. These studies demonstrate at a cellular level that proglumide enhances the effects of opiates. Spinal application of proglumide alone did not cause an inhibition of dorsal horn neuronal responses during noxious heating. These results imply that the potentiation of morphine inhibition is due to a proglumide/morphine interaction and that this interaction is occurring at the level of the spinal cord. It is also important to note that increasing doses of morphine caused a greater degree of inhibition of spinal transmission during noxious heating. Since morphine is a μ-receptor ligand (22), these results confirm and extend the behavioral conclusions (38) of a proglumide/opiate interaction at the μ-receptor.

Clinical applications for proglumide have been suggested (15) in that it could be used for prevention and reversal of opiate tolerance (34,38) and, also, due to its potentiation capabilities, allow physicians to administer lower doses of opiates to manage clinical pain. Another possibility for the clinical use of proglumide is in treating chronic pain. Using the formalin test as a model for tonic pain, our data suggest that low level, tonic pain may induce release of endogenous opiates. In support of this conclusion, naloxone increases pain sensitivity in human subjects experiencing some level of clinical pain yet generally has no effect on normal volunteers (37). Additionally, the use of proglumide may be extended to use in acupuncture, where the prolonged and often discomforting acupuncture needling induces the release of endogenous opiates. Thus, potentiation of the effects of opiates by proglumide has broad biomedical implications, in terms of managing chronic and acute pain in man.

REFERENCES

1. Abbott, F. V., Franklin, K. B. J., Ludwick, R. J., and Melzack, R. (1981): Apparent lack of tolerance in the formalin test suggests different mechanisms for morphine analgesia in different types of pain. *Pharmacol. Biochem. Behav.,* 15:637–640.
2. Abbott, F. V., Melzack, R., and Samuel, C. (1982): Morphine analgesia in the tail flick and formalin pain tests is mediated by different neural systems. *Exp. Neurol.,* 75:644–651.
3. Beinfeld, M. C., Meyer, D. K., Eskay, R. L., Jensen, R. T., and Brownstein, M. J. (1981): The distribution of cholecystokinin immunoreactivity in the CNS of the rat as determined by radioimmunoassay. *Brain Res.,* 212:51–57.
4. Charpentier, J. (1968): Analysis and mechanism of pain in animals: A new concept of pain. In: *Pain,* edited by A. Soluairac, J. Cahn, and J. Charpentier, pp. 171–200. Academic Press, London.
5. Chiodo, L. A., and Bunney, B. S. (1983): Proglumide: Selective antagonism of excitatory effects of cholecystokinin in central nervous system. *Science,* 219:1449–1451.
6. Clark, C. R., Daum, P., and Hughes, J. (1984): Proglumide and cholecystokinin (CCK)-27-32-amide, two reputed peripheral CCK-receptor antagonists, do not compete for central CCK-binding sites. *First International Conference on Neuronal Cholecystokinin Abstr.,* 1:P-16.
7. Collier, H. O. J. (1962): Multiple toe-pinch test for potential analgesic drugs. In: *The Assessment of Pain in Man and Animals,* edited by C. A. Keele and R. Smith, pp. 262–270. Latimer, Trend, Plymouth.
8. D'Amour, F. E., and Smith, D. L. (1941): A method for determining loss of pain sensation. *J. Pharmacol. Exp. Ther.,* 72:74–79.
9. Della-Fera, M. A., and Baile, C. A. (1979): Cholecystokinin octapeptide: continuous picomole injections into the cerebral ventricles of sheep suppress feeding. *Science,* 206:471–473.
10. Dennis, S. G., and Melzack, R. (1980): Pain modulation by 5-hydroxytryptaminergic agents and morphine as measured by three pain tests. *Exp. Neurol.,* 69:260–270.
11. Dubuisson, D., and Dennis, S. G. (1977): The formalin test: a quantitative study of the analgesic effects of morphine, meperidine and brain stem stimulation in rats and cats. *Pain,* 4:161–174.
12. Duggan, A. W., Hall, J. G., and Headley, P. M. (1977): Suppression of transmission of nociceptive impulses by morphine: selective effects of morphine administered in the region of the substantia gelatinosa. *Br. J. Pharmacol.,* 61:65–76.
13. Faris, P. L., Komisaruk, B., Watkins, L. R., and Mayer, D. J. (1983): Evidence for the neuropeptide cholecystokinin as an antagonist of opiate analgesia. *Science,* 219:310–312.
14. Gillis, R. A., Quest, A. J., Pagani, F. D., Dias Souza, J., Traveira Da Silva, A. M., Jensen, R. T., Garvey, T. Z., and Hamosh, P. (1983): Activation of central nervous system cholecystokinin receptors. *J. Pharmacol. Expt. Ther.,* 224(2):408–414.
15. Grumbach, L. (1966): The prediction of analgesic activity in man by animal testing. In: *Pain,* edited by R. S. Knighton and P. R. Dunke, pp. 163–182. Little, Brown, Boston.
16. Hayne, W. F., Jensen, R. T., Lemp, G. F., and Gardner, J. D. (1981): Proglumide and benzotript: members of a different class of cholecystokinin receptor antagonists. *Proc. Natl. Acad. Sci. USA,* 78:6304–6308.
17. Hylden, J. L. K., and Wilcox, G. L. (1983): Effects of spinally-administered morphine and norepinephrine on rat dorsal horn interneurons and spinothalamic tract cells. *Soc. Neurosci. Abstr.,* 9:255.
18. Innis, R. B., Correa, F. M. A., Uhl, G. R., Schneider, B., and Snyder, S. H. (1979): Chole-

cystokinin octapeptide-like immunoreactivity: histochemical localization in rat brain. *Proc. Natl. Acad. Sci. USA,* 76:521–525.
19. Irwin, S., Houde, R. W., Bennett, D. R., Hendershot, L. C., and Seevers, M. H. (1951): The effects of morphine, methadone and meperidine on some reflex responses of spinal animals to nociceptive stimulation. *J. Pharmacol Exp. Ther.,* 101:132–143.
20. Itoh, S., Katsuura, G., and Maeda, Y. (1982): Caerulein and cholecystokinin suppress β-endorphin-induced analgesia in the rat. *Eur. J. Pharmacol.,* 80:421–425.
21. Kinscheck, I. B., Watkins, L. R., Kaufman, E., and Mayer, D. J. (1983): Evidence for a cholecystokinin (CCK)-like endogenous opiate antagonist. *Soc. Neurosci. Abstr.,* 9:792.
22. Lord, J. A. H., Waterfield, A. A., Hughes, J., and Kosterlitz, H. W. (1977): Endogenous opioid peptides: multiple agonists and receptors. *Nature (Lond.),* 267:495–499.
23. Martin, W. R., Eades, C. G., Thompson, J. A., Huppler, R. E., and Gilbert, P. E. (1976): The effects of morphine- and nalorphine-like drugs in the nondependent and morphine-dependent chronic spinal dog. *J. Pharmacol. Exp. Ther.,* 197:517–532.
24. Morley, J. E., and Levine, A. S. (1980): Stress induced eating is mediated through endogenous opiates. *Science,* 209:1259–1261.
25. Morley, J. E., Levine, A. S., Yim, G. K., and Lowy, M. T. (1983): Opioid modulation of appetite. *Neurosci. Biobehav. Rev.,* 7:281–305.
26. Nemeroff, C. B., Osbahr, A. J., III, Bissette, G., Jahnke, G., Lipton, M., and Prangle, A. J., Jr. (1978): Cholecystokinin inhibits tail pinch-induced eating in rats. *Science,* 200:793–794.
27. Rovati, A. L. (1976): Inhibition of gastric secretions by anti-gastrinic and H_2 blocking agents. *Scand. J. Gastroenterol.,* 11(42):113–118.
28. Schiller, P. W., Lipton, A., Horrobin, D. F., and Bodansky, M. (1978): Unsulfated C-terminal 7-peptide of cholecystokinin: a new ligand of the opiate receptor. *Biochem. Biophys. Res. Commun.,* 85:1332–1338.
29. Schmauss, C., Yaksh, T. L., Shimohigashi, Y., Jensen, T. S., Harty, G., and Robard, D. (1983): Studies on the pharmacology of the spinal opiate receptors which modify the rat's response on cutaneous thermal and visceral chemical evoked responses: test selectivity and a disassociation of μ, δ and κ receptors. *Soc. Neurosci. Abstr.,* 9:740.
30. Schmauss, C., and Yaksh, T. L. (1984): *In vivo* studies on spinal opiate receptor systems mediating antinociception. II. Pharmacological profiles suggesting a differential association of mu, delta and kappa receptors with visceral chemical and cutaneous thermal stimuli in the rat. *J. Pharmacol. Expt. Ther.,* 228(1):1–12.
31. Skirboll, L., Hokfelt, T., Dockray, G., Rehfeld, J., Brownstein, M., and Cuello, A. C. (1983): Evidence for periaqueductal gray cholecystokinin substance P neurons projecting to the spinal cord. *J. Neurosci.,* 3(6):1151–1157.
32. Stein, L. J., and Woods, S. C. (1981): Cholecystokinin and bombesin act independently to decrease food intake in the rat. *Peptides,* 2:431–436.
33. Stengaard-Pedersen, K., and Larsson, L. -I. (1981): Localization and opiate receptor binding of enkephalin, CCK and ACTH/β-endorphin in the rat central nervous system. *Peptides,* 2(1):3–19.
34. Tang, J., Chou, J., Iadarola, M. J., Yang, H. -Y. T., and Costa, E. (1983): Possible participation of endogenous cholecystokinin 8 (CCK) in the tolerance to morphine analgesia in the rat. *Soc. Neurosci. Abstr.,* 9:288.
35. Traynor, J. R., Kelly, P. D., and Rance, M. J. (1982): Multiple opiate binding sites in rat spinal cord. *Life Sci.,* 31:1377–1380.
36. Urban, L., Willetts, J., Murase, K., and Randic, M. (1984): Actions of CCK-8 on rat spinal dorsal horn neurons. *First International Conference on Neuronal Cholecystokinin Abstr.,* 1:32.
37. Watkins, L. R., and Mayer, D. J. (1982): The neural organization of endogenous opiate and non-opiate pain control systems, *Science,* 216:1185–1192.
38. Watkins, L. R., Kinscheck, I. B., and Mayer, D. J. (1984): Potentiation of opiate analgesia and apparent reversal of morphine tolerance by proglumide. *Science,* 244:395–396.
39. Watkins, L. R., Kinscheck, I. B., and Mayer, D. J. (1985): Potentiation of morphine analgesia by the cholecystokinin antagonist proglumide. *Brain Res.,* 327:169–180.
40. Watkins, L. R., Kinscheck, I. B., Kaufman, E. F. S., Miller, J., Frenk, H., and Mayer, D. J. (1985): Cholecystokinin antagonists selectively potentiate analgesia induced by endogenous opiates. *Brain Res.,* 327:181–190.

41. Woolfe, G., and MacDonald, A. D. (1944): The evaluation of the analgesic action of pethidine hydrochloride (Demerol). *J. Pharmacol. Exp. Ther.,* 80:300–307.
42. Wüster, M., Schulz, R., and Herz, A. (1980): The direction of opioid agonists towards μ-, δ- and ϵ-receptors in the vas deferens of the mouse and rat. *Life Sci.,* 27:163–170.
43. Wüster, M., Schulz, R., and Herz, A. (1981): Multiple opiate receptors in peripheral tissue preparations. *Biochem. Pharmacol.,* 30:1883–1887.
44. Zieglgansberger, W., and Tulloch, I. F. (1979): The effects of methionine- and leucine-enkephalin on spinal neurones of the cat. *Brain Res.,* 167:53–64.

Advances in Pain Research and Therapy, Vol. 9, edited by H. L. Fields et al. Raven Press, New York © 1985.

Cancer Pain Relief: An Important Global Public Health Issue

Jan Stjernswärd

Cancer Unit, World Health Organization, CH 1211 Geneva 27, Switzerland

World Health Organization (WHO) data show that globally, one out of ten deaths are due to cancer (2). Death, in itself, is unavoidable, but death without pain is surely the right of every individual. Yet in most of the world, cancer victims suffer and die—in far too many cases, inch by inch—with pain, as family and loved ones stand by hopelessly. We must offer them help. Thanks to the work of many experts, we have the knowledge—and the drugs—to prevent pain, to provide relief to cancer patients, and to allow incurable patients to die with dignity. It must weigh heavily on our conscience that, despite our best intentions, what we know is not being applied.

According to a WHO committee on medical research, over half of cancer patients suffer needlessly. Yet there is the knowlege to make sure that virtually all sufferers are spared pain.

We estimate that each year 5.9 million new cancer cases in all forms are diagnosed throughout the world. Of that number, 3 million occur in developing countries. It is also estimated that 4.3 million die annually from cancer, in all forms. Of that number, 2.3 million occur in developing countries (2,6). Indeed, in a number of developing countries, where the overall health situation has improved significantly, cancer is becoming one of the leading causes of mortality.

In the global WHO cancer control program (4), cancer pain relief has been identified as one of the three main priority projects. Our aims are:

1. Preventing: to prevent cancers having known causes;
2. Detecting and curing: to improve early detection of disease while it is still curable and offer adequate therapies;
3. Relieving pain: to offer effective pain relief to all sufferers.

Most of what we know about the extent of the cancer pain problem comes from studies carried out in hospitals and hospices in Western countries, primarily in the United Kingdom and the United States. They have shown that: (a) about 60% of terminally ill patients suffer considerable pain (10); (b) 38% of some 400 nonterminally ill patients suffer significant pain (3);

and (c) almost 30% of cancer patients dying at home, and 20% dying in hospitals, experience severe *unrelieved* pain (5).

In the United Kingdom pain is the most common symptom in patients dying of cancer and it was found to be uncontrolled in 35% (13); and in the United Kingdom and the United States about 25% of all cancer patients die with severe unrelieved pain (7). Last year at least 30,000 individuals in the United Kingdom and 100,000 in the United States died without relief from severe pain (11). This is the experience of the developed world—where non-narcotic drugs such as aspirin, mild narcotics such as codeine, and powerful narcotics such as morphine are relatively inexpensive and obtainable.

If there are undeniable deficiencies in the management of cancer pain among the rich, what about the rest of the world, where the majority of cancer patients are found, where most are incurable at the time of diagnosis, and where drugs are not available? Pain releif is often the only relevant, humane, therapeutic alternative, yet it is, by and large, not offered to millions. Why? We must address such questions squarely and fully.

A WHO-sponsored questionnarie was administered to more than 1,000 cancer patients with pain in three developing countries (Brazil, India, and Sri Lanka) and two developed countries (Israel and Japan). It showed that current treatment brought complete pain relief in less than 10% of patients suffering from severe pain (Table 1). There was little or no relief reported for 29% of the patients with moderate pain. It should be noted that narcotics were given to only 32% of patients from Japan, 23% from Sri Lanka, 6% from Israel, and 3% from India.

The challenge is to share the knowledge that we have and to show how to administer the drugs, or, when not available, help to make them so.

Some of the most important obstacles impeding the implementation of efficient cancer pain relief are patients' lack of awareness that pain can be relieved, their acceptance of pain, fear of drug addiction, underprescribing and underdosing by the profession, wrong timing of drugs given, lack of education of doctors and nurses, poor drug availability and drug legislation.

Little is known about how to manage the treatment of pain. Among health

TABLE 1. *WHO cancer pain questionnaire data*

Pain severity	Patients[a]	Degree of relief (%) Complete	Large	Moderate	Little or none
Mild	53	17	19	42	15
Moderate	172	11	24	35	24
Severe	201	8	15	45	29

[a]Patients reported from single centers in India (*N* = 210, Brazil (*N* = 77), Sri Lanka (*N* = 56), Israel (*N* = 53), and Japan (*N* = 37).

professionals, it would not be an exaggeration to say, that the total sum of knowledge reposes, in the best sense of the word, within a specialists group—the members of the International Association for the Study of Pain.

Because of poor implementation of cancer pain relief, patients endure misery, some without complaint, fearing that to complain might demonstrate a weakness. It is also true that too little training is provided to cancer specialists in how to treat pain. We know that less than 1% of pages in standard oncology texts is devoted to pain (1). Finally, too many patients, in fact the vast majority, are too ill informed about the relief of pain; that is the tragedy, for pain is neither an inevitable nor an unavoidable part of cancer. Freedom from pain should be the right of every cancer victim.

WHO is seeking to expand pain relief from the specialized centers making it an integral part of health care systems, available to communities and reaching all sufferers. In support of overall aims, we need more precise data on the extent of cancer pain worldwide, we need to develop and test guidelines for pain relief, and we need to establish mechanisms for dissemination of the knowledge we have gained. To be specific: There is the need for baseline studies to document the scope of cancer pain, not only in developed countries, but in developing countries as well, and for situation analyses to determine the level of cancer pain and the kind of treatment required.

In response, WHO is developing procedures to help those interested in undertaking such investigations. WHO is testing, for feasibility and effectiveness, guidelines (12) for treating cancer pain in five continents. Probably less than 10% of cancer patients worldwide are treated at specialized cancer centers; our concern extends to the other 90%. The guidelines give a clear plan of how cancer pain can be treated (9).

How can you use your WHO, what are our mechanisms, and what are we planning? The mechanism for the transfer of knowledge from the specialized centers to the community health centers must be solved. There is also the need for more information on the drug registration and legislation, particularly legislation that restricts the availability of medications that relieve pain. However, it has to be balanced and considered in the context of a rise in drug abuse.

In response, WHO is carrying out a survey to collect information, country by country, on measures—legal, administrative and practical—that curtail the availability of drugs. This knowledge must be gathered and also spread. There is the need as well for the establishment of a *network* of supporting individuals, organizations, and countries. Our objective is to provide basic knowledge of the problem of cancer pain and what can be done about it. Our audiences are health policy makers, health care planners, key groups; foremost among them are national and international cancer societies and the general public.

Our aim is to change attitudes about cancer pain management. The need to dispel fears about medications that relieve pain, to make drugs available, to encourage their proper use, and to increase awareness that there are drugs and other therapeutic approaches to manage pain are surely good reasons for such an effort.

WHO welcomes the help of all in completing the unfinished agenda. The relief of pain is one of the greatest challenges in public health today. Pain-relief therapy already exists. This knowledge must be shared with all to make possible freedom from pain as quickly as feasible, certainly by the year 2,000. Those who are in pain cannot wait.

REFERENCES

1. Bonica, J. J. (1980): Cancer pain. In: *Pain,* edited by J. J. Bonica, pp. 335–362, Raven Press, New York.
2. Cancer as a global problem (1984): *Weekly Epidemiological Record (WHO),* 59:125–126.
3. Foley, K. M. (1979): Pain symptoms in patients with cancer. In: *Advances in Pain Research and Therapy, Vol. 2,* edited by J. J. Bonica, and V. Ventafridda, pp. 59–75, Raven Press, New York.
4. World Health Organization, Global Medium Term Programme 13.15, *Cancer* 1984–1989, CAN/MTP/83.12.
5. Parkes, C. M. (1978): Home or Hospital? Terminal case as seen by surviving spouses. *J. R. Coll. Gen. Pract.,* 28:19–30.
6. Parkin, M., Stjernswärd, J., and Muir, C. (1984): Estimates of the worldwide frequency of twelve major cancers. *Bull. WHO,* 62(2):163–182.
7. Saunders, C. M. (1981): Current views of pain relief and terminal care. In: *The Therapy of Pain,* edited by M. Swerdlow, pp. 215–241, MTP Press, Lancaster.
8. Swerdlow, M., and Stjernswärd, J. (1982): Cancer pain relief—an urgent problem. *World Health Forum,* 3(3):325–330.
9. Takeda, F. (1984): WHO cancer pain relief programme—preliminary report from Japan on results of field testing of WHO draft interim guidelines on relief of cancer pain. *Pain* (Suppl. 2)216.
10. Twycross, R. G., and Fairchild, S. (1982): Pain in far advanced cancer. *Pain,* 14:303–310.
11. Twycross, R. G., and Lack, S. A. (1983): Symptom control in far advanced cancer. *Pain Relief,* pp. 1–334. Pitman, London.
12. WHO draft interim guidelines handbook on relief of cancer pain. *WHO Technical Document,* CAN/84.2.
13. Wilkes, E. (1984): Dying now. *Lancet,* 1:950–952.

Advances in Pain Research and Therapy, Vol. 9, edited by H. L. Fields et al. Raven Press, New York © 1985.

Cancer Pain: Psychological Substrates and Therapy

Michael R. Bond

University of Glasgow, Department of Psychological Medicine, Glasgow, G12 OAA, Scotland

There is a widely held view among members of the general public that cancer illnesses are both painful and invariably fatal. Death from cancer is greatly feared, not least because those suffering from it often believe they will experience considerable physical pain at the end of their lives. These feelings are not entirely unjustified. The details of the incidence and prevalence of cancer pain revealed by J. Bonica *(this volume)* do indicate that the number of individuals suffering pain, and the intensity of their pain, tend to increase as illness progresses, however, not all forms of cancer are equally likely to cause pain. In recent years awareness of the emotional problems and needs of cancer patients and their families, promoted by such fears, have received great attention in a drive spearheaded by the Hospice movement. This has led to improvements in patient care; however, scientific evaluation of the contribution of psychological factors to the pain and suffering of cancer has taken place more slowly. In this chapter the latter developments are reviewed.

PREVALENCE AND SEVERITY OF CANCER PAIN

In recent years the prevalence of cancer pain and its severity relative to the pain of other chronic painful diseases has been studied. Daut and Cleeland (6) showed that prevalence rates vary between different forms of cancer as shown in Table 1, and Foley (12) commented that, at the extremes, 85% of patients with primary bone tumors experience pain in contrast to only 5% of patients with leukemia. The extent to which cancer pain is experienced outside hospitals is unknown and prevalence rates within hospitals vary depending on admission policies. Foley (12) gave an overall figure of 29% for admissions to a major cancer center in the United States in 1 week and commented that most patients experienced pain as a direct consequence of the disease process. Foley et al. (13) and, more recently, Twycross and Fairfield (27) have shown that pain may also be due to the effects of treat-

TABLE 1. *Prevalence and severity of cancer pain: Frequency of pain as an early symptom*

Location of carcinoma	% with pain as an early symptom
Ovary	49
Prostate	45
Colorectal	42
Breast	39
Uterus	22
Cervix	18

N = 667.

ment or even unrelated causes (Table 2). Therefore, pain at more than one site is not an uncommon event in cancer patients. These observations are important because there is a relationship between the number and severity of pains patients experience and their levels of emotional distress.

The possible severity of cancer pain should not be underestimated, but it is often not appreciated that chronic pain in nonmalignant disorders, for example, arthritis, may be equally severe and disabling (6). Finally, the prevalence and severity of cancer pain increases in the presence of metastatic disease and this is, in turn, associated with increased levels of emotional distress.

PSYCHOLOGICAL ASPECTS OF CANCER PAIN

In general terms, cancers are illnesses that provoke considerable fear and often the disease gives rise to feelings of helplessness or loss of personal control. If symptoms progress and doctors seem unable to prevent or halt their development the future may seem hopeless and this, combined with helplessness, is known to be a powerful factor in the genesis of depressive states. Anxiety is also a common emotion among cancer patients who worry not

TABLE 2. *Causes of pains in patients with far advanced cancer*

Causes of pains	No. of patients		
	Men	Women	Total
Cancer	42	49	91
Related to treatment	3	9	12
Associated pains	9	10	19
Unrelated pains	15	24	39

only about their fate but also about loss of work, life's goals, and the consequences of their illness for others—particularly family members. However, psychiatric illnesses as opposed to transient changes in emotion are not universal and their time of onset, should they occur, varies with the nature of the disease and rate of its progression. For example, Maguire (21) showed that almost all women who develop breast cancer are anxious from the moment an abnormality is detected, and over half have moderate to severe anxiety at the time of diagnosis. Anger and hostility are common emotions among all chronically ill people and this is true of cancer patients also. These feelings are often particularly acute in patients with chronic pain due to cancer because to them it seems to have no biological purpose.

The physical limitations and debility imposed by illness are increased by the presence of pain and one major consequence is a reduction in patients' social activities and contacts with friends. The way in which individuals cope with their varied physical problems differs. Some become withdrawn and seem to believe that they have an incurable illness, whereas others take an entirely opposite view and behave in a very combative way. Interestingly, the latter attitude may be an advantage (26) because it may prolong life, in contrast to passive acceptance that may actually increase the rate at which the disease progresses. There is considerable anecdotal evidence for this view and Derogatis et al. (8) gave support for it when they examined a group of 35 women with metastatic breast cancer and found that survival was longest in those who were anxious, hostile, and tended to alienate their physicians.

In 1969, Bond and Pearson (4), and later Bond (2) demonstrated that pain in women with carcinoma of the cervix was associated with increased levels of emotionality or susceptibility to emotional breakdown that was reduced if pain was relieved. Pain was also associated with an increased number of physical complaints which, when analyzed in terms of a scale of hypochondriasis (25), revealed increased preoccupation with physical symptoms and fear of disease which patients sought to deny. However, the level of hypochondriasis was lower than that encountered in hypochondriacal psychiatric patients. Bond and Pearson (4) also observed that patients' complaint behavior was directly related to their levels of extraversion or introversion and showed that whereas extraverts tended to complain freely about pain and to seek treatment for it, the opposite was true for introverts.

In the early studies mentioned above, pain was assessed using the analog scale technique for the first time. However, it was soon realized that this method of measurement was unidimensional and, therefore, unsatisfactory because it concerned only the sensory aspect of pain—in other words, its physical severity. The later development of the concept of the multidimensional nature of pain and, on the basis of this concept, of the McGill Pain Questionnaire (MPQ) described by Melzack and Torgerson (23), and later in a more developed form by Melzack (22), provided a means of assessing the sensory, affective, and evaluative aspects of pain experience using word scales. Melzack (22), Dubuisson and Melzack (11) and Graham et al. (16) reported that cancer patients used fewer affective and sensory words than patients with chronic, nonmalignant, painful illnesses, implying that cancer pain was either a less emotionally laden experience than noncancer pain, or that patients denied its effect on their feelings. However, these authors did not differentiate between patients with mild, moderate, and severe levels of pain. By contrast, Kremer et al. (19) compared cancer patients with varying pain levels with noncancer patients who had pain of similar reported intensity. They observed that when pain levels were high both cancer and noncancer patients used similar numbers of affective and sensory words from the MPQ. Under the same conditions women used more affective and evaluative words than men, but this position was reversed when pain levels were low. When the pain levels among cancer patients were low they used significantly more affective words than noncancer patients. In summary, high levels of pain, irrespective of its cause, appears to be associated with increased use of emotionally laden words to describe it, but cancer patients use significantly greater numbers of emotional words than others when their pain is not severe. This difference might indicate a relationship between the number of affective words used and psychiatric measures of mood change. However, Kremer and his colleagues (19) were unable to demonstrate such an association. Although they could not relate psychiatric disturbance to the affective scale of the MPQ, the group did show that cancer and noncancer patients alike do register emotional distress, chiefly on psychiatric scales measuring somatization, depression, and anxiety.

PSYCHIATRIC ILLNESS IN CANCER PATIENTS WITH PAIN

As stated previously, feelings of misery and transient disturbances of emotion and behavior are common in all chronically ill people. Mental illness in cancer patients has been reported by Derogatis et al. (8) who found an overall prevalence rate of 47% for mental disorder among patients with cancer pain in three major centers in the United States. Similar figures were reported earlier by Hinton (18), Hackett and Weissman (17), and Craig and Aboloff (5). The rate is twice that given for general medical inpatients and three times that given for the general population. Derogatis and colleagues (8) showed that there was an association between the amount of psychiatric disturbance and the severity of illness. Using self-report scales and diagnostic criteria of the American Psychiatric Association (DSM III) they revealed that of those patients with a psychiatric disorder 68% had an adjustment reaction, which was a mixture of anxiety and depression. Only 13% had a major depressive illness, and 4% a general anxiety disorder (Table 3). Thus, most psychiatric disturbance was of a reactive nature and over half the

TABLE 3. *DSM-III Psychiatric disorders observed in cancer patients*

Diagnostic category	DSM-III code	Psychiatric diagnosis (%)
Presenile dementia	290.10.	8
Major affective disorder: Unipolar depression	296.20.	13
Adjustment disorder: Depressed mood	309.00.	68
General anxiety disorder	300.02.	4
Personality disorder: schizoid type	301.20.	7

Disorders observed in 101 cancer patients from three cancer centers: John Hopkins Medical Center, Baltimore; Memorial Sloan-Kettering Cancer Center, New York; and University of Rochester Medical Center, New York.

patients studied did not have a measurable emotional disorder. It is important to remember that rates of psychiatric illness do vary between centers depending on the severity of the physical illness of patients admitted to them, and on the type of instruments used for assessment. For example, in relation to the last point it is generally held that self-assessment rating scales give higher prevalence figures than standardized psychiatric interviews. In fact, the prevalence rate quoted by Derogatis and his colleagues (9) is almost certainly too high and a figure between 25 and 30% is probably more accurate.

Ahles et al. (1) in a study of 40 cancer patients with pain and 37 who were pain-free, used a variety of self-report measures of pain, depression, anxiety, and activity to examine the differences between the groups. They showed that the presence of pain was associated with increased levels of depression and anxiety and that patients in hospitals were more anxious than those at home. Within the pain group, those who regarded their pain as evidence of progression of the illness had significantly higher levels of depression and anxiety than those who had not considered this possibility.

There is evidence that psychiatric morbidity is increased by treatment. For example, Peck and Boland (24) reported that radiation therapy for cancer is associated with increased levels of psychiatric illness and that, in part, this may be because patients are so poorly informed about the nature and purpose of the treatment in some cases that they may believe it to be dangerous and even to cause cancer. After treatment only one-third of patients in their study felt treatment had improved their health and, whereas 60% had evidence of symptoms of depression and anxiety beforehand, this figure increased to 80% immediately after treatment. Others have reported that impairment of mental health lasts for a greater period after chemotherapy (20) and it has been estimated that at least 1 in 4 patients who have had a mastectomy or surgery for rectal cancer (10) develop depressive illness, anxiety neurosis, sexual and marital problems in the first year after treatment.

INTERFERENCE OF CANCER PAIN ON THE ACTIVITIES OF DAILY LIFE

Some of the multiple symptoms found in cancer patients, for example, dyspnea and diarrhea, are as distressing, or more so, than pain. Daut and Cleeland (6) examined the specific effect of painful cancer in 667 patients on levels of activity and enjoyment of leisure and personal relationships. They reported that increased levels of pain diminished activity and enjoyment of life and that interference with daily living was marked when pain levels were rated 5 or more on a 0-to-10 scale of pain severity. Moreover, for any given level of pain, patients who believed the symptom represented a worsening of their condition reported the greatest interference with activity and pleasure. The next most affected were those who regarded pain as a result of treatment, and the least affected where those who felt that pain was due to unrelated causes.

ANALGESIC AND PSYCHOTROPIC MEDICATION IN THE MANAGEMENT OF CANCER PATIENTS AND PAIN

In 1966 Bond and Pilowsky (3) reported that the use of analgesics was poorly correlated with reports of pain intensity in cancer patients and that this was owing to a combination of culturally determined attitudes to pain relief and an apparent lack of ability among doctors and nurses to evaluate pain accurately. Since that time there has been a marked improvement in standards of knowledge and care. For example, Daut and Cleeland (6) were able to show a clear correlation between pain intensity and the potency of analgesics prescribed. Nevertheless, only 47% of patients treated achieved at least 70% pain relief and 13% experienced less than 30% relief.

Psychotropic drugs are also given to cancer patients at times to reduce tension and pain and as adjuncts to analgesics. A recent review of the use of such drugs in the treatment of cancer patients by Derogatis (7) shows that they are used chiefly as hypnotics and to control nausea and vomiting (Table 4). Anxiolytics were used less often than antidepressants for psychological distress (57 and 71%, respectively), and drugs in the neuroleptic group were used almost solely to control nausea and vomiting. However, although they are known to potentiate opiate analgesics, this property of the neuroleptics was apparently seldom used.

It is probable that the low level of usage of psychotropic drugs for emotional disturbances is dictated in part by the fact that physicians appreciate that much of the psychological distress experienced by cancer patients in pain is reactive in nature and due to the nature of the illness, its physical and social consequences, and its meaning to those who suffer it. In other words, their distress stems primarily from personal and environmental factors and not from mental illness as such. However, it is also possible that

TABLE 4. *Reasons for prescribing major classes of psychotropic medications as a proportion of the total prescriptions*

Reason for prescribing	All classes	Antianxiety	Antipsychotic	Antidepressant	Hypnotic
Psychological distress	17%	57%	8%	71%	1%
Sleep	44%	7%	1%	23%	85%
Nausea and vomiting	25%	6%	91%	0%	1%
Medical procedure	12%	22%	0%	0%	14%
Pain	1%	4%	1%	6%	0%
Seizure	1%	4%	0%	0%	0%
Total number of prescriptions		405	429	17	814

From ref. 7, with permission.

uncertainty about the mode of action and value of psychotropic drugs in the treatment of chronic physical illnesses coupled with unfamiliary with psychiatric diagnoses contributes to the relatively low rate of prescription.

NONPHARMACOLOGICAL APPROACHES

From the observation that the greater part of psychiatric morbidity in cancer patients is reactive, it should follow that specific psychological techniques are widely used. However, reports in the literature are chiefly confined to advice about the value of counseling and supportive psychotherapy on either an individual or group basis without evidence of their level of effectiveness from well-designed treatment trials. From the information given in this chapter it is clear that there is a need for carefully designed educational programs directed towards relieving the distress felt by patients and their relatives as a result of their lack of knowledge about the cause of pain, its significance, and the effectiveness of treatment. For example, it has been shown that counseling reduces anxiety and depression in breast cancer patients undergoing lengthy treatment. Finer (14) reviewed the possible use of hypnosis for cancer pain and concluded that it may be of value in promoting sleep and well-being in patients with mild pain and emotional distress. Its effectiveness is enhanced by the use of a low concentration of nitrous oxide in oxygen. The use of the technique is severely restricted because only a small proportion of patients are susceptible to hypnosis and it cannot be used when consciousness is impaired for any reason. Treatment based on the use of relaxation without trance should be effective also and have the advantage of wider applicability. Fotopoulos et al. (15) reported that biofeedback is of limited value in the treatment of cancer pain. However, the presence of severe physical illness and metabolic changes in cancer patients does not provide an ideal setting for this form of treatment. Reliable scientific reports of the use of psychological techniques, and, in particular, operant conditioning of behavior and the use of cognitive therapy, have not yet been reported in the literature of cancer pain.

CONCLUSIONS

1. The prevalence of cancer pain varies with disease type. Pain is usually the result of the disease process but may be caused by treatment or other factors. Increasing numbers of pains and increasing severity of pain raises levels of emotional distress.

2. Cancer illnesses provoke a variety of emotional responses which are increased by the presence of pain and severity of illness. Nevertheless, psychiatric disorders occur in less than half the patients and most emotional disturbances are of a reactive nature.

3. Verbal methods of assessment of severe pain reveals that cancer and noncancer patients use an increased vocabulary of affective-laden words to a similar extent. At lower levels of pain cancer patients use a significantly greater number of affective words. However, there does not appear to be a direct relationship between the number of words used and measures of psychiatric illness.

4. The overall prevalence rate for psychiatric illness in cancer patients remains uncertain, but it is known that two-thirds of illnesses are reactive in type and very few are major affective disorders.

5. Analgesics are used with increasing sophistication for pain relief but a small proportion of patients fail to respond to them. Psychotropic drugs are used very little for pain control and only to a moderate extent for the treatment of mental distress and illness. To date, there has been little systematic evaluation of psychological methods of treatment although the use of counseling and supportive psychotherapy is widely advocated and practiced.

REFERENCES

1. Ahles, T. A., Blanchard, E. B., and Ruckdeschel, J. C. (1983): The multidimensional nature of cancer-related pain. *Pain,* 17:277–288.
2. Bond, M. R. (1971): The relation of pain to the Eysenck Personality Inventory, Cornell Medical Index and Whiteley Index of Hypochondriasis. *Br. J. Psychiatry,* 119:671–678.
3. Bond, M. R., and Pilowsky, I. (1966): Subjective assessment of pain and its relationship to the administration of analgesics in patients with advanced cancer. *J. Psychosom. Res.,* 10:203–208.
4. Bond, M. R., and Pearson, I. B. (1969): Psychological aspects of pain in women with advanced cancer of the cervix. *J. Psychosom. Res.,* 13:13–19.
5. Craig, K. D., and Aboloff, M. D. (1974): Psychiatric symptomatology amongst hospitalized cancer patients. *Am. J. Psychiatry,* 131:1323–1326.
6. Daut, R. L., and Cleeland, C. S. (1982): The prevalence and severity of pain in cancer. *Cancer,* 50:1913–1918.

7. Derogatis, L. R. (1982): Psychopharmacologic applications to cancer: An overview. *Cancer,* 50:1962–1967.
8. Derogatis, L. R., Aboloff, M. D., and Melisaratis, N. (1979): Psychological coping mechanisms and survival time in metastatic breast cancer. *JAMA,* 242:1504–1508.
9. Derogatis, L. R., Morrow, G. R., Felting, J., Penman, D., Piasetsky, S., Schmale, A. M., Henrich, M., and Carmicke, C. L. M. (1983): The prevalence of psychiatric disorders among cancer patients. *JAMA,* 249:751–757.
10. Devlin, H. B., Plant, J. A., and Griffin, M. (1971): Aftermath of surgery for rectal cancer. *Br. Med. J.,* 3:413–418.
11. Dubuisson, D., and Melzack, R. (1976): Classification of clinical pain description by multiple group discriminant analysis. *Exp. Neurol.,* 51:480–487.
12. Foley, K. (1979): Pain syndromes in patients with cancer. In: *Advances in Pain Research and Therapy, Vol. 2.,* edited by J. J. Bonica and V. Ventafridda, pp. 59–75. Raven Press, New York.
13. Foley, K., Rogers, A., and Houde, R. (1978): Pain in patients with cancer: A quantative reappraisal. *Proc. Am. Soc. Cancer Res.,* 19:357.
14. Finer, B. (1979): Hypnotherapy in pain of advanced cancer. In: *Advances in Pain Research and Therapy, Vol. 2.,* edited by J. J. Bonica and V. Ventafridda, pp. 223–231. Raven Press, New York.
15. Fotopoulos, S. S., Graham, C., and Cook, M. R. (1979): Psychophysiologic control of cancer pain. In: *Advances in Pain Research and Therapy, Vol. 2.,* edited by J. J. Bonica and V. Ventafridda, pp. 231–245. Raven Press, New York.
16. Graham, C., Bond, S. S., Gerkovich, M. M., and Cook, M. R. (1980): Use of the McGill Pain Questionnaire in the assessment of cancer patients: Replicability and consistency. *Pain,* 8:377–387.
17. Hackett, T. P., and Weissman, A. D. (1969): Denial as a factor in patients with heart disease and cancer. *Ann. NY Acad. Sci.,* 164:802–805.
18. Hinton, J. M. (1963): The physical and mental distress of the dying. *Q. J. Med.,* 32:1–21.
19. Kremer, E. F., Atkinson, J. H., and Ignelzi, R. H. (1982): Pain measurement: The affective dimensional measure of the McGill Pain Questionnaire with a cancer population. *Pain,* 12:153–163.
20. Lee, E. G., and Maguire, P. (1975): Emotional distress in patients attending a breast clinic. *Br. J. Surg.,* 62:162–165.
21. Maguire, P. (1976): The psychological and social sequelae of mastectomy. In: *Modern Perspectives in the Psychiatric Aspects of Surgery,* edited by J. G. Howells, pp. 390–422. Brunner/Mazel, New York.
22. Melzack, R. (1975): The McGill Pain Questionnaire: Major properties and scoring methods. *Pain,* 1:277–299.
23. Melzack, R., and Torgerson, W. S. (1971): On the language of pain. *Anaesthesiology,* 34:50–59.
24. Peck, A., and Boland, J. (1977): Emotional reactions to radiation treatment. *Cancer,* 40:180–184.
25. Pilowsky, I. (1967): Dimensions of hypochondriasis. *Br. J. Psychiatry,* 113:89–94.
26. Silberfarb, P. M. (1982): Research in adaptation to illness and psychosocial intervention. *Cancer,* 50:1921–1925.
27. Twycross, R. G., and Fairfield, S. (1982): Pain in far advanced cancer. *Pain,* 14:303–310.

Advances in Pain Research and Therapy, Vol. 9, edited by H. L. Fields et al. Raven Press, New York © 1985.

Aspects of Psychological Distress and Pain in Cancer Patients Undergoing Radiotheraphy

*'†Henderikus J. Stam, †Connie Goss, †Lorraine Rosenal, †Shirley Ewens, and †Brenda Urton

**Department of Psychology, University of Calgary, Calgary, Alberta, Canada T2N IN4; and †Tom Baker Cancer Centre, Calgary, Alberta, Canada T2N 4N2*

It is frequently observed that the physiologic and psychologic impact of cancer pain is greater than that of nonmalignant chronic pain (e.g., refs. 2,3,11). For example, various authors have reported that cancer patients are more likely to develop reactions of anxiety, depression, hypochondriasis, and somatic focusing than are patients with nonmalignant chronic pain (3,11). Likewise, a number of studies have indicated that the intensity of pain experienced by cancer patients was related to the extent with which it interfered with patients' activities and enjoyment of daily life (5,6). One hypothesis for the relationship between psychological distress and chronic pain is that chronic pain interferes with the activities of daily living to the extent that individuals are no longer able to function in their usual manner leading to increases in distress levels. One purpose of the present study was to determine the interrelationship between pain, psychological distress, and the interference of pain with the activities of daily living.

Very few of the extant surveys of pain in cancer have considered changes in the severity of pain. The severity of pain is critical in assessing the impact on the patient. This study also examined changes in cancer pain and psychological functioning in patients undergoing radiation treatments for cancer.

METHODS

Subjects

Out patients in the Tom Baker Cancer Centre Radiotherapy Department with a self-reported pain problem due to their disease were asked to volunteer for the study. The present report provides the results of 23 patients who took part in the study. Patients were 18 years of age or older and ambulatory.

Materials

All patients completed a modified McGill Pain Questionnaire (8), the Berkman Social Network Scale (BSN; ref. 1), the Centre for Epidemiological Studies Depression Scale (CES-D; ref. 9), the Spielberger State-Trait Anxiety Inventory (STAI; ref. 10), and the Profile of Mood States (POMS; ref. 7). Patients also kept daily records of their levels of pain, depression, anxiety, and drug intake. (These latter variables will not be discussed here for lack of space). Patients also indicated on 0 to 10 scales the extent to which their pain interfered with (a) life in general, (b) their work, (c) their appetite, (d) their ability to sleep, and (e) their sexual functioning.

Procedures

Patients were interviewed at the onset of treatment and again at the completion of, or immediately following, treatment. Patients kept daily records for the duration of treatment. The interval between first and second administration ranged from 2 to 4 weeks.

RESULTS

Interrelationship of Measures

Measures of psychological distress (i.e., depression, anxiety, mood states) were highly correlated with each other within interview 1 and interview 2. Likewise, the pain variables (intensity and frequency) were highly correlated within each interview. The pain variables on the first administration of the questionnaire were only weakly to moderately correlated with the pain variables on the second administration. The psychological variables, however, continued to be consistently and highly correlated across interviews. That this may indicate a change in pain, but not in psychological distress, was confirmed by examining the means of these variables. Although there was a significant reduction in the present pain intensity score from the first (M = 4.14) to the second (M = 2.14) interview, t = 3.37 ($P < 0.05$), there was no such reduction for any of the psychological measures. This is displayed in Fig. 1 for depression (CES-D) and anxiety (trait).

The correlations between the ratings of the interference of pain with the activities of daily living and the rating of pain at its worst are presented in the first row of Table 1. These indicate a relatively high and consistent relationship between pain and interference ratings, replicating the studies of Daut and Cleeland (5,6).

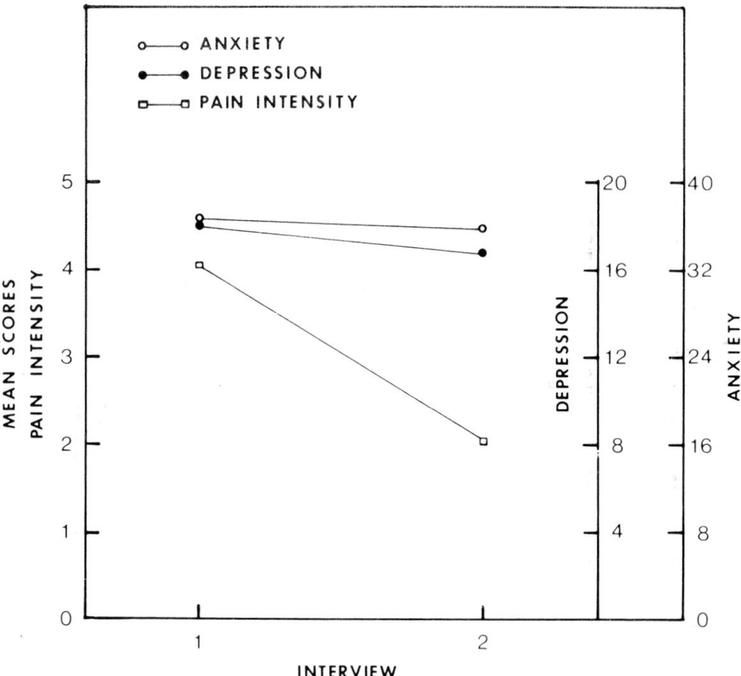

FIG. 1. Changes in present pain intensity, depression (CES-D) and anxiety (trait) from interview 1 to interview 2.

TABLE 1. *Relationship between psychological distress variables and interference of pain with daily living*[a]

	Interference of pain with				
Distress variables	Life in general	Work	Appetite	Sleep	Sexual functioning
Worst pain	0.64[b]	0.57[b]	0.35	0.56[b]	0.55[b]
Depression (CES-D)	0.34	0.41[b]	0.70[b]	0.53[b]	0.45[b]
State anxiety	0.58[b]	0.63[b]	0.67[b]	0.60[b]	0.43[b]
Trait anxiety	0.50[b]	0.53[b]	0.61[b]	0.55[b]	0.43[b]
Profile of mood states					
Depression	0.27	0.29	0.69[b]	0.42[b]	0.37
Vigor	0.16	0.23	−0.02	0.27	0.34
Confusion	0.43[b]	0.54[b]	0.68[b]	0.52[b]	0.42[b]
Tension	0.30	0.40	0.69[b]	0.45[b]	0.29
Anger	0.27	0.27	0.67[b]	0.47[b]	0.49[b]
Fatigue	0.61[b]	0.53[b]	0.70[b]	0.55[b]	0.37
Total POMS	0.40	0.43[b]	0.74[b]	0.52[b]	0.40

[a]All measures reported here were obtained at the outset of radiotherapy.
[b]$p < 0.05$
CES = D, Centre for Epidemiological Studies Depression Scale; POMS, Profile of Mood States.

The relationship between the interference measures and the psychological variables are also presented in Table 1. The table indicates clearly that there is a relatively high relationship between the interference of pain in major areas of people's lives and their subsequent psychological distress. The ratings of the interference of pain with appetite and with sleep are the most highly and consistently related to the distress variables. This may indicate that cancer pain exerts its most severe influence psychologically precisely by interfering with physiological functioning. The index of social networks was only weakly correlated with the interference ratings indicating that relative isolation from others does not necessarily increase the extent to which pain is regarded as intrusive to one's daily life.

CONCLUSIONS

The psychological implications of cancer pain have been well documented (e.g., ref. 4). This investigation provides preliminary evidence that the relationship between psychological distress and cancer pain is not perfect. The amelioration of pain following these patients' course of radiotherapy was not accompanied by an equal reduction in psychological distress. In fact, the distress levels remained constant. Psychological distress variables were highly related with the extent to which the pain interfered with patients' activities of daily life. Although the pain was reduced, it is possible that the inability to lead normal lives due to pain, and/or the cancer itself, may be responsible for the greatest portion of cancer patients' distress levels. Using appropriate controls, this hypothesis could be readily tested in future studies.

ACKNOWLEDGMENTS

This research was supported, in part, by a Canadian Cancer Society Fellowship and an Alberta Heritage Foundation for Medical Research grant to the first author.

REFERENCES

1. Berkman, L. F., and Syme, S. L. (1979): Social networks, host resistance, and mortality: A nine year follow-up study of Alameda County residents. *Am. J. Epidemiol.,* 109:186–204.
2. Bond, M. R. (1979): Psychologic and emotional aspects of cancer pain. In: *Advances in Pain Research and Therapy, Vol. 2,* edited by J. J. Bonica and V. Ventafridda, pp. 81–88. Raven Press, New York.
3. Bonica, J. J. (1980): Cancer pain. In: *Pain,* edited by J. J. Bonica, pp. 335–362. Raven Press, New York.
4. Bonica, J. J., and Ventafridda, V. (editors) (1979): *Advances in Pain Research and Therapy, Vol. 2.* Raven Press, New York.
5. Daut, R. L., and Cleeland, C. S. (1982): The prevalence and severity of pain in cancer. *Cancer,* 50:1913–1918.
6. Daut, R. L., Cleeland, C. S., and Flanery, R. C. (1983): Development of the Wisconsin Brief

Pain Questionnaire to assess pain in cancer and other diseases. *Pain,* 17:197–210.
7. McNair, P. M., Lorr, M., and Drappelman, L. (1971): *POMS Manual.* Education and Industrial Testing Services, San Diego.
8. Melzack, R. (1975): The McGill Pain Questionnaire: Major properties and scoring methods. *Pain,* 1:277–299.
9. Radloff, L. S. (1977): The CES-D Scale: A self-report depression scale for research in the general population. *Appl. Psychol. Meas.,* 1:385–401.
10. Spielberger, C. D., Gorsuch, R. L., and Lushene, R. (1970): *The State-Trait Anxiety Inventory Manual.* Consulting Psychologists Press, Palo Alto.
11. Woodforde, L. M., and Fielding, J. R. (1975): Pain and Cancer. In: *Pain: Clinical and Experimental Perspectives,* edited by M. Weisenburg, pp. 332–336. Mosby, St. Louis.

Advances in Pain Research and Therapy, Vol. 9, edited by H. L. Fields et al. Raven Press, New York © 1985.

Cancer Pain: Neurogenic Mechanisms

P. D. Wall

Cerebral Functions Research Group, Department of Anatomy, University College London, London WC1E 6BT, United Kingdom

John Bonica *(this volume)* has continued to encourage and compliment the basic scientists in their role in the understanding and control of cancer pain. In depressing contrast, Twycross (16) writes in the excellent book he edited on cancer pain:

> Nowhere in this volume has the question of pain transmission within the nervous system been discussed. This is intentional. The practical applications of, for example, the Gate Control Theory, are few both for cancer and non-cancer pain. Likewise, knowledge of the increasing number of central transmitters and of opioid receptors is of little or no value when face to face with the cancer patient in pain.

Even if the truth lies somewhere between Bonica and Twycross, we basic scientists have little reason for the arrogant complacence expressed by some of our distinguished colleagues, nor should we be permitted the escape clause of the coward: "Its all very complicated." To improve our contribution, I believe we badly need advice from the clinician and we need to learn from the patient the real nature of his problem. It has been my contention for some time that we have concentrated, for good reasons, on the wrong location and the wrong time epoch to contribute a helpful understanding of clinical pains (18). The great majority of experimental stimulus sites have been cutaneous, whereas deep tissue is clearly the source of the problem and may well contain different mechanisms. Sudden stimuli and brief responses have been the major target for study, whereas chronic pain may involve at least three modulatory mechanisms to be discussed here which are not revealed by the classical acute studies. The demand is urgent. Even St. Christopher's Hospital with its intense concentration of skill and mercy and its 24-hr monitoring and care is unable to control pain in some 5% of cases, particularly where cancer involves nerve infiltration (1). In more usual situations, some 25% of pains are unrelieved.

The six largest categories of pain causes, according to Twycross and Lack's (17) study of 303 pains in 100 patients are described in Table 1. Pains caused by treatment are a particularly sad challenge. They contributed 5% to Twycross and Lack's series, but for Foley (3) where treatment may have

TABLE 1. *Causes of pain: Largest categories*[a]

Area involvement	%
Bone	19
Nerve infiltration	18.5
Soft tissue infiltration	11.5
Visceral involvement	11
Myofascial syndrome	8
Muscle spasm	5

[a]From a study of 303 pains in 100 patients. From ref. 17, with permission.

been, to put it mildly, more vigorous, there was treatment caused pain in 19% of the inpatients and 25% of the outpatients. In addition to local causes directly attributable to the cancer, we must include systemic changes (Table 2).

Given a systemic tendency to increase or reduce pain, these factors may interact with the local changes produced by the cancer itself. There is an anecdotal belief by many clinicians that cancer pain often surfaces as a recurrence of a previous pain, for example, a low back pain. We need, first, a classical clinical description from the clinicians of the association of particular tumors with particular systemic effects and especially a description of the natural history and time course (13). Modern technology should be able to identify the circulating factors if the relevant serum and cell samples were provided. For over 30 years, hormones have been manipulated by administration or by gland destruction but there remains only sparse information on the relation of these therapies to pain since research has naturally concentrated on tumor regression (2). For example, reports on pain relief following hormone treatment of prostatic carcinoma vary between 10 and 86% with no explanation or even comments on the huge variability. Similarly, after thousands of hypophysectomies, we still do not know which pains are relieved or the time course of relief in spite of the crucial state-

TABLE 2. *Systemic changes attributable to cancer*

Algesic	Analgesic
Neuropathy	Hormonal
Myopathy	CNS
Myositis	
Arthritis [including hypertrophic (Marie-Bamberger) arthritis]	
Hypercoagulation (including embolus, phlebitis)	
Hypocoagulation (including idiopathic thrombocytopenic purpura)	

ment, if true, that some patients are relieved by the time they recover from the anesthetic. Reports on the pain-relieving action of chemotherapeutic agents are even sparser and more difficult to interpret (11–96% relief in prostate and breast cancer) since many of these agents themselves produce pain. The enormously exciting discovery of endogenous opiate systems in man's central nervous system is unfortunately accompanied by a totally chaotic literature on the actual circumstances under which these systems operate (27).

ACUTE PAIN MECHANISMS WITH A GATE CONTROL

Despite the existence of crucial slow onset modulating mechanisms to be discussed, it is simplest to propose that they act on a basic system which operates to generate the pain experienced after acute sudden events (Fig. 1). Small afferent nerve fibers (S) detect tissue damage and excite central cells (T) which project to reflex circuits and to the brain. Influencing this transfer from input to output are families of inhibitory (I) and excitatory neurons (E). It must be emphasized that this is a flow diagram and is not meant to imply anatomical or physiological detail. Similar controlled relays are presumed to exist at each stage along sensory pathways. Particular interest centers on what the factors are that control the effectiveness of firing of the T cells and what operates the inhibitory interneurons. All T cells so far detected are inhibited by excitation of large low threshold afferents (L). It was this discovery that led to our introduction of transcutaneous electrical nerve stimulation (TENS) (24). The majority of T cells are also excited by low threshold afferents. They provide a basis for the appearance of pain produced by light stimulation to normal tissue, allodynia. Cells excited by small visceral afferents also respond to a low threshold input from skin in the rel-

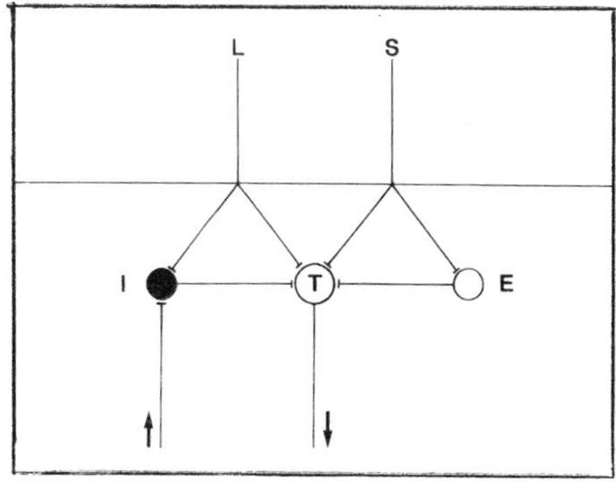

FIG. 1. Basic components of the gate control. (1) Cells excited by nociceptive inputs (S) flanked by excitatory *(open circles)* and inhibitory *(closed circle)* interneurons. (2) Convergent inputs from afferents signaling innocuous events (L) activate inhibitory interneurons. In some cells, these large afferents (L) also excite the cells receiving nociceptive afferents to produce wide dynamic range cells. (3) Descending control systems from the brain (D) may activate inhibitory neurons. This diagram is intended only to illustrate the direction of effects. It should not be taken to imply presynaptic or postsynaptic mechanisms nor should it be taken to imply only monosynaptic pathways.

evant dermatome to give a mechanism for referred pain and tenderness (14). Finally, the last component of the gate mechanism, the descending inhibitory systems from brainstem structures exert a powerful influence on the transmission of afferent impulses from S onto the T cells. We will now describe 3 processes that exert a dominating influence on the effectiveness of this gate control circuitry.

Inflammation Within Damaged Tissue

Direct Effect of Cell Breakdown

The direct effect of cell breakdown (Fig. 2) is characterized by:

1. Invasion by novel cells, e.g., leucocytes, fibroblasts, etc.
2. Further cell breakdown, e.g., mast cells.
3. Vasodilatation.
4. Edema.
5. Sensitization.

Despite a century's effort and the enormous practical importance of identifying the factors responsible for these changes, no clear and definite answer emerges. Favorite algesic candidates are nominated and include histamine, bradykinin, serotonin, substance P, and the prostaglandins. All may play a contributory role but none can yet be assigned a crucial one. The most intense study has been directed at the prostaglandins, particularly PGE_2, but there is an uncoupling of the ability of drugs to inhibit prostaglandin synthesis and their ability to reduce inflammation and pain. For example, the anti-inflammatory MK447 greatly increases PGE_2 but reduces the endoperoxide PGG_2 (6). The leukotrienes that are associated with the PG family are also proposed as algogens, but a recent report suggests they may reduce the sensitivity of some nerve endings (15). The commonest category of cancer pains, the bone pains (19%) must be attributed to local inflammatory changes. Mechanical effects are not the answer because 18% of the bone metastases which respond with a satisfactory analgesia to radiotherapy show no signs of recalcification (4). Therefore, it is necessary to search this lesion for factors which produce the osteolytic effect and the pain. PGE_2 may well be one such factor and may explain the effect of aspirin, but it is likely that the tumor itself may emit direct or indirect pain-producing substances. One tumor, in particular, needs investigation in this respect. The mesotheliomas produced by the carcinogenic effect of asbestos are particularly painful, especially as they involve pleura. It is evident that this pain is not simply due to a nonspecific pleural inflammation because when this highly invasive tumor appears in skin even along a biopsy tract, the small iatrogenic metastasis is extremely painful. Skin tumors, whether primary or metastatic, are not noted for their painful quality, but this tumor is an exception. One may

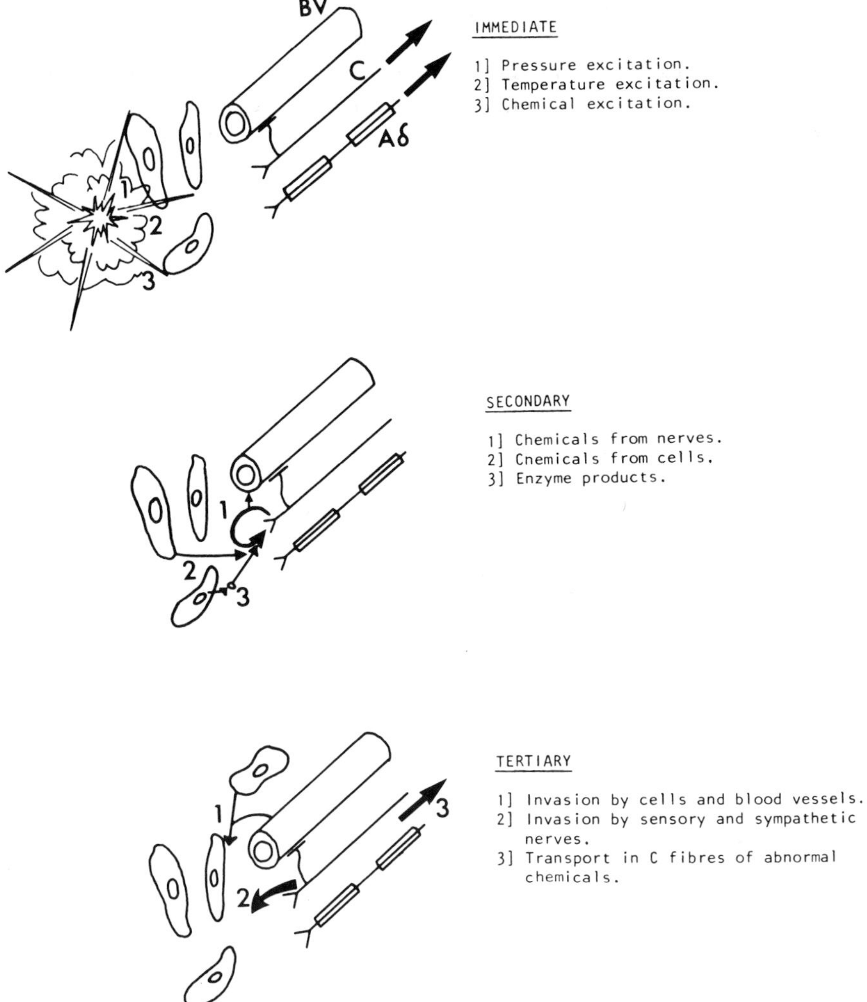

FIG. 2. Sequence of events in tissue and at nerve ends following injury. BV, blood vessel; C, an unmyelinated sensory afferent; Aδ, a small-diameter myelinated afferent. (From ref. 18, with permission.)

suspect either that some pain-producing substance is emitted by the tumor or that the tumor cells may influence nerve fibers or terminals. We need to consider the possibilities widely and freely. For example, the highly effective and specific action of colchicine on gout pain is attributed to its ability to inhibit the migration of a particular leucocyte (10). Modern excellent studies of inflammation have tended to fragment into the examination of particular targets and there is a great need to bring them together in focus on the overriding pain problem.

Indirect Effect by Way of Nerve Fibers in Tissue

The indirect effect of nerve fibers in tissue is characterized by:

1. Vasodilatation.
2. Edema.
3. Sensitization.

Tissue damage fires all types of nerve fibers but interest has naturally focused on the small high threshold afferents that are only activated by injury. Once fired, the peripheral nerve endings change their sensitivity; some increase, some decrease, as reviewed by Campbell *(this volume).* The unmyelinated afferents also emit substances which produce the triple response listed above. Lembeck and Gamse (7) review this neurogenic process which contributes an important faction to inflammation. They emphasize substance P as the peptide responsible for the changes in skin but there must be others (21).

The textbooks treat inflammation as a single general problem produced by tissue damage whether caused by trauma, bacteria, or viruses, or by abnormal chemistry. It is admitted that the presence of foreign cells such as bacteria may accelerate the process. Cancer cells are not foreign in the sense of bacteria and are generally assumed to smash normal cells by brute force and by invasion and occupation of living space where displacement is no longer mechanically possible. This line would suggest that the inflammatory pain effect of cancer is to be equated with slow-onset trauma. Clearly, that simple solution needs to be accepted with the greatest caution. An even simpler extension is to assume that pressure itself whether directly produced by the tumor or indirectly by inflammatory swelling is the actual cause of the pain.

Let us consider the three commonest sites of cancer pain: soft tissue, nerve, and bone. A very simple experiment on yourself immediately suggests that there is something wrong with the straightforward pressure theory. Pump up a blood pressure cuff wrapped around the arm to 200 mm Hg. The sensation is not pleasant immediately after inflation but even this sensation steadily drops. The pressure is far greater than anything that could be produced by a tumor or by inflammation and yet the intensity of the discomfort is clearly very much smaller. This shows us that if pressure plays a part in cancer pain, which it undoubtedly does, it must be acting on a nervous system which is sensitized and not on a normal nervous system. If further evidence of this is needed, try palpating the pressure in a tender tumor and then the pressure in an area under an inflated blood pressure cuff. The question, therefore, moves away from the pressure itself to the sensitization of peripheral nerves and of the central nervous system. Within the damaged tissue, there are two causes to be considered, the sensitization caused by the tissue breakdown itself and the sensitization caused by substances leaking from excited nerves. No doubt different tissues react in different ways. We will examine below the very special case of nerve fibers and it is sufficient here to emphasize that the direct effect of pressure is not enough to produce the severe pains as demonstrated by the experiment of compressing nerve with a blood pressure cuff.

The case of bone needs particular investigation because we do not understand the origin of the pain. Bone is the commonest site of cancer pain. Commonly patients complain of localized bone pain in a situation where metastases are expected but investigation fails to show either X-ray decalcification or isotope absorption. As the situation develops, X-ray and isotope signs appear later as the symptoms increase. It is apparent that some painful process must be in progress in bone with a small lesion which is not sufficiently extensive to produce pain by direct pressure on normal tissue or to produce gross distortion by decalcification, collapse, or fracture. One suspects some inflammatory pain-producing process particularly present in bone tissue about which we know nothing. Research should be directed at three questions: (a) What is the nature of the bone and periosteal tissue which is particularly painful; (b) What is the nature of the tissue in painless bony metastases detected in the course of other investigation; (c) What is the nature of bony metastasis tissue successfully treated for pain by irradiation but where no recalcification has occurred? Answers to these questions might allow an identification of the chemicals responsible for the sensitization which is a crucial aspect of the pain.

The third common site of cancer pain is soft tissue. It is highly unlikely that inflammatory reactions are identical in all types of soft tissue. For example, we have recently compared neurogenic edema in skin and in muscle (11). In skin this is a striking phenomena that can be evoked either by direct stimulation of unmyelinated sensory fibers in skin or by antidromic stimulation of sensory afferents to skin (reviewed in ref. 7). It does not occur in the lining of viscera. In muscle it is sparse and scattered. This led to an investigation of the chemistry of unmyelinated muscle afferents. Rat muscle C fibers fail to contain the characteristic marker of cutaneous C fibers, fluoride-resistant acid phosphatase, and very few fibers contain substance P. It is evident that whereas the same general principles may apply to inflammation in all tissues, the particulars will differ depending on the nature of the damaged cells and their innervation. These differences between tissues could imply different chemistries of inflammatory response and, therefore, different therapeutic possibilities.

Prolonged Central Changes Triggered by Nerve Impulses

It is a common clinical and personal experience that minor deep injuries such as a twisted ankle results in prolonged pain and tenderness which spreads far from the site of injury whereas apparently equivalent cutaneous injuries result in more spatially and temporally restricted sensory disorders. Similar differences have been noted by comparing the effects of experimental noxious stimuli to skin and to deep tissue in man (5,8,9). Skin lesions are associated with pain and tenderness in the immediate region of the damage while deep lesions are, in addition, associated with distant referred areas of pain and tenderness. With an acute experimental lesion such as the injection of 0.2 ml of 6% saline, the cutaneous effect is a rapidly rising pain peaking in less than 1 min and then dying down, although a triple response spreads some centimeters from the punctate lesion. In deep tissue as described in detail by Hockaday and Whitty (5) there is a three-stage time course, immediate local pain followed by distant pain followed by distant tenderness which may persist for a day.

It is evident that there are likely to be central changes as well as peripheral changes of the primary and secondary inflammatory type which must be invoked to explain the widespread effects of peripheral damage. Woolf (26) showed that peripheral thermal injury in decerebrate rats results in a prolonged increase in the excitability of the flexor reflex. Part of this increase has to be attributed to changes within the spinal cord since a delayed peripheral sensory blockade of the area of injury does not abolish the increased excitability. We decided to examine this phenomenon with cutaneous and with muscle afferent barrages (25) (Fig. 3). Twenty conditioning stimuli at C-fiber strength in the sural cutaneous nerve a 1 Hz produced a marked increase in the flexor reflex lasting up to 10 min. However, if the same type of conditioning stimulus originates from muscle nerve, the flexor reflex is enhanced for up to 90 min. Brief tetanic contraction of muscle fibers or nerve section is sufficient to trigger similar prolonged changes. A related phenomenon has been observed in lamina 1 cells when punctate deep skin burns were placed outside the cells' receptive field (12). After 10 to 15 min the excitability of the cells increased and the receptive field of the cells moved to incorporate the area of injury.

C-fiber activity is required to trigger these central changes since they only occur if the conditioning stimuli activate C fibers. Furthermore, they do not occur if the conditioning nerve has been treated with capsaicin, a selective C-fiber neurotoxin. It is important to stress that although triggered by C fibers, the change is not sustained by the continuation of the triggering barrage because local anesthesia of the conditioning nerve fails to abolish the central change once established. These changes may represent a model for the central component of tenderness. There is a particularly evocative clue. If a peripheral nerve is cut, there are prolonged central changes which are discussed later. However, there are three changes relevant to the present phase: (a) short latency or short duration excitation of central cells by C afferents which are cut in the periphery is either normal or increased; (b) the peptide content of the C afferents is decreased; and (c) the prolonged increased excitability of the flexion reflex induced by C afferents is abol-

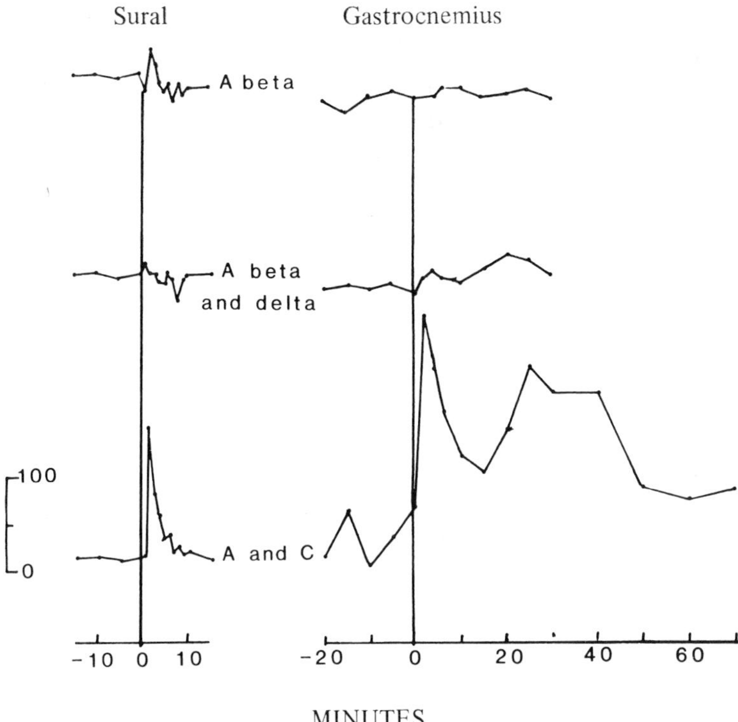

FIG. 3. Plasticity within minutes: Central changes triggered by C afferents. The flexion reflex was measured by recording the discharge of four motor neurons to posterior biceps femoris in a decerebrate spinal rat. The reflex was evoked at the indicated times by a 3-sec pinch to contralateral toes. The total number of spikes in the reflex were recorded (scale, *bottom left*). At time 0, a 20-sec, 1-Hz conditioning stimulus was applied at the indicated strength to either the sural nerve or to the nerve to gastrocnemius. Conditioning stimuli to myelinated fibers produced minimal long-term changes in the height of the flexion reflex. However, when C fibers were included in the conditioning stimulus, the sural conditioning stimulus produced an enhanced reflex for less than 10 min. When the same A and C conditioning stimulus was applied to the nerve to gastrocnemius, there was a marked increase of the reflex for over 60 min.

ished. A possible way to put these three facts together is to propose that peptides are not rapid neurotransmitters but might be responsible for the long-latency, long-duration increased excitability.

Central Reorganization Triggered by Transport in Nerve Fibers

Tissue damage inevitably involves destruction of nerve fibers and in the case of substantial nerve infiltration we recognize this as a major cause of pain in cancer. Pressure on nerves or roots, per se, does not cause pain or excitation. Injury discharges are of brief duration and are followed by a period of silence. If the fiber has been cut across, sprouts grow from the damaged membrane. These sprouts have physiological properties that differ from normal mature membrane in three ways. (a) They are spontaneously active; (b) they are mechanically sensitive; and (c) they are excited by an α-action of the sympathetic system (22,23). These local changes in the region of damage undoubtedly contribute to the pain but there is, in addition, a cascade of changes that sweep centrally from the area of damage and which produce marked central changes (reviewed in ref. 18). The dorsal root ganglion cells whose axons are cut change pharmacologically and become spontaneously active and mechanosensitive (19). The C-fiber central terminals change their peptide content but can still excite central cells often even more effectively than normally. Cut A fibers can no longer evoke dorsal root potentials or primary afferent depolarization (Fig. 4B). In addition to this evidence for a failure of presynaptic inhibition, postsynaptic inhibitory mechanisms normally fired by afferent volleys fail and so excitability rises. The receptive fields of cells which have lost their afferent drive change so that they respond to nearby intact nerves (Fig. 4A). The latency of these changes in rat cord after sciatic nerve section is more than 3 days. It is evident that we should seek the origin of nerve infiltration pain not only at the point of damage, but also in the central nervous system where reactive changes have increased excitability following deafferentation.

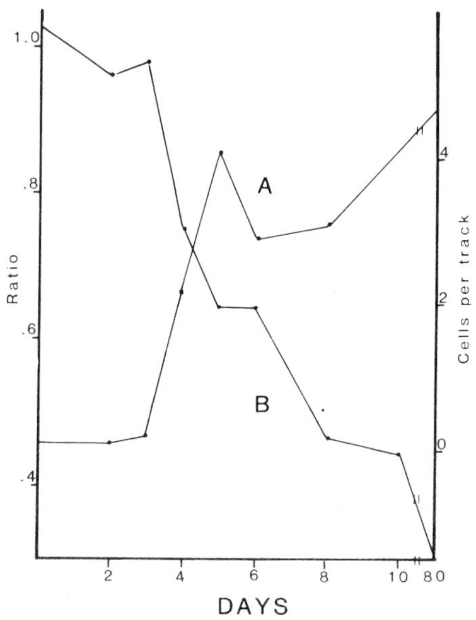

FIG. 4. Plasticity within days: Central changes produced by transport in C fibers. **(A):** Expansion of receptive fields of medial dorsal horn following section of the saphenous and sciatic nerves in the rat. During the first 3 days after nerve section, the medial dorsal horn which normally subserves the foot contained very few cells with peripheral receptive fields. From 4 days onwards, cells with proximal receptive fields began to be recorded in the area where cells previously responded to the now denervated foot. The scale on the *right* shows the average number of cells recorded in each microelectrode track. (Modified from ref. 1a.) **(B):** Decline of dorsal root potential (d.r.p.) evoked by stimulation of the sciatic nerve at the indicated times after sciatic nerve section. The dorsal root potential was recorded in rats on the L5 dorsal root after maximal stimulation of the cut sciatic nerve. The scale on the *left* shows the ratio of the height of the d.r.p. evoked from the chronically cut nerve over that produced on the opposite side by stimulation of the acutely cut side. A marked decline begins 3 days after nerve section. (Modified from ref. 18a.)

The mechanism by which these central changes occur is clearly of great importance for understanding chronic pain states and for proposing possible therapies. Chronic blockade of nerve impulses by tetrodotoxin does not produce them. Crush produces complete peripheral degeneration but fails to induce most of the central changes. There is no evidence of anatomical sprouting of intact afferents to occupy the central territory vacated by peripherally or centrally cut axons. Poisoning of C fibers is sufficient to induce many of the central alterations of A-fiber connectivity (21). Bathing the cut end of the nerve with a steady supply of nerve growth factor decreases at least three of the effects of nerve section: peptide decrease, primary afferent depolarization decrease, and receptive field expansion.

It is clear that some message informs the spinal cord that peripheral axons have been cut. The latency and other properties suggest that chemical transport is involved. The fact that local capsaicin mimics many of the central effects of whole nerve section suggests that C-fiber transport could be the message carrier. That message could be the failure of arrival of a normally transported compound such as the nerve growth factor (NGF), but it is then difficult to understand why crush fails to elicit the effect. An alternative possibility is that C fibers pick up and transport abnormal chemicals from the region of injury and that these induce the central changes. In the absence of any signs of morphological expansion in afferent innervation, the expanded receptive fields seem best explained by the unmasking of normally ineffective inputs which become effective either because of the loss of inhibitions or because of increased postsynaptic excitability. Whatever may be the mechanism, it is clear that peripheral damage induces alterations of central connections so that part of the problem shifts to the central nervous system. The central changes produce abnormal reactions not only to nerve impulses originating in the damaged nerves, but also to nerve impulses in nearby normal nerves which originate in intact tissue.

SUMMARY AND CONCLUSION

Basic science has provided only a minimal understanding of the origins of cancer pain. It has concentrated on the wrong place, the skin, whereas the commonest cancer pains originate from bone, nerve, and deep soft tissue, including muscle. It has concentrated on the wrong time, the first second after an abrupt stimulus, whereas cancer pain is dominated by at least three long-term processes. The three long-term processes are:

1. Inflammation: This process, particularly its neural component, differs in different tissues. The clinician must specify more exactly those conditions which are pain-producing and pain-relieving so that the basic scientist may identify the factors responsible. This applies particularly to bone and muscle.

2. Secondary tenderness: This is induced by changes in the central nervous system triggered by impulses in fine fibers excited in damaged tissue. Investigations must concentrate on specific methods of blocking these impulses and on the chemistry of the long-latency, long-duration changes of central excitability which may be the role of the peptides.
3. Chronic tenderness and pain with deafferentation: This process is also dependent on the fine fibers originating from the area of damage and is produced by the transport of substances in unmyelinated fibers rather than by nerve impulses. Investigations here must concentrate on the manipulation of transported factors.

The future of the problem could be revolutionary since the techniques of basic science should be able to identify the factors responsible for the three long-term processes and to manipulate them with therapeutic advantage.

REFERENCES

1. Baines, M., and Kirkham, S. R. (1984): Carcinoma involving bone and soft tissue. In: *Textbook of Pain,* edited by P. D. Wall and R. Melzack. Churchill Livingstone, Edinburgh.

1a. Devor, M., and Wall, P. D. (1981): Plasticity in the spinal cord sensory map following peripheral nerve injury in rats. *J. Neurosci.,* 1:679–684.

2. Fischer, D. S. (1984): Hormonal and chemical therapy. In: *Clinics in Oncology, Vol. 3, Pain Relief in Cancer,* edited by E. G. Twycross. Saunders, London.
3. Foley, K. M. (1979): Pain syndromes in patients with cancer. In: *Advances in Pain Research, Vol. 2,* edited by J. J. Bonica and V. Ventafridda. Raven Press, New York.
4. Garmatis, C. J., and Chu, F. C. H. (1978): The effectiveness of radiotherapy in the treatment of bone metastases from breast cancer. *Radiology,* 126:235–237.
5. Hockaday, J. M., and Whitty, C. W. M. (1967): Patterns of referred pain in the normal subject. *Brain,* 90:481–496.
6. Kuehl, F. A., Humes, J. L., Egan, R. W., and Ham, E. A. (1977): Role of prostaglandin endoperoxide PGG_2 in the inflammatory process. *Nature,* 265:170–173.
7. Lembeck, F., and Gamse, R. (1982): Substance P in peripheral sensory processes in substance P in the nervous system. *Ciba Foundation Symposium 91,* pp. 35–54. Pitman, London.
8. Lewis, T. (1942): *Pain.* Macmillan, London.
9. Lewis, T. and Kellgren, A. M. (1939): Observations relating to referred pain. Visceromotor reflexes and other associated phenomena. *Clin. Sci.,* 4:47–71.
10. Malawista, S. E. (1968): Colchicine: a common mechanism for its anti-inflammatory and anti-mitotic effects. *Arthritis Rheum.,* 11:191–197.
11. McMahon, S. B., Sykova, E., Wall, P. D., Woolf, C. J., and Gibson, S. J. (1984): Neurogenic extravasation and substance P levels are low in muscle as compared to skin in the rat hindlimb. *Neurosci. Lett.,* 52:235–240.
12. McMahon, S. B., and Wall, P. D. (1984): Receptive fields of rat lamina 1 projection cells move to incorporate a nearby region of injury. *Pain,* 19:235–247.
13. Minna, J. D., and Bunn, P. A. (1982): Paraneoplastic syndromes. In: *Cancer, Principles and Practice of Oncology,* edited by V. T. De Vita, S. Hellman, and S. A. Rosenberg. Lippincott, Philadelphia.
14. Pomeranz, B., Wall, P. D., and Weber, W. V. (1968): Cord cells responding to fine myelinated afferents from viscera muscle and skin. *J. Physiol.,* 199:511–532.
15. Schweizer, A., Bray, M. A., Brom, R., and Glatt, M. (1984): Leukotrienes desensitize the nociceptors to the painful stimulus of bradykinin. *Pain,* (Suppl. 2) 363:S243.
16. Twycross R. G. (1984): Postscript. *Clinics in Oncology Vol. 3, Pain Relief in Cancer.* Saunders, London.

17. Twycross, R. G., and Lack, S. A. (1983): Symptom control in far advanced cancer. In: *Pain Relief*. Pitman, London.
18. Wall, P. D. (1984): *The Textbook of Pain,* edited by P. D. Wall and R. Melzack, pp. 1–16. Churchill Livingstone, London.
18a. Wall, P. D., and Devor, M. (1981): The effect of peripheral nerve injury on dorsal root potentials. *Brain Res.,* 209:95–111.
19. Wall, P. D., and Devor, M. (1983): Sensory afferent impulses originate from dorsal ganglia as well as from the periphery in normal and nerve injured rats. *Pain,* 17:321–339.
20. Wall, P. D., and Fitzgerald, M. (1982): If substance P fails to fulfill the criteria as a neurotransmitter in somatosensory afferents, what might be its function? *Ciba Symposium 91,* pp. 249–266. Pitman, London.
21. Wall, P. D., Fitzgerald, M., Nussbaumer, J. C., Van der Loos, H., and Devor, M. (1982): Somatotopic maps are disorganised in adult rodents treated with capsaicin as neonates. *Nature,* 295:691–693.
22. Wall, P. D., and Gutnick, M. (1974): Ongoing activity in peripheral nerves: II. The physiology and pharmacology of impulses originating in a neuroma. *Exp. Neurol.,* 43:580–593.
23. Wall, P. D., and Gutnick, M. (1974): Properties of afferent nerve impulses originating from a neuroma. *Nature,* 248:740–743.
24. Wall, P. D., and Sweet, W. H. (1967): Temporary abolition of pain in man. *Science,* 155:108–109.
25. Wall, P. D., and Woolf, C. J. (1984): Muscle but not cutaneous C afferent input produces prolonged increases in the excitability of the flexion reflex in the rat. *J. Physiol.,* 356:443–458.
26. Woolf, C. J. (1983): Evidence for a central component of post injury pain hypersensitivity. *Nature,* 306:686–688.
27. Woolf, C. J., and Wall, P. D. (1983): Endogenous opioid peptides and pain mechanisms: a complete relationship. *Nature,* 306:739–740.

Advances in Pain Research and Therapy, Vol. 9, edited by H. L. Fields et al. Raven Press, New York © 1985.

Treatment of Cancer Pain: Current Status and Future Needs

John J. Bonica

Department of Anesthesiology RN-10, University of Washington, Seattle, Washington, 98195

Although the total number of patients with cancer-related pain account for only about 5% of the chronic pain population, cancer pain has special attributes and significance to the patients and their families. Moreover, while some advances have been made in cancer pain research and therapy, these have not been of the same degree as other aspects of pain research and therapy, and certainly they have not been commensurate with the importance of the problem. Consequently, effective control of cancer-related pain has long been and today remains one of the most important and pressing issues in the field of oncology and the health care systems of many countries. This importance stems from the fact that cancer-related pain afflicts millions of people worldwide and, all too frequently, it is inadequately managed. Consequently, many patients spend the last weeks and months or even years of their lives in great discomfort, suffering, and disability which precludes a quality of life that is vital to them.

This chapter includes a brief consideration of: (a) the importance of cancer pain including its incidence and prevalence and its effects on the patient and the family; (b) past and current status of therapy and reasons for past deficiencies; (c) recent advances; and (d) future needs and goals. This chapter represents an update of previous reports (13–16,18,19,21) on this subject and includes special emphasis on recent advances and future needs and goals.

MAGNITUDE OF THE PROBLEM

Incidence and Prevalence

During the past several decades, many countries have developed and maintained highly sophisticated health-related epidemiology and biometry programs that have permitted the acquisition of extensive data on the incidence, prevalence, and most other aspects of every type of cancer. Surpris-

TABLE 1. *Prevalence of cancer pain*

Author (ref.)	Country	Tumor type	Total no. patients studied	Patients with pain No.	Patients with pain %
All stages					
Bassett and Goulston (6)	Australia	Colon-rectal	230	145	63
Birkhahn (9)	Israel	GCP	168	106	39
Carpenter et al. (25)	USA	Hypopharynx	162	87	54
Cornaglia et al. (30)	Italy	STC	814	464	57
Cornee et al. (31)	France	Pancreas	54	36	67
Daut and Cleeland (33)	USA	STC	667	323	48
Descottes et al. (35)	France	Gallbladder	55	41	75
Foley et al. (41)	USA	GCP	540	156	29
Foley (38)	USA	GCP	397	152	38
Greenwald et al. (46)	USA	STC	390	253	65
Gullo et al. (48)	Italy	Pancreas	140	91	65
Minami et al. (63)	Japan	Kidney	81	26	32
Najem et al. (65)	USA	Colon-rectal	220	99	45
Olearchyk (68)	USA	Gastric	243	158	68
Pheils et al. (78)	Australia	Colon-rectal	200	64	32
Reid (83)	USA	Ovary	26	3	11
Ross et al. (84)	UK	Biliary	103	40	39
Weingarten et al. (103)	USA	Pancreas	100	32	32
Totals/mean			4,536	2,276	50
Advanced/terminal					
Aitken-Swan (3)	UK	GCP	200	104	52
Cartwright et al. (26)	UK	GCP	215	187	87
Cukier et al. (32)	Belgium	Kidney	184	115	63
Daut and Cleeland (33)	USA	STC	381	223	59
Ertl (37)	Austria	Gallbladder	40	33	83
Front et al. (42)	Israel	Breast	66	46	70
Foley (38)	USA	GCP	39	23	59
Gilbert et al. (44)	USA	ESCC	235	226	96
Greenberg et al. (45)	USA	Skull metastases	43	30	70
Greenwald et al. (46)	USA	STC	188	131	70
Gullo et al. (48)	Italy	Pancreas	140	98	70
Haran (49)	UK	GCP±	607	401	66
Hinton (50)	UK	GCP	82	55	67
Hui and Chen[a]	Taiwan	Cervix	501	406	81
Kornell (56)	USA	GCP	39	34	86
Kramer (57)	W. Germany	Gallbladder	60	46	77
Lempinen (58)	Finland	Stomach	732	564	77
Martelete[b]	Brazil	GCP	160	136	85
Norton and Lack (67)	USA	GCP	243	99	75
Oster et al. (69)	USA	GCP	43	32	74
Pannuti et al. (71)	Italy	STC	291	186	64
Pannuti et al. (72)	Italy	STC	324	285	88
Parkes (73)	UK	GCP (hospital)	81	51	60
		GCP (home)	61	42	69
Pollen and Schmidt (79)	USA	Prostate	42	23	55
Schutte (87)	Netherlands	a) Breast	160	90	56
		b) Other tumors	67	41	61
Spiegel and Bloom (90)	USA	Breast	86	48	56

TABLE 1. *Prevalence of cancer pain* (continued)

Sun and McLane (93)	USA	ESCC	54	42	78
Sung et al. (98)	Taiwan	Liver	151	113	75
Trotter et al. (96)	UK	GCP	237	171	72
Turnbull (97)	Canada	Lung	280	199	71
Twycross (98)	UK	GCP	500	400	80
Ventafridda and Gallucci (102)	Italy	Lung	145	106	73
Wilkes (105)	UK	GCP	300	174	58
Totals/mean			6,977	4,960	71

[a]Y. Hui and A. Chen, *personal communication.*
[b]M. Martelete, *personal communication.*
GCP, general cancer population; STC, several types of cancer; ESCC, epidural spinal cord compression.

ingly, however, there are no published data from national or international epidemiologic surveys on the incidence and prevalence of *pain* associated with different types of cancer, or their characteristics and their physiologic, psychologic, and economic impact on the patient, on the family, and on society.

This deficiency prompted me, a decade ago, to attempt to obtain rough estimates by extrapolating data on the prevalence of pain obtained from local and regional surveys of the American and world-wide population. As new reports were published, I updated the computations on a biennial interval extrapolating the data in the reports to the data on the incidence of new cancers and cancer deaths, and the estimates of cancer prevalence contained in the reports of the American Cancer Society (ACS) and in the World Health Statistics Annual (WHSA). For this chapter, I have used the 1983 Cancer Statistics published by Silverberg and Lubera (88) for the ACS, which estimated that in the United States the incidence (new cases) of cancer was 820,000, and 440,000 persons were estimated to have died from cancer. The prevalence (new and old cases) is estimated to be 1.95 million. For computation of the prevalence of cancer pain world-wide, the cancer statistics cited by J. Stjernswärd *(this volume)* of the World Health Organization (WHO) were used. These include an incidence of cancer (new cases) of over 5 million, a prevalence of 37 million, and cancer deaths totaled 4.5 million.

To compute the incidence and prevalence of pain among these various cancer populations, I have used data contained in 47 reports published in 15 countries and summarized in Table 1. This number is triple the number of reports used for the last estimate made 2 years ago (20). Some of the reports contain mean data on pain prevalence associated with one specific type of cancer, others report mean data on pain prevalence for the entire cancer population (labeled GCP in Table 1), and still others report mean data on each of several types of tumors as well as the mean prevalence for the entire group of cancer patients studied (STC in Table 1).

The overall means for each of the two stages were obtained by dividing the total number of patients with pain by the total number of patients studied. As noted, the incidence of pain among 4,536 patients presenting with various stages of the disease was 50%, whereas among the 6,977 patients with advanced/metastatic/terminal phase of cancer was 71%.

Table 2 summarizes the data on the incidence of pain with the most common types of tumors in the advanced stage of the disease as derived from data contained in 32 reports (7,25,30,32,33,35,42,44–46,48,57,58,62,63,65,68,69,71,72,78,79,83,84,87,90,93,94,97,102,–105; Yo Hui and A. Chen, *personal communication*). The mean for each specific tumor was obtained by computing data from three to six reports, containing data on each specific lesion. An example is shown in Table 3 for lung cancer. The figures for ranges and means are somewhat different than those previously published because of the larger number of reports included here.

The mean figures in Table 2 were used to estimate the total number of

TABLE 2. *Prevalence of pain with specific (advanced) cancers*

Primary site of cancer	Patients with pain	
	Range	Mean
Oral/pharynx	54–80	66
Stomach	67–77	75
Colon/rectum	47–95	69
Pancreas	72–100	79
Liver/biliary	65–83	77
Lung	57–84	72
Bone (primary)	>70–85	75
Metastasis	55–96	80
Breast	56–94	72
Uterus/cervix	40–100	75
Ovary	49–100	72
Prostate	55–80	70
Urinary organs	62–75	65
CNS	55–83	70
Soft tissue	50–82	60
Lymphomas	20–69	58
Leukemia	5–58	52
Sarcoma	75–89	85

TABLE 3. *Pain with advanced lung cancer*

Author (ref.)	Total no. patients studied	Patients with pain No.	Patients with pain %
Greenwald et al. (46)	99	69	70
Pannutti et al. (71)	40	23	58
Pannutti et al. (72)	84	71	85
Turnbull (97)	280	199	71
Ventafridda and Gallucci (102)	145	106	73
Totals/mean	648	468	72

Americans with advanced or terminal cancer who experienced pain in 1983. The computation entailed multiplying the number of deaths from each specific type of cancer estimated for 1983 by the mean pain prevalence figure for that lesion as shown in Table 4 (e.g., 72% for cancer of the lung, 69% for cancer of the colon/rectum, 72% for cancer of the breast, 70% for cancer of the prostate, etc.). Since not all patients with advanced cancer died in 1983,

TABLE 4. *Prevalence of cancer pain in the United States*[a]

Stage/type of cancer	No. patients (1,000s)	Prevalence (% patients)	Patients with pain (1,000s)
Advanced			
Lung	117	72	84
Colon/rectum	58	69	40
Breast	38	72	27
Prostate	24	70	17
Pancreas	23	79	18
Ovary/cervix/corpus	22	72	16
Lymphomas[b]	21	58	12
Urinary organs	19	65	12
Leukemia[b]	16	52	8
Stomach	14	75	11
CNS	11	70	8
Liver/biliary	10	77	8
Oral/pharynx	9	66	6
Larynx	4	65	3
Bone (primary)	2	80	2
All other	70	20	14
Subtotal	440	68	297
Intermediate therapy/other	1,460	50	730
Total	1,900	53	1,027

[a]1983 estimates rounded to the nearest unit.
[b]Data from children.

the mean figure used is probably conservatively lower than the actual pain prevalence. The computations suggest that of the 440,000 estimated to have died from cancer in 1983, 297,000 or 68% had pain of sufficient severity to require treatment with narcotics or other analgesic therapy. That this figure is probably conservative is suggested by the mean pain prevalence figure (Table 1) of 71% and also by several authors (85,95,97,98) who reported the need for narcotic therapy to control severe pain in 75 to 80% of patients with far advanced or terminal cancer. To compute the prevalence of pain among the remaining 1.51 million Americans with cancer (i.e., the 1.95 million in the prevalence cancer group less the 440,000 persons who died from cancer) the figure of 50% for pain prevalence was used. This suggests that 730,000 Americans with intermediate stage of the disease had pain which, combined with those with advanced lesion, totals 1,027,000.

To compute the prevalence of pain world-wide, the same mean figures for the advanced/terminal and intermediate stage of the disease used for the American population were extrapolated to the aforementioned WHO data. This suggests that world-wide each year, pain is experienced by over 3.0 million patients who die from cancer and over 16 million patients in the remaining cancer population for a total of over 19 million patients. While these computations seem to use an undue or unjustified degree of "epidemiologic" license, there is reason to believe that these data provide reasonable, albeit crude, estimates of the world-wide prevalence of cancer pain. Computation of the death rate per 100,000 patients in some 50 countries reported by WHO reveals that 85% of the countries have death rates which are within 10 to 15% of the United States death rate.

A number of other issues regarding these data need further comments. For one thing, pain in cancer patients may not only be due to direct tumor involvement, but also by: (a) complications of cancer therapy or those of antalgic therapy; (b) cancer-related physiologic and biochemical alterations and those associated with chronic illness such as muscle weakness and other disorders called paraneoplastic syndromes; and (c) painful disorders unrelated to cancer and cancer therapy such as arthritis, osteomyelitis, or osteoporosis. In one study, Foley (38) found that among 143 cancer inpatients referred for pain therapy, the pain was due to the cancer in 78% of the patients, it was associated with cancer therapy in 19% of the patients, and it was unrelated to therapy in 3%. In another study of 80 outpatients referred for pain therapy, the pain was due to the tumor in 62%, it was due to therapy in 28%, and it was unrelated to either in 10% (39). Twycross and Fairfield (99) interviewed 100 consecutive patients with advanced cancer pain referred to their unit for pain therapy and found that this group experienced pain in a total of 303 anatomically distinct sites, with 81 having two or more pains, and 34 having four or more pains. Ninety-one percent had a total of 204 pains caused by cancer, but in only 41% of these was all the pain caused by the cancer itself. Twelve patients had 15 different pain sites due to cancer therapy, 19 had pain caused by paraneoplastic syndromes, while 45 patients also had 65 pains unrelated either to cancer or cancer therapy.

A second point is that although most patients with pain due to the first three categories of etiology have chronic persistent pain, acute pain may be present concurrently caused by a variety of cancer-related conditions. Acute pain due to direct tumor involvement occurs with metastatic fracture of the vertebra or long bone, or with rapid occlusion of a hollow viscus by the tumor. Finally, acute pain frequently occurs during and following various anticancer therapies, particularly postoperative pain following surgical intervention, or acute pain during chemotherapy or radiation therapy, or a combination of these. A retrospective study by my colleagues Sullivan, Chapman, and their associates (92) of patients treated with chemotherapy alone or chemotherapy and radiation therapy at the Fred Hutchinson Cancer Research Center for bone marrow transplantation revealed that 62% of the patients experienced moderate to severe pain, and 22% experienced mild pain for periods of 3 to 4 weeks primarily due to therapy-induced oral mucositis. It should be stressed that the data presented in the foregoing pages do *not* include acute pain among the cancer patient population.

Another problem encountered in attempting to estimate the prevalence of pain is that a number of reports do not indicate the intensity or severity of pain and its duration, periodicity, and other characteristics of pain. However, many of these reports contain data on the percentage of patients who required potent narcotics to relieve severe pain. Moreover, a number of recent surveys report in detail the percentage of patients with mild, moderate, severe, or very severe pain, either using descriptors and/or visual analog scale, and some even have used the McGill Pain Questionnaire.

The final issue that should be discussed is the fact that most of the reports mention the primary site of the cancer in reporting pain but do not specify in what percent of these patients the pain was the result of bony or other distant metastases. However, since tumor invasion of bone (especially the vertebral column, skull, pelvis, ribs, and some of the long bones) is the predominant site of the metastases of cancer of the breast, prostate, colon-rectum, stomach, pancreas, lung, kidney, and sarcomas (104), it may be assumed that bone pain was present in the majority of patients reported. The preeminant role of tumor invasion of bone as a cause of pain is further suggested by the study carried out by Gilbert and associates (44) who noted that in the 235 patients with spinal cord compression caused by metastases to the spine from primary cancer of the lung, breast, prostate, kidney, sarcoma, myeloma, head and neck, and others, pain was a primary symptom in 96% of the patients. Greenberg and associates (45) reported an overall incidence of about 70% pain in patients with metastases to different parts of the skull from various primary sources. Pannuti and associates (72) reported that pain was present in patients with bone metastases in 80% of the patients with primary lung tumors, in 77% of patients with breast cancer, and an average of 67% with various other tumors (ovary, cervix, colon-rectum, stomach, and prostate). Schutte (87) found bone pain in 56% of patients with breast cancer and in 70% of patients with various other tumors. Others have also reported a high incidence of pain with metastatic lesion (79,90).

Summary

In summary, depending on the type and site of the neoplasm, pain is experienced by 20 to 50% of patients when the lesion is diagnosed, by nearly half of the patients in the prevalence group, and by 55 to 95% of the patients with far advanced or terminal cancer with an overall average of approximately 70%. Further analysis of the published reports also suggests that among those cancer patients with pain, the pain is moderate to severe in about 50%, and very severe or excruciating in another 30%. Most patients have two or more types and/or etiologies of cancer-related pain.

Effects of Cancer Pain

Studies carried out during the past decade have duly emphasized that in most patients chronic pain induces physiologic, psychologic, affective, and psychosocial effects that are similar regardless of etiology. However, the physiologic, psychologic, and sociologic impact of cancer pain on patients is greater than that of nonmalignant chronic pain (10,19,20). The physiologic deteriorations are much more severe because these patients have greater problems with sleep disturbances, lack of appetite, nausea, vomiting, and constipation than do patients with nonmalignant chronic pain. In the epidemiologic studies by Daut and Cleeland (32) as well as in our own study (46), it was found that cancer patients with moderate to severe pain [Visual Analog Scale (VAS) rating of 5 or more, on a scale of 0–10] reported significant interference with their activity and enjoyment of life. In addition, 60 to 65% of the patients with advanced cancer pain reported that the pain disrupted their sleep.

Cancer patients with pain also develop greater emotional reactions of fear, anxiety, reactive depression, hypochondriasis, somatic focusing, and neuroticism to the pain when it develops than is found in patients with nonmalignant chronic pain (10,12,74,106). Woodforde and Fielding (106) examined cancer patients with and without pain using the Cornell Medical Index, and demonstrated that the former group was significantly more emotionally disturbed than the latter group, and they responded less well to treatment of their cancer and died sooner. Bond (10) and Bond and Pearson (12) found that cancer patients with pain had raised levels of hypochondriasis and neuroticism while pain-free cancer patients had lower levels than normal. Bond (11) further noted that the scores of patients with high levels of emotionality fell after the pain was relieved by percutaneous cordotomy.

This led Bond to conclude that personality factors are distorted by severe pain and that its relief results in restoration in the direction of normality. For further discussion of this aspect, see chapter by M. Bond *(this volume).*

The social effects of uncontrolled cancer pain are equally devastating. Many patients develop interpersonal problems with members of their family, friends, and the community. The fact that most patients with advanced cancer have to stop working poses not only an economic but also an emotional stress and a feeling of dependency and uselessness. The physical appearance and behavior produced by the patient's pain and suffering stress the family emotionally, which is, in turn, perceived by the patient and results in further aggravating the pain and suffering. Some patients with severe intractable pain become so discouraged and desperate as to contemplate suicide.

PAST STATUS OF CANCER PAIN CONTROL

To effectively evaluate the recent advances, current status, and future needs, it is necessary to consider the status of pain therapy in past years. As early as three decades ago, I reviewed the literature and noted that in many patients with moderate to severe pain due to advanced cancer, the pain was not effectively relieved (13). In the ensuing quarter century, numerous published reports provided impressive evidence that serious deficiency existed not only in this country, but also in other medically advanced countries, including the United Kingdom, Canada, Israel, Italy, the Netherlands, and Germany. Table 5 summarizes the incidence of unrelieved cancer pain as contained in 12 reports.

In his survey, Parkes (73) found that among the hospital patients who had severe or very severe pain, it remained unrelieved during the terminal stage of the disease. Moreover, of patients managed in their home, the incidence of unrelieved severe to very severe pain during the terminal phase increased nearly sixfold over that experienced during the period prior to the terminal phase of the disease. These figures suggest that pain control was inadequate in the hospital and even worse in the home. In another British report, Twycross and Fairfield (99) noted that of the 100 cancer patients referred to their unit for pain management, 73 had pain for more than 8 weeks, and 57 for more than 16 weeks, and that three-fourths of the 73 patients stated that the pain had been severe, very severe, or excruciating—obviously due to inadequate pain control prior to admission to their unit. This problem of inadequate pain relief was the subject of an editorial comment by Cicely Saunders (86). Marks and Sachar (59), of Montefiore Hospital in New York, reported that in three-fourths of patients with moderate to severe or very severe pain, managed with a potent narcotic (meperidine), the pain remained unrelieved through the period of narcotic therapy.

The problem of unrelieved pain occurs not only in patients with advanced

TABLE 5. *Incidence of unrelieved cancer pain*

Author (ref.); year	Country	No. patients studied	No. patients with pain	Pain therapy used[a]	% Pain patients unrelieved by therapy
Aitken-Swan (3) 1959	UK	200	104	Drugs[a]	64
Hinton (50) 1963	UK	82	55	Drugs[a]	48
Cartwright et al. (26) 1973	UK	215	187	Drugs	All unrelieved until death
Marks and Sachar (59) 1973	USA	37	37	Narcotics	73
Parkes (73) 1978	UK	142	93	Drug therapy	Unrelieved until death
Turnbull (97) 1979	Canada	280	199	Palliative cancer rx	45
Pannuti et al. (71) 1979	Italy	291	186	Standard chemotherapy	60
Pannuti et al. (72) 1980	Italy	334	285	Standard chemotherapy	67
				High doses MAP	32
Kornell (56) 1980	USA	39	26	Narcotics	80
Stanley (91) 1982	WHO	433	70	Drug therapy	30PR/40NR
Ventafridda and Gallucci (102) 1985	Italy	145	106	Narcotics	40–50
Greenwald et al. (46) 1982	USA	390	246	Various ACT	50–100

[a]Drugs not specified probably included narcotic and nonnarcotic analgesics.

ACT, anticancer therapy (see text); PR, partial relief; NR, no relief; MAP, medroxyprogesterone acetate.

cancer but also among those receiving anticancer therapy. Greenwald et al. (46) found that during and after cancer therapy, patients continued to have significant pain as follows: Pain was present during and after surgical therapy in 85% of the patients with cancer of the lung, in 100% of the patients with cancer of the pancreas, in 57% of the patients with cancer of the prostate, and in 70% of the patients with cancer of the cervix. The figures for patients treated with chemotherapy were 60% with lung cancer and 50% with prostate cancer, whereas in patients treated with radiation therapy, it was 50% with lung cancer, 75% with prostate cancer, and 60% with cervical cancer. Turnbull (97), of Canada, reported that at the end of palliative therapy, 45% of patients with lung cancer had pain and two-thirds of the patients died with unrelieved pain. Pannuti et al., of Bologna, Italy, in one report (71) stated that among patients treated with chemotherapy during a 4-year period, approximately 60% of patients died in pain. In a second report (72) they stated that with commonly used antiblastic chemotherapy, pain relief was experienced by only 23% of the patients, whereas with high doses of medroxyprogesterone acetate (MAP) pain relief was obtained by 68% of the patients. In another Italian report, Ventafridda and Gallucci (102) of the National Cancer Institute of Milan, reported that in 145 patients who died from cancer of the lung, 40% of those treated in the hospital and over 50% of those treated in the home had unrelieved pain due to insufficient or total lack of narcotic therapy. In their study, Cornaglia et al. (30) also found that in many of the children with moderate to severe pain, the pain was inadequately relieved.

Similar reports of inadequate cancer pain therapy were made by many participants of the International Symposium of Advanced Cancer that was held in Venice, Italy in May 1978 (23). At a workshop on cancer pain sponsored by the WHO and the Floriani Foundation of Milan, Italy, held in Pomerio, Italy in 1982, oncologic authorities from Brazil, India, Israel, Jordan, and Sri Lanka reported that among the 433 patients treated for pain with analgesic drugs, 40% had only partial relief and 30% had no relief. Finally, it should be mentioned that, since its founding in 1977, the National Committee on the Treatment of Intractable Pain has received many thousands of letters from relatives, friends, and doctors describing patients who spent their last months in severe, unrelieved pain (52). Although these are anecdotal reports, reading their contents illustrates more effectively than a statistical study the personal meaning and impact of unrelieved pain, not only for the patient but also for the family.

Reasons for Therapeutic Deficiencies

In view of the great advances in biomedical knowledge and technology and especially the great amount of interest in, and effort devoted to, cancer research and therapy, why is cancer *pain* inadequately relieved? Serious consideration of this important question by this writer in the course of the past three decades (13–16,18,19,21) has repeatedly suggested that it is due to an inadequate appreciation or outright neglect of the problem of *pain* (in contrast to the problem of cancer) by oncologists, medical educators, investigators, research institutions, and national and international cancer agencies. Consequently, there are great voids in our knowledge of clinically relevant aspects of cancer pain, and the knowledge and therapeutic modalities that were available often are improperly applied.

Voids in Knowledge Due to Insufficient Research

Great voids in our knowledge of the mechanisms and pathophysiology of cancer pain exist simply because there has been virtually no research on these important aspects. Review of past research efforts on cancer pain reveals there have been no attempts to develop animal models to permit the study of the substrates of cancer pain. This lack of basic knowledge has prompted some authorities to extrapolate recently acquired data from animal and human studies associated with nonmalignant chronic pain states to explain the neuropathophysiologic mechanisms of cancer pain and to state that "this pathophysiologic pain is therefore, very similar to chronic and recurrent pain states which are initiated by processes other than cancer" (55). Although this may be true, final proof is lacking. Even more surprising is the fact that until 15 years ago, there were no published reports of the psychologic, behavioral, and psychosocial substrates of cancer *pain* and their impact on the patient and the family.

Another glaring deficiency which has had a directly deleterious impact on the management of cancer pain was the lack of pharmacologic studies pertaining to analgesic drugs which are the mainstay of therapy for patients with cancer pain. Although pharmacokinetics of many other drugs were defined and have provided a firm basis for their effective and rational application (76), such studies of analgesic drugs lagged very far behind. Equally important was the lack of controlled clinical trials of analgesics in cancer pain patients in order to define their efficacy, duration, and side effects. The lack of such information has hampered health professionals in their choice of the optimal drug for a particular patient, and the optimal dose and route of administration. Lack of information also caused misconceptions about the development of tolerance and pharmacologic and psychologic dependence which, as is emphasized later, have been responsible for the widespread practice of underdosing patients with severe or very severe pain.

Another research-related deficiency has been the lack of well designed and properly conducted clinical trials to critically evaluate the efficacy, side-effects and complications of various techniques of chemical and surgical interruption of pain pathways. Although nerve blocks have been used with some success for 75 years (13), little or no effort was made to develop or refine new techniques of chemical blockade that would achieve effective relief of pain without side effects inherent in current techniques. The same may be said of various destructive neurosurgical operations (70). Because these procedures for cancer pain have been performed late in the course of the patient's illness, often in debilitated patients, proper evaluation of their efficacy and duration of action has been thwarted by the development of overriding medical problems. Similarly, although some reports have been published on the use of psychologic techniques such as hypnosis, biofeedback, and relaxation, and even the more recent concept of cognitive-behavioral therapies, these have not been subjected to well designed controlled clinical trials (20).

Of the serious deficiencies pertaining to investigation, one of the most important has been the lack of comprehensive data on the incidence and prevalence of cancer pain derived from national and international epidemiologic studies. This neglect of epidemiologic studies has pervaded the entire network of cancer hospitals, cancer centers, and cancer agencies. Until a few years ago, research oncologists did not consider the inclusion of pain in their protocols in evaluating symptomatology and response to various therapeutic modalities. Consequently, in the past and even today, there are many physicians including surgical, radiation, and medical oncologists who believe that pain is not a serious problem because it is not a frequent occurrence in cancer.

Another very important reason for voids in our knowledge about cancer pain has been the lack of sufficient number of scientifically trained persons devoting their time to research in this area. Related to this has been the meager amount of funds for research and research training in cancer pain, even in the most affluent, industrialized nations in the world. For example, during the past decade in the United States, some $2 billion have been spent each year to support the research of tens of thousands of scientists who have investigated the cause, prevention, and treatment modalities of every form of cancer. However, until recently, research on *cancer pain,* per se, which, from the viewpoint of the patient and his family is one of the most important aspects of this dreadful disease (74) was virtually nonexistent. For the period from 1971 to 1976, the National Cancer Institute (NCI) spent a total of nearly $2.5 billion to support its programs and of these only $560,000 or 0.022% was spent for cancer pain research (18,77).

Improper Application of Available Knowledge and Therapeutic Modalities

The improper application of available knowledge and therapeutic modalities has been the most important reason for inadequate cancer pain management. We have drugs and other therapeutic modalities which, if properly applied, would provide good relief to most cancer patients. The blame for this sad state of affairs should not be attributed wholly to the practicing physician, but must be shared by medical educators at the graduate and postgraduate level. Past review of the curricula of medical schools revealed that few, if any, taught students the basic principles of the use of narcotics and other therapeutic modalities that effectively relieve cancer pain. Moreover, many physicians in training for specialization in surgical, medical, or radiation oncology have received little or no teaching about the proper management of cancer pain. Usually, the senior house officer, who has vague and scanty information about cancer pain and its control, teaches the junior house officer how to deal with the problem in a rather empirical way and passes on some of the misconceptions that are mentioned below.

Inadequate or total lack of interest or concern about the problem of pain by oncologists is further attested by the fact that very little, if any, information about the proper management of the *pain* problem is found in the oncology literature. Of the many textbooks on various aspects of cancer, few deal with the problem of pain management, and those do so inadequately. For example, review of the earlier editions of nine important textbooks and monographs on the clinical management of cancer published in the United States prior to 1982 (1,4,7,29,51,52,66,81,85) revealed the startling fact that of a total of 9,300 pages, only 17 were devoted to the symptomatic control of cancer *pain.* Recent editions of these books and a new textbook of oncology (36) contain a total of 12,148 pages, but still only 82 pages are devoted to pain control. Moreover, volumes of the *Yearbook of Cancer* published in the 1970s, as well as numerous journals dealing with various aspects of cancer, contain no papers relevant to pain control (27). Similarly, until recently, in the scientific programs of hundreds of regional, national, and international meetings on cancer research and therapy, pain was not included as a subject for discussion. From these data, the only conclusion that can be drawn is that pain has not been considered important by oncologic scientists and clinicians.

As a result of this lack of education of students and physicians, the pain of cancer has been treated in an empirical manner. Most practitioners have relied on nonnarcotic and narcotic analgesics: Although very useful and having a central role in the control of pain in cancer, for a variety of reasons they have been and continue to be misused. In a small percentage of patients, potent narcotics have been used initially for mild pain which could have been relieved by nonnarcotic analgesics alone or combined with adjuvant drugs. At the other end of the spectrum of the problem, many, if not most, patients with moderate to severe pain of advanced cancer have been given inadequate amounts of narcotics, or the drugs given were weak, or the right drug was given according to circumstances instead of at fixed intervals. In all too many instances, physicians prescribed the analgesics but did not monitor the patient's response, or they failed to titrate the drug dose to the needs of the patient, or failed to use adjuvant drugs when these were indicated. Marks and Sachar (59) found that house officers prescribed amounts of meperidine for patients with moderate to severe pain due to cancer that were about 50 to 65% of the established effective dose, and nurses administered as little as 20 to 30% of the "inadequate dose" prescribed. For example, for patients with severe pain due to abdominal cancer, cancer of the pancreas, or lymphosarcoma, 50 mg meperidine every 4 hr was prescribed and they received only 50 to 75 mg of meperidine *per day*. They followed this finding with a survey of 102 physicians in training in two major New York hospitals and found that, because of inadequate knowledge of the pharmacology of narcotics, most physicians underestimated the effective dose range, overestimated the duration of their action, and had an exaggerated opinion of the dangers of addiction. Similar findings among American nurses were reported by Cohen (28). Apparently this problem of inadequate knowledge of the pharmacology of these drugs and misconception about addiction also prevailed widely in Brazil, Great Britain, France, Germany, Italy, and in many other medically advanced countries (23).

In some instances, inadequate relief with narcotics has been due to misconceptions and/or the philosophy and culture of the patient and/or the family (100). Some patients believe that cancer pain is inevitable and untreatable; others are reluctant to contact their physician or put on a brave face in spite of severe pain; still others believe that analgesics should be taken only as a last resort. Moreover, some patients avoid taking analgesics because of fear of addiction and physical dependence, while others stop taking the drug because of adverse side-effects.

In a small percentage of patients, even properly administered narcotics and other systemic drugs do not produce sufficient relief and other modalities need to be used alone or in combination with drugs (14,15,19,23,24,35,41,100). These include interruption of pain pathways chemically with nerve blocks or with neurosurgical operations, the use of neurostimulating techniques, hypnosis, and other psychologic procedures. Unfortunately, the role of these therapeutic modalities in cancer pain control is not known or appreciated by most practitioners and even by many oncologists. Consequently, for patients whose pain could be relieved more effectively by one or a combination of therapies, they are not considered, or if they are considered, this is done too late.

Inadequate Communication

It is obvious that inadequate or total lack of communication has been an important factor that has impaired the physician's ability to effectively relieve patients with cancer pain. In addition to the obviously poor transfer of information between educators and students, there has been poor communication between research scientists and clinicians, between algologists and oncologists, and between oncologists and general practitioners. This has been due, in part, to the high degree of specialization and subspecialization which has been conducive to publications in highly specialized journals limited to specific fields. Another important problem which has impaired communication and appropriate transfer of information has been the lack of a uniform classification of cancer pain syndromes.

RECENT ADVANCES

Fortunately, during the past decade, but especially during the past 5 years, a number of factors have converged to effect improvement in all of the aforementioned areas. For one thing, a small cadre or nucleus of dedicated individuals with intense interest and involvement with patients with cancer pain has persisted in achieving their objective of improving the care of these patients. Through their unrelenting "drum-beating" in the form of lectures to scientific groups, talks with lay people, publication in scientific journals and books, and active participation in federal research agencies, this small group has been highly effective in encouraging and carrying out research, education, and patient care. These efforts were greatly enhanced by the International Association for the Study of Pain, the journal *Pain,* and their national chapters which have been highly effective in encouraging research and transfer of information.

Advances in New Knowledge

The immense interest in pain research during the past decade has resulted in the acquisition of a vast amount of new information on the anatomic, biologic, and psychologic substrates of acute pain and a modest amount of knowledge on the pathophysiology, neuropathophysiology, and psychology of nonneoplastic chronic pain (20). Equally important have been the studies in cancer patients of the psychologic, behavioral, and sociologic impact of the pain caused by cancer on the patient and the family. A recent study by Ahles and associates (2) demonstrated the multidimensional nature of cancer pain, including sensory, affective, cognitive, and behavioral components and have emphasized that these various facets of cancer pain must be considered if the patients are to be effectively relieved. These and other aspects of this topic are considered in more detail by M. Bond *(this volume).*

One of the most important advances has been the progressive increase in the number of local and regional surveys on the incidence and prevalence of cancer pain. Thus it is noted that a decade ago, only five such studies had been published, but by 1980 the number had increased to 29 reviews and as of mid-1984, I found 47, which are cited to this chapter. Primarily this has been due to increased appreciation of the need for such data and in part to the increased awareness by oncologists to include pain in their protocols for retrospective and prospective studies of cancer and its therapy. The importance of epidemiologic studies pertaining to one type of cancer-related pain was recently emphasized by Berrino (8) who gave guidelines for oncologists to carry out such programs. Another step in this direction was that taken by the NCI of the United States, which provided funds to carry out epidemiologic studies in several comprehensive cancer centers in the United States. These studies involved evaluation of not only the incidence and prevalence of pain, but also correlation with the stage of the disease, age, psychologic and social factors, and many other important aspects of the problem. A summary of two studies has been published, one by Daut and Cleeland (33) and the other by Greenwald et al. (47). Both groups developed and used reliable methods for acquiring comprehensive data on various aspects of cancer pain by personal interviews of patients and by sending questionnaires. Unfortunately, the complete reports have not been published by the NCI staff. As a result of their experience, Daut et al. (34) have published a brief pain questionnaire which was found reliable and valid to acquire data on cancer pain and other types of pain. Because of its simplicity, this should facilitate acquisition of such data.

During the past 5 years or so, significant advances have been made in the study of the pharmacology, pharmacokinetics, and pharmacodynamics of narcotic and nonnarcotic analgesics and, to a lesser extent, of a number of adjuvant drugs which are often combined with systemic analgesics for cancer pain control (5). These advances include the development of well designed clinical assay methods, the development of specific and sensitive analytic techniques to measure exogenous and endogenous opioid analgesics in biofluids, and the development of mathematic models to relate pharmacologic and pharmacokinetic parameters of narcotic, nonnarcotic, and other analgesic drugs (75). These technical advances have now been applied to the evaluation of heroin and morphine revealing that when given in equianalgesic doses, there is no significant difference in analgesic efficacy, side effects, or effects on mood (54). Equally important has been the development of a number of new drugs and of novel drug preparations to reduce undesirable side effects. Other innovations include continuous intravenous and continuous subcutaneous infusions of narcotics, patient-controlled analgesia, and, of course, regional analgesia achieved by intraspinal administration of narcotics. These and other aspects are discussed by K. Foley *(this volume).*

Other new and exciting therapeutic modalities have been developed as a result of recently acquired information about the intrinsic modulatory systems including various neuromodulation techniques. Psychologic/behavioral studies have prompted the clinical application of biofeedback, a cognitive-behavioral training, and reevaluation of hypnosis for cancer pain control (see ref. 20 for review). Unfortunately, many of these procedures have been used clinically based merely on theoretical considerations and laboratory studies. To define more accurately their role in pain control, the extensive psychologic studies of recent years must be complemented with controlled clinical trials. Also important has been the advent of more precise methods of measuring pain both by subjective and objective methodologies.

Advances in Education and Transfer of Information

During the past decade, but especially during the past 5 years, several activities have helped to enhance the diffusion of new information and improve education of physicians, the biomedical scientific community, the staff of regional health agencies, and the public as a whole. These include

TABLE 6. *International symposia on cancer pain*

Date	Place	Subject	Sponsor	Publication	Ref.
Sept. 1975	Florence	Cancer pain research and therapy	NCI, IASP	Proceedings: 160 pp.[a]	Unpublished
May 1978	Venice	Advanced cancer pain	Floriani Foundation, IASP, AISD, NCI, IUCC	Book: APRT Vol. 2 700 pp.	(23)
Feb. 1979	Bethesda	Pain, discomfort, and humanitarian care	NIH, other	Book: 311 pp.	(18)
Oct. 1979	Milan	Continuing care of terminal patients	Floriani Foundation, IASP, IUCC, NCI	Book: 311 pp.	(18)
Nov. 1980	Stockholm	Treatment of cancer pain	Swedish Academy Medical Science	ACTA AN Scand. 150 pp.	(5)
May 1981	Stresa	Superior sulcus syndrome	Floriani Foundation, IASP, IUCC, NCI-Milan	Book: APRT Vol. 4 242 pp.	(24)
May 1982	Heidelberg	Pain in cancer patients	Swiss Cancer League	Book: 238 pp.	(107)
Feb. 1983	Washington, D.C.	Care of terminal patients	USPHS	Summary: *JAMA*	(60)

[a]Proceedings submitted to NCI and participants, but not published.

NCI, National Cancer Institute (USA); IASP, International Association for the Study of Pain; AISD, Associazione Italiana per lo Studio del Dolore; IUCC, Internationale Union Contre Le Cancer; NIH, National Institutes of Health; NCI-Milan, Istituto Nazionale per lo studio e la Cura del Cancro.

eight international symposia listed in Table 6. It is to be noted that the Floriani Foundation of Milan, Italy, which subsidized and was the primary sponsor of three of these symposia, is the only private nonprofit foundation in the world whose funds are used exclusively for the support of research on, and the care of, patients with advanced cancer pain. With the exception of the Stresa Meeting, these symposia were attended by groups of physicians and other health professionals ranging from 200 to 600, including oncologists, basic scientists, clinical algologists, oncologic nurses, and other health professionals.

Through the participation in these symposia and the publication of the proceedings, physicians and other health professionals responsible for the care of cancer pain patients have been provided with the latest research findings and evaluation of therapeutic modalities. Also, the wide publicity in the lay press, consequent to these meetings, has enhanced the appreciation of the importance and magnitude of cancer pain by the public and the staff of research and health care agencies. This factor and the immense efforts of several highly dedicated people have helped to generate the interest and financial support for cancer pain research and therapy.

Another significant advance pertaining to diffusion of clinically relevant information has been an impressive increase in the number of textbooks and journal articles containing information on the management of cancer pain and the inclusion of this subject in national and international cancer congresses. In addition to the aforementioned proceedings, a textbook on the management of cancer pain has been published by Twycross and Lack (100), and by Saunders (86). Equally effective have been the monographs and articles written by Foley and associates (38–40,55,75), by Twycross and co-workers (98–101), Ventafridda and associates (23,24,101), as well as our own group (15–24,46,47).

The increased appreciation of the importance of cancer pain management is reflected, in part, by inclusion of chapters or articles on cancer pain in the oncologic literature. The excellent comprehensive textbook on oncology, edited by V. DeVita, S. Hellman, and S. Rosenberg (36) has 3 chapters that contain ample information on cancer pain control with pharmacologic, neurosurgical, and neurostimulating techniques. *The Manual of Cancer Chemotherapy,* edited by R. Skeele (89), contains a small chapter on pharmacologic therapy, and the two-volume *Textbook on Oncology* edited by Moossa and associates contains a comprehensive overview of all aspects of cancer pain management (22). The increasing interest in cancer pain is further reflected, in part, by the number of citations found in the Medline search that have increased from only 8 in 1978, 36 in 1980, 40 in 1981, 63 in 1982, and 123 in 1983.

Another important achievement related to research and therapy and improvement in communication is development of a taxonomy or classification of cancer pain syndromes. This is based on the classification first proposed by Bonica in 1953 (13), Bonica and associates (17,21,22), Foley and associates (38–40,44,45,80) of the Memorial Sloan-Kettering Cancer Center, Twycross and associates (99,100), and Turnbull (97), among others. A comprehensive classification has evolved that is being widely adopted by many workers in this field (53) (Table 7).

Still another example is the extremely informative brochure on cancer pain developed under the sponsorship of NCI and being distributed by the American Cancer Society to cancer patients and their families. This brochure should do much to allay the fear and apprehension, and rectify mis-

TABLE 7. *Specific pain syndromes related to cancer*

- Direct tumor involvement
  - Tumor infiltration of bone
    - Skull
      - Calvarium syndrome
      - Orbital syndrome
      - Parasellar syndrome
      - Middle fossa (Gasserian ganglia) syndrome
      - Jugular foramen syndrome
      - Clivus syndrome
      - Sphenoid sinus syndrome
      - Occipital condyle syndrome
    - Vertebral column
      - Axis/atlas
      - C_7–T_1 syndrome
      - L_1 metastasis syndrome
      - Sacral syndrome
    - Other bones
      - Pelvic syndrome
      - Hip/femur/knee syndrome
      - Shoulder/arm syndrome
      - Intercostal syndrome
  - Tumor infiltration of nerve
    - Peripheral neuropathy
    - Brachial plexopathy
    - Causalgia syndrome
    - Lumbar plexopathy
    - Sacral plexopathy
    - Epidural spinal cord compression
    - Leptomeningeal carcinomatosis
    - Spinal cord tumors
  - Tumor invasion of hollow viscera
  - Infiltration/compression of major blood vessels
  - Rapid tumor growth in encapsulated organs
  - Inflammation/necrosis/ulceration of mucous membrane and other soft tissue
- Tumor-induced physiologic and biochemical alteration (paraneoplastic syndromes)
  - Muscle dysfunction—disuse atrophy, myofascial syndromes
  - Joint disorders—polymyalgia rheumatic, hypertrophic osteoarthropathy
  - Hypercoagulability—embolism, pain
- Pain syndromes associated with cancer therapy (iatrogenic syndromes)
  - Postsurgical syndromes
  - Postchemotherapy syndromes
  - Postradiation therapy syndromes
  - Postantalgic therapy complications
- Pain unrelated to cancer or cancer therapy
  - Osteoporosis
  - Osteomyelitis
  - Osteoarthritis

conceptions about cancer pain, reassure patients and their families about the efficacy of current therapies, and provide other information that helps the patient and the family actively participate in the pain control program.

Advances in Patient Care

The aforementioned advances in knowledge and the diffusion of information and numerous other factors have helped to improve the care of more and more patients with cancer pain. For one thing, an increasing number of physicians and other health professionals are becoming interested in acquiring the new information and technologies in the management of patients with cancer pain. For another, new and highly specialized methods of diagnosis and therapy provide a more effective and more direct approach by treating and eliminating the cause of pain (75). K. Foley *(this volume)* emphasizes the importance of new knowledge and technology about the pharmacologic approach to cancer pain control. Professor M. Bond *(this volume)* emphasizes the value of new knowledge about the psychologic, affective, and sociologic substrates of cancer pain, the effect on the pain and on helping the patient, the physician, and the family cope with pain.

The advent of new knowledge of the pathophysiologic effects of deafferentation on the function of the dorsal horn and other parts of the neuraxis (see ref. 20 for review) has caused a revision in the use of destructive chemical and surgical procedures including the virtual abandonment of peripheral neurotomy, spinal dorsal rhizotomy, and open cordotomy, and has prompted a decrease in the use of neurolytic blocks. In parallel to this trend has been the refinement of percutaneous cordotomy, the widespread use of stereotactic and microsurgical techniques in producing exquisitely precise ablative lesions in various parts of the neuraxis, and the refinement and wide use of controlled thermocoagulation of the ganglia of the 5th and 9th cranial nerves (70). The new knowledge of the intrinsic modulating mechanism has prompted the widespread use of intraspinal narcotics which have proved to be an effective method of relieving cancer pain, and of such neurostimulating techniques as transcutaneous nerve stimulation, dorsal column stimulation, brainstem and thalamic stimulation (see ref. 62 for review).

Another procedure which is enjoying increasing use is ablation of the pituitary gland, either by chemical or surgical means, for the treatment of hormone-dependent tumors (43,64). In addition to producing objective remission or lack of progression of the tumor in 30 to 40% of patients, this procedure produces pain relief apparently independently of its antitumor effects. Putting aside the current controversy whether pituitary ablation should be achieved with surgical removal, or the injection of alcohol, there is more and more impressive evidence that this procedure is highly effective in relieving severe diffuse pain due to widespread metastases in 45 to 60% of the patients and provides partial relief in another 20 to 25% (43).

The increased appreciation that cancer pain as a complex, multidimensional phenomenon composed of a vast array of sensory, perceptual, emotional, affective, interpersonal, and environmental events has encouraged the increasing use of the multidisciplinary team approach to cancer pain diagnosis and therapy and the hospice concept to the care of patients with terminal disease—two developments that Melzack and Wall (61) believe are the most important advances in the care of patients with cancer pain, and other chronic pain problems. The multidisciplinary team approach to the diagnosis and therapy of complex chronic pain problems, first proposed by this writer over three decades ago (20), has been adopted in a progressively increasing number of medical centers world-wide, including a number of comprehensive cancer centers (47). This has been due, in part, to the increasing realization that the use of multimodal therapy, which for years has been known to be effective in treating cancer, has been found also to be applicable to the management of pain due to cancer. As Payne and Foley (75) have emphasized, the use of selective anesthetic and neurosurgical procedures, and the integration of psychologic and behavioral methods and neurostimulating techniques combined with antitumor therapy and analgesic drug therapy provide the most effective relief in many patients. Equally important has been the widespread adoption of the hospice concept, refined and vigorously advocated by Dame Cicely Saunders (86) and subsequently by Twycross (100) and others, that has proven to be of immeasurable benefit to patients with advanced and terminal disease.

Finally, another very encouraging trend pertaining to patient care has been the activities of the cancer unit of the World Health Organization (WHO), which under the vigorous leadership of Dr. Jan Stjernswärd has developed preliminary plans to improve the management of patients with cancer pain world-wide. In 1982, the WHO Cancer Unit initiated a preliminary survey of the prevalence of cancer pain in Brazil, India, Israel, and Sri Lanka (91). This group developed guidelines for the effective use of systemic analgesics and adjuvant drugs which can be administered by the existing health care personnel in developing countries. These guidelines are being given field trial in several countries and Takeda (95) of Japan has reported that 93% of the patients managed with the prescribed guidelines achieved good pain relief. If others confirm these effective results, these guidelines will be implemented in developing countries world-wide within the next several years and should do much to provide relief of pain and suffering to the millions of patients with cancer pain. I am pleased to announce that a manual or monograph on the management of cancer pain is being written under the editorship of Drs. Ventafridda and Foley, which will be distributed world-wide to compliment the guidelines.

FUTURE NEEDS AND GOALS

In considering future needs and goals, I reviewed my previous reports (14–24) and found that although we have made the aforementioned gains during the past several years, we remain far from the mark of providing effective and lasting relief to all or even the majority of patients with cancer-related pain. To achieve such laudable goals, it will be necessary to sustain and markedly expand current programs and develop new ones pertaining to research, education, and training, and diffusion of information.

The brief overview given in the previous section makes it obvious there remains the urgent need for much greater research on cancer-related pain. Of course current studies on the cause, prevention, and treatment of cancer pain must be sustained and expanded. However, until this dreadful disease can be effectively prevented, it is also essential to find more effective means to relieve cancer pain. Future research should provide much new information on the precise biochemical, neurophysiologic, and psychologic aspects of chronic pain in general, and cancer pain in particular. Once such information becomes available, we can apply the vast knowledge and technology in chemistry, pharmacology, and biochemistry to develop agents that can act specifically to prevent or promptly terminate the various biochemical and neurologic factors that act at molecular and cellular levels and in the nervous system to produce pain. It is hoped such new agents would produce complete relief without significant side-effects. Moreover, future studies should permit more specific definition of the impact of various emotional, psychologic, sociologic, and environmental factors on cancer pain patients and their families, and how this information could be applied more effectively for pain relief.

Clinical research is needed to further evaluate and refine for more precise use currently available therapeutic modalities. In regard to pharmacologic agents, it is necessary to carry out more extensive controlled clinical trials of old and new drugs, using well established principles (75). We also need to apply the same basic principles in evaluating patient-controlled narcotic analgesia, spinal opiate analgesia, regional analgesia with local anesthetics, cognitive-behavioral techniques, and neurostimulating procedures. Finally, and most importantly, is the urgent need to carry out national and international epidemiologic studies on the incidence and prevalence of cancer-related pain, its sociologic and economic impact on the patient, the family, and on society, and the evaluation of the therapies being used including their efficacy, side-effects, and complications. These data are essential to make oncologists, the staff of health agencies, and the public at large appreciate the magnitude of the problem.

Until we acquire new information, we should be able to effectively use the current knowledge and therapeutic modalities to do a much better job in relieving the pain and suffering of cancer patients. To achieve this goal, it is necessary to mount intensive educational and training programs for students of medicine, nursing, and other health professions, as well as family physicians and oncologists. Physicians must be given specific guidelines about proper application of various pain-relieving techniques and the optimal management of the cancer patient. In addition to such programs, it is essential to provide ample sources of information through the oncologic literature, including chapters on the management of pain in *all* the oncologic textbooks and special articles, as well as brochures on cancer pain and its management. It is highly desirable to encourage the activation of hospice units in general hospitals and free-standing hospices, and to have multidisciplinary cancer pain diagnostic and therapy teams in large general hospitals and comprehensive cancer centers.

Finally, it is important to mount a vigorous program for the information and education of the public at large, the leaders of national and regional governments, the staffs of governmental and private agencies that are concerned with biomedical research, education, and patient care related to cancer. Such programs should make the public and the staff of various agencies, as well as the rest of the scientific community, realize the magnitude of cancer pain and the importance of supporting research, research training, and education. An important aspect of public education is to provide information that places cancer-related pain in proper perspective.

To achieve all of these goals, it is desirable, and indeed essential, to develop broad-based, multidisciplinary/interdisciplinary programs in cancer pain research, training, and patient care. Such programs should evolve into "cancer pain centers" as part of large comprehensive cancer centers (47). The centers should include a critical mass of basic and clinical scientists and clinicians including neurooncologists and medical, surgical, and radiation oncologists, clinical algologists (pain specialists), anesthesiologists, clinical pharmacologists, neurosurgeons, psychiatrists, psychologists, social workers, nurses with special knowledge and expertise in pain, theologians, and others with special interest and expertise in cancer pain research and therapy.

SUMMARY

Effective control of pain due to cancer remains an important problem in most countries throughout the world because it affects millions of persons and, in all too many patients, it is inadequately relieved. This chapter contains an updated review of the prevalence of cancer pain, the past status of cancer pain therapy, the reasons for deficiencies that existed, and the advances made during the past several years. Finally, future needs and goals are briefly discussed and recommendations made that may help to markedly improve the welfare of cancer patients.

REFERENCES

1. Ackerman, L. V., and Del Regato, J. A. W. (editors) (1977): *Cancer Diagnosis, Treatment and Prognosis,* 5th ed. Mosby, St. Louis.
2. Ahles, T. A., Blanchard, E. B., and Ruckdeschel, J. C. (1983): The multidimensional nature of cancer-related pain. *Pain,* 17:277–288.
3. Aitken-Swan, J. (1959): Nursing the late cancer patient at home. *Practitioner,* 183:64–69.
4. American Cancer Society, Massachusetts Division (1978): *Cancer: A Manual for Practitioners.* American Cancer Society, Boston.
5. Arner, S., Bolund, C., Rane, A., and Ronnback, L. (editors) (1982): Narcotic analgesics in the treatment of cancer and postoperative pain. *Acta Anaesthesiol. Scand. (Suppl.),* 74(26):1–153.
6. Bassett, M. L., and Goulston, K. J. (1978): Colorectal cancer—a study of 230 patients. *Aust. NZ J. Med.,* 8:669–670 (abstract).
7. Becker, F. (editor) (1982): *Cancer: A Comprehensive Treatise,* 2nd ed. Plenum Press, New York.
8. Berrino, F. (1982): Epidemiology of superior pulmonary sulcus syndrome (Pancoast syndrome). In: *Advances in Pain Research and Therapy, Vol. 4,* edited by J. J. Bonica, V. Ventafridda, and C. A. Pagni, pp. 15–22. Raven Press, New York.

9. Birkhahn, D. (1982): Epidemiology of cancer in Israel. *Proceedings: WHO Workshop on Cancer Pain Relief,* Milan, Italy.
10. Bond, M. R. (1979): Psychologic and emotional aspects of cancer pain. In: *Advances in Pain Research and Therapy, Vol. 2,* edited by J. J. Bonica and V. Ventafridda, pp. 81–88. Raven Press, New York.
11. Bond, M. R. (1979): Psychologic and psychiatric techniques for the relief of pain of advanced cancer. In: *Advances in Pain Research and Therapy, Vol. 2,* edited by J. J. Bonica and V. Ventrafridda, pp. 215–222. Raven Press, New York.
12. Bond, M. R., and Pearson, I. B. (1969): Psychologic aspects of pain in women with advanced cancer of the cervix. *J. Psychosom. Res.,* 13:13–19.
13. Bonica, J. J. (1953): *The Management of Pain.* Lea & Febiger, Philadelphia.
14. Bonica, J. J. (1959): The management of cancer pain. *G.P.,* 10:35–43.
15. Bonica, J. J. (1978): Cancer pain: A major national health problem. *Cancer Nursing J.,* 4:313–316.
16. Bonica, J. J. (1979): Importance of the problem. In: *Advances in Pain Research and Therapy, Vol. 2,* edited by J. J. Bonica and V. Ventafridda, pp. 1–12. Raven Press, New York.
17. Bonica, J. J. (1979): Introduction to the management of cancer pain. In: *Advances in Pain Research and Therapy, Vol. 2,* edited by J. J. Bonica and V. Ventafridda, pp. 115–130. Raven Press, New York.
18. Bonica, J. J. (1980): Pain research and therapy: Past and current status and future needs. In: *Pain, Discomfort and Humanitarian Care,* edited by L. K. Y. Ng and J. J. Bonica, pp. 1–46. Elsevier/North-Holland, Amsterdam.
19. Bonica, J. J. (1982): Management of cancer pain. *Acta Anaesthesiol. Scand. (Suppl.),* 74:75–82.
20. Bonica, J. J. (1983): Pain research and therapy: Achievements of the past and challenges of the future—IASP Presidential Address. In: *Advances in Pain Research and Therapy, Vol. 5,* edited by J. J. Bonica, U. Lindblom, and A. Iggo, pp. 1–36. Raven Press, New York.
21. Bonica, J. J. (1984): Management of cancer pain. In: *Recent Results in Cancer Research, Vol. 89,* edited by M. Zimmerman, P. Drings, and G. Wagner, pp. 13–27. Springer-Verlag, Heidelberg.
22. Bonica, J. J., and Benedetti, C. (1984): Management of cancer pain. In: *Comprehensive Textbook of Oncology,* edited by A. R. Moossa, M. C. Robson, and S. C. Schimpff. Williams & Wilkins, Baltimore *(in press).*
23. Bonica, J. J., and Ventafridda, V. (editors) (1979): *Advances in Pain Research and Therapy, Vol. 2.* Raven Press, New York.
24. Bonica, J. J., Ventafridda, V., and Pagni, C. A. (editors) (1982): *Advances in Pain Research and Therapy, Vol. 4.* Raven Press, New York.
25. Carpenter, R. J., DeSanto, L. W., Devine, K. D., and Taylor, W. F. (1976): Cancer of the hypopharynx. Analysis of treatment and results in 162 patients. *Arch. Otolaryngol.,* 102:716–721.
26. Cartwright, A., Hockey, L., and Anderson, A. B. M. (editors) (1973): *Life Before Death.* Routledge & Kegan Paul, London.
27. Clark, R. L., Cumley, R. W., and Hickey, R. C. (1979–1982): *The Yearbook of Cancer: 1979,* pp. 323–331; *The Yearbook of Cancer: 1980,* pp. 327–337; *The Yearbook of Cancer: 1981,* pp. 301–310. Year Book Medical Publisher, Chicago.
28. Cohen, E. L. (1980): Postsurgical pain relief: Patients' status and nurses' medication choices. *Pain,* 9:265–274.
29. Committee on Professional Education of U.I.C.C. (1982): *Clinical Oncology (A Manual for Students and Doctors),* p. 346. International Union Against Cancer, Springer-Verlag, Berlin.
30. Cornaglia, G., Massimo, L., Haupt, R., Melodia, A., Sizemore, W., and Benedetti, C. (1984): Incidence of pain in children with neoplastic diseases. *Pain,* (Suppl. 2):S28.
31. Cornee, J., Durbec, J.-P., Yoro, J., and Laurats, M. (1974): Statistiques descriptives de la douleur en pathologie pancreatique. *Archives Francaise Maladies Digestives,* 63:375–384.
32. Cukier, J., Pascal, B., and Mangin, P. (1981): Semiology of the cancer of the kidney in adults: review of 184 cases. *Acta Urol. Belg.,* 49:259–262.
33. Daut, R. L., and Cleeland, C. S. (1982): The prevalence and severity of pain in cancer. *Cancer,* 50:1913–1918.

34. Daut, R. L., Cleeland, C. S., and Flanery, R. C. (1983): Development of the Wisconsin Brief Pain Questionnaire to assess pain in cancer and other diseases. *Pain,* 17:197–210.
35. Descottes, B., Cubertafond, P., Catanzano, G., and Caix, M. (1979): Primary cancer of the gallbladder: report of 55 cases. *Sem. Hop. Paris,* 55:1479–1487.
36. DeVita, V. T., Hellman, S., and Rosenberg, S. A. (editors) (1982): *Cancer: Principles and Practice of Oncology.* Lippincott, Philadelphia.
37. Ertl, M. (1976): Das primare Gallenblasenkarzinom. *Chir. Prax.,* 21:609–612.
38. Foley, K. M. (1979): Pain syndromes in patients with cancer. In: *Advances in Pain Research and Therapy, Vol. 2,* edited by J. J. Bonica and V. Ventafridda, pp. 59–78. Raven Press, New York.
39. Foley, K. M. (1982): Clinical assessment of cancer pain. *Acta Anaesthesiol. Scand. (Suppl.),* 74:91–96.
40. Foley, K. M., and Rogers, A. (1981): *Management of Cancer Pain, Vol. 2, The Rational Use of Analgesics in the Management of Cancer Pain.* Hoffman-LaRoche, Nutley, New Jersey.
41. Foley, K. M., Roger, A., and Houde, R. W. (1978): Pain in patients with cancer: A quantitative reappraisal. *Proc. Am. Soc. Cancer Res.,* 19:357.
42. Front, F., Schneck, S. O., Frankel, A., and Robinson, E. (1979): Bone metastases and bone pain in breast cancer: Are they closely associated? *JAMA,* 242:1747–1748.
43. Gianasi, G. (1984): Neuroadenolysis of the pituitary gland. In: *Recent Advances in the Management of Pain—Advances in Pain Research and Therapy, Vol. 7,* edited by C. Benedetti, C. R. Chapman, and G. Moricca. Raven Press, New York.
44. Gilbert, R. W., Kim, J. H., and Posner, J. B. (1978): Epidural spinal cord compression from metastatic tumor: Diagnosis and treatment. *Ann. Neurol.,* 3:40–51.
45. Greenberg, H. S., Deck, D. F., Bikram, B., Chu, F. C. H., and Posner, J. B. (1981): Metastases to the base of the skull: clinical findings in 43 patients. *Neurology,* 31:530–537.
46. Greenwald, H. P., Francis, A., Bergner, M., Perrin, E. B., and Bonica, J. J. (1982): Incidence and natural history of pain in four cancer sites. *Proceedings: XIIIth International Cancer Congress,* Seattle, Abstract 2808.
47. Greenwald, H. P., Bonica, J. J., Chapman, C. R., et al. (1982): Team management of pain in cancer patients. *Proceedings: XIIIth International Cancer Congress,* Seattle, Abstract 2508.
48. Gullo, L., Ventrucci, M., Costa, P. L., Procaccio, L., Nestico, V., and Ripani, R. (1978): Pancreatic cancer. Etiological and clinical observations of 140 cases. *Recent Prog. Med.,* 64:90–97.
49. Haran, B. J. (1978): Facts and figures. In: *Management of Terminal Disease,* edited by C. M. Saunders, pp. 12–18. Edward Arnold, London.
50. Hinton, J. M. (1963): The physical and mental distress of the dying. *Q. J. Med.,* 32:1–21.
51. Holland, J. F., and Frei, E., III (editors) (1982): *Cancer Medicine.* Lea & Febiger, Philadelphia.
52. Horton, J., and Hill, G. J. (editors) (1977): *Clinical Oncology.* Saunders, Philadelphia.
53. International Association for the Study of Pain (1979): Pain terms: A list with definitions and notes on usage. *Pain,* 6:249–252.
54. Janig, W. (1984): Neurophysiological mechanisms of cancer pain. In: *Recent Results in Cancer Research—Pain in the Cancer Patient,* edited by M. Zimmerman, P. Drings, and G. Wagner, pp. 45–58. Springer-Verlag, Heidelberg.
55. Kaiko, R. F., Wallenstein, S. L., Rogers, A., et al. (1981): Analgesic and mood effects of heroin and morphine in cancer patients with postoperative pain. *N. Engl. J. Med.,* 304:1501–1505.
56. Kornell, J. A. (1980): Pain in advanced cancer patients. *Thesis for M.A. of Nursing,* School of Nursing, University of Washington, Seattle.
57. Kramer, A. (1960): Das gallenblasenkarzinom. *Munch. Med. Wochenschr.,* 102:2082–2087.
58. Lempinen, M. (1971): Carcinoma of the stomach. I. Diagnostic considerations. *Ann. Chir. Gynaecol.,* 60:135–140.
59. Marks, R. M., and Sachar, E. J. (1973): Undertreatment of medical inpatients with narcotic analgesics. *Ann. Int. Med.,* 78:173–181.
60. McGivney, W. T. and Crooks, G. M. (1984): Care of patients with severe chronic pain in terminal illness. *JAMA* 251:1182–1188.

61. Melzack, R., and Wall, P. D. (1982): *The Challenge of Pain.* Basic Books, New York.
62. Meyerson, B. A. (1983): Electrostimulation procedures: Effects, presumed rationale and possible mechanisms. In: *Advances in Pain Research and Therapy, Vol. 5,* edited by J. J. Bonica, U. Lindblom, and A. Iggo, pp. 495–534. Raven Press, New York.
63. Minami, T., Masuda, F., and Sasaki, T. (1975): A clinical study on renal cell carcinoma. *Jpn. J. Urol.,* 66:474–484.
64. Moricca, G. (1974): Neuroadenolysis for the antalgic treatment of advanced cancer patients. In: *Recent Advances on Pain,* edited by J. J. Bonica, P. Procacci, and C. Pagni, p. 313. Thomas, Springfield.
65. Najem, A. Z., Hennessey, M., Malfitan, R. C., Cheung, N. K., and Hobson, R. W. (1977): Colon and rectal carcinoma: clinical experience. *Am. Surg.,* 43:583–588.
66. Najerian, J. S., and Delaney, P. (editors) (1976): *Advances in Cancer Surgery,* p. 608. Stratton, New York.
67. Norton, W. S., and Lack, S. A. (1980): Control of symptoms other than pain. In: *Continuing Care of Terminal Patients: Proceedings: International Seminar on Continuing Care of Terminal Cancer Patients.* Pergamon Press, New York.
68. Olearchyk, A. S. (1978): Gastric carcinoma. A critical review of 243 cases. *Am. J. Gastroenterol.,* 70:25–45.
69. Oster, M. W., Vizel, M., and Turgeon, M. S. (1978): Pain of terminal cancer patients. *Arch. Int. Med.,* 138:1801–1802.
70. Pagni, C. A. (1984): Role of neurosurgery in cancer pain: Reevaluation of old methods and new trends. In: *Recent Advances in the Management of Pain—Advances in Pain Research and Therapy, Vol. 7,* edited by C. Benedetti, C. R. Chapman, and G. Moricca. Raven Press, New York.
71. Pannuti, E., Martoni, A., Rossi, A. P., and Piana, E. (1979): The role of endocrine therapy for relief of pain due to advanced cancer. In: *Advances in Pain Research and Therapy, Vol. 2,* edited by J. J. Bonica and V. Ventafridda, pp. 145–166. Raven Press, New York.
72. Pannuti, E., Rossi, A. P., and Marraro, D. (1980): Natural history of cancer pain. In: *Continuing Care of Terminal Patients: Proceedings: International Seminar on Continuing Care of Terminal Cancer Patients,* pp. 75–89. Pergamon Press, New York.
73. Parkes, C. M. (1978): Home or hospital? Terminal care as seen by the surviving spouse. *J. R. Coll. Gen. Pract.,* 28:19–30.
74. Paterson, R., and Aitken-Swan, J. (1954): Public opinion on cancer. A survey among women in the Manchester area. *Lancet,* II:857–861.
75. Payne, R., and Foley, K. M. (1984): Advances in the management of cancer pain. *Cancer Treat. Rep.,* 68(1):173–183.
76. Pazlow, L. K. (1982): Pharmacokinetic aspects of optimal pain treatment. *Acta Anaesthesiol. Scand. (Suppl.),* 74(26):37–43.
77. Perry, S. (1979): *The Interagency Committee on New Therapies for Pain and Discomfort: Report to the White House.* NIH-PHS, Department of Health, Education and Welfare, Washington.
78. Pheils, M. T., Barnett, J. E., Newland, R. C., and Macpherson, J. G. (1976): Colorectal carcinoma: a prospective clinicopathological study. *Med. J. Aust.,* (Suppl.)1:17–21.
79. Pollen, J. J., and Schmidt, J. D. (1979): Bone pain in metastatic cancer of the prostate. *Urology,* XIII:129–134.
80. Posner, J. B. (1977): Spinal cord metastases (including cauda equina): diagnosis and treatment. In: *Neuro-Oncology,* pp. 19–32. Department of Neurology, Memorial Sloan-Kettering Cancer Center, New York.
81. Raven, R. W. (editor) (1977): *Principles of Surgical Oncology.* Plenum Press, New York.
82. Rees, W. D. (1972): The distress of dying. *Br. Med. J.,* 2:105–108.
83. Reid, D. S. (1981): Ovarian cancer at Kent General Hospital during the years 1975–1979. *Del. Med. J.,* 53:399–400;403–405.
84. Ross, A. P., Braasch, J. W., and Warren, K. W. (1974): Carcinoma of the proximal bile ducts. *Lahey Clin. Found. Bull.,* 23:110–120.
85. Rubin, P., and Bakemeier, R. (editors) (1983): *Clinical Oncology for Medical Students and Physicians. A Multidisciplinary Approach.* 6th ed. American Cancer Society, New York.
86. Saunders, C. M. (1978): Editorial note to relief of pain. In: *The Management of Terminal Disease,* edited by C. M. Saunders, pp. 65–66. Year Book Medical Publishers, Chicago.

87. Schutte, H. E. (1979): The influence of bone pain on the results of bone scans. *Cancer,* 44:2039–2043.
88. Silverberg, E., and Lubera, J. A. (1983): Cancer statistics 1983. *CA-A Cancer J. Clin.,* 33:3–26.
89. Skeele, R. T. (editor) (1982): *Manual of Cancer Chemotherapy,* pp. 195–206. Little, Brown, Boston.
90. Spiegel, D., and Bloom, J. R. (1983): Pain in metastatic breast cancer. *Cancer,* 52:341–345.
91. Stanley, K. (1982): Analysis of cancer pain. Questionnaire data. *WHO Workshop on Cancer Pain Relief,* Milan, Italy.
92. Sullivan, K. M., Syrjala, K., Flournoy, N., Chapman, C. R., Storb, R., and Thomas, E. D. (1984): Pain following intensive chemoradiotherapy and bone marrow transplantation (BMT). *Pain,* (Suppl. 2):S215.
93. Sun, H. Y., and McLane, D. G. (1984): Pain in children with spinal cord tumors. *Child's Brain,* 11:36–46.
94. Sung, J. L., Wang, T. H., and Yu, J. Y. (1967): Clinical study on primary carcinoma of the liver in Taiwan. *Am. J. Dig. Dis.,* 12:1036–1049.
95. Takeda, F. (1984): WHO Cancer Pain Relief Program. *Pain,* (Suppl.)2:S216.
96. Trotter, J. M., Scott, R., MacBeth, F. R., McVie, J. G., and Calman, K. C. (1981): Problems of the oncology outpatients: role of the liaison health visitor. *Br. Med. J.,* 282:122–124.
97. Turnbull, F. (1979): The nature of pain that may accompany cancer of the lung. *Pain,* 7:371–375.
98. Twycross, R. G. (1974): Clinical experience with diamorphine in advanced malignant disease. *Int. J. Clin. Pharmacol. Ther. Toxicol.,* 9:184–198.
99. Twycross, R. G., and Fairfield, S. (1982): Pain in far-advanced cancer. *Pain,* 14:303–310.
100. Twycross, R. G., and Lack, S. A. (1983): *Symptom Control in Far Advanced Cancer: Pain Relief.* Pitman, London.
101. Twycross, R. G., and Ventafridda, V. (1980): *The Continuing Care of Terminal Cancer Patients.* Pergamon Press, New York.
102. Ventafridda, V., and Gallucci, C. (1985): Management of cancer of the lung. *Pain (submitted).*
103. Weingarten, L. A., Gelb, A. M., and Fischer, M. (1978): Pancreatic carcinoma: a clinical review and schema for evaluating patients. *Gastroenterology,* 74:1110 (abstract).
104. Weiss, L., and Gilbert, H. A. (editors) (1981): *Bone Metastases.* Hall, Boston.
105. Wilkes, F. (1974): Some problems in cancer management. *Proc. R. Soc. Med.,* 67:23–27.
106. Woodforde, J. M., and Fielding, J. R. (1975): Pain and cancer. In: *Pain, Clinical and Experimental Perspectives,* edited by M. Weisenberg, pp. 332–336. Mosby, St. Louis.
107. Zimmerman, M., Drings, P., and Wagner, G. (editors) (1984): *Recent Results in Cancer Research—Pain in the Cancer Patient.* Springer-Verlag, Heidelberg.

Advances in Pain Research and Therapy, Vol. 9, edited by H. L. Fields et al. Raven Press, New York © 1985.

Comprehensive Treatment in Cancer Pain

V. Ventafridda, M. Tamburini, and F. De Conno

Division of Pain Therapy, Istituto Nazionale per lo Studio e la Cura dei Tumori, 20133 Milan, Italy

The chronic painful experience of cancer reveals itself in the integration of emotional and physical factors (28). This broad concept of pain (physical, psychological, social, and spiritual) lends itself to a comprehensive approach to treatment and care (23).

To be effective, pain treatment must be based on three closely linked operations: (a) pain assessment; (b) therapeutic strategy; and (c) continuing care.

PAIN ASSESSMENT

The evaluation of pain involves the comparison of diagnostic information about the physical cause of pain (e.g., from the neurological examinations, CT scan, X-ray, scintigraphic studies, magnetic resonance imaging, blood chemistry, chemo-radio-hormone sensitivity, etc.) with factors influencing the quality of life of the patient [e.g., the intensity and duration of pain, sleeping hours, Performance Status (Karnofsky), treatment side-effects, etc. (16)]. This comparison should be assessed at every meeting with the patient in order to select the analgesic treatments that offer the maximum effect with the least possible harm. The maintenance of relatively normal activity and psychosocial communication must have priority over the control of pain.

THERAPEUTIC STRATEGY

The therapeutic strategy includes both an immediate attack on pain and continuous control of it. In order to perform this strategy the choice of treatment is based on the concept of a progressive utilization of a sequential pattern starting with the least disabling and traumatic technique.

The primary approach is represented by the use of an oncologic therapy and of nonneurolytic means, mainly represented by analgesic drugs (Fig. 1). As far as specific oncologic treatments, one must consider not only their efficacy with regard to the different histological types of cancer, but also their

PRIMARY THERAPY

PALL. RADIOTHERAPY
PALL. CHEMOTHERAPY
NSAID
ADJUVANT DRUGS
WEAK NARCOTICS
PALL. SURGERY
PERIDURAL BLOCKS
NURSING
PHYSIOTHERAPY

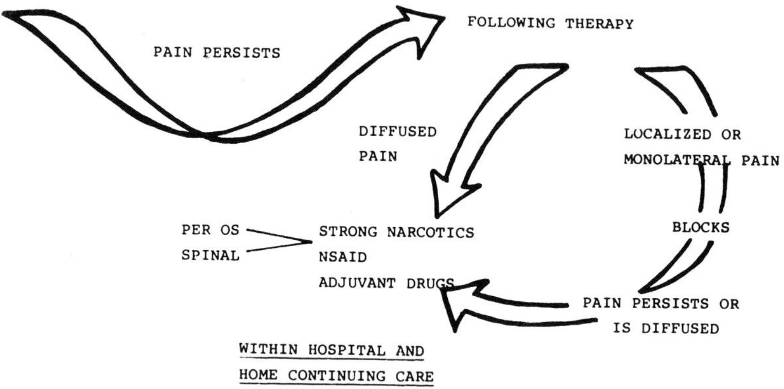

FIG. 1. Therapeutic strategy in cancer pain.

palliative use. For example, radiotherapy can give pain relief ranging from 35 to 95%, according to published literature (1,2,8,10,13,17,26,30,31) (Table 1).

To investigate oncologic alternatives in cancer pain, we processed the medical records of 3,480 patients with pain due to advanced cancer attending the Pain Clinic of the National Cancer Institute in Milan. Forty-one per-

TABLE 1. *Cancer pain treatment by radiotherapy: Survey of literature data (1974–1984)*

Cancer site [Author (ref.)]	No. of patients	% Pain relief	Type of radiotherapy
Pancoast [Hilaris et al. (13), Deeley (8)]	146	69–80	Interstitial, external
Bone metastases [Germatis et al. (10), Benson et al. (1), Bolund (2), Tong et al. (30), Trodella et al. (31)]	1,309	54–90	External
All types [Schlegel (26), Kuttig (17)]	1,200	37.5–75	External, percutaneous

TABLE 2. *Previous history of chronic cancer pain and related effective treatment*[a]

Treatment	Total–partial relief No. patients (%)
Chemotherapy	142 (10)
Radiotherapy	584 (41)
Chemotherapy + radiotherapy	256 (18)
Surgery	85 (6)
Others	185 (13)
Unrelieved[b]	171 (12)

[a]Survey on 3,480 cases. Pain histories reported: 1,423 patients (41%).
[b]Mostly iatrogenic or deafferentation pain.

cent (i.e., 1,423) had a history of chronic pain lasting more than 2 weeks. Seventy-five percent of these patients asserted that their pain was partially or totally controlled by anticancer treatments. In 13%, pain was controlled by other treatments (analgesic drugs and physiotherapy), while in the remainder the pain persisted mostly in those affected by iatrogenic or deafferentation pain (Table 2).

Analgesic drugs should be titrated to the patient and administered according to particular modalities (20,32) following a three-step procedure which goes from nonnarcotic drugs to weak narcotics and lastly to strong narcotics combined, if necessary, with adjuvant drugs such as steroids, psychotropics, and anticonvulsants (Fig. 2).

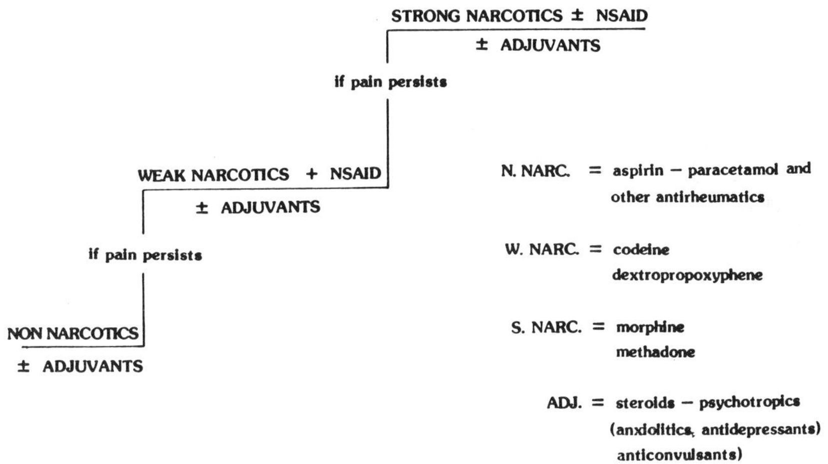

FIG. 2. Analgesic ladder in cancer pain.

In the primary approach, corresponding to the first and second step of the procedure, one has to consider also physiotherapeutic and orthopedic measures, bracing, transcutaneous electrical nerve stimulation (TENS), repeated infiltration or trigger points, or epidurals with local anesthetics or steroids. If pain remains intractable at this stage, with the exception of cases due to iatrogenic syndromes, it is sensible to assume that there is a limited survival time.

Pain persistence determines use of the secondary approach which takes into account two possibilities. Either there is widespread pain due to disseminated metastasis or localized pain in a well-defined area incident to motion. In the first instance, the use of opioids, orally or parenterally and spinally administered, may be considered within the context of a continuous and monitored care. In the second case, neurolytic blocks of pain pathways may be used. If pain still persists, the opioids should be combined with the remaining antalgic effect of the neurolytic blocks. The value of narcotics (if well-tolerated and effective) can be extended by considering neurolytic blocks only as a supplementary approach to the above-mentioned treatments. The control of other symptoms such as weakness, nausea, vomiting, decubitus, ulcers, bladder or oral cavity problems, etc., must be considered within this strategy.

Considerations of Neurolesive Blocks

The neurolesive block is an important tool in cancer pain. To be effective the main requirements are:

1. It must be highly selective for the sensitive pathways.
2. It must not create new functional deficits beyond the already existing ones.
3. It must not be carried out on a preexisting block.
4. It must not be painful.
5. Overall, it must be accepted by the patient.

The great majority of papers dealing with neurolytic techniques show inappropriate follow-up; thus it is difficult to evaluate the efficacy of these treatments. In a survey of 76 major papers on neurolytic blocks published between 1979 and 1983 we observed a lack of follow-up on pain relief regarding its modality and complications in more than 60% of the papers. Furthermore, data on the life activity of the patients and control groups are almost never reported (25).

The percutaneous, chemical, and thermal neurolesions are the most widely used in oncologic routine because they fit the previously mentioned requirements (3,4). In our practice, after a proper titration of analgesics according to the strategy outlined, the need to resort to these techniques has decreased by 80% in the last years and it is now indicated in only about 20% of cases.

Before adopting these techniques it is necessary to consider the cost/benefit ratios as well as ethical factors. In fact, these patients have already undergone many frustrating treatments. Misleading or unreliable information about the duration of the analgesic effect and the possible reduction of performance status would not be ethically acceptable. In considering neurolytic techniques one can see that the indication for their use is limited to well defined clinical situations. Neurolytic blocks, being nonselective on sensitive fibers, may induce motor and other functional impairments and their duration is unpredictable (5,9,34). The main indications are some types of perineal pain with subarachnoid block at L5–S1 (35) and celiac ganglion alcohol block in pancreatic, gastric, hepatic, and renal pains acting on the celiac axis (21).

As far as chemical hypophysectomy is concerned, the antalgic results in case of diffused pain are widely reported in the literature, but the mechanism of action is unknown. Furthermore, the technique of execution and indications are debated and incident pain is not controlled. Our personal experience in 2 groups of patients has shown that treatment with analgesic drugs titrated to patient requirements compares favorably with chemical hypophysectomy in prolonged control of pain (14).

Radiofrequency percutaneous neurolesions are selective and their efficacy in the affected area lasts for a long period. But, unfortunately, the spread of cancer is unpredictable and pain often recurs with violence in the surrounding or contralateral areas.

Thermorhizotomy of the 5th nerve often requires an integration with analgesic drugs because other nerve roots are involved (27).

Percutaneous cordotomy, which is the most useful technique for selectivity, efficacy, and duration, is not free of complications even when correctly performed. It may have painful sequelae and is limited when bilateral lesions are required (15,18,36).

Finally, it is necessary to consider the wide use of chronic administration of opioids by the spinal route. The very encouraging results reported in the literature are counterbalanced by frequent reports of side-effects (12); therefore, this technique requires a careful follow-up. Even though possible tolerance, as in the case of oral administration, should not be considered an impediment, there is, nevertheless, the problem of a foreign body which may be psychologically difficult for patients to accept. Moreover, incident pain is not controlled, thus requiring integration with oral administration of opioids or the use of blocks (11). The chronic infusion by pump or reservoir at spinal or supraspinal levels (6) shows that this technique, although being a valid tool, requires further improvement. Therefore, the chronic use of opioids by spinal route must only be considered as an alternative to oral administration when the latter is not possible or no longer effective.

Clinical Evaluation of the Multimodal Approach

To better understand the actual role of the above-mentioned neurolytic techniques, 2 groups of 100 patients were monitored for over 3 months. The subjects were of both sexes (107 males, 93 females), age ranging from 18 to 87 years, with intractable pain due to the advanced stage of the cancer and not responsive to specific anticancer and symptomatic surgical and X-ray treatments. The first group has been treated by means of the sequential pharmacologic ladder, while the second group, with unilateral pain, was treated with the multimodal approach according to the therapeutic strategy in which the pharmacologic treatment was followed by the use of neurolytic blocks or chronic spinal administration of opioids. In order to gather the second group of patients, it was necessary to consider 218 subjects. One hundred and eighteen of these (45%), after the primary approach, did not require a neurolesive procedure. Patients having blocks were further monitored for 12 weeks from the time of the procedure.

Frequency distribution of the primary pathology showed an incidence of colon-rectum tumors (22.5%), followed by cancer of the breast (20.5%), lung (19%), and head and neck (13.5%). The parameters considered were: (a) primary pathology; (b) sleeping hours; (c) performance status; (d) number, sequence, and duration of analgesic treatment; and (e) pain intensity and duration, expressed by means of an Integrated Score (IS) (37).

The IS is obtained by multiplying the number of hours with pain, which the patient indicates daily on a weekly form, using five key words for the corresponding values of score (mild = 1.0, ... killing = 10.0), and then adding together the partial scores. The IS ranges from 0 to 240, but usually doesn't exceed 100. During a 3-month period 200 patients received a total of 1,530 controls at the Pain Clinic and 2,000 at home (mean 7.6 ± 0.2 SE) with a range of 5 to 17 controls. In this period, information concerning 2,400 values of IS, 800 data on sleeping hours, and 800 on performance status were collected. Statistical analysis was made utilizing Student's *t*-test. All these data were collected daily on a weekly form filled in by the patient at home and reported to the Pain Clinic by the relatives or by the nurse-clinician for those patients receiving Continuing Home Care (22).

Results

If we consider the relief obtained by both groups of patients, at the end of the first week of treatment pain is already reduced by approximately one-half of the baseline values (Fig. 3). Furthermore, pain tends to continue to decrease progressively during the following controls and, in spite of the evolution of the disease, after 12 weeks from the first visit, an average score of approximately one-fifth of the initial value is reached. Patients treated with

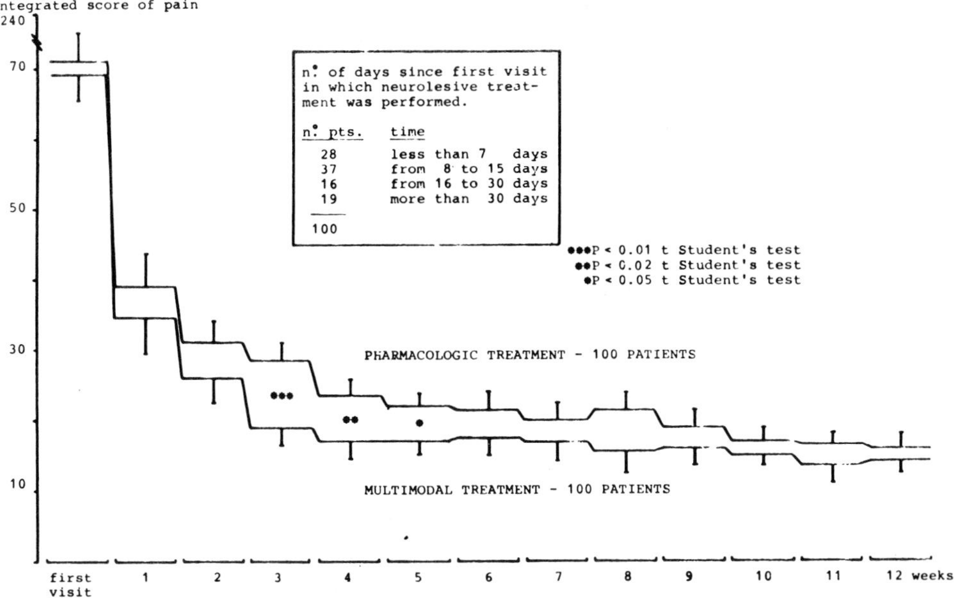

FIG. 3. Analgesic result obtained on 200 patients with advanced cancer pain by means of a sequential pharmacologic ladder compared with multimodal treatment.

neurolytic procedures combined with the pharmacologic ones show a statistically significant and quicker pain relief than those treated with drugs alone, during the first weeks of treatment.

The mean daily sleeping hours increase from the initial 5.30 hours to 8 or more at the fourth, eighth, and twelfth weeks. There is no statistically significant difference between the group treated with drug alone and that treated with the combined techniques. There is a slow reduction of performance status in the course of time. At the first visit about 7% of patients were bedridden and unable to take care of themselves. At the last visit this percentage was slightly more than 20%. In this case also, there are no significant differences between the 2 groups.

A pain-free condition without the need for other analgesic treatment still existed after 3 months in 29% of patients treated with spinal infusions of opioids, in 25% with celiac ganglion alcoholization, in 24% with percutaneous cordotomy, in 12% with chemical rhizotomy, and in 7% with Gasserian thermorhizotomy (Fig. 4). These prospective studies are similar to the retrospective one we carried out on 150 patients and presented at the Seattle World Congress on Cancer in 1982 (38).

All these studies suggest the following: The proper use of analgesic drugs represents the primary therapy. The opium-based drugs represent the most important means. Neurolytic blocks should be thought of only as a supple-

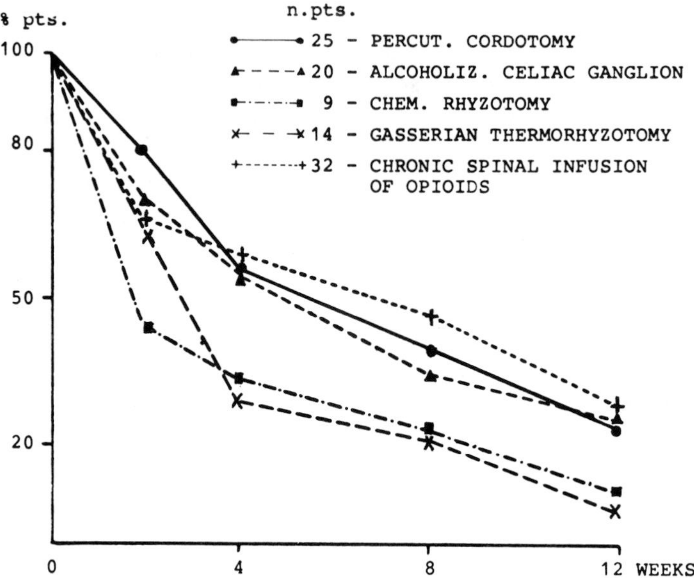

FIG. 4. Duration of pain-free state after neurolytic blocks in 100 patients with advanced cancer pain.

mentary approach. These techniques provide an important respite to pain, but are limited in time. Their indication is specific for pain due to compression of large fibers incident to motion, which can hardly be relieved even by large doses of narcotics. Their primary effect is to reduce the need of analgesics. This was demonstrated in our previous study on cordotomy in Pancoast tumor (7).

CONTINUING CARE

Continuing care is one of the most important factors in cancer pain treatment. The rationale is to offer support to patients who experience the loss of physical, psychologic, and social function, especially when bedridden. In order to be effective, a close monitoring of conditions in the hospital ward or at home is necessary. A positive modification of these conditions is obtained with the help of the medical and nursing staff, and of the relatives and volunteers adequately trained to collect data and to treat the patient. Overall, everyone must be highly motivated in the work. The patient should be aware that pain can always be controlled and that there will always be someone near him until the last day of his life. In order to treat cancer pain optimally, home care resources should be available. The recent introduction of Hospices, Palliative Care Units, and Home Care Service contributes positively to control of pain in terminal cancer patients and represents an important turning point in health policy in cancer (24,33,39).

As Melzack reported, the efficacy of treatments is significantly higher when the socioenvironmental situations are positively modified (19). This has been confirmed in a retrospective study that we carried out on 200 patients followed for 12 weeks. The study compares patients for whom Home Care Service was available to the rest who had no professional home care for whom relatives reported periodically at the Pain Clinic with the weekly chart (Fig. 5). Starting from the eighth week, a significant reduction of pain was observed in the 55 patients on Home Care (21 were on Home Care for less than 15 days). In the last 2 weeks, the difference becomes even bigger and statistically significant ($p < 0.05$). Within this survey, quality of life (according to Spitzer index) (29) and other psychosocial variables have been examined through a questionnaire administered by the visiting nurse in 2 groups of 10 and 15 patients at the first visit (t_0) and at the second- and sixth-week controls (Fig. 6). The mood, anxiety, and sense of weakness were improved significantly more in the patients who received continuing Home Care.

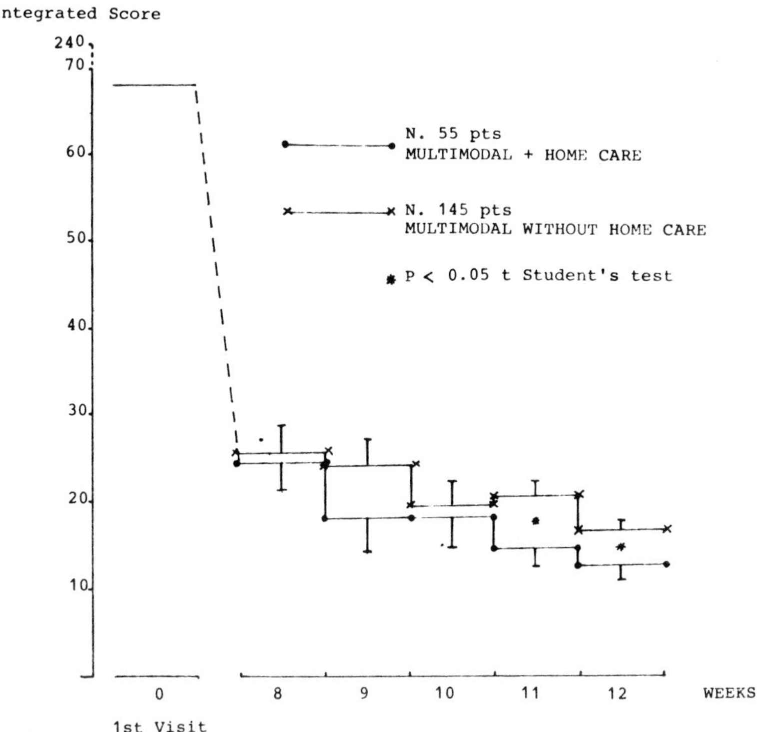

FIG. 5. Analgesic results obtained during the third month of treatment on 200 patients, of whom 55 were able to benefit from Home Care Service.

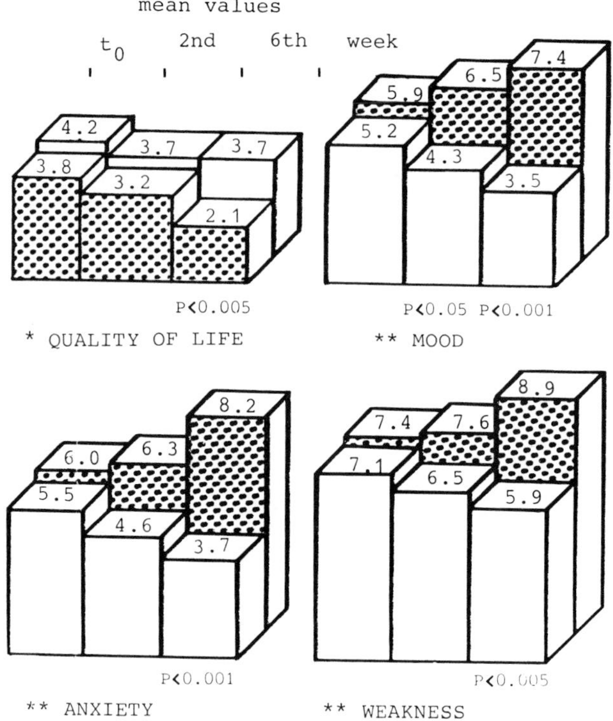

FIG. 6. Quality of life (Spitzer) and other psychosocial parameters in 25 terminal cancer patients. *White bars,* 15 patients with home care; *dotted bars,* 10 patients without home care; *, the higher the score the better it is; **, the higher the score the worse it is.

CONCLUSIONS

If we want to effectively control the suffering of cancer patients it is important to conduct research on new long-lasting analgesic procedures or improve the existing ones. In the meantime, education in the proper administration of analgesic drugs, especially opioids, is essential. These drugs are still underused in developed countries and unavailable in many developing countries. But, above all, it is necessary to evaluate and apply these types of care which are able to preserve the patient's dignity until the last day of life.

ACKNOWLEDGMENTS

This work was supported by grant 83.02874.56 from the Consiglio Nazionale delle Ricerche, Rome. The authors are grateful to the Floriani Foundation for the assistance in preparing the manuscript.

REFERENCES

1. Benson, R. C., Jr., Hesan, S. H., Jones, A. G., and Schlise, S. (1982): External beam radiotherapy for palliation of pain from metastatic carcinoma of the prostate. *J. Urol.,* 127:69–71.
2. Bolund, C. (1982): Pain relief through radiotherapy and chemotherapy. *Acta Anesth. Scand. (Suppl.),* 74:114–116.
3. Bonica, J. J. (1953): *The Management of Pain.* Lea & Febiger, Philadelphia.
4. Bonica, J. J. (1978): Cancer pain. A major national health problem. *Cancer Nurs. J.,* 4:313–316.
5. Clarke, I. M. C. (1984): Nerve blocks. In: *Clinics in Oncology, Vol. 3,* edited by R. G. Twycross, pp. 181–193. Saunders, London.
6. Coombes, D. W., Saunders, R. L., and Pageau M. G. (1982): Continuous intraspinal narcotic analgesia. *Reg. Anesth.,* 7:110–113.
7. De Conno, F., Sganzerla, E., and Ventafridda, V. (1982): Analgesic drugs. In: *Advances in Pain Research and Therapy, Vol. 4,* edited by J. J. Bonica, C. A. Pagni, and V. Ventafridda, pp. 125–132. Raven Press, New York.
8. Deeley, T. J. (1982): Radiation therapy. In: *Advances in Pain Research and Therapy, Vol. 4,* edited by J. J. Bonica, C. A. Pagni, and V. Ventafridda, pp. 87–100. Raven Press, New York.
9. Drechsel, U. (1984): Treatment of cancer pain with neurolytic agents. In: *Recent Results in Cancer Research, Vol. 89,* edited by M. Zimmermann, P. Drings, and G. Wagner, pp. 137–147. Springer-Verlag, Berlin.
10. Garmatis, C. J., and Chu, F. C. H. (1978): The effectiveness of radiotherapy in the treatment of bone metastases from breast cancer. *Radiology,* 126:235–237.
11. Greenberg, H. S., Taren, J., Ensminger, W. D., and Doan, K. (1982): Benefit from and tolerance to continuous intrathecal infusion of morphine for intractable cancer pain. *J. Neurosurg.,* 57:360–364.
12. Gustafson, L. L., Schildt, B., and Jacobsen, K. (1982): Adverse effects of extradural and intrathecal opiates: report of a nation-wide survey in Sweden. *Br. J. Anesth.,* 54:479–485.
13. Hilaris, B. S., Luomanen, R. K., Malian, G. D., and Heuscke, U. K. (1971): Interstitial irradiation of apical lung cancer. *Radiology,* 99(3):655–660.
14. Ischia, S., Lipton, S., and Maffezzoli, G. F. (editors) (1983): *Pain Treatment: Pituitary Neuroadenolysis in the Treatment of Cancer Pain and Hormone-Dependent Tumors.* Cortina International, Verona.
15. Ischia, S., Luzzani, A., Ischia, A., and Maffezzoli, G. F. (1984): Bilateral percutaneous cervical cordotomy: immediate and long-term results in 36 patients with neoplastic disease. *J. Neurol. Neurosurg. Psychiatry,* 47:141–147.
16. Karnofsky, D. A., and Burchenal, J. H. (1949): The clinical evaluation of chemotherapeutic agents in cancer. In: *Evaluation of Chemotherapeutic Agents,* edited by C. M. McLeod, pp. 191–205. Columbia University Press, New York.
17. Kuttig, H. (1984): Radiotherapy of cancer pain. In: *Recent Results in Cancer Research, Vol. 89,* edited by M. Zimmermann, P. Drings, and G. Wagner, pp. 190–194. Springer-Verlag, Berlin.
18. Lipton, S. (1979): Percutaneous cervical cordotomy. In: *Advances in Pain Research and Therapy, Vol. 2,* edited by J. J. Bonica and V. Ventafridda, pp. 425–437. Raven Press, New York.
19. Melzack, R., Ofiesh, J. G., and Mount, B. M. (1978): The Brompton mixture: effects on pain in cancer patients. In: *Psychosocial Care of the Dying Patient,* edited by C. A. Garfield, pp. 386–403. McGraw-Hill, San Francisco.
20. Moertel, C. G. (1980): Treatment of cancer pain with orally administered medications. *JAMA,* 244(21):2448–2450.
21. Moore, D. C. (1979): Celiac plexus block with alcohol for cancer pain of the upper intra-abdominal viscera. In: *Advances in Pain Research and Therapy, Vol. 2,* edited by J. J. Bonica and V. Ventafridda, pp. 357–371. Raven Press, New York.
22. Pozzi, G., Tamburini, M., Corsta, R., and Ventafridda, V. (1979): Costruzione di una cartella di autodescrizione giornaliera del dolore e di parametri di attività di vita. In: *Il Dolore:*

Problemi di Fisiopatologia e Terapia, edited by C. A. Pagni, P. Procacci, and V. Ventafridda, pp. 161–175. Edizioni Libreria Cortina, Verona.
23. Saunders, C. M. (1978): The philosophy of terminal care. In: *The Management of Terminal Disease,* edited by C. M. Saunders, pp. 193–202. Arnold, London.
24. Saunders, C. M. (editor) (1978): *The Management of Terminal Disease.* Arnold, London.
25. Sbanotto, A. (1984): Revisione critica dei risultati antalgici delle tecniche neurolesive. *Thesis,* University of Milan.
26. Schlegel, G. (1982): Die therapie del tumorschmerzes. *Tumordiagnostik,* 3:10–16.
27. Siegfried, J., and Broggi, G. (1979): Percutaneous thermocoagulation of the Gasserian ganglion in the treatment of pain in advanced cancer. In: *Advances in Pain Research and Therapy, Vol. 2,* edited by J. J. Bonica and V. Ventafridda, pp. 463–468. Raven Press, New York.
28. Spiegel, D., and Bloom, J. R. (1983): Pain in metastatic breast cancer. *Cancer,* 52:341–345.
29. Spitzer, W. O., Dobson, A. J., Hall, J., Chesterman, E., Lady, J., Shefferd, R., Battista, R. N., and Catchlove, B. R. (1981): Measuring the quality of life of cancer patients: a concise Q.L. index for use by physicians. *J. Chronic Dis.,* 34(12):585–597.
30. Tong, D., Gillick, L., and Handrickson, F. R. (1982): The palliation of symptomatic osseous metastases: final results of the study of the Radiation Therapy Oncology Group. *Cancer,* 50:839–899.
31. Trodella, L., Ausili-Cefaro, G., Turriziani, A., Marmiroli, N., Cellini, N., and Nardone, L. (1984): Pain in osseous metastases: results of radiotherapy. *Pain,* 18(4):387–396.
32. Twycross, R. G., and Lack, S. A. (editors) (1983): *Symptom Control in Far Advanced Cancer: Pain Relief.* Pitman, London.
33. Twycross, R. G., and Ventafridda, V. (editors) (1980): *The Continuing Care of Terminal Cancer Patients.* Pergamon Press, London.
34. Ventafridda, V., and Martino, G. (1976): Clinical evaluation of subarachnoid neurolytic blocks in intractable cancer pain. In: *Advances in Pain Research and Therapy, Vol. 1,* edited by J. J. Bonica and D. Albe-Fessard, pp. 699–703. Raven Press, New York.
35. Ventafridda, V., Fochi, C., Sganzerla, E., and Tamburini M. (1979): Neurolytic blocks in perineal pain. In: *Advances in Pain Research and Therapy, Vol. 2,* edited by J. J. Bonica and V. Ventafridda, pp. 597–605. Raven Press, New York.
36. Ventafridda, V., De Conno, F., and Fochi, C. (1982): Cervical percutaneous cordotomy. In: *Advances in Pain Research and Therapy, Vol. 4,* edited by J. J. Bonica, V. Ventafridda, and C. A. Pagni, pp. 185–198. Raven Press, New York.
37. Ventafridda, V., De Conno, F., Di Trapani, P., Gallico, S., Guarise, G., Rigamonti, G., and Tamburini, M. (1983): A new method of pain quantification based on a weekly self-descriptive record of the intensity and duration of pain. In: *Advances in Pain Research and Therapy, Vol. 5,* edited by J. J. Bonica, U. Lindblom, and A. Iggo, pp. 891–895. Raven Press, New York.
38. Ventafridda, V., De Conno, F., Tamburini, M., and Pietroiusti, E. (1983): Multimodal approach in management of cancer pain. In: *13th International Cancer Congress, Part D, Research and Treatment* (Progress in Clinical and Biological Research, Vol. 132D), edited by E. A. Mirand, W. B. Hutchinson, and E. Mihich, pp. 17–25. Liss, New York.
39. Zimmermann, J. M. (1981): *Hospice. Complete Care for the Terminally Ill.* Urban & Schwarzenberg, Baltimore.

Advances in Pain Research and Therapy, Vol. 9, edited by H. L. Fields et al. Raven Press, New York © 1985.

Pharmacologic Approaches to Cancer Pain Management

Kathleen M. Foley

Departments of Neurology and Pharmacology, Cornell University Medical College; and Pain Service, Department of Neurology, Memorial Sloan-Kettering Cancer Center, New York, New York 10021

Advances in the diagnosis and treatment of cancer, coupled with advances in pain research and therapy, have improved the quality of care for patients with pain of malignant origin (71). Specialized methods of cancer diagnosis and treatment provide the most direct approach to treating cancer pain by treating the cause of the pain. Advances in cancer pain therapy have allowed for adequate pain control by more effective use of standard drug therapy (non-narcotic, narcotic, and adjuvant analgesic drugs), development of new drugs, use of novel methods and routes of drug administration, use of selective anesthetic and neurosurgical approaches, and integration of cognitive and behavioral approaches to pain control. Application of these therapeutic approaches to cancer patients has offered the unique opportunity to use clinical observations to advance biologic knowledge. Several controversies have developed as each of these approaches has been applied and scrutinized. This chapter will briefly summarize the pharmacologic approaches to cancer pain and address the important controversies (Table 1).

Drug therapy represents the mainstay of treatment for patients with cancer. The choice of the specific drug approach must be based on (a) a full assessment of the type of pain (acute versus chronic), (b) an understanding of the kind of patient with pain, (c) a definition of the specific pain syndrome and its neurophysiologic basis, and (d) an understanding of the clinical pharmacology of the drugs prescribed. Before detailing the pharmacologic approaches to cancer pain, we shall briefly review these components.

In a full assessment of a cancer patient with pain there are certain general principles that should be followed. Lack of attention to these principles (Table 2) is the major cause of misdiagnosis of a specific pain syndrome and inappropriate or inadequate cancer pain management (33).

Equally important, the type of pain and type of patient with pain need to be identified. Cancer patients have both acute pain and chronic pain. This

TABLE 1. *Controversies in cancer pain management*

Choice of the opiate analgesic
Method of drug administration
Route of drug administration
Development of tolerance
Risk of substance abuse and addiction

classification is based on increased understanding of pain mechanisms and recognition that central modulations for acute pain and chronic pain may be different. In the clinical setting, the approaches to management of patients and their responses to treatment are often quite different for the different types of pain. Acute pain is relatively easy to recognize and is more amenable to many of the therapeutic approaches available. In patients with chronic pain, the persistent pain usually has failed to respond to those modalities directed at the cause of the pain. In these patients, pain usually has led to significant changes in personality, life style, and functional ability. Such patients need a treatment approach that encompasses not only treatment of the cause of pain but also treatment of the complications that have arisen in the patient's functional status, social life, and personality. The role of the drug therapy approach is most controversial in this group. In prescribing pharmacologic therapy, evaluation of the psychological impact of pain, coupled with a classification of the patient with pain, provides the best approach to delineating treatment. Five general types of cancer pain patients have been described (Table 3) (34).

Drug therapy plays a major role in management for each of these groups, but there are considerable variations relating to such factors as selection of pharmacologic agents, their administration, and their risk–benefit ratios. Identification of these different types of cancer pain patients is also crucial to gain perspective on the controversies in drug therapy. The risk–benefit ratios for drug use are quite different for patients with acute cancer pain, for

TABLE 2. *General principles*

Believe the patient's complaint
Take a careful history of the pain complaint
Assess the psychosocial status of the patient
Perform a careful medical and neurologic examination
Order and personally review the appropriate diagnostic procedures
Evaluate the patient's extent of disease
Treat the pain to facilitate the diagnostic workup
Consider alternative methods of pain control during the initial evaluation
Reassess the pain complaint during the prescribed therapy

Adapted from Foley (34).

TABLE 3. *Types of patients with cancer pain*

Patients with acute cancer-related pain
Acute pain associated with the diagnosis of cancer
Acute pain associated with cancer therapy, including surgery, chemotherapy, and radiation therapy
Patients with chronic cancer-related pain
Chronic pain associated with cancer progression
Chronic pain associated with cancer therapy, including surgery, chemotherapy, and radiation therapy
Patients with preexisting chronic pain and cancer-related pain
Patients with a history of drug addiction with cancer-related pain
Actively involved in illicit drug use
In a methadone maintenance program
With a past history of drug abuse
Dying patients with cancer-related pain

Adapted from Foley (35).

cancer patients with chronic therapy-related pain without evidence of disease, and for dying patients.

Equally important is the appropriate diagnosis of the specific pain syndrome (31) and differentiation of the underlying mechanism of pain—somatic, visceral, or deafferentation (8,91). Cancer is often associated with several types of pain simultaneously. Both somatic and visceral pain respond to analgesic drug therapy, specifically the non-narcotics and narcotics. Deafferentation pain responds less well to these drugs, whereas the adjuvant drugs are often very useful, pointing up the fact that the choice of the pharmacologic approach must be geared to the specific pain syndrome and its underlying mechanism.

The analgesic drugs commonly used can be divided into three major groups. Group I includes aspirin and the nonsteroidal anti-inflammatory drugs (NSAID), which are believed to act peripherally and to produce analgesia through their ability to inhibit prostaglandin synthesis. Group II includes the narcotic agonists and antagonists, which act both peripherally and centrally by binding to discrete opiate receptors, activating an endogenous pain-suppression system. Group III includes the adjuvant analgesic drugs, such as amitriptyline; they act centrally to produce analgesia in certain pain states through endogenous analgesic systems not fully understood. The knowledge to use these analgesic drugs effectively should be part of every physician's armamentarium in managing patients with cancer pain.

GROUP I: NON-NARCOTIC ANALGESICS

The non-narcotic analgesics are the drugs of choice for mild to moderate pain (4,42,59). The mechanisms of action of their analgesic effects are controversial, but it is believed that they reduce or prevent sensitization of pain

receptors to nociceptive stimuli by preventing or inhibiting prostaglandin synthesis. This class of drugs consists of a heterogeneous group of substances differing in chemical structures and pharmacologic actions. Many of these drugs have analgesic, anti-inflammatory, and antipyretic properties. All of the drugs in this class have analgesic potencies comparable to that of aspirin. However, the analgesic effects of these drugs do have a ceiling: Increasing their dosages beyond certain levels does not produce additive analgesia. The non-narcotic analgesics, when combined with the narcotic analgesics, will produce additive analgesia (30,49). There is experimental evidence to suggest that these drugs may play a special role in pain management for patients with bone metastases (10) because of the documented role of prostaglandins in bone resorption in metastatic bone disease. Aspirin has been shown to have an antitumor effect in an animal bone tumor model (41).
shown to have an antitumor effect in an animal bone tumor model (41).

In clinical practice, this class of drugs represents the primary approach to management of cancer pain, but the choices of non-narcotics and their administration must be individualized. Each patient should be given an adequate trial of one non-narcotic analgesic before switching to an alternative one. Such a trial should include administration of the drug to maximal levels, at regular intervals. Gastrointestinal and hematological side effects often limit their chronic use. These drugs represent the first step in the analgesic ladder advised by the World Health Organization for management of cancer pain. When patients are unable to tolerate the non-narcotic analgesics or have moderate to severe pain that is not controlled by these drugs, which are predominantly for mild to moderate pain, then narcotic analgesics should be used.

GROUP II: NARCOTIC ANALGESICS

The narcotic analgesics, of which morphine is the prototype, vary in potency, efficacy, and adverse effects. These drugs produce their analgesic effects by binding to discrete opiate receptors in the nervous system. This group includes a series of heterogeneous substances with varying chemical structures. In contrast to the non-narcotic analgesics, the narcotic analgesics do not appear to have a ceiling effect; i.e., as the dose is escalated on a log scale, the analgesia increment is linear to the point of loss of consciousness. Effective use of the narcotic analgesics requires balancing the desired effect of pain relief against the undesirable side effects of nausea, vomiting, mental clouding, sedation, constipation, tolerance, and physical dependence. These undesirable effects impose a practical limit on the dosage that can be given to a particular patient. Much of the difficulty encountered in clinical use of these drugs arises from individual variations in responses to a given drug and dosage. This difficulty is compounded by a lack of pharmacologic and pharmacokinetic data on many of the narcotic analgesics. This lack of information on the clinical pharmacology of these drugs and a series of uncontrolled survey-type studies have led to several controversies in drug management of cancer pain. However, there is sufficient pharmacologic information and clinical experience to provide a general outline for practical use of narcotic drugs. Several reviews of oral and parenteral analgesics in the management of cancer pain have suggested guidelines for the use of these drugs (6,32,35,36,38,50,52,64,86,99,100). Table 4 lists those narcotic analgesics that are commonly administered by the oral route for mild to moderate pain. Table 5 lists the properties of the narcotic analgesics commonly used for severe pain. These tables serve as a useful reference point, but individualization of treatment is the rule for management of patients with pain, rather than the exception. Guidelines for rational use of narcotic analgesics are listed in Table 6.

TABLE 4. *Oral non-narcotic and narcotic analgesics for mild to moderate pain*

Drug	Route	Equianalgesic dose (mg)[a]	Duration (hr)	Plasma half-life (hr)	Comments
Aspirin	p.o.	650	4–6	3–5	Standard for non-narcotic comparison; GI and hematologic effects limit use in cancer patients
Acetaminophen	p.o.	650	4–6	1–4	Weak anti-inflammatory effects; safer than aspirin
Propoxyphene	p.o.	65[b]	4–6	12	Biotransformed to potentially toxic metabolite norpropoxyphene; used in combination with non-narcotic analgesics
Codeine	p.o.	32[b]	4–6	3	Biotransformed to morphine; available in combinations with non-narcotic analgesics
Meperidine	p.o.	50	4–6	3–4	Biotransformed to active toxic metabolite normeperidine; associated with myoclonus and seizures
Pentazocine	p.o.	30	4–6	2–3	Psychotomimetic effects with escalation of dosage; available only in combinations with naloxone, aspirin, or acetaminophen in United States

[a]Relative potencies of drugs compared with aspirin for mild to moderate pain.
[b]Some investigators have reported double the stated dose (130 mg and 60 mg) as effective in patients with mild to moderate pain.
Adapted from Foley (35).

TABLE 5. *Oral and parenteral narcotic analgesics for severe pain*

Drug	Route	Equianalgesic dose[a]	Duration (hr)	Plasma half-life (hr)	Comments
Narcotic agonists					
Morphine	i.m. p.o.	10 60	4–6 4–7	2–3.5	Standard for comparison; also available in slow-release tablets
Codeine	i.m. p.o.	130 200[b]	4–6 4–6	3	Biotransformed to morphine; useful as initial narcotic analgesic
Oxycodone	i.m. p.o.	15 30	 3–5	—	Short-acting; available alone or as 5-mg dose in combination with aspirin and acetaminophen
Heroin	i.m. p.o.	5 60	4–5 4–5	0.5	Illegal in United States; high solubility for parenteral administration
Levorphanol (Levodromoran)	i.m. p.o.	2 4	4–6 4–7	12–16	Good oral potency; requires careful titration in initial dosing because of drug accumulation
Hydromorphone (Dilaudid)	i.m. p.o.	1.5 7.5	4–5 4–6	2–3	Available in high-potency injectable form (10 mg/ml) for cachetic patients and rectal suppositories; more soluble than morphine
Oxymorphone (Numorphan)	i.m. p.r.	1 10	4–6 4–6	2–3	Available in parenteral and rectal suppository forms only
Meperidine (Demerol)	i.m. p.o.	75 300[b]	4–5 4–6	3–4 (normeperidine 12–16)	Contraindicated in patients with renal disease; accumulation of active toxic metabolite normeperidine produces CNS excitation

Methadone (Dolophine)	i.m. p.o.	10 20		15–30	Good oral potency; requires careful titration in initial dosing to avoid drug accumulation
Mixed agonist-antagonists Pentazocine (Talwin)	i.m. p.o.	60 180[b]	4–6 4–7	2–3	Limited use in cancer pain; psychotomimetic effects with dose escalation; available only in combination with naloxone, aspirin, or acetaminophen; may precipitate withdrawal in physically dependent patients
Nalbuphine (Nubain)	i.m. p.o.	10 —	4–6	5	Not available orally; less psychotomimetic effects than pentazocine; may precipitate withdrawal in physically dependent patients
Butorphanol (Stadol)	i.m. p.o.	2 —	4–6	2.5–3.5	Not available orally; produces psychotomimetic effects; may precipitate withdrawal in physically dependent patients
Partial agonists Buprenorphine (Temgesic)	i.m. s.l.	0.4 0.8	4–6 5–6	—	Not available in United States; no psychotomimetic effects; may precipitate withdrawal in tolerant patients

[a]Based on single-dose studies in which an i.m. dose of each drug listed was compared to morphine to establish relative potency. Oral doses are those recommended when changing from parenteral to oral routes. For patients without prior narcotic exposure, the recommended oral starting doses are 30 mg morphine, 5 mg methadone, 2 mg levorphanol, 4 mg hydromorphone.

[b]The recommended starting doses for these drugs are listed in Table 4.

Adapted from Foley (35).

TABLE 6. *Guidelines for use of narcotic analgesics in pain management*

Start with a specific drug for a specific type of pain
Know the pharmacology of the drug prescribed:
- The duration of the analgesic effect
- The pharmacokinetic properties of the drug
- The equianalgesic dose for the drug and its route of administration (see Tables 4 and 5)

Adjust the route of administration to the patient's needs
Administer the analgesic on a regular basis after initial titration of the dose
Use drug combinations to provide additive analgesia and reduce side effects, e.g., nonsteroidal anti-inflammatory drugs, antihistamines (hydroxyzine), amphetamine (dexedrine)
Avoid drug combinations that increase sedation without enhancing analgesia, e.g., benzodiazepine (diazepam), phenothiazine (chlorpromazine)
Anticipate and treat the side effects:
- Sedation
- Respiratory depression
- Nausea and vomiting
- Constipation

Watch for the development of tolerance:
- Switch to an alternate narcotic analgesic
- Start with one-half the equianalgesic dose and titrate to pain relief

Prevent acute withdrawal:
- Taper drugs slowly
- Use dilute doses of naloxone (0.4 mg in 10 cc saline) to reverse respiratory depression in the tolerant patient

Do not use placebos to assess the nature of pain
Anticipate and manage complications:
- Overdose
- Multifocal myoclonus
- Seizures

Adapted from Foley (35).

GROUP III: ADJUVANT ANALGESIC DRUGS

Limitations in the use of narcotic analgesics in certain pain states have fostered the use of adjuvant analgesic drugs to manage specific types of cancer pain, e.g., deafferentation pain (9,36,37,45,46). In contrast to the nonnarcotic and narcotic analgesics, for which there are sufficient pharmacologic data to demonstrate their analgesic properties, the use of adjuvant analgesic drugs in management of patients with cancer pain is largely empirical. They have been used primarily to increase the analgesic effects of the narcotic analgesics or to counteract their undesirable side effects. Any attempt to develop guidelines for use of the adjuvant drugs in clinical cancer pain management must be prefaced with certain caveats. These drugs include a wide range of heterogeneous substances developed and approved for clinical uses other than analgesia, including nausea, vomiting, anxiety, mania, depression, and delirium. These drugs are not as effective in relieving pain as the narcotic analgesics, except for methotrimeprazine (Levoprome) (7). With the exceptions of hydroxyzine (5) and amphetamines (39), there have been no efficacy studies of their co-analgesic properties in cancer patients. These drugs have a unique place in the management of cancer pain, and their use has been previously reviewed. The choice from among these drugs should be individualized using the simplest but most potent combinations.

Phenytoin and carbamazepine are anticonvulsant drugs that suppress spontaneous neuronal firing, and they are the drugs of choice for treatment of certain neuropathic pains (89). In cancer pain, carbamazepine has been specifically useful in managing acute shocklike neuralgic pain in the cranial and cervical distributions caused by either tumor infiltration or surgical nerve injury. It has also been effective in patients with stump pain secondary to traumatic neuroma and in patients with lumbosacral plexopathy. The starting dose is 100 mg, slowly titrated up to 400 to 800 mg/day, as tolerated.

Methotrimeprazine, a phenothiazine drug, has definite analgesic properties. Single-dose studies in patients with postoperative pain and chronic cancer pain have demonstrated that 15 mg intramuscularly (i.m.) is equivalent to 15 mg of i.m. morphine (7). This drug is useful in special circumstances (32). In patients who are tolerant, it provides a temporary approach to provide analgesia, presumably by a non-opiate-receptor mechanism. In patients with bowel obstruction and pain, it avoids the constipatory effects of the narcotics. In patients whose respiration is compromised, it avoids the respiratory depressant effects of the narcotics, but it does produce significant sedative effects. In patients with pain and narcotic-induced nausea and vomiting, it acts as both an analgesic and an antiemetic. Chronic administration of this drug in patients with cancer pain has not been fully assessed.

Haloperidol, a butyrophenone, is the first-line drug for management of cancer patients with acute psychosis and delirium, but its role in pain management has been advocated on the basis of animal studies that demonstrated its potentiation of morphine analgesia (46). Several authors have reported its clinical usefulness in cancer patients with pain, suggesting that it works as a co-analgesic, thus allowing for reduction of the narcotic dose. However, this is a controversial area, and certain studies have demonstrated that it produces additive sedative effects without necessarily providing additive analgesic effects. Further studies will be necessary to define its place as a co-analgesic in cancer pain management.

The tricyclic antidepressants may represent the most useful group of psychotropic drugs presently used in pain management. Their analgesic effects are mediated by enhancement of serotonin activity in the central nervous system. Animal studies have demonstrated direct analgesic effects of amitriptyline, as well as its ability to enhance morphine analgesia. Amitriptyline has been reported to be useful for management of patients with chronic pain (103). No control studies in patients with cancer pain have been performed, but there is strong anecdotal evidence to suggest roles for these drugs in management of patients with neuropathic pain and in management of the pain-related sleep disturbances occurring in this population. The analgesic properties of amitriptyline appear to occur independent of its mood-altering effects.

Corticosteroids have been reported to have both specific and nonspecific benefits in managing cancer pain. They can produce euphoria, increase appetite, and reduce bone pain of metastatic origin. Several studies have demonstrated prolonged survival times and control of pain with reduced narcotic dosages in terminal cancer patients receiving steroids (84,85). They are particularly useful in certain pain syndromes such as epidural cord compression and in tumor infiltration of the brachial and lumbosacral plexuses.

Among the antihistamines, hydroxyzine (5) has been demonstrated to have analgesic properties and to provide additive analgesia when combined with morphine. Similarly, dextroamphetamine, when combined with morphine, provides additive analgesia, with reductions in the side effects of morphine in patients with postoperative pain (39). Further studies on these drugs are needed to clarify their usefulness for chronic cancer pain.

Although earlier studies had suggested that cocaine is useful for management of cancer pain, a double-blind crossover study has suggested that cocaine, when combined with morphine, does not potentiate the analgesic effects of morphine but does enhance its mood effects (56). In evaluating the role of cocaine in the Brompton cocktail, it was noted that cocaine, following introduction in 10-mg increments per dose, resulted in a small but statistically significant increase in alertness, whereas stopping cocaine had no detectable effect (97). These studies suggest that cocaine does not play a major role in providing additive analgesic effects.

CONTROVERSIES IN CANCER PAIN MANAGEMENT

Choice of Opiate Analgesic

Several controversies have developed concerning the choices from among the opiate drugs, in part because of a dearth of well-controlled studies comparing the efficacies and side effects of these drugs during chronic administration and in part because of numerous survey data and anecdotal reports that have supported the use of one drug over another. For example, heroin was initially suggested as the drug of choice (79) for management of cancer pain, but morphine is now recognized to be the practical alternative (98). In fact, the World Health Organization (WHO) has requested that oral morphine be part of the essential drug list and made available throughout the world as the "drug of choice." Although its bioavailability varies from 35 to 75%, its short half-life (2–3 hr), its demonstrated efficacy, and its plasma half-life that closely parallels its analgesic half-life make it a drug that can be used without difficulty (76,80,81,83). With repetitive administration, its pharmacokinetics are linear, and there does not appear to be autoinduction following large chronic doses (81,83). As judged by single-dose studies in patients with both acute pain and chronic pain, the relative potency of intramuscular morphine to oral morphine is 1:6 (49). On the basis of a series of survey studies, Twycross has suggested that the relative potency with repeated administration is 1:2 or 1:3 (98,99). This controversy points out the need for methods appropriate to assess relative potency with chronic administration.

As previously noted, oral heroin was considered the drug of choice until Twycross demonstrated that oral morphine could be readily substituted for heroin in the Brompton cocktail (98). More recent studies have demonstrated that heroin is a prodrug. Heroin itself does not bind to the opiate receptor, but must be metabolized to 6-acetyl morphine and morphine to proudce its effect (52). Following oral administration of heroin, only morphine can be measured in the plasma of patients. The use of oral heroin is an inefficient way of delivering morphine to the systemic circulation. Heroin is more soluble than morphine, offering an advantage in patients requiring a parenteral (i.m.) route. However, its solubility advantage is of minor importance, because there are alternative drugs currently available that are either more potent, such as hydromorphone, or more soluble, such as methadone, and there are improved novel methods of drug administration such as subcutaneous morphine infusion (62).

The introduction of continuous subcutaneous opiate infusions (52,57) using a pump attached to a 27-gauge butterfly needle placed in any convenient body site and requiring replacement every 3 or 4 days has further reduced the significance of the solubility issue. More important, the use of subcutaneous morphine reduces the number of i.m. injections to one every 3 to 4 days, as compared with one every 3 to 4 hr. This approach dramatically improves the quality of life for patients requiring parenteral medication at home.

Another controversy concerns the role of methadone in cancer pain management. Methadone's bioavailability is 85%, and from single-dose studies its oral-to-parenteral ratio is 1:2. Its plasma half-life is 17 to 24 hr, but its analgesic half-life is only 4 to 8 hr. Repetitive doses of methadone lead to drug accumulation, and deaths have been attributed to inappropriate use of this drug in cancer patients (28,32,53,82,90). Yet, it is a useful alternative to morphine, requiring greater sophistication in its clinical use as compared with morphine. Methadone should be considered a second-line drug. The controversy over its method of administration will be discussed in the next section.

Clinical pharmacologic studies of meperidine in cancer patients have demonstrated that repetitive dosing can lead to accumulation of a toxic metabolite, normeperidine, that can produce central nervous system (CNS) hyperexcitability characterized initially by subtle mood effects, followed by tremors, multifocal myoclonus, and, occasionally, seizures (55). This CNS hyperexcitability occurs commonly in patients with renal disease, but it can occur following repeated administration in patients with normal renal function. This was more frequent in patients with cancer who were receiving meperidine for treatment of chronic cancer pain. Therefore, the role of meperidine in chronic cancer pain management is limited because of the accumulation of its toxic metabolite.

Lastly, hydromorphone and levorphanol, congeners of morphine, are other alternatives to morphine and methadone. Because of its short half-life, hydromorphone is a useful alternative to methadone in elderly patients who do not tolerate morphine. Levorphanol, with its long plasma half-life, is also a useful alternative to morphine, but it must be used cautiously (27). For patients who are unable to tolerate morphine or methadone, it represents a useful medication with a good oral-to-parenteral ratio of 1:2 (49). However, direct comparisons of these drugs in chronic administration are lacking, and the guidelines for choosing a drug are based on anecdotal reports rather than controlled clinical trials. Careful assessment of the adverse effects of these drugs and their relative merits will be necessary to place these drugs in the appropriate scheme of cancer pain management.

The roles of narcotic partial agonist and mixed agonist-antagonist drugs in cancer pain are quite limited (48). Pentazocine, although widely available, is available in the United States only combined with naloxone. Escalation of the doses of pentazocine produces psychotomimetic effects, limiting the usefulness of this drug in chronic cancer pain management. Buprenorphine, one of the mixed agonist-antagonist drugs, is available in Europe in both sublingual and parenteral forms (77). It is most useful as the starting medication before patients are given narcotic agonist drugs. When used in patients receiving narcotic agonist drugs, its analgesic efficacy will be diminished. Although studies of chronic use of buprenorphine have suggested that it is of value, its clinical use in cancer patients has been limited (101). Both nalbuphine and butorphanol are available only by the parenteral (i.m.) route, thus limiting assessment of their roles in chronic administration, where the oral route is the preferred method.

From this brief discussion of the controversies, one can recognize that there is no "best" analgesic. Rather, individualization of drug choice and dosage is the rule. However, there are pharmacologic reasons to choose one drug over another, and these have been briefly outlined. Studies in the clinical pharmacology of these drugs will be necessary to provide the physician with a better understanding of the principles involved in chronic administration (70).

Method of Drug Administration

This controversy focuses on the issue whether drug should be administered on a fixed basis versus p.r.n. or on-demand basis. In practice, each of these methods has its place. The purpose of using a fixed method of administration is to provide the patient with continuous pain relief, preventing the pain from recurring. The p.r.n. method is based on administration of the drug following recurrence of pain. In chronic cancer pain management there is little to be gained by allowing the patient to have recurrent bouts of pain, particularly if all approaches to treat the cause of the pain have failed. The Hospice movement has strongly advocated the use of a fixed-time approach and has demonstrated its safety and efficacy for morphine and heroin (79,99). The use of a fixed approach has practical value because it prevents the usual medical and nursing delays that occur in the hospital setting when a patient on a p.r.n. schedule requests medication. However, the fixed approach has the potential to be dangerous for patients who have no previous narcotic exposure. This is particularly true with drugs like methadone (half-life 17–24 hr) and levorphanol (half-life 12–16 hr), whose plasma half-lives are much greater than their analgesic half-lives (4–6 hr). Repeated doses of these drugs lead to drug accumulation and side effects. Their titration to effective analgesia is more difficult than with a drug like morphine or hydromorphone, whose half-lives are shorter. Methadone has been implicated in the deaths of several cancer patients because of lack of recognition of its long plasma half-life and potential for accumulation (28).

Of equal importance is the fact that the full effectiveness of these drugs cannot be assessed until they have reached a steady state, which takes approximately four to five half-lives. Therefore, for methadone and levorphanol, it may be 4 to 5 days before a steady-state plasma level of drug is achieved, whereas for morphine or hydromorphone, steady-state levels are achieved in less than 24 hr. Studies by Sawe et al. (82) with methadone demonstrated that when patients titrated their own dosages using a p.r.n. method in the initial titration, they could then be switched to a fixed interval, which in that study was approximately every 8 to 12 hr. We have found that when methadone is administered at these long intervals, patients develop bolus effects, that is, side effects (sedation, most commonly), within 1 hr of dosing. We have noted fewer side effects when the drug is administered every 4 to 6 hr. Therefore, studies comparing fixed and p.r.n. dosing will be necessary to assess the effects of these techniques on patient compliance, patient satisfaction, and the development of side effects. At the current time, the best approach to starting narcotic analgesic therapy is to individualize the timing of administration based on the patient's history of previous narcotic use and medical status. Once the timing interval between doses is established for the patient, drug can be administered on a fixed basis. This approach requires patient, family, nursing, and physician education and can be both efficacious and safe. In a study of oral, patient-controlled analgesia, in which hospitalized patients administered medications to themselves, adequate pain relief without excessive or inappropriate use of the drug was observed. In fact, they required less overall medication than patients on a p.r.n. schedule, because they, rather than the medical staff, were in control (24). Recently, the availability of slow-release morphine preparations for 8- or 12-hr effectiveness has provided patients with greater freedom from repetitive dosing, especially during the night. They appear to be both safe and efficacious (102). Studies assessing this component of effective pain relief will provide insight into the role of control in a patient's degree of pain relief (25,43).

Route of Drug Administration

The limited oral bioavailability of some of the narcotic analgesics, such as morphine, and the fact that these drugs have historically been used to manage acute pain rather than chronic pain have traditionally discouraged the use of these drugs by the oral route. It was the work of Twycross, Saunders, and Houde that led to the use of oral narcotic analgesics in chronic cancer pain (47,79,96,98). There is no longer a controversy. Oral analgesics work effectively if the appropriate equianalgesic doses for the route of administration are used. However, the needs of the cancer patient with pain have provided a strong impetus to develop novel routes of drug administration either to enhance drug activity or to minimize the limiting side effects associated with their acute and chronic administration. For example, sublingual and buccal drug administrations offer the unique advantage of an orally administered drug with the pharmacokinetic profile of an intramuscularly injected drug, avoiding the first-pass effect. Methods for intranasal and transdermal routes are also being developed with this same objective in mind (71).

For some patients, only parenteral administration is possible, and intermittent i.v. bolus or continuous i.v. infusions are used (26,40). Guidelines for continuous infusions have been developed (74), but further information is needed on the relative potencies of drugs by the i.v. route as compared with the i.m. and p.o. routes.

Continuous subcutaneous infusions, using a 27-gauge butterfly needle attached to an infusion pump, also provide an alternative to repetitive i.m. injections (12,62,65). Whether or not continuous infusion offers a special advantage over intermittent bolus injection remains controversial. Pharmacologic and pharmacokinetic studies of patient-controlled analgesia may help to resolve this controversy, but again, the role of this approach in chronic cancer pain management remains undefined, but of major theoretical and practical importance.

Use of epidural and intrathecal routes of administration remains the most controversial issue (13,15,16,18–20,22,23,63,69,72). These approaches are based on the concept that there are opiate receptors in the spinal cord that, when activated, provide selective analgesia without motor, sensory, or autonomic effects (104). Recognition of these selective analgesic sites in this spinal opiate system has led to clinical use of epidural and intrathecally administered opiates to minimize the central effects of these drugs. This approach has been rapidly integrated into the management of patients with postoperative pain and cancer pain without complete assessment of its value. Several questions remain unanswered: What is the best time to start this method of drug administration? What are the relative advantages and disadvantages of epidural and intrathecal administrations? Should the drug be administered continuously or by intermittent bolus? What is the best drug? The answers to these questions will require prospective controlled clinical trials, with measurement of pharmacologic and pharmacokinetic parameters (17).

During our studies of cancer patients we have recognized that prior exposure of the patient to systemic narcotic analgesics (21,44,63,66,67) produces tolerance that limits the effectiveness of spinal opiates. This observation is graphically demonstrated in Fig. 1A, which shows that a patient without significant prior narcotic exposure obtained prolonged pain relief following epidural administration. High levels of drug in the cerebrospinal fluid (CSF) were noted, as well as substantial systemic uptake of drug, as reflected in the plasma levels. In contrast, Fig. 1B illustrates the results for a patient who had a long prior exposure to narcotic analgesics and who obtained no pain relief from 30 mg of epidural morphine, despite high levels of drug in both plasma and CSF. We have concluded that tolerance is a significant factor limiting the use of this approach. Animal studies (104) and limited human data (44,63,66,67) indicate that tolerance develops most rapidly by this route of administration. More important, the concept of selective analgesia has been put in question by pharmacokinetic studies in patients receiving continuous spinal infusions of morphine using an Infusaid pump (66). We have demonstrated that rostral redistribution of drug in the CSF occurs and that at steady state, significant levels of opiate can be measured at the cistern. These data suggest that lumbar epidural or intrathecal administration activates not only spinal sites but also supraspinal sites of analgesia, reducing the advantage of the selectivity of this approach. Clinical studies have confirmed this observation (11). The question concerning the clinical use of this technique is whether or not it offers any special advantages to the cancer patient that outweigh potential complications of placing epidural and intrathecal catheters in the immunosuppressed host. In the United States, where a wide variety of oral analgesics are available for prescription and the treatment of cancer is aggressive, these techniques have been reserved for patients who have failed to obtain relief from systemic analgesic therapy. Although this approach is useful for a limited number of patients, it has not yet made a significant impact in pain control.

In contrast, in those countries in which oral analgesics are not widely available, this technique is often a primary approach, because the anesthesiologist treating pain patients has access to parenteral morphine. When

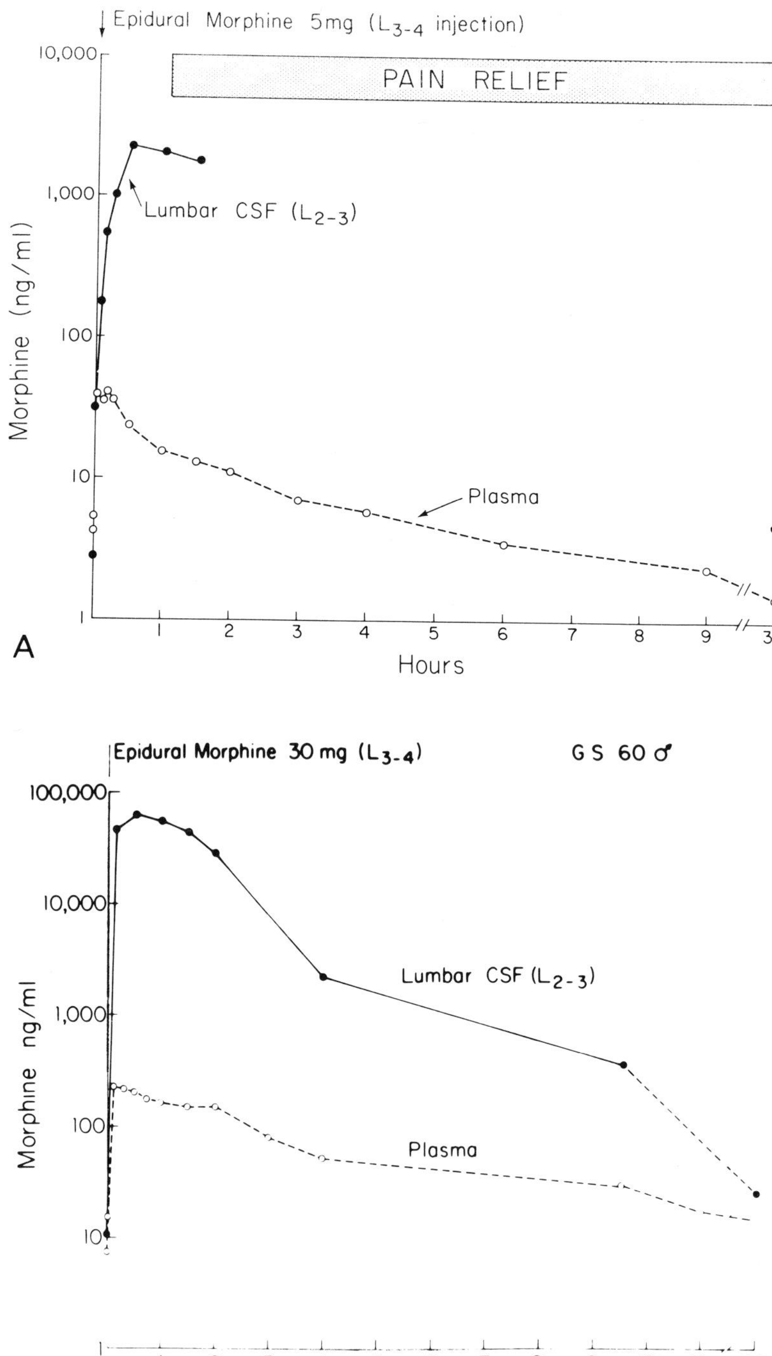

FIG. 1. A: Plasma and CSF levels of morphine following epidural administration in a non-tolerant patient, with associated pain relief. **B:** Plasma and CSF levels of morphine following epidural administration in a tolerant patient, without any associated pain relief or side effects.

used as the initial treatment, it clearly is a useful and successful technique. Prospective studies assessing the quality of life with systemic administration versus epidural and intrathecal administration will be necessary in order to place this technique in the appropriate perspective of cancer pain management. Similarly, as previously discussed, the advantage of a bolus dose versus a continuous infusion requires study. Further studies to develop drugs that will remain localized to spinal cord will expand the usefulness of this approach.

Development of Tolerance

Tolerance is the pharmacologic effect in which with repeated administration, increasing doses are necessary to provide the same effect. Tolerance develops at different rates for the various narcotic effects. Tolerance to respiratory depression develops rapidly, in contrast to the slow development of tolerance (if at all) to the constipatory effects. In the clinical situation, the development of tolerance represents a significant practical management problem. The first sign of tolerance is the patient's report that the analgesic effect is not lasting as long as it once did. This report labels the patient as a clock-watcher, and is often confused by health care professionals as an early sign of "addiction" or psychological dependence. In a controlled study by Houde et al. (49), a shift in the dose–response curve to the right was demonstrated in patients receiving morphine chronically when studied 2 weeks apart. Twycross has stated that tolerance is not a practical problem (99). In our own studies (58) this has been true for patients with stable disease and stable pain. However, in patients with progressive disease and escalating pain, the development of tolerance is associated with the use of increasing doses of analgesics. Inexperienced physicians are often unwilling or afraid to prescribe large doses, resulting in inadequate control of pain. This phenomenon of tolerance is described graphically in Fig. 2. The patient was a 56-year-old woman with pancreatic cancer and a stable pain syndrome who was maintained on oral morphine and intermittent use of aspirin for approximately 50 weeks, when she developed increasing pain, associated with objective tumor progression. Oral doses of morphine were increased, but because of gastrointestinal obstruction she was switched to i.v. opiates, first by i.v. bolus and then by continuous infusion. In the last 4 weeks of life, escalation to 6,000 mg of a continuous i.v. infusion of morphine sulfate per day was necessary to control her pain. She remained awake, without respiratory compromise, until her death from gram-negative sepsis. Tolerance was not a problem when her pain syndrome was stable, but her prior narcotic exposure and increasing pain severity led to larger dosage requirements to provide pain relief. This example suggests that there is no limit to tolerance. She was able to maintain analgesia while tolerant to the sedative and respiratory depressant effects. What is controversial is the relationship

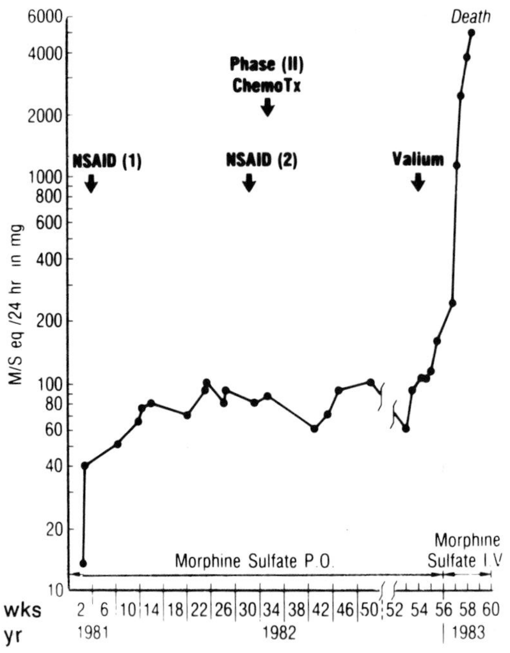

FIG. 2. Pattern of drug intake in a 56-year-old woman with pancreatic carcinoma, with increasing pain and opiate requirements.

of increasing pain severity to increasing narcotic drug requirements. To what extent does pain severity influence or dictate the development of tolerance?

In management of tolerant patients we have also found that cross-tolerance is not complete (47,51). Switching to an alternative narcotic like methadone at one-half the equianalgesic dose in a patient tolerant to the analgesic effect of morphine provides adequate analgesia. Is this phenomenon incomplete cross-tolerance, or does it reflect inherent differences in drugs or specific receptor affinities? Our clinical experience supports the concept of incomplete cross-tolerance, but studies of tolerance development in man will be necessary to clarify the mechanisms inherent in these observations.

The development of drugs for specific receptors offers an opportunity to further study the mechanisms of tolerance and cross-tolerance. Innovative studies of intrathecally administered peptides, such as D-Ala-D-Leu-enkephalin (DADL), that bind selectively to delta receptors important in mediating spinal opiate analgesia (95,104) have provided one approach for obtaining pain relief for some cancer patients tolerant to morphine (67,68). DADL, with selectivity for delta receptors, provided pain relief in patients tolerant to morphine, suggesting that therapeutic approaches based on receptor differences should be tested in the clinical situation.

In summary, in managing tolerant patients, increasing the drug dosages, switching to an alternative drug, or, if these are not fully successful, the use

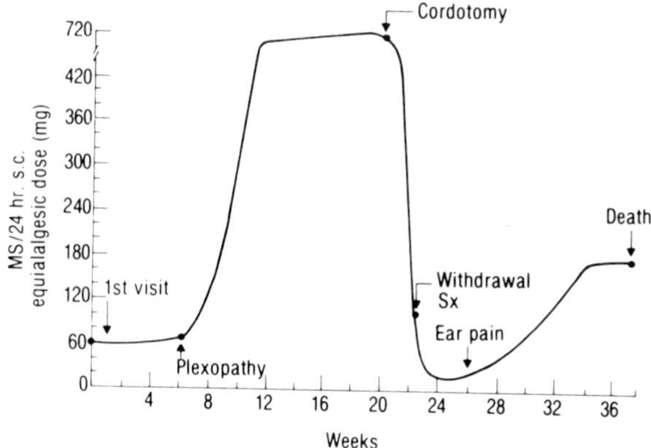

FIG. 3. Pattern of drug intake in a 43-year-old woman with lung cancer, and rapid reduction in opiate drug intake and withdrawal signs. (From Kanner and Foley, ref. 58.)

of combination drug therapy and nondrug approaches may be employed with varying success.

Risk of Substance Abuse and Addiction

Although fear of addiction limits narcotic use by physicians and patients (60,87), there are no published long-term data to support the thesis that chronic use of narcotic analgesics alone causes addiction (1). In fact, there have been very limited published data assessing the degree of physical dependence, substance abuse, or addiction in patients receiving narcotic analgesics for any type of chronic medical illness and pain.

Substance abuse is the use of a drug in a manner that deviates from accepted medical or social patterns. Addiction is a behavioral pattern of compulsive drug use and a preoccupation with securing its supply. These are separate from physical dependence, which is a physiologic effect characterized by the appearance of an abstinence syndrome on abrupt withdrawal of a drug (54). On the basis of a review of patterns of drug use in a cancer pain clinic (58), progression of metastatic disease, with increasing pain severity, is the major factor in the escalation of drug intake. Reduction or elimination of the use of analgesic drugs is associated with successful, specific therapy directed at the cause of the pain. Drug overdose, substance abuse, and psychological dependence did not occur in the population of cancer patients studied (58). Physical dependence did occur, and the distinction between physical dependence and psychological dependence is demonstrated in the case history graphically described in Fig. 3. The patient was a 43-year-old woman with oat-cell carcinoma presenting as a superior sulcus tumor. Pain in the arm and shoulder was initially controlled by codeine (10 mg morphine equivalent per 24 hr). Progessive plexopathy and increasing pain severity led to the use of a combination of levorphanol, oxycodone, acetaminophen, methotrimeprazine, and amitriptyline. Partial relief was obtained, but excessive sedation limited her functional status, and she underwent a high cervical (C1-2) percutaneous cordotomy. The pain relief was dramatic, and the patient discontinued her medications. Within 16 hr she developed a profound withdrawal syndrome characterized by yawning, lacrimation, diarrhea, diaphoresis, and multifocal myoclonus. She refused pain medication and demonstrated no evidence of "purposive behavior" commonly associated with psychological dependence. Withdrawal signs were controlled with reinstitution of 25% of her previous narcotic intake. The surgical procedure was of limited value, with recurrence of pain within 2 weeks requiring dose escalation to treat the new onset of pain. However, these doses of medication were significantly lower than those used prior to the cordotomy, suggesting that the relief of pain by cordotomy had allowed time for reduction of tolerance to medication, and lower doses of drug could be effectively used.

In reviewing the studies on narcotic drug use in chronic cancer pain patients and the risk of addiction one finds a dearth of data. In a prospective study, Porter and Jick (75) monitored the incidence of narcotic addiction among 39,946 hospitalized medical patients. Among 11,882 who received at least one narcotic preparation, there were only 4 cases of reasonably well documented addiction in patients who had no history of addiction. These data, taken from a survey of a general population, suggest that medical use of narcotics is rarely associated with the development of addiction. A series of studies of abuse of analgesics in patients with chronic illness reported that abuse of non-narcotic analgesics or combination drugs was a more common event than was abuse of narcotic analgesics (2,29,61,88). Several recent studies have described the use of chronic narcotic therapy in patients with non-malignant pain and have reported that chronic use is not associated with substance abuse or psychological dependence (73,92–94). The latter studies support the concept that drug use alone is not the major factor in the development of addiction; other medical, social, psychological, and economic conditions seem to play important roles. These conclusions are also supported by studies of U.S. military personnel addicted to narcotics in Vietnam (78). In this group, drug-abuse behavior was strongly dependent on a series of factors, including underlying personality and social, environmental, and economic issues.

Drug therapy is the major approach to manage cancer pain. The development of improved analgesic assay methods, the use of specific and sensitive analgesic techniques to measure drugs in biofluids, and the development of pharmacologic pharmacokinetic models for drug administration are the clinical pharmacologic advances that will help to resolve these issues. However, in the case of cancer patients with pain, successful use of drug therapy is dependent on the knowledge and experience of the health care professional who prescribes it.

Chronic use of narcotics with cancer patients has provided new insight into the concepts of tolerance, physical dependence, and psychological dependence, thereby raising issues that will be resolved only by prospective studies. The cancer pain patient receiving narcotic analgesics provides another type of natural experiment to study the effects of chronic narcotic use in a pain population and offers a unique opportunity to better understand the consequences of chronic drug use.

ACKNOWLEDGMENT

This work was supported in part by a grant from the National Cancer Institute (CA-32897).

REFERENCES

1. Angell, M. (1982): The quality of mercy. *N. Engl. J. Med.,* 302:98–99.
2. Bakewell, W. E., and Wikler, A. (1966): Incidence in a university hospital psychiatric ward. *J.A.M.A.,* 196:710–713.
3. Basbaum, A. I., and Fields, H. L. (1978): Endogenous pain control mechanisms: Review and hypothesis. *Ann. Neurol.,* 4:451–462.
4. Beaver, W. T. (1965): Mild analgesics: A review of their clinical pharmacology. *Am. J. Med. Sci.,* 251:576–599.
5. Beaver, W. T. (1976): Comparison of analgesic effects of morphine sulfate, hydroxyzine and their combination in patients with postoperative pain. In: *Advances in Pain Research and Therapy, Vol. 1,* edited by J. J. Bonica and V. Ventafridda, pp. 553–557. Raven Press, New York.
6. Beaver, W. T. (1980): Management of cancer pain with parenteral medication. *J.A.M.A.,* 244:2653–2657.
7. Beaver, W. T., Wallenstein, S. L., Houde, R. W., et al. (1966): A comparison of the analgesic effect of methotrimeprazine and morphine in patients with cancer. *Clin. Pharmacol. Ther.,* 7:436–446.
8. Bonica, J. J. (1953): *The Management of Pain.* Lea & Febiger, Philadelphia.
9. Breivik, H., and Rennemo, F. (1982): Clinical evaluation of combined treatment with methadone and psychotropic drugs in cancer patients. *Acta Anaesth. Scand.* [*Suppl.*], 74:135–140.
10. Brodie, G. N. (1974): Indomethacin and bone pain. *Lancet,* 1:1160.
11. Bromage, P. R., Camporesi, E. M., Durant, P. A. C., and Nielsen, C. H. (1982): Rostral spread of epidural morphine. *Anesthesiology,* 56:431–436.
12. Campbell, C. F., Mason, J. B., and Weiler, J. M. (1983): Continuous subcutaneous infusion of morphine for the pain of terminal malignancy. *Ann. Intern. Med.,* 98:51–52.
13. Camporesi, E. M., and Redick, L. F. (1983): Clinical aspects of spinal narcotics: Postoperative managements and obstetrical pain. *Clin. Anesth.,* 1:57–70.
14. Chapman, C. R., Casey, K. L., Dubner, R., Foley, K. M., Gracely, R. H., and Reading, A. E. (1984): Pain measurement: An overview. *Pain, (in press).*
15. Chauvin, M., Samii, J., Schermann, J. M., Sandouk, P., Bourdon, R., and Viars, P. (1982): Plasma pharmacokinetics of morphine after IM, extradural and intrathecal administration. *Br. J. Anaesth.,* 54:843–846.
16. Chrubasik, J., Scholler, K. L., Wiemers, K., Weigel, K., and Friedrich, G. (1984): Low-dose infusion of morphine prevents respiratory depression. *Lancet,* 1:793.
17. Colburn, W. A. (1981): Simultaneous pharmacokinetic and pharmacodynamic modeling. *J. Pharmacokinet. Biopharm.,* 9:367–388.

18. Coombs, D. W., Pageau, M. G., Saunders, R. L., and Mroz, W. T. (1982): Intraspinal narcotic tolerance: Preliminary experience with continuous bupivacaine HCL infusion via implanted infusion device. *Int. J. Artifical Organs,* 5:379–382.
19. Coombs, D. W., Saunders, R. L., Block, A., Gaylor, M. S., Colton, T., and Pageau, M. E. (1983): Relief of continuous chronic pain by intraspinal narcotics infusion via an implanted reservoir. *J.A.M.A.,* 250:2336–2339.
20. Coombs, D. W., Saunders, R. L., and Gaylor, M. S. (1982): Epidural narcotic infusion reservoir: Implantation technique and efficacy. *Anesthesiology,* 56:469–473.
21. Coombs, D. W., Saunders, R. L., LaChance, D., Savage, S., Ragnarsson, T. S., and Jensen, L. (1985): Intrathecal morphine tolerance: Use of intrathecal clonidine, DADL, and intraventricular morphine. *Anesthesiology, (in press).*
22. Cousins, M. J., and Bridenbaugh, P. O. (1980): *Neural Blockade.* J. B. Lippincott, Philadelphia.
23. Cousins, M. J., and Mather, L. E. (1984): Intrathecal and epidural administration of opioids. *Anesthesiology,* 61:276–310.
24. Coyle, N. (1979): Self-administration of analgesics in a hospital setting. *Am. J. Nurs.,* 79:1554–1557.
25. Dahlstrom, B., Tamsen, A., Paalzow, L, and Hartvig, P. (1982): Patient-controlled analgesic therapy. IV. Pharmacokinetics and analgesic plasma concentrations of morphine. *Clin. Pharmacokinet.,* 7:266–279.
26. DeChristoforo, R., Corden, B. J., Hood, J. C., Narang, P. K., and Magrath, I. T. (1983): High dose morphine infusion complicated by chlorobutanol-induced somnolence. *Ann. Intern. Med.,* 98:335–336.
27. Dixon, R., Crews, T., Mohacsi, C., Inturrisi, C. E., and Foley, K. M. (1980): Levorphanol: Radioimmunoassay and plasma concentration profiles in dog and man. *Res. Commun. Chem. Pathol. Pharmacol.,* 29:535–548.
28. Ettinger, D. S., Vitale, P. J., and Trump, D. C. (1979): Important clinical pharmacologic considerations in the use of methadone in cancer patients. *Cancer Treatment Reports,* 63:457–459.
29. Ewing, J. A., and Bakewell, W. E.: Diagnosis and management of depressant drug dependence. *Am. J. Psychiatry,* 123:909–917.
30. Ferrer-Brechner, T., and Ganz, P. (1984): Ibuprofen as an analgesic potentiator of methadone in cancer patients. *Am. J. Med.,* 77:78–83.
31. Foley, K. M. (1979): Pain syndromes in patients with cancer. In: *Advances in Pain Research and Therapy, Vol. 2,* edited by J. J. Bonica and V. Ventafridda, pp. 59–75. Raven Press, New York.
32. Foley, K. M. (1981): Current controversies in the management of cancer pain. In: *New Approaches to Treatment of Chronic Pain: A Review of Multidisciplinary Pain Clinics and Pain Centers,* edited by L. K. Y. Ng, pp. 169–181, U.S. Government Printing Office, Washington, D.C.
33. Foley, K. M. (1982): The practical use of narcotic analgesics. In: *Medical Clinics of North America,* edited by M. M. Reidenberg, pp. 1091–1104. W. B. Saunders, Philadelphia.
34. Foley, K. M. (1984): Assessment of pain. In *Clinics in Oncology: Pain Relief in Cancer,* edited by R. G. Twycross, pp. 17–31. W. B. Saunders, London.
35. Foley, K. M. (1985): The treatment of cancer pain. *N. Engl. J. Med., (in press).*
36. Foley, K. M. (1985): Commentary on heroin: Facts and comparisons. *PRN Forum,* 1:2.
37. Foley, K. M. (1985): Adjuvant analgesic drugs in the management of cancer pain. In: *Relief of Chronic Pain,* edited by G. M. Aronoff, pp. 425–433. Addison-Wesley, Reading, Mass.
38. Foley, K. M., and Sundaresan, N. (1984): The management of cancer pain. In: *Cancer Principles and Practices in Oncology,* edited by V. T. DeVita, S. Hellman, and S. A. Rosenberg, 1940–1961. J. B. Lippincott, New York.
39. Forrest, W. H. et al. (1977): Dextroamphetamine with morphine for the treatment of postoperative pain. *N. Engl. J. Med.,* 296:712–715.
40. Fraser, D. G. (1980): Intravenous morphine infusion for chronic pain. *Ann. Intern. Med.,* 93:781–782.
41. Galasko, C. S. B. (1976): Mechanisms of bone destruction in the development of skeletal metastases. *Nature,* 263:507–510.

42. Gerbershagen, H. U. (1979): Non-narcotic analgesics. In: *Advances in Pain Research and Therapy, Vol. 2,* edited by J. J. Bonica and V. Ventrafridda, pp. 255–273. Raven Press, New York.
43. Graves, D. A., Foster, T. S., Batenhorst, R. L., et al. (1983): Patient controlled analgesia. *Ann. Intern. Med.,* 99:360–366.
44. Greenberg, H. S., Taren, J., Ensminger, W. D., and Doan, K. (1982): Benefit from and tolerance to continuous intrathecal infusion of morphine for intractable cancer pain. *J. Neurosurg.,* 57:360–364.
45. Halpern, L. W. (1979): Psychotropics, ataractics and related drugs. In: *Advances in Pain Research and Therapy, Vol. 2,* edited by J. J. Bonica and V. Ventafridda, pp. 275–283. Raven Press, New York.
46. Hanks, G. W. (1984): Psychotropic drugs. *Clin. Oncol.,* 3:135–151.
47. Houde, R. W. (1979): Systemic analgesics and related drugs: Narcotic analgesics. In: *Advances in Pain Research and Therapy, Vol. 2,* edited by J. J. Bonica and V. Ventrafridda, pp. 263–273. Raven Press, New York.
48. Houde, R. W. (1979): Analgesic effectiveness of the narcotic agonist-antagonists. *Br. J. Clin. Pharmacol.,* 7:297S–308S.
49. Houde, R. W., Wallenstein, S. L., and Beaver, W. T. (1966): Evaluation of analgesics in patients with cancer pain. In: *International Encyclopedia of Pharmacology and Therapeutics. Section 6. Clinical Pharmacology,* edited by L. Lasagna, pp. 59–99. Pergamon Press, New York.
50. Inturrisi, C. E. (1982): Narcotic drugs. In: *Medical Clinics of North America,* edited by M. M. Reidenberg, pp. 1061–1071. W. B. Saunders, Philadelphia.
51. Inturrisi, C. E., and Foley, K. M. (1984): Narcotic analgesics in the management of pain. In: *Analgesics: Neurochemical, Behavioral and Clinical Perspectives,* edited by M. Kuhar and G. W. Pasternak, pp. 257–288. Raven Press, New York.
52. Inturrisi, C. E., Max, M. B., Foley, K. M., Schultz, M., Seung-Uon, S., and Houde, R. (1984): The pharmacokinetics of heroin in patients with chronic pain. *N. Engl. J. Med.,* 310:1213–1217.
53. Inturrisi, C. E., and Verebely, K. (1972): Disposition of methadone in man after a single oral dose. *Clin. Pharmacol. Ther.,* 13:923–930.
54. Jaffe, J. H., and Martin, W. F. (1980): Opioid analgesics and antagonists. In: *The Pharmacological Basis of Therapeutics,* edited by A. G. Gilman, L. S. Goodman, and A. Gilman, pp. 494–534. Macmillan, New York.
55. Kaiko, R. F., Foley, K. M., and Grabinski, P. Y. (1983): Central nervous system excitatory effects of meperidine in cancer patients. *Ann. Neurol.,* 13:180–185.
56. Kaiko, R. F., Kanner, R. M., Foley, K. M., et al. (1984): Cocaine and morphine in cancer patients with chronic pain. *Pain,* 2:S203.
57. Kaiko, R. F., Wallenstein, S. L., Rogers, A., et al. (1981): Analgesic and mood effects of heroin and morphine in cancer patients with postoperative pain. *N. Engl. J. Med.,* 304:1501–1505.
58. Kanner, R. M., and Foley, K. M. (1981): Patterns of narcotic drug use in a cancer pain clinic. *Ann. N.Y. Acad. Sci.,* 362:162–172.
59. Kantor, T. G. (1982): Control of pain by nonsteroidal anti-inflammatory drugs. In: *Medical Clinics of North America,* edited by M. M. Reidenberg, pp. 1053–1059. W. B. Saunders, Philadelphia.
60. Marks, R. M., and Sachar, E. J. (1973): Undertreatment of medical inpatients with narcotic analgesics. *Ann. Intern. Med.,* 78:173–181.
61. Maruta, T., Swanson, D. W., and Finlayson, R. E. (1979): Drug abuse and dependency in patients with chronic pain. *Mayo Clinic Proc.,* 54:241–244.
62. Mauskop, A., Coyle, N., Maggard, J., and Foley, K. M. (1985): Continuous subcutaneous narcotic infusions in cancer pain treatment. *ASCO* 4:39.
63. Max, M. B., Inturrisi, C. E., Grabinski, P., Kaiko, R. F., and Foley, K. M. (1981): Epidural opiates: Plasma and cerebrospinal fluid (CSF) pharmacokinetics of morphine, methadone, and beta-endorphin. *Clin. Pharmacol. Therap. (in press).*
64. McGivney, W. T., and Crooks, G. M. (1984): The care of patients with severe chronic pain in terminal illness. *J.A.M.A.,* 251:1182–1188.
65. Miser, A. W., Miser, J. S., and Clark, B. S. (1980): Continuous intravenous infusion of

morphine sulfate for control of severe pain in children with terminal malignancy. *J. Pediatr.,* 96:930–932.
66. Moulin, D. E., and Foley, K. M. (1985): The pharmacokinetics of continuous intrathecal morphine and DADL. *(submitted for publication) Neurology (Minneap.).*
67. Moulin, D. E., Max, M., Kaiko, R. F., Inturrisi, C. E., Maggard, J., Yaksh, T., and Foley, K. M. (1984): The analgesic efficacy of intrathecal D-Ala-D-Leu-enkephalin in the cancer patient with chronic pain. *Pain (in press).*
68. Onofrio, B. M., and Yaksh, T. L. (1983): Intrathecal delta-receptor ligand produces analgesia in man. *Lancet,* 1:1386–1387.
69. Onofrio, B. M., Yaksh, T. L., and Arnold, P. G. (1981): Continuous low-dose intrathecal morphine administration in the treatment of chronic pain of malignant origin. *Mayo Clin. Proc.,* 56:516–520.
70. Paalzow, L. K. (1982): Pharmacokinetic aspects of optimal pain treatment. *Acta Anaesth. Scand.* [*Suppl.*], 74:37–43.
71. Payne, R., and Foley, K. M. (1984): Advances in the management of cancer pain. *Cancer Treatment Reports,* 68:173–183.
72. Poletti, C. E., Cohen, A. M., Todd, D. P., et al. (1981): Cancer pain relieved by long-term epidural morphine with indwelling systems for self administration. *J. Neurosurg.* 55:581–584.
73. Portenoy, R., and Foley, K. M. (1985): Chronic use of opioid analgesics in nonmalignant pain. *(submitted for publication).*
74. Portenoy, R. K., Moulin, D. E, Foley, K. M., Inturrisi, C. E., and Rogers, A. (1985): Continuous intravenous infusions of opiates in cancer pain: Review of 46 cases and guidelines for use. *(submitted for publication).*
75. Porter, J., and Jick, H. (1980): Addiction rate in patients treated with narcotics. *N. Engl. J. Med.,* 302:123.
76. Rane, A., Sawe, J., Dahlstrom, B., Paalzow, L., and Kager, L. (1982): Pharmacological treatment of cancer pain with special reference to use of oral morphine. *Acta Anaesth. Scand.* [*Suppl.*], 74:97–103.
77. Robbie, D. S. (1979): A trial of sublingual buprenorphine in cancer pain. *Br. J. Clin. Pharmacol.,* 7:315S–318S.
78. Robins, L. N., David, D. H., and Nurco, D. N. (1974): How permanent was Vietnam drug addiction? *Am. J. Public Health,* 64:38–43.
79. Saunders, C. M. (1967): *The Management of Terminal Illness.* Edward Arnold, London.
80. Sawe, J., Dahlstrom, B., Paalzow, L., and Rane, A. (1981): Morphine kinetics in cancer patients. *Clin. Pharmacol. Ther.,* 30:629–635.
81. Sawe, J., Dahlstrom, B., and Rane, A. (1983): Steady-state kinetics and analgesic effect of oral morphine in cancer patients. *Eur. J. Clin. Pharmacol.,* 24:537–542.
82. Sawe, J., Hansen, J., Ginman, C., Hartvig, P., Jakobsson, P. A., Milsson, M.-I., Rane, A., and Anggard, E. (1981): Patient controlled dose regimen of methadone for chronic cancer pain. *Br. Med. J.,* 282:771–773.
83. Sawe, J., Svensson, J. O., and Rane, R. (1983): Morphine metabolism in cancer patients on increasing oral doses—no evidence for autoinduction or dose-dependence. *Br. J. Clin. Pharmacol.,* 16:85–93.
84. Schell, H. W. (1966): The risk of adrenal corticosteroid therapy in far advanced cancer. *Am. J. Med. Sci.,* 252:641–664.
85. Schell, H. W. (1972): Adrenal corticosteroid therapy in far advanced cancer. *Geriatrics,* 27:131–141.
86. Shimm, D. S., Logue, G. L., Maltbie, A. A., and Dugan, S. (1979): Medical management of chronic cancer pain. *J.A.M.A.,* 241:2408–2412.
87. Sriwatanakul, K., Weis, B. F., Alloza, J. L., et al. (1983): Analysis of narcotic analgesic usage in the treatment of postoperative pain. *J.A.M.A.,* 250:926–929.
88. Swanson, D. W., Weddige, R. L., and Morse, R. M. (1973): Abuse of prescription drug. *Mayo Clin. Proc.,* 48:359–367.
89. Swerdlow, M. (1982): Anticonvulsant drugs and chronic pain. *Clin. Neuropharmacol.,* 7:51–82.
90. Symonds, P. (1977): Methadone and the elderly. *Br. Med. J.,* 1:512.

91. Tasker, R. R. (1985): Deafferentation. In: *Textbook of Pain,* edited by P. D. Wall and R. Melzack, *(in press).* Raven Press, New York.
92. Taub, A. (1982): Opioid analgesics in the treatment of chronic intractable pain of non-neoplastic origin. In: *Narcotic Analgesics in Anesthesiology,* edited by L. M. Kitahata and D. Collins, pp. 199–208. Williams & Wilkins, Baltimore.
93. Tennant, F. S., and Rawson, R. A. (1982): Outpatient treatment of prescription opioid dependence. *Arch. Intern. Med.,* 142:1845–1847.
94. Tennant, F. S., and Uelman, G. F. (1983): Narcotic maintenance for chronic pain: Medical and legal guidelines. *Postgrad. Med.,* 73:81–94.
95. Tseng, L. (1982): Tolerance and cross tolerance to morphine after chronic spinal D-ala^2-D-Leu^5-enkephalin infusion. *Life Sci.,* 31:987–992.
96. Twycross, R. G. (1974): Clinical experience with diamorphine in advanced malignant disease. *Int. J. Clin. Pharmacol.,* 9:184–198.
97. Twycross, R. G. (1977): Value of cocaine in opiate containing elixers. *Br. Med. J.,* 2:1348.
98. Twycross, R. G. (1977): Choice of strong analgesic in terminal cancer: Diamorphine or morphine? *Pain,* 3:93–104.
99. Twycross, R. G., and Lack, S. A. (1983): *Symptom Control in Far Advanced Cancer: Pain Relief.* Pitman, London.
100. Twycross, R. G., and Ventafridda, V. (1980): *The Continuing Care of Terminal Cancer Patients.* Pergamon, Oxford.
101. Ventafridda, V., DeConno, F., Gaurise, G., et al. (1983): Chronic analgesic study on buprenorphine action in cancer pain—comparison with pentazocine. *Drug Res.,* 4:587–590.
102. Walsh, T. D. (1984): Controlled study of slow release morphine for chronic pain in advanced cancer. *Pain* [*Suppl.*], 2:S202.
103. Walsh, T. D. (1983): Antidepressants in chronic pain. *Clin. Neuropharmacol.,* 6:271–295.
104. Yaksh, T. L. (1981): Spinal opiate analgesia: Characteristics and principles of action. *Pain,* 11:293–346.

Advances in Pain Research and Therapy, Vol. 9, edited by H. L. Fields et al. Raven Press, New York © 1985.

Prospective Evaluation of Treatment Outcome in Patients Referred to a Cancer Pain Center

*Robin S. Cohen, *Theresa Ferrer-Brechner, *Anna Pavlov, and **Anthony E. Reading

**Department of Anesthesiology, UCLA Medical Center; and **Department of Psychiatry and Behavioral Sciences, UCLA, Los Angeles, California 90024*

Estimates of the incidence of pain associated with advanced cancer range from 60 to 80% (1,4). Further, pain syndromes associated with early cancers and cancer-related treatments occur in 5 to 85% of cancer patients (3,4), depending on the type of cancer and treatment. Unrelieved pain is one of the cancer patient's greatest concerns and fears. In a recent needs-assessment survey conducted by Heinrich et al. (5), 30% of the cancer patients sampled reported a need for pain control. Further, studies of cancer patients have revealed that those suffering from pain experience higher rates of emotional problems than those without pain (12). Despite the prevalence and significance of cancer pain, there have been few empirical investigations of the psychological aspects of the syndrome and the efficacy of evaluation and treatment strategies for this specific problem.

The purpose of psychosocial evaluation in a multidisciplinary cancer pain clinic is twofold. First, for practical reasons, a qualitative understanding of the patient's experience is necessary for effective treatment of the individual. Pain occurs in a physical, emotional, cognitive, and behavioral context (11). Thus, understanding the patient's "explanatory model" (2) (that is, one's attitudes, beliefs, and feelings about oneself and the disease and the pain) facilitates an intermeshing of patient and physician approaches to cancer pain and its treatment. By identifying and anticipating patient strengths and barriers to treatment and how the patient makes treatment decisions, the treatment team can work to bring patient and physician expectations into greater alignment, increasing collaboration and trust.

The second purpose of evaluation in a cancer pain clinic is to measure pain and cancer-relevant variables in a quantitative manner to gain an objective understanding of the patient's pain and functioning occurring over time. There are two important goals of quantitative assessment of the cancer pain patient. First, processes that are relevant to the cancer patient's functioning should be measured, in addition to pain sensation. Because treatment of the cancer pain patient, or any pain patient, involves reestablishing higher levels of emotional and behavioral functioning, major components to be measured are sensory, affective, and behavioral aspects of the pain experience.

Because pain is a subjective experience, and actual nociceptive data or physical evidences of injury are difficult to obtain or are uncorrelated with pain experience, it is necessary to quantify data in order to circumvent artifacts and biases associated with verbal reports of a subjective multidimensional experience. Sensitive, accurate, and prospective measurement methods are necessary for formulating treatment plans, monitoring fluctuations in levels of relevant variables over time, evaluating treatment effectiveness, and identifying predictors of treatment response (10).

This descriptive study prospectively evaluated changes in pain, mood, and functional impairment in patients treated at a cancer pain clinic through the use of quantitative multiple measures of these variables over the course of six clinic visits. The purpose of this assessment was to evaluate (a) whether or not cancer pain patients improve over time as a result of treatment in a multidisciplinary cancer pain clinic and (b) whether or not measures used to evaluate these patients are accurate and sensitive.

METHODS

Subjects

Over a 12-month period, 109 consecutively referred patients at the UCLA Cancer Pain Clinic participated in the study. Patients were primarily referred by medical and surgical oncologists in the Southern California area, a majority from UCLA.

Personal demographics. Of the total sample, 45.3% were male and 54.6% were female. The average age was 57.1 years, and the range was from 16 to 84, with 65% falling into the 51 to 70 range.

Cancer-related demographics. Among these patients, 51.2% had metastatic disease, and 48.8% had stable disease. The most common types of cancer were as follows: lung, 24.2%; breast, 11.6%; colorectal, 11.0%; female reproductive, 7.4%; lymphoma, 5.6%; prostate, 5.3%; blood, 5.1%; melanoma, 4.2%; pancreatic, 3.2%; head and neck, 3.0%. A majority of these patients (95.5%) had received conventional cancer therapy before and at the time of referral, such as chemotherapy, radiation, and/or surgery, with 59.6% receiving multiple treatments.

Pain-related demographics. At time of referral to the clinic, these patients had endured cancer pain for a mean of 14 months, with a range from 2 weeks to more than 36 months. Sixty-five percent of the patients had experienced pain for periods ranging from 2 weeks to 1 year. These patients had been taking between 0 and 30 pain-related medications prior to referral, with a mean of 7 medications. The cause of pain was attributed to the cancer itself by 26.6% of patients, to surgery by 23.4%, to radiation by 7.4%, to chemotherapy by 5.3%, and to metastases specifically by 6.4%. Data were analyzed for up to five follow-up visits. Of the total sample, 44 patients attended only the initial consultation, 65 made two visits, 53 made three visits, 41 made four visits, 27 made five visits, and 23 made six visits. The types of treatment received over the course of therapy will not be reviewed; however, a majority (87%) received medication tailoring as a primary approach.

Procedure

During the initial visit the UCLA Pain Profile was administered. This survey elicited information regarding patient demographics, disease-specific data, and concurrent somatic and psychosocial treatment. Data were collected concerning pain, mood, and functional impairment in the form of visual analog scales (VAS) and the McGill Pain Questionnaire (8). The pain VAS was anchored with "no pain" and "the most intense pain imaginable." The mood VAS was anchored with "the most depressed imaginable" and "the most elated imaginable." The functional impairment VAS was anchored with pain "does not interfere at all" and "interferes as much as possible." On follow-up visits, further data on pain, mood, and functional impairment were collected in addition to VAS measurements. The Profile of Mood States (POMS) (7) was used to evaluate mood. This is a scale validated with cancer patients (13) measuring emotional distress using the factors anxiety, depression, anger, vigor, confusion, and fatigue. Activity level (functional impairment) was measured by asking patients to estimate the number of hours spent in various activities, e.g., "working at my job," "household chores," "walking," "exercising," and "doing errands." The McGill Pain Questionnaire was given at every visit to measure pain experience. Thus, over the course of follow-up visits, patient pain experience was measured multiply.

RESULTS

Because visits were at irregular intervals, the use of analysis-of-variance and time-series statistics was inappropriate. For each variable, the slope of the curve of patient scores over time (six visits) was computed. Slopes that were positive implied improvement of condition; negative slopes implied worsening of condition; no slope implied no change [occurred frequently only for pain level (VAS)]. Table 1 illustrates the percentages of patients demonstrating improvement ("better") and worsening ("worse") in pain,

TABLE 1. *Improvement vs. worsening of pain, mood, and functional impairment from initial visit to follow-up 1 and from follow-up 1 through follow-up 5*

Variable	Initial to follow-up 1				Follow-up 1 to 5			
	Better (%)	Same (%)	Worse (%)	χ^2	Better (%)	Same (%)	Worse (%)	χ^2
Pain (VAS)	58	34	8	28.26[a]	50	42	6	34.44[a]
				2.94[b]				0.88[b]
Mood (VAS)	64		35	6.16[c]	50		45	0.31
McGill (Total)	69		20	19.20[a]	58		41	1.99
Functional impairment (VAS)	88		10	23.75[a]	88		10	23.75[a]
Mood (POMS)					61		35	3.45
Activity level (hours/day)					46		42	0.10

[a] $p < 0.001$.
[b] Pearson χ^2 comparing frequencies of "better" (improvement) and "same" (no change).
[c] $p < 0.05$.

mood, and impairment from the initial visit to the first follow-up visit and over subsequent visits. Pearson chi-square statistics comparing obtained frequencies with expected frequencies of improvement and worsening were computed. There were significant differences between frequencies of improvement and worsening for pain level (VAS), pain language (McGill), mood (VAS), and impairment (VAS) from initial visit to first follow-up visit. Over subsequent visits, although the frequency of improvement was consistently greater than the frequency of worsening, this difference was not significant for pain level (VAS), mood level (VAS and POMS), pain language (McGill), and activity level (hours/day). Significantly higher frequencies of improvement were demonstrated for impairment level.

Figures 1, 2, 3, and 4 illustrate mean scores for pain (VAS), emotional distress (POMS), functional impairment (VAS), and activity level over time for patients with progressive (metastatic) disease and stable (nonmetastatic) disease.

In general, improvements in pain level (VAS), impairment (VAS), mood (POMS), and activity level (hours/day) occurred over time for both metastatic and nonmetastatic patients. However, nonmetastatic patients demonstrated lower levels of pain, emotional distress, and functional impairment and differed significantly from metastatic patients in pain level at follow-up visits 3 and 4 ($t = 2.08$, $p < 0.05$; $t = 2.15$, $p < 0.05$), functional impairment at follow-up visit 4 ($t = 2.32$, $p < 0.05$), and activity level at follow-up visit 3 ($t = 1.97$, $p < 0.05$).

DISCUSSION

These data indicate that significant improvements in pain level, mood, and functioning occurred as a result of treatment in this cancer pain center,

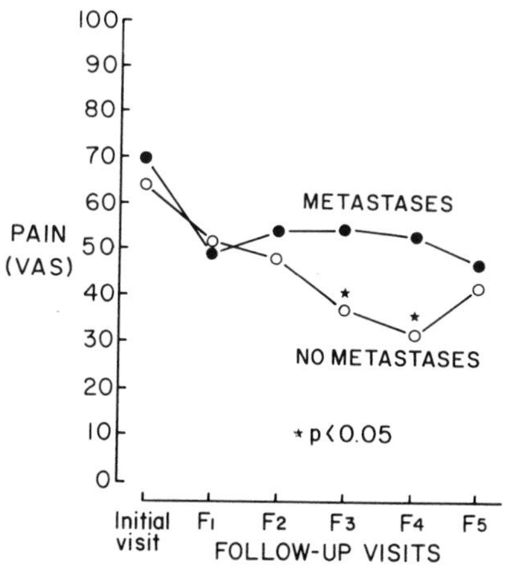

FIG. 1. Mean pain levels, measured by VAS, occurring over six clinic visits for patients with metastatic and nonmetastatic disease.

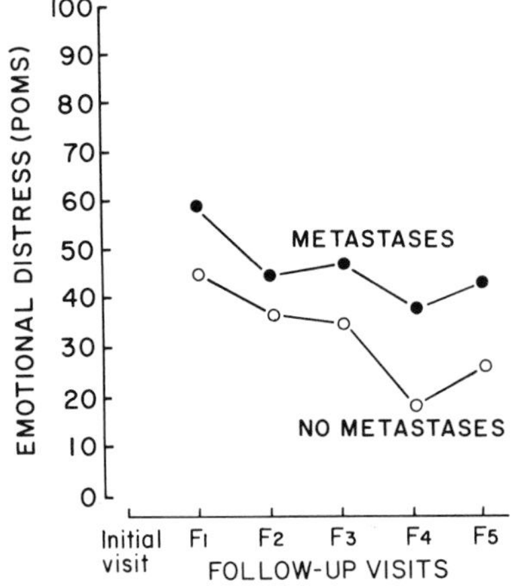

FIG. 2. Mean levels of emotional distress, measured by POMS, occurring over five follow-up visits for patients with metastatic and nonmetastatic disease.

the most dramatic response occurring between the initial visit and the first follow-up, with stabilization over subsequent visits. There are several possible explanations for this effect. First, during the initial period (from initial visit to follow-up 1), 87% of our clinic patients received medication tailoring as treatment of choice. Thus, these findings may support surveys (6,9) indicating that cancer pain is inadequately treated because of physicians' fears of addicting patients and the lack of research and proper education in this area (1). Patients in this sample may have been improperly treated before referral, and therefore the expert medication tailoring afforded in a cancer pain clinic led to striking initial responses. Another plausible explanation for these results is that patients regain hope that their suffering will be alleviated by being seen by a cancer pain specialist, thus improving mood and functioning. A possible artifact, however, is that patients may exaggerate

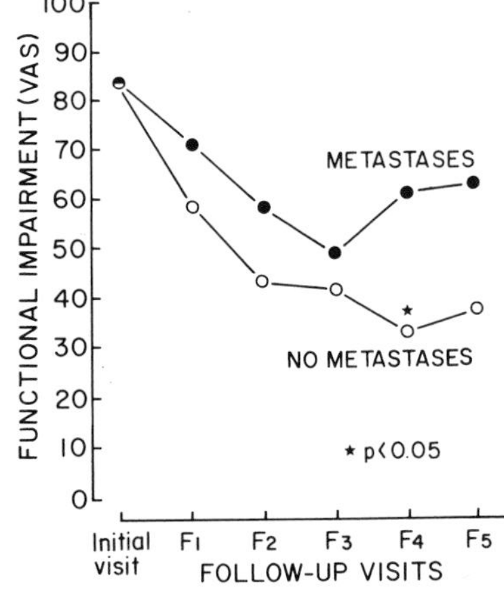

FIG. 3. Mean levels of functional impairment, measured by VAS, occurring over six clinic visits for patients with metastatic and nonmetastatic disease.

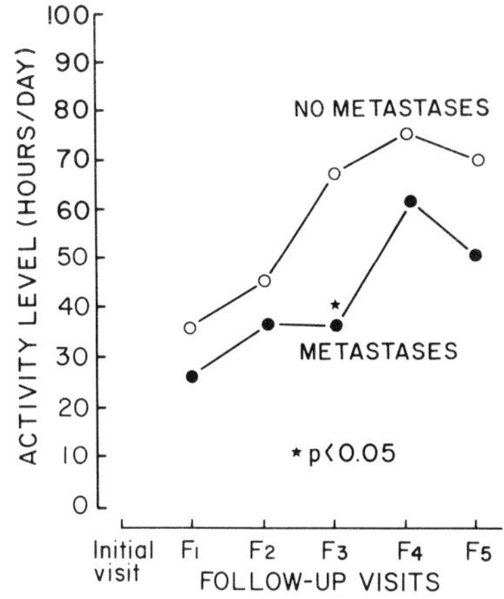

FIG. 4. Mean activity levels, measured by hours per day engaged in physical activities, occurring over five follow-up visits for patients with metastatic and nonmetastatic disease.

their initial pain, impairment, and emotional distress levels to demonstrate their suffering to clinic staff.

This study demonstrates that changes in pain level, mood, and perceived functional impairment can be measured accurately and sensitively over time. Rates of improvement may vary according to the type of treatment measure used and the extent of the cancer. Patients with progressive disease consistently exhibit higher levels of pain, impairment, and emotional distress than stable patients over time. However, patients with progressive disease appear to demonstrate a pattern of improvement similar to that for patients with stable disease, indicating that individuals with advanced cancer can benefit from treatment at a cancer pain clinic.

Further investigation of cancer pain should focus on (a) the effects of specific treatments on pain, mood, and functioning, (b) predictors of treatment response, (c) responses of specific cancer processes to specific treatments, and (d) development of valid, reliable, and sensitive measures specific to the problem of cancer pain.

ACKNOWLEDGMENT

This investigation was supported by the American Cancer Society contract grant number 527-5-E.

REFERENCES

1. Bonica, J. J. (1979): Importance of the problem. In: *Advances in Pain Research and Therapy,* Vol. 2, edited by J. J. Bonica and V. Ventafridda, pp. 1–12. Raven Press, New York.
2. Chapman, C. R. (1979): Psychologic and behavioral aspects of cancer pain. In: *Advances in Pain Research and Therapy,* Vol. 2, edited by J. J. Bonica and V. Ventafridda, pp. 45–56. Raven Press, New York.

3. Daut, R. L., and Cleeland, C. S. (1982): The prevalence and severity of pain in cancer. *Cancer,* 50:1913–1918.
4. Foley, K. M. (1979): Pain syndromes in patients with cancer. In: *Advances in Pain Research and Therapy,* Vol. 2, edited by J. J. Bonica and V. Ventafridda, pp. 59–75. Raven Press, New York.
5. Heinrich, R. L., Schag, C. C., and Ganz, P. A. (1983): Progress in the treatment of cancer patients: Evaluation of rehabilitation needs. *UCLA Cancer Center Bulletin,* 10:8–10.
6. Marks, R. M., and Sachar, E. J. (1973): Undertreatment of medical inpatients with narcotic analgesics. *Ann. Intern. Med.,* 78:173–181.
7. McNair, D., Lorr, M., and Dropplemann, L. (1971): *Manual for Profile of Mood States.* Educational and Industrial Testing Service, San Diego.
8. Melzack, R. (1975): The McGill Pain Questionnaire: Major properties and scoring methods. *Pain,* 1:277–299.
9. Parkes, C. M. (1978): Home or hospital? Terminal care as seen by surviving spouse. *J. R. Coll. Gen. Pract.,* 28:19–30.
10. Reading, A. E., and Cox, D. N. (1979): The measurement of pain. In: *Research in Psychology and Medicine.* Vol. 1. *Physical Aspects: Pain, Stress and Organic Processes,* edited by D. J. Osbourne, M. Gruneberg, and D. R. Eiser, pp. 20–26. Academic Press, London.
11. Turk, D. C., and Kerns, R. D. (1983–84): Conceptual issues in the assessment of clinical pain. *Int. J. Psychiatry Med.,* 13:57–68.
12. Woodforde, J. M., and Fielding, J. R. (1970): Pain and cancer. *J. Psychosom. Res.,* 14:365–370.
13. Worden, J. W., and Weisman, A. D. (1977): The fallacy in postmastectomy depression. *Am. J. Med. Sci.* 273:169–175.

Advances in Pain Research and Therapy, Vol. 9, edited by H. L. Fields et al. Raven Press, New York © 1985.

Relief of Pain by Stabilization of the Spine Affected by Malignancy

*John Miles, **A. J. Banks, and †E. Dervin

**Associated Unit of Neurosciences and Pain Relief Foundation, Walton Hospital, Liverpool; **Bolton General Hospital, Bolton; and †Department of Aeronautical and Mechanical Engineering, Salford University, Manchester, United Kingdom*

Pain is a prominent symptom when malignancy affects the spine (4,7). The true incidence of metastasis of the spine is not known and can only be guessed (18). The relative frequencies at which particular cancers metastasize to the spine have been determined by Stark et al. (21). Spinal deposits from cancer of the lung account for approximately 33% of the total, and those from cancer of the breast approximately 28%. Other cancers contribute 25%, and 14% have no established primary source. Primary malignancy of the spine is much less common, and probably the most common type is the congenital cordoma, and after that, various sarcomas.

ETIOLOGY OF PAIN

The pain experienced may be due to (a) periosteal tension associated with expansion of the involved underlying bone or (b) root compression. Root compression rarely may be purely related to expansion of the bone and trapping of the root in the intervertebral foramen; more commonly there is compression of the root by extradural tumor that usually has grown out from the surrounding bone; in an undetermined proportion of cases there is root compression due to instability of the vertebral spine at the level of the deposit.

The pain due to periosteal tension is that commonly associated with malignancy, namely, a constant, boring "bone" pain particularly bad at night. When there is root compression caused by expansion of the bone or by extradural deposit, the same characteristics may obtain, but that due to instability has its own special associations. This last form of root compression will usually be worse on weight bearing or during maneuvers involving intervertebral joint movement and will be relieved by lying down or not moving. Uncommonly, acute collapse of an involved vertebra will give rise to sudden severe focal spinal pain and/or radical pain, and this is usually associated with minor trauma.

Whereas pain is the most common symptom and almost invariably the earliest symptom, neurological deficit tends to follow over a varying period of time, depending on many factors, not least of all the tissue type of the cancer. The story associated with spinal metastasis from breast and lung tends to be of focal pain and then root pain preceding neurological deficit by 6 to 8 weeks. The period over which radiculopathy or myelopathy then evolves may vary from days to weeks. More slowly growing metastatic malignancy such as that from carcinoma of the prostate and the deposits of multiple myeloma might have a much more protracted story of pain and a more slowly evolving neurological deficit.

PRESENT MANAGEMENT

Any possible treatment directed at the malignancy, be it primary or metastatic, is obviously optimal. This may be endocrinological (10) or chemical (5) or, even more commonly, radiotherapeutic (15). If the type of malignancy is not known, then one is left with the dilemma of either employing these treatments empirically on a presumptive diagnosis or attempting to establish a tissue diagnosis prior to treatment. The commonest method of achieving this is by employing urgent or emergency laminectomy (4), which allows, in addition to establishment of the diagnosis, decompression by removal of accessible extradural tumor. Attempts are being made to establish tissue diagnosis without laminectomy by the use of needle or cannula biopsy, and this method is being currently assessed by our colleague in the Associated Unit of Neurosciences, Liverpool, Mr. Gordon Findlay. The basis for attempting to avoid laminectomy is the well-proven realization that laminectomy itself, in addition to providing decompression for the spinal cord, is bound to render that part of the spine less stable, and because the majority of metastatic deposits affecting the spine are to be found in the vertebral bodies, removal of the posterior structures is very likely to precipitate critical instability (11).

Another approach to the problem is to recognize the factor of instability when it is present and to actively treat it. Because the majority of the malignant deposits are in the vertebral body (16), the logical approach to this problem of vertebral body collapse is to resect the vertebral body, replacing it with either bone graft or a weight-bearing prosthesis (6,8,13,20).

In the cervical region this is not difficult using the now well-established approach for anterior decompression and fusion of the intervertebral discs of the cervical spine. In the thoracic and lumbar regions this is a much more formidable procedure, involving thoracotomy and/or retroperitoneal exploration, and although the results reported (13) are impressive, one is struck by the extremely long survival of these patients, and one is bound to conclude that a high degree of selection is necessary in order to employ such a formidable operation on a fit enough patient whose malignancy has a sufficiently protracted natural history.

In the more common situation of rapidly advancing carcinomatosis with painful involvement of the spine and clinical or radiological evidence of instability, there is much to be said for a simpler posterior approach providing fusion stability of the spinal segment and also allowing for tissue diagnosis and/or spinal decompression laminectomy.

METHOD

Banks and Dervin (2) designed a $\frac{3}{8}$-inch-square stainless-steel rod[1] that can be bent during operation to conform with the contours of the spine (Fig. 1) and can be applied by the posterior approach (Fig. 2). A routine incision is made, and the spinous processes and laminae are exposed as for laminectomy, and if tissue diagnosis or spinal decompression is required, this is conducted over the appropriate segment. Triple laminectomy has been undertaken and stabilization still achieved, but clearly the fewer laminae removed, the less is the adjacent spine needed for fixation, and the less is the surgical trauma inflicted on the patient. The rods are perforated at centimeter intervals to take self-tapping bone screws, and care must be taken to align the positions of these screws with the maximum possibility for screw fixation. The screws are then inserted after fine ($\frac{5}{64}$ to $\frac{7}{64}$) tapping of the cortical bone and screwed through the spinous process base in the line of the opposite lamina (Fig. 3). This gives the longest passage through bone, though we believe that if the screw breaks through onto the posterior surface

[1]The spinal stabilizing rod described is now produced by and is available from Charles F. Thackray Ltd., P.O. Box 171, Park Street, Leeds, United Kingdom, and from Charles F. Thackray (U.S.A.) Inc., New Boston Street, Woburn, Boston, Massachusetts.

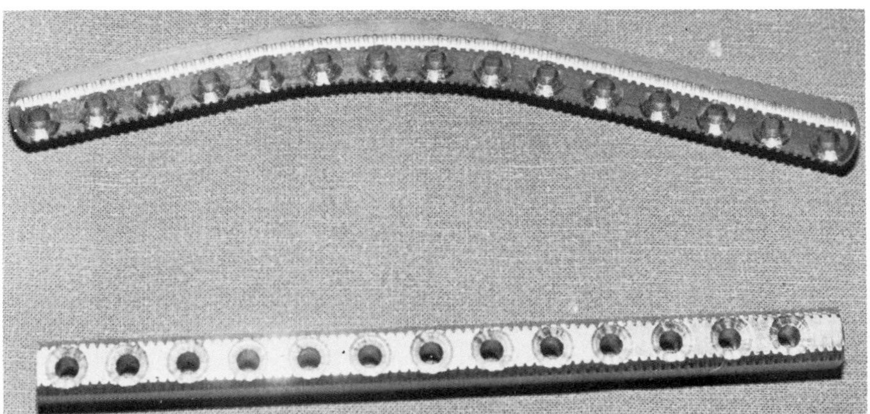

FIG. 1. Stainless-steel spinal stabilizing rod: as supplied (bottom) and as bent to spinal curvature (top).

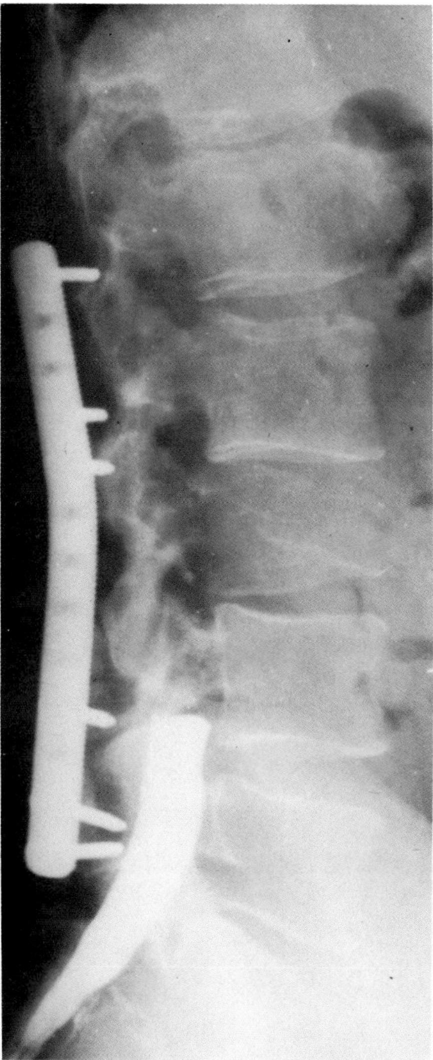

FIG. 2. Lateral lumbar radiograph illustrating the position of the rod fixing an unstable third lumbar vertebra destroyed by a melanoma deposit.

of the cortical bone of the lamina, there is probably an even greater fixation attained. The screws are placed, and an attempt is made to involve at least two vertebrae above and below the level of the instability, but before the final locking of the screws a cyanoacrylate paste is prepared, and small quantities of this are forced in between the rod and the underlying spinous processes and laminae. This material is not used to strengthen the fixation but merely to improve the conformation between the perforated bar and the irregular posterior spinal arches. It can also act as a locking washer on the screws between the inelastic stainless steel and the more elastic bone. This

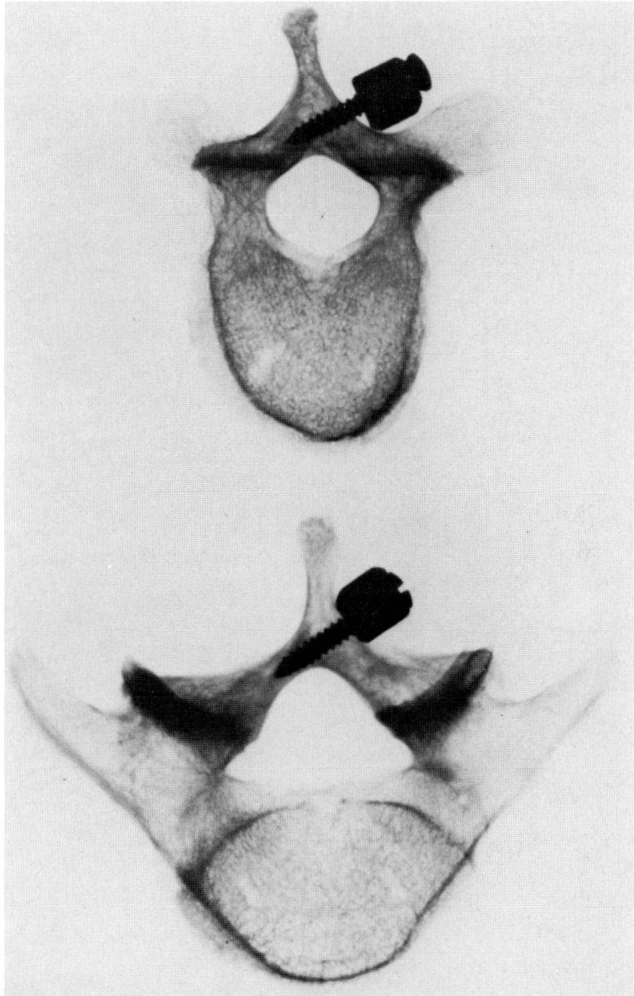

FIG. 3. Axial radiographs of isolated vertebrae, thoracic (top) and lumbar (bottom), illustrating the position of the rod at the spinous process/lamina function and the line of screw fixation.

should help to take up transferred forces between the two structures (2). As the acrylic hardens, the final turns of the screw are made, and a satisfactory firmness or tightness is sought. If the bone appears unsatisfactorily soft, by virtue of either tumor infiltration or osteoporosis, two further steps can be undertaken in order to ensure fixation. First, the screw can be removed, and a small plug of soft cyanoacrylate can be forced into the hole in the rod, and the screw reinserted. This will commonly provide a firm impaction along the bone track. If there are still doubts about the security of the fixation,

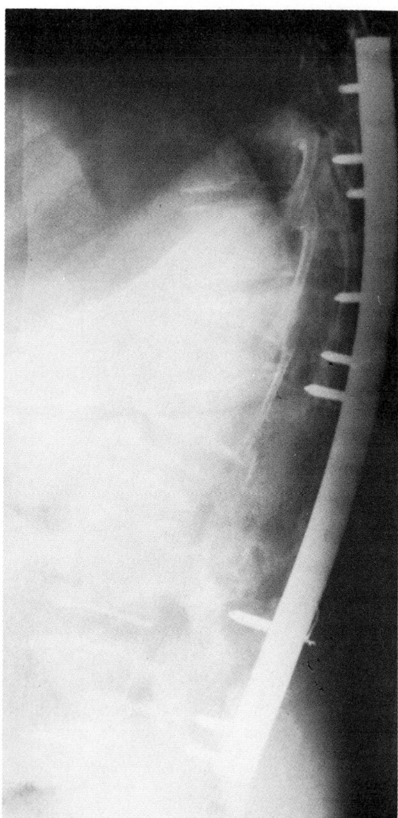

FIG. 4. Radiograph showing a stabilizing bar in the thoracolumbar region covering two collapsed vertebrae with steel wire used to aid in fixation.

standard orthopedic stainless-steel wire can be passed through the remaining holes in the rod and through or around available spinous processes and tightened by a locking knot (Fig. 4).

The stabilizing bar can be applied to any part of the spine from the lower cervical to the sacral, as any kind of curvature can be induced in the bar using a standard bending device during operation. A specialized pair of lightweight bars has been designed and is undergoing trials for application to the cervical region using the same posterior approach. The biomechanical and technical surgical details are available elsewhere (3).

CLINICAL MATERIAL

Thirty patients with painful instability of the spine associated with malignancy have been treated using this method. Three of these patients suffered from primary tumors (cordoma, chondrosarcoma, histiocytoma); 27 patients suffered from metastatic malignancies, of which 13 emanated from the breast and 3 from the prostate, and there were 2 cases of multiple myelomatosis and 2 of melanomatosis.

RESULTS

Figure 5 attempts to illustrate the effect of stabilizing the spine by this technique with regard to relief of pain and also indicates the survival pattern of the group treated. It is clear that the majority of patients treated (particularly the earlier cases) had very advanced malignancy and very limited survival. Twelve survived for 3 months or less, 10 survived for 3 to 6 months, 3 survived for 6 to 12 months, and 5 survived longer than 12 months, of which the longest was 4 years.

Whereas in the majority, pain relief was also around 3 months, in most cases this meant freedom from pain to death. At the other extreme, the patient surviving 4 years remained pain-free from his rather unusual metastatic deposit from carcinoma of the parotid and died of a myocardial

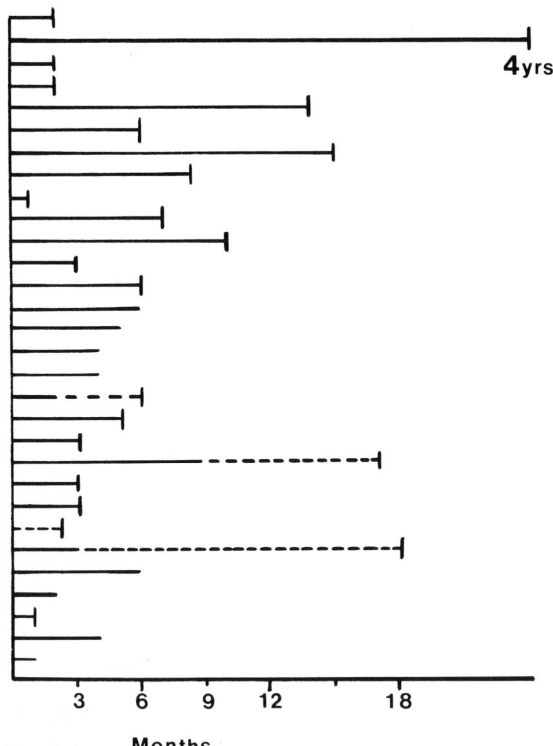

FIG. 5. Line diagrams to illustrate the period of pain relief *(solid lines)* and survival *(to vertical bar)* following stabilization.

infarction. In some cases, whereas pain was relieved, neurological deficit either remained or was only partially relieved or quickly returned. The advantage of pain-free nursing of the incapacitated patient remains, in our opinion, a significant achievement.

In 2 cases, wound infection occurred, but subsequent healing was achieved in 1 case with the prosthesis in place. In the other patient the wound remained open, and the upper screws in the prosthesis loosened and were extruded. This patient had had previous radiotherapy to the site, and whether this played a part in the poor wound healing or whether it was purely a matter of infection or primary loosening of the screws is undetermined. This particular patient had also undergone, simultaneously with the posterior bar fixation, an anterior transthoracic vertebral body replacement with bone grafting, and as we were able to leave the steel bar in place for 2 months, it could then be removed, with firm fixation having been achieved by this anterior fusion. One further patient, following radiotherapy, somehow managed to extrude all his screws, and the prosthesis was removed after 3 months without recurrence of his pain. His instability was due to a lymphoma deposit in the vertebral body, with negligible collapse revealed radiographically.

DISCUSSION

To date, clinical and surgical management of malignancy affecting the spine has been without enthusiasm and largely ineffective (4,15,19). A more careful and critical attitude toward the problem, and particularly the pain involved, will, we believe, allow selection of patients who can be significantly helped, and in this respect stabilization of a clinically or radiologically unstable spine might well prove one of the most useful maneuvers. We would support the use of an anterior approach in the neck when a single vertebral body is involved, and in the chest or perhaps even the lumbar spine when the natural history of the malignancy is sufficiently indolent to suggest that the advantages during prolonged survival will counterbalance the undoubted challenge of major surgery. Stabilization by the posterior approach is much less of a surgical insult, and we believe that the use of the rod described has many advantages over other internal appliances designed to achieve different biomechanical effects, such as in correcting scoliosis (1,9,12,14,17).

The advantages of this method are as follows:

1. The intrinsic strength of stainless steel.
2. The design ability to bend the rod to any spinal configuration.
3. During fixation, the rod is unstressed and is therefore not likely to spring loose or fracture.
4. Multiple fixation points are used, including some close to the site of

instability, again ensuring better fixation and less likelihood of dislocation than if distal fixation points are used.

5. Additional fixation by wires is easily added if thought to be necessary.

CONCLUSION

A method for stabilizing the spine affected by malignancy has been designed and shown to be effective in clinical practice. In addition to effectively relieving the pain associated with instability of the spine, it allows for exploration to obtain tissue diagnosis and/or decompression of the spinal cord and in no way precludes other treatments, including radiotherapy.

ACKNOWLEDGMENTS

We would like to acknowledge the considerable assistance given to E.D. and A.J.B. in the early stage of design by the University of Salford, and more recently the assistance of the Pain Relief Foundation.

REFERENCES

1. Allen, B. L., and Ferguson. R. L. (1982): The Galveston technique for L-rod instrumentation of the scoliotic spine. *Spine,* 7:276–284.
2. Banks, A. J., and Dervin, E. (1980): A simple method for stabilisation of malignant spines. *Engineering in Medicine,* 9:81–83.
3. Banks, A. J., Dervin, E., and Miles, J. B. (1985): Stabilisation of the spine. In: *Persistent Pain,* Vol. V, edited by S. Lipton and J. B. Miles. Academic Press, London *(in press).*
4. Brice, J., and McKissock, W. S. (1965): Surgical treatment of malignant extradural spinal tumours. *Br. Med. J.,* 1:1341–1344.
5. Calman, K. C. (1983): Pain relief by chemotherapy and hormones. In: *Persistent Pain,* Vol. IV, edited by S. Lipton and J. B. Miles, pp. 103–114. Academic Press, London.
6. Cantu, R. C. (1974): Anterior spinal fusion using methyl metha-acrylate. *Int. Surg.,* 59:110–111.
7. Chade, H. O. (1976): Metastatic tumours of the spine and spinal cord. In: *Handbook of Clinical Neurology,* edited by P. J. Vinken and G. W. Bruyn, North Holland, Amsterdam.
8. Cross, G. O., White, H. L., and White, L. P. (1971): Acrylic prosthesis of the fifth cervical vertebra in multiple myeloma. Technical note. *J. Neurosurg.,* 35:112–113.
9. Cusick, J. F., Larson, S. J., Walsh, P. R., and Steiner, R. E. (1983): Distraction rod stabilisation in the treatment of metastatic carcinoma. *J. Neurosurg.,* 59:861–866.
10. Deshpandi, N. (1981): The usefulness and limitations of endocrine treatments in human breast cancer. In: *Persistent Pain,* Vol. III, edited by S. Lipton and J. B. Miles, pp. 34–68. Academic Press, London.
11. Findlay, G. (1985): Adverse effects of the management of malignant spinal cord compression. *J. Neurol. Neurosurg. Psychiatry,* 47:761–768.
12. Galasko, C. S. B., and Sylvester, B. S. (1978): Back pain in patients treated for malignant disease. *Clin. Oncol.,* 4:273–283.
13. Harrington, K. (1981): The use of methyl-methacrylate for vertebral body replacement and anterior stabilisation of pathological fracture dislocations of the spine due to metastatic malignant disease. *J. Bone Joint Surg.,* 63A:36–46.
14. Harrington, P. R. (1962): Treatment of scoliosis corrections and internal fixation by spine instrumentation. *J. Bone Joint Surg.,* 44A:591–603.
15. Hensen, R. A., and Urich, H. (1982): *Cancer and the Nervous System,* p. 149. Blackwell Scientific, Oxford.

16. Kakulas, B. A., Harper, C. G., Shibasaki, K., and Bedbrock, G. M. (1978): Vertebral metastases and spinal cord compression. *Clin. Exp. Neurol.,* 15:98–113.
17. Lugue, E. R., and Cardoso, A. (1977): Segmental corrections of scoliosis with rigid internal fixation. *Orthopaedic Transactions,* 1:136–146.
18. Miles, J. B., Banks, A. J., Dervin, E., and Noori, Z. (1985): Stabilisation of the spine affected by malignancy. *J. Neurol. Neurosurg. Psychiatry,* 47:897–904.
19. Northfield, D. (1973): *Surgery of the Central Nervous System.* Blackwell Scientific, Oxford.
20. Scoville, W. B., Palmer, A. H., Samra, K., and Chong, G. (1967): The use of acrylic plastic for vertebral replacement or fixation in metastatic disease of the spine. *J. Neurosurg.,* 27:274–279.
21. Stark, R. J., Henson, R. A., and Evans, S. J. W. (1982): Spinal metastases: A retrospective survey from a general hospital. *Brain,* 105:189–213.

Advances in Pain Research and Therapy, Vol. 9, edited by H. L. Fields et al. Raven Press, New York © 1985.

Analgesia Elicited by Low-Dose Intraventricular Morphine in Terminal Cancer Patients

*Ramiro D. Lobato, **José L. Madrid, **Lorenza V. Fatela, **Adolfo Gozalo, *Juan J. Rivas, and *Rosario Sarabia

**Neurosurgical Department and **Pain Clinic, Ciudad Sanitaria "1 de Octubre," and Faculty of Medicine, Madrid, Spain*

Bilateral or midline chronic intractable pain caused by advanced orofacial or disseminated cancer may escape control by conventional therapies, and some patients cannot be given adequate doses of oral and parenteral narcotics during the terminal phase because of difficulties with swallowing or because of the sedative and emetic complications.

Evidence that very small amounts of opiate agonists instilled in the proximity of brain and spinal cord neurons involved in pain processing result in a potent and sustained analgesia (1,4,5,10,20,21) led clinicians to attempt pain relief by the "central routes," i.e., epidural, intrathecal, and intraventricular. The experience accumulated shows that low-dose morphine injected into the cerebrospinal fluid (CSF) provides excellent analgesia without dangerous side effects (2,3,8,9,11,15,16,18).

Our observation that low-dose morphine injected into the cisterna magna may suppress pain in any anatomical location without producing concomitant respiratory depression persuaded us to use chronic intraventricular morphine in terminal patients with intractable pain caused by orofacial and disseminated cancer (11). Herein we report our experience with 44 consecutive cases treated during the last 2 years. Because opiate distribution in human CSF following intraventricular administration has not previously been analyzed, we determined morphine kinetics in the CSF compartments during therapy. We also assessed the changes in CSF concentrations of homovanillic and 5-hydroxyindoleacetic acids (HVA and 5-HIAA) and plasma levels of the pituitary hormones.

MATERIALS AND METHODS

Patients with sepsis, coagulopathy, allergy to morphine, or an estimated life expectancy longer than 3 months were excluded. The ages of the selected patients ranged from 17 to 80 years (mean = 56 ± 15 years). Cancer was located in the cephalic region in 19 cases, being disseminated in 12, abdominopelvic in 9, and thoracic in 4. The duration of severe pain before resorting to intraventricular therapy ranged from 1 to 48 months (mean = 7.2 months). Thirty-three patients had antitumor surgery plus radiotherapy and/or chemotherapy, and 9 were treated with antialgic neurosurgery. These measures, together with oral and parenteral analgesics and chronic spinal morphine (used in 22 cases), achieved partial or complete pain relief for variable periods of time.

Oral or parenteral opiates were progressively reduced and then discontinued in patients giving informed consent for intraventricular therapy; prior to initiating it, a morphine bolus was injected into the cisterna magna (36 cases; 0.25 mg average dose, 1 ml total volume) or the lumbar theca (4 cases; 0.5–1 mg total dose) in order to assess the effect and possible risks of subarachnoid morphine. CSF samples were drawn from the cisterna 30 and 60 min after injection to measure local morphine concentrations.

Under local anesthesia, a ventricular reservoir was placed with the catheter tip in the frontal horn of the right lateral ventricle. On the day of surgery, and with the patient under close observation, 0.25 to 1 mg of preservative-free, sterile morphine chloride dissolved in saline solution (1 ml total volume) was administered, and the onset and quality of analgesia, the vital signs, and neurologic function were repeatedly evaluated. In 9 patients, CSF samples were simultaneously drawn from the ventricle and the lumbar subarachnoid space 1, 5, 10, and 24 hr after intraventricular injection to measure morphine, HVA, and 5-HIAA concentrations. To collect samples, 1 ml of CSF was withdrawn and discarded (fluid contained in the reservoir and the lumbar tubing) before taking 2 ml, which were refrigerated at − 70° C until morphine was determined by a solid-phase radioimmunoassay (14) and HVA and 5-HIAA were measured by a chromatographic-fluorometric method (19). In 6 patients, pituitary hormone plasma levels were assayed 1 hr after intraventricular morphine administration.

Chronic intraventricular administration was performed on an outpatient basis by personnel trained in the technique of injection, which consisted in Betadine skin preparation followed by reservoir tapping by means of a tuberculin syringe with a no. 25 needle. To prevent fibrosis of the skin over the reservoir, the site of injection was moved from day to day. Patients were reviewed periodically, and the CSF was cultured repeatedly. Pain relief was conventionally graded as excellent (80–100% reduction), good (60–80%), fair (40–60%), or poor (<40%).

RESULTS

Pain Relief with Cisternal Morphine (Preoperative Test)

All but 1 patient reported powerful pain relief within 6 to 32 min (mean = 17 min) of injection and lasting for 8 to 24 hr (mean = 14 hr). Thirty percent of the patients experienced undesirable side effects, such as nausea, vomiting, facial or generalized pruritus, and urinary retention. Two patients developed naloxone-sensitive respiratory depression 8 and 10 hr after injection. Morphine concentrations in cisternal CSF following administration of 0.25 mg were 1655 ± 112 (SEM) and 750 ± 45 ng/ml at 30 and 60 min, respectively.

Pain Relief with Intraventricular Morphine

Initial morphine doses ranging from 0.25 mg (32 patients) to 0.5 to 1 mg (12 patients) achieved excellent (81% of cases) or good (16% of cases) analgesia lasting for 12 to 58 hr (average duration = 21.7 hr). The onset of pain relief occurred within 2 to 35 min (mean = 15 min) of injection and became complete within 30 min in most patients. Apart from analgesia, the patients reported decreased anxiety and a feeling of overall well-being derived from the absence of chronic pain.

Thirty-six patients (82%) continued to receive one or two doses of intraventricular morphine per day until they died 0.2 to 5 months after initiation of therapy (average survival = 1.8 months). Sixty-five percent of the patients required moderate progressive increases in morphine dosages (usually two to three times the initial amount) in order to maintain adequate pain relief. Tolerance was more marked and appeared sooner in patients who had received large doses of parenteral opiates before initiating intraventricular treatment. During the last week of his life, 1 patient received 16 mg of morphine per day to maintain satisfactory analgesia. In most tolerant patients, however, following twofold to threefold dosage increases, a prolonged phase ensued in which no further dosage escalation was needed.

Eight patients (18%) abandoned therapy for different reasons. One having poor analgesia rejected treatment within the first week. Three more quit during the chronic phase because of protracted nausea, somnolence, and mental clouding. Remarkably, 3 of the 7 patients who gave up treatment during the chronic phase did so because they had permanent resolution of their pain until the basic disease killed them several weeks later. One of these patients developed mild withdrawal.

Side Effects During Acute Phase of Treatment

The incidence of side effects following administration of the initial morphine doses was lower than with intracisternal morphine. However, many patients complained of the collateral effects listed in Table 1. These symptoms subsided spontaneously within hours or a few days without discontinuation of treatment. Three patients developed respiratory depression 4, 8, and 9 hr after receiving the first morphine dose (0.25, 1, and 0.5 mg, respectively), and none of them had had this problem when given 0.25 mg of morphine by the cisternal route. Slowing of respiration was easily reversed by

TABLE 1. *Side effects seen with intraventricular morphine (most patients had more than one symptom)*

Symptoms	Cases
Acute phase	
Nausea and vomiting	7
Somnolence	6
Itching	6
Disorientation	5
Euphoria	3
Visual hallucinations	3
Respiratory depression	3
Urinary retention	1
Dizziness	1
Chronic phase	
Somnolence	2
Mental clouding	2
Disorientation	1
Nausea	2
Euphoria	1

naloxone (0.4–2 mg) without changes in analgesia. Subsequent morphine doses did not cause respiratory depression in these patients. One patient had transient hypotension. Miosis was recorded in 15 patients, and sensory performance and motor function were unaltered in all cases.

Side Effects During Chronic Phase of Treatment

Two patients experienced somnolence and nausea during the chronic phase of treatment, and 2 other patients developed disorientation and mental clouding. One experienced abnormal euphoria.

Complications

Reservoir malfunction occurred in 3 patients who had revision of the implant. Because of defective asepsis during home treatment, 3 patients had reservoir contamination, with secondary CSF reaction.

Morphine Kinetics

Mean CSF morphine levels following intraventricular administration are plotted in Fig. 1. From an initial peak of 14,000 ng/ml, ventricular concentrations fell exponentially, with a two-phase half-life of 2 and 7 hr (K_e = 0.346 and 0.099, respectively). The mean lumbar level within 1 hr of intra-

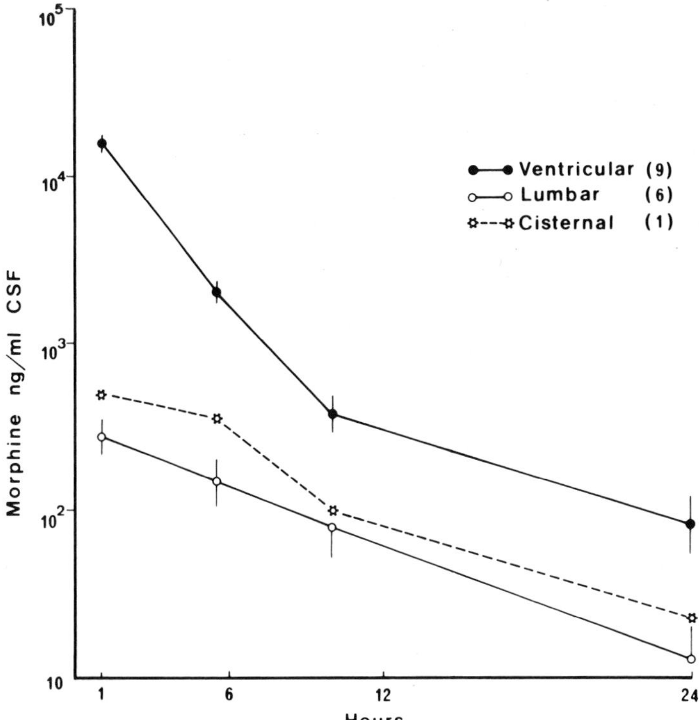

FIG. 1. Morphine CSF concentrations in the lateral ventricle (9 cases), the cisterna magna (1 case), and the lumbar theca (6 cases) following administration of 0.25 mg of morphine through the ventricular reservoir. Points represent mean values ± SEM.

ventricular injection was 287 ng/ml in 6 patients. In 3 other patients not shown in Fig. 1, the lumbar peak occurred about 5 hr after injection. All the patients shown in Fig. 1 enjoyed complete analgesia, which appeared within 40 min of injection and lasted 24 to 48 hr in 6 patients and 16 to 20 hr in 3 patients. These last 3 patients with shorter periods of analgesia had pain located in the inferior part of the body and had received large doses of parenteral narcotics before undergoing intraventricular treatment. They required two to three times the average initial morphine dose to achieve complete analgesia.

Changes in CSF Levels of HVA and 5-HIAA

Ventricular and lumbar CSF levels of these metabolites just before initiation of intraventricular therapy were similar to those found in normal controls. Intraventricular morphine raised HVA and 5-HIAA concentrations in

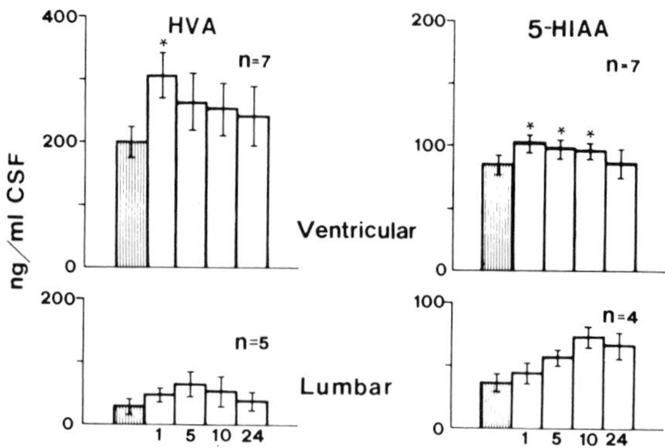

FIG. 2. HVA and 5-HIAA concentrations at ventricular and lumbar levels 1, 5, 10, and 24 hr after instillation of 0.25 mg of morphine into the lateral ventricle. *Shaded bars* are basal levels. *Asterisks* indicate significant increases ($p < 0.05$).

both compartments, but the increases were significant only at the ventricular level (Fig. 2).

Intraventricular morphine significantly increased serum prolactin and decreased antidiuretic hormone within 1 hr of injection. Growth hormone and ACTH were unmodified.

DISCUSSION

We have shown that low-dosage intraventricular morphine may achieve complete and long-lasting pain relief in terminal cancer patients. Analgesia, which appears within a few minutes of injection, whatever the location of pain, is usually accompanied by favorable behavioral responses; our patients were much more relaxed and comfortable than patients receiving parenteral narcotics. Therapy can be safely performed on an outpatient basis without resorting to additional antialgic treatments. The undesirable side effects occurring at the initiation of treatment usually are short-lasting, and the most dreaded (respiratory depression) occurred in only 3 cases, with naloxone restoring respiratory rhythm without interfering with analgesia. The fact that this agent did not reverse analgesia in our patients supports the suggestion that opiate analgesia is mediated by a subpopulation of receptors that are probably located on neurons different from those regulating respiratory depression. It has been found that opiate iontophoresis excites some central gray matter neurons and inhibits others, but only the inhibition is reversible by naloxone (6). Naloxone has also failed to reverse intraventricular-morphine-induced analgesia in the laboratory and stimulation-induced analgesia in humans (13), and it should be borne in mind that opiates may achieve pain relief by activating nonopiate analgesic systems (12).

Respiratory depression never occurred during the chronic phase of treatment in our patients, despite dose escalation. Development of tolerance was not a problem in the present series, probably because of the small doses of morphine employed. A low level of receptor activation may explain why repeated morphine microdoses did not result in the marked and rapid tolerance seen with high-dosage oral and parenteral narcotics. It should be remarked that most patients requiring dosage escalation reached a plateau within days or few weeks, like patients treated with oral opiates (17).

The most awkward problems of chronic intraventricular morphine administration seem to be the risk of infection linked to repeated reservoir tapping and the possibility of the patient developing late mental changes. Multiple reservoir punctures can be circumvented by using refillable continuous-infusion devices instead of conventional reservoirs. The occurrence of late mental clouding seems unpredictable and was observed in 2 terminally ill patients; it is uncertain whether it was caused by the basic disease or by chronic morphine.

The mechanisms and sites of action of intraventricularly injected opiates are not well-known. The question that arises is to what extent the supraspinal and spinal opiate-sensitive systems contribute to the analgesia elicited by intraventricular morphine. The short latencies of the effect (irrespective of the cranial or caudal location of pain) observed in our patients, added to the fact that analgesia in patients with pelvic pain was more rapid following intraventricular than lumbar subarachnoid injection, are consistent with a supraspinal action.

Intraventricularly injected morphine was rapidly distributed into the subarachnoid space in our patients. Drug concentration–time profiles were similar in all cases, indicating that diffusion within the CSF and the CSF bulk flow, which are the major determinants of morphine distribution through the CSF circulation, have little fluctuation between patients. The prolonged elimination of morphine (a drug with a low lipid solubility) from the CSF is consistent with the long-lasting analgesia observed. The relatively low lumbar concentrations as compared with ventricular levels suggest that analgesia is elicited mainly at the supraspinal level. Pain relief was seen to vanish when lumbar morphine concentrations fell below a critical level of 200 ng/ml in patients treated with intrathecal morphine (8), and our patients had such a concentration only for a short time following intraventricular injection. It is likely, however, that simultaneous activation of the spinal opiate-sensitive system also contributes to or reinforces supraspinally induced analgesia.

Finally, we found that intraventricular morphine increases central dopaminergic and serotoninergic turnover, but whether or not these changes relate to analgesia remains unknown (7).

CONCLUSION

Intraventricular administration of morphine seems to be a satisfactory analgesic method that should be reserved for carefully selected patients having otherwise intractable pain and a short life expectancy. The method could be improved by developing new reliable infusion systems and new synthetic drugs liable to retain the analgesic effects of morphine while eliminating the unwanted effects.

REFERENCES

1. Basbaum, A. I., Moss, M. S., and Glazer, E. J. (1983): Opiate and stimulation-produced analgesia: The contribution of monoamines. In: *Advances in Pain Research and Therapy,* Vol. 5, edited by J. Bonica, U. Lindblom, and A. Iggo, pp. 323–339. Raven Press, New York.
2. Coombs, D. W., Saunders, R. L., and Pageau, M. S. (1982): Continuous intraspinal narcotic analgesia. *Reg. Anesth.,* 7:110–113.
3. Chauvin, M., Samii, J., Schermann, J. M., Sandouk, P., Bourdon, R., and Viars, P. (1981): Plasma concentration of morphine after i.m., extradural and intrathecal administration. *Br. J. Anaesth.,* 53:911–913.
4. Fields, H. L., and Basbaum, A. I. (1978): Brainstem control of spinal pain-transmission neurons. *Annu. Rev. Physiol.,* 40:193–221.
5. Gebhart, G. F. (1982): Opiate and opioid peptide effects on brain stem neurons: relevance to nociception and antinociceptive mechanisms. *Pain,* 12:93–140.
6. Gent, J. P., and Wolstencroft, J. H. (1976): Actions of morphine, enkaphalin and endorphine on single neurones in the brainstem, including the raphe and the periaqueductal gray, of the cat. In: *Opiates and Endogenous Opioid Peptides,* edited by H. W. Kosterlitz, pp. 217–224. North Holland, Amsterdam.
7. Ghia, J. N., Mueller, R. A., Duncan, G. H., Scott, D. S., and Mao, W. (1981): Serotoninergic activity in man as a function of pain, pain mechanisms and depression. *Anesth. Analg. (Cleve.),* 60:854–861.
8. Lazorthes, Y., Gouarderes, C., Verdie, J. C., Monsarrat, B., Bastide, R., Campan, L., Alwan, A., and Cros, J. (1980): Analgésie par injection intrathécale de morphine. *Neurochirurgie,* 26:159–164.
9. Leavens, M. E., Hills, C. S., Cech, D. A., Weyland, J. B., and Weston, J. S. (1982): Intrathecal and intraventricular morphine for pain in cancer patients: Initial study. *J. Neurosurg.,* 56:241–245.
10. Le Bars, D., Dickenson, A. H., and Besson, J. M. (1983): Opiate analgesia and descending control systems. In: *Advances in Pain Research and Therapy,* Vol. 5, edited by J. Bonica, U. Lindblom, and A. Iggo, pp. 341–372. Raven Press, New York.
11. Lobato, R. D., Madrid, J. L., Fatela, L. V., Rivas, J. J., Reig, E., and Lamas, E. (1983): Intraventricular morphine for control of pain in terminal cancer patients. *J. Neurosurg.,* 59:627–633.
12. Mayer, D. J. (1979): Endogenous analgesia systems: Neural and behavioral mechanisms. In: *Advances in Pain Research and Therapy,* Vol. 3, edited by J. Bonica, J. C. Liebeskind, and D. G. Albe-Fessard, pp. 385–410. Raven Press, New York.
13. Meyerson, B. A. (1983): Electrostimulation procedures: Effects, presumed rationale, and possible mechanisms. In: *Advances in Pain Research and Therapy*, Vol. 5, edited by J. Bonica, U. Lindblom, and A. Iggo, pp. 495–534. Raven Press, New York.
14. Morris, B. A. (1975): Development of radioimmunoassay for morphine having minimal crossreactivity with codeine. *J. Endocrinol.,* 64:6–7.
15. Onofrio, B. M., Yaksh, T. L., and Arnold, P. G. (1981): Continuous low-dose intrathecal morphine administration in the treatment of chronic pain of malignant origin. *Mayo Clin. Proc.,* 56:516–520.
16. Roquefeuil, B., Benezech, J., Batier C., Blanchet, P., Gros, C., and Mathieu-Daude, J.

(1983): Intéret de l'analgésie morphinique par voie ventriculaire dans les algies rebelles neoplasiques. *Neurochirurgie,* 29:135–141.
17. Twycross, R. G. (1983): Narcotic analgesics in clinical practice. In: *Advances in Pain Research and Therapy,* Vol. 5, edited by J. Bonica, U. Lindblom, and A. Iggo, pp. 534–559. Raven Press, New York.
18. Wang, J. K. (1977): Analgesic effect of intrathecally administered morphine. *Reg. Anesth.,* 2:3–8.
19. Westerink, B. H. C. (1977): Neurochemical methods for the study of putative transmitter metabolism in the nervous system. In: *Manual IBRO-UNESCO Training Course,* edited by Karl-Marx University Press, pp. 84–99. Leipzig.
20. Yaksh, T. L. (1981): Spinal opiate analgesia: Characteristics and principles of action. *Pain,* 11:293–346.
21. Yaksh, T. L., and Rudy, T. A. (1978): Narcotic analgesics CNS sites and mechanisms of action as revealed by intracerebral injection techniques. *Pain,* 4:299–359.

Editorial : Comment on the Use of Nonhuman Animals in Pain Research

The following chapter by Michael Allen Fox was prepared as part of the special symposium on ethics in animal experimentation that was held at the IVth World Congress on Pain, the proceedings of which are presented in this volume. It is important to emphasize that the views expressed by Dr. Fox do not represent those of the International Association for the Study of Pain (IASP) or the organizers of the Congress. It was our original intention to have multiple points of view presented so that readers would receive exposure to the different ideas expressed by philosophers, ethicists, scientists, and laypeople on this important subject. This editorial comment is an attempt to provide an alternative view to that of Dr. Fox.

Dr. Fox presents a point of view that provides philosophical justification for "speciesism," or the exploitation of one species for the benefit of another. He states, "that lacking to various degrees possession of the capacities upon which moral autonomy or agency depends, animals fail to meet the conditions specified for full membership in the moral community and likewise fail to qualify for the having of rights." Although he later points out that the infliction of unnecessary pain and suffering in animals is morally irresponsible, his focus on "rights" differs from other philosophers such as Caplan (1) who focus rather on the status of animals as objects of moral concern. Caplan stresses that we should examine what to do "when the needs of human beings come into conflict with the interests of animals and what principles of morality should govern" in such situations (1). We need to act from a position of moral stewardship in which animals are considered worthy of respect. We have a moral obligation to protect them from excessive pain and suffering in our experimentation. The IASP guidelines (4) are an attempt to develop such an approach. The IASP has accepted the responsibility ". . . to regulate (its) own affairs in such a way as to avoid the charge that (it) is a society dedicated to the infliction of pain" (3). We prefer that we develop our guidelines from a position of moral responsibility rather than debating human versus animal rights. Dr. Fox's views can be used to justify human dominance and exploitation of animals. On the other hand, the views of animal rightists can lead to the prohibition of valuable animal research that is necessary to reduce human pain and suffering. Neither approach will solve our own special dilemma: as pain researchers we need to produce the very sensations that all ethical guidelines for animal experimentation declare must be eliminated or reduced (2).

The Editors

REFERENCES

1. Caplan, A. L. (1983): Animals do have rights. *Nature,* 306:110.
2. Dubner, R. (1983): Pain research in Animals. *Annals N.Y. Acad. Sci.,* 406:128–132.

3. Iggo, A. (1979): Experimental study of pain in animals—ethical aspects. In: *Advances in Pain Research and Therapy, Vol. 3,* edited by J. J. Bonica, J. C. Liebeskind, and D. G. Albe-Fessard, pp. 773–778. Raven Press, New York.
4. Zimmermann, M. (for the Committee for Research and Ethical Issues) (1983): Ethical guidelines for investigations of experimental pain in conscious animals. *Pain,* 16:109–110.

Advances in Pain Research and Therapy, Vol. 9, edited by H. L. Fields et al. Raven Press, New York © 1985.

Ethical Considerations in Painful Animal Research

Michael Allen Fox

Department of Philosophy, Queen's University, Kingston K7L 3N6, Ontario, Canada

In recent years the question of the moral status of nonhuman animals (hereafter, just "animals") has been under fairly intensive and continuous review by a growing number of philosophers and others. Philosophers have, of course, been interested in probing some of the more theoretical issues in this area, such as which ethical theory can best be brought to bear on the question of animals' moral status, and what characteristics may be cited as criteria for designating something as deserving of our moral concern. However, practical applications of their theoretical conclusions have not been wanting, and both philosophers and animal welfarists have focused a good deal of attention on specific areas of large-scale animal use (and, many would hasten to add, abuse), such as animal experimentation. Much of this intellectual ferment and discussion has had salutary effects in terms of increasing awareness on the part of animal users, and this in turn has yielded greater sensitivity to animal suffering and consequently better treatment and care in laboratories and elsewhere. Even antivivisectionist pressures, while exercising a largely negative impact, have played a role in this process. A number of scientific organizations, such as IASP (1), NIH (2), the American Physiological Society (3), and the Society for Neuroscience (4), have reflected carefully and productively on the welfare of laboratory animals and have drafted more enlightened sets of guidelines for workers in the fields concerned.

Though there is no doubt that philosophers involved with animal welfare issues would benefit from greater exposure to scientific research and its methodological requirements and practical constraints, scientists sometimes recognize their need for more solid grounding in the conceptual and ethical considerations that underlie questions of both principle and practice. A brief survey of some of these issues may therefore be in order at this point. In what follows, I shall concentrate on addressing the following questions: (a) What features identify a being as deserving of moral concern in the fullest sense? (b) Are animals our moral equals, i.e., what is the moral status of animals? (c) Does animal experimentation require a moral justification? (d) What is the basis of our moral concern for animals? (e) What does moral concern for animals entail for scientists using laboratory animals? My aim in answering these questions will be to develop a position that will place the ethics of animal experimentation in its proper perspective.

What features identify a being as deserving of moral concern in the fullest sense? A being deserves our fullest degree of moral concern if it possesses those characteristics that we associate with membership in the moral community. My intention in saying this is, of course, not to define animals out of the realm of morality but to indicate that in order to understand what makes a being worthy of our moral concern, we do best to examine first the paradigm case. For while most philosophers will admit that the basis of the moral community is difficult to fathom, they will also agree that the moral status of animals is even more problematic. The paradigm case of moral concern, then, is that for *persons,* or *autonomous beings* like ourselves.

What is an autonomous being, and why is the distinction between things that are autonomous and those that are not so important? An autonomous being is one that is critically self-aware and has the capacity to manipulate concepts in complex ways, use a sophisticated language, reflect, plan, deliberate, choose, and accept responsibility for acting. In other words, an autonomous being can act freely, choose and decide rationally in the fullest sense, and engage in self-making or self-realizing activities. Such a being possesses a range of specialized cognitive abilities that are the essential tools or vehicles by means of which its autonomy evolves, is made known to itself reflexively, and is manifested or expressed to others. We call this kind of being an *agent* or a *person,* because it has the capacity for fully self-conscious, voluntary, and deliberate action—action that can be evaluated, appraised, judged, or otherwise normatively assessed.

Saying that a human is critically self-aware does not simply mean that, ape-like, he (read he or she) can recognize and respond to a mirror image of himself; it implies a whole gamut of qualities. A human being is aware of himself perceptually, to be sure, but also of himself as an object among objects, as a person, as an independent individual with his own integrity, sense of purpose, and worth. He has a concept of his own life—its origin, duration, self-guided direction, and terminus in death—of world history, and of the limitless reaches of time and space beyond the self. He can foresee the possible consequences of his acts and estimate the relative probabilities of each. He can appreciate the necessity for both self-expression and self-regulation. Humans are beings who, because of their acute sense of self, experience anxiety, guilt, despair, shame, remorse, internal conflict, pride, hope, triumph, and so many other emotion-laden states. Initiative, the choice of values, judgment, and role-playing are also expressions of self-awareness in humans. These reflexive acts of consciousness constitute what I call *critical self-awareness,* because humans monitor their own activities, interactions with others, inner states, and levels of self-development on an intermittent basis. We are complicated feedback systems psychologically as well as neurologically. The flow of our conscious life is constantly altered by self-examination, revision, addition, and deletion, and we constantly conduct thought-experiments aimed at improving either mental or physical performance. As a consequence, our behavior is and expresses itself as subject to our own scrutiny, self-direction, and "fine tuning." Each of us has a self-image that is itself a product of our own activity and is open to modification through self-criticism as we express ourselves through various ongoing engagements with the world. It is in this sense that existentialists and those influenced by them have spoken of creative potential, "self-making," or "self-realization."

Only a being with highly evolved cognitive capacities such as the ability to symbolize, think abstractly, reflect, imagine, calculate, invent and solve complex problems, recollect and project could have this kind of awareness and the degree of freedom from and control over the world that it affords. The evolution of complex spoken languages that can serve as vehicles for self-expression and convey the subtleties of human cognitive processes extends the domain of freedom and control manyfold by opening up the possibility of pooled mind-power and cooperative effort. Along with the high degree of freedom from natural necessity possible for *Homo sapiens* come deliberation, choice, and responsibility—the essential ingredients of moral decision-making. Humans' critical self-awareness enables them to envision alternatives, reflect on possible scenarios and outcomes, and optimize benefits through careful selection and organization of appropriate behavior. Each self, then, is essentially expressed in many of its voluntary acts, namely, those governed by deliberation and choice. The context of such acts is that of agency and autonomy, and it is here that we find the assigning of and the willingness to accept responsibility.

Beings that possess the sorts of characteristics I have just been discussing—critical self-awareness; the ability to manipulate complex concepts and to use a sophisticated language (especially for the purpose of communicating wishes, desires, needs, decisions, choices, etc.) (5); the capacity to reflect, plan, deliberate, choose, and accept responsibility for acting—are alone capable of functioning as rational moral agents. It is because they have the capacity for long-range planning, anticipating consequences, choosing among alternative courses of action, taking responsibility, making and following rules, etc., that they can engage in moral behavior, or, in other words, actions that affect others as well as themselves and that are subject to moral appraisal. Furthermore, the possession of these characteristics, plus the capacities to recognize them in others and to care about others, goes a long way toward explaining what we mean by speaking of ourselves as persons. I submit that a moral community is a social group composed of just such interacting autonomous beings, a community within which moral concepts and precepts can evolve and be understood. It is also a social group in which mutual recognition of autonomy and personhood exists. The latter feature is equally important and indeed inseparable from the former, because accountability and the development of moral institutions (6) are contingent on recognition of and respect for persons and their interests.

Are animals our moral equals, i.e., what is the moral status of animals? It follows from the foregoing considerations that only autonomous or self-directed beings (persons or agents) can have full moral status, whether this is defined in terms of membership in the moral community and the possession of rights, as I would define it, or in terms of equal consideration of interests or some other criterion. This is so because: (a) autonomous beings alone are capable of free (self-determining, voluntary), deliberative, responsible action and have the sort of awareness necessary to see this kind of action as essential to their nature, well-being, and development as individuals; (b) autonomous beings alone are capable of recognizing autonomy in others and of full participation in the moral community, as already described. It is neither arbitrary nor arrogant to hold that all and only such beings—beings that have interests that can be harmed if they are not protected—qualify for the possession of rights. Assigning rights to others and claiming them for oneself are tantamount to issuing a declaration of non-intervention in the self-governing lives of others in accordance with an acknowledgment of the sort of beings they are, and acquiring mutual guarantees of this type by tacit agreement. (That is: "All things being equal, I agree to recognize your autonomy and not interfere with its free expression and development if you agree to do the same for me.")

It is for this reason that philosophers have generally regarded rights and obligations as logically connected or inseparably correlated. If I have a right, then others are deemed to have a duty to respect that right, which means either to refrain from interfering with my free exercise of it or to assist me in attaining what I have a right to, as the case may be and as circumstances require and permit.

The conclusion to be drawn, so far as it pertains to animals, is that lacking to various degrees possession of the capacities on which moral autonomy or agency depends, animals fail to meet the conditions specified for full membership in the moral community (7) and likewise fail to qualify for the having of rights. But if they have no rights, and obligations signify the respect for rights, then we have, strictly speaking, no obligations toward animals. Because animals cannot begin to function as equals in a society of autonomous beings, they cannot be counted within the bond of association that makes morality and its institutions viable and gives them vitality.

It is important to underscore here the fact that membership in the moral community is not a cut-and-dried affair. How many and what kinds of affinities with ourselves a creature must exhibit before being counted as autonomous is not something that can be decided in the abstract, but rather has to be examined on a species-by-species basis or even (sometimes) a case-by-case basis. (It will, perhaps, have been noticed that I have spoken of autonomous *beings* or *persons* rather than humans as members of the moral community. Although humans are, so far as we know, the sole members of the moral community, I have avoided excluding *as a matter of principle* the possibility that other species or individuals could also claim membership.) Animals are not an undifferentiated or virtually identical collection of organisms, even if much of the philosophical literature on ethics and animals—regardless of the viewpoint being expressed—persists in generalizing about "animals" in such a way that everything from microorganisms to chimpanzees is indiscriminately embraced.

Utilitarians would object to the line of argument presented thus far, however, because they acknowledge *the capacity to suffer* as the only relevant criterion for membership in the moral community. But whereas it might plausibly be held that this capacity is a *necessary* condition for a being to achieve full moral status, it is not a *sufficient* condition. That utilitarians have thought it is sufficient springs, I believe, from a fundamental mistake in their perception of human nature and motivation, from which they then generalize erroneously to the rest of sentient nature.

What the utilitarians have failed to appreciate concerning human nature is that pleasure and pain (or pleasure and suffering; pleasure and displeasure) are not the sole reference points to which we can appeal when judging of a thing's value or disvalue. Robert Nozick's descriptive account of what it is to be an autonomous agent helps clarify this point. For Nozick, an autonomous being—specifically a human—is

> a being able to formulate long-term plans for its life, able to consider and decide on the basis of abstract principles or considerations it formulates to itself and hence not merely the plaything of immediate stimuli, a being that limits its own behavior in accordance with some principles or picture it has of what an appropriate life is for itself and others, and so on. . . . Such an overall conception, and knowing how we are doing in terms of it, is important to the kind of goals we formulate for ourselves and the kind of beings we are. [8]

The conclusion that should be drawn here, surely, is that humans, as autonomous agents, are beings whose lives have greater value than those of animals because they have almost unlimited potential for self-guided development and growth. This also explains why it is even reasonable to say that human suffering is generally of greater concern than that of animals. The range of possible conditions—to which animals are not subject—that can produce the sense of thwarted agency, diminished selfhood or ineffectualness, from which suffering so often arises, is astronomically high. This is why many philosophers of the past and present have asserted that man is not destined to be happy. Even John Stuart Mill, let us remember, reflected on this problem (9): "It is better to be a human being dissatisfied than a pig satisfied; better to be Socrates dissatisfied than a fool satisfied." If, by being more complex creatures, humans gain significantly in potential sources of pleasure, as the utilitarians too seem prepared to assert, then by the same token they also acquire many more potential sources of suffering. It is because we are the sort of beings that can have a "life plan" at all and, paradoxically, because we can seek ends other than pleasure and the avoidance of suffering that our potential for suffering (and pleasure) is so great.

Does animal experimentation require a moral justification? I have tried to show why we have no strict moral obligations toward animals. And if this is so, it follows that there is no compelling ethical reason why we may not use them for experimentation. Because anything that is not prohibited by a moral imperative of some kind is morally permissible, and because the use of animals for experimentation is not morally prohibited, then this practice falls within the class of actions that are morally permissible. We do not need a correlative *right* to give the seal of approval to everything we do. Animal liberationists frequently talk as if we do, in order to show, allegedly, how shameful our normal practices are. Thus, for example, it is often asked what *right* we have to incarcerate animals or take their lives for the sake of research. If we are forced to speak this way, the correct answer would undoubtedly be that we are "entitled" or have a "justification" to do these things because they are morally permissible, not because we have a "right" to continue doing so.

However, it may still be thought that animal experimentation requires moral justification at least to the extent that it involves suffering. For even if suffering is not *the* central concept of morality, it is certainly an important concern of morality. Not only is suffering deemed to be inherently bad, but we also find repellant the idea of deriving benefits from acts that we know in advance will cause pain to other sentient creatures, whether or not they are members of our own species. But I would nevertheless affirm that animal experimentation is morally permissible even if and to the extent to which it does involve suffering. This is so because the pain animals may be subjected to, although an important matter of concern, is in most cases of lesser moral significance than those things it is weighed against. Animals, not being autonomous agents, lack interests in the moral sense, whereas humans (for example) *do* possess autonomy in the specified sense, and thus have interests, such as an interest in avoiding suffering and securing well-being and health. If it happens to be the case that animal experimentation is an unavoidable means to this end, then the suffering of animals that such research entails may be outweighed by the benefits accruing to the end being sought.

What I have just put forward may be identified as a "lesser evil" argument; but it is more than this. For one may expand it by adding that animal experimentation is *morally imperative* if there is no other way to obtain the kinds of knowledge needed for alleviation of potentially much greater suffering in both humans and animals. If the guiding purposes behind animal experimentation are the alleviation of suffering (in the broadest sense) in both humans and animals and the accumulation of knowledge to the extent that it may conceivably contribute to this end, however, I see no reason why research and humaneness should not be compatible.

What is the basis of our moral concern for animals? Five considerations seem relevant to answering this question. The first is *empathy,* our ability to relate to the sufferings of other creatures. The second is *evolutionary continuity,* our recognition of the degrees of biological and behavioral proximity of other species to our own. The third is the *ecological perspective,* or our sense of belonging to a balanced, self-sustaining system together with other animals and living things on which our lives and the preservation of our species depend. The fourth is the *demeaning nature of cruelty,* the moral corruption we all identify with deliberately harmful or malicious acts and therefore wish to avoid. The fifth is *enlightened collective self-interest,* our desire to guard against the deleterious practical consequences of cruel behavior as experienced by all of us or by its perpetrators. (For example, misleading scientific data may result from experiments on animals that receive substandard care; cruelty, more generally practiced, may bring about the extinction of certain species.) These considerations, taken in conjunction, appear to me sufficient to establish an appropriate level of moral concern on our part for the well-being of other creatures—what we might call a "weak obligation" to treat animals humanely and to limit the ways in which we utilize them to serve our ends. Thus, animals have a kind of limited or adjunct moral status, and we may speak of degrees of ethical continuity (hence concern) depending on their biological and behavioral similarity to us.

There is a tendency in discussions of the ethics of animal research—especially on the part of those associated with the animal welfare movement—to describe excesses as examples of cruelty rather than of inhumaneness. I have myself just been talking about why cruelty to animals is wrong. However, I take it that the word "cruelty" connotes the deliberate or wanton infliction of suffering, whereas "inhumaneness" covers callousness, indifference, or insensitivity toward suffering, as well as neglect, thoughtlessness, and related forms of moral irresponsibility. It seems to me that where moral concerns arise in the context of laboratory animal science, inhumaneness rather than cruelty is more likely to be at issue. Inhumaneness is the cause of what we generally call "unnecessary suffering" (though what this means is seldom spelled out). What kind of suffering is unnecessary, and how is it to be avoided? In the context of animal experimentation, I define suffering as unnecessary when it is *morally unacceptable* because either *excessive* or *preventable,* i.e., dispensable. Moral assessment of experiments on animals has to be done in terms of commonly accepted, reasonable humane standards, and in terms of the salient benefits of the experiments to humans and/or animals, in order to determine that excessive suffering is not being caused.

What does moral concern for animals entail for scientists using laboratory animals? It seems reasonable to require that a research proposal show that the methods or procedures utilized constitute either the *only* way to attack a particular problem or test a key concept or theory, or else the *best* way of all those available. If the latter contention were being advanced, considerations regarding the relative costs of the alternatives, their reliability, the time likely to be consumed by each, and similar factors would be vital to gaining a full picture. A full picture would, as I understand it, show that the degree of animal suffering in question is offset by practical benefits to humans or animals, or else by a contribution to scientific knowledge that most informed persons would judge to be of a significance proportionate to the amount of suffering caused.

Possible modifications of experimental technique that might reduce animal suffering noticeably without affecting the viability of the inquiry should also be considered. This would include such things as increasing the amounts of anesthesia or analgesia employed, reducing the number of animals used, reducing the number of trial runs, altering the animals' diet or housing conditions, shortening the length of time an aversive stimulus is administered or a pathological state is allowed to persist, and changing the method of euthanasia. Ethics committees that review and approve research protocols in advance of an experiment are frequently quite diligent and helpful in this connection.

Clearly, then, an experiment that entails animal suffering and that contravenes the principles inherent in these categories of ethical or moral assessment is one that may be said to produce unnecessary suffering. A scientist who conducts such a piece of research may be judged to be acting inhumanely and to be responsible for causing unnecessary suffering, especially if he has deliberately chosen to disregard available, cost-effective means to reduce suffering that perhaps would not impair in any way the efficiency of his work or undermine the significance of his results.

Feasible alternatives to the use of live or "higher" animals should be explored carefully by a researcher (including the use of human subjects) to further assure that preventable suffering is avoided. Such suffering results, then, when he fails to take advantage of measures (compatible with the given experimental objectives) aimed at reducing either the number of animals used or the number of trials run, or when he overlooks or ignores modifications to experimental design or procedures that are in the interests of minimizing pain and stress.

It seems to me that assuring that animal experiments do not cause unnecessary suffering in either of the two senses specified earlier—that is, that the suffering is neither excessive nor preventable—is quite consistent with and possibly even conceptually inseparable from the overriding notion of stewardship, understood as an attitude that requires the responsible, wise, and prudent use of resources of all kinds.

Inevitably, a position such as the one I have set out here will have some far-reaching consequences for the scientific community. I shall briefly mention a few. First of all, humane education should be a feature of graduate studies and professional degree programs where animal research is essential to the training in question and/or the career to which it leads. Periodic refresher courses emphasizing sensitization to suffering and new humane techniques and alternatives to live animals might also be required of all practicing scientists and laboratory technicians. A thorough and up-to-date review of alternatives should become a standard procedure, where relevant, on all grant applications. These things would obviously add to the costs of training and of carrying out research, as well as to the time these activities consume, and some would no doubt contend that they abridge freedom of inquiry to a certain extent, particularly if legislation rather than professional ethical guidelines is their source. Over time, certain experimental procedures might come to be deemed less acceptable and some species, such as chimpanzees, less appropriate subjects for experimentation from a moral standpoint. All of these results would clearly make many kinds of scientific investigation more difficult, at least in the short term. But no one ever said that doing the morally right thing is easy.

I conclude with a few remarks on pain research. Pain research presents a unique dilemma from a moral viewpoint. For here experimentation often requires the deliberate infliction of pain, which is, of course, the *sine qua non* for any research to take place. This dilemma is heightened by the use of animals for chronic pain studies. By the same token, however, pain research is a kind of ultimate inquiry because of the magnitude of its potential payoff—the control or even the elimination of pain itself. Such research could be warranted or defended on moral grounds if the amount and degree of suffering it produces (which I assume to be great) are not disproportionate to the benefits it is likely to yield. While there is no tidy recipe for performing such an ethical balancing act, pain research appears again to be somewhat unique in that its very existence as a field of knowledge is, as indicated earlier, inseparable from a dedication to practical applications of the most far-reaching sort for both humans and animals. This fact would appear to open the way to a strong argument in its defense.

NOTES

1. Zimmermann, M. (1983): Ethical guidelines for investigations of experimental pain in conscious animals. *Pain,* 16:109–110.
2. NIH guide for grants and contracts. *Laboratory Animal Welfare,* 1984, 13(5):1.
3. Guiding principles in the care and use of animals. *Am. J. Physiol.,* 1984, 246(4):part 2.
4. Ad Hoc Committee on Animals in Research, Society for Neuroscience (1984): *Guidelines for the Use of Animals in Neuroscience Research.* Society for Neuroscience.

5. McCloskey, H. J. (1975): The right to life. *Mind,* 84:413.
6. Such as promise-keeping, truth-telling, the making of contractual agreements, and giving mutual aid in emergencies. For further discussion of this point, see W. T. Blackstone, "Human Rights and Human Dignity," in Ervin Laszlo and Rubin Goetsky, eds., *Human Dignity: This Century and the Next* (New York: Gordon & Breach, 1970).
7. A common rejoinder to the sort of position being advanced here is that it excludes so-called marginal human beings (those who are severely retarded, irreversibly comatose or senile, badly brain-damaged, etc.) from the moral community just as surely as it does animals. For some animals may approach closer to autonomy than these hapless members of our own species. It is then argued that moral concern should depend solely on the capacity to suffer, which is universal among humans, but also establishes animals as deserving of equal moral consideration. However, because *no* capacity is truly universal, the capacity to suffer included (see D. W. Baxter and J. Olszewski, "Congenital Universal Insensitivity to Pain," *Brain,* 83:381–393, 1960), it would seem relevant to consider, when establishing a being's moral status, the capacities possessed by a *typical* member of its species at maturity, given normal development. Looked at in this way, infants and "marginal" humans bear a closer "family resemblance" to us than do even healthy animals.
8. Nozick, R. (1974): *Anarchy, State, and Utopia,* p. 49. Basic Books, New York. Cf. Nozick, R. (1981): *Philosophical Explanations,* pp. 577–578. Belknap Press, Harvard University Press, Cambridge, Mass.
9. Mill, J. S. (1863): *Utilitarianism,* Chapter 2.

Advances in Pain Research and Therapy, Vol. 9, edited by H. L. Fields et al. Raven Press, New York © 1985.

Clinical Pharmacology of Opiate Analgesia

R. A. Boas, N. H. G. Holford, and J. W. Villiger

Section of Anaesthetics and Department of Pharmacology and Clinical Pharmacology, University of Auckland School of Medicine, Auckland, New Zealand

Advances relating to the processes of nociception and analgesia have led to a better understanding of pharmacological treatment of pain. Appropriate choices of individual drugs can now be made together with rational guidelines for their use in normal and disease states. These two issues form the substance of this chapter as they relate to opiate analgesics.

DOSE–RESPONSE RELATIONSHIPS: A FUNCTIONAL CLASSIFICATION

One consideration in making a drug choice depends on the maximum analgesic response that the drug might provide in meeting pain relief. A broad grouping of opiates, as shown in Fig. 1, provides three categories of these drugs based on their limits of analgesic effect at supramaximal doses, i.e., their *efficacy.* This describes the intrinsic pharmacological activities of opiates without consideration of structure, source, receptor binding, or body disposition. Response characteristics for the three groups define the full agonists, the partial agonists, including mixed agonist/antagonist agents, and the opiate antagonists (1).

Agonists are those drugs capable of eliciting a maximum possible response in the system or organism under test, such as fentanyl, morphine, and methadone. The pharmacological analgesic and nonanalgesic responses evoked by these drugs acting at opioid receptors all appear to run in parallel (2). When less than a maximum response is obtained, the intrinsic activity of the drug must be less, producing a result that manifests as a ceiling limit or plateau level of response beyond which further dosing increments generate no further pain relief. Drugs exhibiting these characteristics are termed *partial agonists.* This applies to dextropropoxyphene salts (Darvon, Progesic) and probably to codeine and its various derivatives, though testing of very high doses has not been undertaken experimentally to determine their maximum possible responses.

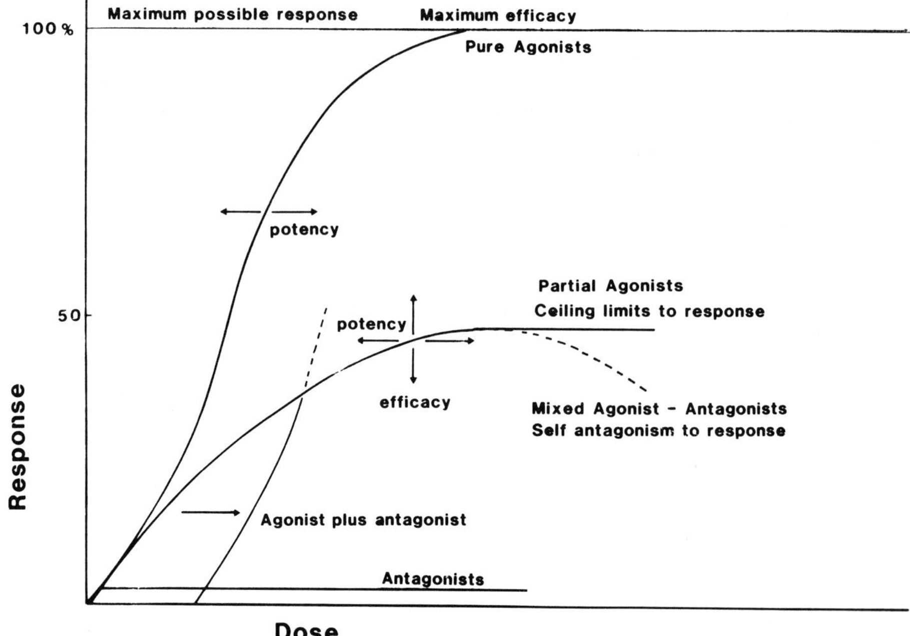

FIG. 1. Dose–response curves depicting differences between classes of opiates. All agonists give the same maximum response, but at different dose levels (potency). Partial agonists show a lesser efficacy, with variable individual peak responses. A subgroup of partial agonists, the mixed agonist/antagonist opiates, show initial partial agonist responses, succeeded by self-antagonism at supramaximal doses. Antagonists exhibit no intrinsic pharmacological activity *(flat line),* but in the presence of other opioids they act to competitively displace them, shifting the dose–response curve to the right.

More recently, new drug developments have focused on a group of partial agonists that also show subsequent reduction in pharmacological action with progressive dosing increments beyond those giving a ceiling response. This is shown by the curved dotted line in Fig. 1. Such drugs as meptazinol, nalbuphine, butorphanol, pentazocine, and buprenorphine manifest this self-antagonism in high doses, giving a type of partial agonist often described as *mixed agonist/antagonist.* The basis for this mixed response probably lies in the type of opioid receptors involved in generating the drug action and the extent to which the cell membrane amplifier systems are activated directly or indirectly by each receptor type. Major advantages arising from this response are the lessened risk of respiratory depression induced with overdosing and the lesser potential for drug abuse and addiction. Respiratory depression occurs, but not to any profound extent, probably running parallel with analgesic efficacy. Whereas efforts and claims have been made for better analgesic selectivity, devoid of these and other untoward responses, no drug in the opiate class has yet been demonstrated to provide analgesia without concomitant opioid side effects.

The drug-receptor complex formed by the clinically used *antagonists* naloxone and naltrexone generates no direct pharmacological effect other than to competitively inhibit the binding of other opioid compounds to the same receptor. Ultimately, the drug effect that dominates will depend on the relative concentrations of the agents at the receptor site as well as their affinities for each of the opioid receptors. These characteristics are also shown in Fig. 1, where increasing shifts in the dose–response curve to the right are brought about with introduction of additional antagonists. Also shown is the property of potency for a drug, indicating that this is the relative dosing needed for agents to attain the same responses. This is differentiated from the maximum response or ceiling limit attainable, which is a lower analgesic efficacy, as discussed for partial agonists.

Within each of the opiate subgroups just discussed, the particular effect that each drug manifests is initially dependent on its access to and concentration at each of the receptor sites. A further determinant is then the drug's affinity for the receptor subgroups. Focusing first on the considerations of drug access to the receptor sites reveals a set of complex kinetic factors that determine differences in drug transfer from sites of delivery to transport in plasma and then to tissue compartments, which all continue as a dynamic process. A common approach to analysis of these kinetic factors is through conceptual models and the study of pharmacokinetics.

DRUG KINETICS AND DRUG ACTIONS

Compartmental models can be described, in part, by using parameters of *volume of distribution* V_D, defining the apparent size of each compartment of drug distribution, and by *clearance* Cl, describing the transfer of drug between and out of each compartment or organ. While there may be limited physical reality in this modeling, such concepts can be used to predict the time course and intensity of drug action from plasma concentration analyses. This is well exemplified in the review of Mather and Meffin (23) in their analysis of intravenous, intramuscular, and oral dosing schedules. Important clinical advances such as the introduction of sublingual buprenorphine and controlled-release morphine were aided by such pharmacokinetic analyses (9,36). Although pharmacokinetic studies in general can give guidance to dosing schedules for patients in chronic pain, further special considerations are needed for the more acutely ill patients who also need effective and safe analgesia. These people often present with abnormal physiological function in terms of cardiac output, organ perfusion, or hepatic and renal function. In these cases it is perhaps more relevant to perceive their dosing needs and variables in a physiological sense of organ mass and its blood flow. The extent of drug extraction from the bloodstream by a particular tissue is then determined by the mass of the tissue, its perfusion, and the tissue:blood partition coefficient (solubility) for that drug. Agents differ widely in their solubility and therefore uptake, especially into fat tissues, and so laboratory indices of solubility (octanol:water partition coefficient) are frequently provided to quantify this characteristic. Though lipid solubility is not the sole determinant of the movement of drugs within the body, there is a close association between solubility and uptake and exit from body compartments. For drugs of high lipid solubility such as fentanyl (octanol:water = 1,000), the concentration–time curves for drug in bloodstream and brain behave very much like those for the anesthetic induction agents. The brain, being a very highly perfused tissue with high lipid content, takes a much higher proportion and total amount of a drug such as fentanyl than with less lipid-soluble agents like morphine (octanol:water = $\sim$1) (22). Thus, fentanyl reaches rapid equilibrium between plasma and brain with little gradient (18). On the other hand, only 1/1,000 of a given dose of morphine enters the entire central nervous system (6,25), taking up to 30 min to peak after intravenous injection, sustaining a concentration gradient of 10:1 between plasma and brain (21). Use of the more soluble but inactive acetylated form of morphine (heroin), as discussed by Foley and associates in the next chapter, gives more rapid drug entry into the brain, where almost immediate enzymatic deacetylation yields active morphine to bring about a more rapid action (19). Another application of morphine's distinctive solubility difference is manifest following its epidural or intrathecal use. Because of its lipid insolubility, morphine is retained within the cerebrospinal fluid (CSF) against high concentration gradients, giving both high potency and extended duration of effect. Functional and anatomical specificity are also retained unless cephalad flow of CSF carries the drug to rostral sites in the brainstem, as discussed by Bromage in this volume.

In practice, the need is to make correct dosing decisions for drug use by either oral or parenteral injection. Oral dosing is subjected to the further variable of *bioavailability,* wherein only a limited proportion of the given drug becomes available for systemic distribution because of hepatic uptake and metabolism during passage from the gut to the systemic bloodstream. Clearly, if 50% of a given pethidine (meperidine) dose is metabolized by the liver following oral ingestion, before the drug is circulated in the body (first-pass metabolism), a dose at least twice the intramuscular or intravenous dose will need to be given over the same time course in order to achieve the equivalent analgesic response. Unfortunately, there is no fixed ratio of metabolism during absorption for all patients. For instance, the bioavailability of morphine varied from 15 to 64% across a group of patients suffering cancer pain (29) because of differences in first-pass metabolism. Although intramuscular and intravenous routes of drug delivery offer 100% bioavailability, the drug is still subject to a sequence of kinetic influences *(vide infra)* that determine the intensity and duration of its pharmacological actions. Furthermore, it is apparent from the foregoing discussion that there are several other inherent drug and patient factors that influence the extent of a patient's response to a given dose of drug.

DRUG KINETICS AND TIME COURSE OF RESPONSE

Onset of Action and Drug Distribution

Absorption of drug raises the plasma drug concentration, leading to rapid uptake into richly perfused brain tissue, as the drug moves along its concentration gradient. The rates at which drugs cross the blood-brain barrier differ markedly. The more readily this process occurs, the more rapid the onset of action.

Peak Effect

The drug dose and its route of administration will determine the rate of entry of drug into plasma and ultimately the maximum clinical response that is produced. However, the peak drug effect occurs at the time when the plasma level begins to decline. This is brought about as a consequence of drug *redistribution,* whereby the drug moves from organs of rich perfusion (brain and heart) to tissues of greater mass, like muscle and fat. The total amount of drug taken up by these tissues then becomes considerable because of the greater proportionate mass of these other tissues. But because blood flow to tissues other than brain and heart is relatively slow at rest, this process of redistribution is quite slow. It may take 30 to 60 min before some tissue levels reach their peaks even after intravenous dosing. Well before this occurs, the decrease in brain concentration will have commenced, beginning as soon as the process of redistribution develops. As the body tissues like muscle take up drug, so plasma concentrations fall, creating a gradient from the brain to plasma, leading to a movement of drug back from richly perfused organs into plasma. It is at this point of reverse movement from the onset phase that the peak effect of opiate analgesia will have been generated. Stated alternatively, the peak effect arises when the rate of drug entering the brain equals the rate of drug exit. Intravenous administration attains peak plasma levels very quickly, but where the processes of drug uptake are sustained following intramuscular, oral, or sublingual use, so the time to peak effect is extended until the balance of drug uptake and drug removal from plasma is achieved. This may occur over an hour or be extended over several hours for slow-absorption drugs like controlled-release morphine or rectal oxycodone.

The rate of drug redistribution is dependent on tissue mass and solubility. The drug moves into tissues to produce large apparent volumes of distribution, resulting in a greater amount of drug in the tissues than in plasma. These processes are concentration-dependent in all phases of drug behavior. Distribution volumes are important clinically in that the duration of response varies directly with the volume of distribution for the drug in use.

Duration of Response: Drug Elimination

The cessation of clinical effect for opiate drugs is brought about by their elimination from the body by metabolic processes, undertaken principally by the liver. That is, total body clearance or the rate of elimination from the body is effectively hepatic clearance for opiate drugs. Clearance is a concentration-dependent process. Hepatic metabolism and subsequent renal excretion of inactive conjugated metabolites begin as soon as drug enters the plasma. It runs in conjunction with drug distribution and redistribution, all these functions being a dynamic process, with the particular dominance of each phase on the plasma concentration determining the pattern of drug response. The process of hepatic extraction is almost complete, and that of metabolic degradation to inactive agents is quite rapid; so the limiting factor of this process is the rate at which blood flow to the liver delivers drug for extraction and metabolism. Even so, elimination to the point of total loss of drug effect from plasma may take many hours, because drugs of high distribution volumes take a long time to achieve full washout from tissues. The exception among opiates in this respect is methadone, which has a much slower metabolic degradation than other agents, with an elimination half-life of 18 to 30 hr. Effective plasma levels are better sustained, allowing for effective twice daily dosing in moderate levels of chronic pain, or single, large intra-anesthetic dosing for treating postoperative pain (14).

In clinical practice it is convenient to express the time course of drug response in terms of plasma half-life, a measure of the time it takes for a drug to fall to a 50% level from its peak following single-dose administration. Average needs for dosing frequency can be guided by this value in stable patients, giving successive doses at the frequency of the half-life for the particular drug in use. Most agents other than methadone have half-lives roughly in the 2- to 4-hr time range. However, these values are derived as a consequence of drug distribution volume and drug clearance, each of which may be altered considerably in certain conditions requiring pain treatment. Safe practice and correct dosing schedules therefore require an examination of the more common deviations from normal function that might bring about untoward response patterns to opiate medication.

CLINICAL STATES INFLUENCING DRUG KINETICS

Tissue Perfusion and Drug Response

Given the importance of blood flow in determining the movement of drugs in the body, there will clearly be major changes in drug action whenever tissue perfusion is restricted or redistributed, as occurs in shock states. Severe pain requiring opiate medication is common in trauma, myocardial infarction, acute bowel disease, and internal hemorrhage, all disorders asso-

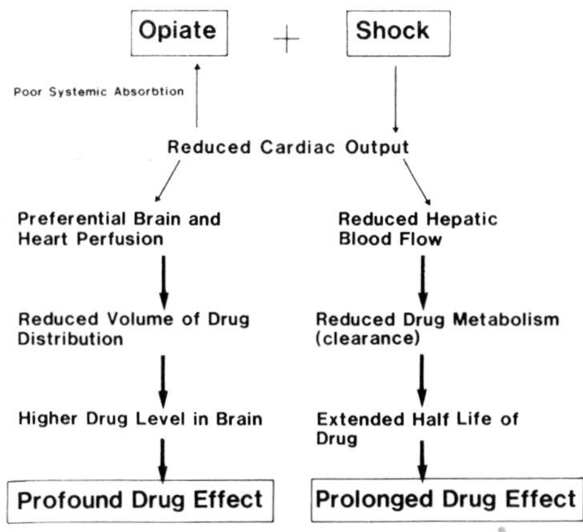

FIG. 2. Physiological disturbances associated with shock induce pharmacokinetic changes that alter drug effects. Limited tissue perfusion leads to poor systemic absorption if drug is ingested or given by intramuscular injection. Preferential perfusion of critical organs such as the brain, heart, and lungs restricts the volume of drug distribution, leading to a higher plasma concentration and a more profound effect for a given dose. This action is also prolonged because of reduced drug clearance associated with hepatic blood flow restriction.

ciated with physiological shock. The critical need in these states is to utilize small and frequent intravenous doses of opiate, titrated to the patient's needs. Drug administration by any other route leads to delayed and unpredictable absorption, with subsequent surges of drug entry into the circulation as perfusion improves under treatment of the disease state. This unregulated return may cause drug overdose and depression. Small doses may be needed because the volume of distribution is smaller than usual on account of poor perfusion to muscle and fat tissues. High plasma concentrations will also be developed more rapidly and sustained longer because of this reduced tissue blood flow, lessening drug distribution, redistribution, and metabolism, as summarized in Fig. 2.

Anesthesia and Opiate Dosing

The physiological and metabolic consequences of anesthesia also bring about a reduction in drug clearance of up to 50% over the time course of an average anesthetic (32). In single small-dose opiate supplementation of anesthesia this is of no practical concern, but the trend to high-dosage narcotic anesthetic techniques lends itself to the potential for opiate overdosing, especially in sustained surgical procedures. Such circumstances require assisted ventilation or close patient monitoring in the postoperative recovery period.

Chronic Opiate Dosing

Several biological changes may alter dosing needs over an extended time of pain management. Alteration in the disease state, for better or for worse, may require either lesser or greater doses, respectively. Treatment of cancer pain in particular can require quite large dosing increases, particularly as a terminal need. Over shorter terms of several weeks, induction of hepatic enzymes by the drug itself or other agents such as barbiturates, alcohol, etc., can lead to greater clearance. Methadone in particular, is subjected to this influence, sometimes necessitating a twofold dosage increase over the first 3 weeks of treatment. The factor of tolerance has sometimes been stated to be a cause of increasing dose demand, but such observations have been based on responses to overdosing, where tolerance to side effects does occur. However, where pain control has been established on the minimum effective dosage, experience indicates stable dosing needs can be sustained over periods of months or years (33,34).

Age Influences on Drug Responses

Age extremes also bring about altered drug handling within the body such that elderly patients and infants show greater responses to given doses of drug. Whereas differences in tissue mass play a small part in modifying the initial response, the greatest influence affecting drug action in the extremes of age are brought about as a result of reduced hepatic metabolism. In a study by Bentley et al. (5), two groups of healthy adults given fentanyl at 10 μg/kg showed plasma levels threefold higher in a group whose mean age was 67 years, as compared with those aged 36. Some of the explanation for the so-called sensitivity of the aged to opiates is provided by this study, which showed the higher plasma levels to be due to reduced drug clearance from metabolic impairment rather than distribution impairment. Neonates similarly have impaired hepatic-based metabolism.

DRUG DOSING

Given this knowledge of drug efficacy, dose–response relationships, and drug handling within the body, it would seem relatively easy to construct accurate dosing guides for virtually all patients needing opiate pain relief. Unfortunately, patients are not uniform in drug needs to obtain acceptable analgesic actions for similar levels of pain. Even within individually tailored dosing by patient-activated demand infusion systems, the amount of drug needed to achieve satisfactory pain relief for the same level of discomfort varies fivefold over a heterogeneous patient group (31). By contrast, the level at which an individual patient achieves comfort occurs over a quite narrow dosing range, representing a threshold level of concentration at which relief occurs (31,32). Thus, attempts to determine dosing levels prospectively, by any system of administration, must be considered as guidelines only, because of the wide range of individual and kinetic variables. In meeting these needs, it is first necessary to establish individual requirements by observed dose–response testing and then setting subsequent dosing regimens on the basis of this response. It also needs to be borne in mind that where changes are made in rates of drug dosage by whatever route, it takes the time of four drug half-lives before the 90% plateau level of peak response is obtained. Thus, if an intravenous infusion rate or 4-hr oral morphine dosage is doubled or increased by any fixed amount to seek better pain control, it will take 12 hr before a new steady state is attained independent of the drug increment itself.

When initiating treatment it is best to give a single or divided intravenous dose at the outset to obtain relief, followed by a steady delivery rate. The actual level that the plasma concentration will achieve is then dose-dependent. Average values of volume of distribution for a given drug times its ED_{50} in humans will guide the initial dose requirement, and clearance values will guide the subsequent infusion rate. For example, in calculating the initial guiding dose for a 70-kg healthy adult with moderate pain, using parenteral pethidine, the usual effective plasma concentration is on the order of 0.5 mg/liter (23). Given the volume of distribution for this individual to be about 200 liters, the standard dose of 100 mg is seen to be quite appropriate. Maintenance dosing needs are harder to provide with precision because of wide individual differences in drug clearance, but if pethidine clearance was 4.8 liter/hr, then 4.8×0.5, i.e., 24 mg/hr of drug would be needed to sustain a steady-state blood level. Although these principles serve as guidelines for patient dosing schedules, the ultimate arbiter is always the response generated by a specific dose in treating pain in an individual patient. In order to further help understand the relationship between plasma concentration and induced pharmacological response, it is necessary to examine the association between drug and receptor site.

RECEPTOR OCCUPANCY AND DRUG EFFECTS: PHARMACODYNAMICS

There is a positive correlation between receptor affinity (*in vitro* binding) and analgesic potency for opiate drugs (22). Using dihydromorphine and sufentanyl binding, these studies also suggest that analgesia is mediated via the mu receptor. However, the relationship between plasma concentration and analgesia does not parallel the drug–receptor-binding curve. First, the analgesic response curve is extremely steep and is perhaps better thought of as the expression of a threshold concentration for pain relief. Below a concentration binding level, pain is present; above it, pain is inhibited, as supported by the clinical studies of Austin et al. (3). Second, in distinction to these tissue binding experiments are the findings from intact animal studies that the plasma concentrations that give relief are sufficient to produce only very low rates of receptor occupancy. For instance, at the analgesic ED_{50} for sufentanyl and morphine, only 2% of the available receptors are occupied (16,28). Drugs of the partial agonist type require much higher receptor occupancy; buprenorphine and pentazocine both need 50% receptor occupancy to achieve comparable levels of analgesia (10,16). The other distinction evident in these same studies is in the steepness of the dose–response curve. Thus, a 50% change in analgesic efficacy required a 10-fold dose increment for buprenorphine, but the same analgesic increment was induced by only a doubling for sufentanyl dosage. This work suggests that in clinical use, partial agonists, with their shallower dose–response curves, are less likely to produce toxic or adverse reactions consequent to dosing errors or inadvertent pharmacokinetic-induced peaks in plasma concentration.

Rates of receptor drug occupancy differ slightly between drugs, equilibrium being established within 10 min for fentanyl but taking up to 30 min for buprenorphine (7). In the course of onset of clinical analgesia, the development of analgesia might be slower to reach maximum but is probably not a limiting factor in its use. In receptor offset studies, buprenorphine was very slow compared with other drugs ($t_{1/2}$ = 166 min), with fentanyl showing rapid and complete dissociation after 1 hr ($t_{1/2}$ = 6.8 min) (7). The clinical observation that established buprenorphine effects are difficult to reverse with naloxone might be explained by this sluggish dissociation. Continuing antagonism by buprenorphine on morphine analgesia, even 12 hr after the last dose of buprenorphine, further supports this prolonged drug receptor association of buprenorphine (10).

Yet a further development in the quest for a more specific relationship between receptor binding and antinociceptive effect has been the finding of stimulus specificity of antinociceptive activity for different drugs (30). These findings suggest that at the spinal level, at least, different opiate analgesics may work at distinct receptor sites, to suppress only particular forms of painful stimuli. If this is pursued it may lead to advances whereby specific forms of pain can be inhibited by the use of highly selective drugs. As a corollary, it may be that the failure of opiates to relieve some forms of pain is due to an absence of antinociceptive function for that particular receptor site or stimulus response that is evoked.

ANALGESIC DRUG COMBINATIONS

Beneficial drug interactions that might facilitate analgesia would allow a reduction in opiate drug dosage and hopefully reduce untoward side effects while still achieving satisfactory pain relief. Two basic approaches have been successful in this quest. One is to use nonopiate analgesics in combination with the weaker agonists or partial agonists. The other employs nonanalgesic psychotropic drugs to supplement analgesia.

Combinations of pain-relieving drugs have been subjected to extensive trial and have stood the test of time. Use of apsirin or paracetamol (acetaminophen) with codeine, dextropropoxyphene, or oxycodone has analgesic superiority over each of the agents alone, the clinical benefit being additive for each of the drugs (4,17). These investigators, Houde and Beaver, have done much to consolidate our knowledge regarding analgesic efficacy of this group of drugs and to identify and quantify the characteristics of placebo responses following the pioneering work of Beecher. Even against this background of well-designed and controlled studies proving quite profound analgesic efficacy for these drug combinations, there is a tendency to seek more potent agents when an increased dosage of the so-called weaker drugs would suffice. The therapeutic ratio of analgesia to side effects is usually better for the various drug combinations, such that they should always be taken to full dosage before transferring to morphine, as might be required in treatment of cancer or nonmalignant chronic pain.

By contrast to the documentation of mixed analgesics, the evidence for additive or beneficial advantages with the use of psychotropic agents is very sparse. Most claims are anecdotal, and few studies have been reported in major journals. An implication, by default, is that the benefits, if any, are few and not very important. Studies with hydroxyzine are a case in point, offering slight analgesic benefit in combination with morphine when used in postoperative pain treatment (11). Both the antihistamines such as hydroxyzine and the phenothiazines offer sedation and tranquilizing actions that may be separately and specifically desirable in short-term use, but run counter to current philosophy in the treatment of most chronic pain. The disturbing and irreversible complication of tardive dyskinesia is also a relative contraindication to their long-term use. Potentiation of sedation and respiratory depression of morphine are said to occur with each of the different groups of psychotropic drugs (34).

Tricyclic antidepressant drugs have also been the subject of many claims and counters as to their analgesic efficacy either alone or in drug combinations. Descending spinal serotonergic and adrenergic inhibitory effects are implicated as possible benefits, at least in terms of segmental antinociception. Animal studies by Goldstein et al. (12) supported this contention, showing rapid potentiation of tail-flick suppression using desipramine-morphine combinations. This additive effect increased further with time, not due to any inherent mechanistic effect but from increased plasma levels of morphine. As has been shown with other drugs undergoing hepatic metabolism via the same cytochrome transformation process, drug levels can accumulate when either tricyclic or antiepileptic drugs are used in combination with opiate analgesics (15). Despite some apparent analgesic effect from tricyclic drugs, their use in well-controlled chronic pain studies proved of no benefit for a group of mixed presentations (27), but they were clearly effective in treatment of postherpetic neuralgia (35).

On balance, drug combinations of analgesics acting via different antinociceptive mechanisms would seem to offer real therapeutic advantage, but there is less evidence to support the inclusion of other agents to enhance pain relief.

OPIATE USE AND DRUG ABUSE

But for concerns of social misuse, the problems of drug choice and availability would be much lessened, allowing for more open-minded drug use and a more humanitarian approach to pain treatment. The public, plus many nursing and medical staff, hold fears of iatrogenically induced dependence to such an extent that opiates are withheld unnecessarily from legitimate and warranted use. However, experience in long-term clinical use suggests that opiates are probably safer than many of the other therapeutic alternatives (32). In fact, addiction rarely occurs with clinical use and the restriction on opiate availability imposed by many national health agencies to limit drug access and therefore abuse almost never curtails the long-term misuse of opiate drugs among addicts. The two issues are not interdependent, one being social and the other medical. Unfortunately, the very occasional medical excesses and the strident calls for action from the drug regulatory agencies have imposed an unfounded emotional fear on our use of these drugs. Little in the way of a counter-response has been mounted on behalf of the consumer need for adequate pain relief, to the extent that regulations are being increasingly enforced throughout the world to restrict legitimate access to opiate medications. It is for this reason that recent drug development and marketing have focused on the partial agonists as alternative "safer" forms of opiate therapy.

CONCLUSIONS

After detailing many, but not all, of the principles of opiate pharmacology applied to clinical treatment of pain, the multitude of issues involved would seem to belie what is essentially a straightforward process for most patients. In practice, treatment proceeds to the benefit of an increasing proportion of patients, particularly in areas of cancer pain treatment (34) and in the relief of postoperative pain (8). Extension of these techniques to other problems of chronic and acute pain states will take these simple measures to an even greater proportion of our patients. However, despite quite major advances in the physiology of nociception, the identification of opioid receptors and their endogenous ligands, and a better understanding of the pharmacology of opiate drugs acting at these receptors, our use of these drugs is hampered by the limits of their low therapeutic ratio. But, we can improve the treatment of pain by selecting the agents of appropriate efficacy, by applying them with greater consistency, and by sustaining individualized dosing schedules. Even so, routine clinical use of opiate drugs holds potential consequences of respiratory depression, nausea, constipation, and sedation. Of equal concern is social abuse of these drugs, which, though essentially independent of legitimate therapeutic use, has led to well-intentioned but misdirected restrictions on their legitimate use while also imposing heavy demands on drug regulatory agencies and law-enforcement officers. Today, our challenge is to understand the scientific basis for correct drug choice and targeted dosing schedules; tomorrow, our hope is for drugs of greater therapeutic specificity in our search for selective analgesia.

REFERENCES

1. Ariens, E. J., and Beld, A. J. (1977): The receptor concept in evolution. *Biochem. Pharmacol.,* 26:913–918.
2. Arndt, J. O., Mikat, M., and Parasher, C. (1984): Fentanyl's analgesic, respiratory and cardiovascular action in relation to dose and plasma concentration in unanaesthetised dogs. *Anesthesiology,* 61:355–361.
3. Austin, K. L., Stapleton, J. V., and Mather. L. E. (1980): Relationship between blood meperidine concentrations and analgesic response. *Anesthesiology,* 53:460–466.
4. Beaver, W. T. (1966): Mild analgesics. A review of their clinical pharmacology. *Am. J. Med. Sci.,* 251:576–604.
5. Bentley, J. B., Borel, J. D., Nenand, R. E., and Gillespie, T. J. (1982): Age and fentanyl kinetics. *Anesth. Analg. (Cleve.),* 61:968–971.
6. Berkowitz, B. A., Ngai, S. H., Yang, J. C., Hempstead, J., and Spector, S. (1975): The disposition of morphine in surgical patients. *Clin. Pharmacol. Ther.,* 17:629–635.
7. Boas, R. A., and Villiger, J. W. (1985): Clinical actions of fentanyl and buprenorphine: The significance of receptor binding. *Br. J. Anaesth.,* 58:192–196.
8. Bonica, J. J. (1983): Current status of postoperative pain therapy. In: *Current Topics in Pain Research and Therapy,* edited by T. Yokota and R. Dubner, pp. 169–189. Excerpta Medica, Amsterdam.
9. Bullingham, R. E. S., McQuay, H. J., Porter, E. J. B., Allen, M. C., and Moore, R. A. (1982): Sublingual buprenorphine used postoperatively: Ten hour plasma drug concentration analysis. *Br. J. Clin. Pharmacol.,* 13:665–673.
10. Dum, J. E., and Herz, A. (1981): In vivo receptor binding of the opiate partial agonist buprenorphine, correlated with its agonist and antagonist actions. *Br. J. Pharmacol.,* 74:627–633.
11. Forrest, W. H., and Beaver, W. T. (1976): Hydroxyzine added to narcotics for analgesia. *Hosp. Pract.,* 11:20–29.
12. Goldstein, F. J., Mojavarian, P., Ossipov, M. H., and Swanson, B. N. (1982): Elevation in analgetic effect and plasma levels of morphine by desipramine in rats. *Pain,* 14:279–282.
13. Goodman, R. R., and Pasternak, G. W. (1984): Multiple opiate receptors. In: *Analgesics: Neurochemical, Behavioural and Clinical Perspectives,* edited by M. Kuhar and G. W. Pasternak, pp. 69–96. Raven Press, New York.
14. Gourley, G. K., Wilson, P. R., and Glyn, C. J. (1982): Methadone produces prolonged postoperative analgesia. *Br. Med. J.,* 284:630–631.
15. Hansen, B. S., Dam, M., Brandt, J., Hvidberg, E. F., Angelo, H., Christensen, J., and Lous, P. (1980): Influence of dextropropoxyphene on steady state serum levels and protein binding of three antiepileptic drugs in man. *Acta Neurol. Scand.,* 61:357–367.
16. Holford, N. H. G. (1984): Drug concentration, binding and effect *in vivo. Pharmaceutical Res.,* 3:102–105.
17. Houde, R. W., Wallenstein, S. L., and Beaver, W. T. (1965): Clinical measurement of pain. In: *Analgetics,* edited by G. de Stevens, pp. 75–122. Academic Press, New York.
18. Hug, C. C., and Murphy, M. R. (1981): Tissue redistribution of fentanyl and termination of its effects in rats. *Anesthesiology,* 53:369–375.
19. Inturrisi, C. E., Max, M. B., Foley, K. M., Schultz, M., Shin, S.-U., and Houde, R. W. (1984): The pharmacokinetics of heroin in patients with chronic pain. *N. Engl. J. Med.,* 310:1213–1217.
20. Inturrisi, C. E., and Foley, K. M. (1984): Narcotic analgesics in the management of pain. In: *Analgesics: Neurochemical, Behavioural and Clinical Perspectives,* edited by M. Kuhar and G. Pasternak, pp. 257–288. Raven Press, New York.
21. Kaiko, R. F., Foley, K. M., House, R. W., and Inturrisi, C. E. (1978): Narcotic levels in

cerebrospinal fluid and plasma in man. In: *Characteristics and Functions of Opioids,* edited by J. M. Van Ree and L. Terenius, pp. 221–222. Elsevier, Amsterdam.
22. Leysen, J. E., Gommeren, W., and Niemegeers, C. J. E. (1983): [^{3}H]sufentanyl, a superior ligand for mu opiate receptors: Binding properties and regional distribution in rat brain and spinal cord. *Eur. J. Pharmacol.,* 87:209–225.
23. Mather, L. E., and Meffin, P. J. (1978): Clinical pharmacokinetics of pethidine. *Clin. Pharmacokinet.,* 3:252–268.
24. Mather, L. E. (1983): Pharmacokinetic and pharmacodynamic factors influencing the choice, dose and route of administration of opiates of acute pain. *Clin. Anaesth.,* 1:17–40.
25. Paalzow, L. K. (1982): Pharmacokinetic aspects of optimal pain treatment. *Acta Anaesth. Scand.* [*Suppl.*], 74:37–43.
26. Perry, D. C., Rosenbaum, J. S., Kurowski, M., and Sadee, W. (1982): [^{3}H]etorphine receptor binding in vivo: Small fractional occupancy elicits analgesia. *Mol. Pharmacol.,* 21:272–279.
27. Pilowski, I., Hallett, E. C., Bassett, D. L., Thomas, P. G., and Penhall, R. K. (1982): A controlled study of amitriptyline in the treatment of chronic pain. *Pain,* 14:169–179.
28. Rosenbaum, J. S., Holford, N. H. G., and Sadee, W. (1984): Opiate receptor binding–effect relationship: Sufentanyl and etorphine produce analgesia at the mu site with low fractional occupancy. *Brain Res.,* 291:317–324.
29. Sawe, J., Dahlstrom, B., Paalzow, L, and Rane, A. (1981): Morphine kinetics in cancer patients. *Clin. Pharmacol. Ther.,* 30:629–635.
30. Schmauss, C., and Yaksh, T. L. (1984): In vivo studies on spinal receptor systems mediating antinociception. II. Pharmacological profiles suggesting a differential association of mu, delta and kappa receptors with visceral, chemical and cutaneous stimuli in the rat. *J. Pharmacol. Exp. Ther.,* 228:1–12.
31. Stapleton, J. V., Austin, K. L., and Mather, L. E. (1979): A pharmacokinetic approach to postoperative pain: Continuous infusion of pethidine. *Anaesth. Intensive Care,* 7:25–32.
32. Tamsen, A., Hartvig, P., Fagerlund, C., and Dahlstrom, B. (1982): Patient controlled analgesic therapy. II. Individual analgesic demand and analgesic plasma concentrations of pethidine in postoperative pain. *Clin. Pharmacokinet.,* 7:164–175.
33. Taub, A. (1982): Opioid analgesics in the treatment of chronic intractable pain of non-neoplastic origin. In: *Narcotic Analgesics in Anesthesiology,* edited by L. M. Kitahata and J. G. Collins, pp. 199–208. Williams & Wilkins, Baltimore.
34. Twycross, R. G. (1983): Narcotic analgesics in clinical practice. In: *Advances in Pain Research and Therapy,* Vol. 5, edited by J. J. Bonica, V. Lindblom, and A. Iggo, pp. 534–559. Raven Press, New York.
35. Watson, C. P., Evans, R. J., Reed, K., Merskey, H., Goldsmith, L., and Walsh, J. (1982): Amitriptyline versus placebo in post herpetic neuralgia. *Neurology,* 32:671–673.
36. Welsh, J., Stuart, J. F. B., Hobeshaw, T., Blackie, R., Whitehall, D., Setanoians, A., Milsted, R. A. V., and Colman, K. D. (1983): A comparative pharmacokinetic study of morphine sulphate solution and MST continuous 30mg tablets in conditions expected to allow steady-state drug levels. *Royal Society of Medicine, International Congress and Symposium Series,* 58:9–13.

Advances in Pain Research and Therapy, Vol. 9, edited by H. L. Fields et al. Raven Press, New York © 1985.

Disposition and Effects of Heroin in Pain Patients

*‡Charles Inturrisi, *†‡Kathleen Foley, †‡Mitchell Max, *Jack Chen, *Michael Schultz, and *‡Raymond Houde

*Departments of *Pharmacology and †Neurology, Cornell University Medical College; and ‡Analgesic Studies Section, Memorial Sloan-Kettering Cancer Center, New York, New York 10021*

For the past several years there has been much debate over the efforts by some groups to persuade the U.S. Congress to change current regulations so as to permit the use of heroin for relief of terminal cancer pain (1,2,9). The supporters of heroin use stress the "unique" chemical and pharmacological properties of heroin, including its rapid onset of action after parenteral administration and greater potency and solubility than morphine (9). In attempting to determine if there is any scientific evidence for uniqueness of heroin as a narcotic analgesic, we have sought to define the relationship between heroin's disposition and certain of its pharmacological effects in patients with pain. Heroin (3,6-diacetylmorphine, diamorphine) is a semisynthetic narcotic analgesic prepared by diacetylating morphine. Heroin is biotransformed into 6-acetylmorphine and morphine. Thus, analytical methods for determination of heroin's disposition must be able to separate and quantitate heroin and its active metabolites. Furthermore, because heroin is susceptible to deacetylation in blood (7,17) the procedure must include provision for stabilization of heroin during collection and sample preparation. The method of solvent-extraction high-performance liquid chromatography (HPLC) developed in this laboratory by Umans et al. (17) meets these requirements and has allowed pharmacokinetic studies of heroin after oral and parenteral doses of heroin.

METHODS

Seven men and 4 women ranging in age from 30 to 65 years (mean = 49.7) with chronic pain who were evaluated by the Pain Service of the Memorial Sloan-Kettering Cancer Center (MSKCC) gave Institutional Review Board (IRB)-approved informed consent to participate in this study. Nine of the patients had advanced cancer, and 2 patients had chronic nonmalignant pain. Each had a clearly defined pain syndrome. All patients had normal hepatic and renal functions and were not receiving chemotherapy at the time of study.

Seven patients received heroin HCl by bolus intravenous injection at doses from 4 to 16 mg depending on their prior narcotic experience. To measure the time course of effects concurrently with the blood concentration–time profiles of heroin and the metabolites, 3 patients received continuous i.v. infusion of heroin for 180 min at rates that ranged from 112 to 333 μg/min. Two patients received a single intramuscular injection of 4 mg of heroin HCl. Three patients received heroin HCl and morphine SO_4 orally in a crossover comparison separated by at least 1 week (Table 1).

Venous blood samples (3 ml) were collected as described (17) by a nurse observer prior to and at selected times during and following drug administration.

During and following the continuous i.v. infusion of heroin, subjective measurements were assessed under "open" (nonblind) conditions. Each patient was asked to estimate pain relief by use of both a visual analog scale (VAS) and a categorical (CAT) scale, as described by Kaiko et al. (8). The patient was also asked to estimate sedation (sleepiness) on a VAS scale, with the extremes being "alert" and "very sleepy." Each scale was presented independent of others and of previously completed scales.

The elimination half-life and blood clearance for heroin were determined using standard pharmacokinetic equations (7). Systemic availability was estimated after an oral dose of heroin or morphine by determination of the AUC (area under the blood concentration–time curve) from time 0 until the last measurable blood concentration at 240 minutes after dosing.

RESULTS

Heroin blood levels decline rapidly and monoexponentially over the first 10 min following i.v. administration and are below the limits of sensitivity

TABLE 1. *Systemic availability of morphine after oral administration of 52.3 mg (as the base) of heroin or morphine*

	Morphine AUC/10 mg[a]		AUC ratio
Patient	Heroin	Morphine	Heroin/morphine
3	1.98	2.16	0.96
4	1.50	1.50	1.00
9	2.34	2.91	0.80
			Mean = 0.92

[a]As morphine equivalents.

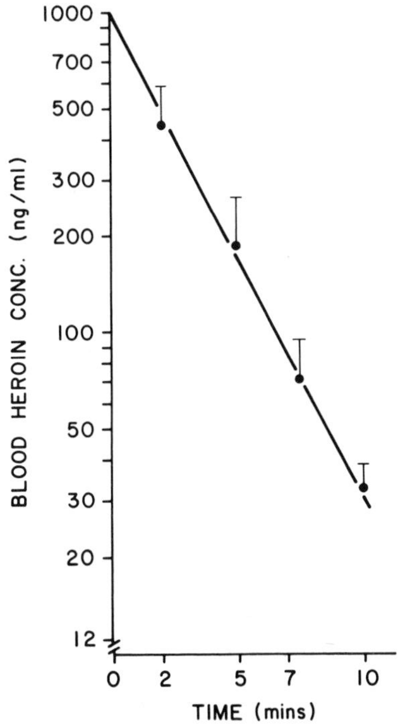

FIG. 1. Mean blood concentration–time profile for heroin after a single i.v. dose of 5 mg (2 patients) or 4 mg (2 patients) of heroin HCl. The points represent mean observed concentration ± SD, and the solid line the theoretical line obtained by fitting the data to a monoexponential equation. (From Inturrisi et al., ref. 7, with permission.)

of the analytical method by 15 min postdrug (Fig. 1). Estimates of heroin's elimination $t_{1/2}$ obtained after i.v. injection or following the cessation of an infusion ranged from 1.7 to 5.3 min, with the mean apparent $t_{1/2}$ equal to 3.0 ± 1.3 (SD) min. Half-life estimates appeared to be independent of dose over the range tested.

Figure 2 shows the blood concentration–time profiles for heroin and metabolites and the measures of pharmacodynamic effect during and following the continuous i.v. infusion of heroin to patient 10. Heroin and 6-acetylmorphine were measured in the first blood sample taken at 5 min into the infusion. Both parent drug and metabolite quickly achieved blood levels that remained constant during the infusion. Heroin achieved an apparent steady-state blood concentration of 57 ng/ml, and 6-acetylmorphine a value of 15 ng/ml. Both parent and metabolite fell rapidly when the infusion was stopped at 180 min. The morphine blood level could be measured only after 45 min into the infusion; it rose to a constant level of 30 ng/ml and slowly declined during the 120-min study period after the infusion was stopped (Fig. 2A). During constant infusion, a doubling of the heroin infusion rate results in a new apparent steady-state blood heroin concentration that is approximately twice the previous level (7). The mean blood clearance of heroin was 30.8 ± 2.1 ml/min/kg.

Figure 2B shows the time course of effects reported during and following the infusion of heroin. This patient reported prompt pain relief on both the

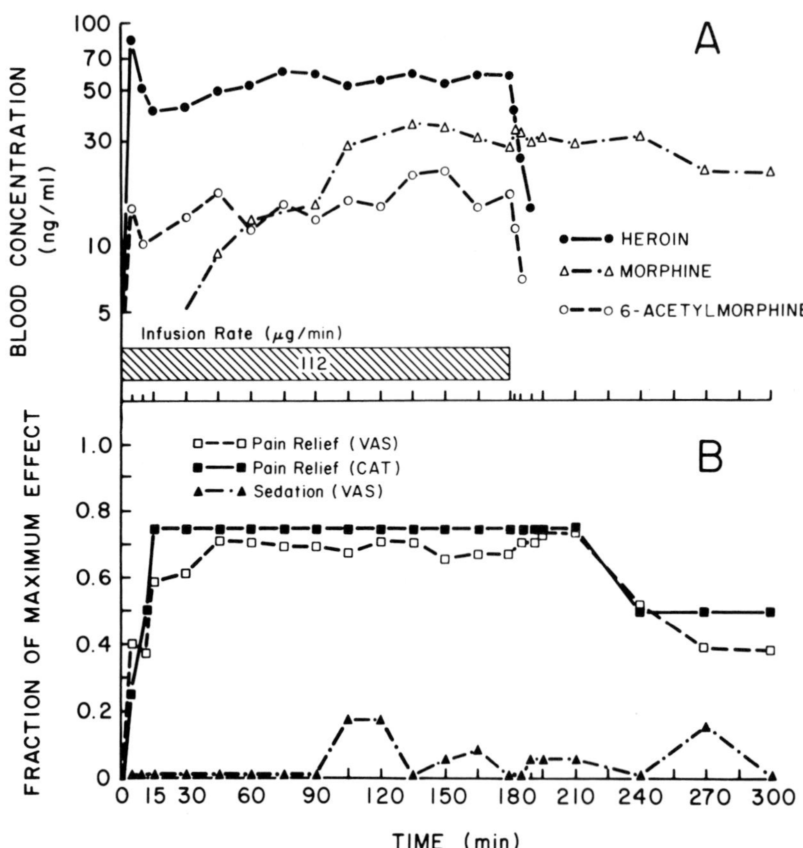

FIG. 2. Blood concentrations **(A)** and effects **(B)** during and following continuous i.v. infusion of heroin to patient 10. The effect data (B) were transformed into "fraction of maximum effect" by dividing the value at each observation time by the maximum possible effect. (From Inturrisi et al., ref. 7, with permission.)

VAS and CAT scales. Approximately the same peak intensity of pain relief (¾ of the maximal possible effect) was achieved with either the VAS or CAT scale. Peak pain relief occurred at 15 to 45 min into the infusion, remained constant during the infusion, and declined when the infusion was stopped.

Figure 3 shows the blood morphine concentration–time profiles after administration of equal oral doses of heroin and morphine to patient 9. In the 3 patients we have studied, neither heroin nor 6-acetylmorphine could be detected in blood following oral administration of heroin. Table 1 compares systemic availabilities of morphine after oral administration of heroin and morphine. The AUC values in Table 1 are given per 10 mg of drug to normalize for the difference in doses administered and corrected to express

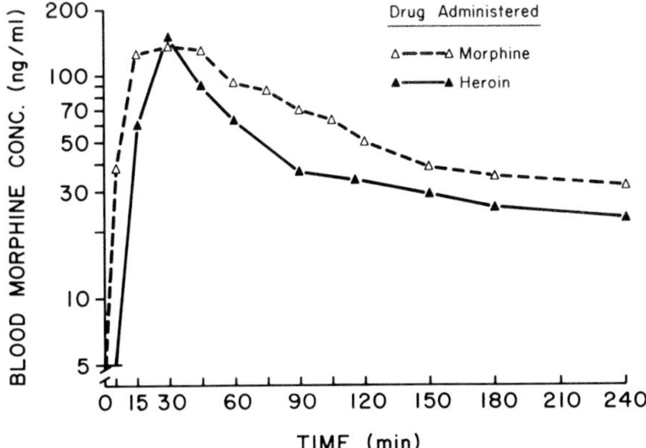

FIG. 3. Blood morphine concentrations following a 52.3-mg oral dose of heroin and the same dose of morphine given 3 weeks later to patient 9. (From Inturrisi et al., ref. 7, with permission.)

the morphine equivalents that can be derived from heroin. The ratio of the AUC values indicates that oral heroin provided an average of 92% as much systemic morphine as an equal oral dose of morphine.

Figure 4 shows blood concentration–time profiles for heroin and metabolites following intramuscular (i.m.) administration of 4 mg of heroin HCl to patient 9. Heroin and 6-acetylmorphine blood levels reached a peak at 10 min after i.m. administration, and thereafter both declined rapidly. Morphine blood concentrations reached a peak at 15 min and declined more slowly than heroin or 6-acetylmorphine blood levels.

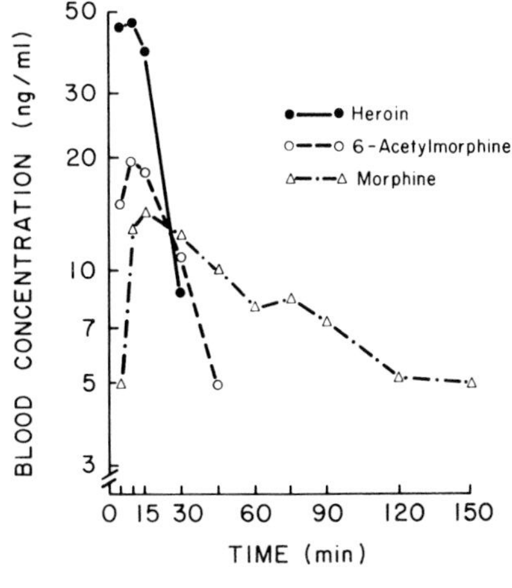

FIG. 4. Blood concentration–time profiles for heroin and metabolites after a single i.m. dose of 4 mg of heroin HCl to patient 9. (From Inturrisi et al., ref. 7, with permission.)

DISCUSSION

We find that heroin is rapidly biotransformed and eliminated in humans. *In vitro* studies by Way et al. (18) demonstrated the ability of human tissue homogenates, including brain, kidney, and liver, as well as human blood, to biotransform heroin into 6-acetylmorphine and morphine. We have found that at 37° C, heroin has a $t_{1/2}$ of approximately 15 min when added *in vitro* to blood from normal human subjects (C. Inturrisi et al., *unpublished observations*). Therefore, whereas degradation in blood may contribute to clearance of heroin from blood, organ clearance would appear to be the main determinant of its rapid disappearance from the systemic circulation.

The continuous-infusion technique resulted in rapid attainment of apparent steady-state blood levels of heroin (Fig. 2) consistent with the short heroin $t_{1/2}$ of 3 min and rapid clearance seen after i.v. injection. The difference between the blood or systemic clearance and renal clearance is often termed nonrenal clearance (7). For a drug like heroin whose renal clearance is negligible (7), we might ask whether or not systemic clearance is equal to hepatic clearance. The blood clearance of heroin is found to average 2,134 ml/min (30.8 ml/min/kg), a value that exceeds the maximum value of 1,500 ml/min for hepatic blood flow in the human (7). Thus, nonrenal clearance of heroin actually exceeds hepatic blood flow, supporting the conclusion that *in vivo* organs other than the liver are capable of biotransforming and eliminating heroin.

The high value for blood clearance of heroin predicts that a significant fraction of orally administered heroin will be cleared by the liver before reaching the systemic circulation. Oral bioavailability studies confirmed this prediction and revealed that within the limits of sensitivity of the analytical methods, oral heroin is subject to complete presystemic or first-pass metabolism to morphine (Fig. 3). When compared in a given patient, equal doses of morphine provide slightly more blood morphine than heroin. Orally administered morphine is subject to a large, but not complete, presystemic elimination, with oral bioavailability averaging only 38% (range 15–64%) (11). In a repeated-dose crossover oral analgesic study, Twycross (14) found that a heroin-to-morphine potency ratio of 1.5 was satisfactory for female patients, but less so for male patients. Our bioavailability studies are consistent with the clinical impression that by the oral route heroin HCl and morphine SO_4 are nearly equipotent. We concur with Twycross that morphine is a satisfactory substitute for orally administered heroin (14). Indeed, we would go further to suggest that, based on our pharmacokinetic studies, administration of oral heroin may be considered a somewhat less efficient means of providing systemic morphine. Furthermore, when the limited shelf life of heroin solutions is considered (13), there would appear to be no reason for selecting oral heroin over oral morphine for pain relief.

Heroin has been reported to be a more potent analgesic, faster in onset of pain relief and of shorter duration, than morphine after i.m. and i.v. administration to humans (6,12). These pharmacodynamic differences have been considered to derive from the more rapid and extensive brain uptake of the more lipid-soluble heroin as compared with morphine (7,10). Our pharmacokinetic studies demonstrate that over the first 10 to 15 min after parenteral administration, heroin and 6-acetylmorphine are present in blood and therefore are available for distribution into the CNS. Figure 2 shows that the onset of pain relief for patient 10 occurred during a time when heroin and 6-acetylmorphine, but not morphine, were present in blood. Because the pharmacokinetics of 6-acetylmorphine have not yet been determined in humans, its volume of distribution relative to heroin is not known. Therefore, the pharmacokinetic significance of the relatively lower blood levels of 6-acetylmorphine compared with heroin cannot be assessed (Figs. 2 and 4). To date, the pharmacodynamics of 6-acetylmorphine also have not been assessed in humans. When administered parenterally to laboratory animals, heroin and 6-acetylmorphine are equipotent, and both are more potent than morphine (3,15,16). Comparison of the apparent partition coefficients for heroin, 6-acetylmorphine, and morphine with the values reported by Herz and Teschemacher (4) for a series of opioids suggests that brain uptake of both heroin and 6-acetylmorphine, but not morphine, is limited only by blood flow. Our pharmacokinetic studies suggest that 6-acetylmorphine formed from biotransformation of heroin in peripheral tissues may contribute to the pharmacodynamic characteristics, rapid onset of action and greater potency, that serve to distinguish heroin from morphine. From Fig. 2 it is also apparent that on cessation of heroin infusion, both heroin and 6-acetylmorphine levels in blood decline rapidly, while morphine blood levels persist, as does some pain relief. Similar kinetic profiles are seen after i.m. heroin (Fig. 4). These results suggest that peripherally formed morphine may contribute to the duration of pain relief obtained after heroin. In this regard it will be of interest to define the pharmacokinetics and pharmacodynamics of 6-acetylmorphine in humans. Because the brain is also capable of the biotransformation of heroin (18), our studies in humans cannot provide direct information on the species that ultimately mediates pain relief at CNS opioid receptors *(vide infra).*

In attempting to place these observations in a clinical perspective it is important to recognize that all of the commonly used narcotic analgesics have significantly higher partition coefficients than morphine (i.e., they are much more lipid-soluble). Following i.m. administration, currently available narcotics such as hydromorphone and meperidine, on the average, appear to reach their peak analgesic effects earlier than morphine and at approximately the same time as heroin (6). Furthermore, hydromorphone HCl is a highly water-soluble salt and more potent than heroin (2,6) and therefore could serve as a parenteral narcotic analgesic in those very tolerant patients in whom the volume limitations imposed by the solubility of morphine SO_4 become an issue. Thus, attempts to identify so-called unique properties for heroin (9) must consider not only whether or not heroin has advantages over morphine but also how it compares with other available narcotic analgesics.

A final consideration derives from experiments with a rat brain opiate receptor binding assay (5) in which we were able to control conditions so as to minimize the hydrolysis of heroin, as well as to account for any binding due to the hydrolysis products of heroin. Under these conditions we found that 6-acetylmorphine and morphine, but not heroin, are capable of binding to the opiate receptor (5).

Thus, our pharmacokinetic and binding results, taken together with the pharmacodynamic studies discussed earlier, lead to the conclusion that heroin lacks intrinsic opioid activity and should be viewed as a lipid-soluble prodrug that serves only to determine the distribution of its active metabolites: 6-acetylmorphine and morphine.

ACKNOWLEDGMENTS

Supported in part by National Institute of Drug Abuse grants DA-01707 and DA-01457 and National Cancer Institute grant CA-32897.

REFERENCES

1. Angell, M. (1984); Should heroin be legalized for the treatment of pain? *N. Engl. J. Med.,* 311:529–530.
2. Brandt, E. M., Jr. (1984): Compassionate pain relief; Is heroin the answer? *N. Engl. J. Med.,* 311:530–532.
3. Eddy, N. B., and Howes, H. A. (1935): Studies of morphine, codeine and their derivatives. *J. Pharmacol. Exp. Ther.,* 53:430–439.
4. Herz, A., and Teschemacher, H.-J. (1971): Activities and sites of antinociceptive action of morphine-like analgesics. *Adv. Drug Res.,* 6:79–119.
5. Inturrisi, C. E., Schultz, M., Shin, S., Umans, J. G., Angel, L., and Simon, E. J. (1983): Evidence from opiate binding studies that heroin acts through its metabolites. *Life Sci.* [*Suppl. I*], 33:773–776.
6. Inturrisi, C. E., and Foley, K. M. (1984): Narcotic analgesics in the management of pain. In: *Analgesics: Neurochemical, Behavioral, and Clinical Perspectives,* edited by M. Kuhar and G. Pasternak, pp. 257–288. Raven Press, New York.
7. Inturrisi, C. E., Max, M. B., Foley, K. M., Schultz, M., Shin, S.-U., and Houde, R. W. (1984): The pharmacokinetics of heroin in patients with chronic pain. *N. Engl. J. Med.,* 310:1213–1217.
8. Kaiko, R. F., Wallenstein, S. L., Rogers, A. G., Grabinski, P. Y., and Houde, R. W. (1981): Analgesic and mood effects of heroin and morphine in cancer patients with postoperative pain. *N. Engl. J. Med.,* 304:1501–1540.
9. Mondzac, A. M. (1984): In defense of the reintroduction of heroin into American medical practice and H. R. 5290—the compassionate pain relief act. *N. Engl. J. Med.,* 311:532–535.
10. Oldendorf, W. H., Hyman, S., Braun, L., and Oldendorf, S. Z. (1972): Blood-brain barrier: Penetration of morphine, codeine, heroin and methadone after carotid injection. *Science,* 178:984–986.
11. Sawe, J., Dahlstrom, B., Paalzow, L., and Rane, A. (1981): Morphine kinetics in cancer patients. *Clin. Pharmacol. Ther.,* 30:629–635.

12. Scott, M. E., and Orr, R. (1969): Effects of diamorphine, methadone, morphine, and pentazocine in patients with suspected acute myocardial infarction. *Lancet,* 1:1065–1067.
13. Twycross, R. G. (1974): Diamorphine and cocaine elixir BPC 1973. *Pharmaceut. J.,* 212:153–159.
14. Twycross, R. G. (1977): Choice of strong analgesic in terminal cancer: Diamorphine or morphine? *Pain,* 3:93–104.
15. Umans, J. G., and Inturrisi, C. E. (1981): Pharmacodynamics of subcutaneously administered diacetylmorphine, 6-acetylmorphine and morphine in mice. *J. Pharmacol. Exp. Ther.,* 218:409–415.
16. Umans, J. G., and Inturrisi, C. E. (1982): Heroin: Analgesia, toxicity and disposition in the mouse. *Eur. J. Pharmacol.,* 85:317–323.
17. Umans, J. G., Chiu, T. S. K., Lipman, R. A., Schultz, M. F., Shin, S.-U., and Inturrisi, C. E. (1982): Determination of heroin and its metabolites by high-performance liquid chromatography. *J. Chromatogr.,* 233:213–225.
18. Way, E. L., Young, J. M., and Kemp, J. W. (1965): Metabolism of heroin and its pharmacologic implications. *Bull. Narc.,* 17:25–33.

Advances in Pain Research and Therapy, Vol. 9, edited by H. L. Fields et al. Raven Press, New York © 1985.

High Systemic Availability of Oral Morphine Sulfate Solution and Sustained-Release Preparation

H. J. McQuay, R. A. Moore, C. J. Glynn, and J. W. Lloyd

Oxford Regional Pain Relief Unit, Abingdon; and Nuffield Departments of Anaesthetics and Clinical Biochemistry, Radcliffe Infirmary, Oxford, United Kingdom

Currently, most people believe that morphine is destroyed in the liver and that two-thirds of an oral dose is removed by the liver before it can get to the nervous system, where it works (23). This "kinetic" belief is supported by the finding in single-dose efficacy studies that an oral dose needs to be several times (up to six) the injected dose to achieve a similar effect (8).

Our knowledge of the metabolism of morphine in man is surprisingly limited, and the reason has been the difficulty in assaying the drug accurately. The "textbook" concept of morphine metabolism is that it is metabolized in the liver to morphine glucuronide, which is then excreted in the urine. This concept has been extended by the classification of morphine as a high-clearance drug (24), a classification that has little support from either *in vitro* or *in vivo* data, and this leads to misleading clinical implications. This chapter reviews the evidence against such a view of morphine metabolism and the clinical sequelae of proposing that morphine metabolism in man involves the kidney rather than the liver at the plasma morphine concentrations seen after oral doses.

The involvement of the kidney in morphine metabolism has historical clinical support. One hundred years ago, a doctor reading *The Family Physician* (Vol. IV, p. 160) would have been told that opium should not be prescribed for patients with Bright's disease or other diseases of the kidney. Since that time, many case reports have appeared (1,2,6,7,19) describing respiratory depression of unexpected degree and duration with drugs of the morphine family in patients with renal impairment (10).

As creatinine clearance falls, so does morphine clearance (11). Cancer pain patients with impaired renal function needed a median dose of only 5 mg oral morphine every 4 hr; those with normal renal and hepatic function and those with normal kidneys but with hepatic impairment needed 20 mg every 4 hr (20). Morphine is more effective in renal failure. Titration of dose to effect is required.

In vitro studies of rabbit proximal tubules have shown that the tubules are capable of morphine glucuronidation at approximately 700 nmol/liter (22), much closer to the observed therapeutic plasma morphine concentrations in man than the K_m for liver glucuronidation. Morphine removal in patients having kidney transplants has supported this finding. The transplant patients, despite normal liver function, could not eliminate morphine at a normal rate until the transplanted kidney started to work (16), suggesting that normal kidney function is important for breaking down morphine.

The problem with classifying morphine clearance as unequivocally high has been the wide range of systemic clearance values reported, from 4 to more than 30 ml/min/kg in a variety of single-dose studies (Fig. 1). This range cannot be attributed simply to assay or methodological error, because

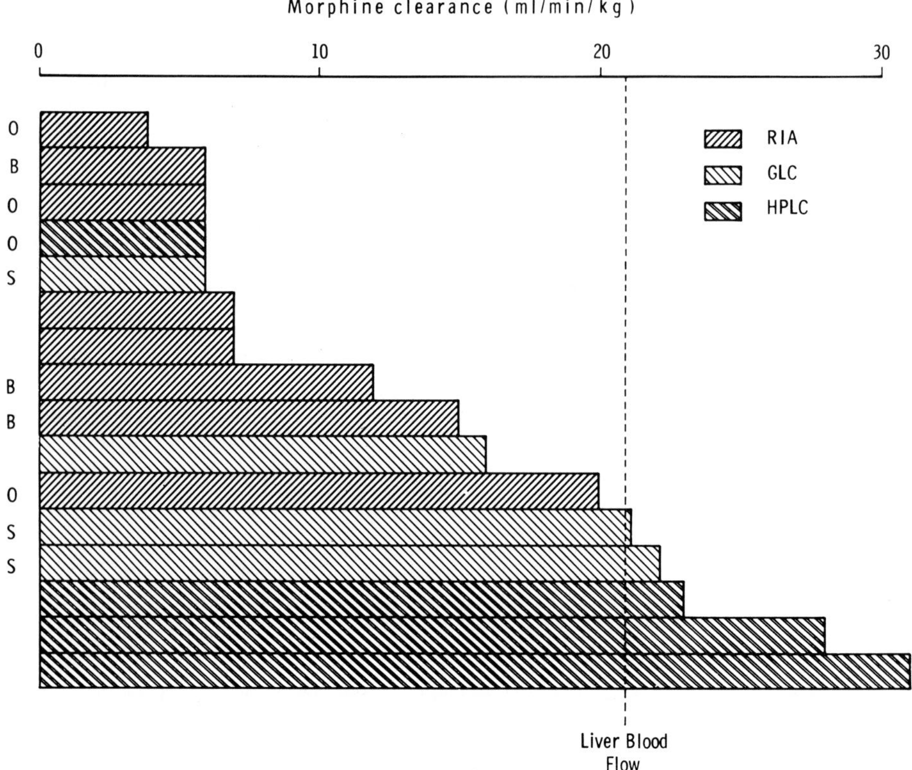

FIG. 1. Morphine clearances from 16 published studies, shaded by method of analysis of plasma morphine concentrations: RIA, radioimmunoassay; GLC, gas-liquid chromatography; HPLC, high-performance liquid chromatography. O, B, and S represent studies done in Oxford, Boston, and Stockholm.

high and low clearance values have been reported from the same laboratories using the same assay method for both high and low clearance studies. In Oxford, using the same assay (15), the range in systemic clearance in single-dose studies was from 4 to 20 ml/min/kg; no clear pathological or physiological differences among these patients were found that were of sufficient magnitude to explain the range. This contrasts with the situation for buprenorphine, for which single-dose clearance estimates have consistently been 900 to 1,200 ml/min (4).

Given the variation in morphine clearance, simple classification as a high-clearance drug is invalid. High-clearance opiates do not show large variations in systemic clearance; they show reduced clearance in liver disease and have low oral availability. The question then arises: What evidence is there that morphine is metabolized in the liver in man?

In human liver homogenate, the Michaelis-Menten constant for glucuronidation of morphine was at a morphine concentration of approximately 2 million nmol/liter (21), whereas in cancer patients therapeutic plasma morphine concentrations are of the order of 200 nmol/liter (12). Rat liver hepatocytes *in vitro* showed uptake of both morphine and nalorphine, but with negligible metabolism of the morphine, compared with 30% seen with nalorphine (9).

In vivo studies in chronically cannulated cows showed that morphine extraction by the liver, far from being constant, actually fell to negligible levels as the portal vein plasma morphine concentrations decreased to levels seen in patients taking oral morphine (5) (Fig. 2).

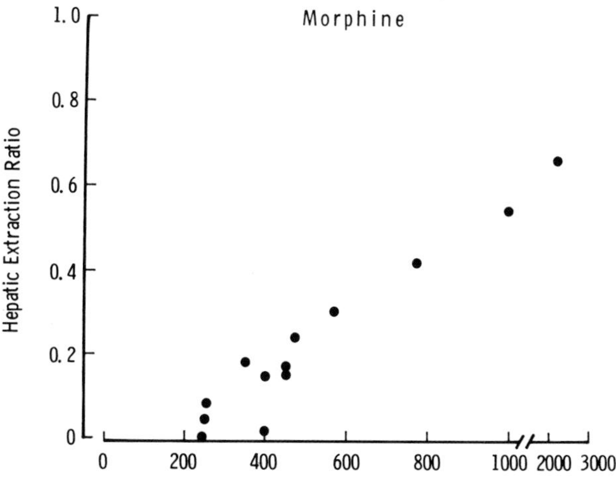

FIG. 2. Hepatic extraction ratios determined in chronically cannulated cows at varying portal vein plasma morphine concentrations. (From Bullingham et al., ref. 5, with permission.)

Indirect clinical evidence that classification of morphine as a high-clearance drug is invalid comes from studies in which drugs known to alter hepatic blood flow were given at the same time as morphine. When cimetidine was given in conjunction with morphine, the reduction in hepatic blood flow caused by cimetidine should have resulted in lower plasma morphine clearance than normal; no difference was found between controls (given morphine alone) and the group given morphine with cimetidine (13). Propranolol, which decreases hepatic blood flow, also failed to produce higher plasma morphine concentrations, and hence lower plasma clearance, when given with morphine (3). Again, this defies the simple classification of morphine as a high-clearance drug.

More directly, impaired liver function should result in higher plasma concentrations and lower clearance for high-clearance drugs. This was shown with pentazocine and pethidine in cirrhotics (17). When plasma morphine concentrations and clearance values in normal volunteers and cirrhotics were compared, no difference was found (18).

The belief that morphine is removed in the liver as a high-clearance drug leads to the prediction that only 30% of an oral dose should survive absorption and passage through the liver and be "available" to the body (23). If the kidney is more important, then the figure should be closer to 100%. The present study measured (rather than estimated) availability to test this hypothesis.

METHODS

Nine patients who required oral narcotic therapy were selected from those attending the Oxford Regional Pain Relief Unit. None suffered from clinically apparent hepatic, renal, cardiac, respiratory, or psychiatric disorder or took drugs known to interfere with the morphine assay. The study was approved by the hospital ethics committee, and informed consent was obtained from the patients.

The study design was open and within-patient crossover. Each of 5 patients [mean age 63.2 ± 7 years (± SEM), weight 73 ± 2 kg, 4F:1M] received an intravenous (i.v.) dose of morphine sulfate pentahydrate, 10 mg (26.4 μmoles Morphine Sulphate Injection BP), on the first study day. On the second day they were given 10 mg of morphine sulfate pentahydrate as an oral slow-release morphine (MST) (MST-1, MST Continus, Napp Pharmaceuticals) with 100 ml of tap water, and on the third day they received oral morphine solution 10 mg (MSS) (Morphine Sulphate Injection BP in 50 ml of tap water). Studies were run on consecutive days when possible. Four other patients (age 66.0 ± 4.5 years, weight 69.0 ± 1.0 kg, 3M:1F) received 20 mg i.v. morphine sulfate on day 1 followed by 20 mg MST on day 2. With both i.v. and oral dosing, samples were taken before injection and at various times between 1 min and 24 hr.

Plasma morphine concentrations were determined by specific radioimmunoassay using ^{125}I-labeled morphine. The antiserum exhibited <1% cross-reactivity with either morphine-3-glucuronide or normorphine (15), and the method has been validated using high-pressure liquid chromatography with electrochemical detection (14). The time to maximum plasma concentration (t_{max}) was determined from individual patient plasma morphine concentration data. The area under the curve to 24 hr (AUC_{24hr}) for plasma morphine concentration against time was obtained using a trapezoidal rule. The relative bioavailability of the oral formulation was calculated by dividing the AUC_{24hr} for the oral dose by the AUC_{24hr} for the intravenous dose. The conversion factor for SI units (nmol/liter) to nanograms per milliliter morphine base was 1/2.64. The paired t-test was used to test for significance of differences; the level of significance was taken as $p < 0.05$.

RESULTS

Mean plasma morphine concentrations following the different oral morphine 10-mg formulations are shown in Fig. 3. By 30 min, the plasma mor-

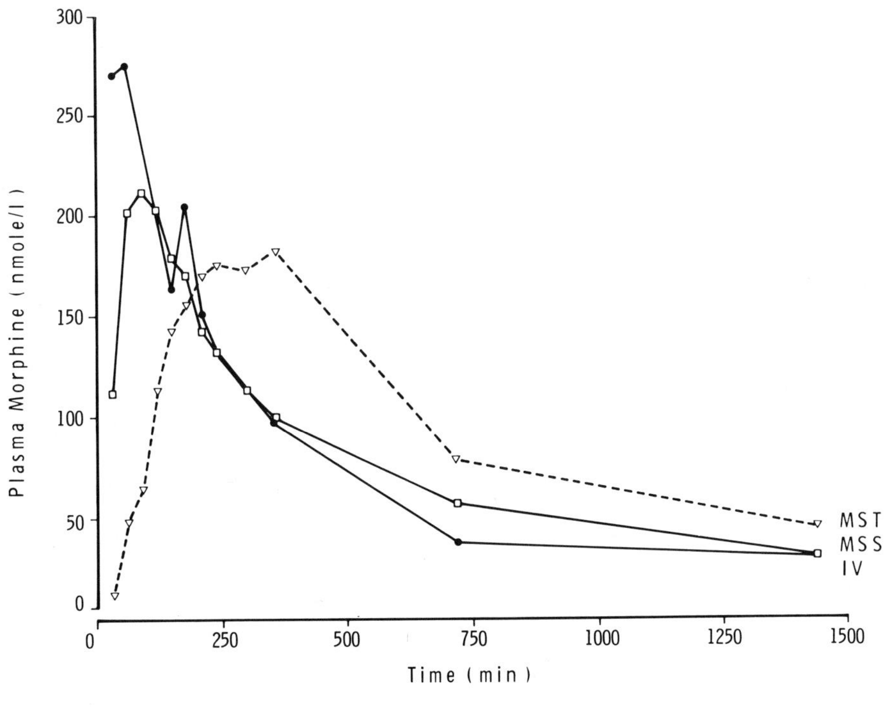

FIG. 3. Plasma morphine concentrations determined at various times after i.v. morphine sulfate 10 mg (IV, *closed circles*), oral morphine sulfate solution 10 mg (MSS, *squares*), and oral sustained-release morphine 10 mg (MST, *triangles*).

TABLE 1. *AUC_{24hr}, time to maximum plasma morphine concentration* t_{max}, *maximum plasma morphine concentration* Cp_{max}, *and relative bioavailability*

Variable	10 mg (*N* = 5)	20 mg (*N* = 4)
Intravenous dose		
AUC_{24hr} (nmol·min/liter)	118,280 ± 15,815	258,865 ± 29,905
Oral solution (MSS)		
t_{max} (min)	102 ± 23	
Cp_{max} (nmol/liter)	272 ± 31	
AUC_{24hr} (nmol·min/liter)	115,870 ± 13,045	
Relative availability (%)	102 ± 13	
Oral sustained-release (MST)		
t_{max} (min)	234 ± 35	210 ± 39
Cp_{max} (nmol/liter)	223 ± 17	419 ± 64
AUC_{24hr} (nmol·min/liter	139,259 ± 16,902	259,488 ± 53,853
Relative availability (%)	122 ± 15	99 ± 14

phine concentrations after MSS were significantly higher than after MST. This significant difference was maintained up to 120 min. From 300 to 1,440 min, plasma morphine concentrations were significantly higher after MST than after MSS. There was no significant difference in AUC_{24hr} values between the i.v. dose and either MSS or MST after the 10-mg doses; the AUC_{24hr} after MST was significantly greater than after MSS, the mean ratio being 1.2 ± 0.03 (SEM, range 1.1–1.25), with significantly greater relative availability of the MST dose (mean 122%) as compared with MSS (mean 100%). There was no significant difference in AUC_{24hr} values between the i.v. dose and MST after the 20-mg doses (Table 1).

DISCUSSION

These results showed that the availability of oral morphine was much higher than had previously been suggested, on average 100% as opposed to the estimate of 30% (23). Taken with the variable extraction ratio data obtained in the cow (5), the simplest interpretation is that at low plasma morphine concentrations in humans, the liver is not the prime site for morphine metabolism.

At portal vein plasma morphine concentrations of approximately 200 nmol/liter, the cow liver removed no morphine. The concentrations after 10 mg oral morphine in this study barely exceeded this level (Fig. 2), so that direct extrapolation from cow to human liver would predict 100% availability. The kidney rather than the liver appears to be responsible for morphine metabolism in this low but therapeutically important concentration range.

At what dose of morphine will the liver contribute to metabolism? Hepatic extraction ratios of greater than 0.5 were seen when portal vein concentrations exceeded 500 nmol/liter; these may be achieved with high single oral doses, chronic oral dosing (>300 mg total daily dose), or rapid i.v. bolus injection. The apparent availability of such doses would be less than 100%. Variable hepatic extraction may be implicated in the variation in published values for morphine clearance. The size of an i.v. dose and the speed with which it is given influence the plasma concentrations; the higher those concentrations, the greater the extent of hepatic metabolism, and the higher the clearance. Variable hepatic extraction may also invalidate calculation of availability using simple AUC_{oral}:$AUC_{i.v.}$ ratios. High peak plasma concentrations following an i.v. bolus engender a different metabolic fate from that encountered by a formulation that sustains plasma concentrations below the level at which no hepatic extraction occurs.

Increasing involvement of the liver in morphine metabolism may also be seen in cancer pain management. The dramatic increase in total oral morphine daily dose requirement beyond a threshold of about 300 mg total oral daily dose probably reflects hepatic involvement in morphine metabolism as plasma concentrations rise. Availability falls as the liver "switches in," and relatively large dose increments are required to achieve increased analgesia.

REFERENCES

1. Barnes, J. N., and Goodwin, F. J. (1983): Dihydrocodeine narcosis in renal failure. *Br. Med. J.,* 286:438–439.
2. Bigler, D., Eriksen, J., and Christensen, C. B. (1984): Prolonged respiratory depression caused by slow release morphine. *Lancet,* 1:1477.
3. Brunk, S. F., Delle, M., and Wilson, W. R. (1975): Effect of propranolol on morphine metabolism. *Clin. Pharmacol. Ther.,* 16:1039–1044.
4. Bullingham, R. E. S., McQuay, H. J., Porter, E. J. B., Allen, M. C., and Moore, R. A. (1982): Sublingual buprenorphine used postoperatively: Ten hour plasma drug concentration analysis. *Br. J. Clin. Pharmacol.,* 13:665–673.
5. Bullingham, R. E. S., Moore, R. A., Symonds, H. W., Allen, M. C., Baldwin, D., and McQuay, H. J. (1984): A novel form of dependency of hepatic extraction ratio of opioids in vivo upon the portal vein concentration of drug: Comparison of morphine, diamorphine, fentanyl, methadone and buprenorphine in the chronically cannulated cow. *Life Sci.,* 34:2047–2056.
6. Don, H. F., Dieppa, R. A., and Taylor, P. (1975): Narcotic analgesics in anuric patients. *Anesthesiology,* 42:745–747.
7. Fine, A., and Churchill, D. N. (1981): Potentially lethal interaction of cimetidine and morphine. *Can. Med. Assoc. J.,* 124:1434–1436 (letter).
8. Houde, R. W., Wallenstein, S. L., and Beaver, W. T. (1965): Clinical measurement of pain. In: *Analgetics,* edited by G. de Stevens, pp. 75–122. Academic Press, New York.
9. Iwamoto, K., Eaton, D. L., and Klassen, C. D. (1978): Uptake of morphine and nalorphine by isolated rat hepatocytes. *J. Pharmacol. Exp. Ther.,* 206:181–189.
10. McQuay, H., and Moore, A. (1984): Metabolism of narcotics. *Br. Med. J.,* 288:237 (letter).
11. McQuay, H. J., and Moore, R. A. (1984): Be aware of renal function when prescribing morphine. *Lancet,* 2:284 (letter).
12. McQuay, H. J., Moore, R. A., Bullingham, R. E. S., Carroll, D., Baldwin, D., Allen, M. C., Glynn, C. J., and Lloyd, J. W. (1984): High systemic relative availability of oral morphine in both solution and sustained release formulation. *Royal Society of Medicine, International Congress and Symposium Series,* pp. 149–154.

13. Mojaverian, P., Fedder, I. L., Vlasses, P. H., Rotmensch, H. H., Rocci, M. L., Swanson, B. N., and Ferguson, R. K. (1982): Cimetidine does not alter morphine disposition in man. *Br. J. Clin. Pharmacol.,* 14:809–813.
14. Moore, R. A., Baldwin, D., McQuay, H. J., and Bullingham, R. E. S. (1984): HPLC of morphine with electrochemical detection: Analysis in human plasma. *Ann. Clin. Biochem.,* 21:125–130.
15. Moore, R. A., Baldwin, D., Allen, M. C., Watson, P. J. Q., Bullingham, R. E. S., and McQuay, H. J. (1984): Sensitive and specific morphine radioimmunoassay with iodine label: Pharmacokinetics of morphine in man after intravenous administration. *Ann. Clin. Biochem.,* 21:318–325.
16. Moore, R. A., Sear, J. W., Baldwin, D., Allen, M. C., Hunniset, A., Bullingham, R., and McQuay, H. J. (1984): Morphine kinetics during and after renal transplantation in man. *Clin. Pharmacol. Ther.,* 35:641–648.
17. Neal, E. A., Meffin, P. J., Gregory, P. B., and Blaschke, T. F. (1979): Enhanced bioavailability and decreased clearance of analgesics in patients with cirrhosis. *Gastroenterology,* 77:96–102.
18. Patwardhan, R. V., Johnson, R. F., Hoyumpa, A., Sheehan, J. J., Desmond, P. V., Wilkinson, G. R., Branch, R. A., and Schenker, S. (1981): Normal metabolism of morphine in cirrhosis. *Gastroenterology,* 81:1006–1011.
19. Redfern, N. (1983): Dihydrocodeine overdose treated with naloxone infusion. *Br. Med. J.,* 287:751–752.
20. Regnard, C. F. B., and Twycross, R. G. (1984): Metabolism of narcotics. *Br. Med. J.,* 288:860 (letter).
21. Sawe, J., Pacifici, G. M., Kager, L., von Bahr, C., and Rane, A. (1982): Glucuronidation of morphine in human liver and interaction with oxazepam. *Acta Anaesthesiol. Scand.* [*Suppl.*], 74:47–51.
22. Schali, C., and Roch-Ramel, F. (1982): Transport and metabolism of [^{3}H]morphine in isolated, nonperfused proximal tubular segments of the rabbit kidney. *J. Pharmacol. Exp. Ther.,* 223:811–815.
23. Stanski, D. R., Greenblatt, D. J., and Lowenstein, E. (1978): Kinetics of intravenous and intramuscular morphine. *Clin. Pharmacol. Ther.,* 24:52–59.
24. Williams, R. A. (1983): Drug administration in hepatic disease. *N. Engl. J. Med.,* 309:1616–1622.

Advances in Pain Research and Therapy, Vol. 9, edited by H. L. Fields et al. Raven Press, New York © 1985.

Clinical Evaluation of Slow-Release Morphine Tablets

T. D. Walsh

Department of Developmental Chemotherapy, Memorial Sloan-Kettering Cancer Center, New York, New York 10021

Oral aqueous solutions of morphine (AQM) or diamorphine (heroin) are often the treatment of choice in experienced units for chronic pain due to advanced cancer. When the dosage is individually titrated against the patient's pain and morphine is given every 4 hr, this approach is safe (5) and extremely effective in relieving pain. Dosage is reviewed regularly (e.g., at 24- or 48-hr intervals) and increased in stepwise increments until the patient is pain-free or pain-controlled. The principles of this approach were described by Saunders (4) two decades ago and were reviewed recently (6). It has been shown in a controlled study (2) to be highly effective in controlling cancer pain. It is self-evident that this approach is time-consuming (five or six drug rounds every 24 hr) and may be difficult to adhere to in hospital practice outside of special hospice units. In domiciliary care it ties patients to a fixed schedule that may necessitate changes in daily routine or sleep disturbance to ensure optimal pain control. The introduction of a slow-release morphine (SRM) tablet thus aroused interest when it was shown to produce plasma levels sustained for 12 hr (1). Such a preparation, if effective, would have considerable convenience value in domiciliary care, and in hospital practice it would save nursing time expended in repeated analgesic rounds every 4 hr. Prolonged plasma levels are not the same as prolonged analgesia, and so we decided to conduct a clinical trial of this preparation. St. Christopher's Hospice has had considerable experience in clinical care, teaching, and research in this field; more than 400 patients per year are given morphine for chronic pain.

CLINICAL EXPERIENCE

Initial evaluation was on a case-by-case basis among patients needing low doses of morphine, e.g., 20 mg/24 hr. We used 10-mg SRM tablets at first—later 30 and 60 mg. The preparation was found to be effective in general use. It became common practice among those stabilized and pain-controlled at a particular dose of AQM to transfer them to an equivalent dosage of SRM (in mg/24 hr) given in two doses every 12 hr. Analgesia was satisfactory, and no apparent differences in side effects were noted. There was a small number of patients whose pain relief was not prolonged; they required the SRM tablet every 8 hr. There were two areas in which the SRM seemed relatively ineffective (compared with AQM): in rapid titration of morphine dose (to achieve initial pain control) and among the minority who required high morphine dosages (>150 mg/24 hr). An advantage of the availability of SRM was that those occasional patients who experienced severe nausea and vomiting with the AQM could be transferred to an equivalent 24-hr dosage of the SRM with improvement in nausea/vomiting and continued satisfactory analgesia. The reasons for this are unclear, but it is of interest that the reverse is also true. In the case of the SRM, it was anticipated that fewer side effects would be experienced, although clinical experience did not support this. Intuitively it seemed that those side effects probably related to peak morphine plasma levels (i.e., nausea, vomiting, sedation) would be less prominent with the SRM. Given the high bioavailability of liquid formulations, the slower rates of release and absorption with the SRM might produce fewer side effects. If should be noted here that the incidence of severe side effects with AQM is low. On clinical grounds, the preparations seemed comparable, and with the introduction of a 100-mg tablet (allowing us to include the higher dose ranges, e.g., 600 mg/24 hr), we decided to evaluate SRM in a controlled trial.

CLINICAL TRIAL

We designed the study to mimic (insofar as possible) clinical practice. A major limitation of conventional clinical analgesic efficacy studies has been the artificial constraints applied to the study design. This has produced confusion concerning a number of issues, such as drug potency and efficacy and equianalgesic dosages. The object was to obtain a realistic picture of the use of SRM in the complex situation of advanced cancer, in which pathological changes in body function are common and polypharmacy is the rule.

MATERIALS AND METHODS

All who participated were hospice inpatients with advanced cancer. All were terminally ill, with a likely life expectancy of weeks or months. None was receiving chemotherapy or radiotherapy. A controlled study designed to fit into established hospice daily routine and practice was employed using a double-blind double-placebo two-way balanced crossover (Table 1). All patients were seen twice daily by an experienced nurse observer. Conventional hospice prescribing practice was adhered to as closely as possible. All decisions concerning drug therapy were made by the patient's personal phy-

TABLE 1. *Study design AQM/SRM Study*

Stabilization period (AQM)	
Randomization (½ AQM:½ SRM)	Day 1
Crossover (all)	Day 3
Crossover (all)	Day 5
Crossover (½)	Day 8
Finish	Day 10

sician, using, insofar as possible (for the purposes of the study), a standardized list of medications, e.g., one nighttime sedative. No restrictions were placed on frequency or magnitude of changes in dosage of any drug. Consecutive patients who were clinically "stable" on static doses of morphine were interviewed to assess suitability for the study. If they were judged likely to have a sufficient life expectancy, were capable of completing visual analog scales (VAS), and were agreeable to participate, they were entered, but only after consultation with the responsible nursing and medical staff. Formal informed consent was not obtained; they were verbally asked to (a) participate in a study of pain, (b) take an extra tablet(s) every 12 hr, and (c) see the nurse interviewer twice daily. If they agreed, they were randomly assigned to continue on the AQM or crossover immediately (day 1) to the same dosage (mg/24 hr) of SRM given in two divided doses every 12 hr. They continued on this for 48 hr before crossover (day 3) and again for a further 48 hr before further (day 5) crossover (Table 1). Crossover took place in both directions, with all finishing on SRM. Morphine dosage was reviewed (according to predetermined criteria) at 24-hr intervals for upward or downward adjustment according to the level of pain. An agreed scheme of analgesics for "breakthrough" pain was agreed in advance so that all could get "as-required" analgesics in addition to morphine liquid/tablets every 4 or 12 hr. Identical SRM placebo/pills were used. Morphine solution and placebo were blindly taste-tested by research, nursing, and medical staff beforehand and were found to be indistinguishable. The aim of the study was to examine both clinical efficacy and side effects; information was collected from patients and nursing staff (Table 2). A standard 10-cm VAS was used for patient measures, with the extremes of each sensation at either end of the scale. Patients self-completed VAS on Saturday and Sunday. Nurse-derived data were collected using a standard recording form completed by the senior nurse on duty for each individual 8-hr period.

RESULTS

Thirty-six patients entered the study, and 30 completed all requirements. There were 22 females and 8 males. There were 60 crossovers from AQM to SRM and 30 from SRM to AQM. Mean age was 67 ± 8 years (68 for

TABLE 2. *AQM/SRM study data collection*

Patient
1. Pain, sedation twice daily: VAS a.m./p.m.
2. Mood, anxiety once daily: VAS a.m.

Nurse[a]
1. Pain, sedation (global measure)
2. Nausea/vomiting (present/absent)
3. Constipation (present/absent)
4. Oriented (yes/no)
5. Pain breakthrough (time/action)
6. Assessment of blindness

[a]Items 1–5 were completed on a standard assessment form for each nursing shift, i.e. three times in 24 hr.

males, 65 for females). Males and females had similar scores for anxiety, mood, pain, and sedation at the base line. Morphine doses were similar at base line for males and females. The morphine dosage range and distribution for the study patients were comparable to those for the general non-study hospice population. Median survival after the study was 22 days (range 0–111 days), compared with a median of 8.0 days (range 0–38) for those withdrawn. All withdrawals were because patients were judged too ill to continue in the study; they were equally distributed between AQM and SRM. VAS scores were analyzed using paired and unpaired *t*-tests. Scores were analyzed within groups (depending on initial randomization) and between groups (to ensure comparability throughout the study). Data on side effects and other nurse-derived data were ranked for nonparametric analysis. This was found to be insensitive, and so data were converted to binomial scores (present/absent) and analyzed using contingency tables. No differences were found in pain, mood, sedation, anxiety, or side-effect scores for any of the crossover points. There was no evidence of carryover or directional effects. Initial randomization did not affect subsequent scoring. Nursing staff were unable to distinguish between the two preparations on the basis on clinical judgment. There was a tendency for those on the SRM to have more nausea and vomiting (as judged by nursing staff), but this was not statistically significant. Adjuvant drug prescribing (e.g., breakthrough analgesics, sedatives) was unaffected by crossover or AQM/SRM use. There was no evidence of pain breakthrough being a problem with SRM; i.e., it seemed to be a true 12-hr preparation.

DISCUSSION

The SRM and AQM formulations of morphine appear comparable in terms of analgesic efficacy and side effects. This applies to the clinical context described (i.e., those already on morphine). The study was not designed to examine the separate issue of whether either was superior in achieving initial pain control. Patients found the tablets acceptable even when several had to be taken at once. There was a bias among nursing staff against the SRM, but they were unable to distinguish the two preparations under double-blind conditions. The tendency toward more nausea and vomiting on the SRM is difficult to explain, but more impressive because of the inability of staff to distinguish the two. An unforeseen feature was the disparity in numbers between males and females. Although the sexes were comparable in terms of age, morphine dosage, and base-line VAS scores, the imbalance was unfortunate given the differences in morphine pharmacokinetics (5) and analgesic requirements between men and women. Aside from the sex imbalance, the study group was representative of the hospice population. Women live longer than men after admission to the hospice; men die quickly from cancer of the common primary site (lung), whereas women appear to have a more protracted terminal phase (3).

It remains possible that the (female) nurse observer identified more closely with female patients. The disparity in frequencies of nausea and vomiting noted partly supports our clinical observations, although in the study this was in one direction, i.e., worse with SRM. We now recommend that patients stabilized on AQM every 4 hr should be transferred to an equivalent dose of SRM (in mg/24 hr) in two 12-hr doses. These results do not usurp the physician's clinical judgment; undoubtedly there will be individual patients who will require SRM given every 8 hr or who will tolerate it better than AQM. However, SRM is clearly acceptable in the majority of cancer patients for long-term control of chronic cancer pain.

CONCLUSIONS

SRM tablets are an acceptable, convenient alternative to AQM. When used in equivalent milligram doses per 24 hr. the preparations are comparable in regard to analgesic efficacy and side effects. We recommend that patients first be stabilized on AQM before transferring to SRM. Clinical judgment must be employed in difficult individual cases.

REFERENCES

1. Leslie, S. T., Rhodes, A., and Black, F. M. (1980): Controlled release morphine sulphate tablets—a study in normal volunteers. *Br. J. Clin. Pharmacol.,* 9:531–534.
2. Melzack, R., Mount, B. M., and Gordon, J. M. (1979): The Brompton mixture versus morphine solution given orally: Effects on pain. *Can. Med. Assoc. J.,* 120:435.
3. St. Christopher's Hospice (1984): Annual statistics. St. Christopher's Hospice, London.
4. Saunders, C. (1963): The treatment of intractable pain in terminal cancer. *Proc. R. Soc. Med.,* 56:195–197.
5. Walsh, T. D. (1984): Opiates and respiratory function in advanced cancer. *Recent Results Cancer Res.,* 89:115–117.
6. Walsh, T. D., and Cheater, F. M. (1983): Use of morphine for cancer pain. *Pharmaceutical Journal,* October 29, 525–527.

Advances in Pain Research and Therapy, Vol. 9, edited by H. L. Fields et al. Raven Press, New York © 1985.

Clinical Aspects of Intrathecal and Epidural Opiates

Philip R. Bromage

Department of Anesthesiology, University of Colorado Health Sciences Center, Denver, Colorado 80262

Narcotic pain control has always been hampered by the fear that effective doses would also produce dangerous respiratory depression. When intraspinal narcotics burst upon the clinical scene in 1979, initial reports suggested that, at last, practical means had been found to circumvent the danger of respiratory depression. These new ways of using old drugs offered a chance to achieve segmental analgesia of great intensity and duration at a spinal level. Implicit in these hopes was the asumption that the intraspinal narcotics would not spread rostrally to any significant degree, and certainly not enough to depress central components of respiratory control. Subsequent work in volunteers and in clinical patients demonstrated that while intraspinal narcotics can indeed confer an improved quality of analgesia, the linkage between pain relef and respiratory depression has not been cut, and ironically the association might be even more dangerous than in the past.

Clinical success with any form of pharmacological therapy depends on working within the margin between toxicity and therapeutic effectiveness, while creating backup systems to minimize the dangers of toxic effects. Intelligent use of the intraspinal narcotics is impossible without some basic understanding of their pharmacokinetics and dynamics. The uptake and distribution of narcotics from the spinal canal are simlar to the movement of intraspinal local anesthetics. In practice, the two classes of agents are often used in combination or alternately, and so it is helpful to review both types of drugs together, remembering, of course, that their sites of action and pharmacokinetics are very different.

Local anesthetics block nerve fibers of all modalities, including sympathetic efferents, whereas narcotics act on opiate receptors at synaptic junctions of small-cell networks throughout the neuraxis, and sympathetic and motor functions remain undisturbed.

PRACTICAL PHARMACOKINETICS

Thirty years ago the dura mater was thought to be impermeable to local anesthetics and similar drugs (24). For this reason, and because the dura fused with the periosteum at the base of the skull, epidural analgesia was considered to avoid the danger of accidental intracranial spread that existed with subarachnoid anesthesia. Today, it is clear that the dura mater is a very poor barrier to the passage of local anesthetics and narcotics. In 1963, studies with ^{14}C-labeled local anesthetics showed that not only was the dura very permeable, allowing a rapid rise of concentration in the cerebrospinal fluid (CSF) after epidural injection, but also these lipid-soluble drugs penetrated the periphery of the cord in a circumferential pattern. They could also spread rostrally to reach the surface of the medulla, and even as far as superficial cortical structures (6). Intrathecally injected local anesthetics had a similar tendency to penetrate the surface of the cord (18). More recent studies have shown that the meninges are also very permeable to narcotics and that dural permeability tends to vary inversely with the square of the molecular weight of the narcotic (45).

The distribution of narcotics within the CSF is very similar to that for the local anesthetics. The narcotics leach out of the CSF into the periphery of the spinal cord, with a speed proportional to their lipid solubility, and then penetrate inward from the surface of the neuraxis (58) to reach opiate receptors lying in their path.

Vascular absorption occurs coincidentally with neuraxial uptake and competes with it, and both local anesthetics and narcotics are transported away from the spinal canal into the bloodstream. Blood levels rise steeply after epidural injection, and then follow a pattern of decline similar to that seen after i.v. or i.m. injection (9,28,46). However, the differential concentrations of narcotics in CSF and blood are very high, ranging from 50:1 to 200:1, thus confirming the enormously high proportion of narcotic delivered to the surface of the spinal cord as the blood-brain barrier is bypassed (21,35,46). Vascular absorption from the spinal canal is slowed by addition of epinephrine 1/200,000 (10,13), and the neural effects are correspondingly enhanced. However, these actions of epinephrine are not entirely due to its local vascular effects, because epidural epinephrine by itself appears to have a primary analgesic action that is independent from its effects on vascular absorption (10,19). Vascular uptake is much less after subarachnoid injection, and then the concentration ratios in CSF and blood are of the order of 1,000:1 to 50,000:1 (47).

PRACTICAL PHARMACODYNAMICS

Spinal narcotics attach to opiate receptors in the small-cell networks of laminae I and II of the dorsal horn and reduce nociceptive input to the cord.

No other afferent or motor activities seem to be affected to any significant degree, expect for the complex mechanism involving initiation of micturition, and retention of urine is a common and troublesome feature of the intraspinal narcotics.

Rostral spread to the upper thoracic, cervical, and medullary regions is associated with a number of other side effects. The most common is a high incidence of nonsegmental itching, which comes on about 3 hr after lumbar injection of epidural morphine (8). Nausea and vomiting occur about 1 hr later, at 4 to 5 hr after injection. Further rostral spread to the medulla is accompanied by varying degrees of respiratory depression. In volunteers, depressed sensitivity to increased inspired concentrations of CO_2 is invariably present within an hour or so of injection (14,38,39). In the case of morphine, this depression reaches its nadir 7 to 10 hr after epidural injection and persists for 16 to 20 hr. However, less respiratory depression is seen in surgical patients, because the increased afferent input of postoperative pain acts as a stimulus that partially compensates for the opiate depression (23). The degree of respiratory depression is intensified by addition of epinephrine 1/200,000 (10). Severe, life-threatening respiratory depression is a relatively common feature of intrathecal administration (22).

A more subtle and rare danger arises if an epidural catheter becomes displaced. Practitioners usually assume that a working epidural will remain a working epidural, and that if all is well, all will continue to be well (11). But this may not be the case if the tip of the catheter accidentally penetrates the dura. Then, a normal epidural dose becomes an overwhelming subarachnoid overdose within the restricted confines of the subarachnoid space. Inadvertent massive overdoses of this nature have occurred on several occasions, one with a fatal result (unpublished), but others with more fortunate outcomes (12,55).

Lipid-soluble agents enter the cord rapidly and tend to exhibit rapid onset and intense and limited segmental analgesia, and then they "wash out" again in a correspondingly rapid fashion. Strong receptor binding may modify this general pattern. For example, the highly lipid-soluble drug sufentanil provides longer duration than its congener fentanyl, which has less lipid solubility, but also less intense binding capability.

PATTERN OF AFFERENT INPUT

Because the mode of action of the spinal narcotics is so different from that of the local anesthetics, it would not be surprising if they exhibited different qualities of pain relief. And indeed they do. The basic action of intraspinal narcotics at small-cell networks seems to control pain of constant ongoing intensity better than pain of a phasic nature, where large numbers of afferent neuronal pools are rapidly recruited and then rapidly decremented. Thus, we see a high success rate with cancer pain, a moderate degree of success with severe postoperative pain, but extremely poor results with the phasic crescendo pain of the late stages of active labor.

PRACTICAL APPLICATIONS OF INTRASPINAL NARCOTICS

The foregoing introductory section is intended to alert the practitioner to three basic constraints in using the intraspinal narcotics.

First, narcotics administered by the intraspinal route are just as dangerous as when given by any other means, perhaps more so, and the side effects are more troublesome. Their attraction lies in their great power. They may be dangerous, but they confer an impressive quality of pain relief unmatched by any other route of medication.

Second, success will differ with different types of pain. Clinical management must recognize and cater for these differences.

Third, a wide range of clinical behavior exists among the various narcotics, depending on their physicochemical characteristics. Successful management depends on rational use of these differences.

In addition, future developments will arise from exploitation of intraspinal mixtures of different classes of agents to achieve optimal analgesic effects. For example, it is already clear that the adrenergic agonist epinephrine has appreciable effects on the modulation of afferent input and on the efficiency of intraspinal narcotics (10,19,62). Other neural transmitters are under intense study for intraspinal applications in pain management.

Chronic Pain

Nonmalignant Pain

Chronic pain that is not fatal and that may persist indefinitely is poorly suited to narcotic control of any sort, because the problems of addiction outweigh the advantages. Cases of this nature are better treated by other methods. However, attempts have been made to use morphine combined with epidural steroids for alleviation of low back pain on a short-term basis, with some interesting results. Huntington et al. (32) treated a series of 25 patients with single epidural injections of 8 to 15 mg of morphine sulfate followed by 80 to 120 mg of methylprednisolone. The authors reported pain relief for more than 3 months. However, there was a high incidence of severe pruritus lasting for up to 5 days, and all diabetic patients in the series experienced pruritus of a particularly severe nature (32).

Malignant Pain

The management of malignant pain must be seen in perspective: Most patients can be kept comfortable by simple means; more complex and heroic measures are needed in only a small minority of cases. The hospice approach to managing terminally ill patients has been immensely successful (60,61). Within this type of organization that covers both inpatient and domiciliary management, large doses of oral narcotic elixirs or "cocktails" such as the old "mistura lethalis," later modified and now known as the "Brompton mixture," have come to be the mainstay of cancer pain therapy. In most patients with terminal pain the oral elixir regimen is remarkably successful, simple to manage, and acceptable to the patients. However, the spinal route offers an excellent alternative to oral or parenteral narcotics in a small minority of patients who have become tolerant to medication and who still suffer severe pain in spite of increasingly large oral doses.

Indwelling spinal catheter techniques offer a variety of ways to bring the opiates close to their receptor targets without the need to achieve high blood and tissue levels throughout the rest of the body. The blood-brain barrier is bypassed, and concentrations of opiates in the surface layers of the cord and medulla can be 10 to 100 times higher than would be possible by oral or parenteral administration.

Initial trials with epidural and intrathecal catheters were carried out by the technically simple lumbar route for control of cancer pain involving lumbosacral and lower thoracic segments. Later, however, attempts were made to control cervical and cranial, and even lumbosacral, pain by placing catheters in the cisterna magna or directly into the cerebral ventricles (40,41,53).

The cranial approaches deliver narcotics close to the periaqueductal gray matter. This region is densely populated with opiate receptor sites and is a strategic center for narcotic pain control (50). On the other hand, the narcotics are also brought in close contact with medullary nuclei concerned with respiratory control (57), and so the margin of safety between effective pain control and dangerous apnea would seem to be very narrow. Nevertheless, in practice, a number of successful series have been reported in which chronic intraventricular cannulation and morphine doses of 100 μg to 4 mg have provided excellent and prolonged relief from severe disseminated cancer pain without apparent respiratory depression (40,41,53).

An explanation for this successful dissociation between pain relief and respiratory depression may lie in the prior habituation or tolerance of brainstem nuclei to increasingly large doses of parenteral narcotics. A striking example of this form of tolerance is seen with *in vitro* isolated brainstem slices from the locus ceruleus (LC). LC cells fire spontaneously and are silenced by morphine. LC cells from animals chronically pretreated with morphine require two to four times more topical morphine to depress activity than cells from narcotically naive animals (1). This suggests that tolerance in the central respiratory mechanisms may equal or perhaps exceed that of nociceptive circuitry in more caudad regions, thus allowing a greater margin of safety in habituated patients than in a normal population.

Transcutaneous epidural catheters provide the simplest and least invasive means for administering intraspinal narcotics over periods of many days or weeks, provided aseptic precautions are observed, with an effective bacterial filter (0.2-μm pore size) incorporated in the system. A number of authors have reported marked success with this method (17,42,65). Domiciliary management can be continued for many months, provided arrangements are made for the catheter to be changed when required, and provided the family, visiting nurses, and the patient are instructed in the basic technicalities of aseptic catheter care.

Epidural dose requirements vary widely, depending on the intensity of pain and the degree of narcotic tolerance that has developed. Magora et al. (42) reported good relief in 8 of 9 patients receiving intermittent doses of only 2 mg morphine. However, in most cases requiring spinal narcotics, much larger amounts are needed, and it may be necessary to increase each intermittent dose up to 40 mg or more every 6 to 12 hr as tolerance develops. In this very high dose range, substantial blood levels will also be achieved, but the amount reaching the circulation will still be less than during high-dose parenteral or oral regimens.

Development of tolerance may be slowed by alternating the mode of analgesia and, as it were, "resting" the opiate receptors (16,64). Thus, substituting epidural local anesthetic injections or infusions for the morphine over a period of 1 or 2 days may "reset" the receptors, and then epidural morphine can be restarted at a somewhat lower dose level.

Totally implanted delivery systems are the next step in technical sophistication and invasiveness. An indwelling Silastic epidural catheter can be tunneled under the skin and attached to an implanted rechargeable reservoir (e.g., "Infusaid" type) delivering a constant metered infusion of morphine into the epidural space. The reservoir can then be recharged at intervals of 2 to 4 weeks depending on the dose requirements of the patient (20). These reservoirs are designed for the relatively high dosage requirements of the extradural route and are necessarily large and may be somewhat uncomfortable for the patient. Smaller reservoirs, greater parsimony of dosage, and lower blood levels of morphine can be achieved by using intrathecal Silastic catheters attached to an implanted Omaya reservoir (40).

At an even more sophisticated and invasive level, intraventricular cannulas may succeed where spinal administration has failed. A cannula is placed under local anesthesia, with the tip in the anterior horn of the lateral ventricle, and is connected to a subcutaneous Omaya reservoir or to a larger exteriorized delivery system (53). Although the danger of respiratory depression with intraventricular systems is likely to be very serious in narcotically naive subjects, the risk appears to be slight in patients who are previously habituated to large doses of morphine by other routes. At the present time, intraventricular delivery seems to offer effective relief in severe intractable pain when more simple delivery systems have failed. However, a larger experience will be needed before the method can be rigorously assessed and evaluated.

Acute Pain

Obstetrical Pain

A number of independent clinical trials have shown that labor pain is poorly controlled by intraspinal narcotics (5,15,31,33,63). Although first-stage labor pain can be adequately managed, second-stage pain is not reliably controlled. Perhaps this failure is due in part to the phasic nature of the sudden and intense but brief pain alternating with periods of uterine relaxation and relief that was alluded to earlier in this chapter.

In addition, rapid blood flow through the extradural venous plexuses at term causes appreciable and sustained narcotic concentrations in maternal blood, thus exposing the fetus to the depressant effects of the circulating narcotics. Because epinephrine reduces vascular uptake and intensifies the analgesic action of narcotics in the epidural space (10), addition of epinephrine 1/400,000 to 1/200,000 may be especially advantageous in the obstetrical context. Two studies of epinephrine added to epidural meperidine during labor have tended to confirm this impression, although neither trial yielded statistically significant results. Perriss (48) and Perriss and Malins (49) found that epinephrine 1/200,000 improved the quality of pain relief from 55% to over 80% when using 50 mg meperidine. Skjoldebrand et al. (56) using only 25 mg meperidine, observed a faster onset of analgesia when epinephrine 1/200,000 was added, together with a smaller degree of vascular uptake.

More practical success has been obtained by adding narcotics to dilute concentrations of local anesthetics used for epidural analgesia in labor. Fentanyl has proved to be especially useful when given in this way. Doses of 80 to 100 μg fentanyl added to 0.3 or 0.5% bupivacaine increased the quality of analgesia and prolonged the duration (36,37). The nagging persistent perineal pain of occipitoposterior positions is well controlled by this type of mixture, and in our practice we have found doses of 60 to 80 μg of fentanyl in 0.25% bupivacaine to be highly effective.

Narcotics relieve labor pain more effectively when given intrathecally than by the epidural route. Subarachnoid doses of 1 to 2 mg morphine provide excellent analgesia throughout the first and second stages of labor (3,4), although supplemental regional anesthesia may be required for delivery and episiotomy (3). However, there is a heavy price to pay in side effects. The duration of action is long and may outlast the labor. Respiratory depression may occur in subarachnoid dose ranges around 1 to 2 mg of morphine; in addition, troublesome pruritus arises in 70 to 90% of patients, and vomiting in 30 to 60%.

Thus, at the present time, labor pain is probably most effectively handled by dilute mixtures of local anesthetics and lipid-soluble narcotics acting together in the epidural space.

Postoperative Pain and Trauma

Opinions differ widely about intraspinal narcotics for acute pain relief. Whereas there is general agreement that they are powerful and extremely effective, there is little agreement on dosage, management regimens, and the importance of side effects. Practice attitudes range from timid underdosage and intense close surveillance to enthusiastic optimism that the practitioner and the patients possess a charmed immunity from hazard, on the assumption that because all has gone well so far in a limited series of cases, all will continue to get well. Unhappily, this assumption is not correct, and the probability that complications will *not* arise in any series with zero numerator (i.e., no complications so far) are as follows (30):

Probability:	95%	99%	99.9%
Betting odds:	3/N	4.6/N	6.9/N

In most series, N is too small to provide comfortable betting odds in a wager in which a patient's life may be the price of losing.

Optimism is borne on two further assumptions: first, that the narcotic has been injected into the right place; second, that pain will override central effects on breathing and provide sufficient afferent input to spur a flagging respiratory control system (23,29). Again, these reasonable suppositions may not be correct under certain circumstances, and then superb analgesia becomes a potential death warrant. There are many published reports of near misses, in which patients have been rescued from profound respiratory depression (64), and clearly the unwanted side effects of spinal anesthesia must be taken very seriously.

This section will examine some of the evidence on both sides, that is, for aggressive pain management as well as for prudent caution, and will attempt to suggest a workable compromise between the two.

Spinal opiates are attractive for management of surgical pain because their relatively pure antinociceptive effect spares sympathetic and motor functions and provides excellent pain relief without the vasodilation, hypotension, and lower-limb weakness that accompanies epidural and subarachnoid block from local anesthetics.

Postoperative tests of respiratory function on the day of upper abdominal surgery show that epidural narcotics produce sufficient analgesia to restore FEV_1 just as effectively as epidural local anesthetics, provided the narcotics are given in sufficient amounts (7,59). The endocrine response to upper abdominal surgery, in terms of plasma cortisol and catecholamine blood levels, is suppressed to about the same degree from the sixth hour onward with either epidural local anesthetics or epidural morphine at doses of 4 to 8 mg (54). Severe muscular skeletal pain is also amenable to the intraspinal narcotics, up to a point. However, extreme phasic pain (for example, from passive movement of major joint implants) may exceed the analgesic capabilities of large doses of spinal narcotics, and then, as in obstetrical pain, local anesthetic blockage may have to be added in order to obtain acceptable relief (51).

Advantages and Disadvantages

Respiratory Depression

Respiratory depression is lilely to arise with intraspinal opiates when the site of injection is close to the head and when the dosage is sufficient to cause high concentrations of drug in the cisternal CSF and brainstem. For example, in one recent study comparing epidural local anesthetic and epidural morphine given in the upper thoracic region for post-thoracotomy pain, 27% of patients receiving 5 mg morphine suffered severe hypopnea and respiratory acidosis that required urgent treatment. On the other hand, in the same study, 23% of patients who received epidural local anesthetic injections at the same spinal level had episodes of severe arterial hypotension to below 60 mm Hg systolic (25). And so the risks of epidural morphine under these circumstances seem to be just as grave and just as frequent as those of epidural local anesthetics. One method flirts with respiratory death, the other with cardiovascular catastrophe, and both are clearly unsafe unless the patients are nursed under appropriately close supervision, where respiratory or cardiovascular complications can be recognized and corrected instantly.

Intrathecal morphine is equally hazardous when used in doses large enough to be effective, and especially when used in conjunction with parenteral narcotics or other respiratory depressant drugs. As with epidural morphine, the danger of respiratory depression is greatest between 6 and 12 hr after administration, and dangerous depression has been reported with doses as low as 1 mg (22). In children, respiratory depression comes on sooner, at about 4 hr. A 22% incidence of respiratory depression has been reported after intrathecal morphine at 0.03 mg/kg in children of 2 to 14 years after open-heart surgery, and a 10% incidence when the dose was reduced to 0.02 mg/kg (34).

Urinary Retention

Urinary retention is a potentially serious complication of intraspinal narcotics, especially after joint replacements of the lower limb, because bladder catheterization may lead to cystitis, bacteremia, and subsequent loss of the prosthesis, accompanied by prolonged hospitalization. Urinary retention is more prevalent in males than in females and appears to be dose-dependent. A 90% incidence was reported in male volunteers receiving 10 mg morphine by the lumbar epidural route (8), and a 100% incidence was reported in a post-thoracotomy series receiving repeated 5 mg boluses up to a total of 40 mg epidural morphine in the first 24 hr after surgery (25). Thus, great technical care must be given to the management of pain after joint prosthetic surgery, and it may be prudent to avoid long-acting intraspinal narcotics in these cases and instead rely on intermittent local anesthetics to provide pain relief and to increase lower-limb blood flow. Then the local anesthetic may be permitted to wear off for brief periods to allow the patient the opportunity for spontaneous micturition. If bladder catheterization becomes necessary in spite of all precautions, it should be carried out by intermittent rather than by continuous insertion.

The other unwanted side effects of intraspinal narcotics are a nuisance rather than a danger in the postoperative period. Pruritus is common and sometimes intense after cesarean section, perhaps because of the high levels of maternal progesterone. The incidence is probably higher than generally recognized, because many patients do not report itching unless directly questioned about it. Nausea and vomiting are relatively common in volunteers (30–40%) (8), but again this complication is difficult to evaluate in postoperative patients.

All side effects of intraspinal narcotics are antagonized by naloxone, and this agent should be kept in constant readiness to combat sudden respiratory depression. However, care must be exercised in its use, because cardiac dysrhythmias and standstill have been reported following bolus i.v. doses of 0.4 mg (2). The drug should be given slowly and in increments of 0.1 mg until the desired effects are obtained. Furthermore, the half-life of naloxone is short (~ 1 hr), and so repeated doses or a constant infusion may be needed to counteract the depression of a long-acting narcotic such as morphine.

Advantages and Technical Aspects

Relief of Pain

All investigators are agreed that intraspinal narcotics produce excellent and prolonged pain relief after trauma (e.g., fractured ribs) and after surgery. However, there is less agreement about choice of drug, dosage and frequency of administration, and whether the narcotics should be given by intermittent bolus or by continuous infusion. These areas of disagreement reflect the large number of variables to be considered and the difficulty of creating a series of well-designed prospective studies to evaluate this powerful but potentially harmful therapy under a wide variety of circumstances.

Restoration of Function

Respiratory function is markedly impaired by reflex responses to pain after thoracic and upper abdominal surgery. Good analgesia helps to restore respiratory function. The epidural opiates perform substantially better than by the parenteral route, and about equally as well as the epidural local anesthetics in terms of restoring a depressed FEV_1 toward preoperative control levels (7). Table 1 summarizes the data from one series in which maximum subjective analgesia and objective restoration of FEV_1 were used as criteria for successful analgesia after upper abdominal or thoracic surgery.

Note that whereas i.v. morphine gave good subjective relief, it did very little to restore FEV_1. On the other hand, a substantially larger increase in FEV_1 occurred when approximately the same dose was given epidurally. The table also shows that whereas the *mean* restoration of FEV_1 was approximately the same for both epidural local anesthetic and epidural narcotics, the standard deviations showed a wider variability of performance with the narcotics. Therefore, one might infer that epidural narcotics restore respiratory function less reliably than epidural local anesthetics and that epidural local anesthetics might be a better choice in patients with pre-existing lung disease. Mixtures of dilute local anesthetic with low concentrations of narcotic permit a low dosage of each component, and these mixtures show some promise of providing the advantages of both while minimizing the disadvantages of each, and they seem well suited to managing postoperative pain in patients with severe obstructive airway disease and compromised lung function. However, the precise pharmacokinetics of these local anesthetic-narcotic mixtures will have to be carefully studied before they can be recommended for general use.

TABLE 1. *Postoperative pain: Restoration of FEV_1 as an objective index of analgesic dose requirements for effective analgesia*

Analgesic intervention	FEV_1 as % of preoperative control	Cumulative dose of analgesic required for effective restoration of FEV_1 (mg)
Nil: pain	40 ± 13.2	—
Intravenous morphine (2-mg increments)	44.5	8.5 ± 2
Epidural lidocaine (1.5%)	68.7 ± 9.1	120 – 210
Epidural narcotics (bolus doses)		
Morphine	67.7 ± 14.0	10.3 ± 2.7
Hydromorphone		1.4 ± 0.5
Methadone		8.6 ± 2
Fentanyl		0.13 ± 0.027

Adapted from Bromage et al. (7).

Early postoperative exercise and ambulation are also facilitated by epidural narcotics, because pain relief is provided without the danger of potential hypotension. However, preservation of sympathetic tone may be a disadvantage when vasodilatation and augmented lower-limb flow might help to prevent deep-vein thrombosis after operations such as hip arthroplasty that are associated with a high incidence of deep-vein thrombosis (43,44). In these cases, intermittent epidural boluses of local anesthetic alternated with narcotic may provide more appropriate vascular dynamics in the lower limb.

Choice of Drug and Dosage

1. Morphine has been the standard against which other opiates have been judged. Dosage regimens have varied widely, with some investigators claiming excellent results from epidural doses as small as 2 to 3 mg (42), whereas others have found 10 mg to be necessary for objective evidence of satisfactory relief from severe postoperative pain (7). The low lipid solubility of morphine encourages rostral spread, and late respiratory depression is a serious hazard in narcotically naive patients (7,14).
2. Hydromorphone (Dilaudid) has greater lipid solubility than morphine, and therefore less tendency to spread rostrally in the CSF. However, we have encountered one case of late respiratory depression with repeated doses of epidural hydromorphone. Doses of 1.0 to 1.3 mg usually provide good pain relief for 6 to 10 hr.
3. Methadone (5–10 mg) and meperidine (25–100 mg) also provide intense postoperative analgesia, but for shorter periods of time, lasting 3.5 to 6 hr.
4. The highly lipid-soluble narcotic fentanyl gives rapid onset of analgesia for shorter periods of 2 to 3.5 hr, depending on dose size in the range of 75 to 150 μg. Excellent analgesia is provided when fentanyl is mixed with a weak concentration of local anesthetic. For example, epidural pump infusions provide deep segmental analgesia without excessive respiratory or cardiovascular depression when set to deliver 6 to 10 ml per hour of a mixture of 0.125 to 0.2% bupivacaine with 30 to 50 μg of fentanyl per hour. The infusion rate of both drugs is reassessed and adjusted at regular intervals depending on subjective pain relief, objective analgesia, and measured respiratory function in terms of FVC and arterial blood gases.

LOGISTICAL CONCLUSIONS

All forms of pain management must be daringly aggressive to be effective, with narcotic dosage pushed to a point where blood and tissue levels are close to the threshold for respiratory depression. In practice this often means that the therapeutic "window" is little wider than an archer's slit in a castle wall. To appreciate the risk–benefit ratio for the spinal narcotics, one must realize that alternative techniques are just as hazardous. For example, sophisticated and pharmacokinetically precise regimens for intravenous narcotics such as meperidine (52) and methadone (26) have therapeutic windows that are alarmingly narrow in narcotically naive patients. Thus, the minimum effective blood concentration (MEC) for i.v. methadone is about 58 ng/ml, and the threshold for clinically obvious respiratory depression is only twice that amount, at about 100 to 110 ng/ml (27). Meperidine, a popular drug for i.v. infusion, has a MEC of about 400 ng/ml, and at that level the slope of the CO_2 response curve is reduced to 50% below control (52).

Thus, in spite of the superior power of the intraspinal narcotics, the basic problems and dangers inherent in aggressive pain control are very similar regardless of the route of administration. While narcotic habituation in malignant pain seems to widen the therapeutic window for all methods of narcotic delivery, in acute pain, close surveillance is essential for safe management. Postoperative patients cannot be made pain-free safely in single hospital rooms without one-on-one nursing coverage, and this sort of close individual care is expensive. Economical solutions to safe pain management require a return to the Victorian ward concept of an open ward, with all patients in view of the central nursing station. Modern intensive-care units (ICU) are based on the Victorian ward concept, but they are staffed and equipped at a very high and costly level. Safe, effective, and economical pain management requires a step-down: an open ward for intermediate-level care, somewhere between the high technology and high cost of the ICU and the dangerous privacy of the single room. Until this concept is widely accepted and shown to be cost-effective, it is unlikely that effective pain control by any method will every become a safe and affordable reality in our hospitals. At present we do not have sufficient grasp of the issues at stake, nor have we instilled the managerial insight to translate the practical necessities of safety and convenience into appropriate hospital design. Until these mundane logistical constraints are addressed, the intraspinal narcotics must remain an exciting, immensely powerful, but costly and underused technique. In the meantime, they will have served to point the way to new fields of neuraxial pharmacology in the elusive quest for pain relief without respiratory depression.

REFERENCES

1. Andrade, R., Vandermaelen, C. P., and Aghajanian, G. K. (1983): Morphine tolerance and dependence in the locus coeruleus: Single cell studies in brain slices. *Eur. J. Pharmacol.*, 91:161–169.

2. Andree, R. A. (1980): Sudden death following naloxone administration. *Anesth. Analg. (Cleve.),* 59:782–784.
3. Baraka, A., Noueihid, R., and Hajj, S. (1981): Intrathecal injection of morphine for obstetric analgesia. *Anesthesiology,* 54:136–140.
4. Bonnardot, J. P., Maillet, M., Colau, J. C., Millot, F., and Deligne, P. (1982): Maternal and fetal concentrations of morphine after intrathecal administration during labor. *Br. J. Anaesth.,* 54:487–489.
5. Booker, P. D., Wilkes, R. G., Bryson, T. H. L., and Beddard, J. (1980): Obstetric pain relief using epidural morphine. *Anaesthesia,* 35:377–379.
6. Bromage, P. R., Joyal, A. C., and Binney, J. C. (1963): Local anesthetic drugs: Penetration from the spinal extradural space into the neuraxis. *Science,* 140:392–394.
7. Bromage, P. R., Camporesi, E., and Chestnut, D. (1980): Epidural narcotics for postoperative analgesia. *Anesth. Analg. (Cleve.),* 59:473–480.
8. Bromage, P. R., Camporesi, E. M., Durant, P. A. C., and Nielsen, C. H. (1982): Nonrespiratory side effects of epidural morphine. *Anesth. Analg. (Cleve.),* 61:490–495.
9. Bromage, P. R., Camporesi, E. M., Durant, P. A. C., and Nielsen, C. H. (1982): Rostral spread of epidural morphine. *Anesthesiology,* 56:431–436.
10. Bromage, P. R., Camporesi, E. M., Durant, P. A., and Nielsen, C. H. (1983): Influence of epinephrine as an adjuvant to epidural morphine. *Anesthesiology,* 58:257–262.
11. Brownridge, P. R. (1983): Epidural and intrathecal opiates for postoperative pain relief. *Anaesthesia,* 38:74–75.
12. Brownridge, P. R., Wrobel, J., and Watt-Smith, J. (1983): Respiratory depression following accidental subarachnoid pethidine. *Anaesth. Intensive Care,* 11:237–240.
13. Burfoot, M. F., and Bromage, P. R. (1971): The effects of epinephrine on mepivacaine absorption from the spinal epidural space. *Anesthesiology,* 35:488–492.
14. Camporesi, E. M., Nielsen, C. H., Bromage, P. R., and Durant, P. A. C. (1983): Ventilatory CO_2 sensitivity after intravenous and epidural morphine in volunteers. *Anesth. Analg. (Cleve.),* 62:633–640.
15. Carrie, L. E. S., O'Sullivan, G. M., and Seegobin, R. (1981): Epidural fentanyl in labour. *Anaesthesia,* 36:965–969.
16. Chayen, M. S., Rudick, V., and Borvine, A. (1980): Pain control with epidural injection of morphine. *Anesthesiology,* 53:338–339.
17. Christensen, F. R. (1982): Epidural morphine at home in terminal patients. *Lancet,* 2:47.
18. Cohen, E. N. (1968): Distribution of local anesthetic agents in the neuraxis of the dog. *Anesthesiology,* 29:1002–1005.
19. Collins, J. G., Kitahata, L. M., Matsumoto, M., Homma, E., and Suzukawa, M. (1984): Spinally administered epinephrine suppresses noxiously evoked activity of WDR neurons in the dorsal horn of the spinal cord. *Anesthesiology,* 60:269–275.
20. Coombs, D. W., Saunders, R. L., Gaylor, M., and Pageau, M. G. (1981): Epidural narcotic infusion: Implantation technique and efficacy. *Anesthesiology,* 55:469–473.
21. Cousins, M. J., Mather, L. E., Glynn, C. J., Wilson, P. R., and Graham, J. R. (1979): Selective spinal analgesia. *Lancet,* 1:1141–1142.
22. Davies, G. K., Tolhurst-Cleaver, C. L., and James, T. L. (1980): CNS depression from intrathecal morphine. *Anesthesiology,* 52:280.
23. Doblar, D. B., Muldoon, S. M., Abbrecht, P. H., Baskoff, J., and Watson, R. L. (1981): Epidural morphine following epidural local anesthetic: Effect on ventilatory and airway occlusion pressure response to CO_2. *Anesthesiology,* 55:423–428.
24. Dogliotti, A. M. (1933): Segmental peridural anesthesia. *Am. J. Surg.,* 20:107–118.
25. El-Baz, N. M. I., Faber, L., P., and Jensik, R. J. (1984): Continuous epidural infusion of morphine for treatment of pain after thoracic surgery: A new technique. *Anesth. Analg. (Cleve.),* 63:757–764.
26. Gourlay, G. K., Wilson, P. R., and Glynn, C. J. (1982): Pharmacodynamics and pharmacokinetics of methadone during the peri-operative period. *Anesthesiology,* 57:458–467.
27. Gourlay, G. K., Willis, R. J., and Wilson, P. R. (1984): Postoperative pain control with methadone: Influence of supplementary methadone doses and blood concentration–response relationships. *Anesthesiology,* 61:19–26.
28. Gustafsson, L. L., Friberg-Nielsen, S., Garle, M., Mohall, A., Rane, A., Schildt, B., and Symreng, T. (1982): Extradural and parenteral morphine: Kinetics and effects in postoperative pain. A controlled clinical study. *Br. J. Anaesth.,* 54:1167–1174.

29. Hanks, G. W., and Twycross, R. G. (1984): Pain, the physiological antagonist of opioid analgesics. *Lancet,* 1:1477–1478.
30. Hanley, J. A., and Lippman-Hand, A. (1983): If nothing goes wrong, is everything all right? Interpreting zero numerators. *J.A.M.A.,* 249:1743–1745.
31. Hughes, S. C., Abboud, T. K., Shnider, S. M., Stefani, S. J., and Norton, M. (1982): Maternal and neonatal effects of epidural morphine for labor. *Anesth. Analg. (Cleve.),* 61:190 (abstract).
32. Huntington, C. T., Cohn, M. L., and Byrd, S. E. (1982): Combined use of epidural morphine and steroid in recurrent postsurgical low back pain syndrome. In: *Abstracts of the International Anesthesia Research Society 56th Congress,* San Francisco, p. 74.
33. Husemeyer, R. P., O'Connor, M. C., and Davenport, H. T. (1980): Failure of epidural morphine to relieve pain in labour. *Anaesthesia,* 35:161–163.
34. Jones, S. E. F., Beasley, J. M., Macfarlane, D. W. R., Davis, J. M., and Hall-Davies, G. (1984): Intrathecal morphine for postoperative pain relief in children. *Br. J. Anaesth.,* 56:137–140.
35. Jorgensen, B. C., Andersen, H. B., and Engquist, A. (1981): CSF and plasma morphine after epidural and intrathecal application. *Anesthesiology,* 55:714–715.
36. Justins, D. M., Francis, D., Houlton, P. G., and Reynolds, F. (1982): A controlled trial of extradural fentanyl in labor. *Br. J. Anaesth.,* 54:409–414.
37. Justins, D. M., Knott, C., Luthman, J., and Reynolds, F. (1983): Epidural versus intramuscular fentanyl. *Anaesthesia,* 38:937–942.
38. Kafer, E. R., Brown, T., Scott, D., Findlay, J. W. A., Butz, R. F., Teeple, E., and Ghia, J. N. (1983): Biphasic depression of ventilatory responses to CO_2 following epidural morphine. *Anesthesiology,* 58:418–427.
39. Knill, R. L., Clement, J. L., and Thompson, W. R. (1981): Epidural morphine causes delayed and prolonged ventilatory depression. *Can. Anaesth. Soc. J.,* 28:537–543.
40. Leavens, M. E., Stratton Hill, C., Jr., Cech, D. A., Weyland, J. B., and Weston, J. S. (1982): Intrathecal and intraventricular morphine for pain in cancer patients: Initial study. *J. Neurosurg.,* 56:241–245.
41. Lobato, R. D., Madrid, J. L., Fatela, L. V., Rivas, J. J., Reig, E., and Lamas, E. (1983): Intraventricular morphine for control of pain in terminal cancer patients. *J. Neurosurg.,* 59:627–633.
42. Magora, F., Olshwang, D., Eimerl, D., Shorr, J., Katzenelson, R., Cotev, S., and Davidson, J. T. (1980): Observations on extradural morphine analgesia in various pain conditions. *Br. J. Anaesth.,* 52:247–252.
43. Modig, J., Hjelmstedt, Å., Sahlstedt, B., and Maripuu, E. (1981): Comparative influences of epidural and general anaesthesia on deep venous thrombosis and pulmonary embolism after total hip replacement. *Acta Chir. Scand.,* 147:125–130.
44. Modig, J., Borg, T., Karlström, G., Maripuu, E., and Sahlstedt, B. (1983): Thromboembolism after total hip replacement: Role of epidural and general anesthesia. *Anesth. Analg. (Cleve.),* 62:174–180.
45. Moore, R. A., Bullingham, R. S. J., McQuay, H. J., Hand, C. W., Aspel, J. B., Allen, M. C., and Thomas, D. (1982): Dural permeability to narcotics: In vitro determination and application to extradural administration. *Br. J. Anaesth.,* 54:1117–1128.
46. Nordberg, G., Hedner, T., Mellstrand, T., and Dahlström, B. (1983): Pharmacokinetic aspects of epidural morphine analgesia. *Anesthesiology,* 58:545–551.
47. Nordberg, G., Hedner, T., Mellstrand, T., and Dahlström, B. (1984): Pharmacokinetic aspects of intrathecal morphine analgesia. *Anesthesiology,* 60:448–454.
48. Perriss, B. W. (1980): Epidural pethidine in labour. *Anaesthesia,* 35:380–382.
49. Perriss, B. W., and Malins, A. F. (1981): Pain relief in labour using epidural pethidine with adrenaline. *Anaesthesia,* 36:631–633.
50. Pert, C. B., Kuhar, M. J., and Snyder, S. H. (1976): Opiate receptor: Autoradiographic localization in rat brain. *Proc. Natl. Acad. Sci. U.S.A.,* 73:3729–3733.
51. Pierrot, M., Blaise, M., Dupuy, A., Hugon, S., and Cupa, M. (1982): Analgésie péridurale à dose élevée de fentanyl: Échec de la méthode pour la kinésithérapie post-opératoire précoce avec chirurgie du genou. *Can. Anaesth. Soc. J.,* 29:587–592.
52. Rigg, J. R. A., Ilsley, A. H., and Vedig, A. E. (1981): Relationship of ventilatory depression to steady-state blood pethidine concentrations. *Br. J. Anaesth.,* 53:613–620.
53. Roquefeuil, B., Benezech, J., Blanchet, P., Batier, C., Frerebeau, P., and Gros, C. (1984):

Intraventricular administration of morphine in patients with neoplastic intractable pain. *Surg. Neurol.,* 21:155–158.
54. Rutberg, H., Håkanson, E., Anderberg, B., Jorfeldt, L., Mårtensson, J., and Schildt, B. (1984): Effects of the extradural administration of morphine, or bupivacaine, on the endocrine response to upper abdominal surgery. *Br. J. Anaesth.,* 56:233–238.
55. Sidi, A., Davidson, J. T., Behar, M., and Olshwang, D. (1981): Spinal narcotics and central nervous system depression. *Anaesthesia,* 36:1044–1047.
56. Skjoldebrand, A., Garle, M., Gustafsson, L. L., Johansson, H., Lunell, N.-O., and Rane, A. (1982): Extradural pethidine with and without adrenaline during labor: Wide variation in effect. *Br. J. Anaesth.,* 54:415–420.
57. Taveira, A. M., Silva, D., Souza, J. D., Quest, J. A., Pagani, F. D., Moerschbaecher, J. M., Buller, A., Hamosh, P., and Gillis, R. A. (1983): Central nervous system site of action for the respiratory depressant effect of diacetylmorphine (heroin) in the cat. *J. Clin. Invest.,* 72:1209–1217.
58. Teschemacher, H. J., Schubert, P., and Herz, A. (1973): Autoradiographic studies concerning the supraspinal site of the antinociceptive action of morphine when inhibiting the hindleg flexor reflex in rabbits. *Neuropharmacology,* 12:123–131.
59. Torda, T. A., and Pybus, D. A. (1984): Extradural administration of morphine and bupivacaine. A controlled comparison. *Br. J. Anaesth.,* 56:141–146.
60. Twycross, R. G. (1977): Choice of strong analgesic in terminal cancer: Diamorphine or morphine? *Pain,* 3:93–104.
61. Walsh, T. D. (1984): Oral morphine in chronic cancer pain. *Pain,* 18:1–11.
62. Welchew, E. A. (1983): The optimum concentration for epidural fentanyl. *Anaesthesia,* 38:1037–1041.
63. Writer, W. D. R., James, F. M., III, and Wheeler, A. S. (1981): Double-blind comparison of morphine and bupivacaine for continuous epidural analgesia in labor. *Anesthesiology,* 54:215–219.
64. Yaksh, T. L. (1981): Spinal opiate analgesia: Characteristics and principles of action. *Pain,* 11:293–346.
65. Zenz, M., Schappler-Scheele, B., Neuhaus, R., Piepenbrock, S., and Hilfrich, J. (1981): Long-term peridural morphine analgesia in cancer pain. *Lancet,* 1:91.

Advances in Pain Research and Therapy, Vol. 9, edited by H. L. Fields et al. Raven Press, New York © 1985.

Pain Treatment on Long-Term Basis Using Extradural Opiates

J. Eriksen and H. B. Andersen, representing the Danish Epidural Opiate Study Group

The Pain Clinic, Department of Anaesthesia, Bispebjerg Hospital, University of Copenhagen, DK-2400 Copenhagen, Denmark

Clinical use of extradural opiates dates back only to 1979 (1). In an earlier retrospective study, we described our experience with outpatients (2). The Danish Epidural Opiate Study Group consists of 26 anesthesiology departments that in a prospective multicenter study evaluated benefits and risks in the use of extradural opiates for long-term pain treatment.

The study was performed during the period from November 1, 1981, to December 31, 1983. An "on-line" registration was made of relevant data concerning patients treated with extradural opiates for more than 7 days. The data are presented here.

RESULTS

The patients involved are categorized in Table 1. Practically all kinds of cancer diagnoses were represented in the malignant group (711 patients). The group with nonmalignant diseases (224 patients) included mainly conditions such as fractures of the pelvis and ribs, herpes zoster, and ischemic pain in the lower limbs. The postoperative group (136 patients) consisted of patients with a protracted postoperative course. Both malignant and nonmalignant diseases were represented in this group.

The mean durations of treatment for inpatients and outpatients are shown in Table 2. One hundred eighty-three patients with malignant diseases and 33 patients with nonmalignant diseases were periodically treated as outpatients for a mean period of 65 days in the malignant group and 147 days in the nonmalignant group. Medically unskilled persons were involved in extradural opiate instillation in 4% of cases. No specific problems emerged among these patients.

Most patients (95%) received morphine, and 5% received buprenorphine extradurally, as seen in Table 3. The total daily doses of morphine were 12 to 13 mg initially and 12 to 21 mg terminally. The corresponding figures for

TABLE 1. *Patients*

Patients treated > 7 days	Malignant diseases (M/F)	Nonmalignant diseases (M/F)	Postoperative treatment (M/F)
Number of patients	365/346	139/85	91/45
Mean age (years)/(range)	62(5–89)/60(9–93)	55(15–93)/63(18–90)	59(18–91)/56(23–90)

TABLE 2. *Duration of treatment (inpatients and outpatients)*

	Malignant diseases (M/F)	Nonmalignant diseases (M/F)	Postoperative treatment (M/F)
Number of patients	365/346	139/85	91/45
Mean duration of treatment (days)/(range)	49(3–292)/54(1–250)	37(3–732)/25(1–434)	12(11–34)/24(3–63)
Number of patients periodically treated as outpatients	149/34	19/14	
Mean duration of treatment as outpatients (range)	65(1–237)/71(1–372)	147(7–228)/44(3–372)	

TABLE 3. *Numbers of patients receiving morphine and buprenorphine*

	Malignant diseases (M/F)	Nonmalignant diseases (M/F)	Postoperative treatment (M/F)	All groups (M/F)
Morphine				
Number of patients	354/330	134/77	89/45	488/407
Total daily dose (mean)				
Initially	13/14	12/12	11/11	12/12
Terminally	21/44	10/10	9/10	13/21
Number of daily doses (mean)				
Initially	2/2	2/2	2/2	2/2
Terminally	3/3	2/2	3/3	3/3
Buprenorphine				
Number of patients	11/16	5/8	2/0	16/24
Total daily dose (mean)				
Initially	1.3/1.4	0.9/0.8	1.0/0	1.0/1.1
Terminally	1.7/1.8	1.3/0.8	0.9/0	1.3/1.3
Number of daily doses (mean)				
Initially	2/2	2/2	2/0	2/0
Terminally	3/3	2/2	2/0	2/0

buprenorphine were 1.0 to 1.1 and 1.1 to 1.3 mg. Except for the postoperative group, our data show an increasing need for both morphine and buprenorphine during the treatment period. This could be partly due to increased pain intensity and partly due to tolerance development.

Pain relief was evaluated by the doctors involved in the study according to patients' pain complaints and total situation. As can be seen in Table 4, good to fair pain relief was achieved in 395 patients (60%) in the malignant group. In the nonmalignant group, 199 patients (95%) had good to fair pain relief. The corresponding figures in the postoperative group were 118 patients (97%).

Side effects are shown in Table 4. Nausea and pain on injection were the most common side effects in the malignant group, being 41 and 25%, respectively. In the nonmalignant group, urinary retention was seen in 40% and nausea in 24% of patients. Urinary retention and nausea were the most common side effects seen among postoperative patients (33%). In all groups, nausea was the most common side effect, being seen in 83 patients (39%). Urinary retention was seen in 60 patients (27%) and pain on injection in 48 patients (22%). Respiratory depression was seen in 3 patients in the malignant group, 2 patients in the nonmalignant group, and 1 postoperative patient. Bacteriological examination of catheter tips revealed contamination with *Staphylococcus albus* in 37 patients and *S. aureus* in 39 patients.

Treatment was terminated in 97 patients (11%) because of ineffective analgesia (Table 5) and in 55 patients (6%) because of intolerable side effects.

TABLE 4. *Pain relief from and side-effects in treatment with extradural opiates*

Pain relief	Malignant diseases (M/F)	Nonmalignant diseases (M/F)	Postoperative treatment (M/F)	All groups (M/F)
Pain relief				
Good	209/186	98/62	71/36	307/248
Fair	99/111	24/15	6/5	123/126
Inadequate	22/27	5/5	2/1	27/32
Total	330/324	127/82	79/42	457/406
Side effects				
Number of patients	80/94 (711)	28/17 (224)	6/6 (136)	108/111 (935)
Nausea	26/46	3/8	2/2	29/54
Vomiting	16/28	1/4	0/1	17/32
Pruritus	3/9	2/3	1/2	5/12
Dizziness	7/5	1/1	0/0	8/6
Constipation	13/15	0/1	0/0	13/16
Pain on injection	15/28	4/1	0/1	19/29
Urinary retention	32/10	15/3	3/1	47/13
Respiratory depression	1/2	0/2	0/1	1/4

Numbers in parentheses represent total number of patients.

TABLE 5. *Causes of termination*

	Malignant diseases	Nonmalignant diseases	Postoperative treatment	All groups
Patient dead	319	30		349
Patient terminal	59	6		65
Patient cured	124	126	25	275
Ineffective analgesia	57	7	33	97
Side effects	28	7	20	55
Other reasons	90	33	34	157
Total	677	209	112	898

However, only patients treated for more than 7 days were included in the study. Some of the patients for whom the treatment was otherwise indicated may have stopped the extradural treatment earlier because of unknown problems. In Denmark, the total number of newly detected cancer cases is about 20,000 per year. Twelve thousand of these patients will experience pain through their remaining life (3). In this investigation only 356 patients (2.9%) per year needed treatment with an extradural catheter.

In the postoperative group the number of patients was 136. Only patients with a protracted postoperative course were included. In Denmark, an estimation of these operations is 2,500 operations out of the total number of 150,000 operations (16%).

CONCLUSION

Long-term treatment with extradural opiates is a good alternative to conventional pain treatment in selected cases. Serious side effects seldom occur, and the treatment can in many cases, especially within the malignant group, be handled by the patients or relatives on an outpatient basis.

REFERENCES

1. Behar, M., Olshwang, D., Magora, F., and Davidson, J. T. (1979): Epidural morphine in treatment of pain. *Lancet,* 1:527–528.
2. Crawford, M., Andersen, H. B., Augusterborg, G., Bay, J., Beck, O., Benveniste, D., Larsen, L. B., Carl, P., Djernes, M., Erikser, J., Grell, A. M., Henriksen, H., Johansen, S. H., Jørgenson, H. O. K., Møller, I. W., Pedersen, J. E. P., and Raulo, O. (1983): Pain treatment on outpatient basis utilizing extradural opiates. A Danish multicenter study comprising 105 patients. *Pain,* 16:41–49.
3. Twycross, R. G. (1984): Pain relief in cancer. *Clin. Oncol.,* 3:6–10.

Advances in Pain Research and Therapy, Vol. 9, edited by H. L. Fields et al. Raven Press, New York © 1985.

Differential Effects of Fenfluramine and Dextroamphetamine on Acute and Chronic Pain

*Nicholas G. Ward, *John A. Bokan, *Jesse Ang, and **Stephen H. Butler

*Departments of *Psychiatry and Behavioral Sciences and **Anesthesiology, University of Washington Seattle, Washington 98195*

Fenfluramine (Fen), a selective releaser of serotonin (3,4,17), may be useful in exploring the serotonin hypothesis of chronic pain. Varying degrees of depression frequently accompany chronic pain (29). Sternbach et al. (27) hypothesized that a deficit in central serotonergic activity might underlie coexisting chronic pain and depression. If depressed chronic pain patients have a functional reduction in serotonergic activity, then these patients might experience an acute hypoalgesic response to Fen. Demonstration of this response could have research and clinical utility.

Evidence for the serotonergic hypothesis comes from both animal and human studies. Most animal studies (5,11,15,35) have reported that increases in serotonergic activity result in hypoalgesia (the term *hypoalgesia* is being used to mean a relative decrease in pain, as opposed to *analgesia,* the absence of pain), whereas decreases result in hyperalgesia. Further support comes from studies in humans reporting hypoalgesic responses to L-tryptophan, a precursor of serotonin (13,23,24), and to the presumed serotonergic antidepressants such as chlomipramine (27) and zimelidine (12).

Two other studies, however, did not appear to support the serotonergic hypothesis. Almay et al. (1) reported that cerebrospinal fluid (CSF) 5-hydroxyindoleacetic acid (5-HIAA) in psychogenic pain patients was non-significantly higher than in organic pain patients. Ghia et al. (7) similarly found that CSF 5-HIAA was significantly higher in pain patients than in those with no pain and was the same in acute and chronic pain patients. However, high serotonin turnover resulting in high 5-HIAA may be a response to low serotonergic receptor function, rather than being a marker of high functional serotonergic activity.

Other studies have suggested that a broader biogenic amine hypothesis should be considered. In animals, increases in dopaminergic activity usually result in hyperalgesia, and decreases result in hypoalgesia (28). Gonzalez et al. (9) concluded that hyperalgesia is more specifically caused by stimulation of D-1 but not D-2 receptors. Thus, bromocriptine, a D-1 antagonist, but a D-2 agonist, has hypoalgesic activity (21). Reports on norepinephrine (NE) have been more mixed, with NE appearing to have inhibitory effects on pain at the spinal cord level (19,36) but excitatory effects at levels above the locus ceruleus (22).

In humans, presumed noradrenergic antidepressants have been reported to be as effective in relieving pain as serotonergic ones (14). Furthermore, high initial urinary concentrations of 3-methoxy-4-hydroxyphenethyleneglycol (MHPG), a metabolite of NE, have been reported to be predictors of pain response to antidepressant medication (32). To account for the newer data, it has been proposed that either low serotonergic activity or high noradrenergic activity or both underlie chronic pain with depression (32). Antidepressants might relieve pain by down-regulating NE as well as by increasing serotonergic activity. According to the same theory, serotonin and NE play lesser roles in acute pain regulation, whereas endogenous opiates play a greater role.

In support of this modified theory, von Knorring et al. (31) reported that CSF β-endorphin levels in patients with chronic pain were significantly correlated with acute pain thresholds. Furthermore, patients with "functional" pain and more depression had high β-endorphin levels and were relatively hypoalgesic to acute pain. Any possible abnormalities in biogenic amine function that might have decreased acute pain tolerance were clearly overshadowed by increased β-endorphin activity. In another study of patients with chronic pain and depression, CSF β-endorphin levels were not found to correlate with severity of chronic pain (33). Thus, β-endorphin appears to modulate acute pain but not chronic pain in patients with chronic pain and depression.

Most of the positive and negative studies used to test the original serotonin hypothesis and the subsequent biogenic amine hypothesis of chronic pain suffer from significant limitations. The animal studies involved acute pain, not chronic pain. The positive and negative studies involving metabolites were limited by their inability to measure net serotonergic or noradrenergic activity. The antidepressant studies were limited by the very mixed pharmacologic effects of the antidepressants used (20). The use of precursors such as tryptophan is limited by possible deficits in their conversion to serotonin. A pharmacologic challenge with a relatively pure serotonergic agent such as Fen might circumvent most of these problems.

Brownell and Stunkard (2) have argued that because Fen is easily differentiated from placebo, a placebo-controlled trial is not meaningful. This problem allows the opportunity to compare Fen with a pharmacologically related drug, dextroamphetamine (Dex). Dex is principally a mixed releaser of NE and dopamine (DA). Thus, it is not a pure enough agent to test the biogenic amine hypothesis of chronic pain. Its stimulant activity appears to be secondary to dopaminergic receptor stimulation, possibly of D-2 receptors (8,25). In controlled trials it has been reported to have analgesic activity in acute laboratory-induced pain (34) and to augment the effects of morphine in postsurgical pain (6). There have been no controlled studies reporting the effects of Dex on chronic pain. A controlled replication of its effects on acute pain and a controlled demonstration of its effects on chronic pain are needed.

Based on the theories and data presented, we hypothesized that in patients with chronic pain and depression, Fen would not have hypoalgesic effects on acute pain, but would on chronic pain. On the other hand, based on previous research, we predicted that Dex would have hypoalgesic effects on both acute and chronic pain. Because mood and pain are frequently related and both Fen and Dex affect mood, the relationships between drug-induced changes in mood and changes in pain were examined.

METHODS

Because chronic pain might affect acute pain thresholds, a depressed group not presenting with pain was used for the study of acute pain thresholds, and a separate group complaining of chronic back pain and depression was used for the study of chronic pain. All subjects were recruited by means of newspaper advertisements. Subjects were included if they gave informed consent, met research diagnostic criteria (RDC) (26) and DSM III criteria for unipolar major affective disorder, depression, nonpsychotic, or DSM III criteria for a dysthymic disorder, and received ratings of 18 or higher on a 24-item Hamilton Depression Rating Scale (HRS) (10). All subjects had been free of psychoactive drug use for at least 30 days prior to test drug administration and had not abused alcohol or drugs at any time during the past year. A double-blind crossover design counterbalanced between patients for order of drug administration was used. Each drug-free subject received either Dex 15 mg or Fen 40 mg p.o. at 9:00 a.m. on two separate days at least 48 hr apart. Immediately prior to drug administration and again at 12 noon, subjects completed the Profile of Mood States (POMS, "now" version) (16). Because 85% of subjects can discriminate Fen from placebo, a placebo was not used in this study (2). We reasoned that a direct comparison of two psychoactive drugs might ultimately prove to be more worthwhile.

Acute Pain Study

Sixteen subjects, 12 females and 4 males, ages 27 to 64 years (mean age 39.2 $\pm$ 4.4), with mean HRS score 24.9, were included in this part of the study. All had a chief complaint of depression, but not pain, and were medically healthy by history. On each day prior to and 3 hr after drug administration, an ice-water tolerance test was performed. Subjects were instructed to put the entire right hand in ice water (0° C) up to a line drawn on the wrist. Pain sensation was then rated verbally every 10 sec on a 0-to-10 scale (with 0 = no pain and 10 = unbearable pain). A pain tolerance threshold was determined by the number of seconds the subject left the hand in the ice water before spontaneously pulling it out. Because we had determined in preliminary testing that anyone who could leave a hand in 2 min could keep the hand in indefinitely, 2 min was used as the maximum time for each trial.

Chronic Pain Study

Fifty subjects, 26 females and 24 males, ages 20 to 64 years (mean age 40.8), with mean HRS score 26.2 ± 6.8, were included in this part of the study. All had responded to a newspaper advertisement asking for people who suffered from both back pain and depression. In addition to meeting the previously described depression criteria, all candidates accepted for this part of the study had to have had persistent chronic back pain for 40% or more of their waking hours, lasting 6 months or longer, with an average severity rating of 4 or greater on a 0 (no pain) to 10 (worst pain imaginable) rating scale, and not be involved in any litigation regarding their pain. Furthermore, following a back exam by an orthopedic surgeon specializing in back pain, no person accepted could be a candidate for back surgery or have a physical abnormality that completely explained the location and/or severity of the pain reported. Only one candidate had entirely "functional" pain as defined by von Knorring et al. (31), and none had entirely physiologically based pain. Immediately preceding drug administration and again at noon, subjects rated their pain on a visual analog scale (10-cm line with opposite poles marked "no pain" and "pain as bad as it could be").

RESULTS

As can be seen in Table 1, Dex, but not Fen, significantly increased acute pain tolerance. In fact, there was a nonsignificant trend toward decreased pain tolerance with Fen. As seen in Table 2, both Dex and Fen significantly reduced chronic pain ratings, with no significant differences between the two drugs.

Both drugs significantly decreased POMS depression, fatigue, and confusion-bewilderment ratings and increased POMS vigor ratings (paired *t*-test, $p < 0.02$). As seen in Tables 3 and 4, Fen's effects on depression, confusion-bewilderment, and fatigue were also correlated with a decrease in chronic pain, whereas none of Dex's effects on mood were correlated with a decrease in pain.

These results did not appear to be confounded by age, sex, weight, or

TABLE 1. *Acute pain: seconds in ice water*

	Pre	Post	P
Dex	50	67.5	<0.014
Fen	52.1	44.1	N.S.

TABLE 2. *Chronic pain: visual analog scale*

Drug	Pre	Post	*p*
Dex	43.8	32.6	<0.029
Fen	37.5	24.5	<0.006

Fen versus Dex: paired *t*-test: $t = -0.42$; $p < 0.679$.

TABLE 3. *Correlation of percent change POMS vs. pain rating: Fen*

Poms subscale	Acute pain	Chronic pain
Vigor	0.37	−0.18
Tension/anxiety	−0.10	0.22
Depression	−0.03	0.60[a]
Anger/hostility	−0.40	0.08
Confusion/bewilderment	−0.22	0.41[a]
Fatigue	−0.35	0.46[a]

[a] $p < 0.005$.

TABLE 4. *Correlation of percent change POMS vs. pain rating (all nonsignificant)*

POMS subscale	Acute pain	Chronic pain
Vigor	0.18	−0.13
Tension/anxiety	−0.08	−0.09
Depression	−0.20	0.19
Anger/hostility	−0.05	0.13
Confusion/bewilderment	−0.11	0.11
Fatigue	−0.19	0.24

order of drug administration. There were no significant differences between males and females on pain measures (time in ice water or visual analog rating), either at base line or after using either drug. There were also no significant correlations between age or weight and base-line or postdrug pain ratings. The order of administration of drugs did not significantly affect changes in pain ratings. There were also no significant differences between the two groups in age, severity of depression, or sex distribution.

DISCUSSION

This study supports the hypothesis that Fen can significantly reduce chronic pain but not acute pain in patients with chronic back pain and depression and that serotonin modulates these functions. Fen's positive effect on pain is significantly related to its positive effects on mood. Because Fen is a relatively pure releaser of serotonin, we assume that a net increase in serotonergic activity has caused the improvement in mood and chronic pain. This study indirectly supports the theory of Sternbach et al. (27) that a serotonin deficit underlies both chronic pain and depression. Because an increase in serotonergic function decreased pain and depression in a subgroup of patients in this study, we conclude that there was a relative deficit in serotonin function in these patients.

This study also supports the hypothesis that Dex can decrease both acute experimental pain and chronic clinical pain in depressed individuals. Dex's effects on pain appear to be independent of its effects on mood. These data suggest that biogenic amines such as NE and DA are important in the modulation of both acute and chronic pain in humans. Because increasing evidence suggests that Dex's stimulant/euphoriant effects are a result of D-2 receptor stimulation (25), perhaps its analgesic effects are mediated by another receptor system. Purer agonists and antagonists of each receptor system (e.g., D-1, D-2, α-1, α-2, etc.) would be necessary to determine which system or systems are producing Dex's analgesic effects and whether or not different systems are modulating chronic and acute pain. If Dex's euphoriant and analgesic effects are independent, this opens up the exciting possibility that testing of such agonists and antagonists could lead to a nonstimulating, nonaddicting, nonopiate analgesic drug.

If NE postsynaptic agonists prove to have consistent analgesic properties, the biogenic amine hypothesis of pain would need to be modified. The hypothesized high noradrenergic activity underlying chronic pain and depression depends on the observation that high MHPG is a predictor of hypoalgesic response to antidepressants (32). High MHPG, however, may not be indicative of high net noradrenergic activity, but rather indicative of low postsynaptic NE receptor function. High NE turnover, with resulting high MHPG, thus may be a result of mechanisms compensating for the low NE sensitivity.

In regard to their effects on chronic pain, Fen and Dex may share common mechanisms of action with the tricyclic antidepressants (TCA). Because there is increasing evidence that TCAs effectively reduce pain in a variety of nondepressed patients with chronic pain (33), Fen and Dex might be expected to have similar effects in these patients. Further research with nondepressed pain patients is needed to determine if findings from this study can be generalized to this broader patient group.

Acute responses of chronic pain to Fen and Dex might also be used as predictors of pain responses to antidepressants. Dex has been used successfully as a predictor of antidepressant response to presumed noradrenergic TCAs (30). Similarly, an analgesic response to Dex might successfully predict an analgesic response to noradrenergic TCAs, and an analgesic response to Fen might successfully predict an analgesic response to serotonergic TCAs. Because only 50 to 55% of pain patients get significant pain reduction from TCAs, and this usually takes several weeks, with multiple side effects, improved prediction of response with acute drug challenges would considerably enhance clinical practice.

In summary, results from this study suggest further modifications of our biogenic amine hypothesis of chronic pain. The catecholamines (DA and/ or NE) appear to have a pain-inhibiting role in both acute and chronic pain, whereas serotonin appears to be inhibitory only in chronic pain. Other studies suggest that β-endorphin has a significant pain-inhibiting role in acute pain but not chronic pain. On the other hand, transmitters like serotonin have a role in the modulation of chronic pain (18). Further studies examining the roles and interactions between biogenic amines and endorphins in chronic pain may help clarify chronic pain mechanisms and may lead to new, more effective treatments for chronic pain.

REFERENCES

1. Almay, G. L., Johansson, F., von Knorring, L., Sedval, G., and Terenius, L. (1980): Relationships between CSF levels of endorphins and monoamine metabolites in chronic pain patients. *Psychopharmacologia,* 67:139–142.
2. Brownell, K. D., and Stunkard, A. J. (1982): The double-blind in danger: Untoward consequences of informed consent. *Am. J. Psychiatry,* 139:1487–1489.
3. Clineschmidt, B. V., Zacchei, A. G., Totaro, J. A., Pflueger, A. B., McGuffin, J. C., and Wishousky, T. I. (1978): Fenfluramine and brain serotonin. *Ann. N.Y. Acad. Sci.,* 305:222–241.
4. Clineschmidt, B. V., and Bunting, P. R. (1980): Differential effects of pharmacological agents acting on monoaminergic systems on drug-induced anorexia. *Prog. Neuro-Psychopharmacol.,* 4:327–339.
5. Fibiger, H. C., Mertz, P. H., and Campbell, B. A. (1972): The effect of para-chlorophenylalanine on aversion thresholds and reactivity to foot shock. *Physiol. Behav.,* 8:259–263.
6. Forrest, W. H., Jr., Brown, B. W., Jr., Brown, C. R., Defalque, R., Gold, M., Gordon, E., James, K. E., Katz, J., Mahler, D. L., Schroff, P., and Teutch, G. (1977): Dextroamphetamine with morphine for the treatment of postoperative pain. *N. Engl. J. Med.,* 296:712–715.
7. Ghia, J. N., Mueller, R. A., Duncan, G. H., Scott, D. S., and Mao, W. (1981): Serotonergic activity in man as a function of pain, pain mechanisms, and depression. *Anesth. Analg. (Cleve.),* 60:854–861.
8. Goeders, N. E., and Smith, J. E. (1983): Cortical dopaminergic involvement in cocaine reinforcement. *Science,* 221:773.
9. Gonzalez, J. P., Sewell, R. D. E., and Spencer, P. S. J. (1981): Evidence for central selective dopamine receptor stimulation in the mediation of nomifensine-induced hyperalgesia and the effects of opiate antagonists. *Neuropharmacology,* 20:1039–1045.
10. Hamilton, M. (1960): A rating scale for depression. *J. Neurol. Neurosurg. Psychiatry,* 23:56–62.
11. Harvey, J. A., Schlosberg, A. J., and Yunger, L. M. (1974): Effect of *p*-chlorophenylalanine and brain lesions on pain sensitivity and morphine analgesia in the rat. *Adv. Biochem. Psychopharmacol.,* 10:233–245.
12. Johansson, F., and von Knorring, L. (1979): A double-blind controlled study of a serotonin uptake inhibitor (zimelidine) versus placebo in chronic pain patients. *Pain,* 7:69–78.
13. King, R. B. (1980): Pain and tryptophan. *J. Neurosurg.,* 53:44–52.
14. Lindsay, P. G., and Wycoff, M. (1981): The depression-pain syndrome and its response to antidepressants. *Psychosomatics,* 22:571–577.

15. Lints, C. E., and Harvey, J. A. (1969): Altered sensitivity to footshock and decreased brain content of serotonin following brain lesions in the rat. *J. Comp. Physiol. Psychol.,* 67:23–31.
16. McNair, M. D., Lovr, M., and Droppleman, L. F. (1971): In: *Profile of Mood States.* Educational and Industrial Testing Service, San Diego, Ca.
17. Pinder, R. M., Brogden, R. N., Sawyer, P. R., Speight, T. M., and Avery, G. S. (1975): Fenfluramine: A review of its pharmacological properties and therapeutic efficacy in obesity. *Drugs,* 10:241–323.
18. Przewlocka, B., Stala, L., Lason, W., and Przewlocki, R. (1984): The role of dynorphin in spinal mechanisms of analgesia. Presented at the 14th Collegium Internationale Neuro-Psychopharmacologica, Florence, Italy.
19. Ramana Reddy, S. V., and Yaksh, T. L. (1980): Spinal noradrenergic terminal system mediates antinociception. *Brain Res.,* 189:391–401.
20. Richelson, E. (1983): Are receptor studies useful for clinical practice? *J. Clin. Psychiatry,* 44:4–9.
21. Robertson, J., Weston, R., Lewis, M. J., and Barasi, S. (1981): Evidence for the potentiation of the antinociceptive action of morphine by bromocriptine. *Neuropharmacology,* 20:1029–1032.
22. Sagen, J., Winker, M. A., and Proudfit, H. K. (1983): Hypoalgesia induced by the local injection of phentolamine in the nucleus raphe magnus: Blockage by depletion of spinal cord monoamines. *Pain,* 16:253–263.
23. Seltzer, S., Marcus, R., and Stoch, R. (1981): Perspectives in the control of chronic pain by nutritional manipulation. *Pain,* 11:141–148.
24. Seltzer, S., Stoch, R., Marcus, R., and Jackson, E. (1982): Alteration of human pain thresholds by nutritional manipulation and L-tryptophan supplementation. *Pain,* 13:385–393.
25. Silverstone, T. (1980): Psychopharmacology of anorectic drugs in man. *Prog. Neuro-Psychopharmacol.,* 4:371–374.
26. Spitzer, R. L., Endicott, J., and Robins, R. (1977): *Research Diagnostic Criteria (RDC) for a Selected Group of Functional Disorders.* Biometrics Research, New York State Psychiatric Institute, New York.
27. Sternbach, R. A., Janowsky, D. S., Huey, L. Y., and Segal, D. S. (1976): Effects of altering brain serotonin activity on human chronic pain. In: *Advances in Pain Research and Therapy, Vol. 1,* edited by J. J. Bonica and D. Albe-Fessard, pp. 601–606. Raven Press, New York.
28. Tulunay, C., Sparber, S. B., and Takemori, A. E. (1975): The effect of dopaminergic stimulation and blockade on the nociceptive and antinociceptive responses of mice. *Eur. J. Pharmacol.,* 33:65–70.
29. Turner, J. A., and Romano, J. (1984): Review of prevalance of coexisting chronic pain and depression. In: *Advances in Pain Research and Therapy,* Vol. 7, edited by C. S. Benedetti, G. Moricca, and C. R. Chapman, pp. 123–130. Raven Press, New York.
30. Van Kammen, D. P., and Murphy, D. L. (1978): Prediction of imipramine antidepressant response by a one-day *d*-amphetamine trial. *Am. J. Psychiatry,* 135:1179–1184.
31. von Knorring, L., Almay, B. G. L., Johansson, F., and Terenius, L. (1978): Pain perception and endorphin levels in cerebrospinal fluid. *Pain,* 5:359–365.
32. Ward, N. G., Bloom, V. L., Dworkin, S., Fawcett, J., Narasimhachari, N., and Friedel, R. O. (1982): Psychobiological markers in coexisting pain and depression: Toward a unified theory. *J. Clin. Psychiatry,* 43:32–39.
33. Ward, N. G., Bokan, J. A., Phillips, M. R., Benedetti, C., Butler, S., and Spengler, D. (1984): Antidepressants in concomitant chronic back pain and depression: Doxepin and desipramine compared. *J. Clin. Psychiatry,* 45:54–57.
34. Webb, S. S., Smith, G. M., Evans, W. O., and Webb, N. C. (1978): Toward the development of a potent, nonsedating, oral analgesic. *Psychopharmacologia,* 60:25–28.
35. Yaksh, T. L., and Wilson, P. R. (1979): Spinal serotonin terminal system mediates antiociception. *J. Pharmacol. Exp. Ther.,* 208:446–453.
36. Yaksh, T. L., and Ramana Reddy, S. V. (1981): Studies in the primate on the analgetic effects associated with intrathecal actions of opiates, α-adrenergic agonists and baclofen. *Anesthesiology,* 54:451–467.

Advances in Pain Research and Therapy, Vol. 9, edited by H. L. Fields et al. Raven Press, New York © 1985.

Doxepin Effects on Chronic Pain and Depression: A Controlled Study

*Stuart R. Hameroff, *Randall C. Cork, *Julie L.Weiss, *B. Robert Crago, and **Thomas P. Davis

*Departments of *Anesthesiology and **Pharmacology, University of Arizona Health Sciences Center, Tucson, Arizona 85724*

Chronic pain and depression often coexist. Chronic pain states can cause clinically significant reactive depression, and primary depression can also manifest chronic pain behavior (4,6,12). Depression and chronic pain may share common pathophysiology and potentiate negative effects on patients' coping and pain tolerance. Accordingly, tricyclic antidepressants are commonly prescribed for the combination of chronic pain and depression. Tricyclics lack the dependency problems of opiate drugs and are empirically helpful, but their mechanisms are unclear, and documentation of their clinical benefits for pain is scarce (5,7,ll,l4). Chronic pain mechanisms have been theoretically explained by both overactivity of pain perceptive and cognitive neuronal pathways and underactivity of endogenous analgesic pathways. Tricyclic effects are usually attributed to blockade of synaptic membrane uptake of neurotransmitters. Potentiation of adrenergic, serotonergic, and opioid pathways has been theoretically linked to a clinical tricyclic effect. Latency in tricyclic therapeutic onset may result from enzyme-dependent active metabolites, or blockade of neuronal uptake causing trophic feedback and enhanced turnover of neurotransmitter precursors, enzymes, membrane proteins, and other factors (9).

The present study was designed to evaluate the clinical effects of the tricyclic doxepin hydrochloride on measurable aspects of chronic pain and related depression. Doxepin was studied because it reportedly has good sedation and anxiolytic properties and few cardiovascular effects (10). The purposes of the study included an attempt to document the effectiveness and required plasma levels of the tricyclics in treating coexisting chronic pain and depression and to correlate mood and depression indices with chronic pain perception and plasma opioids.

METHODS

With informed consent of patients and approval of the Human Subjects Committee, 60 consecutive patients with chronic cervical and/or lumbar spine pain and coexisting clinical depression were studied (Table 1). These patients had been followed in our outpatient clinic for several months or more and had had no change in physical condition or pain complaints for at least 2 months. Diagnoses included chronic disc disease, posttraumatic or degenerative arthritis, myofascial syndromes, and postsurgical conditions such as arachnoiditis and epidural scarring. Some patients were receiving concomitant therapies, including trigger-point injections, biofeedback, and other medications, and these treatments were maintained at their regular frequency. No patients received tricyclics for at least 2 weeks prior to the study. Depression was defined by a Hamilton Depression Scale score of 18 or greater on a 24-item scale.

Physical examination, clinical laboratory blood tests, electrocardiogram, and chest X-ray were used for all patients entering the study. At the study outset, base-line values were obtained for all parameters, and all patients received placebo for the first week ("washout"). On completion of washout, patients were randomly assigned to one of two treatment groups. Physicians and evaluators were blind to group assignment. Dosage began at 50 mg h.s. and increased to 300 mg unless marked improvement (by Global Assessment) or side effects were encountered. The following parameters were monitored at washout, base line, 1 week, 2 weeks, 4 weeks, and 6 weeks:

1. The Hamilton Depression Scale, a formalized interview that allows for some interpretation by the clinical evaluator but results in a quantitative index of depression. Throughout the study, each patient was evaluated by the same interviewer, who was blind to whether patients were receiving active drug or placebo.
2. The Clinical Global Assessment Scale, which gives numerical values to patient status to indicate mild, moderate, or marked improvement.

TABLE 1. *Patient population*

	Doxepin		Placebo	
	Enter	Complete	Enter	Complete
Male	17	15	15	12
Female	13	12	15	12
Age	48.9 ± 2.4		48.4 ± 2.0	
Number previous lumbar or cervical spine surgeries	2.8 ± 1.4		1.1 ± 0.4	

3. Visual analog scales of 0 to 100, used to measure seven subjective dimensions of pain and related factors: average pain (pain severity), percentage of time pain was felt (pain incidence), effect of pain on activity, effect of pain on sleep, effect of pain on mood, effect of pain on muscle tension, and effect of pain on consumption of other drugs. Analog scales were arranged so that higher numbers always indicated worsened condition.
4. Quantitative determinations of plasma doxepin and its metabolite nordoxepin using gas chromatography and mass spectrometry (GC/MS). Refinements in sample preparation permitted sensitive measurements (2). Many analytic methods have been used to measure tricyclics in general and doxepin in particular. These include gas-liquid chromatography (GLC) with flame-ionization detection, capillary GLC with nitrogen-phosphorus detection, high-performance liquid chromatography, and GC/MS with mass-fragmentography detection (3). Our methods, using GC/MS, permitted precision, selectivity, and low sample volume (1.0 ml) at extremely low concentrations (2 ng/ml). Sensitivity was enhanced by purifying samples by organic extraction, thus eliminating extraneous and potentially cross-reacting substances. To further improve sensitivity, sample tubes were made of special plastic to which peptides do not adhere (1,13).
5. Standing and supine blood pressures, heart rate, temperature, and weight.
6. Endogenous opioids: Plasma beta-endorphin was measured using the New England Nuclear radioimmunoassay kit. Nonspecific opioids, including enkephalins, were assessed based on the ability of patients' plasma to displace weakly bound, radiolabeled opiate from opiate receptors (enkephalin-like activity) (13). Nonspecific substances measured by this assay could include dynorphin and a variety of enkephalins and nonpeptide opioids.

Data were analyzed by multivariate discriminant analysis and grouped and paired *t*-tests. Statistical significance was set at the $p<0.05$ level.

RESULTS

Of the 60 patients entering the study, 6 were discontinued because of side effects (Table 1). When the code was broken, it was found that 3 of these patients (one man with chest pain, 2 women with dry mouth) had been receiving placebo, and 3 patients (dry mouth) had been on doxepin. Three other patients (all on placebo) left the study for nonmedical reasons. During the study, it was impossible, based on side effects, to distinguish between patients taking placebo and those taking drug.

Daily Dose, Plasma Doxepin, and Nordoxepin

Oral doses were increased until patients demonstrated marked improvement or side effects. Figure 1 shows average daily doses (mg/kg) for both groups. In the doxepin group, plasma levels (Fig. 1) suggest that a plateau reached at week 1 was maintained through week 4, with a subsequent increase at week 6 in both doxepin and desmethyldoxepin levels. At 6 weeks, the sum of the doxepin and desmethyldoxepin plasma levels was approximately 70 ng/ml. Most clinically significant effects occurred at week 6, when plasma doxepin and desmethyldoxepin totaled a mean of 70 ng/ml, at an average dose of 2.5 mg/kg.

Global Assessment

Global assessment scores (Fig. 2) were constant through washout and base line for both groups and did not significantly improve in the placebo group. By grouped *t*-test, doxepin patients were improved as compared with placebo patients at weeks 1, 2, 4, and 6. By paired *t*-test, doxepin patients at week 6 were significantly improved as compared with doxepin patients at base line. By paired *t*-test, placebo patients at week 6 were also improved as compared with placebo patients at base line.

Hamilton Depression Scores

Washout and base-line Hamilton scores did not differ between the two groups (Fig. 2). By grouped *t*-test, the doxepin-treated patients had better (lower) Hamilton depression scores than placebo patients at weeks 2, 4, and 6. By paired *t*-test, placebo-treated patients showed some improvement at week 6 compared with base line; however, the doxepin-treated patients had significant improvement compared with base line at weeks 1, 2, 4, and 6. Doxepin-patient mean Hamilton values of week 6 were below the entry level for depression (18). Note that improvement on Hamilton scores (and all subsequent variables) is downward on the *y* axis.

Pain severity. Pain severity scores (Fig. 3) were lower (better) in the doxepin patients at week 6 by grouped *t*-test.

Percentage time pain felt. Percentage time pain was felt ("pain incidence," Fig. 3) was lower in doxepin patients than in placebo patients by grouped *t*-test at weeks 4 and 6. Percentage time pain was felt was also lower in doxepin patients at weeks 4 and 6 compared with doxepin patients at base line by paired *t*-test.

Pain effect on activity. Pain effect on activity (Fig. 4) was less in doxepin patients than in placebo patients at weeks 4 and 6 by grouped *t*-test.

Pain effect on mood. Pain effect on mood (Fig. 4) was not significantly different between the two groups.

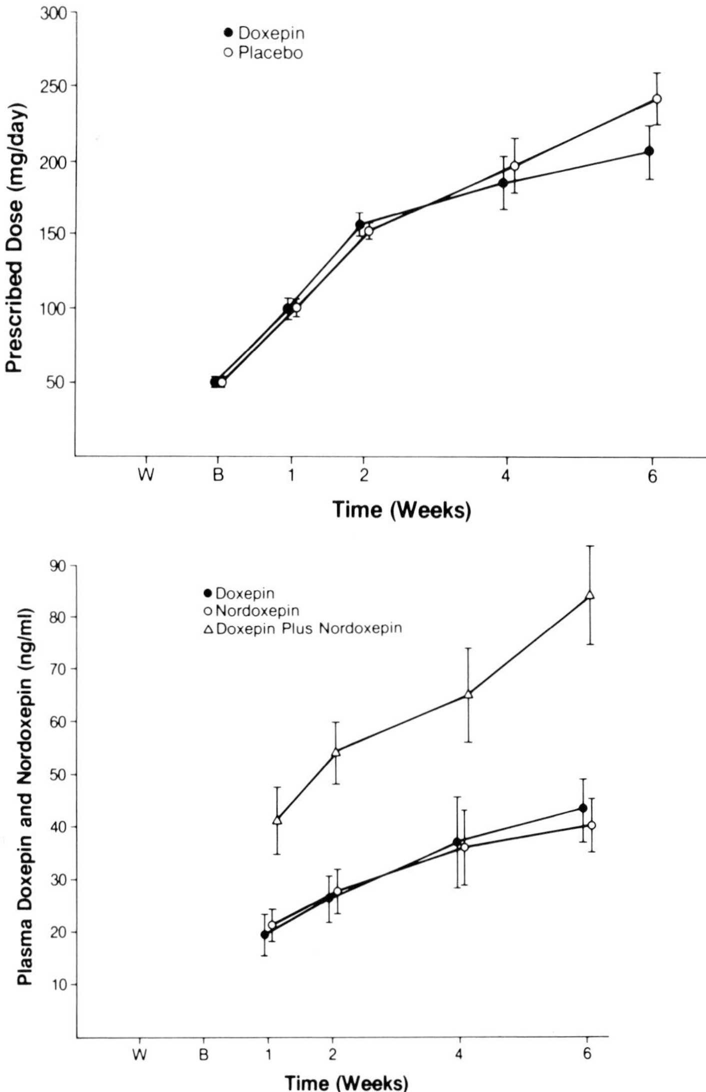

FIG. 1. Top: Daily oral doses of doxepin and placebo (simulated capsules) showed no significant differences between the groups. **Bottom:** Plasma doxepin, nordoxepin (desmethyldoxepin), and the sum of both (ng/ml).

Pain-related muscle tension. Pain-related muscle tension (Fig 5) was lower in doxepin patients than in placebo patients at week 4 by grouped *t*-test. By paired *t*-test, pain-related muscle tension was lower in doxepin patients at week 4 than in doxepin patients at base line.

Pain effect on sleep satisfaction. Pain effect on sleep satisfaction (Fig. 5)

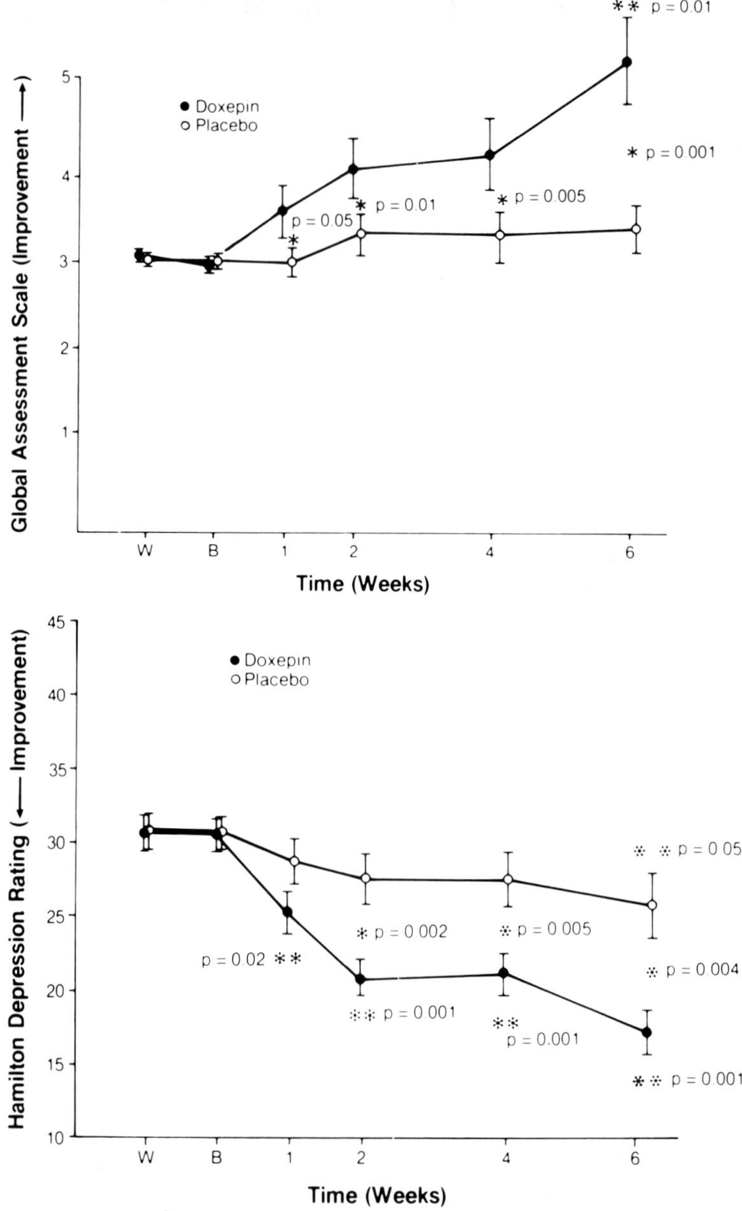

FIG. 2. Top: Global Assessment scores. By grouped *t*-test (*), doxepin patients were improved as compared with placebo patients at weeks l, 2, 4, and 6. By paired *t*-test (**), doxepin patients at week 6 were significantly improved as compared with doxepin patients at base line. By paired *t*-test, placebo patients at week 6 were also improved as compared with placebo patients at base line. **Bottom:** Hamilton depression scores. By grouped *t*-test (*) doxepin patients had better (lower) scores than placebo patients at weeks 2, 4, and 6. By paired *t*-test (**) placebo patients at week 6 were improved as compared with base line. Doxepin patients were improved as compared with base line at weeks 1, 2, 4, and 6.

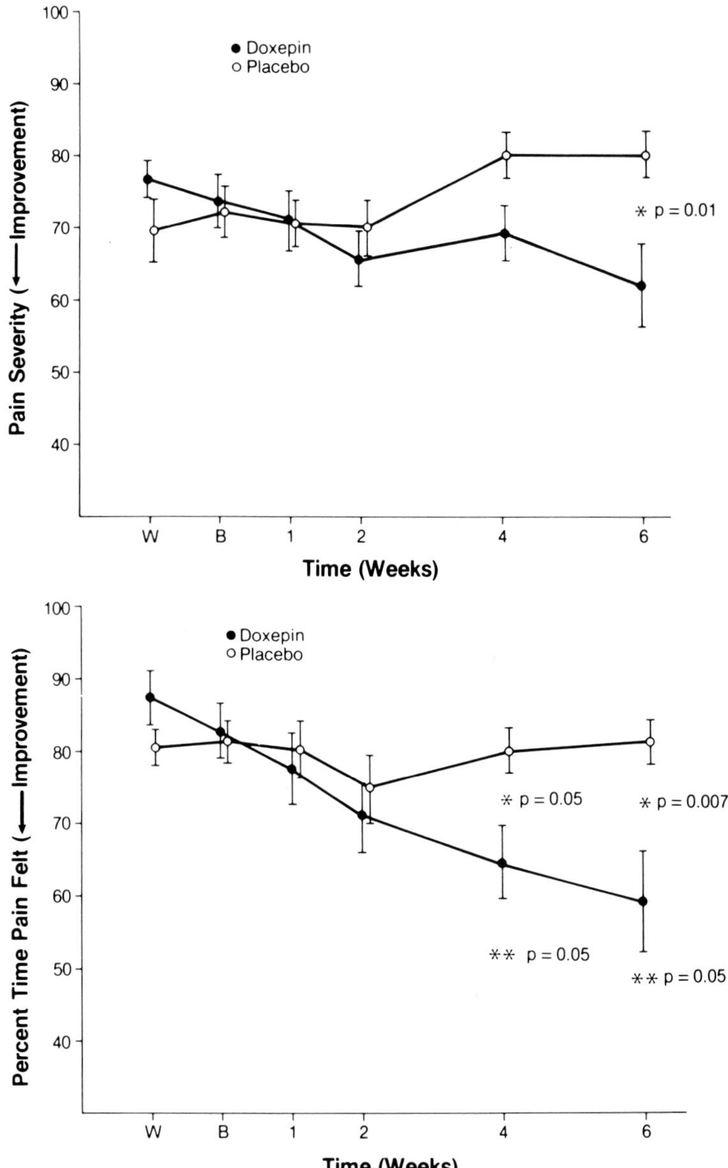

FIG. 3. Top: Pain severity scores were better in doxepin patients at week 6 by grouped *t*-test (*). **Bottom:** Percentage time pain was felt was better in doxepin patients than in placebo patients by grouped *t*-test (*) at weeks 4 and 6. By paired *t*-test (**) scores were better in doxepin patients at weeks 4 and 6 as compared with base line.

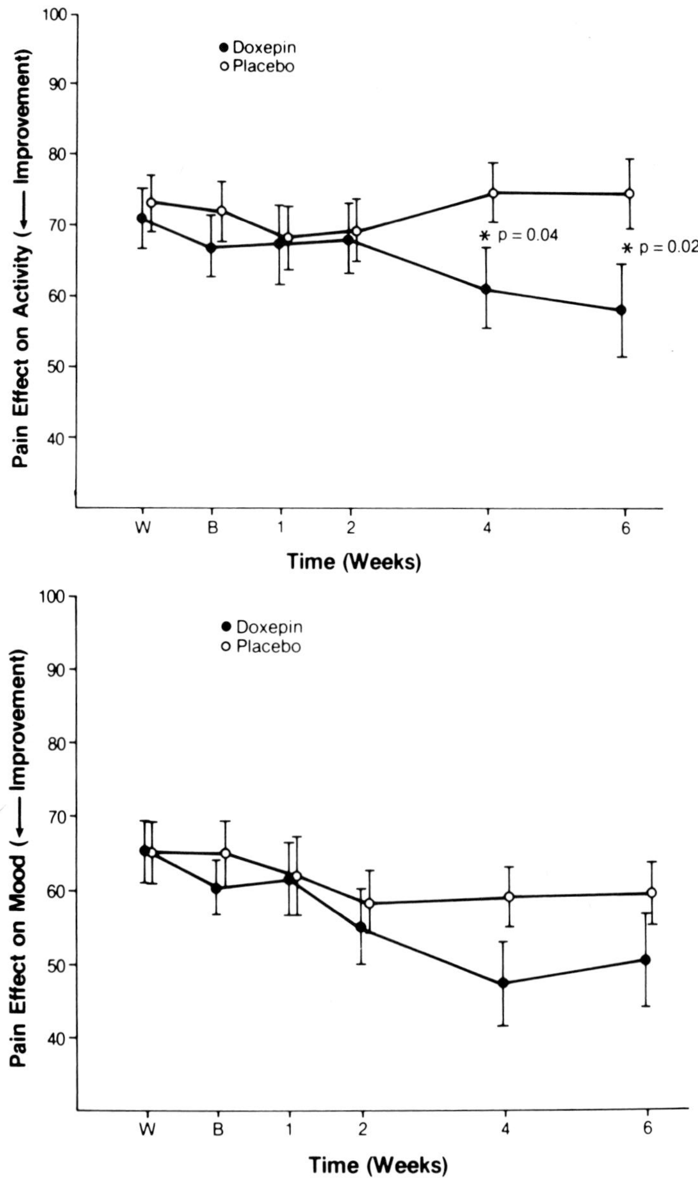

FIG. 4. Top: Pain effect on activity was better in doxepin patients than in placebo patients at weeks 4 and 6 by grouped *t*-test (*). **Bottom:** Pain effect on mood was not different between the two groups.

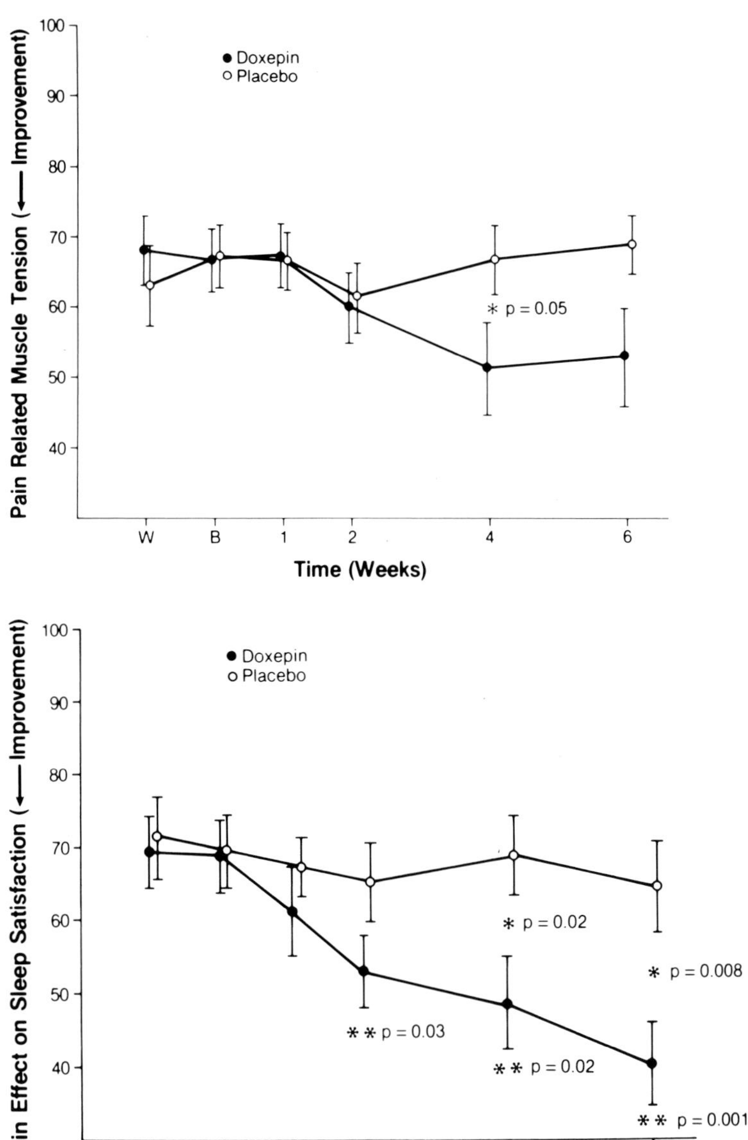

FIG. 5. **Top:** Pain-related muscle tension was better in doxepin patients than in placebo patients at week 4 by grouped *t*-test (*). By paired *t*-test (**) scores were better in doxepin patients at week 4 as compared with base line. **Bottom:** Pain effect on sleep satisfaction was better in doxepin patients than in placebo patients at weeks 4 and 6 by grouped *t*-test (*). By paired *t*-test (**), scores were lower in doxepin patients at weeks 2, 4, and 6 as compared with base line.

was lower in doxepin patients than in placebo patients at weeks 4 and 6 by grouped *t*-test. By paired *t*-test, pain effect on sleep satisfaction was lower in doxepin patients at weeks 2, 4, and 6 than in doxepin patients at base line.

Pain-related drug consumption. No significant differences in pain-related consumption of other drugs occurred (not shown).

Supine and standing blood pressure. Supine and standing blood pressure (not shown) showed no statistically significant differences between the doxepin and placebo groups, nor were there statistically significant differences between supine and standing pressures ("orthostatic effect") in either group.

Heart rate, respiratory rate, temperature, weight, height. No statistically significant differences in any of these parameters were observed, although heart rate in the doxepin group was slightly higher than in the placebo group.

Plasma beta-endorphin immunoreactivity. Plasma beta-endorphin immunoreactivity (not shown) showed high variability and no significant differences between the two groups.

Plasma enkephalin activity. Plasma enkephalin activity (not shown) showed high variability and no significant differences between the two groups.

DISCUSSION

Patients with chronic pain and depression often have accompanying problems, including sleep disorders, muscle tension, and analgesic drug dependency, as well as emotional and social maladjustment. Empirical use of tricyclic antidepressants in this situation is common, although the vagaries and elusiveness of chronic pain and depression symptoms make documentation and quantification difficult. In the study reported here we attempted to document and quantify chronic pain/depressive symptoms in outpatients referred to and followed in our Chronic Pain Clinic. Doxepin, a tricyclic with reportedly good sedation, muscle relaxation, antihistaminic and antidepressant value, with minimal cardiovascular effects, was compared with placebo. The results demonstrate the efficacy of doxepin for depression as well as pain-related parameters in patients in whom other treatment modalities had been exhausted and indicate that doxepin is a valuable treatment for chronic pain and depression.

REFERENCES

1. Brunswick, D. J., and Mendels, J. (1977): Reduced levels of tricyclic antidepressants in plasma from vacutainers. *Comm. Psychopharmacol,* 1:131–134.
2. Davis, T. R., Veggeberg, S. K., Hameroff, S. R., and Scherer, K. L. (1983): A sensitive and quantitative determination of plasma doxepin and demethyldoxepin by chromatography and mass spectrometry: a correlation with oral dosage and chemical effects in depressed chronic pain patients. *J. Chromatogr.*, 273:436-441.
3. Friedel, R. O., and Raskind, M. A. (1975): Relationship of blood levels of Sinequan to clinical effects in the treatment of depression in aged patients. In: *Sinequan Doxepin: A*

Monograph of Recent Clinical Studies, edited by J. Mendels. Excerpta Medica, Lawrenceville, N.J.

4. Ibor, J. J. L. (1972): Masked depressions. *Br. J. Psychiatry,* 120:245–258.
5. Lee, R. and Spencer, P. S. J. (1977): Antidepressants and pain: A review of the pharmacological data supporting the use of certain tricyclics in chronic pain. *J. Int. Med. Res.* [*Suppl. 1*] 5:146–156.
6. Merskey, H. (1965): The effect of chronic pain upon the response to noxious stimuli by psychiatric patients. *J. Psychosom. Res.*, 8:405–419.
7. Moore, D P. (1980): Treatment of chronic pain with tricyclic antidepressants. *South. Med. J.*, 73:1585–1586.
8. Naber, D., Picker, D., Dionne, R. A., et al. (1980): Assay of endogenous opiate receptor ligands in human CSF and plasma. *Substance and Alcohol Actions/Misuse*, 1:83–91.
9. Oswald, I., Brezinova, V., and Dunleavy, D. L. F. (1976): On the slowness of action of tricyclic antidepressant drugs. *Br. J. Psychiatry*, 120:673–677.
10. Pender, R. M., Brogden, R. N., Speight, T. M., et al. (1977): Doxepin up-to-date: A review of its pharmacological properties and therapeutic efficacy with particular reference to depression. *Drugs*, 13:161–218.
11. Pilowsky, I., Hallett, E. C., Bassett, D. L., Thomas, P. G., and Penhall, R. K. (1982): A controlled study of amitriptyline in the treatment of chronic pain. *Pain*, 14:169–180.
12. Sternbach, R. A. (1974): *Pain Patients' Traits and Treatments.* Academic Press, New York.
13. Veith, R. C., Raisys, V. A., and Perera, C. (1979): The clinical impact of blood collection methods on tricyclic antidepressants as measured by GC/MS-SIM. *Comm. Psychopharmacol.*, 2:491–494.
14. Ward, N., Bloom, V., and Friedel, R. O. (1979): Effectiveness of tricyclics in the treatment of coexisting pain and depression. *Pain*, 7:331–341.

Advances in Pain Research and Therapy, Vol. 9, edited by H. L. Fields et al. Raven Press, New York © 1985.

Effects of Two Tricyclic Antidepressants on Behavior, Arthritis, and Response to Noxious Stimulus in Rats with Adjuvant-Induced Arthritis

Stephen H. Butler, Jeanne Weil-Fugazza, Françoise Godefroy, and Jean-Marie Besson

Unite de Recherches de Neurophysiologie Pharmacologique, INSERM U 161, 75014 Paris, France

Tricyclic antidepressants (TCAs) have been used to treat chronic pain of various causes for several years without adequate explanation of their activity. Some have postulated that the therapeutic effect could be related to their antidepressant effects (2,15,18), whereas others have proposed that TCAs may possess analgesic properties (2,15). Although in one study TCA analgesia could not be demonstrated in normal human volunteers with acute pain (3), some animal studies indicate that acute or subchronic administration of TCAs increases the response threshold to acute noxious stimuli (5,9,13,17,19,21). However, these results do not adequately explain the efficacy of TCAs in chronic pain, because in clinical studies, the pain reduction after TCA administration is seen only after several days to weeks of treatment.

The purpose of the present study was to examine this problem by investigating the effect of *chronic* administration of TCAs in an animal pain model.

Rats with adjuvant-induced arthritis (8,16) were chosen for this study because it has recently been reported that the scratching observed in these animals could be considered as a parameter for study of chronic pain (4). In addition, neuronal responses recorded at various levels of the nervous system are significantly modified in arthritic rats (6,10,12,14).

Dr. Butler's present address is Department of Anesthesiology, University of Washington, Seattle, Washington 98195.

METHODS

Ninety Sprague-Dawley rats with adjuvant-induced polyarthritis were used in this study. They were randomly divided into three groups of 30 animals. Base-line assessments of weight, clinical signs of arthritis, pain responses to acute noxious stimuli, and behavioral parameters took place 21 days after induction of the polyarthritis (predrug evaluation period). Then animals received double-blind daily intraperitoneal injections of amitriptyline (10 mg/kg), imipramine (10 mg/kg), or saline for 4 weeks. At the end of this period, the same parameters were assessed. Because the dosages of TCAs used in our experiments induced sleepiness, all the observations were made at least 24 hr after the last injection.

Nociception

The effects on nociception were evaluated by the pain response obtained by applying graded pressure to the hind paw with a Randall-Selitto apparatus up to the threshold for vocalization and by behavioral observations according to De Castro Costa et al. (4) based on a 30-min observation period. During this period the following parameters were recorded:

Scratching. The rat starts by licking some part of its body or by vibrating its elevated hind paw near or on its ear, then changes to biting its skin or pulling its fingers or toes between its clenched teeth. This behavioral activity was recorded in seconds over 30 min.

Exploratory activities. These activities included the numbers of incidences of rearing or sniffing, running, and climbing, these latter three activities being recorded in seconds over 30 min.

Polyarthritis

The effects on polyarthritis were evaluated by measuring the circumference of the ankle joint bilaterally, by estimating different clinical signs such as deformities of the paws or the tail, conjunctivitis, bleeding from the nose, and balanitis, and by evaluating mobility. Each criterion was assigned a number that permitted us to establish a numerical arthritic score (maximum = 18) (Table 1) and a mobility score (maximum = 4) (Table 2).

RESULTS

When considering the evolution of clinical signs, some differences were observed in our experiment performed on Sprague-Dawley rats as compared with the study of De Castro Costa et al. (4) performed on Wistar rats.

First, in the nontreated rats, we did not observe a spontaneous regression of arthritic signs between 3 weeks and 7 weeks after administration of

TABLE 1. *Arthritis number scale*

Anatomy	Score	Description
Limbs (each scored separately)	3	Marked deformity with edema involving toes
	2	Moderate to marked deformity
	1	Edema does not involve toes, mild deformity only
Tail	3	Marked deformity with ulcers
	2	Marked deformity without ulcers or moderate deformity with ulcers
	1	Mild deformity only
Eyes	1	Conjunctivitis
Penis	1	Inflammation and/or discharge
Mucosa	1	Blood discharge from nose

Freund's adjuvant (numerical arthritis score 10.1 ± 3 at the predrug evaluation period and 9.6 ± 2.3 at 4 weeks later), whereas such a decrease was observed in the De Castro study. This allows us to evaluate clearly the effects of chronic TCAs on arthritis.

Second, close scrutiny of the data from the predrug evaluation period revealed that in each group there were animals that, despite having advanced arthritis, exhibited little or no scratching. Because the definitive description of this model for chronic pain indicates scratching as a primary manifestation of pain (4), the statistical analysis of the results was performed on subgroups triaged by the level of scratching at the predrug evaluation period. For this purpose, each group of rats (saline-treated, amitriptyline-treated, and imipramine-treated rats) was divided into two subgroups: those for which the duration of scratching at the predrug evaluation period was more than 100 sec over the 30-min period of observation and those for which the duration of scratching was less than 100 sec. We found that the duration of scratching in this latter group at the predrug evaluation period was not significantly different from that observed in a group of 30 normal rats run in parallel (duration of scratching 26 ± 7 sec).

TABLE 2. *Mobility scale*

Score	Description
0	No movement (lying down only)
1	Crawling only
2	Walking only
3	Walking and running with difficulty
4	Walking and running normally

The results show no significant variation in scratching duration in the group of saline-treated arthritic rats triaged for their high level of scratching, but both TCAs significantly decreased this behavior in arthritic rats triaged with the same criteria (Fig. 1). In the group of rats for which scratching was less than 100 sec per 30 min, a significant increase in the duration of this behavioral pattern was observed in the saline-treated rats, whereas TCAs counteracted this increase. These observations strongly support the idea that chronic TCAs reduce pain behavior in arthritic rats. This is reinforced by the observations summarized in Fig. 1. Such treatment enhanced the duration of exploring activity and the frequency of rearing.

On the other hand, chronic TCA treatment was associated with significant reductions in clinical signs of arthritis (decrease in arthritis score and increase in mobility score) (Fig. 1). This latter observation suggests that amitriptyline and imipramine may exhibit, at least in some pathological states, peripheral anti-inflammatory activity. Such a hypothesis is supported by our previous observation that the rise in plasma free tryptophan levels observed in arthritic rats (22) is decreased by chronic administration of phenylbutazone and also by chronic administration of amitriptyline and imipramine (7). This seems to confirm that TCAs may possess some common properties with anti-inflammatory drugs. This hypothesis also agrees with the observation that TCAs depress *in vitro* prostaglandin synthetase (11) and therefore would interfere with the inflammatory process. This is a possible explanation for our results, but, in fact, many additional tissue processes are involved in the inflammatory and autoimmune responses (23), and consequently other mechanisms may play a part in the observed reduction of arthritis by TCAs. These remain to be determined precisely by further studies.

Whatever the mechanisms involved in these peripheral processes, one is obliged to consider that this effect has an important role in the reduction of pain behavior. However, a central site of effects for TCAs cannot be excluded, because these drugs interact with the activity of serotonergic systems within the CNS, and the role of these systems has been well-established (1,20).

The lack of effect of chronic amitriptyline and imipramine on the threshold for vocalization in response to acute noxious stimuli (Fig. 1) brings into question the hypothesis of an analgesic effect of these drugs. However, this latter observation is not surprising if we consider that this analgesic test is based on application of acute noxious stimuli, whereas TCAs seem to affect clinical signs (scratching, rearing, exploring) that reflect chronic pain in relation to the disease. This assertion corresponds to clinical studies that did not reveal an analgesic effect of these compounds on acute pain in normal volunteers (3), whereas their efficacy has been reported on pain and pain behavior in chronic pain patients (2).

	SALINE	AMITRIPTYLINE	IMIPRAMINE
SCRATCHING	→	↘ ***	↘ *
EXPLORING	→	↗ **	↗ **
REARING	→	↗ *	↗ n.s.
THRESHOLD for VOCALIZATION (acute noxious stimulus)	→	→	→
NUMERICAL ARTHRITIS SCORE	→	↘ *	↘ *
NUMERICAL MOBILITY SCORE	→	↗ *	↗ *
ANKLE CIRCUMFERENCE	↗ **	→	→

* P < 0.05 _ ** P < 0.01 _ *** P < 0.001

FIG. 1. Effects of chronic administration of amitriptyline (10 mg/kg, i.p.) and imipramine (10 mg.kg, i.p.) daily over 4 weeks on behavioral parameters and clinical signs of arthritis in rats triaged for their high level of scratching (> 100 sec/30 min).

In conclusion, the present results indicate that scratching is a crucial criterion for preselection of arthritic rats for pharmacological studies related to the eventual effects of various compounds on chronic pain. These results also indicate that chronic amitriptyline and imipramine reduce clinical signs of arthritis and underline the usefulness of further systematic clinical investigations in patients suffering from chronic pain associated with inflammatory processes.

ACKNOWLEDGMENTS

This research was supported by grants from Caisse Nationale d'Assurance Maladie des Travailleurs Salaries (CNAMTS) and la Direction des Recherches et Etudes Techniques (DRET). S. H. Butler was supported by the University of Washington and by a grant from the French Foreign Minister.

REFERENCES

1. Besson, J. M., Oliveras, J. L., Chaouch, A., and Rivot, J. P. (1981): Role of the raphe nuclei in stimulation producing analgesia. In: *Serotonin: Current Aspects of Neurochemistry and*

Function, edited by B. Haber, S. Gabay, M. R. Issidores, and S. G. A. Alivisatos, pp. 153–176. Plenum Press, New York.

2. Butler, S. H. (1984): Present status of tricyclic antidepressants in chronic pain therapy. In: *Recent Advances in the Management of Pain: Advances in Pain Research and Therapy,* Vol. 7, edited by C. Benedetti, C. R. Chapman, and G. Moricca, Raven Press, New York.
3. Chapman, C. R., and Butler, S. H. (1978): Effects of doxepin on perception of laboratory-induced pain in man. *Pain,* 5:253–262.
4. De Castro Costa, M., De Sutter, P., Gybels, J., and Van Hees, J. (1981): Adjuvant-induced arthritis in rats: A possible animal model of chronic pain. *Pain,* 10:173–186.
5. Gaillard-Plaza, G., Lopez-Timoneda, F., and Montastruc, J. L. (1983): Endomorphines et action analgesique experimentale de l'amitriptyline. *Rev. Neurol. (Paris),* 139:529–530.
6. Gautron, M., and Guilbaud, G. (1982): Somatic responses of ventrobasal thalamic neurons in polyarthritic rats. *Brain Res.,* 237:459–477.
7. Godefroy, F., Weil-Fugazza, J., Besson, J.-M., and Butler, S. H. (1984): Effects of antirheumatic drugs and tricyclic antidepressants on total and free serum tryptophan levels in arthritic rats. In: *Progress in Tryptophan and Serotonin Research,* edited by H. G. Schlossberger, W. Kochen, B. Linzen, and H. Steinhart. Walter de Gruyter, Berlin.
8. Gouret, C., Mocquet, G., and Raynaud, G. (1976): Use of Freund's adjuvant arthritis test in anti-inflammatory drug screening in the rat: Value of animal selection and preparation at the breeding center. *Lab. Anim. Sci.,* 26:281–287.
9. Guiol, C., Tran, M. A., Blanc, M., Charlet, J. P., Eschalier, A., Cotonat, J., and Montastruc, J. L. (1983): Is there any relationship between antinociception, doses and plasma levels of chlomipramine during subchronic treatment in rats? *Biomed. Pharmacoth.,* 17:59–62.
10. Iggo, A., Guilbaud, G., and Tegner, R. (1984): Sensory mechanisms in arthritic rat joints. In: *Advances in Pain Research and Therapy,* Vol. 6, edited by L. Kruger and J. C. Liebeskind, pp. 83–93. Raven Press, New York.
11. Krupp, P., and Wesp, M. (1975): Inhibition of prostaglandin synthetase by psychotropic drugs. *Experientia,* 31:330–331.
12. Lamour, Y., Guilbaud, G., and Willer, J. C. (1983): Altered properties and laminar distribution of neuronal responses to peripheral stimulation in the SmI cortex of the arthritic rat. *Brain Res.,* 273:183–187.
13. Larsen, J. J., and Arnt, J. (1984): Spinal 5-HT or NA uptake inhibition potentiates supraspinal morphine antinociception in rats. *Acta Pharmacol. Toxicol. (Kbh.),* 54:72–75.
14. Menetrey, D., and Besson, J. M. (1982): Electrophysiological characteristics of dorsal horn cells in rats with cutaneous inflammation resulting from chronic arthritis. *Pain,* 13:343–364.
15. Montastruc, J. L., Tran, M. A., Charlet, J. P., Gaillard-Plaza, G., David, J., Cotonat, J., Guiraud, B., and Rascol, A. (1983): Etude des proprietes analgesiques et des concentrations plasmatiques de chlomipramine dans les douleurs chroniques. *Rev. Neurol. (Paris),* 139:583–587.
16. Newbould, B. B. (1963): Chemotherapy of arthritis induced in rats by mycobacterial adjuvant. *Br. J. Pharmacol. Chemother.,* 21:127–130.
17. Ogren, S. O., and Holm, A. C. (1980): Test-specific effects of the 5HT-reuptake inhibitors alaproclate and zimelidine on pain sensitivity and morphine analgesia. *J. Neurol. Transmission,* 47:253–271.
18. Pilkowsky, I., Chapman, R., and Bonica, J. J. (1977): Pain, depression and illness behaviour in a pain clinic population. *Pain,* 4:183–192.
19. Rigal, F., Eschalier, A., Devoize, J. L., and Pecharde, J. C. (1983): Activities of five antidepressants in a behavioural pain test in rats. *Life Sci.,* 32:2965–2971.
20. Rivot, J. P., Weil-Fugazza, J., Godefroy, F., Bineau-Thurotte, M., Ory-Lavollee, L., and Besson, J. M. (1984): Involvement of serotonin in both morphine and stimulation-produced analgesia: Electrochemical and biochemical approaches. In: *Advances in Pain Research and Therapy,* Vol. 6, edited by L. Kruger and J. C. Liebeskind, pp. 135–150. Raven Press, New York.
21. Uzan, A., Kabouche, M., Rataud, J., and Le Fur, G. (1980): Pharmacological evidence of a possible tryptaminergic regulation of opiate receptors by using indalpine, a selective 5-HT uptake inhibitor. *Neuropharmacology,* 19:1075–1079.
22. Weil-Fugazza, J., Godefroy, F., Bineau-Thurotte, M., and Besson, J. M. (1984): Plasma

tryptophan levels and 5-hydroxytryptamine synthesis in the brain and the spinal cord in arthritic rats. In: *Progress in Tryptophan and Serotonin Research,* edited by H. G. Schlossberger, W. Kochen, B. Linzen, and H. Steinhart, pp. 405–408. Walter de Gruyter, Berlin.
23. Willoughby, D. A., Dunn, C. J., and Giroud, J. P. (1977): Nouvelles methodes experimentales d'etude des anti-inflammatoires et anti-rhumatismaux. In: *Actualites Pharmacologiques,* XXeme serie, pp. 25–48. Masson, Paris.

Advances in Pain Research and Therapy, Vol. 9, edited by H. L. Fields et al. Raven Press, New York © 1985.

Influence of Acetylsalicylic and Salicylic Plasma Levels on Psychophysical Measures of Long-Standing Natural Pain Stimuli

*F. Anton, *H. O. Handwerker, *A. Kreh, *P. W. Reeh, **E. Walter, and **E. Weber

**Second Physiological Institute and **Laboratory of Clinical Pharmacology, University of Heidelberg, D-6900 Heidelberg, Federal Republic of Germany*

It is difficult to provide reliable measures for the effects of non-narcotic analgesics using experimental algesimetry. According to Beecher's still relevant criticism, these problems are due to the fundamental differences between clinical and experimental pain: The noxious stimuli used in the laboratory are generally too short (ranging from milliseconds to seconds) and too weak, and they always have the same, predictable time course (3). The "submaximum effort tourniquet technique" developed by Beecher's group was designed to avoid these disadvantages (9). Unfortunately, this method can be applied only once in a session, thus imposing narrow limits on the experimental design. More recent algesimetric methods based on evoked potentials and "signal detection theory" ignore again the discrepancy between clinical and experimental pain. In addition, the nature of the measured parameters is still controversial (4,6).

We have previously examined two simple methods of noxious stimulation that largely fulfill Beecher's requirements but can be repeated in one session (1,2). The aim of the present study was to validate this algesimetric approach in a double-blind crossover study applying two doses of aspirin and placebo; our particular concern was the possible correlation between the acetylsalicylate and total salicylate plasma levels and the subjective magnitude estimates of the pain sensation.

METHODS

Two methods of noxious cutaneous stimulation that induced continuously increasing strong pain sensations during 2 min of application were used.

Mechanical Stimulation

A feedback-controlled constant force of 12 N was applied to the interdigital web between the fourth and fifth fingers of the left hand by a motor-driven forceps having faces of 30 mm^2 each.

Thermal Stimulation

Starting from an adaptation temperature of 30°C, the surface of the left index was cooled to 0° C by a thermode that was perfused with a thermostatically controlled glycerol-water mixture. During the stimulus, the blood flow was occluded by a tourniquet at the base of the finger.

These stimuli did not induce lasting damage of the skin when repeatedly applied.

Assessment of Pain Intensity

The subjects were cued by an acoustic signal at 10-sec intervals to assess their current pain intensity by moving a lever that controlled a vertically displayed electronic visual analog scale (VAS) consisting of 32 LEDs. On this scale, the following points were defined: The lower end was the pain threshold, the upper end was the tolerance limit, and a point at the lower third was the "intervention point." The latter corresponded to a pain level that would cause the subject to intervene in a nonexperimental situation.

Figure 1 illustrates the sequence of an algesimetric session. The pain ratings increased in the course of each stimulus. The time courses and the intensities of the pain sensations were fairly reproducible during repetitive stimulation.

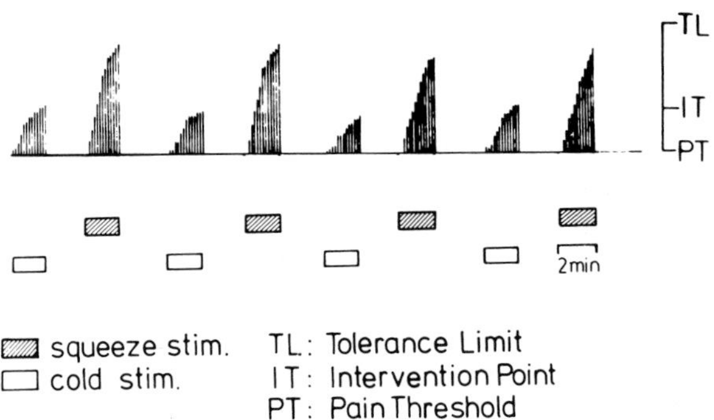

FIG. 1. Sequence of an algesimetric session: Pain ratings on a VAS are represented as vertical bars.

Experimental Protocol

The double-blind crossover study was carried out with 12 male subjects (ages 19–29). Each subject took part in one training session and in three medication sessions separated by 7 to 10 days. The subjects gave informed consent. They received a commensurate payment.

The subjects were explicitly informed that they would receive placebo and two doses of aspirin in random order. After each session they were asked to guess which medication had been administered ("presumed medication").

The drug was given 2.5 hr after the last intake of food and drink consisting of a standarized snack at noon. With 100 ml of water, three seemingly identical tablets were swallowed that contained 1,500 mg, 500 mg, or no aspirin.

Each algesimetric session consisted of 13 mechanical and 13 thermal stimuli alternatively applied at 5-min interstimulus intervals (Fig. 1). The medication was given at the end of the second stimulus. In each experiment, 14 blood samples (2 prior to and 12 following drug administration) were taken from a venous catheter to measure the plasma levels of acetylsalicylic acid (ASA) and total salicylic acid (SA) by high-performance liquid chromatography.

Data Evaluation

The stimulus parameters and the pain ratings were recorded on-line and stored on floppy disks by a microcomputer. The mean rating score during each stimulus was used as the basic pain measure. Two other psychological parameters were derived from it: (a) The differences between each mechanical stimulus and the mean of the two temporally related cold stimuli were calculated and called *pain rating differences.* The cold stimuli were generally perceived much weaker than the squeeze stimuli. This provided the possibility to take the cold pain rating as an intraindividual standard and to relate the mechanically induced pain to it. (b) The differences between the individual squeeze pain ratings under aspirin medication and the corresponding ratings under placebo were calculated and labeled as *placebo-related pain ratings.* Together with the plasma level parameters, these data were analyzed at the university computer center using the general linear models (GLM) of SAS (statistical analysis system, SAS Institute Inc., Cary, North Carolina).

RESULTS

The following analyses were confined to the squeeze pain ratings and derived parameters described earlier, because the cold pain ratings were generally much lower and less sensitive to the experimental effects.

Analysis of Mean Pain Ratings

A four-way analysis of variance was computed with the mean squeeze pain ratings averaged over the time of 30 to 120 min following drug intake. In this period, medication effects were expected. The factors were (a) real medication, (b) presumed medication *(vide supra),* (c) succession of sessions, and (d) subjects. The analysis was computed with 11 subjects, because the twelfth abstained from a presumption (factor b). This model covered 91% of the variance ($R^2 = 0.91$). Two factors yielded significant effects: (b) the differences between subjects ($p < 0.001$) and (d) the presumed medication ($p < 0.006$). These presumptions concerning the received medication were correct only by chance. The subjects tended to gradually lower their ratings depending on their conviction of having received placebo or one of the two doses of aspirin (Fig. 2).

One main purpose of the study was to relate the pain ratings to the ASA and SA plasma concentrations, the time courses of which are shown in Figs. 3C and 3D. The averaged ASA level (1,500 mg aspirin intake) reached a sharp peak after some 40 min and then declined; the concentrations of SA continuously increased throughout the 120-min session.

An analysis of covariance was computed with the plasma level parameters different from zero and the temporally related squeeze pain ratings. This model ($R^2 = 0.77$) revealed a highly significant covariance with the ASA plasma concentrations ($p < 0.002$), whereas that with the SA levels was not

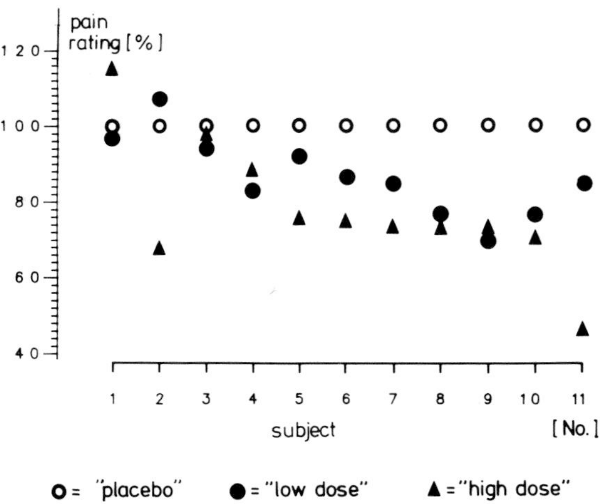

FIG. 2. Effects of presumed medication on the squeeze pain ratings of 11 subjects. The mean responses under the "placebo" hypothesis were taken as 100%: "placebo' ratings < "small-dose"ratings ($p = 0.01$), "small-dose" ratings < "large-dose" ratings ($p = 0.01$), "placebo" ratings < "aspirin" ratings ($p = 0.001$). (From Handwerker, ref. 5.)

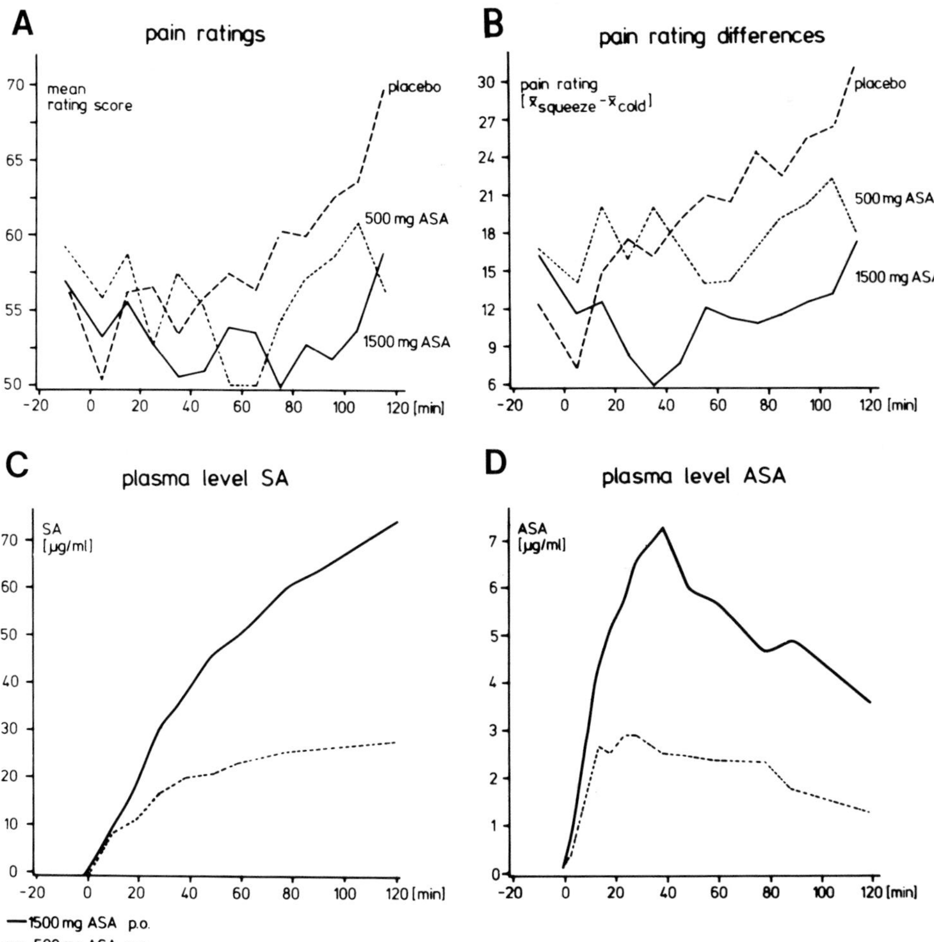

FIG. 3. A: Squeeze pain ratings averaged over each stimulus; drug administration at time 0. The range of the scores lies between "intervention point" (40 points) and pain tolerance level (128 points). **B:** Mean rating differences between each squeeze stimulus and the neighboring cold pain stimuli. **C** and **D:** Time courses of SA and ASA plasma concentrations following oral administration of aspirin tablets.

significant. After partialling out other significant effects (sequence of sessions and differences between subjects), only the high ASA plasma levels following 1,500 mg aspirin were significantly correlated with the squeeze pain rating ($r = -0.38$, $p < 0.0001$). Partial cross-correlations showed that there were no phase shifts between plasma concentrations and changes in pain ratings.

Analysis of Mean Pain Rating Differences

Pain rating differences were calculated between mechanical and thermal stimuli, as described earlier. Figure 3B shows the time course of this derived parameter under the different experimental conditions. A five-way analysis of variance was computed with the factors (a) real medication, (b) presumed medication, (c) succession of sessions, (d) subjects, and (e) succession of stimuli within the session. In this model ($R^2 = 0.65$), all factors were found to be significant. In particular, there was a highly significant effect of the real medication ($p = 0.0001$). A consecutive test (Scheffe) showed that this was due to a strong effect of the high aspirin dose, whereas the effect of the low dose was not significantly different from placebo. This is also indicated by comparison of Figs. 3B and 3D showing that the early depression of the pain measure is closely related to the peak of the ASA plasma concentration in the case of the 1,500-mg aspirin dose. The corresponding analysis of covariance ($R^2 = 0.74$) revealed a significant effect of the ASA plasma level ($p < 0.03$), whereas the SA plasma levels showed no significant effects. The respective partial correlation coefficients between the ASA levels following the high dose of aspirin and the pain rating differences were $r = -0.3$, $p < 0.001$. The ASA levels after intake of the low dose and the total SA plasma concentrations did not show this correlation.

Analysis of Mean Placebo-Related Pain Ratings

The repeated noxious mechanical stimulation of the same interdigital web induced continuously increasing pain ratings when placebo had been administered (Fig. 3A). Aspirin seemed to influence this trend, because

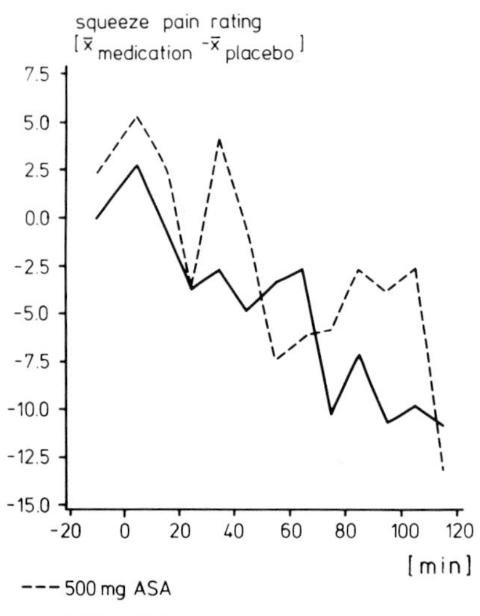

FIG. 4. Mean squeeze pain ratings, plotted as difference between medication and corresponding placebo time scores.

especially in the second hour following drug administration, the squeeze pain ratings remained below the respective values under placebo.

Correspondingly, the differences between sequeeze pain ratings under aspirin and under placebo became more negative (Fig. 4). When these placebo-related pain ratings were entered into an analysis of covariance (R^2 = 0.54) together with the plasma level parameters, a highly significant effect of the SA concentration was found ($p < 0.0001$), whereas the ASA level did not play a significant role. This is illustrated by the negative correlation between the placebo-related pain ratings and the SA plasma levels, which was highly significant for both aspirin doses (Fig. 5).

DISCUSSION

In double-blind assays, administration of placebo has become a major tool to assess the influence of suggestion. Under our experimental conditions, all the subjects but one tried to guess which drug they had received, and after the sessions they revealed their opinions on request. These presumptions, which were correct only by chance, significantly influenced the squeeze pain ratings. This shows that in a double-blind design, the placebo effect will still have an impact on the experimental outcome. When testing drugs without any perceivable effects or side effects, the variance of the data will be increased by the random distribution of the hypothesis effect. This additional variance might be reduced by giving the subjects as little information as ethically justifiable about the medication schedule or by providing some misleading information.

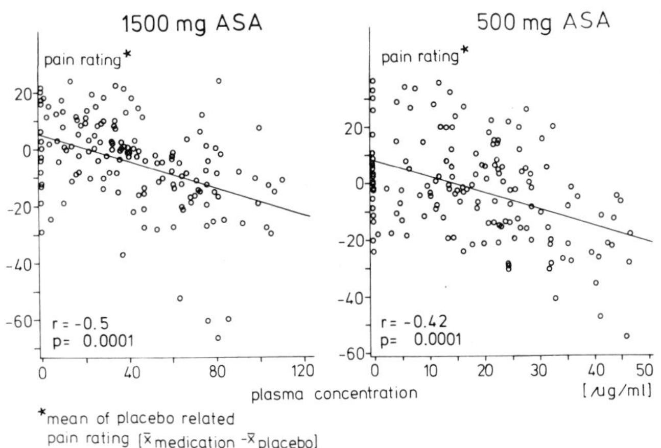

FIG. 5. Correlation of the placebo-related squeeze pain ratings with the SA plasma levels (N = 12). **A:** 1,500 mg aspirin. **B:** 500 mg aspirin. Correlation parameters: $r = -0.5$, $p = 0.0001$ for 1,500 mg aspirin; $r = -0.42$, $p = 0.0001$ for 500 mg aspirin. For interpretation of the correlation plots, consider the different scales of the abscissa.

It is known that the large variance of algesimetric data may completely mask the hypoalgesic effect of a tested drug. In this study we used two ways to overcome this problem. One approach was to reduce the variance by relating the pain ratings to an intraindividual standard that was affected by the same interfering variables. In this study the cold pain ratings were used as such a standard because they reflected the individual rating habits, but neither showed the drug effects nor the hyperalgesic time trend of the squeeze pain ratings. The derived parameter "pain rating differences" revealed a significant effect of the high aspirin dosage.

Another approach was to compute an analysis of covariance with the actual plasma levels of the tested drug. The analysis of variance can take account only of the drug dose applied. Especially after oral administration, this dose may, however, lead to rather variable effective plasma concentrations in variable time courses. The use of plasma concentrations in the analysis of covariance reduces the variance due to bioavailability even if plasma was not the relevant compartment for the analgesic action of the drug. This approach revealed a significant negative correlation between ASA plasma levels and the pain ratings.

Under placebo medication, the pain ratings continuously increased as a sign of hyperalgesia in the repeatedly squeezed interdigital webs. Our interpretation that this was due to inflammatory processes has recently been supported by means of infrared thermography of the stimulated site *(unpublished results).* We observed a hyperthermic focus up to 4° C warmer than the surrounding skin for several hours after the stimulus. The slowly developing hyperalgesia was not observed under aspirin medication, as revealed by the "placebo-related" squeeze pain ratings. This parameter was sensitive even for the small aspirin dose. It was correlated with the plasma concentrations of SA but not of ASA.

The relative analgesic and anti-inflammatory potencies of ASA and of SA have been discussed in the literature (7,8,10). Previously, correlations between analgesic effects and plasma levels have been demonstrated only for SA (7,10). However, such correlations might be fortuitous, because ASA and SA are not measured in the compartment relevant for analgesic actions.

In our study, an early effect (maximal 40 min after drug intake) was correlated with the ASA plasma levels. A distinct, slowly increasing effect was correlated with the SA levels. Whether the first action reflects ASA-induced hypoalgesia and the second the reduction of inflammatory hyperalgesia by either ASA or SA remains to be studied.

ACKNOWLEDGMENTS

We wish to thank all our subjects, E. Schumacher, E. Welk, and W. Ruf for technical assistance, and Mrs. P. Roth for carefully editing this manuscript.

This work was supported by the DFG, grant HA 831/8 and by Bayer AG.

REFERENCES

1. Adriaensen, H., Gybels, J., Handwerker, H. O., and Van Hees, J. (1984): Nociceptor discharges and sensations due to prolonged noxious mechanical stimulation—a paradox. *Human Neurobiol.,* 3:53–58.
2. Anton, F., Kreh, A., Reeh, P. W., and Handwerker, H. O. (1984): Algesimetry using natural stimuli of long duration. In: *Pain Measurement in Man,* edited by B. Bromm, Chapter 33. Elsevier, Amsterdam.
3. Beecher, H. K. (1953): Limiting factors in experimental pain. *J. Chronic Dis.* 4:11–26.
4. Coppola, R., and Gracely, R. H. (1983): Where is the noise in SDT pain assessment? *Pain,* 17:257–266.
5. Handwerker, H. O. (1984): Some aspects of pain measurement in man. *Drug Res.,* 34(11):1093–1095.
6. Harkins, S. W., Price, D. D., and Katz, M. A. (1983): Are cerebral potentials reliable indices of first or second pain? In: *Advances in Pain Research and Therapy,* Vol. 5, edited by J. J. Bonica, U. Lindblom, A. Iggo, L. E. Jones and C. Benedetti, pp. 185–191. Raven Press, New York.
7. Seymour, R. A., and Rawlins, M. D. (1982): Efficacy and pharmacokinetics of aspirin in post-operative dental pain. *Br. J. Clin. Pharmacol.,* 13:807–810.
8. Seymour, R. A., Rawlins, M. D., and Clothier, A. (1984): The efficacy and pharmacokinetics of sodium salicylate in postoperative dental pain. *Br. J. Clin. Pharmacol.,* 17:161–163.
9. Smith, G. M., Egbert, L. D., Markowitz, R. A., Mosteller, F., and Beecher, H. K. (1966): An experimental pain method sensitive to morphine in man: The submaximum effort tourniquet technique. *J. Pharmacol. Exp. Ther.,* 154:324–332.
10. Ventafridda, V., and Martino, G. (1976): Observations on the relationships between plasma concentration and analgesic activity of a soluble acetylsalicylic acid derivate after intravenous administraiton in man. In: *Advances in Pain Research and Therapy,* Vol. 1, edited by J. J. Bonica and D. Albe-Fessard, pp. 529–536. Raven Press, New York.

Advances in Pain Research and Therapy, Vol. 9, edited by H. L. Fields et al. Raven Press, New York © 1985.

Effect of Epidural Steroids in the Cervical and Lumbar Region on Surgical Intervention for Diskogenic Spondylosis

*,†Ronald P. Pawl, *Warren Anderson, and †Morton Shulman

**Pain Treatment Centers, Lake Forest Hospital, Lake Forest, Illinois 60045; and † Illinois Masonic Medical Center, University of Illinois, Chicago, Illinois 60657*

Surgical decompression of nerve roots in an attempt to relieve neck and arm or low back and leg pain associated with degenerative disk disease is carried out quite frequently in the United States and represents a significant proportion of the surgery performed by most neurosurgeons and some orthopedic surgeons. A criticism of many such surgical procedures has been that the patient probably would have improved spontaneously if adequate time were allowed to lapse, or if other, nonsurgical or less invasive procedures were added to the treatment regimen prior to surgery. In carefully selected series of patients who have arm or leg pain emanating from a single root entrapped by a herniated disk, the statistical results from surgical decompression are quite gratifying, in the range of 90% or better. However, perhaps the majority of root decompression surgeries are performed on patients whose symptoms are not so clearly defined. As a consequence, the [reported] results of decompressive surgery falls far below an acceptable level, in the range of 50 to 60%.

In 1961, Gardner and his colleagues reported on the use of steroid preparations introduced into the spinal epidural space, and later into the subarachnoid space, in the treatment of patients with painful radiculopathy (2,3). Even though the initial results in the patients treated were quite positive, the technique was not readily adopted, especially by surgeons. On the other hand, Winnie began using epidural and subarachnoid steroid injections in his nerve block pain clinic, and subsequently reported a high degree of relief in patients with painful radiculopathies, similar to the results noted by Gardner and his group (4,10,11). The mechanism whereby steroids relieve radicular pain is not understood, but then the mechanism of pain production by a herniated disk is also poorly understood. Winnie has speculated that an inflammatory reaction is set up by the spinal derangement resulting from disk herniation, and that the anti-inflammatory action of the injected steroid relieves the pain (11). Epidural and intrathecal steroids are absorbed slowly after injection, mostly locally and with little systemic effect, making this mode of administration superior to other oral or parenteral modes of administration (7,9). Although the mode of action is still unclear, by the second half of the 1970s, epidural steroid injections were becoming a popular therapy for painful radiculopathies, particularly among anesthesiologists who were involved in the management of chronic pain patients (5). Little or no complications have been reported using the loss of resistance technique for injecting the steroid preparations in either the lumbar or cervical spinal canal epidurally, but the preservative used for the steroids has been thought to cause nerve root damage when injected intrathecally (1,8). The latter technique, therefore, has been discontinued by most therapists.

TECHNIQUE

The epidural steroid injection was introduced into the pain treatment center regimen by Anderson at Lake Forest Hospital, and by Shulman [at Illinois Masonic Medical Center] (6), both anesthesiologists. Pawl, a neurosurgeon at both institutions, is also director of a multidisciplinary pain treatment center at each hospital. The technique of injection is based on the concept that as a needle tip passes through tissues such as muscle and ligament, the turgor of the tissue will occlude the needle orifice. When the needle tip enters the epidural space, the loose fatty tissue does not effectively occlude the needle orifice. The resistance of the tissue against the needle orifice is checked periodically as the needle is advanced toward the epidural space by thumb pressure on a syringe, half-filled with sterile saline or air. If the needle orifice is occluded by tissue, the air or saline will be compressed by thumb pressure on the syringe plunger, and the plunger will be forced outward by the compressed fluid or gas when the thumb is removed. As soon as the needle tip enters the epidural space, pressure on the plunger forces the air or saline into the loose tissues and the plunger will not rebound when the thumb pressure is released. The procedure is carried out on inpatients or outpatients for either cervical or lumbar injections, and under sterile precautions. Usual external anatomical landmarks are used to localize the level of the injection, and an attempt is made to place the steroid and local anesthetic mixture at the level and on the side clinically involved. Forty to 80 mg of methylprednisolone (Depomedrol) is suspended in approximately 5 cc of low-dose local anesthetic solution for injection after the needle has been checked to see whether or not cerebrospinal fluid escapes from the needle after placement using the above technique. If spinal fluid does escape the needle, it is removed and the epidural space is reentered from a different angle. Patients with lumbar syndromes are placed at complete bed rest for 3 days after the injection, either at home or in the hospital, whereas those with cervical syndromes are put in light, comfortable cervical traction, at home if the apparatus is available there, or in the hospital. All patients are asked to restrict their activities for another week thereafter, and at that time a decision is made regarding an additional injection. If there is nearly complete or complete relief, or no relief at all, further injections are not recommended. In those patients with definitive partial, but unacceptable, pain relief, a second—rarely a third—injection is recommended. Although previous studies have indicated little systemic absorption from steroids injected epidurally (7,9), we have not allowed any patient to have more than three injections in a 6-month period.

An analysis of approximately 100 patients so treated at the Lake Forest facility was carried out in 1979 *(unpublished).* These patients, with mixed cervical and lumbar syndromes, appeared to have an accelerated recovery if their symptoms were not so severe, but in those patients with severe radicular symptoms the injection did not prevent the need for ultimate surgical decompression. Over the last 4 years, Pawl has observed that the routine use of epidural steroid injections as part of the management of painful spinal syndromes was reducing the number of surgical decompressions being performed by him, and the present study was carried out to investigate that impression.

EFFECT OF EPIDURAL STEROID INJECTIONS ON INCIDENCE OF SURGERY

The surgical records for cervical and lumbar decompressive surgery of Pawl and his two colleagues were reviewed for the years 1974 to 1976 (Table 1), the 3 years prior to the year Pawl began to use epidural steroid injections as routine treatment. A total of 229 lumbar laminectomies were performed by the group, or an average of 76 per year. Of these surgeries, 134 were performed by Pawl, or an average of 45 per year. One hundred and fifty-three cervical procedures, mostly anterior cervical diskectomies and fusions were performed by the group in the same period, for an average of 51 per year; 89 such procedures were carried out by Pawl, an average of 30 per year. These figures were compared to similar data from the years 1981 to 1983. During this time Pawl recommended epidural steroid injections as part of the routine management of spinal diskogenic pain problems before consideration of surgical decompression. Pawl's two partners, however, recommended the steroid injection only rarely and sporadically during this interval. In 1982 and 1983, chemonucleolysis was added to the surgical armamentarium and is included in the surgical series, since the indications for chemonucleolysis are identical to those for laminectomy for herniated disk syndromes. The group performed 229 lumbar spinal surgeries including 47 chemonucleolyses, for an average of 76 cases per year. Pawl performed 137 of these including 40 chemonucleolyses, for an average of 45 per year.

TABLE 1. *Spinal surgeries*

Year	Surgical area	Pawl	Surgeon 2	Surgeon 3	Total
1974	Cervical	26	8	5	39
	Lumbar	42	8	15	65
1975	Cervical	33	10	15	58
	Lumbar	46	19	26	91
1976	Cervical	30	18	8	56
	Lumbar	46	9	18	73
Average	Cervical	30			51
	Lumbar	45			76
1981	Cervical	17	5	15	37
	Lumbar	39	8	17	64
1982	Cervical	18	5	6	29
	Lumbar	57	15	13	85
1983	Cervical	15	3	20	43
	Lumbar	40	20	16	80
Average	Cervical	17			36
	Lumbar	45			76

In the same interval, the group performed 109 cervical surgeries, an average of 39 per year, and 53 were carried out by Pawl, for an average of 18 per year. Thus, the number of surgical procedures carried out for painful lumbar spinal problems was not altered in spite of the addition of epidural steroid injections to the therapeutic regimen, whereas the number of cervical surgical procedures was reduced by 40% in Pawl's series and reduced in the entire group's series by the same number as the reduction in Pawl's series, after introduction of the epidural steroid technique preoperatively.

RETROSPECTIVE REVIEW OF THE RESULTS OF EPIDURAL STEROID INJECTIONS

In an effort to determine how effective epidural steroid injections were in the management of painful spinal problems, the records of 247 patients treated with this technique in 1981 and 1982 were reviewed. In addition, those patients who were not operated on were questioned by telephone regarding the outcome of their epidural steroid injections. This provides a minimum of 18 months follow-up in each case. A total of 103 patients with cervical syndromes were seen and treated with epidural steroid injections in those 2 years. Thirty-five of those patients, or roughly one-third, ultimately required surgical intervention. Of the 68 patients who were not considered for or refused surgical consideration, only 36 were considered to have typical radicular syndromes of the type usually considered appropriate for surgical intervention, that is, more upper extremity pain than neck pain, and some objective or subjective neurological deficit such as weakness of a major muscle group or paresthesias in a radicular dermatomal distribution

TABLE 2. *Results of epidural steroid injections in patients with cervical syndromes*[a]

Relief[b]	With radiculopathy[c]	Without radiculopathy[d]
5	9	1
4	9	7
3	10	7
2	5	2
1	1	2
0	0	3
Patients with litigation		
5	1	0
4	0	0
3	0	2
2	1	2
1	0	2
0	0	4
Total	36	32

[a]Patients who were referred by Pawl but did not undergo surgery (1981 and 1982).
[b]Relief rates: 5 = 100%; 4 = 75–90%; 3 = 50–75%; 2 = 25–50%; 1 = 5–25%; 0 = 0.
[c]Averages: 28/34 (82%); 6/34 (18%). Averages of patients with litigation: 1/2 (50%); 1/2 (50%).
[d]Averages: 15/22 (69%); 7/22 (31%). Averages of patients with litigation: 2/10 (20%); 8/10 (80%).

(Table 2). Twenty-nine of the 36 patients, or 80%, indicated that the relief of pain from the epidural steroid injection was 50% or more, and the other 7 patients did not feel they had enough pain to consider surgical decompression. We conclude that patients with a cervical syndrome of radicular pain in the upper extremity and a neurological deficit, subjectively or objectively, half can expect relief from nonsurgical management that includes an epidural injection of steroids.

The other 32 patients treated with cervical epidural steroid injections in this period, but not considered for surgical intervention by either the patient or the surgeon or both, were patients primarily with neck and interscapular or headache pain, or in whom the arm or shoulder pain was secondary and not typical of radicular pain, and there was no clear-cut objective or subjective neurological problem. Seventeen, or 53%, of these patients noted 50% or better relief of their symptoms. Ten of these patients were in litigation over their condition, and 8 claimed the injection gave them no relief. Of the patients who were not in litigation, 15 of 22, or 70%, noted 50% or more relief of pain. Patients who have diskogenic or other spinally originating cervical pain without serious compromise of their nerve roots can therefore expect relief from an epidural steroid injection.

Patients with lumbar syndromes were similarly analyzed, and 96 patients who underwent surgical decompression in 1981 and 1982 after nonsurgical treatment, including epidural steroid injections, had their records reviewed. Only the data from 1982 regarding patients treated without surgery were available at the time of this review, consequently comparative data similar to that analyzed above in patients with cervical spine disorders is available only for that year (Table 3).

Fifty-seven surgical decompressions, including 30 chemonucleolysis procedures, were carried out in 1982 after epidural steroid injections failed to give the patients significant relief. In the same time frame, 48 other patients were treated with epidural steroid injections and did not consider surgery for further relief of pain. Of those 48 patients, only 26 had radicular syndromes that included sciatica and objective or subjective neurological deficit of such a magnitude that surgical intervention might be recommended. Of 83 patients initially evaluated with sciatica and a neurological deficit at that time, 57, or nearly 70%, ultimately required surgical decompression.

Among the 26 patients with radicular syndromes who were treated with epidural steroid injections, but were not considered surgical candidates by either the physician or the patient or both, were 9 patients who were in litigation over their condition. Of these patients, 5 reported less than 50% relief of pain. In the group of patients without such litigation, 12 of 17, or 70%, reported more than 50% relief of pain.

Other lumbar syndromes treated with epidural steroid injections included low back and diffuse sciatic pain, without definitive root compression syndromes, but including patients with spinal stenosis syndromes without neurological compromise. Only approximately 50% of those patients received 50% or more relief of their pain from epidural steroid injections, and if the

TABLE 3. *Patients with lumbar epidural steroid injections*[a]

Relief[b]	With radiculopathy[c]	Without radiculopathy[d]
5	2	1
4	4	3
3	6	5
2	1	1
1	1	1
0	3	3
Patients with litigation		
5	1	1
4	1	1
3	2	1
2	3	3
1	1	0
0	1	2

[a]Patients who were referred by Pawl but did not undergo surgical decompression (1982).

[b]Relief rate same as in Table 2.

[c]Averages: 12/17 (70%); 5/17 (30%).

[d]Averages: 9/14 (68%); 5/14 (36%). Averages of patients with litigation: 7/17 (41%); 10/17 (59%).

poor results in cases involving litigation are removed, the results increase to about 65%. No objective complications were recorded in this series. Approximately 15% of patients who were interviewed by telephone indicated that they did not like the thought of being injected deep into the spinal column, or disliked the pain or paresthesia they experienced during the injection.

CONCLUSIONS

Corticosteroid preparations injected into the epidural space using the loss of resistance technique have benefit in the treatment of painful syndromes resulting from degenerative disk disorders including radiculopathy from herniated disks. Although 50% of patients with cervical radicular syndromes and 30% of patients with lumbar radicular syndromes were able to avoid surgery with the help of epidural injections, the treatment appears to have effectively reduced the need for spinal surgery in the cervical region only. Although this result is gratifying, it is much less than the results reported by Winnie and Hartmann and their colleagues (4,10,11), and puts the use of this technique in a different light. The incidence of surgical decompression carried out in both the lumbar and cervical cases somewhat surprised us. We have considered ourselves to be conservative with regard to recommending spinal decompressive surgery, and regularly utilize a pain management program instead of surgery for our patients. Generally, it has been thought by the authors that only 25% or 30% of patients with cervical radiculopathies and about 50% of those with lumbar radiculopathies require surgical decompression. In this series, 50% of patients with cervical radiculopathy and 70% of those with lumbar radiculopathy ultimately underwent surgery for their condition. This is in spite of the additional management with epidural steroid injections. Because the addition of epidural steroid injections to the therapeutic regimen has significantly reduced cervical spine surgeries, it is possible that the incidence of surgical intervention prior to this treatment program was even higher than 50% in cervical cases.

Epidural steroid injections have also proven of therapeutic benefit in those patients whose cervical or lumbar spondylosis syndromes are not associated with significant radiculopathy, and thus would not be considered for surgical intervention. The lack of significant complications in this series bespeaks the benign nature of the treatment.

REFERENCES

1. Dougherty, J. H., Jr. Fraser, R. A. (1978): Complications following intraspinal injections of steroids: report of two cases. *J Neurosurg.,* 48:1023–1025.
2. Gardner, W. J., Goebert, H. W., Jr., and Sehgal, A. D. (1961): Intraspinal corticosteroid in the treatment of sciatica. *Trans. Am. Neurol. Assoc.,* 86:214–215.
3. Goebert, H. W., Jr., Jallo, S. J., Gardner, W. J., et. al. (1961): Painful radiculopathy treated

with epidural injections of procaine and hydrocortisone acetate: Results in 113 patients. *Anesth. Analg.,* 40:130–134.
4. Hartmann, J. T., Winnie, A. P., Ramamurthy, S., Mani, M. R., and Meyers, H. L. (1974): Intradural and extradural corticosteroids for sciatic pain. *Orthoped. Rev.,* 3(12):21–24.
5. Pawl, R. P. (1979): *Chronic Pain Primer,* p. 74. Yearbook, Chicago.
6. Shulman, M., Nimmagadda, U., Valenta, A. (1984): Cervical epidural steroid injection of pain control of cervical spine origin. *Proceedings: American Society of Anesthesiology,* New Orleans.
7. Sehgal, A. D., Tweed, D. C., Gardner, W. J., et. al. (1963): Laboratory studies after intrathecal corticosteroids. *Arch. Neurol.,* 9:64–68.
8. Sugar, O. (1983): Steroid injections (editorial). *Surg. Neurol.,* 19:91.
9. Swerdlow, M., and Sayle-Creer, W. (1970): A Study of extradural medication in the relief of the lumbosciatic syndrome. *Anaesthesia,* 25:341–345.
10. Winnie, A. P., Hartman, J. T., Meyers, H. L., Ramamurthy, S., and Barangan, V. (1972): Pain clinic II: Intradural and extradural steroids for sciatica. *Anaesth. Analg.,* 51(6):990–999.
11. Winnie, A. P., and Ramamurthy, S. (1976): Steroids for discogenic pain. *Proceedings: World Congress of Anesthesiology,* Mexico City.

Advances in Pain Research and Therapy, Vol. 9, edited by H. L. Fields et al. Raven Press, New York © 1985.

Surgical Approaches to the Primary Afferent and the Spinal Cord

Ronald R. Tasker

Division of Neurosurgery, Toronto General Hospital, Toronto, M5G 1L7, Canada; and Department of Surgery, University of Toronto, Toronto, Ontario, Canada M5S 1A1

"To every action there is an equal and opposite reaction." The time-honored observation is about as applicable to the physiology of pain as it is to physics. In the normal state our bodies enjoy somatosensory homeostasis whereby we are comfortable and free from pain. This biochemical and electrophysiological state is constantly being challenged by perturbing inputs at all levels of the peripheral and central nervous systems. The offending effects of these perturbations set in motion modulating activities capable of quieting them up to the level of some unknown threshold, beyond which the perturbing influences prevail and set in motion the substrate for conscious awareness of pain. Though we understand it so poorly, we recognize three levels at which perturbing inputs can occur which are capable of producing the conscious awareness that we call pain. The first is peripheral, where activation of nociceptors results in nociceptive pain and where, possibly, other disturbances, caused by neural damage, may produce some instances of deafferentation pain. The second level of input is at the site of the largely incomprehensible central neuronal disturbance responsible for most examples of deafferentation pain. The third level of input is also central, probably cortical, and responsible for psychogenic pain. Surgical attempts to treat intractable pain can be characterized either as attempts to interrupt the perturbing input or to enhance the suppressive modulatory effects the perturbing input is thought to produce, either reversibly or permanently, by open or percutaneous means.

Interruption of peripheral nociceptive input can be aimed at the receptor, nerve, dorsal root, dorsal root entry zone, spinothalamic tract, reticulothalamic system, and their cranial nerve equivalents. Presumably similar strategies would prove effective in certain deafferentation syndromes caused by peripheral derangement, if they exist; and they must be rare. In deafferentation pain it is theoretically possible to interrupt the input derived from the deranged activity of the responsible central neurons, or else to destroy those neurons themselves, either in the spinal cord or brainstem, wherever they occur.

These introductory comments are developed in the light of surgical manipulations of the primary afferents and the spinal cord, carried out in an attempt to exploit growing scientific knowledge. Inevitably, this chapter includes a critique of available techniques, reflecting the author's personal bias that progress in surgery is manifest by simplification with enhanced precision. Translated into currently available expertise, this means the substitution of percutaneous techniques for open techniques, with physiological localization wherever possible.

PAIN SYNDROMES AND SURGICAL TECHNIQUES

Pain Syndromes

It is useful to list the common pain problems neurosurgeons are called on to treat and the surgical techniques in regular use for their management, aimed at the primary afferents and spinal cord.

Common pain syndromes consist of: (a) tic douloureux; (b) chronic nociceptor activity caused by cancer; (c) chronic nociceptor activity caused by noncancerous disease; (d) deafferentation syndromes; and (e) the pain of chronic degenerative, usually lumbar, disk disease.

Examples of nociceptive activity caused by noncancerous disease are those associated with osteoarthritis and some traumatic cauda equina lesions with intractable radicular pain. The pain of chronic degenerative disk disease is usually a "mixed bag" of nociceptive, deafferentation, and psychogenic factors.

Nociceptive Versus Deafferentation Pain

Of the various pain syndromes described it is essential to differentiate nociceptive and deafferentation pain (99,101,103). By nociceptive pain is meant the conscious awareness of pain dependent on chronic stimulation of nociceptors and continual transmission in nociceptive afferent pathways, essentially, the spinothalamic tract. Though there is no consensus, and there may be subgroups of differing pathophysiologies, most deafferentation pain syndromes behave as if the conscious awareness of the pain were dependent on some diffuse central abnormal neuronal activity induced by the deafferentation not involving the primary afferent systems, which has become independent of peripheral input and which continues despite isolation from the periphery.

Deafferentation syndromes include the pain caused by peripheral nerve, root, and cord damage, the causalgias, postherpetic neuralgia, postcordotomy dysesthesia, postthoracotomy and other iatrogenic and posttraumatic pain syndromes, "thalamic pain," and other syndromes caused by brainstem lesions, and phantom and stump pain. They have in common the features that the pain is often dysesthetic or causalgic, is usually associated with areas of raised threshold for one or more modalities of somatosensory input, is usually relieved by local anesthetic blockade, but not by permanent neurosurgical interruption at the same level. The pain may be accompanied by hyperpathia (allodynia) or sympathetic dystrophy. Moreover, although the hyperpathia can be relieved by completion of deafferentation in the somatotopically appropriate area, for it occurs only in areas of preserved somatosensory input, the accompanying pain usually is not. Similarly, sympathetic dystrophy, but usually not the pain it accompanies, is relieved by sympathetic interruption. By the term hyperpathia or allodynia is meant the perception of non-noxious stimuli as noxious and/or the perception of noxious stimuli as excessively noxious in an area of elevated sensory threshold to at least one modality.

SURGICAL TECHNIQUES AIMED AT THE PRIMARY AFFERENT AND CORD

Nociceptive Pain

Nociceptive pain is usually treated by permanent interruption of nociceptor input or by modulating nociceptive input electrically or chemically. Common procedures include:

1. Percutaneous neurectomy.
2. Percutaneous rhizotomy.
3. Percutaneous cordotomy.
4. Epidural morphine instillation.
5. Chronic periventricular-periaqueductal gray (PVG-PAG) stimulation.
6. ? Pituitary ablation.
7. Compression-decompression procedures in tic.

PVG-PAG stimulation is thought to inhibit access of nociceptor input to spinothalamic tract in the dorsal horn by means of a naloxone-reversible descending pathway from nucleus raphe magnus. There is evidence, however, of other descending modulatory pathways from medial upper brainstem that are not naloxone-reversible and which may or may not be involved in the reported instances of relief of *deafferentation* pain syndromes by PVG-PAG stimulation. Amano et al. (2) found no relation between pain relief and third ventricular β-endorphin levels during PVG-PAG stimulation. The role of pituitary ablation in the relief of pain caused by nonhormone-dependent cancer is unknown but is suspected of being modulatory.

Deafferentation Pain

Deafferentation pain is usually treated by, presumably, modulating abnormal neuronal activity or destroying implicated neurons. Common procedures at the afferent or cord level include: (a) chronic stimulation of peripheral nerve; (b) chronic stimulation of dorsal column-lemniscal system; and (c) lesions in the region of the dorsal root entry zone.

Destructive lesions such as cordotomy, mesencephalic tractotomy, and medial thalamotomy relieve less than half, usually no more than one-quarter to one-third, of patients with deafferentation pain through an unknown mechanism that could include placebo effect, reticulothalamic interruption, or elimination of abnormally active neurons.

Lesions in the region of the dorsal root entry zone (DREZ) are a puzzle. Originally intended to relieve nociceptive pain through interruption of Lissauer's tract or of nociceptive fibers coursing away from the dorsal roots just after cord entrance, such lesions made by Nashold and his associates (55) by impaling and coagulating the sites of entry of dorsal rootlets are reported to relieve deafferentation pain preferentially, and more successfully than other destructive procedures. The mechanism by which this comes about is unknown, input interruption, elimination of abnormal neuronal activity, and exploitation of some peculiar property of Lissauer's tract all being possibilities. So-called DREZ lesions could reasonably be expected to relieve hyperpathia but their success in spontaneous deafferentation pain is surprising.

PERMANENT DESTRUCTIVE TECHNIQUES AIMED AT AFFERENTS

Sympathectomy

Sympathectomy, preferably performed percutaneously with phenol as introduced by Boas et al. (6), though useful in controlling sympathetic syndromes, usually fails to control intractable pain including deafferentation pain, even when the latter is accompanied by certain features that resemble sympathetic dystrophy. Rarely, after partial lesions of, particularly, the sciatic nerve, the procedure may achieve dramatic relief of a syndrome that resembles ordinary deafferentation pain syndromes, consisting of pain, hyperpathia, and reflex sympathetic dystrophy. This observation, and the fact that local anesthetic blockade of the sympathetic system often relieves deafferentation pain temporarily, tempts the surgeon to resort unsuccessfully to sympathectomy in a wide variety of deafferentation pain states.

However, the situation with pain arising in such viscera as the pancreas is different in that nociceptive fibers travel with the sympathetic system to reach the spinal cord and sympathetic interruption, therefore, also interrupts primary nociceptive afferents. Hardy (23) described 70% incidence of relief of pain associated with cancer of the pancreas in 56 patients after bilateral open splanchnicectomy associated with T9-T12 sympathectomy. Partial recurrence of pain was observed in 23 patients and the mortality was 7%. Other complications mentioned without statistics were empyema and pneumothorax, paraplegia having been reported by other authors. Moore (49) reported 94% excellent or good results with 186 alcohol blocks of the celiac plexus in 168 patients with pain caused by cancer of the upper abdominal viscera. Complications, again mentioned without statistics, included hypotension, postoperative pain, damage to somatic nerves, subarachnoid injection, and the hypothetical possibility of visceral injection.

Neurectomy and Rhizotomy

Indications

Neurectomy and rhizotomy may be useful in the treatment of nociceptive pain by interrupting the primary afferent nociceptive pathway, but rarely give lasting relief in deafferentation pain. In a series of 35 cases of deafferentation pain of the chest wall, most consisting of postthoracotomy syndrome, only 25% derived lasting significant relief after percutaneous intercostal neurectomy. Early pain relief was usually followed by recurrence at an increased level (99).

In nociceptive pain caused by cancer, neurectomy and rhizotomy are seldom useful either because the pain is so rarely restricted to the distribution of one or a few nerves or roots. When indicated, these procedures should be performed by the percutaneous radiofrequency technique to minimize the impact of surgery and to increase precision through the ability to employ physiological localization. Eventual regeneration of severed nerves is probably the rule after many of these techniques, accompanied by recurrence of pain.

Technique

The technique consists of identifying the target structure by surface landmarks and image intensification as necessary. During brief general anesthesia without paralyzing agents or neuroleptanalgesia and local anesthesia, a suitable needle electrode with a bare tip of appropriate size is introduced. Threshold slow (about 2 Hz) and fast (30–100 Hz) stimulation is performed and electrode position adjusted to obtain a suitable threshold and quality of response, based on experience, whereupon a radiofrequency lesion is made. Stimulation should then be repeated and lesioning repeated as well, if the threshold is not greater than it was before.

"Facet Rhizotomy"

This procedure attempts to identify and interrupt the posterior ramus of, usually, a lower lumbar or the first sacral root or the articular branch. It may be useful in reducing nociceptive spondylogenic pain in patients with degenerative disk disease. Such pain should be confined to the lumbosacral area, buttock, and upper thigh, preferably aggravated by activity and relieved by rest. The procedure is usually performed at two to three levels bilaterally, seeking out particular sites where stimulation produces sensory effects in the area of the patient's pain. This electrically-induced sensory effect is often described in the literature as reproducing the patient's pain, but in the author's experience always consists of paresthesiae, never pain; the induction of pain by electrical stimulation of the nervous system is achieved only under special circumstances in certain patients with deafferentation syndromes (102).

Originally popularized by Rees (73) using a knife, the procedure was performed percutaneously by Shealy (82) making it possible to identify the target site physiologically. Reported improvement varies from 50 to 60% (30). Obviously only spondylogenic pain responds and presumably nerve regeneration limits duration of relief. Oudenhoven (60) reported 74% excellent and 15% good results in 66 patients who had not had previous spinal surgery; and 35% excellent, 24% good results in 48 who had been previously operated upon. Burton (10) obtained excellent results in 42% of 126 patients overall, 67% in those not previously exposed to spinal surgery. McCulloch (40) also reported 67% success in 82 previously unoperated patients. Dunsker et al. (18), however, reported only 20% overall satisfactory results, patients with previous spinal surgery never gaining relief. He could increase the incidence of good results to 40% by selecting those patients in whom diagnostic local blockade of the facet nerve relieved the pain.

Occipital Neurectomy

A similar approach has been applied by Blume (4) and Blume and Fromm (5) in the treatment of pain at the cervicocranial junction with a reported 75% improvement over a 1- to 4-year follow-up in 114 and 250 patients, respectively.

Trigeminal Neurectomy and Rhizotomy

Percutaneous radiofrequency coagulation of the divisions, ganglion or roots of the trigeminal nerve can be used either with the selective microcoagulation technique or with the conventional larger straight needle to treat nociceptive pain other than tic douloureux. Based on Kirschner's original work (32), the technique was refined by Sweet et al. (94), making it safer, more effective, and enhanced by the possibility of physiological corroboration of target site. The latter is considerably enhanced by the use of a small curved electrode introduced through a fine hollow needle which can be progressively extruded in various directions to locate discrete groups of fibers or neurons which can then be more or less selectively lesioned to produce analgesia without anesthesia, as shown by Nugent et al. (57) and Tew and Tobler (104). It is difficult to find sufficient series of patients exclusive of those suffering from tic douloureux to evaluate the procedure in other pain syndromes. The complications, of course, are similar regardless of the cause of pain. Tew and Tobler (104) in a study of 700 patients treated with the conventional straight-needle technique, found the incidence of weakness of the masseter to be 24%, of unpleasant paresthesiae 27%, diplopia 2%, and keratitis 4%. These problems were diminished when a curved electrode was used in 200 subsequent patients when there was a 9% incidence of masseter weakness, 11% of paresthesiae, 0% diplopia, and 2% keratitis.

In treating the pain caused by cancer it is wise to produce total denervation of the trigeminal nerve to minimize recurrence, preferably at the level of the gasserian ganglion or preganglionic rootlets in order to minimize regeneration. Incomplete or peripheral denervations are usually of little value. Siegfried and Broggi (86) obtained good lasting pain relief in half their 20 patients.

Denervation of the trigeminal nerve may be utilized cautiously in noncancerous nociceptive conditions other than tic such as facial migraine. The technique is not only useless in deafferentation pain but also increases pain severity. Maxwell (39) reported relief of pain in all 8 of his patients with chronic migrainous neuralgia, which he distinguished from facial migraine, without any complications.

The basic principles of percutaneous radiofrequency trigeminal neurectomy can also be applied to the lower cranial nerves (9,104). Pagura et al. (62) report 11 out of 15 patients with cancer pain relieved completely at the expense of glossopharyngeal dysfunction in all.

Intercostal Neurectomy

Intercostal neurectomy, useless in postthoracotomy and other deafferentation syndromes, may have a role in the relief of localized nociceptive pain in the chest wall usually caused by cancerous involvement. It may be particularly useful in patients in whom percutaneous cordotomy is contraindicated because it would have to be done on the side of a solitary functioning lung and achieve a relatively high level of analgesia, risking interruption of the ipsilaterally distributed pathway responsible for unconscious respiration (98). It can be used to eliminate the hyperpathia, *but not the spontaneous pain,* of postherpetic neuralgia.

Dorsal Rhizotomy

The same indications and limitations apply to dorsal rhizotomy as to neurectomy. One additional indication is the elimination of hyperpathia, *but not pain,* in deafferentation syndromes such as those found in postherpetic neuralgia and after spinal cord lesions. However, if the spontaneous pain of these deafferentation syndromes cannot be controlled, it is probably unwise to attack the accompanying hyperpathia by further denervation for fear of further aggravation of the pain.

The early experience was, of course, with open dorsal rhizotomy. McLaurin (41), in a literature review, found the procedure successful in 28 to 56% of cases. Loeser (36) reported 28% long-term, 63% short-term relief in 46 patients with various pain syndromes, and 43% long-term and 54% short-term relief in those with cancer. Onofrio (58) found that none of 23 patients with incisional pain, 5 out of 18 with cancer pain, 1 out of 5 with postherpetic neuralgia, and 23% of 78 patients with pain associated with lumbar disk disease were relieved by dorsal rhizotomy. Sindou et al. (90) reviewed the literature describing 585 patients undergoing dorsal rhizotomy for pain caused by cancer, of whom 153 were followed up long-term. Fifty-nine percent enjoyed early, 47% late pain relief, with an average mortality of 5%, though the range in different series was from 0 to 20%.

Smith (91) advocated the excision of the dorsal root ganglion for the relief of intractable pain, a suggestion followed up by others in an attempt to improve results by elimination of ventral root afferents and/or of elements altered by deafferentation. This procedure requires more extensive scrutiny.

The introduction of the percutaneous radiofrequency technique for dorsal rhizotomy in 1971 apparently by Uematsu et al. (107) was a major step forward and makes open rhizotomy obsolete. Caution is required, however, in avoiding injury to indispensable radicular arteries, particularly at T1 to T4 and T11 and L1; Uematsu considers lower cervical and lumbar rhizotomy ill-advised in patients with normal neurological function of the related extremities (106). An initial report quoted 7 excellent and 2 good results in 17 patients with mixed pain syndromes (107). Pagura (61) reported a 76% incidence of pain relief in 50 patients, 13 with cancer, 37 with lumbar disk disease; 2 patients suffered temporary paresis after upper lumbar rhizotomy.

Injection of Phenol, Alcohol, and Other Sclerosing Agents

The injection of phenol, alcohol, or other noxious or sclerosing chemical agents into nervous tissue or subarachnoid space (31) is less satisfactory than the use of radiofrequency lesion-making, except in the case of sympathectomy because of the unpredictable spread of the agent, the difficulty of controlling lesion location and extent, the difficulty of physiological verification of the target structure, and the impermanence of the result (44). Thus, the percutaneous technique should completely replace the use of nerve and root blocks, including subarachnoid blocks, with neurolytic agents. Moore (50) states:

> Treatment of cancer pain of the pelvic viscera with neurolytic drugs is a 'trade-off' between pain relief and complications—with or without pain relief. Percutaneous or surgical cordotomy, myelotomy and lobotomy usually are more accurate and effective. They are preferred to neurolytic, chemical sectioning techniques for they seldom require repeating as is the rule with neurolytic drugs.

Ventafridda and Martino (110) reported the following results with subarachnoid neurolytic root blocks:

1. C7 to T5: 132 blocks in 89 patients with 47% good results, 21% complications.
2. T5 to T12: 68 blocks in 53 patients with 45% good results, 28% complications.
3. L1 to S5: 119 blocks in 85 patients with 74% good results and 67% complications.

Mean duration of pain relief was 15.4 days.

Papo and Visca (64) observed 40% good results in 290 phenol subarachnoid rhizotomies, the best results (70–75% pain relief) occurring with abdominal, lumbar, inguinal, saddle, and bone pain. Leg weakness occurred in 6.8% and was severe in 3.8%. Arm weakness affected 1.7% significant in 0.3%, and bladder disturbance affected 5.4%, severely in 1.7%.

Swerdlow (95) found published records of 1,151 patients treated with subarachnoid alcohol and 1,387 with phenol root blocks with good results reported in 46 to 60% and 48 to 68%, respectively. In his personal experience with 300 patients, there were 44% good results. In a further series of 130 patients, there were 62% good results, the improvement being attributed to increasing experience. Complications which persisted for more than 1 week included 4% paresis, 7% bladder disturbance, 1% bowel disturbance, 1% headache, 4% "paresthesiae and numbness."

Despite reported success rates of 67 to 86% with subarachnoid hyperbaric phenol and glycerine injected into the L5–S1 interspace for the management of pain caused by cancer, Ventafridda et al. (109), in 39 patients with cancer, encountered a 49% incidence of bladder dysfunction postoperatively.

Subarachnoid Injection of Cold and/or Hypertonic Saline

A number of investigators have reported pain relief in patients with cancer after the subarachnoid injection of cold and/or hypertonic saline. Presumably this technique acts by way of nociceptor input interruption. There seems little to recommend such procedures, however, because of the uncertain result, the need to perform them under general anesthesia because of the discomfort the injections produce, and the side-effects such as tremor, weakness, fasciculation, paresthesiae, hypertension, tachycardia, tachypnea, and sometimes pulmonary edema.

Ventafridda and Spreafico (111), in reviewing the technique, found cold isotonic saline useless in 21 patients and differing concentrations (5,7.5,10%) of cold hypertonic saline variously effective, producing long-term pain relief in 0 to 40% of similar groups of patients. Hypertonic saline at room temperature was marginally successful.

Swerdlow (95) observed 1 month's relief of pain in fewer than 50% of patients with cancer with 11% temporary, 1% serious complications.

PERMANENT DESTRUCTIVE TECHNIQUES AIMED AT THE SPINAL CORD

A variety of destructive techniques directed towards the spinal cord have been proposed for the relief of intractable pain:

1. Percutaneous cordotomy
    - Lateral high cervical approach
    - Anterior low cervical approach
2. Open cordotomy
    - High cervical
    - High thoracic
    - Anterior low cervical
3. Commissurotomy
    - Percutaneous high cervical
    - Open
    - Open microsurgical
4. Percutaneous section of trigeminal descending tract and/or caudal nucleus
5. Cordectomy

Cordotomy

Surgical interruption of the spinothalamic tract in the cord, introduced by Spiller and Martin (93), is one of the most popular surgical procedures used for the control of pain. With the introduction of the radiofrequency percutaneous technique by Mullan et al. (53) and Rosomoff et al. (79), cordotomy by the open technique became obsolete. The percutaneous technique is simpler, safer, and because of physiological corroboration, more precise and, when performed at the high cervical level by the lateral approach, produces analgesia more effectively than cordotomy by any other means. In this author's opinion, it is the treatment of choice for nociceptive pain below the

C4 dermatome. Though most suitable candidates suffer from cancer, occasional patients with noncancerous pain such as the lancinating radicular pain associated with cauda equina lesions can also be benefited. Patients with deafferentation pain, whether or not caused by cancer, such as those suffering from burning, dysesthetic pain associated with wasting, and sensory loss in the C8–T1 dermatomes caused by bronchogenic carcinoma, are seldom benefited.

The technique consists of introducing a needle electrode into either the occipital–C1 or the C1–C2 lateral spinal interspace under X-ray control, confirming position in the cord by myelography, recording of impedance, and by electrical stimulation. The spinothalamic tract is recognized by the induction of isolated somatotopically organized contralateral hot or cold sensations during 100 Hz stimulation. Too anterior a position in anterior horn results in tetanization of ipsilateral muscles in the cervical dermatomes, too posterior a position, in or near the corticospinal tract, ipsilateral tetanization anywhere in the body when the stimulation is applied. When all criteria of proper electrode position have been satisfied, a radiofrequency lesion is made.

Contraindications, other than deafferentation pain and pain above the C5 dermatome, include the absence of a functioning lung contralateral to the intended cord lesion when analgesia above the lower thorax is required, for such a lesion would interrupt the ipsilaterally distributed pathway for automatic respiration. Midline lower trunk pain, especially in the perineum (44), caused by cancer is better treated by chronic epidural morphine instillation than by bilateral cordotomy. Bilateral cordotomy can be safely performed at the high cervical level as long as high levels of analgesia are not achieved bilaterally, but at the expense of a 22% chance of impairment of bladder function. The chief role for the low anterior percutaneous approach is the performance of a cordotomy on the second side when a high level of analgesia is not required and must be absolutely avoided for fear of respiratory complications. This can still be accomplished by careful graded lesioning at the high cervical level as well, by avoiding making lesions at sites where stimulation causes contralateral warm or cold sensations in the hand, arm, or neck. Percutaneous cordotomy can also be performed under general anesthesia in the uncooperative patient as long as muscle relaxants are not used, all the criteria of lesion placement other than the sensory effects still being observed. In the author's experience in 244 cases (98), the procedure can be accomplished in 99% of patients, achieving spinothalamic interruption in 92.4%, effective pain relief at the time of discharge from hospital in 94.4%, at longer term follow-up in 82.3%. Pain relief after bilateral surgery obeys the *p*-squared rule and is therefore, overall, lower than for unilateral surgery. Complications are minimal in contrast to the frequently repeated published statements to the contrary (70). Recurrence of pain after successful cordotomy occurs in most patients with deafferentation pain. In those with nociceptive pain, recurrence is unusual for several years in areas of adequate analgesia. However, pain ipsilateral to the lesion appears or is intensified in 41% of patients postoperatively and a further 6% develop contralateral pain at a level higher than before and out of the range for which the cordotomy was performed. Rosomoff in a review of 789 patients (78) reported similarly satisfactory experience.

Complications in our 244 cases were 0.5% mortality, 0.5% transient respiratory failure, 0.5% permanent significant paresis, 4% bladder dysfunction for unilateral procedures, 22% for bilateral procedures, and temporary paresis in 21%. Roughly 24% developed postoperative Horner's syndrome, but in most cases this passed off by the time of longer-term follow-up.

Commissurotomy

Introduced by Armour in 1927 (3) as a substitute for cordotomy by which spinothalamic and presumably reticulothalamic fibers are interrupted as they cross in the anterior commissure of the cord by an incision at the segmental level of the pain and up to three segments above it, commissurotomy produces bilateral pain relief usually with transient analgesia in the appropriate dermatomes bilaterally. Theoretically, it spares respiratory pathways. The mechanism of pain relief is obscure, since pain relief does not appear to be related to the production of analgesia in dermatomes corresponding to decussating spinothalamic fibers at the level of the lesion, nor even to section of the anterior commissure. These issues are lucidly reviewed by Cook et al. (13). It would seem to this writer that open commissurotomy has little to recommend it, the same effects being possible in most patients by other means which spare the need for laminectomy.

Wertheimer and Lecuire (114) reported a 65% success rate in 93 patients with various pain syndromes, 7 of whom died. Piscol (70), advocating a microsurgical open technique, still produced 6 patients with paresis out of 23. Payne (65) reports 75% relief of perineal and lower body pain caused by cancer in 24 patients, with lower limb paresthesiae in 71% of which 8% were permanent. He observed a 50% incidence of transient loss of position sense and 45% pain recurrence. Adams et al. (1) report 88% satisfactory pain relief with the open operation in 24 patients suffering mainly from cancerous nociceptive pain. Bladder dysfunction occurred in 12%, paresis in 8%, dyesthesia temporarily in most, and persistently in 6%. McLaurin (41) reported 16 long-term excellent results out of 34 patients with 1 death, 2 instances of dysesthesia, and temporary paresthesiae and bladder disturbances. Broager (8) reported 16 long-term excellent results in 34 patients, all but 3 of whom had cancer, with 1 death, dysesthesia in 2, temporary loss of deep sensation and sphincter disturbance in others. Sourek (92) reported 36 thoracic and 3 cervical commissurotomies with 79% incidence of pain relief and 1 death.

Pain tended to recur after cervical section. Nearly all his patients experienced transient dysesthesia, bladder disturbance, and difficulty walking. Girdle analgesia usually faded, but loss of touch, vibration, and position sense persisted.

The introduction of the percutaneous technique for commissurotomy by Hitchcock (24) is of considerable interest. Always performed in the occipital–C1 interspace, it appears to relieve pain at any level in the body without inducing analgesia, as if it were interrupting some extralemniscal pain pathway rather than effecting a segmental commissurotomy (81). Hitchcock (24) reported 10 excellent and 2 good results out of 14 patients with pain caused by cancer, and excellent results in all 3 patients treated for deafferentation pain. There was no clinically demonstrable sensory loss, but bizarre patterns of analgesia occurred. By the percutaneous method, Eiras et al. (20) reported good initial results in all their patients with advanced cancer that they were able to follow, though pain recurred in 3, at the expense of dysmetria and gait disturbance of up to 2 weeks' duration in all of them. Schvarcz (81) reported 78% satisfactory results in 79 patients with midline and bilateral pelvic cancer pain. Postoperative gait unsteadiness was "common" in his patients, but there were no persistent motor or autonomic side effects. Papo (63), however, found the pain relief short-lived.

Cordectomy

"Cordectomy," in reality retransection of the cord or excision of a segment above the level of a functionally complete spinal cord lesion, has been advocated for the treatment of pain in paraplegics, which is nearly always of the deafferentation type. A deafferenting procedure, it is not surprising that it is ineffective in most patients (19,42,99). Jefferson's experience (29) is interesting in that he found cordectomy very effective in relieving the pain associated with traumatic lesions of the spinal column below D10, particularly pain located in the anterior thighs and over the knees, and especially episodic pain. His clinical descriptions of successfully treated patients resemble closely those of the author's patients responding to percutaneous cordotomy.

Tractotomy of the Descending Tract of the Trigeminal Nerve

Hitchcock (25), Crue et al. (14), and Schvarcz (80) have developed and exploited a percutaneous technique for the radiofrequency coagulation of the descending trigeminal tract in the upper cervical cord based on the same principles as percutaneous cordotomy. The trigeminal tract is recognized by the induction of ipsilateral facial paresthesiae during 100 Hz stimulation. Relatively few patients have been subjected to this procedure, most of them suffering from deafferentation syndromes. The mechanism of pain relief is obscure as it is in the case of so-called DREZ lesions, to which the same considerations apply.

Schvarcz has recorded his growing experience in a series of publications. In 100 patients (80) there was 87.5% relief of postherpetic neuralgia, 57% of anesthesia dolorosa, 72% of "dysesthesia," and 83.8% of pain caused by cancer. Transient ipsilateral ataxia and occasional contralateral hypalgesia were the only complications reported.

Cord Lesions in the Vicinity of the Entry of the Dorsal Roots

Hyndman (28) attributed the several dermatomes' discrepancy between the level of cordotomy and that of the resulting analgesia to the ascent of pain fibers in Lissauer's tract before decussation and utilized a 2-mm wide incision of the cord to a depth of 2 mm across the dorsal root entry line at the same level to raise the level of analgesia after cordotomy. Inspired by anatomical studies demonstrating the separation ventrolaterally of small fibers from large at the site of entry of dorsal root into spinal cord, presumably en route to Lissauer's tract, Sindou proposed (87) and performed (88,89) microscopic selective section of these ventrolaterally located small fibers by cutting to a depth of 1 mm at a 45° angle with a razor blade just lateral to the root entry, in an attempt to control certain pain syndromes. Sindou and his associates use the technique primarily for the relief of pain caused by cancer, and that associated with spasticity. In the former, 65% of 20 patients enjoyed satisfactory pain relief, with 5% mortality. The advantage of the procedure over other more conventional operations is the avoidance of sensory loss in important roots (cf. rhizotomy), of respiratory complications in pain in the cervical dermatomes (cf. cordotomy) though C4 lesions must be avoided for respiratory reasons, and the ability to achieve high levels of analgesia. Leg hypotonia is a troublesome complication, however (89). In another report (88), however, 2 patients out of 13 died. The operation is deemed most appropriate for cancer pain in the cervical dermatomes, especially that of the Pancoast syndrome. M. Sindou *(personal communication)* also has found the procedure of value in relieving allodynia, or hyperpathia, associated with such deafferentation pain syndromes as that following amputation, myelopathy, multiple sclerosis, and thalamic pain.

Nashold and Ostdahl (55) devised a similar procedure in 1979 in which they impaled the exposed cord at the site of avulsed or deafferented dorsal rootlets somatotopicographically related to chronic pain of the deafferentation type, using an electrode similar to that used for percutaneous cordotomy. Multiple radiofrequency lesions, which they referred to as dorsal root entry zone or DREZ lesions, were made until the entire painful area had been covered. The procedure was used first in patients with pain caused by brachial plexus avulsion, with success in 78% of the original 18 patients. The initial relatively high neurological morbidity has been reduced by subsequent refinement of technique using more carefully defined lesions and monitoring cord evoked potentials. Subsequent publications (22,54) have reported 11 of 13 patients relieved of pain associated with paraplegia, 10 at the level of the conus or cauda, and 8 out of 12 cases of postherpetic neuralgia. Of the latter, 4 developed ipsilateral leg weakness and hypesthesia, 1 developed dysesthesia, and 8 developed minor degrees of ipsilateral leg weakness. In a review (56), good results were reported in 67% of 21 patients with brachial plexus avulsion, 50% of 13 paraplegics, 50% of 12 patients with postherpetic neuralgia, the follow-up being too short for evaluation of results in 5 patients with phantom pain. Dieckmann and Veras (16) report relief of pain in 61% of 18 patients undergoing this procedure, with 1 death and 2 significant complications.

Despite the reduced level of morbidity, the need for laminectomy makes this procedure, in the author's opinion, one to be considered only after the simpler and safer techniques of peripheral nerve or epidural cord stimulation have failed to relieve deafferentation pain.

MODULATING PROCEDURES

Repeated Local Anesthetic Blockage

Repeated local anesthetic blockade in the management of deafferentation pain as advocated by Livingston (35) has not been successful in this author's experience.

Epidural Morphine Instillation

The first attempt to control pain pharmacologically with a permanent indwelling epidural cannula was apparently that of Pilon and Baker (69) using local anesthetics. However, attention was directed to the use of opiates with the demonstration that morphine is taken up in the dorsal horn where it blocks nociceptive access to the spinothalamic tract, as reviewed by Yaksh (115). This observation prompted Wang et al. (113) to inject morphine intrathecally achieving many hours of relief of pain caused by cancer. Epidural injections of morphine then became popular for the relief of acute, particularly postoperative, pain and a number of groups such as Ventafridda et al. (108) studied the use of intrathecal morphine for the relief of chronic pain such as that caused by cancer. In 41 patients with cancer, Ventafridda et al. (108) injected morphine both into the cervical and lumbar intrathecal space with striking relief of pain. Cervical injections produced significant nausea, but no better analgesia than lumbar injections. These authors noted the development of tolerance when morphine was given daily, but others did not. These observations led naturally to the implantation of intrathecal and epidural cannulae attached either to pumps or refillable reservoirs for the longer-term instillation of morphine in patients with chronic pain. Onofrio et al. (59) first utilized a constant rate perfusion pump. Poletti et al. (71) used a refillable system successfully in 2 patients maintained on 2 mg morphine every 8 to 12 hrs without the development of tolerance. Penn et al. (66) reported 8 excellent and 5 good results with intrathecal or epidural instillation using a programmable pump in 14 patients with pain caused by cancer. Meyerson et al. (44) reported 62% and D'Annunzio et al. (15) 60% satisfactory results. In Meyerson's experience there were no complications, in D'Annunzio's 60% of patients suffered minor though annoying side-effects.

Although the use of spinal morphine instillation is still under review, it has an obvious place in the treatment of cancer pain. The advantages are that it is technically simple, particularly using an epidural cannula attached to a refillable subcutaneous reservoir, the dosage of morphine is less than that required by administration through other routes thus avoiding unwanted central effects, and the risks are low. The disadvantages are that the drug is most effective delivered over the appropriate dorsal horns, making its use in patients with high levels of pain questionable because of the risk of respiratory depression. Respiratory depression can occur in delayed fashion even after low injections and must be cautiously watched for. Fortunately, tolerance is not inevitable, with dosages of morphine usually plateauing at no more than four times the initial level used. The nuisance of repeated injections, the risk of infection, and the inevitability of equipment failure remain problems requiring solution.

Nevertheless, the technique has become a useful means of treating, in particular, patients with bilateral and midline pain in the lower trunk and perineum, as well as certain other patients unsuited for cordotomy, constituting a simple substitute for "anterior" commissurotomy, PVG-PAG stimulation, or hypophyseal alcohol injection. It is occasionally effective in deafferentation pain.

Hypophyseal Alcohol Injection

Though not strictly a neurosurgical procedure aimed at the primary afferent or cord, alcohol injection into the hypophysis is mentioned here because the unknown mechanism of its action in relieving the pain of nonhormone-dependent cancer may involve some unrecognized modulation of peripheral nociceptive input. This is not related to pituitary destruction, hypothalamic involvement, alteration in the levels of any as yet demonstrated blood or cerebrospinal fluid (CSF) substances, and is not reversed by naloxone (12). The concept was originally introduced for the endocrinological effects open hypophysectomy brought to bear on, usually, hormone-dependent cancer of the breast and prostate along with the pain that accompanied it (37,67,85,105). Tindall et al. (105) reported 76% pain relief in hormone-dependent tumors with a 5% mortality, a 14% incidence of CSF rhinorrhea, and 4% of meningitis.

A variety of percutaneous and stereotactic techniques were devised to circumvent open operation in patients requiring hormonal manipulation which will not be reviewed here. Pituitary destruction by alcohol was more recently popularized by Morrica (51) for the relief of cancer pain, not only in hormone-dependent but also in hormone-independent disease. This simple technique, requiring a minimum of experience and equipment, appears to offer pain relief to a large percentage of cancer patients at the expense of pain recurrence in 3 to 4 months, the frequent need for repetition of the procedure, a mortality of up to 2%, the risk of rhinorrhea, up to a 2% risk of visual complications, and transient postoperative headache, diabetes insipidus, hyperthermia, and polyphagia (33,34,48,52). Miles (47) achieved 43% excellent results in 122 patients, with 8 deaths, 5 instances of visual and oculomotor disturbance, 2 of hypothalamic disturbance, and a 10 to 20% incidence of CSF leak, 1% of meningitis, 60% of diabetes insipidus, most of the complications being transient. Madrid (38) achieved 67% complete immediate pain relief with a 3% incidence of CSF rhinorrhea, 0.3% meningitis, and 3% visual-oculomotor disturbances. Takeda et al. (96,97), as part of an organized study of the mechanism and role of ethanol adenolysis, obtained 80% immediate pain relief in 102 patients with pain caused by cancer. In the 43 patients with hormone-dependent tumors relief was 95%, whereas in the 59 with nonhormone-dependent disease, it was 69%. Some of the former tumors regressed. Most patients experienced transient euphoria and polyphagia and there was a 10% incidence of visual field disturbance, 4% temporary ophthalmoplegia, and 50% diabetes insipidus. Curiously, Yanagida et al. (116) found correlation between pain relief and electrical stimulation of the pituitary in subsequent ethanol adenolysis in 25 patients with cancer.

The injection of alcohol into the pituitary is a useful method for controlling nociceptive pain in cancer where more specific techniques are either unsuitable or the necessary facilities are unavailable.

Chronic PVG-PAG Stimulation

Though not strictly a surgical procedure aimed at the primary afferent or cord, medial mesencephalic–diencephalic chronic stimulation is mentioned here since its known function consists of activating a descending serotoninergic pathway from nucleus raphe magnus that inhibits the entry of nociceptive impulses into the spinothalamic tract. Conceived by Richardson and Akil (77) based on the observations of Reynolds in animals (74), this procedure has been widely used in the treatment of chronic pain. Though most surgeons recognize it as a treatment for nociceptive pain (27,72,75–77), achieving up to 80% relief of pain with an 11% risk of neural trauma, 4 to 15% of infection, 3 to 9% of device failure, 11% of lead breakage, and 7% of electrode migration, relief of deafferentation syndromes has also been reported. The pain relief achieved by PVG-PAG stimulation is not always reversible by naloxone, even in patients with cancer (7). The technique, particularly in the case of terminal cancer patients using long-term percutaneous electrodes as advocated by Meyerson et al. (45), is a therapeutic alternative in patients unsuited for or failing to respond to simpler techniques. Infection in Meyerson's experience was apparently not a problem.

This type of stimulation, dependent as it is, at least in many patients, on opiate pathway activation, is prone to induce tolerance, requiring restriction of duration of stimulation and enhancement of its effect with tryptophan or disulfiram. However, Boivie and Meyerson (7) did not observe tolerance in their patients.

Chronic Stimulation of Nerves and Cord

Hoping to exploit the Melzack-Wall (43) gate theory of pain, Wall and Sweet (112) proposed the use of chronic stimulation of peripheral nerves for the control of pain by stimulation-induced large fiber suppression of pain activity in small fibers. Carrying the conceptual process one step rostrally, Shealy et al. (83) introduced cord stimulation. Lemniscal pathway stimulation in the brain presumably has similar effects. Chronic stimulation was used initially in patients with various pain syndromes, but it was gradually seen to be more effective in patients with deafferentation pain than in those with nociceptive pain. Most observers agree that in order to relieve pain, large nerve fibers or the dorsal columns must be activated and that, for relief to occur, paresthesiae must be induced in the area of pain. Apart from technical problems such as inability to achieve appropriate paresthesiae because of neural damage, or inability to produce them in the proper location, still only some 60% of patients with deafferentation pain, who would seem to be suitable candidates, achieve initial pain relief. There is no adequate selection technique available other than a trial of test percutaneous stimulation.

Peripheral Nerve Stimulation

Since most pain syndromes cover the distribution of more than a single peripheral nerve, chronic nerve stimulation requires an open procedure to implant the electrode, and since nerves appropriate for stimulation may have already been traumatized to cause the deafferentation pain in the first place, dorsal cord stimulation is usually preferred to peripheral nerve stimulation. Reported success in peripheral nerve stimulation varies from 30 to

50% (11,68) and according to Picaza et al. falls to zero after 2 years (68). The following complications have been reported: nerve damage, 1%; infection, 3 to 5%; tissue reaction, 3%; tenderness over incision, 3 to 8%; ineffective stimulation, 15%; displacement of electrode, 3%; and equipment failure, 3%.

Dorsal Cord Stimulation

The introduction of the percutaneous technique for epidural cord stimulation by Erickson (21), Hoppenstein (26), and Dooley (17) has introduced two advantages to the field of chronic stimulation: (a) the avoidance of laminectomy and (b) the ability to test the effects of stimulation simply, prior to implantation. In the author's opinion, because of the low success rate overall and the inability to predict which patient will respond, preliminary percutaneous testing is mandatory and open surgery for implantation of electrodes should be reserved for patients in whom percutaneous insertion has failed or proven impossible. Electrodes should always be placed in the epidural space; electrodes implanted in the original way intra- or subdurally carry a 1 to 4% risk of cord compression, 0.5 to 17% of CSF leak, and 5 to 20% of seroma. In most series (100), 40 to 50% of patients "pass" the trial stimulation test. The subsequently implanted stimulators then yield a 60 to 84% incidence of pain relief. Complications of the percutaneously implanted device consist of electrode migration in up to 61%, infection in 1 to 7%, incisional pain in up to 58%, electrode breakage in 4 to 23%, receiver failure in 0.5%, transmitter failure in 5%, skin erosion or breakdown in 1 to 5%. Unfortunately, despite adequate continued technical performance of the stimulator, the incidence of pain relief falls off with time for no known reason.

In the author's opinion, chronic epidural dorsal cord stimulation by percutaneously introduced electrodes following a preimplantation trial of test stimulation is the treatment of choice for all deafferentation syndromes, including those caused by brainstem lesions, before more complex techniques such as nerve or brain stimulation, destructive cord or brain lesions are considered.

Trigeminal Stimulation

Meyerson and Håkansson (46) have popularized the use of chronic stimulation of the trigeminal nerve, originally conceived by Sheldon (84), in patients with deafferentation pain. Following successful test stimulation with a straight epidural spinal electrode introduced percutaneously through the foramen ovale, permanent implantation is done usually by the Frazier, middle fossa approach. This procedure should be considered prior to brain stimulation in patients with anesthesia dolorosa or other trigeminal deafferentation

entation syndromes. Meyerson and Håkansson found that 56% of their patients "passed" the stimulation test and 75% of those subsequently implanted continued to get satisfactory relief.

CONCLUSIONS

A variety of pain-relieving procedures have been discussed. These can best be summarized by presenting a "flowsheet" showing the author's preference for treating common pain syndromes.

Nociceptive Pain Caused by Cancer

Percutaneous radiofrequency neurectomy or rhizotomy of somatic or cranial nerves is rarely a superb technique in those very few patients in whom the pain is sufficiently localized. For unilateral or bilateral pain below the C4 dermatome, percutaneous cordotomy by the lateral high cervical technique is the treatment of choice. An absolute contraindication is the presence of a solitary functioning lung ipsilateral to the intended lesion when a high level of analgesia is required. In bilateral pain, bilateral high levels of analgesia must be avoided. For relatively localized midline and bilateral pain, especially in the pelvic area, the installation of a device for the chronic epidural administration of morphine is preferred. In the relatively small percentage of patients with pain above the C5 dermatome or in those with a solitary lung requiring a high level of analgesia, no thoroughly suitable solution is available. Intercostal neurectomy or rhizotomy may be considered if the pain is sufficiently localized, or else hypophyseal alcohol injection, chronic PVG-PAG stimulation, percutaneous commissurotomy, mesencephalic tractotomy, or medial thalamotomy.

"Failed Back" Pain

The pain of chronic degenerative disc disease is more difficult to treat. It often consists of a variety of nociceptive, deafferentation and psychogenic processes, each requiring separate strategies in a patient already jaded by a long, unsuccessful contact with medicine. It is most important first to rule out treatable pain syndromes such as root compression, spinal instability, and spinal stenosis. Next, the existing intractable pain must be dissected into spondylogenic nociceptive, other nociceptive, and deafferentation elements. Spondylogenic pain may be reduced, at least temporarily, by facet rhizotomy, but percutaneous dorsal rhizotomy is rarely effective in intractable radicular nociceptive pain. Deafferentation responds to chronic stimulation, commonly employed at the dorsal cord level. A number of surgeons utilize lemniscal pathway and/or PVG-PAG stimulation in their patients with failed back syndrome, a choice justifiable to this author's thinking only in extreme situations in which simpler techniques have failed.

Deafferentation Pain

All deafferentation syndromes, whether peripheral or central, justify a trial of test stimulation with percutaneous epidural electrodes going on to permanent implantation in patients who "pass the test." One exception is trigeminal pain, best investigated with percutaneous stimulation of the trigeminal nerve through the foramen ovale. Contraindications to dorsal cord stimulation include atrophy of the appropriate dorsal columns caused by the deafferenting process or obliteration of the epidural space by previous surgery. When cord stimulation fails or is impossible, peripheral nerve or lemniscal pathway brain stimulation, lesions in the region of the dorsal root entry, or trigeminal tractotomy are alternatives. Epidural electrodes may be inserted by open laminotomy when the epidural space is obliterated by scar.

SUMMARY

One must know the patient, dissect his pain syndrome, evaluate his disability, and, only then, embark on a program of surgical therapy beginning with the simplest measures and proceeding to the more complex, as far as the patient's disability warrants.

REFERENCES

1. Adams, J. E., Lippert, R., and Hosobuchi, Y. (1982): Commissural myelotomy. In: *Operative Neurosurgical Techniques. Indications, Methods, and Results,* edited by H. H. Schmidek and W. H. Sweet, pp. 1155–61. Grune & Stratton, New York.
2. Amano, K., Tanikawa, T., Kawamura, H., Iseki, H., Notani, M., Kawabatake, H., Shiwabu, T., Suda, T., Demura, H., and Kitamura, K. (1982): Endorphins and pain relief. Further observations on electrical stimulation of the lateral part of the periaqueductal gray matter during rostral mesencephalic reticulotomy for pain relief. *Appl. Neurophysiol.,* 45:123–135.
3. Armour, D. (1927): Surgery of the spinal cord and its membranes. *Lancet,* 2:691–697.
4. Blume, H. G. (1976): Radiofrequency denervation in occipital pain: a new approach in 114 cases. In: *Advances in Pain Research and Therapy, Vol. 1,* edited by J. J. Bonica and D. Albe-Fessard, pp. 691–698. Raven Press, New York.
5. Blume, H., and Fromm, S. (1977): Radiofrequency denaturation in occipital pain: a new approach. *Sixth International Congress of Neurological Surgery,* pp. 221–222. Excerpta Medica, Amsterdam.
6. Boas, R. A., Hatangdi, V. S., and Richards, E. G. (1976): Lumbar sympathectomy—a percutaneous chemical technique. In: *Advances in Pain Research and Therapy, Vol. 1,* edited by J. J. Bonica and D. Albe-Fessard, pp. 685–689. Raven Press, New York.
7. Boivie, J., and Meyerson, B. A. (1982): A correlative anatomic and clinical study of pain suppression by deep brain stimulation. *Pain,* 13:113–126.
8. Broager, B. (1974): Commissural myelotomy. *Surg. Neurol.* 2:71–74.
9. Broggi, G., and Siegfried, J. (1979): Percutaneous differential radiofrequency rhizotomy

of glossopharyngeal nerve in facial pain due to cancer. In: *Advances in Pain Research and Therapy, Vol. 2,* edited by J. J. Bonica and D. Albe-Fessard, pp. 469–473. Raven Press, New York.
10. Burton, C. V. (1976): Percutaneous radiofrequency facet denervation. *Appl. Neurophysiol.,* 39:80–86.
11. Campbell, J. N., and Long, D. M. (1976): Peripheral nerve stimulation in the treatment of intractable pain. *J. Neurosurg.,* 45:692–699.
12. Capper, S. J., Conlon, J. M., Lahuerta, J., Miles, J. B., and Lipton, S. (1984): Peptide concentrations in the C.S.F. following injection of alcohol into the pituitary gland. *Pain,* Suppl.2:S316.
13. Cook, A. W., Nathan, P. W., and Smith, M. C. (1984): Sensory consequences of commissural myelotomy. A challenge to traditional anatomical concepts. *Brain,* 107:547–568.
14. Crue, B. L., Todd, E. M., and Carregal, E. J. (1970): Percutaneous radiofrequency stereotactic trigeminal tractotomy. In: *Pain and Suffering,* edited by B. L. Crue., pp. 69–79. Thomas, Springfield, Illinois.
15. D'Annunzio, V., Denaro, F., and Meglio, M. (1984): Personal experience with intrathecal morphine in the management of pain from pelvic cancer. *Acta Neurochir.,* Suppl. 33:421–425.
16. Dieckmann, G., and Veras, G. (1984): High frequency coagulation of dorsal root entry zone in patients with deafferentation pain. *Acta Neurochir.,* Suppl. 33:445–450.
17. Dooley, D. M. (1975): A technique for the epidural percutaneous stimulation of the spinal cord in man. Presented at the *Annual Meeting of American Association of Neurological Surgeons,* 1975, Miami Beach.
18. Dunsker, S. B., Wood, M., Lotspeich, E. S., and Mayfield, F. H. (1977): Percutaneous electrocoagulation of lumbar articular nerves. In: *Pain Management,* edited by J. F. Lee, pp. 123–127. Williams & Wilkins, Baltimore.
19. Durward, Q. J., Rice, G. P., Ball, M. J., Gilbert, J. J., and Kaufmann, J. C. E. (1982): Selective spinal cordectomy: clinicopathological correlation. *J. Neurosurg.,* 56:359–367.
20. Eiras, J., Garcia, J., Gomez, J., Carcavalla, L. I., and Ucar, S. (1980): First results with extralemniscal myelotomy. *Acta Neurochir.,* Suppl. 30:377–381.
21. Erickson, D. L. (1975): Percutaneous trial of stimulation for patient selection for implantable stimulating electrodes. *J. Neurosurg.,* 43:440–444.
22. Friedman, A. H., Nashold, B. S., Jr., and Ovelinen-Levitt, J. (1984): Dorsal root entry zone lesions for the treatment of postherpetic neuralgia. *J. Neurosurg.,* 60:1258–1262.
23. Hardy, R. W., Jr. (1982): Surgery of the sympathetic nervous system. In: *Operative Neurosurgical Techniques. Indications, Methods, and Results, Vol. 2,* edited by H. H. Schmidek and W. H. Sweet, pp. 1045–1061. Grune & Stratton, New York.
24. Hitchcock, E. R. (1970): Stereotactic cervical myelotomy. *J. Neurol. Neurosurg. Psychiatry,* 33:224–230.
25. Hitchcock, E. R. (1970): Stereotactic trigeminal tractotomy. *Ann. Clin. Res.,* 2:131–135.
26. Hoppenstein, R. (1975): Percutaneous implantation of chronic spinal cord electrode for control of intractable pain. Preliminary report. *Surg. Neurol.,* 4:195–198.
27. Hosobuchi, Y. (1980): The current status of analgesic brain stimulation. *Acta Neurochir.,* Suppl. 30:219–227.
28. Hyndman, O. R. (1942): Lissauer's tract section. A contribution to chordotomy for the relief of pain. (Preliminary report). *J. Int. Coll. Surgeons,* 5:394–400.
29. Jefferson, A. (1983): Cordectomy for intractable pain. In: *Persistent Pain, Vol. 4,* edited by S. Lipton and J. Miles, pp. 115–132. Grune & Stratton, New York.
30. Johnson, I. (1974): Radiofrequency percutaneous facet rhizotomy. *J. Neurosurg. Nursing,* 6:92–96.
31. Katz, J. (1974): Current role of neurolytic agents. In: *Advances in Neurology, Vol. 4,* edited by J. J. Bonica, pp. 471–476. Raven Press, New York.
32. Kirschner, M. (1932): Elektrokoagulation des Ganglion gasseri. *Zentralbl. Chir.,* 47:2841–2843.
33. Lipton, S. (1978): Percutaneous cervical cordotomy and the injection of the pituitary with alcohol. *Anaesthesia,* 33:953–957.
34. Lipton, S., Miles, J., Williams, N., and Bark-Jones, N. (1978): Pituitary injection of alcohol for widespread cancer pain. *Pain,* 5:73–82.

35. Livingston, W. K. (1976): *Pain Mechanisms: A Physiologic Interpretation of Causalgia and Its Related Causes.* Plenum Press, New York.
36. Loeser, J. D. (1974): Dorsal rhizotomy: indications and results. In: *Advances in Neurology, Vol. 4,* edited by J. J. Bonica, pp. 615–619. Raven Press, New York.
37. Luft, R., and Olivecrona, H. (1953): Experiences with hypophysectomy in man. *J. Neurosurg.,* 10:301–316.
38. Madrid, J. L. (1979): Chemical hypophysectomy. In: *Advances in Pain Research and Therapy, Vol. 2,* edited by J. J. Bonica and V. Ventafridda, pp. 381–391. Raven Press, New York.
39. Maxwell, R. F. (1982): Surgical control of chronic migrainous neuralgia by trigeminal ganglio-rhizolysis. *J. Neurosurg.,* 57:459–466.
40. McCulloch, J. A. (1976): Percutaneous radiofrequency lumbar rhizolysis (rhizotomy). *Appl. Neurophysiol.,* 39:87–96.
41. McLaurin, R. L. (1977): Neurosurgical approaches to pain in cancer. In: *Pain Management,* edited by J. F. Lee, pp. 186–194. Williams & Wilkins, Baltimore.
42. Melzack, R., and Loeser, J. D. (1978): Phantom body pain in paraplegics: Evidence for a central pattern generating mechanism for pain. *Pain,* 4:195–210.
43. Melzack, R., and Wall, P. D. (1965): Pain mechanisms—a new theory. *Science,* 150:971–979.
44. Meyerson, B. A., Arnér, S., and Linderoth, B. (1984): Pros and cons of different approaches to the management of pelvic cancer pain. *Acta Neurochir.,* Suppl. 33:407–419.
45. Meyerson, B. A., Boëthius, J., and Carlsson, A. M. (1978): Percutaneous central gray stimulation for cancer pain. *Appl. Neurophysiol.,* 41:57–65.
46. Meyerson, B. A., and Håkansson, S. (1980): Alleviation of atypical trigeminal pain by stimulation of the gasserian ganglion via an implanted electrode. *Acta Neurochir.,* Suppl. 30:303–309.
47. Miles, J. (1979): Chemical hypophysectomy. In: *Advances in Pain Research and Therapy, Vol. 2,* edited by J. J. Bonica and V. Ventafridda, pp. 373–380. Raven Press, New York.
48. Miles, J. (1983): Neurological advances in the relief of pain. *Br. J. Hosp. Med.,* 30:348–353.
49. Moore, D. C. (1979): Celiac (splanchnic) plexus block with alcohol for cancer pain of the upper intra-abdominal viscera. In: *Advances in Pain Research and Therapy, Vol. 2,* edited by J. J. Bonica and V. Ventafridda, pp. 357–371. Raven Press, New York.
50. Moore, D. C. (1979): Role of nerve block with neurolytic solutions for pelvic visceral cancer pain. In: *Advances in Pain Research and Therapy, Vol. 2,* edited by J. J. Bonica and V. Ventafridda, pp. 593–596. Raven Press, New York.
51. Morrica, G. (1974): Chemical hypophysectomy for cancer pain. In: *Advances in Neurology, Vol. 4,* edited by J. J. Bonica, pp. 707–714. Raven Press, New York.
52. Moricca, G. (1976): Neuroadenolysis for diffuse intractable cancer pain. In: *Advances in Pain Research and Therapy, Vol. 1,* edited by J. J. Bonica and D. Albe-Fessard, pp. 863–869. Raven Press, New York.
53. Mullan, S., Harper, P. V., Hekmatpanah, J., Torres, H., and Dobbin, G. (1963): Percutaneous interruption of spinal pain tracts by means of a strontium 90 needle. *J. Neurosurg.,* 20:931–939.
54. Nashold, B. S. Jr., and Bullitt, E. (1981): Dorsal root entry zone lesions to control central pain in paraplegics. *J. Neurosurg.,* 55:414–419.
55. Nashold, B. S., and Ostdahl, R. H. (1979): Dorsal root entry zone lesions for pain relief. *J. Neurosurg.,* 51:59–69.
56. Nashold, B. S., Jr., Ostdahl, R. H., Bullitt, E., Friedman, A., and Brophy, B. (1983): Dorsal root entry zone lesions: A new neurosurgical therapy for deafferentation pain. In: *Advances in Pain Research and Therapy, Vol. 5.,* edited by J. J. Bonica, U. Lindblom, and A. Iggo, pp. 739–750. Raven Press, New York.
57. Nugent, G. R., and Berry, B. (1974): Trigeminal neuralgia treated by differential percutaneous radiofrequency coagulation of the gasserian ganglion. *J. Neurosurg.,* 40:517–523.
58. Onofrio, B. M. (1974): Rhizotomy: What is its place in the treatment of pain. In: *Advances in Neurology, Vol. 4,* edited by J. J. Bonica, pp. 621–623. Raven Press, New York.
59. Onofrio, B. M., Yaksh, T. L., and Arnold, P. G. (1981): Continuous low-dose intrathecal

morphine administration in the treatment of chronic pain of malignant origin. *Mayo Clin. Proc.,* 56:516–520.
60. Oudenhoven, R. C. (1974): Articular rhizotomy. *Surg. Neurol.,* 2:275–278.
61. Pagura, J. R. (1983): Percutaneous radiofrequency spinal rhizotomy. *Appl. Neurophysiol.,* 46:138–146.
62. Pagura, J. R., Schnapp, M., and Passarelli, P. (1983): Percutaneous radiofrequency glossopharyngeal rhizolysis for cancer pain. *Appl. Neurophysiol.,* 46:154–159.
63. Papo, I. (1979): Spinal posterior rhizotomy and commissural myelotomy in the treatment of pain. In: *Advances in Pain Research and Therapy, Vol. 2,* edited by J. J. Bonica and V. Ventafridda, pp. 439–447. Raven Press, New York.
64. Papo, I., and Visca, A. (1979): Phenol subarachnoid rhizotomy for the treatment of cancer pain: A personal account on 290 cases. In: *Advances in Pain Research and Therapy, Vol. 2,* edited by J. J. Bonica and V. Ventafridda, pp. 339–346. Raven Press, New York.
65. Payne, N. S. (1984): Dorsal longitudinal myelotomy for the control of perineal and lower body pain. *Pain,* Suppl.2:S320.
66. Penn, R. D., Paice, J. A., Gottschalk, W., and Ivankovich, A. D. (1984): Cancer pain relief using chronic morphine infusion. *J. Neurosurg.,* 61:302–306.
67. Perrault, M., LeBeau, J., Klotz, B., Sicard, J., and Clavel, B. (1952): L'hypophysectomie totale dans le traitement du cancer du sein; premier cas français; avenir de la méthode. *Therapie,* 7:290–300.
68. Picaza, J. A., Hunter, S. E., and Cannon, B. W. (1977): Session in peripheral nerve and neuromuscular stimulation. Pain suppression: chronic effects. *Neurology,* 1:226–227.
69. Pilon, R. N., and Baker, A. R. (1976): Control of chronic pain by means of an epidural catheter. *Cancer,* 37:903–905.
70. Piscol, K. (1976): Die "offenen" spinalen Schmerzoperationen (anterolaterale Chordotomie und kommissurale Myelotomie) in der modernen Schmerzbekämpfung. *Langenbecks Arch. Chir.,* 342:91–99.
71. Poletti, C., Cohen, A. M., Todd, D. P., Ojemann, R. G., Sweet, W. H., and Zervas, N. T. (1981): Cancer pain relieved by long-term epidural morphine with permanent indwelling systems for self-administration. *J. Neurosurg.,* 55:581–584.
72. Ray, C. D., and Burton, C. V. (1980): Deep brain stimulation for severe chronic pain. *Acta Neurochir.,* Suppl. 30:289–293.
73. Rees, W. E. S. (1974): Multiple bilateral percutaneous rhizolysis in the treatment of the slipped disc syndrome. Presented at the *Annual Meeting of AANS,* St. Louis.
74. Reynolds, D. V. (1969): Surgery in the rat during electrical analgesia induced by frontal brain stimulation. *Science,* 164:444–445.
75. Richardson, D. E. (1982): Long-term follow-up of deep brain stimulation for relief of chronic pain in the human. In: *Modern Neurology,* edited by M. Brock, pp. 449–453. Springer-Verlag, Berlin.
76. Richardson, D. E., and Akil, H. (1977): Long term results of periventricular gray self-stimulation. *Neurosurgery,* 1:200–202.
77. Richardson, D. E., and Akil, H. (1977): Pain reduction by electrical brain stimulation in man. Part 2. Chronic self-administration in the periventricular gray matter. *J. Neurosurg.,* 47:184–194.
78. Rosomoff, H. L. (1977): Percutaneous radiofrequency cervical cordotomy for intractable pain. *Sixth International Congress of Neurological Surgery, International Congress Series,* 148:110–111. Excerpta Medica, Amsterdam.
79. Rosomoff, H. L., Carroll, F., Brown, J., et al. (1965): Percutaneous radiofrequency cervical cordotomy: Technique. *J. Neurosurg.,* 23:639–644.
80. Schvarcz, J. R. (1978): Spinal cord stereotactic techniques re trigeminal nucleotomy and extralemniscal myelotomy. *Appl. Neurophysiol.,* 41:99–112.
81. Schvarcz, J. R. (1984): Stereotactic high cervical extralemniscal myelotomy for pelvic cancer pain. *Acta Neurochir.,* Suppl. 33:431–435.
82. Shealy, C. N. (1975): Percutaneous radiofrequency denervation of spinal facets. *J. Neurosurg.,* 43:448–451.
83. Shealy, C. N., Mortimer, J. T., and Hagfors, N. R. (1970): Dorsal column electroanalgesia. *J. Neurosurg.,* 32:560–564.
84. Sheldon, C. H. (1966): Depolarization in the treatment of trigeminal neuralgia: evaluation

of compression and electrical methods; clinical concept of neurophysiological mechanism. In: *Pain,* edited by R. S. Knighton and P. R. Dumke, pp. 373–386. Little, Brown, Boston.

85. Shimken, H. R., Ortega, P., and Naffziger, H. C. (1952): Effects of surgical hypophysectomy in a man with malignant melanoma. *J. Clin. Endocrinol. Metab.,* 12:439–453.
86. Siegfried, J., and Broggi, G. (1979): Percutaneous thermocoagulation of the gasserian ganglion in the treatment of pain in advanced cancer. In: *Advances in Pain Research and Therapy, Vol. 2,* edited by J. J. Bonica and V. Ventafridda, pp. 463–468. Raven Press, New York.
87. Sindou, M. (1972): Etude de la jonction radicellomédullaire postérieure. La radicellotomie postérieure sélective dans la chirurgie de la douleur. *Medical thesis,* Lyon.
88. Sindou, M., and Lapras, C. (1982): Neurosurgical treatment of pain in the Pancoast-Tobias syndrome: selective posterior rhizotomy and open anterolateral C2-cordotomy. In: *Advances in Pain Research and Therapy, Vol. 4,* edited by J. J. Bonica, pp. 199–206. Raven Press, New York.
89. Sindou, M., Fischer, G., Goutelle, A., and Mansuy, L. (1974): La radicellotomie postérieure sélective. Premiers résultats dans la chirurgie de la douleur. *Neurochirurgie,* 20:391–408.
90. Sindou, M., Fischer, G., and Mansuy, L. (1976): Posterior spinal rhizotomy and selective posterior rhizidiotomy. *Prog. Neurol. Surg.,* 7:201–250.
91. Smith, F. P. (1970): Trans-spinal ganglionectomy for relief of intercostal pain. *J. Neurosurg.,* 32:574–577.
92. Sourek, K. (1977): Mediolongitudinal myelotomy. In: *Progress in Neurological Surgery, Vol. 8,* edited by H. Krayenbühl, P. E. Maspes, and W. H. Sweet, pp. 15–34. Karger, Basel.
93. Spiller, W. G., and Martin, E. (1912): The treatment of persistent pain of organic origin in the lower part of the body by division of the anterolateral column of the spinal cord. *JAMA,* 58:1489–1490.
94. Sweet, W. H., and Wepsic, S. G. (1974): Controlled thermocoagulation of trigeminal ganglion and results for differential destruction of pain fibers. *J. Neurosurg.,* 29:143–156.
95. Swerdlow, M. (1979): Subarachnoid and extradural neurolytic blocks. In: *Advances in Pain Research and Therapy, Vol. 2,* edited by J. J. Bonica and V. Ventafridda, pp. 325–327. Raven Press, New York.
96. Takeda, F., Fujii, T., Uki, J., Fuso, Y., Tozawa, R., Kitani, Y., and Fujita, T. (1983): Cancer pain relief and tumor regression by means of pituitary neuroadenolysis and surgical hypophysectomy. *Neurol. Med. Chir. (Tokyo),* 23:41–49.
97. Takeda, F., Uki, J., Fujii, T., Kitani, Y., and Fujita, T. (1983): Pituitary neuroadenolysis to relieve cancer pain: Observations of spread of ethanol installed into the sella turcica and subsequent changes of the hypothalamopituitary axis at autopsy. *Neurol. Med. Chir. (Tokyo),* 23:50–54.
98. Tasker, R. R. (1982): Percutaneous cordotomy—the lateral high cervical technique. In: *Operative Neurosurgical Techniques. Indications, Methods, and Results, Vol. 2,* edited by H. H. Schmidek and W. H. Sweet, pp. 1137–1153. Grune & Stratton, New York.
99. Tasker, R. R. (1985): Deafferentation. In: *Textbook of Pain,* edited by P. D. Wall and R. Melzack, pp. 119–132. Churchill Livingstone, Edinburgh.
100. Tasker, R. R. (1985): Safety and efficacy of chronic neural stimulators. Contract with Canada Department of Health and Welfare *(in preparation).*
101. Tasker, R. R., Organ, L. W., and Hawrylyshyn, P. (1980): Deafferentation and causalgia. In: *Pain,* edited by J. J. Bonica, pp. 305–329, Raven Press, New York.
102. Tasker, R. R., Organ, L. W., and Hawrylyshyn, P. A. (1982): *The Thalamus and Midbrain of Man. A Physiological Atlas Using Electrical Stimulation,* pp. 154–157, 167–172. Thomas, Springfield, Illinois.
103. Tasker, R. R., Tsuda, T., and Hawrylyshyn, P. A. (1983): Clinical physiological investigation of deafferentation pain. In: *Advances in Pain Research and Therapy, Vol. 5,* edited by J. J. Bonica, U. Lindblom, and A. Iggo, pp. 713–738. Raven Press, New York.
104. Tew, J. M., Jr., and Tobler, W. D. (1982): Percutaneous rhizotomy in the treatment of intractable facial pain (trigeminal, glossopharyngeal, and vagal nerves). In: *Operative Neurosurgical Techniques. Indications, Methods, and Results,* edited by H. H. Schmidek and W. H. Sweet, pp. 1083–1100. Grune & Stratton, New York.

105. Tindall, G. T., Christy, J. H., Nixon, D. W., Williams, A. M., and Patton, J. M. (1977): Trans-sphenoidal hypophysectomy for pain of disseminated carcinoma of the breast and prostate gland. In: *Pain Management,* edited by J. F. Lee, pp. 172–185. Williams & Wilkins, Baltimore.
106. Uematsu, S. (1982): Percutaneous electrothermocoagulation of spinal nerve trunk, ganglion, and rootlets. In: *Operative Neurosurgical Techniques. Indications, Methods, and Results, Vol. 2,* edited by H. H. Schmidek and W. H. Sweet, pp. 1177–1198. Grune & Stratton, New York.
107. Uematsu, S., Udbarhelyi, G. B., Benson, D. W., and Siebens, A. A. (1974): Percutaneous radiofrequency rhizotomy. *Surg. Neurol.,* 2:319–325.
108. Ventafridda, V., Figliuzzi, M., Tamburini, M., Gori, E., Palolaro, D., and Sala, M. (1979): Clinical observation on analgesia elicited by intrathecal morphine in cancer patients. In: *Advances in Pain Research and Therapy, Vol. 3,* edited by J. J. Bonica, J. C. Liebeskind, and D. Albe-Fessard, pp. 559–565. Raven Press, New York.
109. Ventafridda, V., Fochi, C., Sganzerla, E. P., and Tamburini, M. (1979): Neurolytic blocks in perineal pain. In: *Advances in Pain Research and Therapy, Vol. 2,* edited by J. J. Bonica and V. Ventafridda, pp. 597–605. Raven Press, New York.
110. Ventafridda, V., and Martino, G. (1975): Clinical evaluation of subarachnoid neurolytic blocks in intractable cancer pain. In: *Advances in Pain Research and Therapy, Vol. 1,* edited by J. J. Bonica and D. Albe-Fessard, pp. 699–703. Raven Press, New York.
111. Ventafridda, V., and Spreafico, R. (1974): Subarachnoid saline perfusion. In: *Advances in Neurology, Vol. 4,* edited by J. J. Bonica, pp. 477–484. Raven Press, New York.
112. Wall, P. D., and Sweet, W. H. (1967): Temporary abolition of pain in man. *Science,* 155:108–109.
113. Wang, J. K., Nauss, L. A., and Thomas, J. E. (1975): Intrathecally applied morphine in man. *Anesthesiology,* 50:149–151.
114. Wertheimer, P., and Lecuire, J. (1953): La myelotomie commissurale postérieure. *Acta Chir. Belg.,* 52:568–574.
115. Yaksh, T. L. (1981): Spinal opiate analgesia: characteristics and principles of action. *Pain,* 11:293–341.
116. Yanagida, H., Corssen, G., Trouwborst, A., and Erdmann, W. (1984): Relief of cancer pain in man: alcohol-induced neuroadenolysis vs. electrical stimulation of the pituitary gland. *Pain,* 19:133–141.

Advances in Pain Research and Therapy, Vol. 9, edited by H. L. Fields et al. Raven Press, New York © 1985.

Premorbid MMPI Profiles of Low-Back Pain Patients: Surgical Successes Versus Surgical Failures

Steven D. Hagedorn, Toshihiko Maruta, David W. Swanson, and Robert C. Colligan

Department of Psychiatry and Psychology, Mayo Clinic and Mayo Foundation, Rochester, Minnesota 55905

The Minnesota Multiphasic Personality Inventory (MMPI) has been a major tool for investigating the psychological dimensions of the patient with chronic low-back pain. In his pioneering paper, Hanvik (3) reported that patients with "functional" low-back pain had significantly higher scores on MMPI scales 1 (Hs), 2 (D), 3 (Hy), 4 (Pd), 7 (Pt), and 8 (Sc) than did patients with medically verified, "organic" low-back pain. The group of patients with "functional" low-back pain demonstrated a classic "conversion V" on the MMPI, with elevation of scales 1 (Hs) and 3 (Hy) and a relative depression of scale 2 (D).

However, Sternbach et al. (11) found no significant differences in MMPI profiles between a group of 44 patients with physical findings and a group of 24 patients without physical findings. In a further study, Sternbach et al. (10) found that patients with low-back pain of less than 6 months in duration had significantly lower scores on scales 1 (Hs), 2 (D), and 3 (Hy) than did patients with pain of more than 6 months in duration.

Gentry et al. (1), like Hanvik, found that patients with low-back pain had elevations on scales 1 (Hs), 2 (D), and 3 (Hy). Patients with low-back pain for more than 10 years had significantly higher scores on scale 2 (D) than did patients with low-back pain for less than 10 years.

Phillips (8) compared the MMPI profiles of patients who had low-back pain with profiles of patients who had fractures. Both groups had elevations on scales 1 (Hs), 2 (D), and 3 (Hy), but the scores from patients with low-back pain were significantly higher.

McCreary et al. (5) studied patients who had conservatively treated low-back pain and found that scales 1 (Hs) and 3 (Hy) were elevated more than 2 standard deviations over those of normal persons.

More recent investigators have attempted to use the MMPI as a predictor of outcome in low-back surgery. Oostdam and Duivenvoorden (6) showed that scales 1 (Hs) and 3 (Hy) could discriminate those patients in whom low-back surgery was likely to fail.

Waring et al. (13) found that elevations of scales 1 (Hs) and 3 (Hy) were of no value in predicting surgical success. However, Pheasant et al. (7) found that scales 1 (Hs) and 3 (Hy) were "inversely related to rated surgical outcome" and that a "conversion-V pattern (Hs and Hy above 70, with D relatively lower) appears to be associated with relatively poor surgical outcome."

Long (4) found that patients with the following four characteristics tended to be surgical failures: elevated scale 1 (Hs); elevated scales 1 (Hs) and 3 (Hy) in the conversion V configuration; elevated scales 1 (Hs), 3 (Hy), and 4 (Pd); and elevated scale 4 (Pd).

All of these investigators have used MMPIs from patients who took the MMPI after the onset of their chronic pain. Our study uses MMPIs obtained before the onset of their back pain. All of these patients subsequently required surgical management. The MMPI data, obtained before the onset of back pain, were examined to determine if any premorbid personality characteristics differentiated the patients rated as surgical successes from those described as surgical failures.

METHODS AND DESCRIPTION OF PATIENT POPULATION

Swenson et al. (12) have provided MMPI norms based on a sample of 50,000 Mayo Clinic medical outpatients. These 50,000 patients were then cross-matched with all patients who received a diagnosis of low-back pain or who underwent low-back surgery at the Mayo Clinic from 1966 to 1981. It is possible that the surgeon's clinical estimate regarding probable benefit from surgery may have introduced an unknown degree of selection bias since they may have temporarily excluded some patients with significant psychological disorders until appropriate psychological treatment had been provided. Sixty-two patients fulfilled the following criteria necessary for inclusion in this study: (a) no complaint of low-back pain before, and at the time of, completing the MMPI, (b) subsequent onset of low-back pain, (c) confirmation of anatomic lesions by neurologic examination and myelography, (d) low-back surgery, with identification of a surgical lesion, and (e) sufficient follow-up data to justify designation as a surgical success or surgical failure.

Of the 62 patients, all of whom had surgery, 41 (66%) were rated as surgical successes (26 men, 15 women) and 21 (34%) as failures (17 men, 4 women). No significant demographic differences (sex, marital status, age at onset, age at surgery, percentage with positive myelogram) were found between the success and failure groups. At surgery, all patients were shown to have had a herniated disk or spondylolisthesis. Postsurgical follow-up periods ranged from 6 months to 15 years.

The prepain MMPI profiles were retrieved from the computer data banks, and the 3 validity scales and the 10 clinical scales were utilized for comparison. The following comparisons were carried out (utilizing the two-tailed *t*-test): (a) female failure group versus the female general medical population (12), (b) female success group versus the female general medical population, (c) female failure group versus the female success group, (d) male failure group versus the male general medical population (12), (e) male success group versus the male general medical population, and (f) male failure group versus the male success group.

RESULTS

No statistically significant differences were found between the female failure group and the female general medical population (Fig. 1, top). When the female success group was compared with the female general medical population, the success group had significantly lower scores on scales 2 (D) and 0 (Si). A significantly higher mean score on scale 2 (D) for the failure group was found when the female success and failure groups were compared.

No statistically significant differences were found when the male success and failure groups were compared with the male general medical population or when the male success and failure groups were compared with each other (Fig. 1, bottom).

DISCUSSION

Because of the small sample size, clinicians should exercise caution in using these data. Certain trends, however, can be speculatively identified.

Women who suffered from low-back pain and who failed to improve after surgery had no statistically elevated MMPI scales compared with the female general medical population. In contrast, females who showed definite postsurgical improvement had significantly ($p < 0.01$) lower scores on scales 2 (D) and 0 (Si) than did the female general medical population. However, the female success and failure groups could not be statistically differentiated on the basis of the premorbid MMPI, although this may be due to the small size of the failure group.

For males, no significant differences in mean scores were noted when the success and failure groups were compared or when each of these groups was compared with the male general medical population. Thus, no premorbid traits, as defined by the MMPI, characterized these patients, regardless of the surgical outcome.

In summary, these data suggest that the differences in MMPI configurations reported by other researchers, based on MMPIs obtained after the onset of pain, reflect the psychological effect of the chronic pain state rather than the premorbid personality traits. That these patients had their baseline MMPI before developing back pain was both an asset and a limitation on

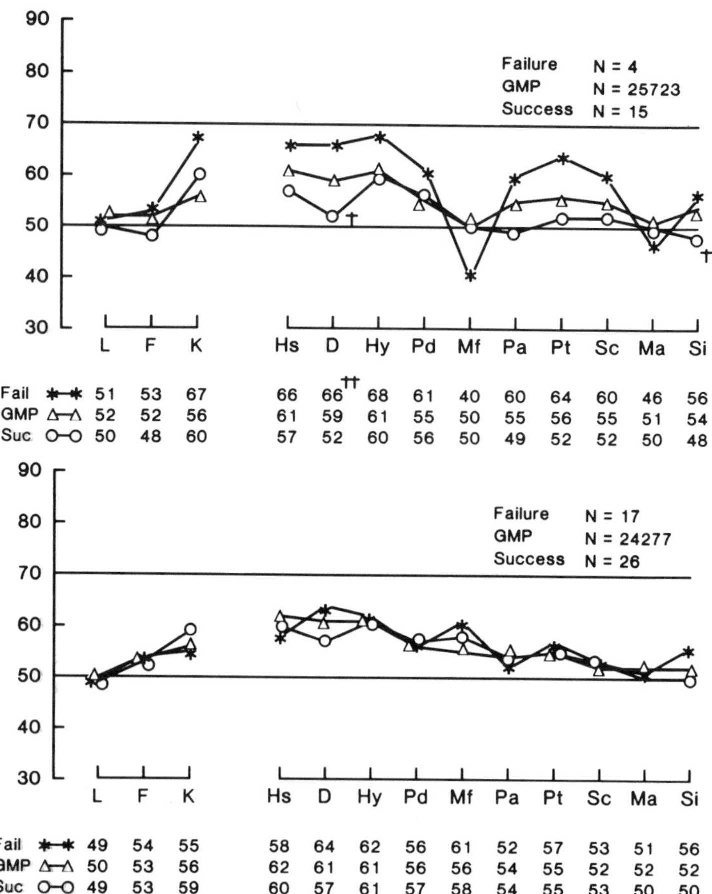

FIG. 1. Premorbid MMPI profiles. **Top:** Females; + = $p < 0.01$ comparing female successes versus GMP; ++ = $p < 0.01$ comparing female successes versus female failures. **Bottom:** Males; GMP = general medical population at Mayo Clinic.

this study. It permitted us to address the question of whether there is an MMPI personality pattern predisposing a person to chronic low-back pain. However, since we did not have MMPIs from the time of surgery or follow-up, we could not define subsequent psychological changes in these patients—changes perhaps occurring after an injury, after the onset of their pain, or after other physically or mentally stressful life experiences.

We hope to clarify this issue in a further study and have identified 240 subjects who developed "functional" or musculoskeletal low-back pain of greater than 2 years in duration, subsequent to completing premorbid MMPIs. Our subsequent research also will make use of some of the special MMPI scales developed specifically for use with patients having low-back pain (2,9).

REFERENCES

1. Gentry, W. D., Shows, W. D., and Thomas, M. (1974): Chronic low back pain: a psychological profile. *Psychosomatics,* 15:174–177.
2. Hanvik, L. (1949): Some psychological dimensions of low back pain. *Thesis,* University of Minnesota, Minneapolis.
3. Hanvik, L. J. (1951): MMPI profiles in patients with low-back pain. *J. Consult. Psychol.,* 15:350–353.
4. Long, C. J. (1981): The relationship between surgical outcome and MMPI profiles in chronic pain patients. *J. Clin. Psychol.,* 37:744–749.
5. McCreary, C. P., Turner, J., and Dawson, E. (1980): Emotional disturbance and chronic low back pain. *J. Clin. Psychol.,* 36:709–715.
6. Oostdam, E. M. M., and Duivenvoorden, H. J. (1983): Predictability of the result of surgical intervention in patients with low back pain. *J. Psychosom. Res.,* 27:273–281.
7. Pheasant, H. C., Gilbert, D., Goldfarb, J., and Herron, L. (1979): The MMPI as a predictor of outcome in low-back surgery. *Spine,* 4:78–84.
8. Phillips, E. L. (1964): Some psychological characteristics associated with orthopaedic complaints. *Curr. Pract. Orthop. Surg.,* 2:165–176.
9. Pichot, P., Perse, J., Lebeaux, M. O., Dureau, J., Perez, C., and Ryckewaert, A. (1972): La personnalité des sujets presentant des douleurs dorsales fonctionnelles: valeur de linventaire multiphasique de personnalité du Minnesota (M.M.P.I.). *Rev. Psychol. Appl.,* 22:145–172.
10. Sternbach, R. A., Wolf, S. R., Murphy, R. W., and Akeson, W. H. (1973): Aspects of chronic low back pain. *Psychosomatics,* 14:52–56.
11. Sternbach, R. A., Wolf, S. R., Murphy, R. W., and Akeson, W. H. (1973): Traits of pain patients: the low-back "loser." *Psychosomatics,* 14:226–229.
12. Swenson, W. M., Pearson, J. S., and Osborne, D. (1973): *An MMPI Source Book: Basic Item, Scale, and Pattern Data on 50,000 Medical Patients.* University of Minnesota Press, Minneapolis.
13. Waring, E. M., Weisz, G. M., and Bailey, S. I. (1976): Predictive factors in the treatment of low back pain by surgical intervention. *Adv. Pain Res. Ther.,* 1:939–942.

Advances in Pain Research and Therapy, Vol. 9, edited by H. L. Fields et al. Raven Press, New York © 1985.

Nerve Block for Herpetic Pain

K. Dan, K. Higa, and B. Noda

Department of Anesthesiology, School of Medicine, Fukuoka University, Fukuoka 814-01, Japan

Lipton (3) stated in his *Relief of Pain in Clinical Practice* in 1979 that there is no treatment that can reliably relieve the pain and discomfort present in the developed condition of postherpetic neuralgia. Such relief remains a difficult problem and prevention in the early stage of the disease is the most effective approach. Nerve block therapy for herpetic pain has been used since 1969 when Colding (1) reported the effects of this method. However, little efficacy in trigeminal I and other regions has been reported, even with early induction of nerve block therapy.

We investigated the effect of nerve block therapy on 1,000 patients, 700 within 2 weeks after eruption, and 300 patients with postherpetic neuralgia treated at Fukuoka University Hospital from 1973 to 1983.

SUBJECTS AND METHODS

Among the 1,000 Japanese patients seen in our clinic, 356 complained of severe pain and these patients were hospitalized. The other 644 with moderate or mild pain were treated on an out-patient basis.

One or a combination of the following nerve blocks was prescribed:

1. Local infiltration or conduction block.
2. Regional sympathetic ganglion block.
3. Epidural block (mainly continuous and sometimes intermittent single).

Mepivacaine (1%) was mainly used for nerve block treatment. In those with postherpetic neuralgia lasting over 1 to 3 months, imipramine 50 mg or amitriptyline 50 mg daily, imipramine or amitriptyline and Neurotropin[R]3 tablets were prescribed for at least 3 weeks. Nerve block therapy was continued three times weekly and oral medication was given.

For evaluation of nerve block therapy, the patient self-rating score was adopted. Taking the subjective pain before initiation of nerve block therapy as 100%, patients were frequently asked to state the severity of pain during the course of treatment. In some patients, it was often difficult to obtain an exact rating of the residual pain. Almost complete pain relief with some residual sensation such as slight numbness or a low grade of dysesthesia was rated as 10% or less; with slight pain but no disturbance of active daily life and if patients were sometimes not conscious of pain while working, it was rated 20%. The reply of patients with residual pain in over 30% was recorded as correctly as possible. Final rating of the residual pain was made by questionnaire sent to the patients 6 months after the completion of treatment.

To investigate the residual pain after nerve block therapy, questionnaires were sent to all patients who visited our pain clinic. Of the 1,000 patients, 749 patients responded.

RESULTS

Statistical Observations of Herpes Zoster Patients

Morbidity as a Function of Age

Morbidity in those over 50 was high; 73% of our patients were over 50, and 52% were over 60 (Fig. 1).

Morbidity by Anatomical Distributions

Eruption of herpes zoster extended over several segments of dermatomes. A careful sensory test on the affected skin revealed that a certain area was less sensitive to temperature and pain. This area was located in a single innervated region of skin. Consequently, the affected dermatome in a patient was determined to be the single sensory innervated area. The highest rate of morbidity was seen in trigeminal I in 198(19.8%), next were upper thoracic regions (T2–T4), T4 in 83 cases, T3 in 70 cases, T2 in 60 cases, and the other 589 were included in the other 28 dermatomes.

Results of Nerve Block Therapy

Starting Periods

Seven hundred and forty-nine patients who responded to questionnaires were divided into groups, depending on the starting periods of nerve block treatments (Fig. 2, left).

Group 1: 529 patients for whom block treatments were started within 2 weeks after skin eruption.
Group 2: 96 patients from 2 weeks to 1 month.
Group 3: 69 patients from 1 month to 3 months.
Group 4: 33 patients from 3 months to 12 months.
Group 5: 22 patients over 1 year.

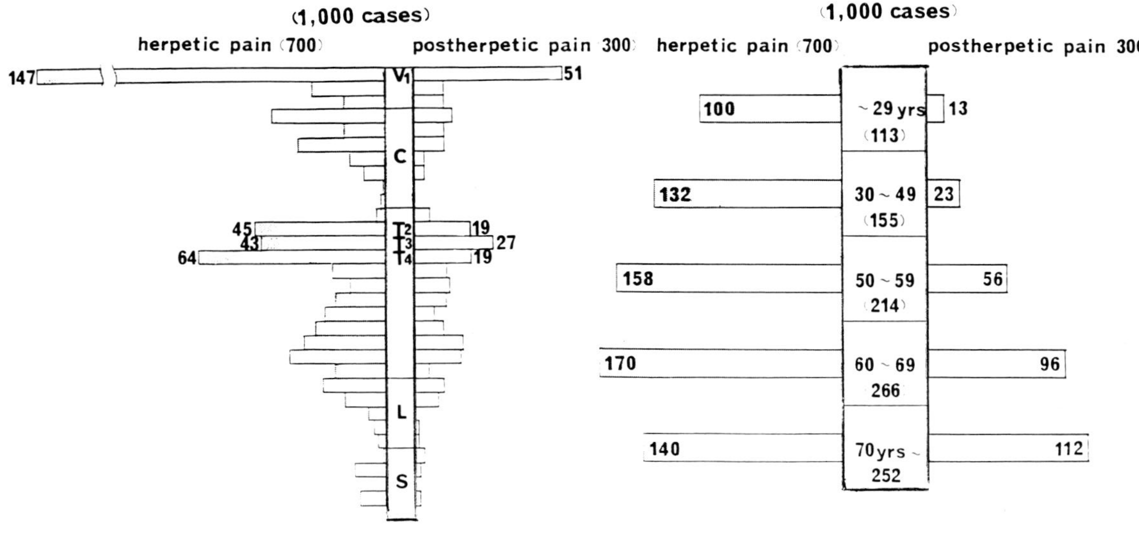

FIG. 1. Herpes zoster: Anatomical **(left)** and age distribution **(right)**.

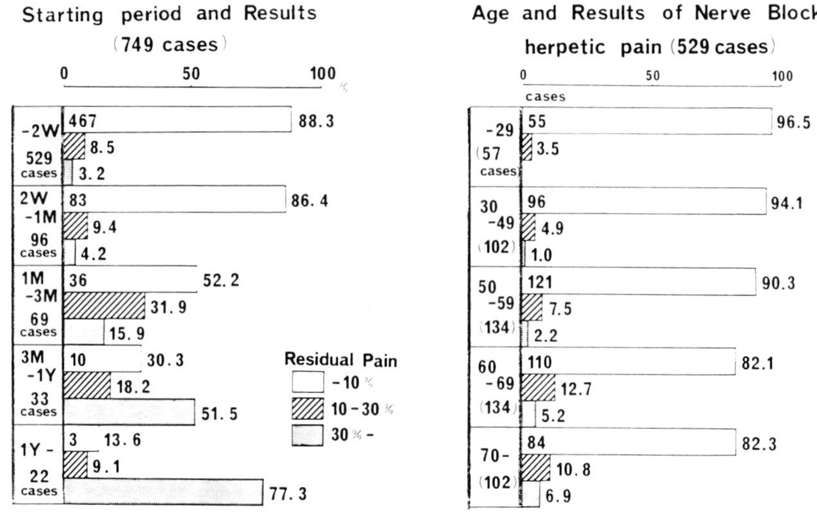

FIG. 2. Results of nerve block therapy.

Four hundred sixty-seven (88.3%) out of 529 patients (Group 1) responded to nerve block therapy and did not progress to postherpetic neuralgia. In 86.4% of 96 (Group 2), the result was good. In Group 3, 52.2% of 69 had good results; but in 30% of 33 in Group 4 and only 13.6% of 22 in Group 5 were the results good. In contrast, the proportion of patients with residual pain over 30% abruptly increased when the treatment had been begun 3 months after skin eruption.

Age

Fifty-five (96.5%) out of 57 patients under 29 responded well to nerve block therapy and did not progress to postherpetic pain (Fig. 2; right). The rate of excellent results very gradually decreased with advancing age, that is, 94.1% in their 30s and 40s, 90% in their 50s, 82% in their 60s, and 82% in those over 70 years of age. On the other hand, the rate of patients with residual pain over 30% increased gradually with advancing age.

Anatomical Distribution

Fifteen (14.2%) out of 106 patients in whom the eruption was located in trigeminal I region did not respond well to nerve block therapy, and 12.5% in T2, 11.1% in T3, and 10.3% in T4 (Fig. 3). Sixty-two (11.7%) out of 529, including all regions, herpetic patients for whom block treatment started

	Herpetic Pain	
	cases	residual pain over 10%
V_1	106	15 (14.2%)
2	22	3 (13.6%)
⋮		
C_2	27	3 (11.1%)
⋮		
T_2	32	4 (12.5%)
3	36	4 (11.1%)
4	39	4 (10.3%)
⋮		
T_9		
10		
11	26	4 (15.4%)
⋮		
L	40	4 (10.0%)
S	18	3 (16.7%)
Total	529	62 (11.7%)

Fukuoka Univ. Hospital Aug.1973 – June 1983

FIG. 3. Anatomical distribution and effects of nerve block in 529 patients for whom block started within 2 weeks after eruption.

within 2 weeks after eruption did not respond well to nerve block therapy. These results indicate that the effect of nerve block therapy on each affected anatomical dermatome is almost the same according to questionnaires sent 6 months after termination of the nerve block treatment.

Durations Required for Complete Pain Relief

To investigate the time required for complete pain relief in each region, the percentage of patients with complete pain relief is plotted as a function of number of treatment days on the abscissa, and these are delineated for each group. Figure 4 shows an example of the result of the thoracic affected region. All crossed marks represent the days of therapy and the rate of patients with complete pain relief. This can be expressed by

$$Y = 2.21 \log X - 3.00$$

where Y = rate of complete relief of herpetic pain and X = therapeutic days for complete relief.

The duration of nerve block treatment required to obtain complete relief of pain for 50% of patients in each group was 20 days in case of the lumbosacral region, 25 days for the thoracic or cervical, and 35 days for the trigeminal area. The duration for 90% of patients was 55 days in case of the lumbosacral region, 85 days for the thoracic, 115 days for the cervical, and 130 days in case of trigeminal affected areas (Fig. 5).

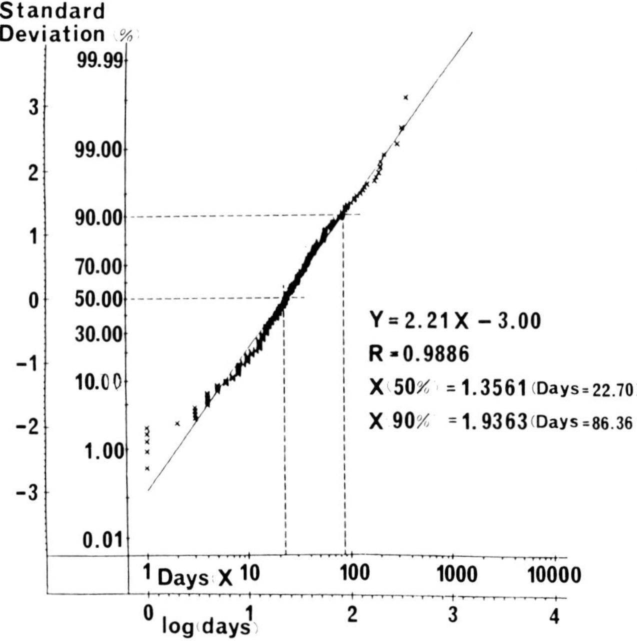

FIG. 4. Herpetic pain in thoracic region in 230 cases.

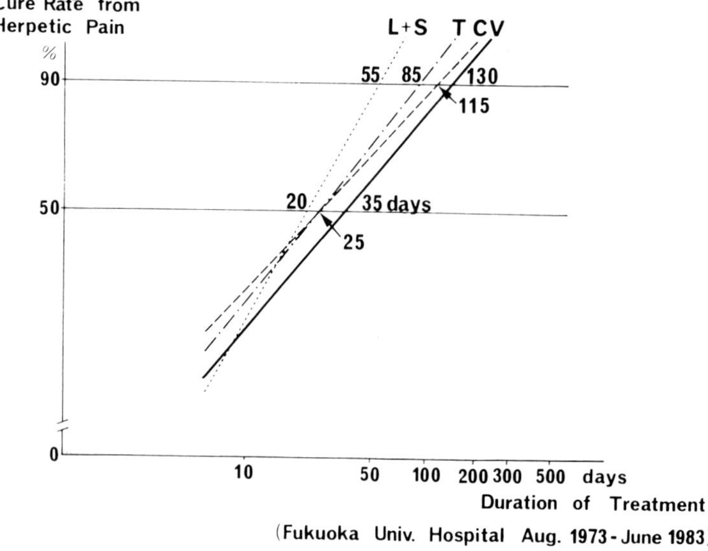

FIG. 5. Duration of nerve block treatment for complete cure.

DISCUSSION

Early nerve block therapy for herpetic pain is a well-recognized treatment for prevention of postherpetic neuralgia. Colding (1) reported that sympathetic ganglion blocks, three to four times on the average, are effective for herpetic pain and prevent progression to postherpetic neuralgia. However, severe pain was difficult to treat with this frequency of nerve blocks. To alleviate severe zoster pain, continuous epidural block has to be applied all night, each night for several weeks. There is still no established regimen for effective treatment.

Which symptoms of herpes zoster will be the most reliable for estimation of a possible postherpetic neuralgia? Observation of the grade of serial changes of eruption is needed. Attention should be directed to the time required for recovery of skin eruption.

Delayed type hypersensitivity reactions to varicella-zoster virus antigen and duration of pain show a good relation, and stimulation index to varicella-zoster virus antigen and duration of pain have a close relation in patients treated with nerve blocks (2). These two parameters of cellular immunity must show a good correlation to the period of recovery of skin eruption. However, the duration of burning sensation in the affected area and the grade of postherpetic neuralgia could not be inferred from the severity of skin eruptions. It seems more likely that serial changes of skin eruption indicate only the dermal pathological changes of varicella-zoster virus infection and do not express the degenerative state of posterior ganglion which is likely to be responsible for the herpetic and postherpetic pain. Therefore, whenever nerve block therapy is prescribed for zoster patients, first attention should be directed to the grade of pain and its nature during the treatment. The principle for nerve block treatment is to produce complete pain relief and maintain it as long as possible.

Next, the sensory test on the affected area is another important device for estimation of postherpetic neuralgia. Each patient has some degree of sensory disturbance on the affected area, even in the initial state of skin eruption. Attempts should be made to decrease the intensity and area of hypesthesia to temperature and pain in the affected region during nerve block treatment. This is a good sign and has no sequela. But despite early and frequent nerve block treatment, a persistent analgesia or hypesthesia of the affected area with some residual pain suggests that some degree of postherpetic neuralgia will remain and that nerve block treatment has to be continued.

The relationship between starting periods and nerve block therapy show that nerve block treatment for patients initiated between 2 weeks and 1 month after skin eruption was effective, as compared to the effect of nerve block treatment for patients within 2 weeks. However, nerve block therapy should be applied as soon as possible when skin eruption and pain become evident, because the sooner the block treatment after skin eruption, the shorter the duration of treatment. This is not a statistical evaluation, but rather our clinical findings in a 10-year experience.

The anatomical distribution of herpes zoster showed that the incidence of herpes zoster in trigeminal I and upper thoracic (T2–T4) regions was higher than that in the other regions, but the overall results of nerve block therapy did not differ in the anatomical dermatome. No difference was found even in the trigeminal region according to questionnaires sent to our patients at least 6 months after the completion of treatment. However, apparent differences were found in the duration of nerve block treatment required to obtain complete relief of pain for 50% of patients in each group. The duration of treatment correlated well with the order of innervation from lumbosacral to trigeminal, the higher the innervation the longer was the duration of treatment.

REFERENCES

1. Colding, A. (1969): Effect of regional sympathetic blocks in the treatment of herpes zoster. *Acta Anaesthesiol. Scand.,* 13:133–141.
2. Dan, K., Higa, K., Tanaka, K., and Mori, R. (1983): Herpetic pain and cellular immunity. In: *Current Topics in Pain Research and Therapy,* edited by T. Yokota and R. Dubner, pp. 293–305. Excerpta Medica, Amsterdam.
3. Lipton, S. (1979): Post-herpetic neuralgia. In: *Relief of Pain in Clinical Practice,* pp. 231–248. Blackwell, Oxford.

Advances in Pain Research and Therapy, Vol. 9, edited by H. L. Fields et al. Raven Press, New York © 1985.

Plasma Lanthanides and Local Anesthetic Therapy in Localized Inflammatory Condition

*Mauro Esposito, **Massimo Oddone, *Paola Collecchi, and †Maurizio Cutolo

**National Institute for Cancer Research, 16132 Genoa; **Department of General Chemistry, University of Pavia, 27100 Pavia; and †Rheumatological Center, University of Genoa, 16148 Genoa, Italy*

Lanthanides, or rare-earth metals, constitute a series of fifteen transition-elements (group 3b) starting with lanthanum (atomic number 57) and ending with lutetium (atomic number 75). Competition of lanthanum for calcium (Ca^{2+}) binding sites and its ability to depress electric potentials of nerves and neuromuscular function are well known (9,21). Moreover, recent studies suggest that lanthanum has a stronger influence on the cell membrane characteristics than the local anesthetic procaine (1,2).

Local anesthetics are drugs, that, when applied locally to nerve tissue in appropriate concentrations, block nerve impulse propagation (17,20). Although the molecular mechanism of action of these drugs is not fully understood, it is widely accepted that they act on the cell membrane, presumably by increasing their permeability to osmotically active particles (10,18,19). Membrane-bound Ca^{2+} can be stoichiometrically displaced by local anesthetics (16,19), and this is thought to happen at some site that controls the permeability of sodium (4).

Procaine hydrochloride is commonly used as a local anesthetic, and data obtained with mammalian cells in culture show an enhancement of hyperthermic killing by this drug (6); the potential usefulness of this effect in cancer therapy has been suggested (7,8,22).

In light of these findings, the principal purpose of this chapter is the evaluation of the effect of local procaine therapy on plasma lanthanides levels as measured by Neutron Activation Analysis.

MATERIALS AND METHODS

Subjects

Two groups of subjects were considered; Group I—30 apparently normal individuals, aged 30 to 70 years (mean ± SD: 54.6 ± 18.0) were analyzed in order to obtain the reference values for basal plasma lanthanides levels; group II—8 patients aged 45 to 58 years (mean ± SD: 52.7 ± 5.0) suffering from epicondylitis at the elbow.

The patients were treated with local injections of the anesthetic procaine hydrochloride 1% (Bioindustria, Novi Ligure, Italy) at times 0, 3, and 7 days after initial observation. Total volumes of 5 to 7 ml (50–70 mg) of local anesthetic were injected into the junction of the muscle and its fibrous attachment to the bone of the affected epicondyle. No other treatment with analgesic, steroidal, and nonsteroidal antiinflammatory drugs had been given for at least 15 days.

Samples

Blood samples of 10 ml each were always drawn from antecubital veins of the affected elbow in fasting human subjects, before local anesthetic injection. All samples were collected with plastic syringes, between 7 and 9 a.m., then transferred to plastic tubes containing 50 μl of K_3-ethylenediaminetetracetic acid (K_3-EDTA) as an anticoagulant (Sclavo, lot no. 81800); plasma was separated from red blood cells by centrifugation at 2,000 × g for 15 min and kept at 4° C until analyzed. Great care was taken to avoid contamination of samples during either collection or storage prior to analysis. No metal tools were used, only utensils made from Perspex or other plastics. One-ml plasma samples were oven-dried in Petri dishes and stored inside "snap-on"-type quartz bags. In order to minimize air-borne contamination, all samples were kept inside a dust-free cabinet installed inside a clean room far from the laboratory (3,12–14).

Radiochemical Neutron Activation Analysis

The choice of the proper nuclear reaction was made according to Meloni et al. (15). Some nuclear characteristics of the lanthanides studied are shown in Table 1.

Standard reference materials nos. 1571 [Orchard Leaves; National Bureau of Standards (NBS), Certificate of Analysis, Standard Reference Material 1571 Orchard Leaves] and 1577 (Bovine Liver; NBS, Certificate of Analysis, Standard Reference Material 1577 Bovine Liver), were prepared according

TABLE 1. *Nuclear data of lanthanides determined by radiochemical neutron activation analysis*

Element	Abundance of stable nuclide (%)	Activation cross-section (barn)	Produced radionuclide	Half-life	Measured γ-ray energy (KeV) and relative intensities
La	99.9	8.9	^{140}La	1.68 days	1,595(100), 487(48)
Ce	88.48	0.6	^{141}Ce	32.5 days	145(100)
Nd	17.18	2	^{147}Nd	11.1 days	91(100), 531(45)
Eu	47.7	5,900	^{152}Eu	12.2 years	344(100), 1,408(90)
Gd	0.2	125	^{153}Gd	236 days	98(100)
Yb	0.14	11,000	^{169}Yb	32.6 days	64(100), 198(85)
Lu	2.6	2,100	^{177}Lu	6.75 days	208(100)

to the method recommended by the NBS. Standard Kale samples were also used in the analysis (11).

Irradiation of samples and standards was carried out with a thermal flux of about 8×10^{12}n cm^{-2}s^{-1}, for 1 week, at the University Research Reactor of Pavia, Italy. Induced radioactivity was measured by γ-ray spectrometry at the Radiochemistry Laboratory of the University of Pavia, using an 18% efficiency Ge(Li) detector coupled to an analyzer-computer system.

After irradiation and cooling, the samples were dissolved with a 12 M HCl/14 M HNO_3 solution; the solution was dried and treated with the same mixture, again dried and finally treated with 0.5 M HCl solution.

Known amounts of the lanthanides to be determined were added as carriers. The solution was then passed through a chromatographic column filled with Dowex W 50 × 8(100–200 mesh, H^+ form, 2.5 height, and 0.1 cm I.D.) previously equilibrated with distilled water. Most of the metals, lanthanides included, are thus adsorbed on the column. After washing with H_2O, a first elution with a 0.01 M $H_2C_2O_4$ solution in 0.5 M HCl was performed to remove interfering elements such as Sc, Co, and Fe from the column; a second elution with 2 M HNO_3 was then carried out to remove interfering alkaline metals, alkaline-earth metals and As; finally the lanthanides group was eluted from the column with 6 M HCl. The determination of lanthanum (La), cerium (Ce), neodymium (Nd), europium (Eu), gadolinium (Gd), ytterbium (Yb), and lutetium (Lu) on the eluate was then made by γ-ray spectrometry.

Statistical Method

The two-sample *t*-test (comparison of two means, unpaired case) was used to test the significance of differences in mean concentrations of healthy volunteers and patients.

TABLE 2. *Lanthanide content of the Standard Reference Material*[a]

Element	Orchard leaves NBS-SRM 1571		Bovine liver NBS-SRM 1577	
	This work: (μg/g ± SD)	Gladney (ref. 11)	This work: (μg/g ± SD)	Gladney (ref. 11)
La	1.4100 ± 0.0200	1.200	0.0310 ± 0.0040	0.028
Ce	1.1800 ± 0.0300	1.000	0.0510 ± 0.0050	0.046
Nd	0.450 ± 0.040	0.400	0.1600 ± 0.0300	0.170
Eu	0.0930 ± 0.0030	0.090	0.0041 ± 0.0003	0.002–3.100
Gd	0.0140 ± 0.0060	0.00164–0.100	0.0014 ± 0.0004	< 0.001
Yb	0.0290 ± 0.0050	0.027	0.0028 ± 0.0006	0.005–0.830
Lu	0.0086 ± 0.0003	0.0061–0.010	0.0064 ± 0.0007	< 0.001

[a]Lanthanide: μg/g.

RESULTS

Table 2 shows the lanthanide content of the Standard Reference Material compared with the values reported by Gladney (11). The sensitivities for La, Ce, Nd, Eu, Gd, Yb, and Lu are reported in Table 3. Table 4 shows the results of plasma lanthanides levels in all considered subjects.

Basal values of plasma levels of all lanthanides in patients suffering from epicondylitis at the elbow were significantly higher as compared to the 30 healthy controls. Although mean plasma La level 3 days after first procaine treatment was higher than that observed before the local anesthetic injection (20.5 ± 11.9 versus 13.8 ± 4.5, respectively), this difference did not reach statistical significance. However, a significant increase ($p < 0.02$) was observed at the 4th day after second procaine treatment, the 7th day after starting therapy.

On the contrary, during procaine therapy, the variations from the basal

TABLE 3. *Sensitivities for lanthanides determined by radiochemical neutron activation analysis*

Element	Radionuclide used	Measured γ-ray (KeV)	Sensitivity (ng)[a]
La	^{140}La	1,595	0.200
Ce	^{141}Ce	145	0.100
Nd	^{147}Nd	91	0.090
Eu	^{152}Eu	1,408	0.005
Gd	^{153}Gd	98	0.010
Yb	^{169}Yb	198	0.020
Lu	^{177}Lu	208	0.004

[a]Evaluated under the experimental conditions described in this paper.

TABLE 4. *Mean plasma levels of lanthanides in all considered subjects*[a]

Element	Normal condition	Inflammatory condition	3rd day after I procaine treatment	4th day after II procaine treatment
La	5.5 ± 1.2	13.8 ± 4.5[b]	20.5 ± 11.9	26.4 ± 8.3[d]
Ce	54.0 ± 7.9	98.6 ± 7.5[b]	82.5 ± 23.1	85.2 ± 14.1
Nd	46.0 ± 2.9	91.0 ± 2.0[b]	85.5 ± 12.8	83.6 ± 8.3
Eu	4.8 ± 1.0	15.6 ± 4.5[b]	17.0 ± 6.0	16.2 ± 4.7
Gd	1.5 ± 0.2	7.7 ± 1.3[b]	8.3 ± 3.3	7.6 ± 1.5
Yb	4.1 ± 1.5	6.5 ± 1.6[c]	6.4 ± 1.1	6.9 ± 0.6
Lu	0.5 ± 0.1	1.0 ± 0.5[b]	1.1 ± 0.3	1.2 ± 0.3

[a]The concentration values of lanthanides are expressed as ng/ml plasma, mean ± SD.
[b]Statistically significant $p<0.001$, compared to normal condition.
[c]Statistically significant $p<0.025$, compared to normal condition.
[d]Statistically significant $p<0.02$, compared to inflammatory condition.

inflammatory condition of plasma levels of the other lanthanides studied, were not statistically significant (Table 4).

CONCLUSIONS

The reported sensitivities (Table 3) clearly indicate that radiochemical neutron activation analysis (RNAA) procedure can be safely applied to the determination of low levels of rare earth elements in biological materials.

Elements of the rare earth series (lanthanides) occur in only trace amounts in organisms and play no known biochemical role (9). As observed of other trace metal elements (e.g., copper, iron), plasma lanthanide concentrations could also be altered during inflammatory processes following modified influences of redox reactions (5). This preliminary study suggests that endogenous plasma levels of lanthanides are significantly affected by inflammatory conditions, and that local procaine therapy could significantly influence only La plasma concentrations. To our knowledge, this is the first *in vivo* study of plasma lanthanide levels before and after procaine therapy in patients suffering from localized inflammatory condition.

Nerve and muscle cells are highly sensitive to procaine and La, and it has been suggested that both agents might act by displacing Ca^{2+} from the cell membrane, blocking transport and inhibiting functions which depend on this mechanism (4,9). In particular, the observed increase in plasma La concentration during procaine treatment could be due to a selective competitive displacing action for La determined by the local anesthetic drug.

In addition, the ability of procaine and La to enhance cell killing by hyperthermia (2) may suggest a similar mechanism of action on the cell membrane, and, indeed, a potential therapeutic usefulness of both agents in malignancies. Further studies of lanthanides status and of the effect of procaine therapy on plasma La concentrations are now in progress.

ACKNOWLEDGMENTS

We thank Dr. Paolo Bruzzi for his assistance in the statistical analyses. This work was supported in part by the National Research Council (CNR, Rome, Italy) within the "Progetto Finalizzato: Preventive and Rehabilitative Medicine. Sottoprogetto SP 8: Control of Pain," contract 82.02043.53

REFERENCES

1. Anghileri, L. J., Marchal, C., and Robert, J. (1982): Enhancement of hyperthermia effects on cancer cells by cell membrane interaction with La^{3+}. *Proceedings: 13th International Cancer Congress,* Seattle, Washington.
2. Anghileri, L. J., Marchal, C., Crone, M. C., and Robert, J. (1983): Enhancement of hyperthermia lethality by Lanthanum. *Arch. Geschwulstforsch.,* 53:335–339.
3. Bowen, H. J. M. (1974): Problems in the elementary analysis of standard biological materials. *J. Radioanal. Chem.,* 19:215–226.
4. Covino, B. G., and Vassalio, H. (1976): Pharmacodynamic aspects of local anesthetic agents. In: *Local Anesthetics: Mechanism of Action and Clinical Use,* pp. 13–39. Grune & Stratton, New York.
5. Cutolo, M., Rovida, S., Samantha, E., and Accardo, S. (1980): Effect of drugs on serum copper and its correlation with other humoral factors in rheumatoid arthritis. In: *Inflammation: Mechanisms and Treatment,* edited by D. A. Willoughby and J. P. Giroud, pp. 453–458. M.T.P., Lancaster.
6. Djordjevic, B. (1979): Differential effect of procaine on irradiated mammalian cells in culture. *Radiology,* 131:515–519.
7. Djordjevic, B., and Szechter, A. (1981): Potentiation of radiation lethality in HeLa cells by mild hyperthermia and procaine. *Radiology,* 141:533–535.
8. Djordjevic, B. (1983): Variable interaction of heat and procaine in potentiation of radiation lethality in mammalian cells of neoplastic origin. *Int. J. Radiat. Biol.,* 43:399–409.
9. Evans, C. H. (1983): Interesting and useful biochemical properties of lanthanides. *TIBS,* 8:445–449.
10. Feinstein, M. B., Fernandez, S. M., and Sha'Afi, R. I. (1975): Fluidity of natural membranes and phosphatidylserine and ganglioside dispersion: Effects of local anesthetics, cholesterol and protein. *Biochem. Biophys. Acta,* 413:352–370.
11. Gladney, E. S. (1980): Elemental concentration in NBS Biological Environmental, Standard Reference Materials. *Anal. Chim. Acta,* 118:385–396.
12. Hudnik, V., Marolt-Gomiscek, M., and Gomiscek, S. (1984): The determinations of trace metals in human fluids and tissues. Part 1. *Anal. Chim. Acta,* 157:143–150.
13. Hudnik, V., Marolt-Gomiscek, M., and Gomiscek, S. (1984): The determinations of trace metals in human fluids and tissues. Part 2. *Anal. Chim. Acta,* 157:183–186.
14. Hudnik, V., Marolt-Gomiscek, M., and Gomiscek, S. (1984): The determinations of trace metals in human fluids and tissues. Part 3. *Anal. Chim. Acta,* 157:303–311.
15. Meloni, S., Oddone, M., Cecchi, A., and Poli, G. (1982): Destructive neutron activation analysis of REE in geological samples: A comparison between two methods. *J. Radioanal. Chem.,* 71:429–446.
16. Papahadjopoulos, D. (1970): Phosopholid model membranes. III. Antagonistic effects of Ca^{2+} and local anesthetics on the permeability of phosphatidylserine vesicles. *Biochem. Biophys. Acta,* 211:467–477.
17. Ritchie, J. M. (1975): Mechanism of action of local anesthetic agents and biotoxins. *Br. J. Anaesthesiol.,* 47:191–198.

18. Roth, S., and Seeman, P. (1971): All-lipid soluble anesthetics protect red cells. *Nature (New Biol.),* 231:284–285.
19. Seeman, P. (1972): The membrane actions of anesthetics and tranquilizers. *Pharmacol. Rev.,* 24:583–655.
20. Strichartz, G. (1976): Molecular mechanisms of nerve block of local anesthetics. *Anesthesiology,* 45:421–441.
21. Switzer, M. E. (1978): The lanthanide ions as probes of calcium ion binding sites in biological systems. *Sci. Prog.,* 65:19–30.
22. Yatvin, M. B. (1977): The influence of membrane lipid composition and procaine on hyperthermic death of cells. *Int. J. Radiat. Biol.,* 32:513–521.

Advances in Pain Research and Therapy, Vol. 9, edited by H. L. Fields et al. Raven Press, New York © 1985.

Cognitive Techniques for Controlling Pain: Generality and Individual Differences

*Georgina Harris and **Gary B. Rollman

**Department of Psychological Services, University Hospital, London, Ontario N6A 5A5; and **Department of Psychology, University of Western Ontario, London, Ontario N6A 5C2, Canada*

There has been a great deal of interest in the last few years in psychological approaches to pain control. In particular, cognitive-behavioral strategies have been investigated as providing a means whereby a person's tolerance to pain can be increased.

Most of the research in this area has been done in the laboratory, using experimentally induced pain. These studies have suggested that tolerance levels can indeed be enhanced through the use of cognitive techniques. The evidence for the efficacy of these strategies in controlling clinical pain is meager. The number of studies is comparatively small and the results have been equivocal [see Tan (6)].

What of the research using experimentally induced pain? Is it possible that in the search for positive evidence as to the efficacy of cognitive-behavioral techniques for pain control, important problems go unnoticed? A perusal of the literature shows that cognitive-behavioral interventions do apparently result in subjects increasing their pain tolerance levels, but the data are averaged over many subjects and the variability is great. What this variability reflects is that some subjects benefit from the interventions, but others do not. If the work of the laboratory is to be translated into the treatment of the clinician, this is of the first importance.

Some recent research attempted a preliminary look at the individual differences which may be associated with the ability to use cognitive interventions effectively. A second question which was explored was whether cognitive techniques are effective *across* stressors. Interventions which would only modify certain kinds of pain, cold, for example, could not be expected to be useful clinically. The generality of pain measures across stressors was addressed in an earlier paper by Harris and Rollman (3) where both generality and discriminant validity were demonstrated.

METHOD

Subjects

Forty students, 20 male and 20 female, served as subjects. The age range was from 18 to 30, with a mean of 20 years.

Apparatus

Three stressors were used to obtain measures of pain threshold and tolerance.

1. Electrical stimulation: A constant current stimulator delivered trains of 40 1-msec monophasic square wave pulses at 100 Hz to the left volar forearm through a pair of Grass silver electrodes filled with Grass electrode paste. Stimulation was increased in discrete steps of 0.15 mA, beginning at 0.075 mA. An upper limit of 7.5 mA was used, but the subjects were not informed of this.

2. Cold water pressor: Observers inserted their right arm into a tank of circulating ice water. The temperature of the water was constantly monitored by a thermistor with a digital display. The mean water temperature was 1.8° C with a standard deviation of 0.29° C. The tank was furnished with a handle which subjects held lowered to the bottom, so that the angle of their arms in relation to the flow of water was identical. The ice was kept behind a wire mesh to prevent it from touching the skin. A 300-sec, unannounced, upper limit was used.

3. Pressure: A Forgione and Barber (2) pressure algometer applied a 2,000-g weight to the first phalanx of the subject's left forefinger. Individuals placed and removed the weight themselves. Again, the maximum exposure was limited to 300 sec.

Procedure

Each subject was exposed to the three stressors in one of the six possible random orders. Estimates of pain threshold and pain tolerance levels were obtained. For cold and pressure, pain threshold was defined as the amount of time elapsed between the beginning of stimulation and the point at which it became painful. Pain threshold for shock was the current level at which the subject reported that its quality first changed from touch to faint pain.

Tolerance for cold and pressure was defined as the amount of time between the beginning of stimulation and withdrawal from the apparatus. For shock, tolerance was the intensity at which the subject indicated that he or she did not wish to receive the next higher stimulus.

After these initial measures were made, subjects were presented with cognitive strategies similar to those used by Scott and Barber (4). These strategies were presented via a tape recording and began with the suggestion that the subject relax, followed by four tactics for coping with pain. The four strategies included attention diversion, dissociation, transformation of the sensation, and imaginative diversion. After listening to the tape, subjects were again presented with the three stressors and threshold and tolerance measures were obtained for each. Finally, the subjects took part in a brief interview and filled out a questionnaire about the use of strategies. During the interview they were asked about the sorts of thoughts they had had during the testing. This was done in order to explore the possibility of catastrophizing thoughts having occurred. The questionnaire was aimed at discovering which of the strategies, if any, the subject had used and whether they had used any strategy of their own during the pretest. There have been occasional suggestions in the literature that the failure of some subjects to increase their tolerance level after the introduction of a cognitive strategy might be due to the fact that they were already using a self generated strategy during the pretest and so could not be expected to improve further. This possibility does not appear to have been tested, however.

RESULTS

The group means suggested that subjects increased their tolerance levels significantly after the introduction of the cognitive strategies. The intervention appeared to be effective for all three stressors, the change being significant at the $p < 0.001$ level for shock and $p < 0.05$ for cold and pressure. As in earlier studies, however, these data showed considerable variability.

There is some evidence that subjects whose initial pain measures are high appear to be able to increase them significantly more than subjects with low initial measures, [Spanos et al. (5), Vallis (7)]. In the present study, the data from the pretest measures were divided by a median split into high and low pain sensitivity range (PSR) groups for each stressor. The PSR is defined as being the range between pain threshold and pain tolerance. When the pre- and postintervention measures were compared for these two groups within each of the three stressors, only the high PSR groups had significantly increased their tolerance levels for shock and cold, while the low groups had not. Both groups, however, increased their tolerance levels for pressure significantly (Table 1).

The answers to the questionnaire showed that approximately half of the subjects had been using a self-generated coping strategy during the pretest. With all three stressors, the group of subjects who had used these strategies increased their tolerance measures beyond those achieved by subjects who had not used a strategy during the pretest. These differences approached but failed to meet significance for shock and cold. For pressure the differences are significant, $p < 0.05$, and indeed only the group of subjects who used an original strategy increased their tolerance levels for pressure after the inter-

TABLE 1. *Mean changes in tolerance, compared to baseline, after cognitive intervention: high and low PSR groups*

	Tolerance change		
	Shock (mA)	Cold (sec)	Pressure (sec)
High PSR	0.98[a]	28.73[a]	23.66[b]
Low PSR	0.67	4.94	25.92[b]

[a] $p < 0.001$.
[b] $p < 0.01$.

vention (Table 2). Therefore, it was not the case that using a coping strategy in the pretest precluded an increase in tolerance level in the posttest.

A survey of the individual data suggested the following. Subjects who used a coping strategy during the pretest and were in the high PSR group always increased their tolerance levels. The subjects who failed to increase their tolerance for any stressor had all reported not using a strategy in the pretest. Some subjects actually decreased their tolerance levels for some stressors but the variables associated with this were not clear cut, though having a low tolerance measure and failing to use coping strategies were clearly important. If subjects reported catastrophizing thoughts during the test, tolerance levels did not improve and were invariably below the median PSR for the stressor involved. This was the case even if they reported that they were trying to use a coping technique.

DISCUSSION

It was demonstrated that the cognitive strategies could be effective for all three stressors and it is useful to know that there is a general rather than a

TABLE 2. *Mean changes in tolerance, compared to baseline, after cognitive intervention*[a]

Pretest strategy	Tolerance change		
	Shock (mA)	Cold (sec)	Pressure (sec)
Yes	0.92[b]	25.77[b]	44.27[b]
No	0.72[b]	9.22[b]	−3.86

[a] Subjects who used a coping strategy in the pretest (Yes) and those who did not (No).
[b] $p < 0.05$.

stressor-specific response. At the same time, however, the variability of the data reflect individual differences which need to be pursued. A subject's PSR or pain tolerance measures may have some predictive power as to the likelihood that a cognitive coping strategy will be effective. It is clear, however, that this variable can be modified by other factors. Indeed, it was the high PSR group which showed the greatest variability of response. Having the habit of using coping strategies, measured here by the presence or absence of use of these techniques in the pretest, also appeared to be a potential predictor of effectiveness of a cognitive intervention. When questioned, subjects who reported that they had used coping tactics in the pretest said that listening to the intervention tape had enabled them to organize their strategies and use them more effectively in the posttest.

The ability to cope with pain must be a function of many interacting variables. There is not as yet a clear understanding of how this occurs, nor is it known which of the variables might be the most amenable to modification and change or even if it is always wise to attempt to do so. It is possible that the subjects who did not benefit from the use of a cognitive coping strategy are similar to the people identified as "avoiders" by Cohen and Lazarus (1). These were the patients who, when given preparatory information for surgery and postoperative pain, did relatively worse than similar patients who were not given such information. If this is the case then one must consider the possibility that to use cognitive strategies wholesale, without regard to individual differences, may mean that some people will suffer more pain than would otherwise have been the case. Clearly, if cognitive strategies are to be used clinically, this is an important ethical, as well as scientific, consideration.

REFERENCES

1. Cohen, F., and Lazarus, R. W. (1979): Active coping processes, coping disposition and recovery from surgery. *Psychol. Rep.,* 45:867–873.
2. Forgione, G. A., and Barber, T. X. (1971): A strain-gauge pain stimulator. *Psychophysiology,* 8:102–106.
3. Harris, G., and Rollman, G. B. (1983): The validity of experimental pain measures. *Pain,* 17:369–376.
4. Scott, D. S., and Barber, T. X. (1977): Cognitive control of pain: Effects of multiple cognitive strategies. *Psychol. Rec.,* 2:373–383.
5. Spanos, N., Horton, C., and Chaves, J. (1975): The effects of two cognitive strategies on pain threshold. *J. Abnorm. Psychol.,* 84:677–681.
6. Tan, S. Y. (1982): Cognitive and cognitive behavioural methods for pain control: A selective review. *Pain,* 12:201–228.
7. Vallis, M. (1979): A component analysis of stress inoculation: Application to analogue pain. *Master's thesis.* University of Western Ontario.

Advances in Pain Research and Therapy, Vol. 9, edited by H. L. Fields et al. Raven Press, New York © 1985.

Transcutaneous Electrical Nerve Stimulation in Severe Angina Pectoris: A Controlled Long-Term Study

*C. Mannheimer, **C.-A. Carlsson, *A. Vedin, and *C. Wilhelmsson

**Department of Medicine, Östra Hospital, S-416 85 Göteborg; and **Department of Neurosurgery, Sahlgren's Hospital, S-413 45 Göteborg, Sweden*

Transcutaneous electrical nerve stimulation (TENS) has developed as a noninvasive means of therapy for the control of pain of various etiology. Furthermore, the field of application of TENS now includes functional disturbances of autonomic systems (2). Thus, TENS used to control delivery pain, has been shown to increase placental blood flow (4) and Kaada (3) has shown that TENS can induce peripheral vasodilatation in patients with peripheral arterial diseases.

In a previous study the short-term effects of TENS were tested on patients with angina pectoris provoked by atrial pacing during cardiac catheterization (6). Stimulation had a pain-reducing effect manifested by an increased tolerance to pacing, improved myocardial lactate metabolism, and less pronounced ST-segment depression during TENS treatment compared to the control recordings at identical pacing rates. These beneficial results were due mainly to a decreased afterload, indicated by a drop in systolic blood pressure.

The aim of the present study was to evaluate in a controlled long-term study the effects of TENS on patients with severe angina pectoris.

PATIENTS

Twenty-three patients between the ages of 41 and 71 years were selected. All patients had severe angina pectoris. The antianginal pharmacological treatment taken at the beginning of the study was regarded as optimal. All patients had been considered for coronary bypass surgery.

METHODS

The present study consisted of 3 parts.

1. A run-in period of 3 weeks to get the patients used to the test situation and to establish the average working capacity of each patient through repeated exercise testing.
2. A treatment period where the patients were randomly allocated to TENS treatment (12 patients) and to a control group (11 patients). The treatment period lasted 10 weeks with one exercise test every second week.
3. A posttreatment period which was identical for both groups with one exercise test every week. During this period no TENS treatment was used.

Each patient always performed the exercise tests at the same time of the day throughout the whole study. An electrically braked bicycle ergometer was used. The initial workload was increased stepwise every minute so that the patients reached the maximal workload within 4 to 9 min. The increment was either 5 or 10 W. Once the starting levels and the per-minute increments were established, they remained unchanged in each patient throughout the study. The exercise test was run to maximally tolerable symptoms and thus only stopped because of severe chest pain or severe dyspnea. All patients were asked to abstain from short-acting nitrates and those belonging to the treatment group from TENS 2 hr before the exercise tests.

The following variables were used:

1. Maximal total work during exercise (Wmin).
2. Pulse rate, blood pressure, and the product of pulse rate and blood pressure before, during, and after the exercise tests.
3. Chest pain and dyspnea reported by the patient were recorded during and after exercise testing according to a scale ranging from 0 to 5 where 0 meant no discomfort and 5 meant maximal discomfort. To reach maximal discomfort the patients were urged to continue the exercise to levels producing grade 4 or 5 of either pain or dyspnea.
4. ST-segment changes during and after exercise. The electrocardiograms were recorded by a 12 channel ECG recorder. Roughly the ST-segment depression represents ischemic changes in the myocardium.
5. Recovery time (minutes after maximal work is defined as the time elapsed until disappearance of pain or dyspnea (stage 0)).
6. The frequencies of anginal attacks and the consumption of short-acting nitroglycerine per week were registered.

A commercially available transcutaneous nerve stimulator was used. The stimulator delivers constant current 0.2 msec pulses and the pulse frequency was set to 70 Hz. The intensity of the stimulation was individually adjusted to a level immediately below that producing pain (15–50 mA). The electrodes were placed on the patient's chest at the site of the most intense pain. The patients carried the electrodes in this way during day time. They were instructed to take 3 TENS treatment sessions per day: morning, noon, and evening. Each treatment should last for at least 1 hr. In addition to this the patients were asked to use TENS treatment for 1 to 10 min at anginal attacks. The safety aspects concerning TENS on the chest had been carefully studied.

STATISTICAL METHODS

The treatment group and the control group were compared with respect to run-in values, differences between run-in values and treatment values and, finally, as differences between run-in values and posttreatment values by means of Fisher's permutation test. All *p*-values concern two-sided test.

RESULTS

Mean exercise tolerance in the two groups is shown in Table 1. The mean exercise tolerance during the treatment period was significantly higher in the treatment group.

During the treatment period the mean ST-segment depression at highest comparable workload and immediately after exercise in the treatment group decreased compared to run-in (Table 2). These differences between the groups persisted during the posttreatment period.

At highest comparable workload no differences were found with respect to heart rate, blood pressure, and the product heart rate/blood pressure.

Mean recovery time decreased in the treatment group both during the treatment period and during the posttreatment period compared to the run-in period (Table 3).

The frequency of anginal attacks and the consumption of short-acting nitrates decreased in the treatment group both during the treatment period

TABLE 1. *Mean exercise tolerance (Wmin)*

	Run-in	Treatment period	Posttreatment period
Treatment (N = 11)			
Mean	555	637	523
SD	277	308	231
Control (N = 10)			
Mean	588	564	532
SD	186	179	139
	NS	$p < 0.001$	NS

TABLE 2. *Mean ST-segment depression (mm) at highest comparable workload during and immediately after maximal exercise*

	Run-in		Treatment period		Posttreatment period	
	During exercise	After exercise	During exercise	After exercise	During exercise	After exercise
Treatment (N = 11)						
Mean	3.6	3.7	2.3	2.5	2.8	3.0
SD	1.6	1.6	1.1	1.3	1.3	1.2
Control (N = 10)						
Mean	2.9	2.9	2.9	3.0	3.0	2.8
SD	1.5	1.7	1.4	1.6	1.4	1.5
	NS	NS	$p < 0.001$	$p < 0.001$	$p < 0.001$	$p < 0.01$

TABLE 3. *Mean recovery time after maximal exercise (min)*

	Run-in	Treatment period	Posttreatment period
Treatment (N = 11)			
Mean	5.2	3.6	4.0
SD	2.4	2.4	2.2
Control (N = 10)			
Mean	3.0	3.2	3.1
SD	0.7	0.6	0.7
	$p < 0.01$	$p < 0.001$	$p < 0.05$

and during the posttreatment period compared to the run-in period (Table 4).

All but one of the patients in the treatment group wanted to continue the TENS treatment after the end of the trial and reported beneficial effect in reducing anginal attacks and increased physical activity (Table 5).

DISCUSSION

The results of this study are well in agreement with the previous study of the short-term effects of TENS (6). The mechanisms of action have not been explored, but four possible mechanisms may be considered: an unspecific placebo effect, pain inhibition with secondarily sympathetic inhibition, pain inhibition and sympathetic inhibition as parallel phenomena, and sympathetic inhibition with secondary pain inhibition.

It is virtually impossible to design a blind study of treatment with TENS since there is no placebo equivalent for the sensation of stimulation. There-

TABLE 4. *Mean frequency of angina attacks and the consumption of short-acting nitroglycerin per week*

	Run-in		Treatment period		Posttreatment period	
	Frequency of angina per week	Nitroglycerin consumption per week	Frequency of angina per week	Nitroglycerin consumption per week	Frequency of angina per week	Nitroglycerin consumption per week
Treatment ($N = 11$)						
Mean	27	39	15	21	19	31
SD	22	53	13	28	23	43
Control ($N = 10$)						
Mean	19	13	22	15	23	14
SD	18	11	20	11	19	11
	NS	NS	$p < 0.01$	$p < 0.05$	$p < 0.05$	$p < 0.05$

TABLE 5. *Patients' own estimate of the treatment*

Patient no.	Effect of TENS on anginal attacks	Physical activity after TENS treatment	Wish to continue TENS treatment
1	+	+	Yes
4	−	−	No
5	+	+	Yes
7	+	−	Yes
10	+	+	Yes
11	+	+	Yes
16	+	−	Yes
19	+	+	Yes
20	+	+	Yes
21	+	−	Yes
22	+	+	Yes

fore, an unspecific placebo effect in studies with TENS must be anticipated. Recent data suggest that placebo analgesia can be reversed by naloxone indicating that the effect might be exerted via neuronal systems using endorphins (5). This implies that TENS and placebo may employ a common mechanism and that unspecific placebo effects in an unpredictable way can influence the "real" effect of stimulation. However, the effect of TENS on ST-segment depressions and myocardial lactate metabolisms indicate that other mechanisms are of major importance than unspecific placebo effect.

In accordance with the second alternative it is quite possible that the pain-reducing effect of TENS also may inhibit the segmental sympathetic outflow since in the dorsal horn of the spinal cord there are connections between pain fibers and sympathetic neurons.

With respect to the third alternative it is well-known that visceral pain, as in angina pectoris, is localized to the body surface. The elicitation of visceral effects by stimulation of the skin is well documented in animal and human experiments (6). A recent study showed that low frequency stimulation of the sciatic nerve gave a significant decrease of the blood pressure in hypertensive rats (7). This effect could be reversed by naloxone. These studies support the assumption that electrical stimulation can influence various organs probably by changes in the reflex mechanisms and that this effect can be elicited without influencing the pain-transmitting system.

Finally, with respect to the fourth alternative it is quite possible that electrical stimulation blocks sympathetic activity peripherally or centrally and that this sympathetic blockade may be responsible for the produced analgesia. Upper thoracic sympathectomy has been used to treat patients with severe anginal pain (1). Although the operation was devised to cut afferent pain fibers, it seems possible that the pain-reducing effect was due to the removal of the efferent sympathetic innervation of the heart. β-Adrenergic blockade has an effect similar to that of surgical sympathectomy. This is in accordance with the concept that the pain reduction and the increased effort tolerance following sympathectomy is primarily a result of interruption of the efferent innervation of the heart rather than section of sensory pathways.

Preliminary results from a pacing study show that arterial levels of epinephrine and norepinephrine were lower during TENS treatment at identical pacing rate compared to control levels indicating a decreased sympathetic activity ($p < 0.01$ and $p < 0.05$, respectively).

CONCLUSIONS

The present study shows that TENS has a pain-relieving effect on patients with severe angina pectoris. This effect is associated with a decreased degree of myocardial ischemia as evidenced by the reduction of ST-segment depression. The observed effects are consistent with a lowered cardiac work and myocardial oxygen consumption during TENS probably connected with a decreased sympathetic activity.

REFERENCES

1. Apthorp, G. H., Chamberlain, A., and Haywood, G. W. (1964): The effects of sympathectomy on the electrocardiogram and effort tolerance in angina pectoris. *Br. Heart J.,* 26:218–25.
2. Augustinsson, L. E., Carlsson, C. -A., and Fall, M. (1982): Autonomic effects of electro-stimulation. *Appl. Neurophysiol.,* 45:185–9.
3. Kaada, B. (1982): Vasodilatation induced by transcutaneous nerve stimulation in peripheral ischemia (Raynaud's phenomenon and diabetic polyneuropathy). *Eur. Heart J.,* 3:303–14.
4. Kubista, P., Philipp, K., and Boschitsch, E. (1980): Verbässerung der Placentaren Durchströmung durch Transkutane Nervenstimulation. *Wien Med. Wochenschr.,* 18:595–7.
5. Levine, J. D., Gordon, N. C., and Fields, H. L. (1978): The mechanism of placebo analgesia. *Lancet,* ii:654–7.

6. Mannheimer, C. (1984): Transcutaneous electrical nerve stimulation (TENS) in angina pectoris. *Thesis,* University of Göteborg.
7. Yao, T., Andersson, S., and Thorén, P. (1982): Long-lasting cardiovascular depressor response following sciatic stimulation in spontaneously hypertensive rats. Evidence for the involvement of central endorphine and serotonin systems. *Brain Res.,* 244:295–303.

Advances in Pain Research and Therapy, Vol. 9, edited by H. L. Fields et al. Raven Press, New York © 1985.

Spinal Cord Stimulation for the Treatment of Peripheral Vascular Disease

Karl E. Groth

Medtronic Europe, 75008 Paris, France

Spinal cord stimulation (SCS) performed by a percutaneously inserted epidural electrode is a nondestructive and accepted therapeutic modality for the control of chronic pain. The best results with SCS have been obtained in the treatment of the intractable pain of low back syndrome and in the treatment of phantom limb pain (17,18,21,22,24,25). The risks of implantation are well-known because of the extensive use of this method for the relief of pain (3,4,5,12,23). These risks, including persistent pain at receiver site, infection, and cerebral spinal fluid leak, occur in a very small percentage of patients.

Recently, spinal cord stimulation has been suggested as an alternative method of managing patients with peripheral vascular disease who have difficult clinical problems that cannot be solved by conventional methods. This recommendation is based on clinical experience with pain relief produced by therapeutic spinal cord stimulation which has shown an effect on peripheral blood flow. Experience with this therapy indicated that symptoms and signs of ischemic peripheral vascular disease have improved (1,2,8,10,19).

The presence of vasodilator fibers in the dorsal spinal cord roots has been known for many years. Stimulation of the posterior roots produces regional vasodilation and was used by Foerster to map regional dermatomes (11). Later, when SCS came into therapeutic use, Cook described some autonomic changes which occurred in the legs of patients with multiple sclerosis (7). These included regional increase in blood flow such as elevated skin temperature, change in skin color, and improved tissue integrity. Based on this experience, Cook used direct stimulation of the posterior roots in the spinal cord by implanted electrodes with coupled radio frequency activation of electrodes for peripheral vascular disease and pain (8). His patients had obstructive arteriosclerotic peripheral vascular disease unresponsive to sympathectomy and arterial bypass. He described relief of pain associated with increased skin temperature, improved plethysmographic blood flow, and improved tissue integrity. He considered these changes in circulation to be beyond that which could be achieved by sympathectomy and postulated that the benefits were due to activation of vasodilator fibers in the posterior roots. He thought it probable that persistent spinal cord stimulation would avoid the need for amputation in some patients.

Dooley and Pasprak (10) studied 16 patients who had electrical stimulation of the spinal cord or of selected nerve roots and found that electrical stimulation produced arterial dilatation in the extremities by antidromic stimulation of fibers in the posterior root of the spinal cord and by stimulation of sympathetic fibers within the spinal cord. Therefore, he concluded that electrical stimulation of the spinal cord or of selected posterior roots would seem to be an appropriate therapy in individuals with peripheral vascular disease not amenable to conventional methods of treatment.

Meglio et al. described the treatment of excruciating foot pain in a 58-year-old man who had a complete obstruction of the right femoral artery due to arteriosclerotic disease (19). There were trophic ulcers on the right foot. Drug treatment, lumbar sympathectomy, and endarterectomy were ineffective. Following percutaneous implantation of the two epidural electrodes at T7 and T8 vertebral levels, bipolar stimulation performed at 60 Hz 0.5 msec provided immediate pain relief. Stimulation was applied for 1 hr every 2 hr. Two months later the ulcers were healing and pain control was complete. A substantial increase in blood flow was evident on noninvasive measurements (photoplethysmography and rheography). Cessation of the stimulation was followed by recurrence of pain and worsening of the ulcers but this was reversed again when SCS was resumed.

Meglio and Cioni, in 1982, reported 44 patients treated for pain of diverse causes (20). They stated that pain relief and increased circulation occur to a significant degree after epidural spinal cord stimulation and urged that others consider this alternative to conventional therapy early in the treatment of peripheral vascular disease.

Augustinsson et al. (2), reviewing the autonomic effects of electrical stimulation in different pathophysiologic conditions, showed that the technique was a useful tool in the treatment of various autonomic disturbances. According to Augustinsson, there are three possible explanations for the underlying physiological mechanisms of vasodilating effects: antidromic activation of C fibers in the posterior roots, activation of ascending pathways to supraspinal autonomic centers, and segmental inhibition of vasoconstriction fibers.

Augustinsson regards segmental inhibition of vasoconstriction fibers as the most plausible explanation and says that the SCS may evoke reflexes that inhibit the discharge of descending vasoconstrictive fibers, thus causing vasodilatation. He acknowledged that the operating mechanism to improve blood supply by SCS was still unclear but stated that the effects were not secondary to pain relief. Augustinsson used epidural stimulation in 6 patients with marked circulatory disturbances. Four patients had atherosclerotic disease and 2 had vasospastic disease.

Substantial improvement, including healing ulcers, was achieved in 5 patients. Measurements showed improvement in arterial toe pressure, skin temperature, and skin circulation. In his opinion, the main criterion for selection of patients with vascular disease for SCS was a decreased arterial blood pressure in the affected limb. He thought the main therapeutic indications were vasospastic disease and arteriosclerosis.

To understand better the role of SCS in the patient with peripheral vascular disease, 117 patients from five different centers were studied. The objective of this study was to evaluate the efficacy of SCS in controlling ischemic pain, improving walking capacity, and increasing peripheral blood flow.

METHODS

Patients

Patients selected for SCS had disabling ischemic pain not amenable to therapy by any other means. Standard assessment methods, including angiography, were performed to verify the presence of obstructive vascular disease which was not amenable to surgical reconstruction. Patients who had previous surgical treatment, including endarterectomy, sympathectomy, and arterial bypass, were included for study. All patients received the customary advice regarding the care of their illness, the benefits of exercise and the deleterious effects of continued smoking of tobacco. Vasodilating drugs were not used in these patients. Details of the patients studied are given in Table 1.

TABLE 1. *Patients selected for SCS*[a]

Etiology	Stage II: Intermittent claudication	Stage III: Rest pain and no tissue involvement	Stage IV: Rest pain with tissue involvement	Total
ASO (without diabetes)	5	29	29	63
ASO (with diabetes)	1	23	15	39
Vasospastic disease		4	3	7
Buerger's disease	3	3		6
Other		2		2
Total	9	61	47	117

[a]Male: N = 96; female: N = 21; age: mean = 63.1 years, range = 34–91 years.

Epidural Spinal Cord Stimulation

The patients were implanted with commercially available spinal cord systems (PISCES® Medtronic, Minneapolis, Minnesota). The system applies pulsed electrical stimuli via implanted electrodes to the dorsal aspect of the spinal cord. The use of the system requires that electrodes be placed in the epidural space under fluoroscopic control to identify the pathway that the lead will take. The electrodes were inserted through a needle of appropriate size and positioned over the lower thoracic region (T9/T11). When satisfactory position was obtained, the electrodes were connected to an external screener for test stimulation over a 3- to 5-day period. The patient should feel paresthesias and a sensation of warmth in the affected area in order to obtain positive clinical results. Once the patient was selected for chronic stimulation the system was internalized with a totally programmable internal power generator. The stimulation was adjusted to produce paresthesias and a feeling of warmth in the limbs.

Pain Assessment

The degree of pain control was compared to prestimulation pain levels. The patient was asked to evaluate his/her pain as a percent of control with 0% being no relief and 100% being total relief. Increments of 25% were used to evaluate partial pain control.

Walking distance was estimated at preimplant and last follow-up. Patients were asked to describe in city blocks how far they could walk before pain began. The estimates were evaluated on three levels: 0 to 100 meters, 100 to 500 meters, and 500 to 1,000 meters.

Blood Flow

Blood flow was evaluated by: ankle to brachial pressure ratios, toe pressure, skin temperature, and ^{133}Xe clearance. The local systolic arterial ankle and brachial blood pressures were measured by a pulse detection method. The recording device consisted of a strain gauge, cuffs, and recorder. The toe pressure was measured in a similar manner. The error in pressure measurement was estimated to be 7 to 10 mm Hg.

Skin temperature was measured by a conventional thermistor bridge. The display is divided in tenths of degrees centigrade. The accuracy is 0.5° C.

^{133}Xe skin flow measurements were taken at two sites of each leg; just below the head of the fibula and on the dorsum of the foot. The technique for measurement was the same as described by Daly and Henry (9).

Before testing, patients were off stimulation for 24 hr. In all cases, the patients first rested for 30 min in a supine position before testing.

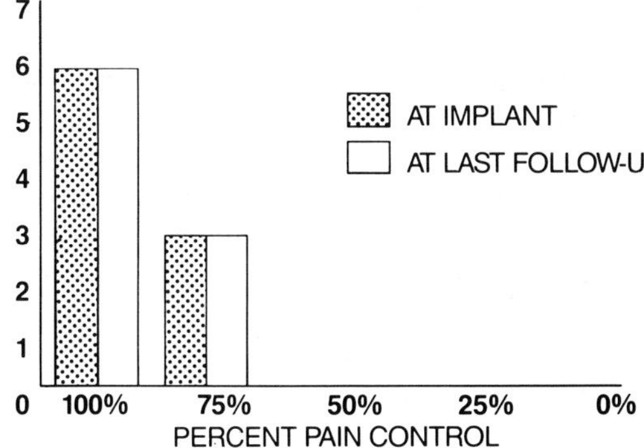

FIG. 1. Pain control. Patients with intermittent claudication, stage II (*N* = 9).

RESULTS

Pain Control

One hundred and one (86%) of the 117 patients implanted received sufficient pain control to justify chronic stimulation. Of the 16 patients who received no pain control, 7 presented with rest pain and no tissue involvement, and 9 presented with rest pain with tissue involvement. Pain control at implant and last follow-up by disease stage is shown in Figs. 1, 2, and 3. All patients in stages II and III maintained pain control throughout the follow-up period. Seven patients in stage IV lost control of their pain during the follow-up period and discontinued use of their system. In the last follow-up, 94 (93%) of 101 patients had clinically significant control of their ischemic pain.

Improvement in walking capacity is illustrated in Fig. 4. Sixty patients had a claudication distance of less than 100 meters before stimulation. After stimulation, all but 16 showed significant improvement. Fifty-seven had a

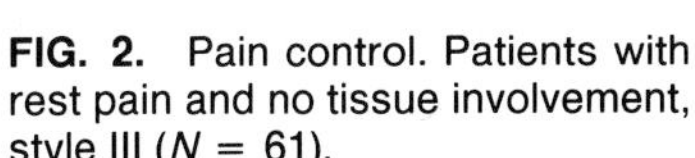

FIG. 2. Pain control. Patients with rest pain and no tissue involvement, style III (*N* = 61).

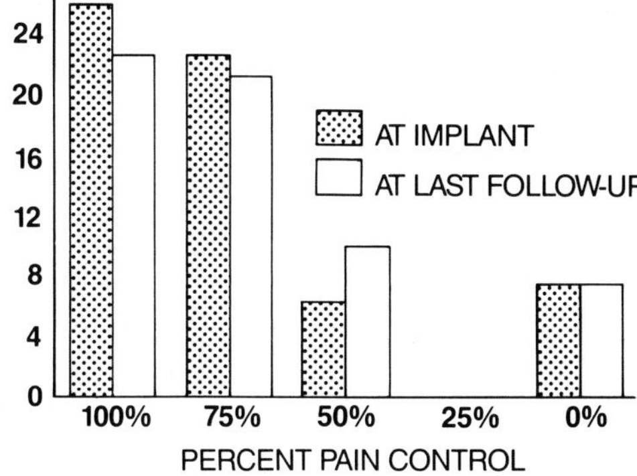

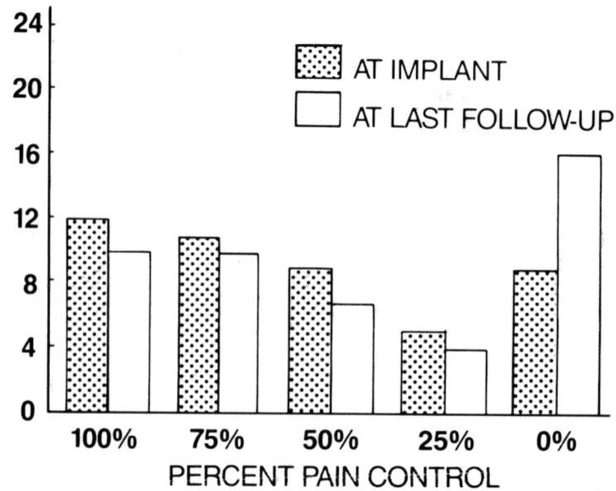

FIG. 3. Pain control. Patients with rest pain and tissue involvement, stage IV (N = 47).

claudication distance of between 100 and 500 meters before stimulation. All but 6 patients from this group showed improvement. Of the 117 patients that demonstrated an impairment in walking distance, 95 (81%) showed significant improvement following stimulation.

Blood Flow

The effects of electrical stimulation on blood flow are summarized in Table 2. Significant changes were observed in toe pressure, skin temperature, skin flow in the foot, and muscle flow at rest. Increases were observed in the ankle to brachial pressure ratios and muscle flow during exercise, but these were not significant.

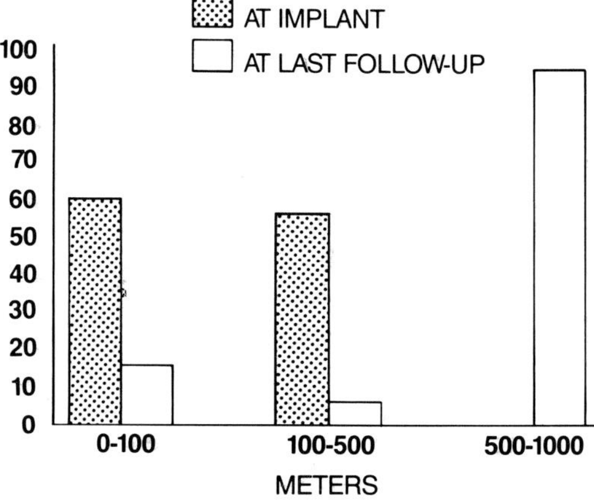

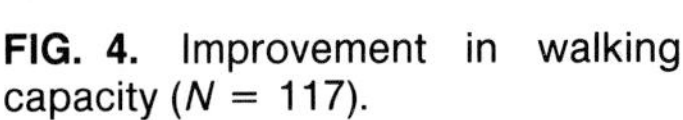
FIG. 4. Improvement in walking capacity (N = 117).

TABLE 2. *Effect of electrical stimulation on blood flow*

Test	No. of patients	Results before SCS	Results at last follow-up	p[a]
Ankle to brachial pressure ratio	28	0.53	0.75	NS
Toe pressure	22	20 ± 7 mm Hg	60 ± 10 mm Hg	0.005
Skin temperature	17	27° C ± 0.5° C	31° C ± 0.5° C	0.01
^{133}Xe (ml/min/100 g)				
Skin flow				
Left foot	4	5.45 ± 1.13	6.90 ± 1.64	0.02
Left leg	4	3.33 ± 1.86	3.23 ± 0.70	NS
Muscle flow				
At rest	4	1.10 ± 0.68	2.20 ± 1.13	0.05
Exercise	4	3.68 ± 1.45	5.24 ± 2.93	NS

[a]Mean and standard deviation given.

Discussion

The spectrum of symptoms due to peripheral vascular disease includes intermittent claudication in the relatively early stages, rest pain as the disease progresses and, finally, gangrene of the extremity leading to major tissue loss (6,14). The treatment varies with the stages of the disease. In early stages of the disease, which features intermittent claudication, surgical treatment is usually not indicated; but, instead, there is emphasis on patient education, principally relative to tobacco smoking, exercise programs, and on nonsurgical measures. Vasodilating drugs have not been useful. Conservative measures control the symptoms in most patients, but arteriosclerosis is a progressive disease and about 10% of patients with intermittent claudication develop more serious and disabling symptoms over a long period of time.

Patients with rest pain have severe arterial disease and inadequate collateral blood flow. Pain at rest indicates that the blood flow to the leg is so impaired that even minimal nutritional requirements of the skin cannot be met. In patients with rest pain, which comprise about 10% of the patients, trophic ulcers may occur on the feet and ankles. Gangrenous changes in the toes are a common manifestation. If untreated, most patients with rest pain will require amputation, usually above the knee because lower levels of amputation often do not heal. The severe symptoms and threat of tissue loss dictates treatment to restore blood supply to the legs. After noninvasive diagnostic measures in the clinic, angiography is commonly performed in order to detect the location and nature of the obstructive disease. Surgical relief of the obstruction by appropriate bypass operations is practiced if feasible. The long-term results are affected by the progressive nature of the disease. After reconstruction with a graft or vascular prosthesis, the patency rate of the bypass is about 60% after 5 years of use.

In patients with gangrene of the foot, which comprise about 10% of the patients seen in the hospital, amputation is necessary. Commonly, the status of the arterial circulation is studied by noninvasive techniques and by angiography in order to be certain that surgical relief of the obstruction would not permit conservation of part of the leg.

Sympathectomy has not proven to be of value in improving intermittent claudication and it does not appear to increase blood supply to the muscles. However, sympathectomy, by enhancing percutaneous vasodilatation, may lead to an increase in cutaneous blood flow and therefore is sometimes used in those people who have trophic cutaneous ulcers and is occasionally performed in combination with an amputation in order to improve the blood supply to the amputation stump.

All patients selected for SCS in this review had severe symptoms and had either failed to respond to conventional surgical and medical treatment or were not suitable for such therapies. Of the total group of 117 patients, 101 had a sufficiently marked clinical response to SCS to justify permanent stimulation. The clinical results lasted for as long as stimulation continued. The procedure carries few risks and is relatively uncomplicated.

Several mechanisms may be involved in explaining the clinical results. The most obvious reason for increased blood flow is the control of the pain itself which may break the reflex vasoconstriction/pain cycle. However, the increase in blood flow continues beyond the period of stimulation and this indicates actions other than breaking the pain-vasoconstriction cycle. Increase in sympathetic nervous system activity is an unlikely mechanism because of the fine balance that would be required to inhibit α-adrenergic vasoconstrictor fibers while stimulating cholinergic vasodilator fibers. It is very unlikely that SCS could achieve such a balance.

A more likely mechanism may involve vasodilatory substances. In the past two decades many studies have provided evidence of active vasodilation through a cholinergic, histaminergic, purinergic, dopaminergic, and possibly a β_2-adrenergic mediator, as well as the involvement of prostaglandins (15), plasma-kinins, and one, as yet unidentified, mediator, all operating through sympathetic nerves (16). By employing selective pharmacological antagonists of any of these mediators, except prostaglandins, vasodilation is not blocked. Recently Hilton and Marshall (13) have demonstrated vasodilation in muscle following dorsal root stimulation. They felt this was due to antidromic stimulation of small-diameter fibers. The effect was not blocked by sympathetic blocking agents but could be blocked by prostaglandin inhibitors. From this they inferred that the effect was mediated by the release of prostaglandins in the muscle.

Another active vasodilator possibly involved is vasoactive intestinal polypeptide (VIP) (16). Preliminary observations appear to be of interest, but the causal relationship between stimulation, increases in VIP, and vasodilation remains to be determined.

CONCLUSION

Based on the clinical experience presented we can conclude that ischemic pain is successfully managed by SCS, walking capacity increases during SCS, and significant increases in blood flow follow SCS. Further investigation is needed to determine the mechanisms involved.

Spinal cord stimulation appears to be an appropriate therapy for individuals with peripheral vascular disorders not amenable to conventional methods of treatment. The principal indication is ischemic pain without extensive tissue involvements.

SUMMARY

One hundred and seventeen patients with various peripheral vascular disorders were implanted with commercially available spinal cord stimulation systems (Medtronic). Patients were evaluated for pain control, improvement in walking distance, and increases in blood flow. The follow-up period ranged from 4 months to 5.4 years (mean 12.7 months). Sixteen of the 117 patients failed to demonstrate improvement of symptoms and were not considered for chronic stimulation. In the last follow-up, 94 (93%) patients had clinically significant control of their ischemic pain; 95 (94%) showed improvement in walking distance, and significant increase in blood flow was demonstrated in some patients by toe pressure, skin temperature, and ^{133}Xe measurements.

ACKNOWLEDGMENTS

I am very grateful to A. Fluks, Kerkrade, Netherlands; and Drs. L. E. Augustinsson, Göteberg, Sweden; Y. Karavel, Creteil, France; D. Fiume, Rome, Italy; and M. Meglio, Rome, Italy for their assistance in gathering clinical information on their patients.

REFERENCES

1. Augustinsson, L. (1981): Indications for spinal cord stimulation. *Proceedings: Seventh International Congress of Neurologic Surgery,* Munich.
2. Augustinsson, L. E., Carlsson, C. A. and Fall, M. (1982): Autonomic effects of electrostimulation. *Appl. Neurophysiol.,* 45:185–189.
3. Burton, C. V. (1975): Dorsal column stimulation: Optimization of application. *Surg. Neurol.,* 4:171–179.
4. Burton, C. V. (1975): Implanted devices for electronic augmentation of nervous system function. *Med. Instru.,* 9:221–223.
5. Burton, C. V. (1977): Safety and clinical efficacy, *Neurosurgery,* 1:214–215.

6. Coffman, J. D. (1979): Intermittent claudication and rest pain: Physiologic concepts and therapeutic approaches. *Prog. Cardiovasc. Dis.,* 22:53–72.
7. Cook, A. W., and Weinstein, S. (1973): Chronic dorsal column stimulation in multiple sclerosis. *NYS J. Med.,* 73–2868.
8. Cook, A. W. (1976): Vascular disease of extremities. Electrical stimulation of spinal cord and posterior roots. *NYS J. Med.,* 76:366–368.
9. Daly, J. M., and Henry, R. E. (1980): Quantitative measurement of skin perfusion with Xenon-133. *J. Nucl. Med.,* 21:156–160.
10. Dooley, D., and Pasprak, M. (1976): Modification of blood flow to the extremities by electrical stimulation of the nervous system. *South. Med. J.,* 69(10):1309–1311.
11. Foerster, O. (1933): The dermatomes in man. *Brain,* 56:1.
12. Fox, J. L. (1975): Dorsal column stimulation for relief of intractable pain: Problems encountered with neuropacemakers. *Surg. Neurol.,* 2:59–64.
13. Hilton, S. M., and Marshall, S. M. (1980): Dorsal root vasodilatation in cat skeletal muscle. *J. Physiol. (Lond.),* 299:277–288.
14. Imparato, A., Kim, G., Davidson, T., and Crowley J. (1975): Intermittent claudication: its natural history. *Surgery,* 78:795–802.
15. Kaada, B. (1982): Vasodilation induced by transcutaneous nerve stimulation in peripheral ischemia. *Eur. Heart J.,* 3:303.
16. Kaada, B. (1983): Promoted healing of chronic ulceration by transcutaneous nerve stimulation. *Vasa,* 12:262–269.
17. Long, D. M., and Hagfors, N. (1975): Electrical stimulation in the nervous system: the current status of electrical stimulation of the nervous system for relief of pain. *Pain,* 1:109–123.
18. Long, D. M. (1977): Electrical stimulation for control of pain. *Arch. Surg.,* 112:884–888.
19. Meglio, M., Cioni, B., Bal Lago, A., DeSantis, M., Pola, P., and Serricchio, M. (1981): Pain control and improvement of peripheral blood flow following epidural spinal cord stimulation. *J. Neurosurg.,* 54:821–823.
20. Meglio, M., and Cioni, B. (1982): Personal experience with spinal cord stimulation in chronic pain management. *Appl. Neurophysiol.,* 45:195–200.
21. Neilson, K. D., Adams, J. E., and Hosobuchi, Y. (1975): Experience with dorsal column stimulation for relief of chronic intractable pain: 1968–1973. *Surg. Neurol.,* 4:148–152.
22. Shealy, C. N., Mortimer, J. T., and Hagfors, N. R. (1970): Dorsal column electroanalgesia. *J. Neurosurg.,* 32:560–564.
23. Shealy, C. N. (1975): Dorsal column stimulation: Optimization of application. *Surg. Neurol.,* 4:142–145.
24. Sweet, W. H., and Wepsic, J. G. (1974): Stimulation of the posterior columns of the spinal cord for pain control: indications, technique, and results. *Clin. Neurosurg.,* 21:278–310.
25. Urban, B. J., and Nashold, B. S., Jr. (1978): Percutaneous epidural stimulation of the spinal cord for relief of pain. *J. Neurosurg.,* 48:323–328.

Advances in Pain Research and Therapy, Vol. 9, edited by H. L. Fields et al. Raven Press, New York © 1985.

Defining the "Chronic Pain Syndrome": An Epidemiological Method

*J. Crook and **E. Tunks

*School of Nursing and **Department of Psychiatry, Faculty of Health Sciences, McMaster University, Hamilton, Ontario, Canada*

A number of efforts have been made to create a composite picture of the "typical chronic pain patient," from the point of view of biological psychiatry (2,3), clinical presentation (1), psychological characteristics (10), or psychodynamic mechanisms (7). Such composite pictures, and the theoretical models drawn from them, are derived from experiences with patients who have been referred to pain clinics. However, patients who have been thus selected through the referral process may not actually be representative of individuals in the general population who suffer persistent pain. For example, Chapman et al. (4), in a nonrandomized survey, found considerably more emotional disturbance in patients attending a pain center, than in patients attending a private anesthesiology practice specializing in pain management. A parallel to this might be seen in a study by Pond and Bidwell (9) comparing epileptics attending hospital clinics to those managed in a general practice; even though both groups had a comparable number of epileptic seizures, those attending the hospital clinics showed more social and psychological disturbance.

The question is important for several reasons. First, the factors affecting the likelihood of becoming a chronic pain clinic patient should be identified, if clinical management is to be correctly focused. Second, treatments that are found appropriate and efficacious for chronic pain clinic patients may not necessarily be the most appropriate for persistent pain sufferers in the general population, and vice-versa. Third, for the purpose of planning health care delivery, it would be important to have some basis to determine if the clinical resources and organization such as are found in chronic pain clinics should be made available to the general population, and in what quantity. It is necessary to use the techniques of epidemiology to answer the above questions.

PAIN SUFFERERS IN THE COMMUNITY

This epidemiological study was carried out in the region of Burlington, Ontario, Canada (5). Five hundred households were selected randomly from the register of a group family practice. Because of the practically universal health insurance, the group was likely representative of the population of the city as a whole. Analysis of the age distribution of the study group showed that it was similar to the distribution in ages of all of the patients registered with the family practice group. Of the 500 households selected randomly, 394 were eligible for the study (living within the survey area reached by local telephone, and having no serious language barrier). These households represented 827 individuals total. The survey was carried out by a standardized telephone interview by trained interviewers using a pretested questionnaire.

The initial key questions of the interview were the following: "Are you or any member of your family over 18 years of age often troubled with pain?" The second was: "Have you or any family members experienced any noteworthy pain within the last 2 weeks?" If a pain sufferer was identified in the family by the first question, this individual was then interviewed. If the answer to both the above two questions was the affirmative, the individual was deemed to suffer "persistent pain." If an individual affirmed that they did not usually suffer pain, but that they had suffered during the last 2 weeks, they were deemed to have experienced "acute pain." The breakdown of subjects into the "persistent," "acute," and "no pain" groups can be seen in Table 1.

It was found that the prevalence of "persistent pain" is very high. Twenty-four percent of households surveyed identified a family member who suffered persistent pain, giving a total calculated prevalence rate for the survey population of 11%.

TABLE 1. *Family practice survey*[a]

"Pain in last 2 weeks?"	"Often suffering pain"? Yes [*N* (%)]	No [*N* (%)]
Yes	Persistent pain group: [90 (11%)]	Acute pain group: [43 (5%)]
No	Not interviewed: [25 (3%)]	No pain group: [669 (81%)]

[a]*N* = 827.

SURVEY OF PAIN CLINIC PATIENTS

The same telephone questionnaire was used in a survey of individuals who had attended active treatment in a nearby university pain clinic during the previous 6 months. Of 165 names retrieved from the pain clinic, 56 were eligible (because they lived within the same local telephone exchange region, and had no serious language barrier).

Using the same questionnaire, the pain clinic patients were grouped into the same categories of "persistent pain," "acute pain," and "no pain" groups (Table 2).

COMPARISON OF THE TWO SURVEY GROUPS

The details of the complete study are reported elsewhere (5,6). This chapter is concerned specifically with those patients endorsing "persistent pain" (often suffering pain, and experiencing noteworthy pain within the previous 2 weeks).

No significant difference was found between the family practice or pain clinic groups on the variables of sex or age distribution, marital status, educational level, religion, ethnic background, income level, or occupation. The employment status however, was significantly different, with 2% of the family practice group being unemployed on account of pain disability compared to 38% of the pain clinic group, a highly significant difference ($p = 0.000$). Patients from either group ranked the most common sites for pain similarly, most frequently reporting back or lower back pain, and less frequently, lower extremity, head and face, neck and shoulder, and upper extremity pain. Length of pain history was also similar in both groups with two-thirds reporting a pain history of 3 years or longer. A significant difference was found between the groups in the nature of the reported precipitating event, with 34% of the pain clinic group reporting work accident compared to only 7% of the family practice group, and 36% of the pain clinic group reporting

TABLE 2. *Pain clinic survey*[a]

"Pain in last 2 weeks?"	"Often suffering pain"?	
	Yes [*N* (%)]	No [*N* (%)]
Yes	Persistent pain group: [48 (86%)]	Acute pain group: 0
No	Not interviewed: [4 (7%)]	No pain: [4 (7%)]

[a] $N = 56$.

spontaneous onset compared to 68% of the family practice group. This difference is significant at $p = 0.000$ (Table 3).

Both the length of pain attacks and the frequency of recurrences were reported as higher among the pain clinic group. Pain clinic patients showed a significantly higher utilization of family physicians ($p = 0.008$) and other health professionals ($p = 0.001$), and if hospitalized, their hospital stays were much longer. In the 2 weeks preceding the survey, 68% of the chronic pain clinic patients had consulted a physician, whereas only 30% of the family practice patients had done so. The family practice patients reported self-initiated self-care activities to deal with their pain. In the study no direct attempt was made to distinguish patient-initiated versus clinician-initiated visits to health professionals. However, it was noted that during the previous year, the pain clinic patients had triple the mean number of family physician visits, the same mean number of emergency room visits as the

TABLE 3. *Comparison of family practice and pain clinic groups*

	Family practice		Pain clinic		
	No.	%	No.	%	X^2 df
Employment					
Full-time	36	42	7	16	32.9 5 df $p = 0.000$
Part-time	9	10	3	7	
Housewife	22	25	11	24	
Student	2	2	1	2	
Retired	16	19	6	13	
Disabled/unemployed	2	2	17	38	
Length of pain history					
Less than 6 months	7	8	1	2	2.9 3 df NS
7–12 months	7	8	2	4	
1–3 yr	20	23	13	28	
3+ yr	52	61	31	66	
Precipitating event					
Accident					
Work	6	7	16	34	22.3 4 df $p = 0.0002$
Home	3	3	1	2	
Other	14	16	6	13	
Postsurgery/illness	5	6	7	15	
Spontaneous	59	68	17	36	
Body locations (top 5 ranks) (multiple answers)					
Back/lower back	28 (1)		25 (1)		
Lower extremity	23 (2)		16 (2)		
Head/face	20 (3)		13 (4)		
Neck/shoulder	14 (4)		16 (3)		
Upper extremity	13 (5)		6 (5)		

Numbers in parentheses represent rank.

community patients, and that the mean hospital stay doubled for pain clinic patients compared to community patients.

From the questionnaire, several indices were constructed, and these were used to compare the two groups. These indices were as follows. The "global function index" comprised six items tapping self-assessments of social, emotional, and physical functioning, and life satisfaction. The "physical difficulty index" was constructed from "yes-no" responses to eight questions related to common daily activities: walking, climbing stairs, traveling, dressing and undressing, bending, walking one mile, etc. The "pain on activity" index had the patients rate their pain on a scale of 0 to 10 on the specific common daily activities. The "emotional index" required patients to rate depression and anxiety on a variety of standard indicators of mental status. The "attitude index" assessed the patient's assessment of the seriousness of his or her pain as well as his perceived ability to control it. The "behavioral index" identified actions taken by the respondent to avoid, prevent, or reduce pain. The "social consequences" index included items such as job change, law suits, disability claims, and drug or alcohol addiction. The pain clinic group was significantly worse on every one of these indices (p = 0.000). In examining the relationship between these indices, it was found that there was a low correlation between "physical difficulty" and "pain on activity" on the one hand, and the emotional and behavioral indices on the other. This suggests that these represent two major independent variables important to the condition of being a chronic pain patient. Neither is the cause of the other, but both are essential factors.

Summarizing the above, the most striking differences between the two groups were; the reported origin of the pain (with the pain clinic patients frequently reporting work accident); the psychosocial and functional impairment which was reportedly much higher among the chronic pain clinic patients; evidence that pain clinic patients endorse more pain and more impairment; lack of evidence that pain locations (and presumably diagnoses) or pain durations differ between the groups.

This study indicates that persistent pain sufferers who are likely to be referred to chronic pain clinics are more likely to demonstrate the following characteristics: The onset of the pain is most often linked to a precipitating event, often involving injury at work. They report a greater intensity and constancy of pain, with more difficulty in activities of daily living. They experience somatic symptoms such as loss of appetite, reduced energy, and diminished libido along with more typical depressive feelings. They frequently choose social withdrawal as a response to pain. The long-term consequences of their problem include job loss, litigation, occupational disability, and alcohol or drug abuse. They are frequent users of health services including family physician as well as other health care personnel.

Follow-up of the "persistent pain sufferers" in the two survey groups this year demonstrates a further interesting finding. Using the same questionnaire and criteria, two-fifths of those in the family practice group, and one-fifth of the chronic pain patients, no longer report this problem (J. Crook; *unpublished data*). Whatever the reasons for this, it suggests that the chronic pain patients are a prognostically more difficult group, notwithstanding specialized pain clinic input which the other family practice patients likely did not receive.

DISCUSSION

This study suggests that persistent pain sufferers attending chronic pain clinics are not typical of individuals in the general population who suffer persistent pain but who are not referred to such clinics. Out of the relatively large number of people in the community who suffer persistent pain, there is probably a subgroup of individuals who are more likely to be identified by primary health workers for referral to specialty clinics. This is consistent with the findings of the nonrandomized study carried out by Chapman et al. (4), and the work of Merskey (8). (This is not to suggest a stereotypy that all chronic pain clinic patients are alike, but rather to say that certain factors are more common in such clinic patients, and that this has implications for health care and treatment strategy.)

It is no surprise that patients with chronic pain are likely to suffer psychological and social disturbances. The question has arisen, however, whether such disturbance leads to the symptom of pain (7,12) or whether the persistence of a painful disorder may lead to psychological changes (11). Although persistent pain likely constitutes a significant stress on psychological and social well-being, this study indicates that the duration of pain, or the body locations of pain, by themselves do not necessitate the development of psychological and social disorder.

This study found that the pain clinic patients scored higher on indices tapping self-assessments of physical, emotional, and social functioning, but that there was at the same time a lack of correlation between the pain-related and the psychosocial-functional indices; our interpretation is that it is the individuals who suffer the coincidence of both psychosocial disturbance and also painful symptoms who are more likely to become chronic pain clinic patients. They likely are deficient in coping skills, and having greater adaptive problems with regard to work and social roles, and suffer greater emotional distress. Because their pain is more often related to work injuries, and there is a greater probability of litigation or compensation claim, the factors of adversary relationships and resentment, and the attendant sense of dissatisfaction, may be etiologically significant.

We believe that in matters of prognosis, there is an interaction between the painful medical disorder on the one hand, and the psychosocial and adaptive difficulties on the other hand. The latter includes the elements of adversary relationships (which may tend to undermine the therapeutic relationship), and lack of psychological and social coping repertoires (management of which would require reeducative and rehabilitative measures and environmental change.). When these different classes of problem are associated, the presenting clinical problem as stated by the patient is likely to be centered on the pain complaint, but attention to the medical disorder alone is unlikely to result in a satisfied patient, because of the other major complications.

There are two major implications of this for health-care planning. One is that management of chronic pain problems at the specialty clinic level often cannot be based on single approaches such as nerve blocks alone, but rather on multidisciplinary intervention, especially environmental and psychosocial. The other is that not all persistent pain problems necessarily are associated with such complications, although they are more likely at the pain clinic setting. It would be prudent to develop and to put in place screening procedures to specifically target those patients who suffer pain associated with serious psychosocial dysfunction, concentrating the more specialized and expensive multidisciplinary intervention on them.

REFERENCES

1. Black, R. G. (1980): The clinical syndrome of chronic pain. In *Pain, Discomfort and Humanitarian Care,* edited by L. K. Ng and J. J. Bonica, pp. 207–219. Elsevier/North-Holland, Amsterdam.
2. Blumer, D., and Heilbronn, M. (1982): Chronic pain as a variant of depressive disease: the pain-prone disorder, *J. Nerv. Ment. Dis.,* 170:381–406.
3. Blumer, D., Zorick, F., Heilbronn, M., and Roth, T. (1982): Biological markers for depression in chronic pain, *J. Nerv. Ment. Dis.,* 170:425–428.
4. Chapman, C. R., Sola, A. E., and Bonica, J. J. (1979): Illness behavior and depression compared in pain center and private practice patients, *Pain,* 6:1–7.
5. Crook, J., Rideout, E., and Browne, G. (1984): The prevalence of pain complaints in a general population, *Pain,* 18:299–314.
6. Crook, J., Tunks, E., and Rideout, E. (1985): An epidemiological comparison of persistent pain sufferers and chronic pain patients *(submitted).*
7. Engel, G. L. (1959): Psychogenic pain and the pain-prone patient, *Am. J. Med.,* 26:899–918.
8. Merskey, H. (1980): The role of the psychiatrist in the investigation and treatment of pain. In *Pain: Research Publications: Association for Research in Nervous and Mental Disease, Vol. 58,* edited by J. J. Bonica. Raven Press, New York.
9. Pond, D. A., and Bidwell, B. H. (1959): A survey of epilepsy in 14 general practices, *Epilepsia,* 1:285–298.
10. Sternbach, R. A. (1974): *Pain Patients: Traits and Treatment.* Academic Press, New York.
11. Sternbach, R. A., and Timmermans, G. (1975): Personality changes associated with reduction of pain. *Pain,* 1:177–181.
12. Walters, A. (1969): Psychogenic regional sensory and motor disorders, alias hysteria, *Can. Psychiatr. Assoc. J.,* 14:573–590.

Advances in Pain Research and Therapy, Vol. 9, edited by H. L. Fields et al. Raven Press, New York © 1985.

Denial in the Depressive and Pain-Prone Disorders of Chronic Pain

A. J. Bouckoms, R. E. Litman, and L. Baer

Department of Psychiatry, Massachusetts General Hospital, Boston, Massachusetts 02114

The relationship of depression to chronic pain is obscure. Depressed mood, depressive symptoms, and despondent behavior are found in up to 100% of chronic pain patients (4). The diagnosis of major depression with neurovegetative symptoms is less common, being present in 20% of chronic pain patients (5). Variable diagnostic criteria and their validity are thus implicated as obstacles for diagnostic classification and as the basis for rational treatment.

There are advocates of chronic pain as masked neurovegetative depression to be treated with antidepressants (2). Some see the depression as the manifestation of a personality style that draws from early developmental conflicts of guilt, anger, and masochism (2,3,6). Others see the depression as reactive, subsiding when the pain is relieved. These three formulations of depression and pain have dramatically different causes, treatments, and prognoses which justify their study.

A valid assessment of the pain patient's unhappiness might be evident if measures of neurovegetative depression, pain-prone personality disorder, and early developmental stability were ascertained in a group of chronic pain patients.

AIMS

1. The frequency and nature of depression in chronic pain patients were ascertained by assessing the global clinical impression of mood, the number of neurovegetative symptoms of major depressive illness, and dexamethasone suppression of 4 p.m. cortisol.

2. The frequency of the individual features of pain-prone disorder (2) was documented to establish the critical content items in pain-prone disorder.

3. The relationship between outcome at the end of the hospitalization, depression and pain-prone disorder was ascertained to determine if any of these parameters are related to prognosis.

4. The developmental history of chronic pain patients, patients having attempted suicide, and normal controls were compared (1). Developmental stability examines the quality of the person's early interpersonal relationships, particularly with their parents.

METHOD

Sixty-three consecutive patients with chronic pain referred to the neurosurgery service at Massachusetts General Hospital were studied. These pain patients were selected for inpatient treatment because of intractable pain. They were not primarily psychiatric patients nor those with abnormal pain behavior. Massachusetts General Hospital is a tertiary inpatient center for the treatment of chronic pain, where it is routine for the neurosurgeon, neurologist, anesthesiologist, and psychiatrist to see almost every patient. The only patients the psychiatrist did not see, and hence were not included in this sample of 63 patients, were patients with a definite diagnosis of trigeminal neuralgia. The patients were interviewed by the psychiatrist (A.B.) at first in an open-ended manner and then using a semistructured format. The semistructured interview consisted of:

1. Diagnostic and Statistical Manual for Mental Disorders (DSM-III) symptoms of major affective disorder or other psychiatric diagnosis.
2. A Global Impression (yes/no) by the doctors as to whether the patient was depressed.
3. Review of 17 symptoms of pain-prone disorder as described by Blumer and Heilbronn (2).
4. Global Impression (yes/no) by the doctors as to whether the patient was pain-prone, that is, demonstrating prominent pain behavior.
5. Family history of chronic pain, alcoholism, chronic illness, depression, or other psychopathology.
6. Developmental history that examines separation from parents, physical and emotional deprivation, overt and covert conflict, and a global rating of stability. The focus is on the quality of the child's early life rather than historical facts alone. The assessments are made according to the history, the patient's subjective evaluation, and the psychiatrist's examination.

Data from these 62 pain patients was compared with identically gathered data on 98 attempted suicide patients and 102 matched controls previously published (1).

Pain at the time of discharge from hospital was rated on a forced choice categorical scale as either greatly improved, slightly improved, or no better. The developmental histories of the pain patients were compared to normals and attempted suicide patients. The same semistructured questionnaire was used. Age, education, and occupation (Hollingshed-Redlich Scale) were documented. Four p.m. plasma cortisol levels were measured the day after a 1-

mg oral dosage of dexamethasone was ingested at 11 p.m. Analysis of results consisted of: (a) frequency distributions of the parameters measured; and (b)χ-square analysis of contingency tables for variables thought to be related.

RESULTS

Sixty-three patients with chronic pain (present more than 6 months) were evaluated over the course of 2 years. One person refused the complete consultation.

Demographics

The mean age of the subjects was 52 years, 52% were female and 48% male. Thirty-three percent worked at levels 1, 2, 3 of the Hollingshed-Redlich Scale, while the remaining 67% were between levels 4 and 6. Forty percent were educated at level 1, 2, or 3, and the remaining 60% were between levels 4 and 6. These results indicate that the patients were predominantly of middle and upper-middle class by both education and occupation.

Diagnoses

The principal physical diagnoses are listed in Table 1. The principal anatomical sites of pain were back, limb, and face. The history, physical find-

TABLE 1. *Principal physical diagnosis in chronic pain patients*[a]

	No. patients
Posttraumatic neuropathy	15
Rhizopathy	10
Unknown	9
Arachnoiditis/low back pain	6
Cluster headache	3
Postherpetic neuralgia	3
Atypical trigeminal neuralgia	2
Metastatic cancer pain	2
Amputation pain	2
Poststroke pain	2
Osteoarthritis	2
Psychopathology alone	2
Diabetic neuropathy	2
Spasmodic torticollis	1
Anesthesia dolorosa	1

[a] *N* = 62.

TABLE 2. *Principal psychiatric diagnosis in chronic pain patients*[a]

	No.	%
Psychological factors affecting physical condition	19	30
No psychiatric diagnosis	16	26
Major depression	15	24
Personality disorder	6	11
Somatoform disorder	3	5
Dementia	3	5

[a]*N* = 62.

ings, and character of the pain were consistent with deafferentation pain in 41% of patients. The typical patient has had previous surgery without pain relief, seen several different specialists and had modest physical findings with marked suffering. The principal psychiatric diagnosis is listed in Table 2. The commonest psychiatric diagnosis was psychological factors affecting physical condition (DSM III 316). This diagnosis subsumes those with adjustment disorders, and minor depression (RDC) associated with their pain. Twenty-six percent had no psychiatric symptoms of any kind despite their pain.

Prognosis

At the time of discharge from this hospitalization pain was rated as greatly improved in 33%, slightly improved in 19%, and no better in 48%. The degree of improvement in pain did not correlate with any of the variables measured.

Pain-Prone Features

The frequency distribution of pain-prone features and depression symptoms are presented in Table 3. Although an impression of being pain-prone was present in 43% of subjects, only 5% had more than 10 of 17 pain-prone symptoms. Global impression of pain-prone behavior correlated with specific pain-prone criteria ($p < 0.001$). Table 4 defines the frequency of individual pain-prone symptoms assessed. Continuous pain with depressive symptoms, either present or past, was most common. Denial of feelings about the suffering was common. Anger was frequently denied (44%) even though the patients appeared clearly upset. Early work onset, absence of words for feelings, ergomania, overt masochism, and an unrealistic desire for surgery were individually present in less than 20% of patients.

Family history was notable for 37% of subjects having family history of chronic illness and 29% having a family history of pain. Family history of

TABLE 3. *Depression/pain-prone: Frequency distribution*

	No. symptoms	%
Pain-prone (global)		43
Pain-prone	2–5	68
	6–10	27
	>10	5
Depression (global)		44
DSM-III depression	≤2	63
	3–4	16
	≥5	21

TABLE 4. *Pain-prone symptoms: Frequency*[a]

	%
Continuous pain	64
Depressive symptoms	60
Past history depressive symptoms/alcoholism	60
Denial of anger	44
Chronic family suffering	40
Hypochondriacal traits	32
Idealization of others	28
Chronic privation	24
Suffering of depression worse than pain	24
Strong aggressive drive unfulfilled	20
Inability to recognize internal feelings	20

[a]Early work onset, absence of words for feelings, ergomania, overt masochism, and an unrealistic desire for surgery were present in less than 20% of patients.

depression at 10% and alcoholism at 8% are no higher than the general population. Family history of chronic illness correlated with a family history of chronic pain ($p < 0.01$). Family history of alcoholism correlated with family history of unspecified psychopathology ($p < 0.001$). There were no other significant correlations between the family history parameters.

Depression

A global impression of depression was seen in 44% of patients. Twenty-one percent of all patients had more than 4 of the DSM-III symptoms for major affective disorder. Global depression correlated with DSM-III rated depressive symptoms ($p < 0.001$). A 4 p.m. post-dexamethasone cortisol of greater than 5 mcg/dl was used as a marker of an abnormal hypothalamic pituitary axis. One-third of patients failed to suppress their cortisol below 5 mcg/dl. There was no correlation between dexamethasone suppression results and global impressions of depression, DSM-III criteria for depression, pain-prone disorder, or pain at discharge. DSM-III symptoms of depression correlated ($p < 0.05$) with the global developmental stability of subjects' childhood. There was no correlation between DSM-III depression, pain-prone features, or pain at discharge. There was no correlation between specific DSM-III rated depression and specific pain-prone features. Similarly, there was no correlation between global depression and global pain-prone features.

Developmental History

Developmental stability was rated according to the presence of overt or covert conflict, separation from parents during childhood, physical or emotional deprivation, and overall global stability. Forty-nine percent had a globally unstable or chaotic background, 31% were subject to physical or emotional deprivation, and 54% had conflict with parents (Table 5). χ-square comparisons of normals, pain patients, and attempted suicide patients were calculated from the information in Table 5. Global stability was not significantly different between pain and control patients. However, covert conflict is seen with almost identical frequency in pain (37%) and attempted suicide patients (36%). The corollary is that increased covert conflict in pain compared to control patients is significant at the $p < 0.01$ level, identical to the significant difference between AS and controls. Pain patients

TABLE 5. *Developmental stability of pain vs. attempted suicide vs. control patients*

	Pain (%)	AS (%)	Controls (%)
Conflict			
Overt	17[a,d]	53[a]	39[d]
Covert	37[b]	36	17[b]
Separation	40	31	51
Deprivation			
Physical	6	3	3
Emotional	25	44	41
Global			
Stable	51	9[c]	60[c]
Unstable	39	53	34
Chaotic	10	38[c]	6[c]

[a] $p < 0.001$ highly significant.
[b] $p < 0.01$ significant.
[c] $p < 0.001$ highly significant.
[d] $p < 0.01$ significant.

claim less overt conflict than attempted suicide patients or controls. This supposed lack of overt conflict in pain compared to AS patients is highly significant at the $p < 0.001$ level. Likewise there is a significant difference between controls and pain patients on overt conflict ($p < 0.01$). Global stability is highly significantly different between attempted suicide patients and controls ($p < 0.001$) as previously demonstrated (1).

Inter-rater reliability was checked. Four hundred and twenty items of data on 10 patients were checked for inter-rater reliability between the 2 psychiatrists evaluating these patients. Twenty-five items were inconsistent. This gives an interreliability of 94%.

DISCUSSION

The 63 chronic pain patients reviewed are an upper-middle class group with persistent severe pain. Referral to a tertiary neurosurgery service with severe treatment failures behind them reflects selection for help-seeking that makes generalizations to all pain patients speculative. However, they are long-suffering refractory cases of pain that were not specially selected for abnormal pain behavior or depression. We estimate they reflect a wider group of chronic pain patients rather than patients selected for psychological disorders that get referred for study to pain units. The present study was exploratory in nature, and aimed to investigate the characteristics of and relationships between a large number of little-studied variables. Because of the large number of statistical comparisons, it is possible that some of the significant differences reported occurred by chance. These data will therefore require replication in future studies.

The Global Impression of depression was not substantiated in most patients with only one-fifth showing evidence of a neurovegetative depression. This is consistent with other recent studies showing this same 20% prevalence of major depression in chronic pain. Whether this is truly major biological affective disorder is still in doubt. There is a remarkably low incidence of family history of depression (10%), and no correlation with failure to suppress cortisol in the dexamethasone test. The 20% of patients who have more than four neurovegetative symptoms may be severe cases of demoralization, anxiety, and conservation withdrawal rather than true biological depression. Furthermore, the higher frequency of family history of chronic illness and pain suggests that these patients' depressed mood is related more to chronic long suffering than major depressive illness as defined by DSM III. The correlation between global developmental stability and the DSM-III symptoms of depression supports this contention.

The frequency distribution of pain-prone symptoms defines the common elements of this entity. Depressive symptoms are the core entity. However, the lack of correlation between pain-prone symptoms, DSM-III symptoms of depression, and dexamethasone suppression of cortisol pose a question as to whether pain-prone disorder is truly a biological depressive equivalent. Depressive symptoms are common along with chronic family and personal suffering and strong denial of affect, particularly anger. The lack of fulfillment of strong aggressive drive, inability to recognize internal feelings, idealization of others while feeling chronically deprived are individually found in only one-fifth to one-quarter of patients. Taken together they suggest a developmental disorder of the narcissistic type. Narcissistic personality style is characterized by a superficially aggressive style and apparently good coping based on denial of feelings. The pain patients describe themselves as aggressive, successful copers, despite chronic family illness and psychological stress. Angry, depressed feelings may be present, but an idealized view of the situation is usually foremost. A pseudo-healthy state based on denial of feelings is striking by the dissonance between what the patient claims and the physician observes face to face with the patient and in the disruption of the patient's life. The presence of pain seems to threaten this brittle competence. We propose that the narcissistic injury of the pain may be more damaging than the physical injury. The narcissistic psychological pain can be equally disabling as the original physical problem. Denial of this psychological problem is characteristic of the problem, therefore making it particularly insidious. Validation of these extrapolations requires examination of the developmental history information. Overall, pain patients' developmental stability is similar to controls, not like suicide attempters. Although there is a trend towards pain patients having unstable global development, there is no statistically significant difference between them and control patients. The major developmental instability in pain patients is in covert conflict where they are similar to attempted suicide patients. The pain patients claim less emotional deprivation than controls, suggesting that denial is operative. The high frequency of covert conflict relative to overt conflict is notable. There is no significant difference between the frequency of separation in pain patients versus attempted suicide patients. This lack of difference between pain patients and controls is similar to what was found with attempted suicide patients, suggesting it is not physical separation, per se, that is important, but the quality of emotional life irrespective of the exact physical circumstances of the person's childhood.

The implications of these findings are as follows:

1. Major depression is present in 24% of chronic pain patients, although depressive symptoms are present in 60%. There is growing evidence that major depressive illness is less common than was previously thought in chronic pain conditions (5). A prospective longitudinal study looking at affective symptoms, combined with a life-time history of affective disease with validated family history data will be necessary to examine this problem more closely.

2. The diagnosis of pain-prone disorder as a masked depressive equivalent is on equally uncertain ground as the diagnosis of major depression. The lack of correlation with depressive symptoms may be simply a reflection of denial of affect, but this is a circular line of reasoning that requires validation. Our findings of lack of correlation with specific DSM-III symptoms, dexamethasone suppression test, and global developmental stability detract from the proposition that pain-prone disorder is a biological depressive equivalent. Most of the symptoms of pain-prone disorder are quite uncommon, and this brings the specific content validity of some features of pain-prone disorder into question. The common features of depression and denial characterize the disorder. Pain-prone disorder may not be an affective or behavioral entity in its own right. Pain-prone disorder appears to be a set of symptoms that identifies a group of unhappy people with psychiatric distress best explained by other etiologies such as major depression and covert developmental narcissistic deficits.
3. Covert conflict in 37% of the chronic pain patients suggests a developmental deficit in the childhood of these patients. The significance of this figure is emphasized by the inverse relationship of overt to covert conflict between chronic pain patients and controls. This covert conflict, combined with the frequent denial of feelings, unfulfilled aggressive drive, and unrealistic idealization of others in the face of deprivation provides evidence that developmental conflict is the single most common finding in chronic pain patients. It is more common than major depression. It provides a concept from which the common pain-prone symptoms may be derived and understood. Denial of developmental conflict may be the precursor to the frequently described denial of affective symptoms or masked depression.

SUMMARY

Covert developmental psychological conflict is the most common index of psychopathology in chronic pain, more common than depression or pain-prone disorder. The denial of conflict despite severe developmental instability was present in 37% of pain patients, 36% of attempted suicide patients, and 17% of normal controls. Denial of current affect, particularly anger, was present in 44% of pain patients. The implication is that denial of anger and psychological conflict be sought as a key marker of psychopathology in chronic pain patients.

ACKNOWLEDGMENT

Our thanks to K. Adam, W. Sweet, and D. O'Brien.

REFERENCES

1. Adam, K. S., Bouckoms, A., and Streiner, D. (1982): Parental loss and family stability in attempted suicide. *Arch. Gen. Psychiatry,* 39(9)1081–1085.
2. Blumer, D., and Heilbronn, M., (1982): Chronic pain as a variant of depressive disease. The pain-prone disorder. *J. Nerv. Ment. Dis.,* 170(7)381–392.
3. Engel, G., (1959): "Psychogenic" pain and the pain-prone patient. *Am. J. Med.,* 26:899–918.
4. Lindsay, P., and Wycoff, M. (1981): The depression-pain syndrome and its response to antidepressants. *Psychosomatics,* 22(7)571–577.
5. Reich, J., Tupin, J., and Abramowitz, S. (1983): Psychiatric diagnosis of chronic pain patients. *Am. J. Psychiatry,* 140(11)1495–1498.
6. Tinling, D. C., and Klein, R. F. (1966): Psychogenic pain and aggression: The syndrome of the solitary hunter. *Psychosom. Med.,* 28:738–748.

Advances in Pain Research and Therapy, Vol. 9, edited by H. L. Fields et al. Raven Press, New York © 1985.

Effects of Spouse Abuse and/or Sexual Abuse in the Development and Maintenance of Chronic Pain in Women

Joel D. Haber and Cindy Roos

Pain Center, University of Alabama in Birmingham, Birmingham, Alabama 35294

Within the last decade the abuse of females in our society has become a problem of widespread interest. Political figures, national interest groups, and professionals from various disciplines have been instrumental in exposing this violent phenomenon. Despite these attempts, abuse often goes undetected because of its taboo and hidden nature.

The incidence and prevalence of women who have been physically and/or sexually abused is astonishingly high. Conservative estimates of this problem suggest that abuse occurs in 17% of American couples (18), while more liberal estimates place violence as occurring in 50 to 60% of all marriages (4). The victims in these close relationships are most often women (5,17). Strauss (17) reported that at least 3 to 4 million women are battered each year in the United States. Furthermore, women are three times more likely to become involved in an abusive relationship if they were victimized as children (8). Incest, for example, is much more prevalent among females than males (6). Whereas incest requires that the victim be related to the abuser, other offenses such as rape in which the parties typically are not blood related and often involve single encounters, is also an offense committed primarily against females (3). Regardless of the type of abuse, often there are long-term, devastating effects on these women.

The widespread variability between statistics exposing the incidence and prevalence of abuse in women indicates that detection and documentation of this problem is difficult. Few studies have systematically evaluated the varying types of abuse cases whose presentation may appear solely in the medical system. These cases most frequently enter the system through the family practitioner or the emergency room (9,15). Due to the physical injuries and chronic health problems that often develop secondary to abuse (19), the medical system has often been considered the primary source of detection and help for these women. Unfortunately, without formal training geared at detecting abuse, physicians detect abuse and seek proper treatment avenues in a very small percentage of cases (10,13). Data currently suggest, then, that the medical system has had difficulty identifying abuse cases.

In the above studies, the abuse suffered by women was typically severe in nature and not just a one-time occurrence. Over 50% of the women who were identified as abused in one study had received medical attention from the same hospital department for physical ailments related to abuse on more than one occasion (13). Compounding the problem of detection and severity of abuse is the reluctance on the part of abused women to discuss their victimization unless directly asked about it (12). Further, when the abuse is particularly severe, and women are hospitalized for injuries related to abuse, the percentage of abuse detected is still relatively low (1). Regardless of the severity of the abuse, researchers consistently note that their figures clearly underestimate the magnitude of the problem. The ultimate outcome of the abused women who remain undetected in the medical system is unclear; however, it has been found that they continue to seek medical attention for physical problems (16).

The previous discussion has illuminated the difficulties of abused women in obtaining appropriate care and the difficulty of the medical profession in identifying cases for intervention. Since early detection of abuse has important implications for treatment, addressing these problems is central to helping these victimized women.

Current research in the area of abuse has not focused on prospective research. What happens to a woman who has not received adequate treatment early in the abuse chain is unknown. Although women do continue to seek medical attention, the duration and frequency of these visits remains uncertain. Further, the possibility exists that women find another entry into the medical system once the abuse related to the acute problems has not been addressed adequately. A very surprising finding has been the high percentage of chronic pelvic pain patients with sexual abuse (including incest). Although statistics vary, estimates in this population have been as high as 65% (11). Given this incidence of sexual abuse in chronic pelvic pain patients, the likelihood that some type of abuse exists in women with other forms of chronic pain seems high. Therefore, we hypothesized that physical and/or sexual abuse might be present in a larger chronic pain population. The initial purpose of this study was to document the incidence and prevalence of abuse in this population, and to gather demographic information related to the problem. A second goal was to view the potential relationship between abuse and the development and maintenance of chronic pain.

METHOD

Subjects

The subjects were 151 women who presented to the University of Alabama—Birmingham Pain Center for evaluation between October 1983 and

May 1984. These women were all referred to the Pain Center by their primary physicians for various chronic pain problems that were of at least 6 months duration.

Procedure

All women referred to the Pain Center were evaluated by a multidisciplinary pain team including a licensed clinical psychologist. The psychologist conducted or supervised two graduate assistants training in medical psychology during these interviews. The psychological assessment included an interview centered around a standard questionnaire prepared by the senior author of this chapter. The questionnaire explored the psychological, social, and medical aspects of the patient's chronic pain problem and obtained demographic information. A specific section of this questionnaire examined the possibility of sexual and physical abuse across the patient's life span. If a patient evidenced or reported experiencing abuse, this area was explored in detail. All evaluations lasted for approximately 1 hr. Based on each interview, subjects were identified as abused or nonabused. If abuse was present, this was delineated into physical, sexual, or both types of abuse.

In addition to the categoreis of abuse, subjects were subclassified into pain site groups, which included four groupings: low back pain, headache, abdominal, or other. The "other" category encompassed specific syndromes, (e.g., leg pain) or multiple pain sites (e.g., leg, back, and headache). Multiple pain sites were included in the "other" category when the patient could not identify one pain area as a primary complaint. The "low back pain" and "other" categories accounted for 82% of the total sample, and were evenly matched for subjects in the abused and nonabused groupings. Equal numbers of headache and abdominal pain subjects could not be matched for abuse and nonabuse at the time of the study.

RESULTS

The results of this study revealed that 53% of the women evaluated at this multidisciplinary pain center were physically and/or sexually abused. In this sample 90% of the women reported that abuse occurred during adult years (greater than 18 years of age) with women experiencing a mean of 12 years of abuse. Spouses accounted for 71% of all abuse incidents reported. Of the 17% of abuse reported during childhood and adolescent years, under 10% involved incestuous relationships with a parent. Of women experiencing abuse, 16% evidenced sexual abuse, 43% revealed physical abuse, and 41% were victims of both types of abuse. In all cases the abuse preceeded the onset of pain.

The abused group ranged in age from 19 to 68, with a mean age of 42.5 years. The nonabused group ranged from 20 to 76 years, with a mean age of 44.6. There were no statistical differences between the age of the abused and nonabused groups. In this sample, only 15% of the women seen were black. A smaller percentage of the black subjects were abused (39%, $N = 23$), as compared to a much higher percentage of white subjects (56%, $N = 128$). The differences between the nonabused and abused groups on the racial variable were nonsignificant. Socioeconomic status (SES) differences were not significant between abused and nonabused groups across low, middle, or high income groupings. Although a greater percentage of abused women appeared in the low SES (income below $10,000/year) grouping (49 and 20%, respectively), only 37% of the total sample fell into a low SES category. Additionally, racial differences did not differentiate the higher percentage of abused women in the low SES group.

The site of the chronic pain in relation to the abused and nonabused groups appears in Table 1. The largest part of the sample was distributed into "low back pain" or "other pain." Abdominal (pelvic pain) and headache subjects revealed the largest percentages of abused women, although these groupings contained a small number of subjects. Interestingly, abdominal pain accounted for 75% of the sexual abuse cases ($p < 0.04$). No other location of abuse was significantly differentiated by the physical or sexual type of abuse.

Psychologically, the abused women used somatization and denial as their primary coping style compared to the nonabused group (61 versus 21%, respectively). The nonabused chronic pain women reported symptoms of major depression as their primary coping style (50 versus 29%, respectively). Even though abused women had vegetative signs of depression (i.e., appetite, sleep disturbance, etc.), their denial of psychological problems was highly significant compared to the nonabused group ($p < 0.001$).

Review of medical records and clinical interview data revealed that abused women were twice as likely as nonabused women to have spontaneously arising pain (spontaneous pain refers to pain that could not be linked to any specific antecedent) and no injury-related pain ($p < 0.001$). Additionally, abused women had significantly more medical problems in their history for which they sought treatment than did nonabused women ($p < 0.005$).

TABLE 1. *Abuse as a function of pain location*

	Low back	Abdominal	Headache	Other
Abused women	$N = 30$ 45%	$N = 8$ 67%	$N = 11$ 73%	$N = 31$ 53%
Nonabused women	$N = 36$ 55%	$N = 4$ 33%	$N = 4$ 27%	$N = 27$ 47%

DISCUSSION

A surprising finding in this study is the high incidence of physical and sexual abuse in women experiencing chronic pain. These results place abuse in a chronic pain sample at the upper end of previous estimates of this problem in the general population. The heavy representation of abuse in this population includes women of all ages and social classes. This study is consistent with recent research that suggests that abuse is not solely a lower SES phenomenon, but includes upper class women as well (5). Racial variables do not account for any differences in abused and nonabused women. Contrary to what one might expect, abuse occurred in a smaller percentage of black women than white women.

Another surprising finding of this study is the extensive number of years women reported experiencing abuse. This supports research which found that victimized women presenting to an emergency room are generally involved in longstanding abusive relationships (14). The lengthy nature of the abuse in our sample suggests that these women may suffer long-term difficulties and adjustment problems.

Although the majority of women in the present study were not involved in an abusive relationship at the time of their chronic pain, they tended to be very reluctant to discuss their abusive incidents. Many women reported that they had never discussed this abuse with anyone. Also, numerous victims reported that their abuse was difficult for them to deal with emotionally, and chose to "block it out" instead. The tendency on the part of abused victims to deny psychological problems is supported by the large percentage of individuals in this group that use somatization as their primary coping style. On the other hand, the majority of nonabused women with chronic pain do not use denial as a style of coping, and were instead classified as evidencing major depression.

The heavy reliance of abused subjects on somatization as a coping style provides support for their greater use of the medical system for physical problems. A significant difference in the number of medical problems in the abused women as compared to the nonabused women was found in the present study, thus revealing that abused women are seen frequently in the medical system for physical problems and are not likely to admit to abuse (2). Additionally, we found that chronic somatic complaints of abused women may not have a specific cause. Abused women with chronic pain were significantly more likely to have pain of spontaneous origin as opposed to an injury-related onset.

The denial, lack of a defined event precipitating pain, and increased number of medical problems in the abused group, suggest that the development of chronic pain in women may be related to severe abuse. Some women reported that their pain kept their spouses from abusing them more often. Several women directly admitted that the lack of treatment early in their abusive history led to the development of their pain problems. The high correlation of sexual abuse in abdominal pain patients highlights this issue.

The implications of this study must be viewed with caution and await further research. However, physicians need to be sensitive to abuse, and detect its occurrence early in women, when help may be possible. During the chronic pain stage women have already sought repeated medical attention for a "pain cure" that reinforces a denial of previous psychological difficulties. Chronic pain, which is a very reinforcing event, may be maintained with many secondary gains. Avoidance of psychological problems with a corresponding increase in "sick" behavior may provide the outlet women need for professional treatment.

In summary, abused women appear to utilize the health care system to a greater extent than nonabused women due to their greater number of medical problems and somatic complaints. With health care costs escalating to phenomenal levels, it is important that abused women be detected early and referred to professionals dealing with these cases. Although the percentage of abused women identified in this study is high, we believe that our figures may actually underestimate the true extent of this problem (7). In many of our cases women initially denied abuse, but were more willing to admit to victimization during follow-up treatment. Approaching this problem in a caring manner may expose and lessen the continued emotional and physical trauma for many women.

ACKNOWLEDGMENTS

This research was supported by the Department of Anesthesiology, University of Alabama, Birmingham. Thanks to Lurene Bentley for devoted editing and typing.

REFERENCES

1. Brismar, B., and Tuner, K. (1982): Battered women: a surgical problem. *Acta Chir. Scand.,* 148:103–105.
2. Brown, B., Carpio, B., and Martin, D. S. (1982): Wife abuse: An old family problem, a new health problem. *Can. Nurse,* 78:23–28.
3. Burgess, A. W., and Holmstrom, L. L. (1974): *Rape: Victims of Crisis.* Brady, Bowie, Maryland.
4. Davidson, T. (1978): *Conjugal Crime: Understanding and Changing the Wife Beating Pattern.* Ballantine, New York.
5. Egger, S. J., and Crancher, J. (1982): Wife battering: analysis of the victim's point of view. *Aust. Fam. Physician,* 11:830–832.
6. Finkelhor, D. (1979): What's wrong with sex between adults and children? Ethics and the problem of sexual abuse. *Am. J. Orthopsychiatry,* 49:692–699.
7. Geer, J., Heiman, J., and Leitenberg, H. (1984): *Human Sexuality.* Prentice-Hall, Englewood Cliffs.
8. Harris, L. A. (1979): A survey of spousal violence against women in Kentucky. *Kentucky Commission on Women,* Study #792701.

9. Kirkland, K. (1982): Assessment and treatment of family violence. *J. Fam. Pract.,* 14:713–718.
10. Mandel, J. B., and Marcotte, D. B. (1983): Teaching family practice residents to identify and treat battered women. *J. Fam. Pract.,* 17:708–716.
11. Murphy, T. M. (1981): Profiles of pain patients, including chronic pelvic pain: University of Washington Clinical Pain Service. In: *New Approaches to Treatment of Chronic Pain: A Review of Multidisciplinary Pain Clinics and Pain Centers.* United States Government Printing Office, Washington, D.C.
12. Post, R. D., Willett, A. B., Franks, R. D., House, R. M., Back, S. M., and Weissberg, M. P. (1980): A preliminary report on the prevalence of domestic violence among psychiatric inpatients. *Am. J. Psychiatry,* 137:974–975.
13. Rounsaville, B., and Weissman, M. M. (1977): Battered women: a medical problem requiring detection. *Int. J. Psychiatry Med.,* 8:191–202.
14. Rounsaville, B. J. (1978): Battered wives: barriers to identification and treatment. *Am. J. Orthopsychiatry,* 48:487–494.
15. Shipley, S. B., and Sylvester, D. C. (1982): Professionals' attitudes toward violence in close relationships. *Journal of Emergency Nursing,* 8:88–91.
16. Stark, E., Flitcraft, A., and Frazier, W. (1979): Medicine and patriarchal violence: the social construction of a "private" event. *Int. J. Health Serv.,* 9:461–493.
17. Straus, M. A. (1978): Wife beating: how common and why? *Victimology: Int. J.,* 2:443–458.
18. Straus, M. A., and Hotaling, G. T. (1980): *The Social Causes of Husband-Wife Violence.* University of Minnesota Press, Minneapolis.
19. Viken, R. M. (1982): Family violence: Aids to recognition; *Postgrad. Med.* 71:115–122.

Advances in Pain Research and Therapy, Vol. 9, edited by H. L. Fields et al. Raven Press, New York © 1985.

Spouse's Perception of the Chronic Pain Patient: Estimates of Exercise Tolerance

*Andrew R. Block, **Sara L. Boyer, and *R. K. Silbert

**Indiana Center for Rehabilitation Medicine, Indianapolis, Indiana 46202; and **Purdue University, Indianapolis, Indiana 46223*

There is a growing recognition among both researchers and clinicians that the symptom reports and levels of functional disability displayed by patients with complaints of chronic pain can be influenced by interpersonal factors. Fordyce (7), for example, has speculated that "significant others", such as the patient's spouse, parents, or even health care providers may respond towards the patient in ways which reward pain complaints and low activity levels. For example, the spouse might provide the patient with a great deal of solicitous attention whenever the patient complains of exhaustion or pain, while withholding attention for behavior other than symptomatic complaints. With the passage of time such solicitous responding, by providing operant reinforcement for illness behavior, could be expected to maintain low levels of physical activity and high levels of symptom complaint. Support for such an operant conceptualization of interpersonal response underlying pain behavior has been obtained both in our own laboratory (4) and by others (5).

Although it appears that many spouses may respond to patients in ways which reinforce disability and pain behavior, the basis for such maladaptive response patterns by the spouse has received scant attention. There appear to be two possible lines of explanation for spouses systematically rewarding pain behavior. First, it has been speculated that family members' *emotional responsiveness* to illness displays may be quite intense, and thus care-giving responses may be easily elicited (10). A great deal of laboratory analog research points to the veridicality of such emotional underpinnings for solicitous responding. Berger (1), for example, demonstrated that when viewing a confederate who appears to be experiencing pain, observers experience increases in autonomic activity. Further, Krebs (9) showed that the level of autonomic activity elicited in an observer when viewing emotional displays was positively associated with observer's altruistic behavior towards the subject. In a more directly applicable study, we found that some spouses of chronic pain patients, especially spouses reporting high levels of marital satisfaction, showed intense psychophysiological response (GSR) while watching patients' facial pain displays (4).

A second but not necessarily opposed explanation for solicitous responses may lie in the spouses' *cognitive interpretation* both of patients' illnesses and of the significance of symptoms. A number of writers have provided suggestions similar to that of Weakland (14), which point to a consideration of the family's "conception of the disease." Certainly, if spouses believe that even low levels of physical activity will produce further injury, they will be likely to prevent the patient from engaging in such activity. Support for the influence of cognitive factors was obtained in research of Swanson and Maruta (13) who found that if spouses and patients closely agreed on their interpretations of the patient's pain experience, the patient was unlikely to benefit from treatment.

The present study examines both cognitive and emotional factors which may underlie the spouse's response to chronic pain. Spouses received a questionnaire, the Spouse's Perception of Disease (SPOD-II), which was designed to assess several aspects of their cognitive interpretation of and emotional adjustment to the patients' pain syndrome. Emotional adjustment was additionally assessed by the SCL-90 (6). In order to examine the natural response tendencies of the spouses towards patients, spouses viewed a videotape of physical therapy exercises which constitute a major portion of each patient's rehabilitation treatment. Each spouse then made estimates of the patient's ability to engage in these exercises. Instructional conditions for these estimates were varied across subjects in order to influence judgments of exercise abilities. Half the spouses were instructed to make the exercise tolerance estimate based on the assumption that the patient would only put in a minimal treatment effort, and the other half of the spouses were instructed to assume that the patient would put in maximal effort. We predicted that (a) exercise tolerance estimates would be related to spouse's cognitive interpretation and emotional adjustment, and (b) instructional conditions would affect exercise tolerance estimates depending upon the spouse's interpretation of the patient's pain syndrome.

METHOD

Subjects

Subjects were spouses of 30 patients having chronic pain complaints. All patients were receiving comprehensive rehabilitation services on an outpatient basis at the Indiana Center for Rehabilitation Medicine. Characteristics of the patients are displayed in Table 1.

TABLE 1. *Patient characteristics*

	Mean (years)	SD
Chronicity	1.1	0.6
No. surgeries	1.3	0.4
Age	42.1	18.9
Marriage duration	10.3	8.6

Overview of Procedure

Within 2 weeks from their referral, all married patients and their spouses were approached for their participation in the study. After agreeing to participate, the spouse completed the SPOD-II and the SCL-90. After completion of the paper and pencil measures, spouses were taken to an adjoining room for further instructions and for observation of the exercise videotape. All spouses viewed the same videotape. However, the instructions for viewing the tapes varied across subjects such that one-half of the spouses were assigned to the *minimal effort* condition and one-half were assigned to the *maximal effort* condition. The observation instructions for the two conditions were as follows:

1. *Minimal effort condition.* "You will be viewing a videotape of five standard physical exercises. These exercises are designed to strengthen the back and stomach muscles. Your husband (wife) will be learning and practicing each of these exercises as part of his (her) treatment here. On each of the five exercises the individual you see will "hold" the exercise, at the point of maximal exertion, for a period of 60 sec. We do not expect that your husband (wife) can now hold these exercises for that length of time. However, in order to strengthen the back and stomach muscles it is important that each patient learn to hold all of these exercises and increase holding times.

After you view each of these exercises, we are going to ask you three questions:

a. Estimate the length of time which your husband (wife) would be able to hold the exercise at present.
b. Estimate how much pain your husband (wife) would experience while performing the exercise. You will give your pain ratings on a scale from 0 to 10 where 0 = no pain and 10 = the worst possible pain imaginable.
c. Estimate the length of time which your husband (wife) will be able to hold the exercise after 4 weeks of treatment here. In making this final estimate it is important that you choose a holding time which your husband or wife *can achieve easily.* That is, *for how long a time do you*

think your husband (wife) will be able to hold the exercise, even if he (she) only puts a minimum amount of effort during treatment here?"

2. *Maximal effort condition.* The instructions for this condition were identical to those given in the minimal effort condition with the exception of the instructions for estimates of holding time at the end of treatment. For the maximal effort condition the instructions for making the final exercise tolerance ratings read as follows:

c. "Estimate the length of time which your husband (wife) will be able to hold the exercise after 4 weeks of treatment here. In making this final estimate it is important to choose a holding time which your husband (wife) can *only achieve with difficulty. That is, for how long a time do you think your husband (wife) will be able to hold the exercise if he (she) pushes himself (herself) to put in the maximum possible amount of effort during treatment here?"*

Paper and Pencil Measures

SPOD-II

The SPOD-II (Fig. 1) is a 20-item questionnaire, based on previous research in our laboratory (3), which was designed to be used in a wide variety of disability syndromes. Four particular dimensions of the spouse's interpretation are assessed: *Pessimism* (PM) assesses feelings of optimism versus pessimism about the future course of the patient's illness; the *psychological* (P) dimension assesses the perception that psychological or attitudinal factors contribute to the patient's difficulties; *limitations* (L) assesses the perception that the patient's activity level is severely limited; *distress* (D) determines the extent to which spouses feel physiological arousal or emotional upset when they know the patient is experiencing pain. Answers to all questions were given on a six-point Likert-type scale with the anchor points: 1 = strongly disagree to 6 = strongly agree.

SCL-90

The SCL-90 is a self-report clinical rating scale which has been used with a wide variety of psychiatric and medical patients. Its use with chronic pain patients and their spouses was reported by Shanfield et al. (11). Although the SCL-90 provides a wealth of information regarding specific areas of psychological disturbance, an overall measure of emotional disturbance, the Global Symptom Index (GSI), was used in the present context.

Please answer the following questions using the scale provided. Place your answer on the line to the left of each item.

1	2	3	4	5	6
strongly disagree	moderately disagree	mildly disagree	mildly agree	moderately agree	strongly agree

L +	1.	There are many activities which the patient should avoid so that he/she can escape further harm.
D +	2.	I feel better when the patient feels better.
P +	3.	The patient is moody.
L +	4.	I often feel the patient is overexerting.
PM +	5.	No one knows the solution to the patient's problem.
D +	6.	When the patient's symptoms get worse I feel very disturbed.
PM −	7.	I feel that recovery is just a matter of time.
L −	8.	I think the patient takes more naps than he/she needs to.
P +	9.	The patient worries too much about minor aches and pains.
PM −	10.	I am optimistic that the patient will regain full ability to function.
L +	11.	I often tell the patient to slow down.
P +	12.	The patient cannot do as much when he/she is under stress.
P +	13.	The patient's problems become worse when he/she is upset or nervous.
D −	14.	I am not bothered when the patient complains of physical problems.
PM −	15.	With the correct treatment I'm sure the patient will show great improvement.
P +	16.	A big part of the pateint's problems is that he/she is depressed.
PM −	17.	I have given up hope that the patient will be able to recover.
D +	18.	Sometimes it seems that the patient's problems are my own.
D +	19.	I cannot relax when the patient is having a bad day.
L +	20.	I have been doing more housework lately because the patient is not able to do as much.

FIG. 1. SPOD-II questionnaire. Letters on line to left of each question indicate original SPOD-II scale: D = Distress, P = Psychological, PM = Pessimism, L = Limitations. Directionality of question indicated by + or − to form total scale score. The value for each "−" item is subtracted from 6 then all + and − items are added.

RESULTS

Table 2 displays the means and standard deviations for each of the four dimensions of the SPOD-II, for the SCL-90, and the exercise tolerance estimates.

Table 3 displays the correlations of paper and pencil measures with each other and with exercise tolerance estimates. Examination of this table reveals *limitations* and *distress* are closely related, as are *psychological* and *pessimism.* Several SPOD-II dimensions are related to exercise tolerance estimates. The SCL-90 GSI score, however, appears related neither to the SPOD-II responses nor to exercise tolerance estimates.

Figure 2 displays further data on the relationship of SPOD-II responses to exercise tolerance estimates. In developing this figure, summary scores for each subject were created by adding the total for both *psychological* and

TABLE 2. *Results*

Measures	Mean	SD
SPOD-II scales		
Limitations	22.3	5.4
Distress	17.8	6.3
Psychological	21.8	6.4
Pessimism	23.7	5.8
SCL-90		
GSI	0.53	0.21
Exercise tolerance		
Present	27.3	12.8
1 month	40.5	11.7
Pain	8.6	4.1

pessimism items. Spouses were then divided into two groups based on a median split of these summary scores. That is, spouses in Group 1 were relatively optimistic about the patient's recovery and believed that the patient had relatively few psychological problems. Group 2, alternatively, was pessimistic and believed the patient had many psychological problems. The differences between exercise tolerance estimates for the two groups is most striking under the maximum effort condition. In this condition group 1 spouses estimated a major increase in exercise tolerance, whereas group 2 estimated almost no increase in tolerance: $t(13) = 2.26$, $p < 0.05$.

TABLE 3. *Intercorrelations of all paper and pencil measures and exercise tolerance estimates*

	SPOD-II				SCL-90	Exercise tolerance			
	Lim	Dist	Psych	Pess	GSI	Pres	1 mo	Pain	Chron
Lim	1.00								
Dist	0.49[a]	1.00							
Psych	0.18	0.22	1.00						
Pess	0.21	0.21	0.58[a]	1.00					
GSI	0.12	0.16	0.27	0.23	1.00				
Pres	0.07	−0.14	0.01	0.06	0.12	1.00			
1 Mo	−0.13	−0.18	0.06	−0.03	−0.10	0.74[a]	1.00		
Pain	0.26	0.29	−0.33	−0.35	−0.13	−0.63[a]	−0.58[a]	1.00	
Chron	0.03	0.15	0.07	0.19	0.04	−0.04	−0.21	0.04	1.00

[a] $p < 0.01$

Abbreviations: Lim = limitations; Dis = distress; Psych = psychological; GSI = Global Symptom Index; Pres = present; 1 Mo = 1 month; Chron = chronic.

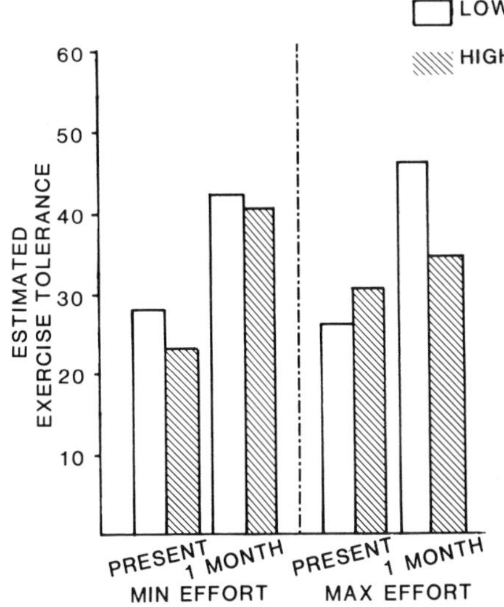

FIG. 2. Spouse's present and 1-month exercise tolerance estimates under the minimum and maximum effort instructions. *Open bars* are spouses low in "Negativism" and *stippled bars* are spouses high in "Negativism."

DISCUSSION

Even though the numbers of subjects involved in this preliminary investigation is small, the results point in some intriguing directions. First, spousal perceptions of the chronic pain patient, at least as measured by the SPOD-II, appear to have two underlying dimensions. In our questionnaire, measures of distress experienced by the spouse upon viewing patient pain displays are highly correlated with the spouse's belief that the patient's functional ability ought to be extremely restricted. The close relationship of these two sets of measures is predicted from research by Krebs (9) and thus, we shall term these combined measures the "Empathy" dimension. On the other hand, SPOD-II responses assessing pessimism about the patient's prognosis are correlated strongly with a belief that the patient has major psychological problems. This dimension, which we term "Negativism," appears to be relatively independent of the Empathy dimension. Of course, further research will be needed to establish the consistency and orthogonality of these dimensions.

A second interesting result of this study is that Negativism appears to be affected by the effort instructions. That is, spouses who score high on Negativism predict almost no increase in exercise tolerance across the course of treatment, especially under the maximum effort condition. These spouses' negative attitude towards the patient, one might therefore expect, would translate into little support for the patient's efforts at treatment. Since a sense of support by significant others has been shown in many studies to be associated with higher health status (12), the patients with negative spouses might be expected to show smaller gains in treatment than patients whose spouses are more positive.

A somewhat unexpected result obtained in this study is that the Empathy dimension appears unrelated to exercise tolerance estimates. Empathic and unempathic spouses did not differ greatly in estimates, regardless of effort instructions. Perhaps, empathic spouses are able to separate their own distress from the patient's pain experience. If this is true, however, one would expect that *distress* would not be highly correlated with the *limitations* scale. It will take further research, therefore, to determine whether Empathic spouses as predicted by Krebs research would behave in a more solicitous fashion than unempathic spouses.

The current study demonstrates the initial utility of the SPOD-II as an instrument for assessing the spouse's perception of the chronic pain patient. It appears that spousal interpretations also may apply to expectations for the progress of rehabilitation. Greater numbers of subjects in the present study and more in depth investigations into family dynamics (cf. ref. 8) will be required to determine the full extent to which family members modulate the patient's pain and illness behavior.

REFERENCES

1. Berger, S. M. (1962): Conditioning through vicarious instigation. *Psychol. Rev.,* 69:450–466.
2. Block, A. R. (1981): An investigation of the response of the spouse to chronic pain behavior. *Psychosom. Med.,* 43:415–422.
3. Block, A. R., and Boyer, S. L. (1984): The spouse's adjustment to chronic pain: Cognitive and emotional factors. *Soc. Sci. Med.,* 19:1313–1317.
4. Block, A. R. Kremer, E. F., and Gaylor, M. (1980): Behavioral treatment of chronic pain: The spouse as a discriminative cue for pain behavior. *Pain,* 9:243–252.
5. Cairns, D., and Pasino, J. A. (1977): Comparison of verbal reinforcement and feedback in the operant treatment of disability due to chronic low back pain. *Behav. Ther.,* 8:621–630.
6. Derogatis, L. R., Rickels, K., and Rock, A. F. (1976): The SCL-90 and the MMPI: A step in the validation of a new self-report scale. *Br. J. Psychiatry,* 128:280–289.
7. Fordyce, W. E. (1976): *Behavioral Methods for Chronic Pain and Illness.* Mosby, St. Louis.
8. Hafstrom, J. L., and Schram, V. R. (1984): Chronic illness in couples: Selected characteristics, including wife's satisfaction with the perception of marital relationships. *Fam. Relat.,* 33:195–203.
9. Krebs, D. (1975): Empathy and altruism. *J. Pers. Soc. Psychol.,* 32:1134–1146.
10. Meissner, W. M. (1980): The family and psychosomatic medicine. *Psychiatr. Ann.,* 10:35–49.
11. Shanfield, S. B., Heiman, E. M., Cope, D. N., and Jones, J. R. (1979): Pain and the marital relationship: Psychiatric distress. *Pain,* 7:343–351.
12. Steidl, J. H., Finkelsten, F. O., Wexler, J. P., Feyerbaum, H., Kitsen, J., Kliger, A. S., and Quinlan, D. M. (1980): Medical condition, adherence to treatment regimens and family functioning: Their interactions in patients receiving long-term dialysis treatment. *Arch. Gen. Psychiatry,* 37:1025–1027.
13. Swanson, D. W., and Maruta, T. (1980): The family's viewpoint of chronic pain. *Pain,* 8:163–166.
14. Weakland, J. H. (1977): Family somatics—A neglected edge. *Fam. Process,* 16(3):263–272.

Subject Index

O

Q

R